Farm Animal Surgery

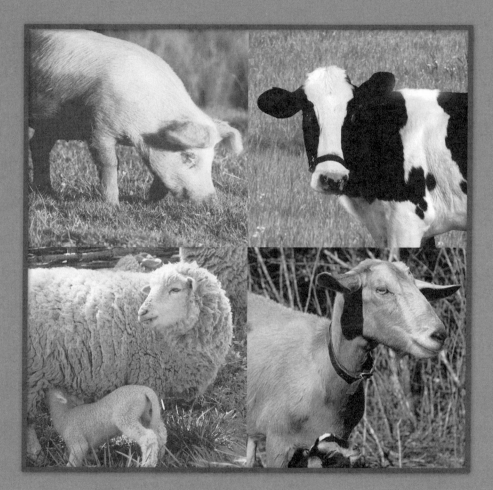

Susan L. Fubini, DVM, Dipl ACVS

Professor of Large Animal Surgery

Department of Clinical Sciences

Cornell University, Ithaca, New York

Norm G. Ducharme, DMV, MSc, Dipl ACVS

Professor of Large Animal Surgery

Department of Clinical Sciences

Cornell University, Ithaca, New York

With 726 illustrations

SAUNDERS

An Imprint of Elsevier

SAUNDERS
An Imprint of Elsevier

11830 Westline Industrial Drive
St. Louis, Missouri 63146

Notice

Pharmacology is an ever-changing field. Standard safety precautions must be followed, but as new research and clinical experience broaden our knowledge, changes in treatment and drug therapy may become necessary or appropriate. Readers are advised to check the most current product information provided by the manufacturer of each drug to be administered to verify the recommended dose, the method and duration of administration, and contraindications. It is the responsibility of the treating veterinarian, relying on experience and knowledge of the patient, to determine dosages and the best treatment for each individual patient. Neither the publisher nor the editor assume any liability for any injury and/or damage to persons or property arising from this publication.

International Standard Book Number

0-7216-9062-9

Senior Editor: Elizabeth M. Fathman
Managing Editor: Teri Merchant
Publishing Services Manager: Pat Joiner
Project Manager: Keri O'Brien
Designer: Amy Buxton

Printed in the United States of America

Last digit is the print number: 9   8   7   6   5   4   3   2

To our parents and our families:
Debbie, Ricky, Mike, and Marc
and
Rory, Logan, Jimmy, Rebel, and Mason
for their love and support.

CONTRIBUTORS

David E. Anderson, DVM, MS, Dipl ACVS
Associate Professor, College of Veterinary Medicine
The Ohio State University, Columbus, Ohio

Gary M. Baxter, VMD, MS, Dipl ACVS
Associate Professor, Department of Clinical Sciences
Veterinary Teaching Hospital
Colorado State University, Fort Collins, Colorado

William H. Crawford, MVSc, DVM, BSA, BA.S
Young-Crawford Veterinary Clinic
Innisfail, Alberta, Canada

André Desrochers, DMV, MS, Dipl ACVS
Associate Professor
Département de sciences cliniques
Faculté de médecine vétérinaire
Université de Montréal
St-Hyacinthe, Quebec, Canada

Thomas J. Divers, DVM, Dipl ACVIM, ACVECC
Professor, Department of Clinical Sciences
College of Veterinary Medicine
Cornell University, Ithaca, New York

Earl M. Gaughan, DVM, Dipl ACVS
Department of Clinical Sciences
College of Veterinary Medicine
Auburn University, Auburn, Alabama

Robert O. Gilbert, BVSc, MMed Vet, Dipl ACT, MRCVS
Professor and Associate Dean
Clinical Programs and Professional Service
College of Veterinary Medicine
Cornell University, Ithaca, New York

Scott R. R. Haskell, DVM, MPVM
Assistant Clinical Specialist
Department of Animal Science
College of Veterinary Medicine
University of Minnesota, St. Paul, Minnesota

Bruce L. Hull, DVM, Dipl ACVS
Professor, College of Veterinary Medicine
The Ohio State University, Columbus, Ohio

Nita L. Irby, DVM, Dipl ACVO
Lecturer, Department of Clinical Sciences
College of Veterinary Medicine
Cornell University, Ithaca, New York

Jennifer M. Ivany, DVM
Clinical Instructor
Department of Veterinary Clinical Sciences
The Ohio State University, Columbus, Ohio

William W. Muir, DVM, PhD, Dipl ACVA, ACVECC
Professor
Section of Perioperative Medicine, Anesthesia and Pain Management
Department of Veterinary Clinical Sciences
The Ohio State University, Columbus, Ohio

Charles W. Nydam, DVM
Nydam Veterinary Clinic, PC
Stamford, New York

Daryl Van Nydam, DVM, PhD
Senior Extension Associate
Department of Population Medicine and Diagnostic Science
College of Veterinary Medicine
Cornell University, Ithaca, New York

Stephanie Nykamp, DVM
Resident
College of Veterinary Medicine
Cornell University, Ithaca, New York

Anthony P. Pease, DVM
Resident, Department of Clinical Sciences
College of Veterinary Medicine
Cornell University, Ithaca, New York

Gillian A. Perkins, DVM, Dipl ACVIM
Lecturer, Department of Clinical Sciences
College of Veterinary Medicine
Cornell University, Ithaca, New York

Paul J. Plummer, DVM
Resident, College of Veterinary Medicine
University of Tennessee, Knoxville, Tennessee

Judy Provo-Klimek, DVM, MS
Department of Anatomy and Physiology
College of Veterinary Medicine
Kansas State University, Manhattan, Kansas

Peter C. Rakestraw, DMV, MS, PhD, Dipl ACVS
Assistant Professor
Department of Large Animal Medicine and Surgery
College of Veterinary Medicine
Texas A&M University, College Station, Texas

Jerry R. Roberson, DVM
Professor, Department of Surgery and Medicine
College of Veterinary Medicine
Kansas State University, Manhattan, Kansas

Allen J. Roussel, Jr., DVM, MS, Dipl ACVIM
Professor and Associate Department Head
Large Animal Medicine and Surgery
College of Veterinary Medicine
Texas A&M University, College Station, Texas

Guy St. Jean, DMV, MS, Dipl ACVS
Professor of Surgery and Head
Department of Veterinary Clinical Sciences
School of Veterinary Medicine
Ross University, West Farm, St. Kitts, West Indies

Donald F. Smith, DVM, Dipl ACVS
Professor and Dean
College of Veterinary Medicine
Cornell University, Ithaca, New York

Susan M. Stehman, MS, VMD
Extension Veterinarian
Department of Population Medicine and Diagnostic
    Science
College of Veterinary Medicine
Cornell University, Ithaca, New York

Adrian Steiner, FVH, MS, Dipl ECVS
Professor, Wiederkäuerklinik
Universität Bern, Switzerland

Ahmed Tibary, DMV, MS, DeS, PhD
Diplomate American College of Theriogenologists
Associate Professor of Large Animal Theriogenology
Department of Veterinary Clinical Science
College of Veterinary Medicine
Washington State University, Pullman, Washington

Ava M. Trent, DVM, MVSc
Associate Professor
College of Veterinary Medicine
University of Minnesota, St. Paul, Minnesota

Steven S. Trostle, DVM, MS, Dipl ACVS
San Luis Rey Equine Hospital
Bonsall, California

Beth Valentine, DVM, PhD
Associate Professor
Department of Biomedical Sciences
College of Veterinary Medicine
Oregon State University, Corvallis, Oregon

David Van Metre, DVM
Assistant Professor
Department of Clinical Sciences
College of Veterinary Medicine and Biomedical
    Sciences
Colorado State University, Fort Collins, Colorado

Richard Wheeler, DVM, Dipl ACT
Poudre River Veterinary Clinic
Fort Collins, Colorado

Eugene C. White, DVM
Assistant Professor
School of Veterinary Medicine
Tufts University, North Grafton, Massachusetts

J. Brett Woodie, DVM, MS, Dipl ACVS
Assistant Professor, Department of Clinical Sciences
College of Veterinary Medicine
Cornell University, Ithaca, New York

Amy Yeager, DVM
Instructor, Radiology
College of Veterinary Medicine
Cornell University, Ithaca, New York

FOREWORD

If it is the duty of this current generation of veterinary scholars to stand on the shoulders of their predecessors, then surely Professors Fubini and Ducharme have met their obligation admirably.

The advent of bovine medicine in North America is often traced to Professors James Law and D.H. Udall of Cornell University, and their students, Walter J. Gibbons and Myron G. Fincher. Later, Francis H. Fox (Cornell University) and William Boucher (University of Pennsylvania) became recognized as the most learned and influential professors of modern bovine medicine.

However, as the pace of advances in farm animal medicine started to moderate in the 1960s and 1970s, the development of surgery as a clinical specialty—and the embracing of farm animal surgery as a full participant in this effort—catapulted the understanding of abdominal disorders and other diseases to new levels. Surgical intervention offered a dynamic perspective on pathophysiological processes in real time, while correction and repair were still possible Moreover, it offered new possibilities for the advancement of diagnostics and therapeutics that otherwise would not have been available to internists.

What Bruce Hull calls the *golden age of food animal surgery* would not have been possible without the determined efforts of a handful of dedicated surgeons. Individuals such as Bruce Hull (The Ohio State University), William Donawick (University of Pennsylvania), Dale Nelson (Illinois State University), and the late Donald Horney (University of Guelph) worked closely with their internal medicine counterparts and, importantly, with a creative and energetic cadre of private practitioners. While farm animal surgery was progressing in North America, parallel advances were being made overseas, led by such people as A. Weaver (Glasgow University), F. Nemeth (Utrecht University), A. De Moor (University of Gent), G. Dirksen (Munich University), M. Stöber (Hannover Veterinary University), and Jit Singh (Haryana Agricultural University). Through their combined efforts, and the efforts of their students, they did more to advance the understanding of important illnesses of the dairy cow over two decades than any group in the history of bovine medicine.

Farm animals are unusually suited to the successful surgical repair of a multitude of interesting and challenging conditions. Combining an unusually docile demeanor with an extraordinary tolerance to major intervention, surgery on these animals can be as rewarding as any in the veterinary profession.

Although orthopedic, reproductive, and mammary gland surgery present many challenges for the large animal surgeon, abdominal surgery in the dairy cow is in a class by itself. The practitioner or surgical specialist who frequents the bovine abdomen for more than the most routine procedures must have a clear and unambiguous understanding of surgical anatomy and of related anatomic pathology to ensure a consistently successful outcome. Equally important is a good working knowledge of fluid and electrolyte therapy, and of contemporary medical management of the metabolically impaired dairy cow.

The usefulness of any textbook depends on the credibility and experience of the authors and editors. Professors Fubini and Ducharme bring as much experience to the table as any in the country, with the possible exception of Hull.

Through frequent reference to what is recorded here, as well as liberal sharing of improvements and new challenges, farm animal surgery will continue to prosper as a discipline to the betterment of the food animal industry and the society it serves.

Donald F. Smith

PREFACE

During our professional careers, we have been fortunate to interact with many talented large animal clinicians. In addition, we have had our share of complications in our surgical endeavors. To quote Rick Hackett (a saying apparently passed down from Al Gabel), "If you are not having a problem, you are not doing enough." We want to share the knowledge we have gained, including what we are still learning from our failures. Our aim in *Farm Animal Surgery* is to document and illustrate our collective experiences so it is useful for large animal veterinarians, veterinary students, and residents-in-training.

Farm animal surgery as a specialty has become more sophisticated, and many techniques are being adapted for use in cattle or small ruminants. A clinician must decide on a range of management options when facing a surgical problem. These options must consider the medical problem as well as practical and financial limitations. Our intent was to publish a comprehensive description of the various surgical procedures available in farm animals. References are provided for related medical conditions and very specialized procedures. Many colleagues have assisted us, and we hope we have accomplished this task. European and Canadian authors have provided a vital, more global perspective. Many figures were generously provided by colleagues from different institutions and different departments at Cornell.

We would like to recognize those individuals largely responsible for our career development and farm animal knowledge base. These include Dr. Donald Smith, our current Dean and an outstanding food animal surgeon, Dr. Richard Hackett, our department chair and steadfast friend, and Dr. Francis Fox, a legendary food animal and ambulatory clinician. We lost two very close colleagues in recent years whose meaningful assistance were instrumental in our specialty development: Dr. Don Horney, a food animal surgeon from the University of Guelph, and our beloved friend and colleague, Dr. Bill Rebhun, an internist whose footsteps we follow every day while caring for dairy cattle in the northeast.

We would also like to thank our current colleagues at Cornell, many of whom contributed to the book and make coming to work here every day a pleasure: Lisa Fortier, Laurie Goodrich, Alan Nixon, Brett Woodie, Michael Schramme, Gillian Perkins, Tom Divers, Dorothy Ainsworth, and Julia Flaminio. We would like to acknowledge our excellent residents, many of whom are wonderful friends, and our students, who teach us much more than they know.

We are grateful to Elsevier and Teri Merchant, especially for her patience and advice, and to Anne Littlejohn for her secretarial and editorial expertise, and for her attention to detail.

Susan L. Fubini
Norm G. Ducharme

CONTENTS

Farm Animal Surgery

HISTORY OF FARM ANIMAL SURGERY

Bruce L. Hull

Early records indicate that sheep were domesticated as early as 7000 BC and that cattle have been domesticated since 6000 BC. Cave art in the Upper Paleolithic period in the Franco-Cantabrian region depicts horses and ruminants. Bovine castration was practiced as far back as 7000 BC. The 539 BC code of rules for veterinary work specifically referred to surgery of the ox. Although the domestication of horses lagged behind other species, much of the early surgeries described in domestic species were for horses, not other species. Early literature suggests that this fact was due to the horse's value in battle, whereas cattle, sheep, and goats were salvaged for food. Castration was the only early surgery performed in cattle. Ancient Romans did not castrate cattle younger than 2 years of age. Castration and tail docking has been documented in early Africa (exact date is unknown). At a similar time, limb amputation and lancing of abscesses was talked about in Africa.

The American Indians had no domestic animals. The discoverer Columbus brought cattle to the New World on his second voyage in 1493. In 1523 brain surgery to remove hydatid cysts in cattle was described. There was an "expert cow doctor" practicing in Virginia as early as 1625. Although it can hardly be considered surgery, shoeing oxen was recorded in 1780. There were six veterinary schools in Germany before 1800, and by 1802 Thomas Jefferson had his ewes' tails docked. In 1805 Richard Peters recommended using a trocar for bloat and also called for the establishment of a veterinary profession in America.

George Dadd was the first veterinary surgeon to use general anesthesia (ether or chloroform) in about 1850.

However, general anesthesia use for veterinary surgery did not occur with much frequency until 40 years later. Dadd also advocated spaying cattle in 1832. This practice began in the United States and was later taken to Europe. In the 1800s, Louis Pasteur suggested aseptic surgery by stating, "If I had been a surgeon, I would never introduce an instrument into the human body without having passed it through boiling water."

In the early 1700s, 200 million cattle died in Europe from rinderpest. As a result of this great plague, two schools of veterinary medicine were established in France (Lyon in 1761 and Alfort in 1765) during the 1760s. The United States did not establish its first school of veterinary medicine until 1852, when the Veterinary College of Philadelphia was formed. From this beginning until World War I veterinary colleges flourished. Schools seemed to close almost as fast as they opened, and by 1933 only 12 remained in North America, including one college in Canada.

Aside from castration, there was little mention of bovine surgery before the late 1800s. In 1894, *Moller's Operative Veterinary Surgery* (Dollar's translation into English) textbook first described details about food animal surgery. Moller's book described at great length personal communications about food animal surgeries originating in Europe, many of which still have variations used worldwide today. The book described surgery for lumpy jaw, trephination of sinuses, and esophageal surgery. Tapping the pleural and peritoneal cavities was discussed, as were hernia repair, rumenotomy, and intestinal resection without the benefit of anesthesia. Moller

1

described amputation of the prolapsed rectum as well as uterine and udder amputation.

Moller's work was initially carried to the United States by W. L. Williams in *Surgical and Obstetrical Operations*, and later by such classic texts as *Veterinary Surgery* by E. R. Frank and *Surgical Principles and Techniques* by W. F. Guard. However, these textbooks and many of the earlier works were primarily equine. Frank mixes equine and bovine surgery within chapters devoted to organ systems, whereas Guard devotes 30 out of 240 pages to bovine surgery. The *Textbook of Large Animal Surgery* (1974), *Techniques in Large Animal Surgery* (1982), *Atlas of Large Animal Surgery* (1985), and *Food Animal Surgery* (1994) were more recent contributions regarding food animal surgery. There have undoubtedly been other contributions not mentioned here, as well as more specialized books, such as *Ruminant Urogenital Surgery*, that have greatly expanded our knowledge of surgery in the food animal species.

Since the middle 1900s, food animal surgery has become a recognized specialty. The American Association of Bovine Practitioners and American College of Veterinary Surgeons were founded in 1965. The European College of Veterinary Surgeons was established in 1991. These three organizations have helped focus on the need for specialists in bovine medicine and surgery and to advance the specialty of bovine practice. Although the American and European Colleges of Veterinary Surgeons are composed primarily of small animal and equine surgeons, they have greatly enhanced all veterinary surgery and advanced surgery specialties in all animal species.

A review of veterinary surgery from the beginning indicates many procedures have been tried for 100 years or more. However, recent advances in anesthesia have allowed food animal surgeons to be more meticulous in their approach and to practice aseptic technique more easily. Surgeons can perform more delicate surgery and more exacting tissue apposition using the newer suture materials, which leads to improvements in healing and better cosmetic results. Advancements in antimicrobials and fluid therapy have helped improve aftercare and have provided superior results. Most recently, improvements in pain medications and increased use of pain management has increased patients' well-being.

Economics is still the major deterrent to precise and extensive surgery in the various food animal species, as it has been for much of the history of veterinary surgery. Cattle value has increased as a result of artificial insemination and, more recently, embryo transfer techniques, which have spurred new interest in bovine surgery. The future of commercial cloning is presently uncertain but may drive the development of future surgical techniques.

It has been a privilege during my 40 years associated with farm animal surgery to experience the hand of the great masters and witness the breaking of the "golden age" of food animal surgery.

RECOMMENDED READINGS

Directory of the American Veterinary Medical Association, 39th edition. Schaumburg, 1990, The American Veterinary Medical Association.

Dollar JAW: *Moller's Operative Veterinary Surgery.* New York, 1894, William R. Jenkins Company.

Dunlop RH, Williams DJ: *Veterinary Medicine, an Illustrated History.* St. Louis, 1996, Mosby.

Frank ER: *Veterinary Surgery.* Minneapolis, 1939, Burgess Publishing Company.

Guard WF: *Surgical Principles and Techniques.* Columbus, Ohio, 1953, WF Guard.

Hofmeyr CFB: *Ruminant Urogenital Surgery.* Ames, Iowa, 1987, Iowa State University Press.

Kersjes AW, Nemeth F, Rutgers LJE: *Atlas of Large Animal Surgery.* Baltimore, 1985, Williams and Wilkins.

Liautard A: *Animal Castration.* New York, 1884, William R. Jenkins Company.

Merillat LA, Campbell DM: *Veterinary Military History of the University States.* Kansas City, 1935, The Haver-Glover Laboratories.

Noordsy JL: *Food Animal Surgery.* Trenton, NJ, 1994, Veterinary Learning Systems.

Oehme FW: *Textbook of Large Animal Surgery.* Baltimore, 1972, Williams and Wilkins.

Smithcors JF: *The Veterinarian in America (1625-1975).* Santa Barbara, Calif., 1975, American Veterinary Publications, Inc.

Schwabe CW: *Cattle, Priests and Progress in Medicine.* St. Paul, 1978, University of Minnesota Press.

Swabe J: *Animals, Disease and Human Society.* New York, 1999, Routledge.

Turner SA and McIlwraith CW: *Techniques in Large Animal Surgery.* Philadelphia, 1982, Lea and Febiger.

Williams WL: *Surgical and Obstetrical Operations.* Ithaca, N.Y., 1906, published by author.

PART I

General Considerations

CHAPTER 1

EXAMINATION OF THE SURGICAL PATIENT

Gillian A. Perkins

Physical Examination

This section focuses on examination of the cow abdomen. Examination of the other body systems is discussed in the relevant chapters. Every good physical examination begins with a good history. The basic information consists of the cow's lactation number, days in milk, diet, and pregnancy status. The herd person typically provides an accurate history—including any fever, previous medications or surgery, feed intake, changes in ration, and manure production.

The physical examination should begin with an evaluation of the overall well-being of the cow and her attitude. Many diseases in the cow present as merely a decrease in milk production and appetite (e.g., left-displaced abomasum, right-displaced abomasum, and ruminal distention), and the cow often appears quiet yet somewhat normal. The more acute, severe disorders such as lactic acidosis, abomasal volvulus, cecal volvulus, and hardware disease will show evidence of dehydration (mild to severe shock), abdominal pain, and general malaise. A history of colic and/or presence of abdominal pain at the time of physical examination should alert the veterinarian to act quickly and suspect causes such as indigestion or diseases that require surgical attention, such as intestinal obstruction or cecal disease.

Hydration can be estimated by evaluating a palpebral or cervical skin tent, moistness of the nose, and depth of the eye within the socket. A packed cell volume (PCV) and total protein quantitates the hydration status of the cow. The temperature, pulse, and respiratory rates will indicate the systemic health of the patient. One must also look for evidence of hypocalcemia, such as muscle fasciculations, weakness, sluggish papillary light reflexes, and cold extremities (e.g., the pinna), which could result in rumen and intestinal hypomotility.

The paralumbar fossas and the right paramedian abdomen should be evaluated for evidence of previous surgery or toggle-pin fixation. A quick oral examination should be performed to check for oral ulceration and abnormal breath (ketosis or lung abscess). Concurrent periparturient disorders such as mastitis and ketosis often exist. Therefore an examination of the udder that includes palpation, a California mastitis test (CMT), and strip plate analysis, along with urine ketone test, includes is necessary.

Examination of the gastrointestinal tract includes evaluation of the abdominal shape for evidence of distension or bloat, auscultation of the rumen and intestinal motility, simultaneous auscultation and percussion (pinging), ballottement, and rectal examination. Ancillary diagnostic tests such as abdominocentesis, rumen fluid analysis, and passage of an ororumen tube can be performed to help differentiate the exact diagnosis. This chapter will now be divided into two main categories preceded by discussion of ancillary diagnostic tests: disorders that cause abdominal distension and those that cause tympanic resonance.

Diagnostic Procedures

RUMEN FLUID ANALYSIS

Rumen fluid can be obtained by passing an ororumen (stomach tube into the rumen) tube, weighted tube, or by rumenocentesis. The smell and color of the fluid obtained can be evaluated subjectively. Rumen fluid is generally aromatic, and, depending on the diet of the cow, the color can range from green to yellow to brown. A milky-to-brown color with a very pungent sour or acidic odor indicates grain engorgement (Figure 1-1). The presence of multiple small bubbles giving rise to a "frothy" appearance defines a frothy bloat. Depending on the diet, the normal pH ranges from 5.5 to 7.5; pH below 5.5 indicates rumen acidosis. Contamination of the rumen fluid with bicarbonate-rich saliva is the most common reason for a high rumen fluid pH. Pathologic reasons for a pH greater than 7.0 include decreased activity of the rumen flora, whereas a pH greater than 8.0 suggests urea toxicity. Other special tests—such as a

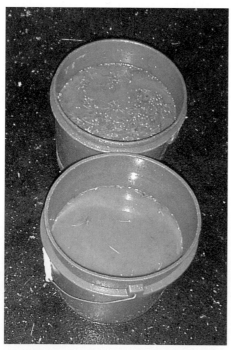

Figure 1-1   Rumen fluid from a Brown Swiss steer that ingested excessive amounts of bagels three days before. The pH of the fluid was <5. It had a very pungent odor and was a chocolate milk consistency and color.

Gram stain and direct microscopic examination for protozoa, methylene blue test, and sediment activity test—have been described but often do not have a practical application for the veterinarian in the field and provide little information other than what can be gained from a good physical assessment of the cow. A high rumen chloride (>30 mEq/L, normal <25-30 mEq/L) is consistent with reflux of chloride from the abomasum into the forestomachs and supports a diagnosis of pyloric outflow obstruction (posterior functional stenosis).

Ororumen Tube

With a cow in a stanchion or head-gate, an ororumen tube can best be passed by the operator standing beside the cow's head. The arm closest to the cow is placed over the bridge of the nose, and the hand is placed in the oral cavity (dental space) by opening the mouth and lifting dorsally. The opposite hand (furthest away from the cow) is free to gently pass the Fricke speculum into the mouth along the hard palate. The hand that is holding the mouth open can be used to guide the speculum caudally by placing the speculum between the hard palate and the cup of the hand. A slight resistance is palpated as the base of the tongue is reached. With continued gentle pressure, the speculum is advanced slightly into the oropharynx. The speculum is then stabilized by the hand that restrains the mouth and head. At this point, the tube can be passed through the speculum into the pharynx and advanced into the esophagus and the rumen. Simultaneously distending the esophagus with gas by blowing into the tube as it advances may make passing the tube easier. Once the rumen is entered, a characteristic odor and rush of gas is usually heard. To confirm placement of the tube, one can blow into the tube and have someone auscultate over the left paralumbar fossa for bubbling sounds in the rumen. Palpation of the tube in the cervical esophagus also confirms correct placement. The tube can be manipulated back and forth and manual pressure applied to the left paralumbar fossa to try to obtain fluid or gas. At this point, samples should be obtained and any therapy administered. This may include intraruminal fluids, rumenotorics, transfaunate, or electrolytes. Should the cow begin to regurgitate around the tube, the head should be flexed and lowered to prevent aspiration of rumen contents, and the tube should immediately be occluded and pulled with a steady stroke moving outward and ventrally. Kinking the end of the tube to prevent back flow of rumen contents into the pharynx of the cow decreases the risk of aspiration pneumonia. Unkinking the tube and holding the dependent aspect over a collection device (fecal cup, bucket, etc.) may permit retrieval of fluid from within the tube lumen.

The Kingman tube is a large-diameter tube that is used to evacuate abnormal rumen contents or for rumen

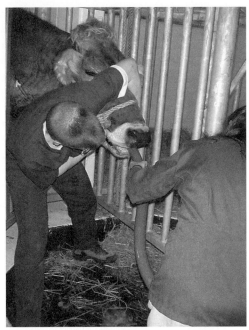

Figure 1-2 Passing a Kingman tube in a Brown Swiss steer with carbohydrate overload. The head should be kept straight to minimize pharyngeal trauma.

lavage to alleviate the need for surgery or decrease abdominal distension in preparation for surgery. The cow's head must be held straight, forward, and slightly raised above horizontal. A speculum is placed in the oral cavity; copious lubrication is applied to the tube, and with gentle pressure, it is passed down the esophagus to the rumen (Figure 1-2).

Abdominocentesis

Peritoneal fluid can be helpful in establishing a diagnosis and determining a prognosis for many gastrointestinal disorders. Two sites are recommended for abdominocentesis in cattle. The first evaluates the right cranial abdomen and is most helpful in cases in which a localized peritonitis is suspected secondary to perforation of an abomasal ulcer. This area runs from the midline to the right milk vein just caudal to the xiphoid. The second site is located just above the udder on the right side under the fold of the flank. The site is clipped and prepared for an aseptic procedure. A tail-jack is used for restraint and an 18-gauge, $1\frac{1}{2}$ needle is inserted through the skin and slowly advanced into the peritoneal cavity. Alternatively, the area can be infused with lidocaine, a small stab incision made in the body wall with a 15 blade, and a teat cannula used to obtain the abdominal fluid. Cattle have very strong abdominal musculature that can move the needle or teat cannula; therefore they should be held carefully and kept at a 90-degree angle to the ground (see Figure 10.5-4). If available, ultrasono-graphic evaluation of the abdomen may reveal free peritoneal fluid, and if the fluid is not near any vital structures at risk of being perforated, then the abdominocentesis can be done at that particular site. Because cows produce copious amounts of fibrinogen, the fluid may be difficult to obtain and preparation of both sites for abdominocentesis may be more efficient. A normal abdominal fluid analysis in one location and an inflammatory tap in the other may indicate a localized problem. The fluid should be clear and colorless to yellow. The total protein should be <3.0 g/dL and the nucleated cell count <10,000/μL, consisting of neutrophils and mononuclear cells.

LABORATORY WORK

Gastrointestinal disorders of cattle, whether they are forestomach, abomasal, intestinal, or cecal in origin, most commonly show hypochloremic metabolic alkalosis accompanied by hypokalemia caused by inappetence. This means that electrolyte levels may help confirm clinical suspicions and help formulate a therapeutic plan, but they are not all that helpful in localizing a specific problem.

A paradoxic aciduria often develops in cows with hypochloremic alkalosis. It is paradoxic because one would expect that the alkalotic cow would retain hydrogen ions to counteract the alkalosis. However, because of dehydration, the kidney retains sodium. Chloride is not available; therefore another positive ion needs to be excreted. Hypokalemia in these patients makes the hydrogen ion the only positive ion available, which is excreted in the urine in exchange for sodium, resulting in a low urine pH. Hypocalcemia is also commonly observed.

Strangulating lesions of the abomasum, cecum, or small intestine can result in bowel necrosis and accumulation of lactic acid. This can cause a high anion gap, hypochloremic acidosis indicating a poor prognosis. Infrequently, a moderate to severe case of ketosis may result in a high anion gap acidosis caused by ketoacidemia. On a practical basis, easy-to-use cow-side tests such as the I-stat* can determine plasma electrolyte levels, ionized calcium, and creatinine in less than 2 minutes per test.

Complete blood cell counts can quantitate the degree of inflammation and be run sequentially to monitor the patient's response to a disease entity. A persistent lymphocytosis and clinical signs of pyloric obstruction could make the clinician suspicious that the cow is infected with bovine leukosis virus (BLV) and may have abomasal lymphoma. However, very few cattle infected

---

*I-STAT Corporation, East Windsor, NJ 08520, USA, *http://www.istat.com.*

with BLV (<4%) actually develop tumors. Increased concentrations of fibrinogen, an acute phase protein along with globulins, contribute to an overall increase in total plasma protein and are typical of an inflammatory process such as an intraabdominal abscess or peritonitis. An increased PCV and total protein supports dehydration.

ABDOMINAL ULTRASONOGRAPHY

Use of ultrasound equipment on the farm is becoming more commonplace. Clients are requesting pregnancy diagnosis with the aid of ultrasound. The same rectal 3.5 MHz ultrasound probe can be used to explore the abdomen either transrectally or transabdominally. A 5 MHz probe gives deeper penetration but may not be cost-effective. The ultrasound has helped the author in the diagnosis of intraabdominal abscess associated with hardware disease, liver abscesses, abomasal ulceration, and other causes of gastrointestinal disturbances, including neoplasms, peritoneal effusion, omental bursitis, and intestinal disorders, such as intussusceptions and strangulating small intestinal obstruction. Ueli Braun has published numerous papers on ultrasonography of bovine abdomen, which the reader should refer to for more detailed information.

Disorders Causing Abdominal Distension in Cattle

VAGUS INDIGESTION

Vagus indigestion (VI) is rumen atony caused by damage or inflammatory changes to the vagus nerve as it courses through the pharynx, thoracic cavity, and perireticular and pyloric regions. The vagus nerve provides both sensory and motor innervation to the bovine forestomach compartments and abomasum. Like other neurologic disorders, the cause of VI is determined after localizing the lesion and four types of vagal indigestion have been defined: 1) failure of eructation; 2) omasal transport failure or anterior functional stenosis; 3) pyloric outflow obstruction or posterior functional stenosis; and 4) indigestion of late pregnancy based on the site that the vagal nerve has been affected. The editors have modified this classification (see Section 10.3). In Types II and III, the term *stenosis* is not entirely correct because there is no true narrowing of the tract; however, there is a functional blockage or paralysis and relaxation whereby ingesta is unable to traverse the omasum to the abomasum or the abomasum to the pylorus and duodenum, respectively. Alternatively, one could approach a cow with VI by examining the pharynx, neck, thorax, and cranial abdomen for lesions that may involve the nerve as it courses through those respective locations. Cows with VI may have low heart rates (40 to 60 beats per minute), and the rumen, on auscultation, will have frequent, small, uncoordinated

contractions. Feces tend to be scant and pasty with larger particulate matter due to inappropriate passage of feedstuffs. The most common causes of VI include traumatic reticuloperitonitis or hardware disease, reticular abscess (usually involving the medial wall of the reticulum), liver abscesses (right cranial and ventral aspect of the liver), pneumonia, postabomasal volvulus, and abomasal ulcers.

A great deal of information can be gained from standing behind a cow and observing the abdominal contour. Viewing the cow from either side and evaluating the shape of the paralumbar fossa and rib cage can also be helpful. The "papple" shape is classic for a cow with rumen distension in which the distended dorsal sac of the rumen occupies the dorsal left flank and the ventral sac of the rumen distends to not only fill the left ventral abdomen but also to distend over into the right ventral abdomen, thus giving an apple shape to the left side and a pear shape to the right side (Figures 1-3 and 1-4). The challenge is to determine the type and cause of the distention (Table 1-1). Auscultation of rumen motility, palpation of the rumen in the paralumbar fossa, accompanied by simultaneous auscultation and percussion (pinging) and succession, rectal examination, and rumen fluid analysis can be helpful in differentiating between these disorders. Other less common rule outs for distension of the entire left abdomen and right ventral abdomen include advanced pregnancy, hydrops, and abomasal impaction.

I—Failure of Eructation

With ruminal distension caused by free gas, a large ping can be heard dorsally on the left side of the abdomen

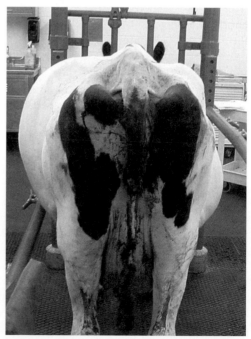

Figure 1-3 Classic papple-shaped abdomen in a cow with rumen distention.

TABLE 1-1

Differential Diagnosis for Cows with a Papple-Shaped Abdomen

PAPPLE-SHAPE			
VAGAL INDIGESTION			OTHER
TYPE I FAILURE OF ERUCTATION	TYPE II FAILURE OF OMASAL TRANSPORT	TYPE III PYLORIC OUTFLOW OBSTRUCTION	

Free gas bloat
Esophageal obstruction
Obstruction at the cardia
Right lateral recumbency
	Hardware disease
	Liver abscess
	Reticular abscess, adhesion,
	  peritonitis (without foreign body)
	Diffuse peritonitis
	Neoplasia of rumenoreticular
	  fold and esophageal groove
	Inflammatory disease of
	  reticular and rumen wall
	Papilloma or mass at
	  reticulomasal orifice
	Herniation of reticulum through
	  diaphragm
		Volvulus of the abomasum
		Right or left displacement of the abomasum
		Inflammation or adhesions involving the
		  reticulum and/or fundus of the
		  abomasum
		Advanced pregnancy with a large fetus
		Abomasal impaction
			Frothy bloat
			Lactic acidosis
			Diffuse peritonitis
			Hydrops

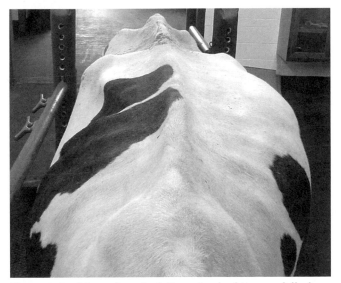

Figure 1-4   View of ruminal distention looking caudally from the withers region. Notice the marked distention of the left paralumbar fossa.

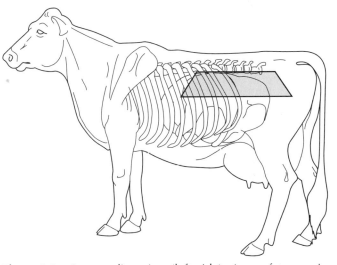

Figure 1-5   Rumen distention (left side). Area of tympanic resonance *(shaded)* heard with ruminal tympany.

beginning in the caudal left paralumbar fossa (as far back as the tuber coxae) and extending cranially to the eighth to tenth intercostal spaces (ICSs). The ping can also be heard dorsally over the midline (above the transverse processes of thoracic and lumbar vertebrae) with free gas rumen bloat. The ventral border of a rumen ping commonly has a very distinct horizontal line that distinguishes it from the tympanic resonance of a left-displaced abomasum (Figure 1-5). The rumen tends to be static in cows with free gas bloat, and the area of the ping corresponds to a palpably taut elastic tension on the external abdomen. The dorsal sac of the rumen on rectal

examination will feel tight and rebounds when indented. The dorsal sac of the rumen can extend to the right past the midline, whereas the ventral sac may also be palpable because it is distended with feed material. An ororumen tube (if passed in a manner that successfully reaches the trapped gas) can relieve the gas, and the ping and rumen distension palpated on rectal examination will decrease, thus confirming suspicion of free gas bloat.

II—Failure of Omasal Transport
Omasal transport failure results from impairment of the flow of ingesta from the reticulum through the omasal

canal into the abomasum and is considered true forestomach disease. This is the most common form of VI; perireticular or liver abscesses and traumatic reticuloperitonitis are the most likely causes. Toxic rumenitis, papilloma, and neoplasms of the rumenorectiular fold and esophageal groove have also been reported. The abomasum and omasum are empty in cows with omasal transport failure, and the forestomach compartments become progressively distended with the rumen taking on an L shape or as defined from external evaluation a papple shape. A mild to moderate amount of gas may accumulate dorsally in the rumen and multiple small (secondary) uncoordinated rumen contractions can be heard. Traumatic reticuloperitonitis deserves particular attention as a primary rule-out during examination of cows with VI. Cattle affected with hardware disease may stand with the elbows abducted, back arched, and the abdominal wall tensed. Other signs include a dramatic drop in milk production and complete anorexia. Improvement in uncomplicated cases may be seen in 3 to 5 days and manifests as less obvious pain and improvement in appetite and milk production. Chronic cases may have prolonged decreases in feed intake, fecal output, and milk production. Rumen motility may be decreased to absent, and the rumen can be somewhat small from inappetence to enlarged and bloated in more chronic cases in which the vagus nerve is involved.

Evaluating the cow for pain in the left cranial midabdomen should be performed by using the withers pinch or grunt test. Firm pressure can be applied over the withers (withers pinch) with both hands. A normal cow will drop in response to this, whereas a cow with cranial abdominal pain may wince, become somewhat agitated, throw her head around, stand tall, and resist while arching the back ventrally. This is not a sensitive test, and further evidence for hardware disease may be needed. The clinician can perform the grunt test by kneeling beside the cow on the left cranial aspect near the xiphoid and placing one knee under the cow with the fist resting on the knee. The fist and knee are lifted together and pressed into the cow's cranial and ventral abdominal wall. The cow's head and neck are observed for signs of discomfort, and any movement away from the pressure should be noted. A stethoscope can also be held under the cow's trachea during the grunt test to listen for a grunt. Alternatively, a pole about 1- to 1.5-m long can be placed under the cow and held at each end by two assistants. Beginning at the xiphoid and moving caudally, the pole is pulled upward slowly and then allowed to fall suddenly. An area of tenderness near the reticulum would suggest traumatic reticuloperitonitis. To determine whether a magnet is already in place, the operator, facing caudally and holding a compass at the level of the elbow, stands beside the cow's left shoulder. The

compass should be observed for deflection while the operator walks caudally beside the cow at the level of the elbow. If the compass passes a magnet, it will deflect but will maintain its bearing if no magnet is present. Ultrasonographic examination (3.5 or 5 MHz linear probe) of the cranial left paramedian abdomen and along the left thoracic wall to the point of the elbow between the 6th and 7th (ICSs) can be done to evaluate the perireticular region. The reticulum appears half-moon–shaped and has biphasic contractions that occur at a rate of approximately 1 cycle per minute. The reticulum moves about 8 cm (ventral to dorsal) for the first incomplete contraction and then greater than 17.5 cm (ventral to dorsal) for the second contraction. The amplitude, speed, and frequency of these contractions are diminished in cases of traumatic reticuloperitonitis. Displacement of the reticulum, accompanied by inflammatory changes and/or abscesses, is visualized as echogenic structures with or without capsules and echolucent fluid. Neither free foreign bodies nor foreign bodies are able to be imaged within the reticulum because of the interference of air. A free foreign body has been visualized in one cow because of the anechoic fluid surrounding the foreign body. Lateral reticular radiographs can help locate a foreign body and magnet, outline the contour of the reticulum, show the presence of abscesses (gas accumulation or gas/fluid interface), and demonstrate involvement of other abdominal or thoracic structures. Repeat radiographs can be used if the foreign body appears to rest in the lumen of the reticulum to determine whether it is adhered in that position or is the result of a reticular contraction. A serum total protein measurement often is helpful in diagnosing inflammatory conditions, particularly internal abscesses in the bovine when the value is increased (>7.5 g/dL). A normal total protein does not rule out the possibility of an internal abscess and hardware disease.

Failure of Abomasal Outflow

Pyloric stenosis results from damage to the vagus nerve that affects passage of feed material from the abomasum into the intestines. In this case the abomasum and omasum fill initially, and no forestomach distension is observed. Then, as a result of overdistension of the abomasum, "internal vomiting"—in which abomasal contents back-up into the rumen, distension of the rumen results, and a papple-shaped abdomen may be observed. As a result, the rumen chloride concentrations may increase above 30 mEq/L. The lesions that contribute to this syndrome include abomasal lymphoma, inflammation, and adhesions of the reticulum and abomasal fundus as well as compression of the pyloric region by a large fetus and secondary to right-sided abomasal volvulus.

Other Causes of Ruminal Distension

FROTH ACCUMULATION IN THE RUMEN

Cows with frothy bloat will have a papple shape, but will not have a significant dorsal gas cap and, therefore, will not ping like the free gas bloat. The rumen will be palpably enlarged and doughy both externally and internally (per rectum), but when an ororumen tube is passed, the distension remains and the ingesta retrieved during evacuation of the tube will appear as its name suggests — "frothy" with lots of small bubbles. A recent history of ingestion of a ration high in legumes may suggest a true frothy bloat. However, cows with vagal syndrome and improper mixing and fermentation of feedstuffs within the reticulorumen can also develop frothy type ingesta.

RUMEN ACIDOSIS

The cow with ruminal acidosis or grain overload has a decreased-to-absent appetite, general malaise, and dehydration and may have a dorsal accumulation of gas that results in variably sized rumen pings. The classic telltale sign is the remarkable sloshing of fluid in the rumen heard when succussion of the left abdomen is performed. Collection of a rumen fluid sample for pH is diagnostic. A metabolic acidosis caused by the absorption of volatile fatty acids from the rumen is observed along with evidence of dehydration with an increased PCV and total protein and prerenal azotemia. An abrupt change in ration or intake of high carbohydrate feedstuffs is often determined from a complete history.

ABOMASAL ULCERS

Abomasal ulcers most commonly occur in cows in the first 60 days after calving. They are associated with high-carbohydrate or concentrated feeds, stress, nonsteroidal antiinflammatory drug (NSAID) use, and bovine leukosis virus and can be secondary to abomasal displacement and prolonged accumulation of acid in the abomasum. Abomasal ulcers can be classified as nonperforating, nonperforating with severe blood loss, and perforating ulcers that result in either diffuse or localized peritonitis and sometimes omental bursitis. Nonperforating abomasal ulcers involve the mucosa and some of the submucosa. The cow may be asymptomatic or have partial anorexia and decreased rumen motility. Involvement of the submucosal blood vessels by the ulcer results in hemorrhage into the abomasum, and melena may be observed. Severe hemorrhage will result in signs of hemorrhagic shock with pale mucous membranes, tachycardia, anemia, and cool extremities. A localized peritonitis can occur secondary to an acute leakage of abomasal contents, generally from an ulcer along the ventral body of the abomasum. These usually become walled off by fibrinous adhesions that adhere to the abomasum, to the parietal peritoneum, and/or to the omasum. Acutely affected cows are anorexic, with a fever and decreased rumen motility; some may exhibit bruxism. The cow responds to deep palpation of the ventral cranial right abdomen and shows abdominal pain in this region. Ultrasonographic examination may show an area of variable echogenicity consistent with peritonitis. An abdominocentesis with an increased white blood cell count, and total protein will confirm the diagnosis. Perforation of the abomasum with leakage of abdominal contents into the omental bursa results in a more chronic disease, in which a septic purulent process accumulates within the omental bursa but does not involve the intestines. The cow often will have a decreased appetite, weight loss, progressive abdominal distension bilaterally from rumen stasis, and accumulation of fluid in the omental bursa. The total serum protein may be low because of loss of protein into the third space. Perforation of the abomasum with massive leakage of abdominal contents will result in diffuse peritonitis and a cow with peracute signs of shock, such as tachycardia (100-120 bpm), tachypnea, and cool extremities. Complete anorexia, fever, rumen and intestinal atony, and scant manure will be noticed initially. As the inflammatory response ensues within the abdomen and the leakage of ingesta continues, the ventral abdomen will become distended, and sometimes a fluid wave can be balloted. The rumen may become distended secondary to atony. Rectal examination may reveal a pneumoperitoneum, and ingesta may be palpable. Free fluid with a variable echogenicity and sometimes echodense spots consistent with gas are seen on ultrasonographic examination. An abdominocentesis with a foul odor that contains visible as well as cytological evidence of plant material engulfed by macrophages and bacteria can confirm the diagnosis.

Disorders that Cause Tympanitic Resonance (Pings) in Cattle

Areas of tympanitic resonance caused by a gas-fluid interface, gaseous distension of abdominal viscera, and free air in the abdomen can be detected by simultaneous auscultation and percussion of the abdomen. This is done by placing the stethoscope on the abdomen and snapping the index or middle finger of the opposite hand to tap on the cow's abdominal wall around the stethoscope at variable distances. The finger must be tapped aggressively to elicit a detectable tympanic resonance. The stethoscope is moved systematically around the abdomen while the finger is snapped against the abdominal wall. Once an area of tympanic resonance is heard, the area of

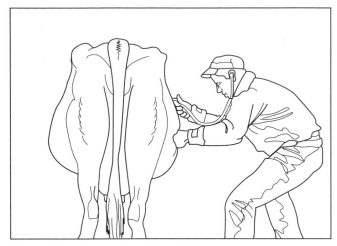

Figure 1-6   Succussion of the abdomen.

TABLE 1-2
Etiology of Right- and Left-sided Tympanic Resonances

LEFT-SIDED PING	RIGHT-SIDED PING
Rumen tympany	Gas distension of the proximal colon
Rumen collapse or void	Cecal dilatation +/− volvulus
Left displaced abomasum	Right displacement +/− volvulus of
Pneumoperitoneum	the abomasum
	Small intestinal distension
	Pneumoperitoneum
	Pneumorectum
	Ventral sac of rumen
	Physometra

the entire ping should be carefully determined to differentiate the viscera involved. Simultaneous auscultation and succussion (ballottement) should be performed to elicit a splashing or wave sound, which confirms the presence of a distended viscus with a gas and fluid interface. Ballottement involves placing the bell of the stethoscope over an area of tympanic resonance and simultaneously applying pressure with the opposite arm in a repeated motion (somewhat of a smooth punching motion) in the paralumbar fossa as close as possible to the ping (Figure 1-6). The fluid wave can sometimes be difficult to hear in less distended viscera, and repeated attempts should be performed to confirm the presence of a fluid wave.

LEFT-SIDED PINGS
Causes of a left-sided tympanic resonance include rumen tympany (discussed earlier), rumen collapse or void, left displacement of the abomasum, and pneumoperitoneum (Table 1-2).

LEFT DISPLACEMENT OF THE ABOMASUM
The classic tympanic resonance consistent with a left-displaced abomasum (LDA) is on the dorsal one third of

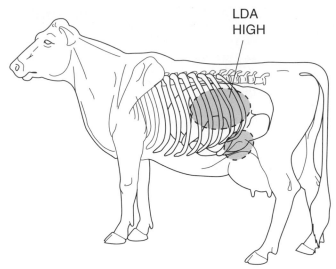

Figure 1-7   LDA—high and low (left side). Area of tympanic resonance *(shaded)* heard with a typical LDA. Note that the pings can be heard at different levels on the left side of the abdomen.

the left abdomen extending from the eighth to ninth ICS to a hand's width into the paralumbar fossa. The ping of an LDA commonly forms a somewhat circular pattern (Figure 1-7), which helps differentiate it from a distended rumen ping (see Figure 1-5). Ballottement accompanied by auscultation will confirm the presence of a large, fluid-filled viscus under the rib cage as a fluid wave creates a splashing sound with this technique. The location of the LDA often displaces the rumen medially, and the abomasum balloons under the rib cage giving the "sprung rib cage" appearance at the last two ribs. One can sometimes visualize a half-moon shape extending beyond the last rib into the paralumbar fossa. The entire left side of the cow should be evaluated for tympanic resonances because the abomasum has been heard displaced in a variety of places, including a much more caudoventral location along the costochondral junction. If the cow does not ping during the examination and no other illness is determined, the examination should be repeated after providing the cow with food and water. An LDA is not palpated per rectum except in the smallest cow, although the astute observer may feel the dorsal sac of the rumen somewhat displaced medially and pushing the left kidney beyond midline further to the right of the abdomen.

RUMEN VOID PING
A rumen void ping, or rumen collapse, is heard in the dorsal half to third of the abdomen on the left from the cranial paralumbar fossa extending forward to the tenth and eleventh ICSs. This ping is thought to be caused by the vacuum produced in the peritoneum by the

collapse of the dorsal sac of the rumen when the cow is anorexic and has poor rumen fill. The affected cow tends to have a sunken paralumbar fossa, and fluid cannot be detected when ballottement is performed. On rectal palpation, the left kidney is pulled ventrally and to the left, and a collapsed dorsal sac of the rumen is felt. The clinician should search for an underlying disease entity, such as bronchopneumonia, metritis, or mastitis to explain the rumen collapse.

PNEUMOPERITONEUM

Pneumoperitoneum is defined as free air or gas in the peritoneal cavity, most commonly found after exploratory laparotomy. Other causes of pneumoperitoneum include a ruptured viscus, such as a perforating abomasal ulcer, ruptured uterus, or progression of pneumothorax and pneumomediastinum. Mild to marked bilateral dorsal abdominal distension is observed (apple shape), and a tympanic resonance can be heard bilaterally in the top third of the abdomen to the midline. Ballottement and auscultation does not reveal a fluid wave. The rumen motility is difficult to auscultate because free air lies between the parietal peritoneum and the visceral peritoneum of the rumen. On rectal examination, pneumoperitoneum can be very obvious in some cases in which the air in the abdomen causes the rectum to collapse around the clinician's hand, thus making palpation of abdominal structures frustrating and difficult. Crepitus and/or feed material can also be palpated in some instances in which the underlying disease is a ruptured or leaking intestinal viscus.

RIGHT-SIDED PINGS

The right side of the cow is very complex. Pings on the right can be associated with a right-displaced abomasum (RDA), abomasal volvulus (RVA), cecal dilation and/or volvulus, distension of the proximal colon, pneumorectum, pneumoperitoneum, distension of small intestine, ventral sac of rumen, and physometra (see Table 1-2). Careful anatomic differentiation of these conditions must be made to pursue appropriate treatment.

RIGHT DISPLACEMENT AND/OR VOLVULUS OF THE ABOMASUM

An RDA is heard by simultaneous percussion and auscultation along a line from the tuber coxae to the right elbow extending cranially to the ninth ICS. The ping of an RDA extends cranially to the ninth rib (Figure 1-8). The caudal border of the viscus may reach the 13th rib or may extend slightly into the paralumbar fossa, creating a half-moon–shaped distension and a sprung rib cage, which can be seen when viewed from behind. A more caudal ping may be evident when the omentum has been torn and the abomasum is located more caudally.

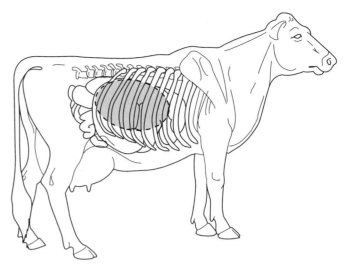

Figure 1-8 Abomasal volvulus (RVA). Area of tympanic resonance heard with RDA and RVA *(shaded)*.

Ballottement and auscultation will confirm a fluid wave underneath the ribs. The right side of the abdomen will appear distended, and sometimes ruminal tympany may occur secondary to mechanical outflow obstruction created by the abomasal displacement or volvulus and/or concurrent hypocalcemia. The area of tympanic resonance tends to be somewhat larger with greater fluid accumulation when the cow has an abomasal volvulus. An abomasal volvulus is more likely to be palpated per rectum at arm's length near the cranial aspect of the paralumbar fossa. It feels like the outer surface of a partially inflated inner tube that is covered by omentum. The dairy cow today is large, and often the right displaced abomasum is beyond reach. The systemic condition of the cow can allow one to predict, before surgery, whether the abomasum is displaced or twisted. Signs of hypovolemic shock (increased heart rate and dehydration) and endotoxemia, along with evidence of a shift from hypokalemic hypochloremic metabolic alkalosis to a high anion gap metabolic acidosis (lactic acidosis), are common indicators of abomasal volvulus with a less favorable prognosis and a need for prompt intervention.

CECAL DILATATION AND/OR VOLVULUS

A cecal dilatation and volvulus will have a tympanic resonance heard on the right midabdomen that extends cranially to the tenth or eleventh ICS and involves part or all of the paralumbar fossa (Figure 1-9 A and B). The ping may vary considerably, depending on the amount of distension of the incredibly elastic cecum. Ballottement of the involved area reveals a splashy "washing machine–type" sound as a result of the fluid accumulation in the cecum. The distension of the right paralumbar fossa is noted from behind and from the side of the

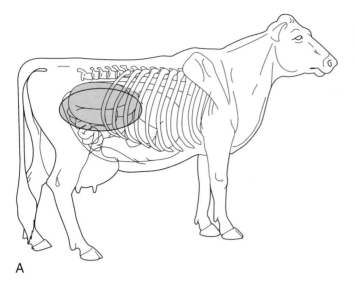

A

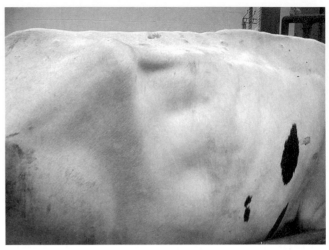

Figure 1-10   Right side of cow displaying distended cecum and proximal colon in a Holstein cow with cecal volvulus.

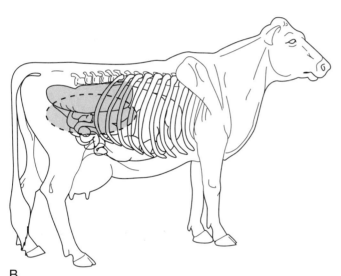

B

Figure 1-9   A. Cecal volvulus (right side). Area of tympanic resonance *(shaded)* heard in cows with a cecal volvulus. **B.** Cecal dilatation (right side). Area of tympanic resonance *(shaded)* heard in cows with cecal dilatation.

cow. The outline of the distended cecum in cases of dilatation and/or proximal colon with cecal volvulus can sometimes be visualized in the paralumbar fossa (Figure 1-10). On rectal examination, determining whether the cecum is dilated or progressed to a volvulus can be difficult. The distended cecum is easily palpable in the middle right and caudal abdomen lying horizontally in front of the pelvis in either instance, as a viscus that is about 6 to 9 inches in diameter and somewhat watermelon in shape and size (cylindrical/tubular). Sometimes the apex of the cecum is directed into the pelvic inlet so that it is obvious at the start of a rectal

examination. A cecal volvulus is suspected if more than one loop of the cecum/proximal colon (folded tube) is palpable per rectum in the right central and caudal abdomen in the region of the paralumbar fossa because the apex has rotated cranially and because the body is palpable. Small intestinal distension may accompany cecal disorders and may be palpable as small bicycle-tire tubes on rectal examination in the right cranial and mid-abdomen. The differentiation between cecal distension and volvulus is important because cecal distension does not necessarily require surgery. Cattle with a normal heart rate, some manure production, mild dehydration, and mild to moderate distension of the cecum on rectal examination may be considered to have cecal dilatation and treated, at least initially, conservatively with fluids and cathartics. Cecal volvulus typically causes more severe systemic signs including colic, hypotension, tachycardia, little or no manure production, dehydration, and palpation per rectum of the apex of cecum rotated cranially. These findings are indications for surgical intervention. Findings often are not straightforward, and the decision whether to operate is not easy. In most instances a right-sided standing exploratory laparotomy should be performed because the risk of further compromise of a volvulus of the cecum outweighs the benefits of medical management of a moderate to severe cecal distension.

DISTENSION OF THE PROXIMAL COLON
An area of tympanitic resonance in the dorsal paralumbar fossa the width of a hand extending cranially for two to three rib spaces is caused by moderate distension of the proximal colon and is clinically insignificant. Neither abdominal distension nor succussible fluid is present.

PNEUMORECTUM

Distension of the rectum and distal colon with air can cause a variably sized linear tympanic resonance in the right dorsal third of the caudal abdomen from the tuber coxae along the dorsal paralumbar fossa and—infrequently—cranial to the paralumbar fossa. Abdominal distension is not present and fluid cannot be heard on succession. Rectal examination will reveal an air-filled rectum, making palpation of abdominal viscera difficult until the air is evacuated.

DISTENSION OF THE SMALL INTESTINE

Small intestinal distension with fluid and gas occurs in simple indigestion, small intestinal obstruction, and secondary to cecal disorders. The most common small intestinal obstructive disorders have an acute onset of anorexia, decrease in milk production, abdominal pain, and gastrointestinal stasis. Differential diagnosis includes indigestion, volvulus of the small intestine, intussusception, and the more recently reported jejunal hemorrhage syndrome (JHS). *Clostridium perfringens* type A has been isolated from cows with JHS, although the etiology is debatable. Cows with small intestinal obstructive lesions often display signs of colic, such as kicking at their abdomen and preferring recumbency. The cow will have progressive abdominal distension as the small intestines proximal to the obstruction become enlarged in the right middle and ventral abdomen, followed by decreased pyloric outflow and subsequent abomasal and forestomach enlargement and left-sided distension. Variable tympanic resonances may be heard on the right side of the abdomen. Ballottement and simultaneous auscultation of the right lower abdomen will reveal tinkling and splashing sounds associated with fluid pooling in the small intestines. Feces are scant to absent. It is difficult to impossible to distinguish between intestinal volvulus and JHS before exploratory laparotomy. A history of JHS on the farm can be helpful. Frequently affected cows are profoundly dehydrated with blood in the manure. Cows with intussusception also pass small amounts of sticky, dark-red material that consists of blood from the sloughed mucosal surface of the intussusceptum (raspberry jam), mixed with mucus from the distal part of the gastrointestinal tract. Rectal examination in cows with intestinal disorders reveals multiple loops of small intestine that feel like bicycle inner-tube tires and range from 4 to 8 cm in diameter without any distension of the cecum. It has been reported that only 50% of cows with intussusception had distended loops of small intestine palpable per rectum, and in only half of those could a firm mass, presumed to be the intussusception, be palpated. Ultrasonographic examination in some cases can reveal a bull's eye sign (loop within a loop) consistent with an intussusception and small intestinal distension

with poor motility. Thick intestinal walls can be seen in cows with primary small intestinal surgical lesions. The author has seen variable echogenicity structures, like thrombi, within the intestinal lumen of cows with JHS.

PHYSOMETRA

Endometritis that results in fluid and gas accumulation in the uterus (physometra), in particular the right horn, can cause a small tympanic resonance in the lower right paralumbar fossa. This is a very uncommon cause of right-sided ping in a cow. Abdominal distension is not present, and a fluid wave is difficult to elicit with ballottement. Rectal and vaginal examinations will confirm the diagnosis.

VENTRAL SAC OF RUMEN

Gas in the distended ventral sac of the rumen to the point at which it causes a right-sided ping occurs infrequently. It can be confusing when present and can cause a clinician to do a right-sided exploratory laparotomy when it is not indicated. The general appearance of the cow should be that of a distended rumen—papple-shaped. The ping may be fairly consistent to indiscrete and rests in the midabdomen in the right paralumbar fossa. A rectal examination will reveal a markedly enlarged ventral sac of the rumen, which is taut and gas-distended.

RECOMMENDED READINGS

Belknap EB, Navarre CB: Differentiation of gastrointestinal diseases in adult cattle. *Vet Clin of North Am: Food Animal Pract* 16: 59-86, 2000.

Blikslager AT, Bristol DG, Hunt EL: Abomasal impaction in cattle. *Compend Contin Educ* 15: 1571-1575, 1993.

Braun U: Ultrasonographic examination of the liver and gallbladder in cows: normal findings. *Compend of Contin Educ* 18: 561-573, 1996.

Braun U, Amrein E: Ultrasonographic examination of the caecum and the proximal and spiral ansa of the colon of cattle. *Vet Rec* 149: 45-48, 2001.

Braun U, Eicher R, Hausammann K: Clinical findings in cattle with dilatation and torsion of the caecum. *Vet Rec* 125: 265-267, 1989.

Braun U, Fluckiger M, Gotz M: Comparison of ultrasonographic and radiographic findings in cows with traumatic reticuloperitonitis. *Vet Rec* 135: 470-478, 1994.

Braun U, Fluckiger M, Nageli F: Radiography as an aid in the diagnosis of traumatic reticuloperitonitis in cattle. *Vet Rec* 132: 103-109, 1993.

Braun U, Gansohr B, Fluckiger M: Radiographic findings before and after oral administration of a magnet in cows with traumatic reticuloperitonitis. *Am J Vet Res* 64: 115-120, 2003.

Braun U, Gotz M: Ultrasonography of the reticulum in cows. *Am J Vet Res* 55: 325-332, 1994.

Braun U, Hermann M, Pabst B: Haematological and biochemical findings in cattle with dilatation and torsion of the caecum. *Vet Rec* 125: 396-398, 1989.

Braun U, Iselin U, Lischer C, Fluri E: Ultrasonographic findings in five cows before and after treatment of reticular abscesses. *Vet Rec* 142: 184-189, 1998.

Braun U, Wild K, Guscetti F: Ultrasonographic examination of the abomasum of 50 cows. *Vet Rec* 140: 93-98, 1997.

Cable CS, Rebhun WC, Fubini SL, Erb HN, Ducharme NG: Concurrent abomasal displacement and perforating ulceration in cattle: 21 cases (1985-1996). *J Am Vet Med Assoc* 212: 1442-1445, 1998.

Constable PD, St. Jean G, Hull BL, Rings DM, Hoffsis GF: Preoperative prognostic indicators in cattle with abomasal volvulus. *J Am Vet Med Assoc* 198: 2077-2084, 1991.

Constable PD, St. Jean G, Hull BL, Rings DM, Morin DE, Nelson DR: Intussusception in cattle: 336 cases (1964-1993). *J Am Vet Med Assoc* 210: 531-536, 1997.

Fubini SL, Ducharme NG, Hollis HN, Smith DF, Rebhun WC: Failure of omasal transport attributable to perireticular abscess formation in cattle: 29 cases (1980-1986). *J Am Vet Med Assoc* 194: 811-814, 1989.

Fubini SL, Erb HN, Rebhun WC, Horne D: Cecal dilatation and volvulus in dairy cows: 84 cases (1977-1983). *J Am Vet Med Assoc* 189: 96-99, 1986.

Fubini SL, Grohn YT, Smith DF: Right displacement of the abomasum and abomasal volvulus in dairy cows: 458 cases (1980-1987). *J Am Vet Med Assoc* 198: 460-464, 1991.

Fubini SL, Yeager AE, Mohammed HO, Smith DF: Accuracy of radiography of the reticulum for predicting surgical findings in adult dairy cattle with traumatic reticuloperitonitis: 123 cases (1981-1987). *J Am Vet Med Assoc* 197: 1060-1064, 1990.

Garry FB, Hull BL, Rings DM, Kersting K, Hoffsis GF: Prognostic value of anion gap calculation in cattle with abomasal volvulus: 58 cases (1980-1985). *J Am Vet Med Assoc* 192: 1107-1112, 1988.

Godden S, Frank R, Ames T: Survey of Minnesota dairy veterinarians on the occurrence of and potential risk factors for jejunal hemorrhage syndrome in adult dairy cows. *The Bovine Pract* 35: 104-116, 2001.

Grohn YT, Fubini SL, Smith DF: Use of a multiple logistic regression model to determine prognosis of dairy cows with right displacement of the abomasum or abomasal volvulus. *Am J Vet Res* 51: 1895-1899, 1990.

Grymer J, Johnson R: Two cases of bovine omental bursitis. *J Am Vet Med Assoc* 181: 714-715, 1982.

Rebhun WC: The medical treatment of abomasal ulcers in dairy cattle. *Compend Contin Educ* 4: S91-S98, 1982.

Rebhun WC: Abdominal Diseases. In Rebhun WC: *Diseases of Dairy Cattle*. Philadelphia, 1995, Lippincott, Williams & Wilkins, pp 106-154.

Underwood WJ: Rumen lactic acidosis. Part II. Clinical signs, diagnosis, treatment, and prevention. *Compend Contin Educ* 14: 1265-1270, 1992.

Van Metre DC, Fecteau G, House JK, George LW: Indigestion of late pregnancy in a cow. *J Am Vet Med Assoc* 206: 625-627, 1995.

Ward JL, Ducharme NG: Traumatic reticuloperitonitis. *J Am Vet Med Assoc* 204: 874-877, 1994.

CHAPTER 2

DIAGNOSTIC IMAGING IN THE FOOD ANIMAL

Anthony Pease, Stephanie Nykamp, Amy Yeager

Diagnostic imaging, such as radiographs and ultrasound, is an invaluable and underused tool for the food animal practitioner. Other infrequently used modalities include nuclear medicine, computed tomography (CT), and magnetic resonance imaging (MRI). Because of the variety of available imaging modalities, the proper imaging study must be selected to maximize the chance of detecting lesions while minimizing time and cost to the client. This section will provide an outline for general techniques and indications of when to use various imaging modalities in the food animal.

Radiology

Survey radiography, including digital and computed radiography, is considered the mainstay of diagnostic imaging. The various views that can be acquired have been described in detail in other publications (Bargai et al, 1989; Pharr and Bargai, 1997). A table has been provided to illustrate a general guide—a starting point—for techniques to acquire different radiographic studies in various species (Table 2-1). Unfortunately, the nature of ambulatory work does not allow practitioners the luxury of developing the film, evaluating the radiograph, adjusting the technique, and retaking radiographs if the exposure is unsatisfactory. For this reason, all recommendations assume an average-sized animal and a film-to-tube focal distance of no greater than 40 inches (or as close as possible in regard to thorax and abdomen). If the patient appears thin or obese, decreasing or increasing the kilovolt peak (kVp) by no less than 15% adjusts the technique. Alternatively, the milliamps per second

(mAs) can be changed by no less than 50%, depending on the radiographic study required.

In general, increasing the kVp will provide greater penetration of the X-ray photons and give an overall gray appearance, which is desirable for thoracic radiographs. In contrast, increasing the exposure time (mAs) will increase the contrast of a film, thus making it more black and white. This technique provides good bone detail that is desirable when radiographs of the extremities are obtained.

Proper technique will aid in providing a quality film; however, appropriate measures must be taken to provide adequate radiation safety to the practitioner, patient, and technicians. The basic principle of ALARA—an acronym for *As Low As Reasonably Achievable*—should always be used. This means using a cassette holder, lead gloves, and lead aprons when exposing a film. The minimum exposure time should be used, and all personnel should be kept as far from the primary beam as possible. It should always be remembered the cassette, lead gloves, and lead apron do not stop the primary X-ray beam. Therefore people or body parts in line with the primary beam receive a radiation dose similar to that of the structure being imaged.

In addition to survey radiographs, contrast radiography can also be performed to provide additional information about soft tissue structures. Contrast procedures that examine the esophagus, digits, mammary gland, and urinary bladder have been described. Positive contrast mammography can be performed on the mammary gland; however, to the author's knowledge, no milk withdrawal times for iodinated contrast media have been

TABLE 2-1

Suggested Radiographic Techniques for the Species Indicated

SPECIES/LOCATION	KVP	MAS	SPECIES/LOCATION	KVP	MAS
Adult Bovine			**Adult Porcine**		
Head (sinus/mandible*)	75/85*	10	Head	80*	12
Neck	75	10	Neck	80*	12
Thorax			Thorax		
Cranioventral	120	40	Craniolateral	80*	6.3
Craniodorsal	120	10	Caudolateral	80*	6.3
Caudodorsal	120	4.4	Ventrodorsal	80*	6.3
Caudoventral	120	10	Abdomen		
Cranial abdomen	120	60	Craniolateral	85*	12
Extremity			Caudolateral	85*	12
Carpus	70	6.3	Ventrodorsal	85*	12
Stifle	85*	20	Extremity		
Tarsus	70	6.3	Carpus	63	8
Digit	60	5	Stifle	75*	200
Pelvis			Tarsus	63	8
Ventrodorsal	100	1000 × 2 exp	Digit	63	6.3
Lateral	100	1000 × 2 exp	Pelvis		
Teat (fine screen)	80	1-5	Ventrodorsal	85	200
Quarter (fine screen)	80	20	Lateral	85	200
Calf			**Piglet**		
Head	70	10	Head	60*	10
Neck (bone/soft tissue)	65/60	24/10	Neck	55*	10
Thorax			Thorax	75*	3.6
Ventrodorsal	80	3.6	Abdomen	75*	6.8
Lateral	70*	3.6	Extremity	60	3
Abdomen	70*	8	Pelvis		
Extremity	55	5	Ventrodorsal	75*	32
Pelvis			Lateral	75*	32
Ventrodorsal	70*	32			
Lateral	70*	36			
Caprine/Ovine					
Head	70	8			
Neck	65	10			
Thorax	70*	3.6			
Abdomen	70*	6.8			
Extremity	60	2.5			

All techniques assume an average-sized animal and regular or medium screen films except for teat and quarter films (fine screen).
*indicates an 8:1 grid is required, and exp = exposure (pelvic radiographs require a second exposure for a 2 second total exposure time). (Courtesy of Renea L. McNeill, LVT; Patricia Homer, LVT; and Barbara Chapman, RT).

published. In addition, intravenous sodium iodine is not for use in the lactating dairy cow; thus no inferred withdrawal time can be made. Therefore if iodinated contrast media is used in the lactating cow, the recommendation is to strip the teat thoroughly and observe a withdrawal time of approximately 5 days. In the United States, this withdrawal time is only a suggestion, and the authors recommend contacting the local state regulatory commission before performing the procedure. To perform positive contrast mammography, a small volume (10-30 ml) of iodinated contrast media (Hypaque-76*) is

infused into the affected and a nonaffected teat via a teat cannula. Lateral radiographic projections are then acquired of each mammary gland separately. Structural lesions of the papillary duct and lactiferous sinus can be detected (Figure 2-1).

Positive contrast urethrography is difficult to perform in goats because of the urethral process. In the pig, it is also difficult to pass a urinary catheter in a retrograde fashion because of the spiral nature of the penis. For this reason, positive contrast, normograde urethrography via a tube cystotomy is recommended. This procedure entails placing a percutaneous cystotomy tube and approximately 50-200 milliliters of iodinated contrast medium (e.g. Hypaque-76) into the urinary bladder.

*Diatrizoate Megalumine and Diatrizoate Sodium, Nycomed Inc., Princeton, NJ.

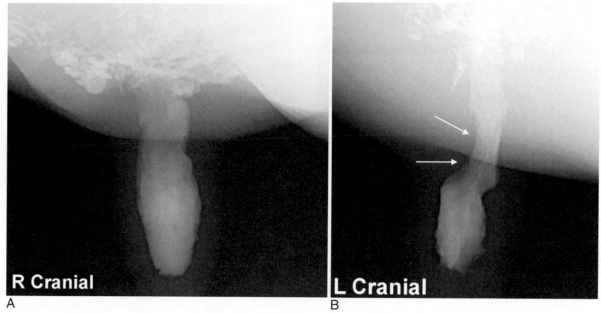

Figure 2-1   Contrast lateral radiographs of the unaffected right cranial quarter **(A)** and the left cranial quarter **(B)** in an adult cow. Note the filling defect *(arrows)* in the lactiferous sinus of the left cranial quarter **(B).**

The bladder is filled with sterile saline until the urine overflows into the urethra or the urinary bladder is palpable. A liter of saline may be required before urination occurs and the urethra is opacified. Gentle pressure can be placed on the urinary bladder to promote emptying. This procedure provides a positive contrast cystogram and a positive contrast urethrogram.

Thoracic and abdominal radiography, especially in large food animals, requires specialized equipment generally found only in teaching or referral hospitals. The reticulum can be imaged with a portable unit if the cow is first placed in dorsal recumbency. This moves the reticulo and abomasal contents toward the back of the animal, and the air rises to outline the ventral position of the reticulum (see Figure 10.3-4). Alternate imaging modalities, such as ultrasonography, should be considered for evaluating the thorax and abdomen.

Ultrasound

For ultrasound the thorax or abdomen of a large animal, the major requirement is a low-frequency (MHz) probe. This is because the lower the frequency of the sound waves emitted, the deeper the penetration of the probe. However, the depth of penetration is inversely proportional to resolution, which means the deeper the structure being imaged, the less clear it will appear.

Ultrasound works by sending high-frequency sound waves into the structure being imaged. The sound waves are then attenuated, absorbed, scattered, or reflected back to the transducer. The transducer detects the sound waves reflected back and determines the depth of the sound wave based on the time that passes from the initial pulse. This assumes that the structure imaged is soft tissue, which conducts sound at 1540 m/s. The intensity of the reflected sound wave is converted to a gray scale. Based on the time and intensity of the sound waves returned to the transducer, an image is produced. The images are then described based on the echogenicity, margin, and size. Echogenicity is a relative term and is usually described based on the surrounding parenchyma or another structure (for example, spleen is hyperechoic in comparison to liver, and kidney is hypoechoic to spleen).

The convention to display images is to have the patient's left side on the right side of the video screen or print (much like viewing a radiograph). In addition, dorsal or cranial is oriented on the left of the video monitor and ventral or caudal is on the right. Images are described based on the plane on which they were acquired. Generally this involves transverse (cross-section), longitudinal (long-axis) or oblique image planes. These planes can be related either to the patient as a whole (transverse sonogram of the cranial abdomen) or to the organ or structure being imaged (longitudinal image of the abomasum).

In a standard large animal (bovine) abdomen, a 2- to 5-MHz probe generally is used. The sonographer can use

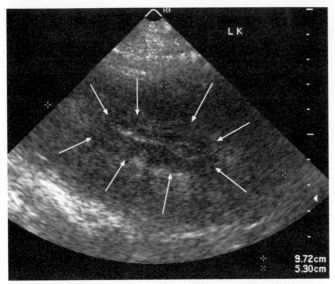

Figure 2-2 Transverse sonogram of the left kidney with a 5-3-MHz phased array sector probe in an adult Rambouillet sheep with a history of weight loss. Note the hypoechoic medulla of the kidney *(arrows)* in comparison to the cortex. This patient was diagnosed with immune-mediated glomerulonephritis secondary to chronic *Corynebacterium pseudotuberculosis* infection.

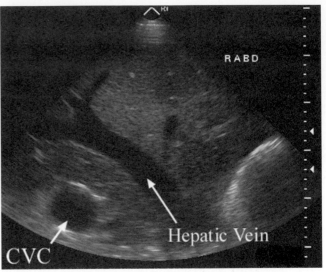

Figure 2-3 Oblique sonogram of the liver using a 3-2-MHz phased array sector probe in an adult Holstein cow with a history of anorexia and diarrhea for 7 days. Note the large hepatic vein and caudal vena cava (CVC). The patient had right-sided heart failure with secondary passive congestion of the liver and gallbladder.

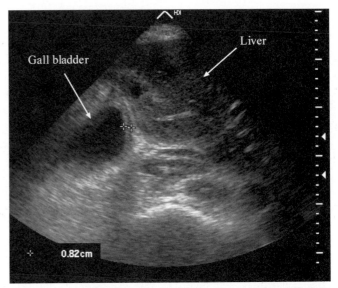

Figure 2-4 Oblique sonogram of the liver with a 3-2-MHz phased array sector probe in an adult Holstein cow with a history of anorexia and diarrhea for 7 days. Note the thick wall of the gallbladder (8 mm), attributed to edema. The patient had right-sided heart failure with secondary passive congestion of the liver and gall bladder.

any approach as long as it is systematic and thorough. At the Farm Animal Hospital at Cornell University, the general abdominal ultrasound examination begins at the paralumbar fossa of either the right or left side, progresses cranially between intercostal spaces, and continues to the level of the thoracic cavity (lungs and heart). Then the opposite side is imaged. The technique described can be used for any farm animal but is different than the organ system approach used in small animals. For the left abdominal window of the bovine, the rumen and reticulum are the most notable structures. The liver and spleen can also be evaluated. In the right abdominal window, the right and left kidneys (Figure 2-2), omasum, liver (Figure 2-3), gallbladder (Figure 2-4), and intestines can be seen. In the ventral abdomen, the intestines, abomasum and reticulum can be seen. During transrectal ultrasound, evaluation of the reproductive tract and potentially of the urinary bladder and left kidney can be performed.

No established technique has been reported for evaluating the thorax. In the authors' hospital, thoracic ultrasonography generally begins cranially and progresses caudally while using the intercostal spaces. This is done until lung is no longer detected. Because the lung is relatively superficial, a higher-frequency probe (8- to 5-MHz) can be used for normal lung. A low-frequency probe is required to evaluate the heart, large pleural fluid accumulations, and large pulmonary or mediastinal lesions. During thoracic ultrasonography, only the surface of aerated lung (Figure 2-5) can be seen because

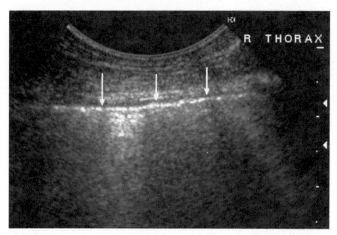

Figure 2-5 Transverse sonogram of the right thorax using an 8-5-MHz curved array probe in an 8-month-old pigmy goat with post-anesthetic hypoxia. Note the bright hyperechoic line *(arrow)* with no returning echoes deep to the structure. This line should move with respiration and represents the interface of lung and pleural space. No abnormality is detected.

air interface reflects 99% of the sound waves back towards the transducer. In doing so, the air interface prevents detection of deeper structures. Pulmonary lesions must extend to the surface of the lung to be detected. Thoracic ultrasound is most useful for detecting pleural fluid, pleural masses, and body wall lesions (Figure 2-6 and 2-7A and B). Ultrasound-guided fine needle aspirates for cytology and culture can be obtained to aid in making a diagnosis.

Ultrasound of specific locations—including: neck, umbilicus, mammary glands, subcutaneous tissues, joints, limbs, and perineum—can be performed. These sites are generally used to evaluate lymph nodes, foreign bodies, masses, abscesses, or urinary calculi.

The use of ultrasound to evaluate fractures of the shoulder, proximal thoracic and pelvic-limbs, or pelvis has also been suggested. This is because, as described previously, the techniques required for radiography of these structures are generally beyond the capabilities of the ambulatory practitioner. In addition, ultrasonography gives real-time images in a method that is anatomically intuitive and can be a means to acquire a diagnosis using fine-needle aspirates or biopsies.

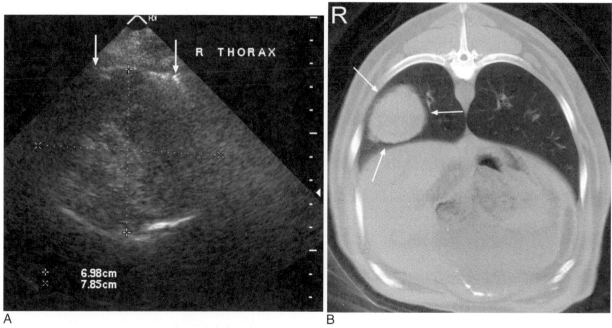

A

B

Figure 2-6 Longitudinal sonogram using a 5-3-MHz phased array sector probe **(A)** and transverse CT **(B)** of the right thorax in an adult Rambouillet sheep with a history of weight loss. In the sonogram, note the large, hyperechoic mass in the right caudal lung lobe. The ribs *(arrows)* cast acoustic shadows that obscure the cranial and caudal aspects of the mass. On CT **(B),** note the large, soft tissue dense mass within the right caudal lung lobe *(arrows)*. This mass was a pulmonary abscess that cultured positive for *Corynebacterium pseudotuberculosis.*

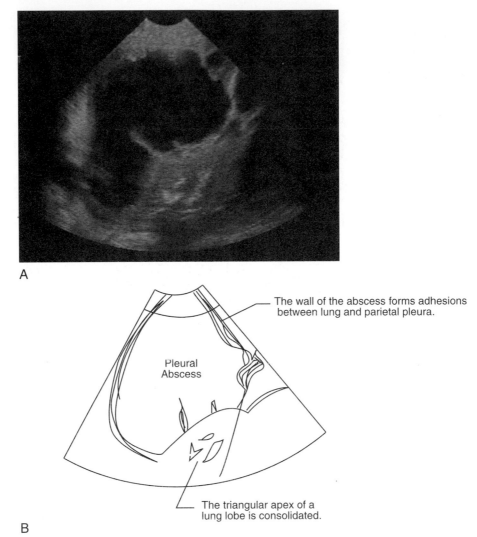

A

B

The wall of the abscess forms adhesions between lung and parietal pleura.

Pleural Abscess

The triangular apex of a lung lobe is consolidated.

Figure 2-7   *A,* Transverse sonogram of left thorax using an 8-5 MHz convex linear probe in a 6-year-old Suffolk ewe with a pleural abscess. The right side of the sonogram is ventral. *B,* Schematic representation of sonogram.

Nuclear Medicine, CT, and MRI

Other imaging modalities infrequently used in food animal practice include nuclear medicine, CT, and MRI. Nuclear medicine is not recommended in food animals in the United States. The United States Nuclear Regulatory Committee states that no radiopharmaceuticals are approved for use in animals intended for the human food supply. However, the use of Technetium methylene diphosphonate (^{99m}Tc-MDP) for bone scintigraphy can be useful for diagnosing lameness or other skeletal abnormalities (see Figure 2-7). Use of radiopharmaceu-

ticals is off-label in the food animal; therefore consultation with the Food and Drug Administration is recommended if the procedure is attempted. Computed tomography and MRI have been used in a very limited fashion in food animals. Generally, the size of the animal (bovine) limits evaluations to the head (including brain and sinuses) and distal extremities (Figure 2-8). The cost of these modalities keeps them reserved for animals with high value, such as transgenic cattle. The requirement for general anesthesia and specialized equipment make these modalities unlikely to become universally used or recommended for the food animal.

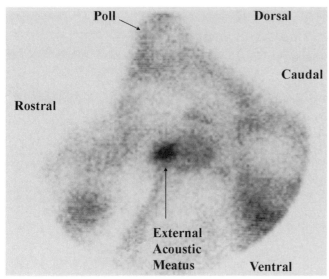

Figure 2-8   Left-lateral bone scintigraphy of the head in a 1-year-old Holstein cow with cervical pain. Technetium methylene diphosphonate—110 milliCuries—was administered intravenously, and images were acquired 2 hours after injection. No abnormality is detected. Note the high activity detected in the petrous temporal bone. This is considered a normal finding because of superimposition of dense bone; therefore a large amount of activity is present in that area.

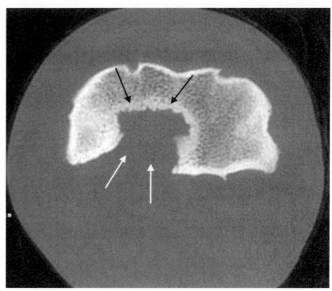

Figure 2-9   Transverse CT of the left thoracic-limb in a 3-year-old bull with left thoracic-limb lameness. In the distal metaphysis of the left third metatarsal bone, there is a focal area of bone lysis *(arrows)*. The bull was euthanized, and the necropsy disclosed a bone abscess at this site.

RECOMMENDED READINGS

Bargai U, Pharr JW, Morgan JP: The need for radiology in the bovine practice. In Bargai U, Pharr JW, Morgan JP: *Bovine radiology*, Ames, Iowa, 1989, Iowa State University Press.

Bargai U, Pharr JW, Morgan JP: Views and positioning in radiography of cattle. In Bargai U, Pharr JW, Morgan JP, eds: *Bovine radiology*, Ames, Iowa, 1989, Iowa State University Press.

Bargai U, Pharr JW, Morgan JP: The Esophagus. In Bargai U, Pharr JW, Morgan JP, eds: *Bovine radiology*, Ames, Iowa, 1989, Iowa State University Press.

Braun U, Fohn J, Pusterla N: Ultrasonographic examination of the ventral neck region in cows. *Am J Vet Res* 55: 14-21, 1994.

Gogoi SN, Nigam JM, Singh AP: Angiographic evaluation of bovine foot abnormalities. *Vet Rad* 23: 171-174, 1982.

Kofler J, Edinger HK: Diagnostic ultrasound imaging of soft tissues of the bovine distal limb. *Vet Radiol Ultrasound* 36: 246-252, 1995.

Pharr JW, Bargai U: Radiology. In Greenough P, editor: *Lameness in cattle*, ed 3, Philadelphia, 1997, WB Saunders.

Singh AP, Nigam JM: Radiography of bovine esophageal disorders. *Mod Vet Pract* 61: 867-869, 1980.

Singh G, Singh J, Williamson HD et al: Radiographic visualization of the ruminant upper urinary tract by a double contrast technique. *Vet Rad* 24: 106-111, 1983.

Singh G, Vig MM, Kumar R: Contrast radiography in the diagnosis of teat affections. *J Am Vet Radiol Soc* 16: 11-12, 1975.

CHAPTER 3

NEOPLASIA

Beth A. Valentine

The description of neoplastic disorders and incidence of neoplasia in farm animals has historically relied heavily on surveys conducted on animals at slaughter houses. The incidence of tumors reported in such surveys indicates that tumors are most common in cattle (0.23%) and are uncommon in sheep (0.002%), goats (0.009%), and pigs (0.004%).

Far fewer clinical descriptions of neoplasia in farm animals exist than do clinical reports of neoplastic diseases in dogs, cats, and horses. Reports of surgical treatment of tumors of farm animals are even less common. The changing face of livestock husbandry—with the increase in small "hobby" farms, sanctuaries, and petting zoos—will likely result in earlier detection of clinical signs associated with neoplastic disease and increased owner interest in pursuing surgery. With the advent of improved diagnostic procedures—in particular, ultrasound—detecting internal tumors at early stages is possible.

The following chapter describes neoplastic disorders of cattle, sheep, goats, and pigs that might present for surgical biopsy or surgical excision. As such, tumors of organs such as the heart and brain have been excluded. In many cases of farm animal neoplasia, extrapolation from information available on results of surgery on similar tumors in cats, dogs, and horses is the best that can be provided at this time. It is hoped that future editions of this or similar texts will be able to incorporate what should be a growing body of literature regarding surgical treatment of farm animal tumors.

Tumors of the Skin and Soft Tissue

Skin tumors are the most common neoplasms in farm animals. This is in large part caused by the high incidence of papillomavirus-induced lesions in the skin of cattle. Other tumors occur less frequently, and skin tumors in general are less common in sheep, goats, and pigs. Tumors of the soft tissue (subcutis and skeletal muscle) are uncommon and are included in this section because they are likely to present as mass lesions visible and palpable on external physical examination.

PAPILLOMA AND FIBROPAPILLOMA (PAPILLOMATOSIS)

Papillomas, commonly called *warts,* are the most common skin tumor of cattle. Shorthorn cattle appear to be predisposed to development of cutaneous papillomatosis. These tumors in cattle result from bovine papillomavirus infection and most often occur in animals less than 2 years of age. Viral infection of skin is thought to occur most often after trauma, infections, ectoparasites, or ultraviolet light exposure that damages the skin. Virally-induced cutaneous papillomatosis occurs less commonly in sheep and goats of any age, and a viral cause is suspected in affected goats. Papillomatosis is rare but can occur in pigs of all ages. Piglets can be born with congenital papillomas that may or may not be virally induced. Papillomas can also involve the eyes of cattle and the genitalia of cattle and pigs and are discussed in the sections on tumors of the eye and tumors of the female and of the male genital tract. Papillomas of the udder and teats in cattle, sheep, and goats are discussed in the section on tumors of the udder and mammary gland.

Bovine papillomas can become quite large and multinodular. They may be broad-based or pedunculated. They are alopecic and surface hyperkeratosis is typical. Exophytic growths are most common, although flat plaque-like growths are also possible. Lesions can occur anywhere on the body, but the head, neck and dewlap are common sites (Figure 3-1). In sheep, papillomatosis most often involves the skin of the face and legs. Goat papillomas most often occur on the head, neck, shoulders, and upper forelegs.

Raised lesions of the interdigital skin of adult cattle are a unique entity. These lesions have previously been called *interdigital papillomas,* but this disorder is now thought most likely to be induced by bacterial spirochetes rather than by papillomavirus. *Papillomatous digital dermatitis* is a more appropriate term, and these lesions are typically single, raised, painful growths often with surface finger-like projections of epithelium. Lameness, weight loss, and decreased milk production occur in cattle with interdigital papillomatous dermatitis. These growths can occur only in individual animals or can apparently spread to involve multiple animals.

Histologic evaluation of papillomas reveals two main types of proliferative lesions. Those with entirely squamous epithelial proliferations are classified as squamous papillomas, and those with proliferation of underlying fibrous connective tissue as well as of epithelium are classified as fibropapillomas. Papillomaviruses are known to be capable of inducing proliferation of both epithelial cells and fibroblasts. Identification of the spirochetes associated with bovine papillomatous digital dermatitis requires silver stains.

Papillomas in farm animals can be contagious, with an incubation period of about 2 to 6 months. Most papillomas that develop in young animals will spontaneously regress. Surgical excision of one tumor or use of immunostimulants have been said to speed the regression, but whether these procedures actually alter the

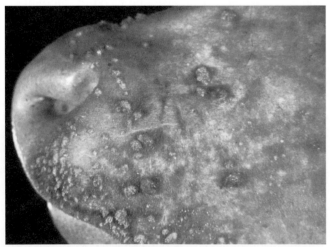

Figure 3-1   Multiple papillomas caused by bovine papillomavirus on the muzzle and lips of a young cow.

(Courtesy of Dr. Stan Snyder.)

natural course of the disease is not clear. Papillomas in adult sheep and goats less commonly regress spontaneously, and persistent tumors can undergo malignant transformation to squamous cell carcinoma (see Squamous Cell Carcinoma). Congenital papillomas in piglets can grow rapidly after birth. Surgical excision or cryotherapy of cutaneous and interdigital papillomas of cattle and of papillomas of sheep, goats, and piglets is often curative. In dairy cattle, treatment of interdigital papillomas with parenteral penicillin, ceftiofur, or topical oxytetracyline resulted in resolution of the lesions, which is good evidence that bacteria play an important pathogenic role in this disorder. Recurrence or subsequent development of new lesions, however, occurred in almost 50% of cases.

SQUAMOUS CELL CARCINOMA

Squamous cell carcinoma is the second most common skin tumor in almost all farm animals. Swine are the exception, as cutaneous squamous cell carcinoma is very rare in pigs. This is interesting, as the development of cutaneous squamous cell carcinoma has been linked to ultraviolet light exposure of thinly haired unpigmented skin, which most pigs have in abundance. Viral papillomas can progress to cutaneous squamous cell carcinoma, especially those on the udder (see Tumors of the Udder and Mammary Gland). Squamous cell carcinoma typically occurs in adult animals. In cattle, Herefords and Ayrshires are predisposed to squamous cell carcinoma, most likely because of their large areas of unpigmented skin. Aged ewes and Merino sheep are predisposed to development of squamous cell carcinoma, and both ultraviolet light exposure and exposure to photosensitizing plants are proposed etiologic factors. Saanen, Saanen cross, and Angora goats with white- or gray-haired areas appear to be predisposed to cutaneous squamous cell carcinoma. This tumor in goats has been reported to be more common in females, most likely because of the syndrome of udder papillomatosis and squamous cell carcinoma (see Tumors of the Udder).

Cutaneous squamous cell carcinoma causes a raised, proliferative, and ulcerated lesion and in cattle is most common at mucocutaneous junctions, such as the periocular skin and skin of the vulva. Squamous cell carcinoma in the skin of Merino sheep most often occurs on the ears and less commonly involves the muzzle, lower lip, and vulva. Those on the vulva occur primarily in sheep in which perineal surgery has been performed to reduce fly strike. Tumors in sheep are often multicentric. Squamous cell carcinoma of the ears of sheep can begin as a cutaneous horn, as a hyperkeratotic plaque, or can occur at the site of ear trauma such as from an identification punch. This tumor is rare in sheep less than 4 years of age. Squamous cell carcinoma in sheep can also occur in periocular skin. Cutaneous squamous cell carcinoma in goats is most common on the ears, udder, vulva, and perineum. Tumors in pigs can be single or multiple.

Histologic features are of well differentiated to poorly differentiated invasive squamous epithelium with associated sclerosis and inflammation. Atypical squamous cells indicative of neoplasia can be seen on cytologic preparations.

Metastasis of cutaneous squamous cell carcinoma can occur, most commonly to local lymph nodes. Metastasis is, however, typically a late event, preceded by a long period of local invasion. Immunotherapy of ovine squamous cell carcinoma has been shown to actually increase the rate of metastasis. Wide surgical excision, cryotherapy, hyperthermia, or radiation therapy of tumors before metastasis can be curative.

CUTANEOUS HORN

Cutaneous horn occurs in cattle, sheep, and goats. These growths can be single or multiple and consist of firm hornlike projections up to 10 cm long. Histologically, cutaneous horn is formed by compacted laminated keratin. Surgical excision is usually curative, although histopathologic evaluation of the base of the lesion to rule out underlying papilloma or carcinoma is warranted.

MELANOCYTIC TUMORS

Both benign and malignant melanocytic tumors occur in farm animals. Melanoma is most common in Sinclair miniature and Duroc-Jersey swine and is thought to be inherited in these breeds. Melanoma also occurs with some frequency in Hampshire and Iberian pigs. Melanoma does not occur in white swine and does not appear to be related to ultraviolet light exposure. Melanomas occur in the skin of cattle with some frequency, are relatively uncommon in goats, and are rare in sheep.

Melanomas in cattle occur most often in young animals. Tumors are either present at birth or develop within the first 2 years. Melanoma most commonly occurs in gray-haired cattle and in black-, or red-haired cattle, such as Angus. Melanoma in sheep occurs in the skin or the base of the horn in adult to aged animals, and Suffolk and Angora sheep are predisposed breeds. Melanoma in goats occurs in adult to aged animals. Angora goats may be predisposed, as is any goat of gray or brown coat color. Melanoma in predisposed swine breeds can develop at any age but are most often present at birth or develop within 1 year of age.

Melanoma is recognized clinically by areas of gray to black pigmentation within a solid fleshy raised mass. Melanomas occur within the dermis, the subcutis, or both. The overlying skin is often darkly pigmented, smooth, and partially to completely alopecic. Melanomas

in cattle occur on the head (especially the jaw), neck, trunk, or legs. Most tumors arise in areas of pigmented hair. Size of tumors in cattle vary widely, from less than 5 cm to up to 25 cm. Melanoma in cattle most often occurs as a solitary lesion with intact overlying skin. Melanomas in sheep are often multiple and occur in the subcutis under areas of pigmented skin. Melanomas of goats occur most often in the perineum, with rare involvement of other sites such as the udder, coronary band, ear, and base of the horn. Melanomas in goats can be single or multicentric. Tumors of the perineum in goats vary from infiltrative to pedunculated and often are ulcerated. Affected goats often rub and lick the area, and secondary infection is common. Enlargement of local lymph nodes and poor body condition are also common in goats with melanoma. Melanomas in predisposed pigs can be either solitary or multiple, and occur as either flat plaquelike tumors or larger raised tumors, most often on the trunk (Figure 3-2).

Histologic and cytologic examination of samples from melanocytic tumors reveals the characteristic melanin-containing neoplastic cells, often admixed with heavily pigmented melanophages. Cellular pleomorphism and mitotic activity are variable. Those tumors with high mitotic indices are most often malignant. Evidence of local or epidermal invasion is also a good indicator of malignancy.

Melanocytic tumors that occur in young cattle are almost always benign and cured by wide surgical excision. Melanomas in older cattle can, however, develop metastases to local lymph nodes or internal organs. Melanomas of sheep and goats are most often malignant, with frequent metastases. Perineal melanomas of goats can exhibit widespread metastases to multiple lymph

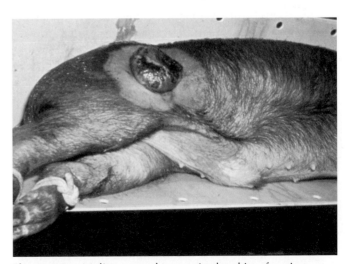

Figure 3-2 Malignant melanoma in the skin of a pig. (Courtesy of Dr. Danny Scott.)

nodes; to bone; and to internal organs, including lungs, liver, adrenal glands and kidneys. Surgical excision of cutaneous melanomas in goats can be attempted, but death from metastatic tumors is common. The melanomas of predisposed breeds of pigs have an interesting behavior that has made them a useful animal model for the study of melanocytic tumors of people. The flat tumors typically spontaneous regress starting as early as 1 month of age, often leaving a halo of depigmented skin and hair. Larger, raised tumors often metastasize within the first year of life.

MAST CELL TUMORS

Mast cell tumors are most common in cattle and often involve the skin. Age of affected cattle ranges from 2 months to 12 years. Holstein and Holstein crosses may be predisposed. Cutaneous mastocytosis occurs in pigs 6 to 18 months of age. No reports were found of mast cell tumors in sheep or goats.

Mast cell tumors in the skin of cattle can be single or multiple. These tumors are raised, firm, tan nodular masses that can be ulcerated. Tumors can be discrete or infiltrative. Histologic and cytologic preparations are characterized by sheets of well differentiated to pleomorphic mast cells with admixed eosinophils. Mitoses are rare. Tumor necrosis, fibrosis and mineralization are common histologic findings in cattle. Porcine mastocytosis results in multiple nodular solid gray-white skin lesions that can be ulcerated. Tumors in pigs contain relatively homogeneous neoplastic mast cells admixed with eosinophils. Cutaneous mastocytosis in pigs may or may not have associated widespread visceral involvement.

Cutaneous mast cell tumors in cattle are associated with a relatively high rate of metastasis. Spread to lung and lymph node is most common, and metastasis to liver and muscle is also reported. Tumor cell morphology (i.e., well-differentiated vs. pleomorphic) does not appear to predict metastatic behavior, as even very well-differentiated mast cell tumors in cattle have undergone widespread metastasis. Wide surgical excision is the treatment of choice, and a guarded prognosis following surgery is warranted.

CUTANEOUS LYMPHOMA

Cutaneous lymphoma occurs most commonly in cattle and is extremely rare in sheep, goats, and swine. Most cases of cutaneous lymphoma in cattle occur in young adults 1 to 3 years of age. Lymphoma involving the skin of cattle is associated with the sporadic form of bovine leukosis and is not associated with bovine leukemia virus (BLV) infection.

Skin lesions are most often multifocal and commonly involve the neck and trunk. Onset is sudden, and initial lesions resemble an urticarial reaction. The initial lesions progress to form variably sized firm nodules within the skin and/or subcutis. The overlying skin may be normal, variably alopecic, hyperkeratotic, or ulcerated. Lesions often regress spontaneously, only to reappear. Histologic and cytologic preparations reveal sheets of a relatively homogeneous population of neoplastic lymphocytes. Effacement of tissue architecture is seen on histologic preparations.

Surgical excision of cutaneous bovine lymphoma is only useful as a diagnostic procedure. No effective treatment has been reported, and eventual death caused by involvement of internal organs is typical.

CUTANEOUS VASCULAR TUMORS

Cutaneous vascular tumors are most common in cattle but also occur in sheep, goats, and pigs. Tumors can be congenital or acquired. Congenital tumors may actually be hamartomas rather than true neoplasms.

Calves can be born with multiple cutaneous vascular lesions. Those that involve gingiva and tongue are described in Tumors of the Oral Cavity and Jaw. Cutaneous vascular lesions in neonatal calves are often described by owners as appearing to be "blood blisters." Vascular lesions in neonatal calves can be disseminated throughout the skin and can also involve internal organs. In adult cattle, a syndrome known as *bovine cutaneous angiomatosis* occurs. Lesions can be single or multiple and often occur on the dorsum of the trunk. These tumors are soft, pink to reddish gray, can be sessile or pedunculated, and often bleed sporadically. Cutaneous vascular neoplasms occur in goats of all ages and are most often single, raised pink to red lesions that often bleed. In pigs, hemangiomas occur in the scrotal skin, especially of Yorkshire and Berkshire boars. Scrotal hemangiomas in pigs are often multicentric and progress from tiny purple papules to raised, hyperkeratotic lesions.

Cytologic evaluation of vascular tumors most often reveals only blood. Histologic evaluation is necessary to identify the proliferative endothelial cells lining vascular channels in these lesions. These channels vary from capillary (most common in congenital neoplasms of calves) to cavernous, and can contain a mixture of vascular structures. Very well differentiated lesions may be classified as hamartomas. Abnormal vascular channels lined by well-differentiated endothelium are hemangiomas, whereas tumors with cellular pleomorphism and mitotic activity are hemangiosarcomas.

Vascular lesions of all types can exhibit local invasion and recurrence after incomplete excision. Wide surgical excision of tumors, when possible, is often curative, as even cutaneous hemangiosarcomas rarely metastasize.

OTHER TUMORS OF THE SKIN

Uncommon skin tumors of farm animals include basal cell and sebaceous tumors, histiocytoma, and organoid nevus.

A basal cell tumor in the lacrimal pouch of a 2.5-year-old intact male Hampshire sheep has been reported, and a basosquamous tumor was reported in the tail of an adult cow. Sebaceous hyperplasia occurs rarely in adult goats. Basal cell and sebaceous tumors are raised, alopecic exophytic growths that can be ulcerated. Histologic features are of circumscribed nodular growths of relatively orderly basal-type epithelial cells with a variable amount of admixed stroma (basal cell tumor) or of proliferative but well-differentiated sebaceous glands (sebaceous hyperplasia). These tumors are benign and surgical excision is curative.

Histiocytoma occurs on the scrotum of buck goats. Tumors are circumscribed raised lesions that are formed by sheets of histiocytic cells with a high mitotic index. Spontaneous regression of histiocytoma can occur in goats.

Organoid nevus is a nonneoplastic hamartomatous lesion composed of a localized zone of increased dermal collagen with admixed enlarged and often disarrayed follicles and adnexa. Organoid nevus occurs rarely in cattle and pigs. Organoid nevi can be flat, plaquelike lesions or can be elongated and pedunculated. The latter are often also called *skin tags*. Surgical excision of organoid nevus is curative.

CYSTS

Cysts of the skin are uncommon lesions of cattle, sheep, goats and swine. They can be single or multiple, and can be congenital or acquired. Epidermal cysts (epidermal inclusion cysts), dermoid cysts, and follicular cysts are most common. Cysts are most common in Merino and Suffolk sheep, in which a hereditary basis is suspected. Cysts within the udder skin of older ewes involve mammary glandular epithelium and contain milk. Epidermal and dermoid cysts are less common in cattle. Cysts within the wattle of Nubian and Nubian cross goats are developmental anomalies present at or soon after birth that are suspected to arise from branchial cleft remnants. A hereditary basis for wattle cysts in goats is suspected.

Cystic skin lesions in farm animals are most often asymptomatic, although their presence will adversely affect hide quality. Cysts can rupture and develop secondary inflammation with ulceration of overlying skin or can be discrete and nodular with normal overlying skin. Wattle cysts in goats are soft and fluctuant with normal overlying skin (Figure 3-3). Cystic skin lesions in sheep have been associated with development of carcinoma and with systemic illness.

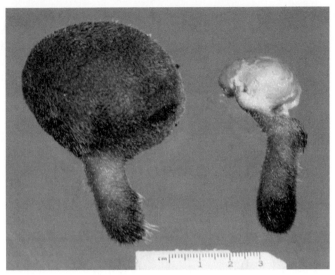

Figure 3-3   Wattle cysts in goats.

(Courtesy of Dr. John King.)

Cytologic evaluation of epidermal, dermoid, and follicular cyst contents will reveal keratin, often admixed with cholesterol clefts and macrophages. Milk can be aspirated from udder cysts in sheep. Wattle cysts contain clear liquid. Surgical excision and histopathologic evaluation to identify the type of cells and structures within the cyst wall will allow for classification of the type of cyst present. Epidermal cysts are lined by keratinizing epithelium lacking adnexal structures. Dermoid cysts are lined by keratinizing epithelium with associated adnexa. Follicular cysts consist of dilated and keratin-filled hair follicles. Wattle cysts are lined by a single to double layer of cuboidal to columnar epithelial cells. When either a single or a small number of cysts are present, surgical excision is curative. Excision of udder cysts of sheep is neither necessary nor recommended.

SOFT TISSUE TUMORS

Soft tissue tumors are less common in farm animals than are tumors of the skin. Included in this group of tumors are fibroma, fibrosarcoma, neurofibroma, lipoma, smooth muscle tumors, and rhabdomyosarcoma.

Fibroma and fibrosarcoma occur rarely in the skin and subcutis of cattle, sheep, goats, and pigs. Cutaneous neurofibromas are most common in Holstein cattle, in which a syndrome that resembles human neurofibromatosis—in which multiple cutaneous tumors composed of admixed Schwann cells and fibroblasts occur in people with genetic defects in the neurofibromatosis gene—occurs. Neurofibromas of cattle associated with large nerve trunks such as the brachial plexus, intercostal nerves, and cardiac nerves also occur. Subcutaneous lipomas occur occasionally in cattle and are rare in sheep, goats, and pigs. Smooth muscle tumors are very rare. A subcutaneous leiomyosarcoma has been reported in a cow, and a fibroleiomyoma occurred in the skin of a pig. Rhabdomyosarcoma within skeletal muscle has been reported in cattle, sheep, and pigs. Most soft tissue tumors occur in adult to aged animals. Rhabdomyosarcoma is an exception, as it can occur in young as well as older animals. In piglets, rhabdomyosarcomas can occur associated with a genetic defect. Intramuscular rhabdomyosarcoma has also been reported in a 1-year-old sheep.

Soft tissue tumors present as progressively enlarging masses or swellings. Fibroma, fibrosarcoma, leiomyosarcoma, and leiomyoma usually occur as single masses. Neurofibroma and rhabdomyosarcoma are often multicentric. Rhabdomyosarcoma in farm animals typically arises within skeletal muscle. Cattle with neurofibromas involving large peripheral nerve trunks can develop signs of lameness and denervation atrophy.

Soft tissue tumors vary from fleshy to fatty to myxoid, depending on the tumor cell type. Cytologic evaluation will distinguish lipoma from other mesenchymal tumors. Histologic evaluation—and possibly immunohistochemistry—is needed to distinguish fibroma, fibrosarcoma, neurofibroma, leiomyosarcoma, and rhabdomyosarcoma.

Subcutaneous lipoma in farm animals is most often an isolated and discrete tumor. Other soft tissue tumors are typically locally invasive but rarely metastasize. Wide surgical excision of these tumors, when possible, could be curative.

Tumors of the Eye

Tumors involving the eyelids, conjunctiva, cornea, and orbit are relatively common in cattle and less common in other farm animal species. Ocular squamous papilloma, squamous cell carcinoma, and orbital lymphoma of cattle are most common. Ocular squamous cell carcinoma can also occur in sheep, especially those at high altitudes. Ocular dermoids are developmental anomalies present at birth that occur sporadically in calves and pigs. Ocular lymphangiosarcoma in cattle is rare.

Cutaneous papillomas caused by bovine papillomavirus occur on the eyelids or corneoscleral junction of young cattle and can predispose to development of ocular squamous cell carcinoma. Bovine squamous cell carcinoma is most common in the limbal and eyelid conjunctiva but can also arise in the cornea. Squamous cell carcinoma that involves the orbit and retrobulbar tissue is much less common. Bovine ocular squamous cell carcinoma occurs in all breeds, but Herefords appear to be predisposed to this tumor. Ocular squamous cell

carcinoma usually occurs in cattle over 5 years of age. Lack of eyelid pigmentation and ultraviolet light are etiologic factors, although a genetic predisposition is also suspected. Ocular squamous cell carcinoma occurs much less commonly in sheep. Lymphoma can involve the orbit of adult cattle as part of a more generalized neoplastic process associated with BLV infection. Ocular dermoid is not a true tumor but presents as an ocular mass lesion in neonatal calves and piglets. Ocular dermoid is a developmental defect in which a zone of skin, often haired, is present at birth on the cornea or conjunctiva (Figure 3-4). Ocular dermoids are most common in polled Herefords and also occur in pigs. Lymphangiosarcoma of the limbus has been reported in an 8-year-old Holstein cow. Ocular tumors have not been reported in goats.

Tumors of squamous epithelium often begin as a smooth raised plaque that progresses to form an exophytic squamous papilloma. Some ocular papillomas will spontaneously regress. Persistent papilloma can progress to noninvasive and then to invasive squamous cell carcinoma. Not all ocular squamous tumors exhibit this sequential development, and invasive carcinoma may be the first clinically noted lesion. Squamous cell carcinoma is a raised proliferative lesion that is often ulcerated and often is secondarily infected (Figure 3-5). Squamous cell carcinoma of the conjunctiva can spread to involve the globe, and corneal squamous cell carcinoma can spread to involve conjunctiva. In advanced cases, determining the initial site of malignant transformation is often

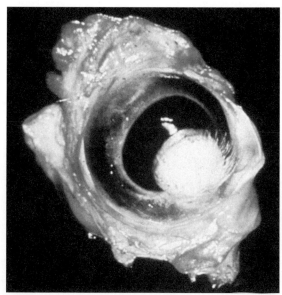

Figure 3-4   Ocular dermoid in a piglet.

(Courtesy of Dr. Howard Gelberg.)

impossible. Neoplastic squamous cells are seen on histologic and cytologic preparations.

Lymphoma of the orbit and retrobulbar space most often causes progressive exophthalmos of the affected eye. In dairy cattle, early signs of exophthalmos may not be noticed, as many dairy breeds normally have mild exophthalmos. When protrusion of the globe becomes severe enough to interfere with eyelid closure, rapid development of exposure keratitis occurs. The lymphoma is most often deep within the orbit, thus precluding diagnostic procedures such as biopsy or cytology. Complete physical examination for other affected organs or serologic testing for bovine leukemia virus infection are useful diagnostic procedures. Evaluation of tumor tissue by cytology or histopathology after removal of the globe reveals sheets of relatively homogeneous lymphocytes, and marked invasion and obliteration of normal architecture are seen in tissue sections.

Ocular dermoids do not enlarge, but the presence of hairs often results in irritation of the lids or cornea that can become secondarily infected. The ocular lymphangiosarcoma reported presented as a progressively enlarging subconjunctival mass at the limbus. Biopsy revealed irregular vascular channels devoid of blood, consistent with origin from lymphatics.

Ocular squamous cell carcinoma is locally invasive and destructive but metastasis is uncommon. Rarely, ocular squamous cell carcinoma in cattle undergoes spontaneous remission. Surgical removal of the affected globe and lids in cattle and sheep can be curative, although in predisposed cattle carcinoma can develop in the other eye. Other successful therapies for ocular squamous cell

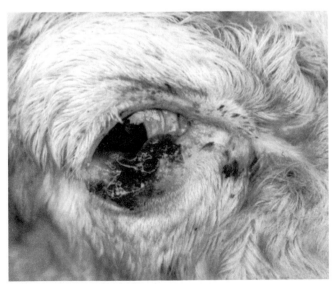

Figure 3-5   Bovine periocular squamous cell carcinoma. (Courtesy of Dr. Barry Cooper.)

carcinoma include cryosurgery, hyperthermia, radiation, and immunotherapy. Removal of exophthalmic globes because of orbital or retrobulbar lymphoma should be considered only as a palliative measure to make the animal more comfortable. Complete excision of orbital lymphoma is not possible, and the involvement of other organs leads to eventual death, usually within 6 months of diagnosis. Surgical excision of dermoids is curative. Removal of the affected globe was apparently curative in the cow with ocular lymphangiosarcoma.

Tumors of the Oral Cavity and Jaw

Tumors involving oral mucosa and bones of the jaw are most common in cattle, less common in sheep, and rare in goats and pigs. Epithelial, odontogenic, vascular, osseous, and fibroblastic tumors occur.

MUCOSAL TUMORS

Papilloma caused by bovine papillomavirus can occur in the oral mucosa of calves. Exophytic polypoid to sessile growths are seen, and tumors can be multicentric. In contrast, oral squamous cell carcinoma occurs in older animals and is an invasive destructive tumor. Vascular tumors of the gingiva and tongue occur in young calves and can be present at birth. Most often these are single fleshy masses that can be superficially ulcerated.

Histologic examination will distinguish the relatively orderly epithelial proliferation of papilloma from the pleomorphic and invasive epithelium of squamous cell carcinoma. Vascular tumors are characterized by clusters of well-differentiated capillary-type blood vessels in a fibrous stroma. Whether these tumors represent benign neoplasia (hemangioma) or vascular hamartomas is unclear. Their presence at birth suggests that the latter is most likely.

Viral papillomas are benign lesions that most often regress spontaneously. Surgical excision of these masses is also curative. Squamous cell carcinoma is not likely to be recognized in farm animal species until a relatively late stage of development, when wide surgical excision is difficult or impossible. Vascular tumors often exhibit some degree of local infiltration and slowly enlarge as the animal grows. Wide surgical excision is often necessary for cure, and cryotherapy has been reported to be an effective treatment.

BONE TUMORS

Tumors of bones of the jaw include odontogenic tumors, osteoma, fibroma, fibrosarcoma, and myxomatous tumors. Odontogenic tumors occur most often in cattle and sheep and rarely in pigs. Odontogenic tumors are most often evident in young to young adult animals but have also been diagnosed in older animals. Presumably, odontogenic tumors identified in adults had been present for some time before diagnosis. Tumors of odontogenic origin have a variety of histologic features that result in various—often confusing—classifications that are prone to change. Tumor types identified in farm animals include odontoma (including ameloblastic, compound, and complex odontoma), ameloblastoma, and ameloblastic fibroodontoma. Osteoma and fibroma also occur in the jaws of adult cattle. Fibrosarcoma of the jaw occurs in adult sheep grazing bracken fern. Myxomatous tumors (myxoma and myxosarcoma) occur in adult cattle.

Tumors of the jaw most often present as slowly enlarging firm to bony growths. These tumors often arise at or near tooth roots and can cause loosening and malalignment of adjacent teeth. Radiographic evaluation is useful to determine the site and extent of the tumor. Histologic evaluation is necessary to distinguish the various types of odontogenic and mesenchymal tumors that occur in the jaws of farm animals. Odontogenic tumors consist of varying elements of odontogenic epithelium with or without induction of dental or mesenchymal tissue. Biopsy diagnosis of osteoma often relies on the clinical and radiographic description of the lesion, as it is not possible to distinguish the histologic features of small samples of osteoma from those of normal bone. Myxomatous tumors are characterized by proliferation of spindle to dendritic cells in a loose myxoid stroma.

Fibroma, osteoma, and odontogenic tumors of the jaw are noninvasive and can be cured by wide surgical excision. For tumors located rostrally, mandibulectomy or maxillectomy is advised. Myxomatous tumors of the jaw, however, are typically locally invasive and difficult or impossible to completely excise. Recurrence is common, although metastasis has not been reported.

Tumors of the Gastrointestinal System

Tumors of the esophagus, stomachs, and intestines are relatively common in farm animals, particularly cattle. Various benign and malignant tumors can occur. Tumors of associated exocrine glands (pancreatic and salivary) also occur but are rare.

ESOPHAGUS

Esophageal tumors are uncommon and occur mostly in cattle. Esophageal papilloma in cattle may be associated with bovine papillomavirus. In areas with high bracken fern exposure (see Forestomach section) esophageal papillomas and squamous cell carcinoma can occur. Gross and histopathologic features of esophageal papilloma and squamous cell carcinoma are similar to those in the forestomachs (see Forestomach section). Esophageal tumors can result in clinical signs of bloat, excessive salivation, or esophageal obstruction or can be incidental findings.

FORESTOMACH

Tumors of the omasum, reticulum, and rumen occur most often in cattle but are uncommon in most parts of the world. Papilloma, fibropapilloma, and fibroma are the most common tumors in the forestomach of cattle. Although a viral etiology has been proposed, immunohistochemical studies of a small number of cases did not find evidence of papillomavirus. These tumors are less common in sheep, and no reports of forestomach neoplasia were found in goats. Papillomas can occur at any age. Squamous cell carcinoma occurs in older cattle and sheep and often results from malignant transformation of a papilloma. In cattle in Kenya and northern England, the interaction between bovine papillomavirus infection and the mutagens present in bracken fern is suspected to be the cause of a high incidence of forestomach papillomas and of malignant transformation of papilloma to squamous cell carcinoma. Lymphoma can involve the rumen and reticulum of older cattle as part of a more generalized neoplastic process associated with BLV infection. Fibrosarcoma of the rumen has been seen in an adult sheep.

Forestomach papilloma, fibropapilloma, and fibroma in cattle most often occur in the rumen near the ruminoreticular groove, thus causing recurrent bloat. Squamous cell carcinoma occurs at these sites and, in sheep, can also occur in the reticulum and omasum. Abdominal pain, bloat, and excessive salivation often accompany forestomach squamous cell carcinoma in cattle. Clinical signs have not been reported in sheep with forestomach neoplasia. Forestomach lymphoma is typically associated with concurrent abomasal involvement, as well as other organs, and generalized ill-thrift. Involvement of the omasum by lymphoma is less common. Leiomyoma of the omasum has been seen as an incidental finding in a goat.

Fibroma, fibropapilloma, and papilloma of the forestomach are benign, localized tumors that form exophytic nodular or multinodular smooth-surfaced, firm, tan masses (Figure 3-6). Tumors may be sessile or pedunculated. These tumors are readily excised via rumenotomy, but they can be multiple, especially in areas with a high incidence. Histopathologic evaluation is necessary to differentiate those tumors that have epithelial proliferation (papilloma), both epithelial and fibroblastic proliferation (fibropapilloma), or only fibroblastic elements (fibroma). Histopathologic evaluation is also needed to identify evidence of malignancy in the rare cases of forestomach fibrosarcoma. The fibrosarcoma seen in the rumen of a sheep had metastasized to the liver.

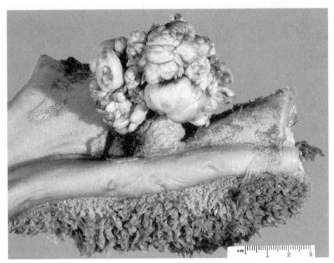

Figure 3-6 Fibropapilloma in the rumen of a cow.

(Courtesy of Dr. Stan Snyder.)

Squamous cell carcinoma is an invasive and destructive tumor. Mucosal ulceration caused by squamous cell carcinoma is common. Histopathologic evaluation reveals nests of invasive squamous epithelial cells in dense collagenous stroma. Neoplastic squamous cells may be seen on cytologic preparations, but the degree of sclerosis often results in poor exfoliation of epithelial cells. Surgical excision of early and localized forestomach squamous cell carcinoma might be possible, but in most cases the extent of tumor at the time of diagnosis precludes surgical intervention.

Lymphoma most often results in locally extensive firm and nonulcerated thickening of the forestomach wall by pale tan solid tissue. Rarely, forestomach lymphoma may involve only the serosa. Sheets of relatively homogeneous lymphocytes are seen on cytologic and histopathologic preparations, and transmural involvement with obliteration of normal architecture is characteristic.

Abomasum and Stomach

Abomasal tumors occur in older cattle, usually those over 5 years of age. The vast majority are lymphomas associated with BLV infection. Abomasal lymphoma also occurs sporadically in goats. Adenocarcinomas occur in cattle but are uncommon. Abomasal mast cell tumor in cattle and gastric lymphoma and squamous cell carcinoma in swine are rare tumors. Abomasal tumors can result in clinical signs of outflow obstruction, but often generalized ill-thrift is the only sign. An abomasal adenocarcinoma in a cow was associated with abdominal distention from peritoneal effusion.

Lymphoma causes a locally extensive to diffuse thickening of the abomasal wall (Figure 3-7). Borders are

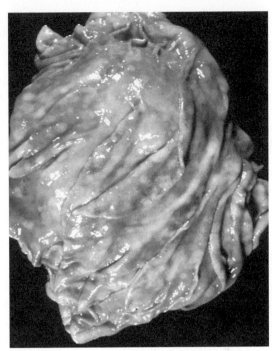

Figure 3-7 Lymphoma causing pale areas of thickening visible on the mucosal surface of the abomasum of a goat.

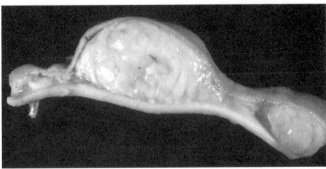

Figure 3-8 Transverse section demonstrating submucosal thickening by pale tissue characteristic of abomasal lymphoma in a cow.

(Courtesy of Dr. Barry Cooper.)

often difficult to discern. Abomasal lymphoma can be soft to firm. Mucosal ulceration is rare. Solid pale tan to white solid tissue is seen on section (Figure 3-8). Sheets of relatively homogeneous lymphocytes are seen on cytologic and histopathologic preparations, and this tumor is invasive and causes obliteration of tissue architecture. Adenocarcinoma is a very firm tumor often with extensive mucosal ulceration. Invasive nests of neoplastic epithelial cells are embedded in dense stroma. Mucin can also be prominent. Because of the sclerotic nature of this tumor, epithelial cells can be difficult to identify on cytologic preparations.

Lymphoma is often an insidious disorder with gradual onset of organ dysfunction and cachexia. Lymphoma isolated to the abomasum is rare. In most cases of abomasal lymphoma tumor is also found at other sites, such as in the heart and uterus. Adenocarcinoma can be localized or can exhibit marked invasion. Adenocarcinoma can undergo widespread metastasis through lymphatics to the abdominal and thoracic cavities. Spread to peritoneum and pleura results in carcinomatosis.

INTESTINE

Small intestinal adenocarcinoma is relatively common in sheep, usually affecting those 4 years of age or older. Primary intestinal tumors are uncommon in other farm animal species. Intestinal adenocarcinoma occurs sporadically in older cattle and goats, and occurs rarely in older pigs. Papillomas occasionally occur in the small intestine of cattle. Lymphoma can involve the intestine of older cattle as part of a more generalized neoplastic process. Ileal lymphoma occurs in pigs and is most common in pigs less than 1 year of age. Leiomyoma and leiomyosarcoma are sporadic intestinal tumors of cattle and pigs. Ganglioneuromatosis involving the colon has been seen in a steer and carcinoid tumor can involve either the small intestine or the colon of cattle. Most cases of small intestinal adenocarcinoma in sheep are found at necropsy or at slaughter, and ascites caused by tumor metastasis is the most common clinical sign before death. Carcinoma cells may be visible in cytologic preparations of ascites fluid. Diarrhea and weight loss occur in cattle with carcinoid tumors. Large tumors of any type within the intestinal tract can result in signs of intestinal obstruction or recurrent bloat. Involvement of the intestinal wall by neoplasms of any type often results in extensive adhesions. Clinical signs have not been reported in pigs with ileal lymphoma.

Firm thickening of the involved intestinal segment is characteristic of neoplasia (Figure 3-9). Adenocarcinoma and carcinoid tumors arise in the mucosa, thus resulting in extensive mucosal involvement and often ulceration. Transmural growth to involve the serosa is common. Adenocarcinoma often causes annular intestinal stenosis and is characterized by invasive nests of glandular epithelium with marked associated sclerosis. Carcinoid tumors are composed of closely packed nests of round cells often with fine cytoplasmic granules. Carcinoid tumors in cattle can be multiple and can metastasize to mesenteric lymph nodes. Leiomyoma, leiomyosarcoma, and ganglioneuromatosis arise within the outer intestinal wall and involve mucosa only by extension. These tumors are firm and smooth and may become quite large before clinical signs are apparent. Smooth muscle tumors form nodular masses formed by interlacing bundles of elongate smooth muscle cells.

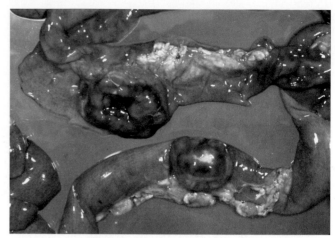

Figure 3-9   Localized lymphoma of the wall of the small intestine in a cow.

Ganglioneuromatosis is a more diffuse lesion that causes locally extensive mural thickening without a focal mass lesion. Nerve fibers admixed with ganglion cells are characteristic histopathologic features. Solitary intramural nodular masses within the terminal ileum are typical of intestinal lymphoma in pigs. These tumors arise within Peyer's patches and consist of sheets of small to large lymphocytes effacing architecture. Metastasis of ileal lymphoma to mesenteric lymph nodes or to serosal surfaces is common in pigs. Metastasis of intestinal adenocarcinoma in sheep to mesenteric lymph nodes and serosal surfaces is common. In cattle, metastasis of intestinal adenocarcinoma is most often to mesenteric lymph nodes and liver.

If detected at an early stage, surgical excision of intestinal adenocarcinoma could be curative. Given the high metastatic rate, however, a guarded prognosis would be warranted. Similarly, excision of a solitary intestinal carcinoid might be successful, but the potential for metastasis would warrant a guarded prognosis. Surgical excision of intestinal leiomyoma, leiomyosarcoma, and ganglioneuromatosis is more likely to be successful, as these tumors rarely metastasize. Resection of intestinal lymphoma is unlikely to be curative, as the neoplastic process is likely to be either multicentric or to have metastasized.

PANCREAS

Pancreatic exocrine tumors are rare. All reported pancreatic exocrine tumors have been in adult to aged cattle and were identified at slaughter. Proliferative lesions of the exocrine pancreas include nodular hyperplasia, adenoma, carcinoma, neural tumors (neurofibroma and neurofibrosarcoma), and fibrosarcoma.

Clinical signs in cattle with pancreatic carcinoma may be inapparent, or affected cattle may present as downer cattle. Exocrine pancreatic carcinoma is associated with peripancreatic and intraabdominal fat necrosis and mineralization and fibrosis and thickening of the mesentery. Tumors are very firm, pale, tan, and nodular. Metastatic lesions may be more obvious than the primary tumor. Exocrine pancreatic tumors are often poorly differentiated, with a high mitotic index and extensive sclerosis. Metastasis to mesenteric lymph nodes, liver, and other abdominal organs is common.

Neurofibroma, neurofibrosarcoma, and fibrosarcoma are not associated with clinical signs. These tumors form discrete nodular masses of firm, pale, tan to white tissue. Characteristic interlacing fascicles and whorls of spindle cells are seen histopathologically. Metastasis of neural tumors or of pancreatic fibrosarcoma has not been reported.

SALIVARY GLAND

Salivary gland tumors in farm animals are rare. Adenoma and carcinoma occur occasionally in cattle. Salivary gland tumors are rare in sheep and are not reported in goats or pigs. Tumors result in firm swelling of the affected gland. Neoplastic proliferation of epithelial cells with a variable amount of associated fibrous stroma is seen histopathologically. In cattle, metastasis to local lymph nodes can occur.

Tumors of the Respiratory Tract

Tumors of the respiratory tract occur in the nasal passages and sinuses, the ethmoid region, and in the lung. Respiratory tumors are most common in cattle and sheep and are much less common in pigs and goats.

TUMORS OF THE NASAL PASSAGES AND SINUSES

Papillomavirus can cause proliferative lesions in the nasal skin at sites of bull rings in cattle. Apparently infective nasal papillomas also occur in goats. Nasal adenocarcinoma occurs most commonly in sheep (Figure 3-10) but can also occur in cattle and pigs. Squamous cell carcinoma of the horn core in adult cattle, sheep, and goats often presents as a cutaneous tumor, but origin from sinus epithelium is suspected. Osteoma of the nasal/sinus bone occurs in adult cattle. Ethmoid tumors that include epithelial, mesenchymal, and mixed tumors occur endemically in cattle and sheep in various areas worldwide and can involve young adult animals as well as older animals. A viral cause—most likely a retrovirus—is suspected.

Clinical signs of tumors within nasal passages and sinuses include nasal discharge and respiratory stridor and dyspnea. Large tumors can result in expansion of overlying bone to form an externally visible lesion.

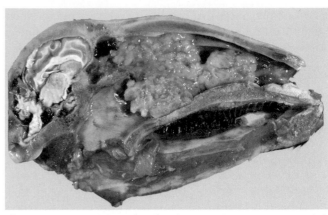

Figure 3-10 Invasive nasal adenocarcinoma in an adult sheep.

(Courtesy of Dr. John Schmitz.)

Squamous cell carcinoma of the horn core often results in loosening and/or distortion of the horn. Tumors of the ethmoid region can result in exophthalmos.

Histologic evaluation will distinguish the various types of tumors. Cytologic evaluation of material collected during nasal flushing can distinguish the atypical epithelial cells of carcinoma from reactive cells caused by inflammatory lesions. Papillomavirus infection at the site of a nasal ring in bulls can mimic fibrosarcoma due to abundant mesenchymal proliferation.

Papillomas are benign lesions that often regress spontaneously. Surgical excision is also curative. Osteoma of the nasal/sinus bone is a benign lesion, but surgical excision is not often possible. Carcinomas, sarcomas, and mixed tumors of the nasal passage, sinus, and ethmoid region are locally invasive malignant tumors. Curiously, metastasis to lymph nodes and lung has been reported in cattle with nasal tumors but not in sheep. Surgical excision of these tumors is not likely to be an option because of the extent of the lesion and cost of surgery.

TUMORS OF THE LUNG

Lung tumors are uncommon in cattle and goats. Tumors and tumorlike lesions occur most often in the lungs of sheep and goats due to retroviral infection. Pulmonary tumors have not been reported in pigs. Tumors of pulmonary epithelium are most common, although rare cases of rhabdomyosarcoma of the lung have occurred in lambs and calves. Multiple pulmonary papillomas have been described in the diaphragmatic lobes of Angora goats.

Pulmonary adenomatosis (Jaasiekte) is a retroviral-associated neoplastic disorder that affects adult sheep and occurs endemically in many parts of the world. Pulmonary adenomatosis must be distinguished from ovine progressive pneumonia (maedi), also a retroviral-associated disorder that results in nonneoplastic proliferative lung lesions. Proliferative pulmonary lesions similar to those in ovine progressive pneumonia occur in goats with caprine arthritis-encephalitis virus (CAEV).

Most lung tumors in cattle and goats have been found as incidental findings at necropsy or slaughter. Rhabdomyosarcoma in lambs can cause severe dyspnea and death. Pulmonary adenomatosis, ovine progressive pneumonia, and caprine interstitial pneumonia caused by CAEV result in progressive dyspnea and cachexia. Metastasis of carcinomas and of ovine pulmonary adenomatosis is possible.

Tumors are fleshy to firm, depending on the degree of associated sclerosis. Solitary, discrete adenomas and invasive carcinomas occur. Multiple coalescing zones of pulmonary consolidation by pale slightly firm tissue are typical of ovine pulmonary adenomatosis and progressive pneumonia. Histologic evaluation will distinguish benign and malignant epithelial tumors based on cell morphology and degree of invasion. Rhabdomyosarcoma consists of interlacing bundles of striated muscle cells, and invasion of adjacent parenchyma is typical. Pulmonary adenomatosis in sheep is characterized by proliferation of type 2 alveolar lining cells forming invasive masses. Ovine progressive pneumonia and pulmonary lesions in goats with CAEV result in profound interstitial thickening that can mimic neoplasia, but associated chronic inflammation, particularly of lymphocytes, is a distinguishing feature.

Tumors of the Thoracic Cavity

Tumors of the thoracic cavity are not uncommon in farm animals. Thymic lymphoma occurs in calves 3 months to 2 years of age as a form of sporadic bovine leukosis and also occurs in sheep and pigs. Mediastinal lymphoma has been reported in goats, but it is not clear whether these tumors were true lymphoma or lymphocyte-rich thymomas. Thymoma is most common in adult goats but has also been reported in adult cattle, sheep, and pigs. Saanen goats may be predisposed to development of thymoma. Localized mesothelioma occurs within the thoracic cavity of adult cattle and pigs.

Clinical signs are most often progressive respiratory difficulty associated with both growth of the tumor and frequent associated pleural effusion. Progressive cachexia is common. Palpable enlargement of the brisket region can occur in cases of thymic lymphoma and intrathoracic mesothelioma. Enlargement of peripheral lymph nodes can accompany thymic lymphoma.

Cytologic evaluation of pleural fluid or of mass aspirates can distinguish the atypical lymphocytic proliferation of lymphoma from the mesothelial proliferation of mesothelioma. Thymoma can be more difficult to

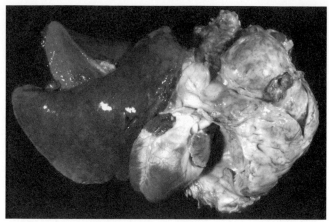

Figure 3-11   Mediastinal mass typical of thymoma in a goat. (Courtesy of Dr. Barry Cooper.)

diagnose on cytologic preparations, as the thymic epithelial cells that are the neoplastic population may be obscured by large numbers of associated nonneoplastic small lymphocytes. Histologic evaluation is often necessary for definitive diagnosis of thymic lymphoma, thymoma, and mesothelioma.

Thymic lymphoma in calves is not amenable to surgical excision, and metastasis is common. Intrathoracic mesothelioma is generally widespread on pleural surfaces, and surgical excision is not possible. Thymoma can get quite large but is typically still a localized mediastinal mass (Figure 3-11). Although no reports of surgical excision of thymoma in farm animals were found, extrapolation from results of thymoma surgery in dogs and cats would suggest that surgical excision could be curative.

Tumors of the Udder and Mammary Gland

Udder skin tumors are relatively common in farm animals. Mammary gland neoplasia, however, is uncommon. Inflammatory and hyperplastic lesions and benign and malignant tumors of epithelial or mesenchymal cells are possible.

UDDER

Papillomas can involve the skin of the udder and teats. Papillomavirus has been shown to cause skin growths in cattle, and a viral etiology is suspected in sheep, goats, and pigs. In cattle, papillomas occur in young animals, usually less than 2 years of age, and involvement of the teat is common. A syndrome of papillomatosis that involves teats and nonpigmented skin of the udder occurs in goats of any age (Figure 3-12), especially white

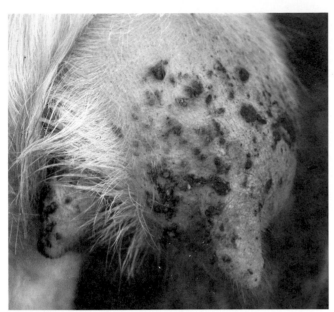

Figure 3-12   Multiple papillomas on the udder of a goat.

(Courtesy of Dr. Mary Smith)

Saanen or Saanen cross goats, and these lesions are prone to malignant transformation to squamous cell carcinoma. The growths appear to be infective, at least to other Saanen goats, with appearance of multiple affected animals within 4 to 6 months of introduction of an infected animal. Exposure to sunlight may also be an etiologic factor. A similar syndrome occurs less commonly in sheep. Papillomas on the teats are often secondarily infected and can interfere with nursing or milking.

Papillomas are exophytic and often pedunculated skin growths that are often multinodular. Surface ulceration can result from mechanical trauma. In cattle, viral-induced skin growths can be composed entirely of proliferative epithelium (papilloma) or can contain both epithelial and fibrous proliferation (fibropapilloma). Papillomas in goats are characterized by epithelial proliferation without a fibrous component. Bovine cutaneous papillomas typically undergo spontaneous regression. Udder papillomas in goats can undergo spontaneous regression without recurrence, can regress in winter and reoccur in summer, or can be persistent. The latter tumors are prone to malignant transformation to squamous cell carcinoma. Squamous cell carcinoma of the skin of the udder occurs less commonly in sheep. Squamous cell carcinoma is a spreading ulcerative lesion that is often firm because of associated sclerosis. Invasive cords and nests of neoplastic squamous epithelium are seen on histopathologic evaluation. Neoplastic cells can be difficult to obtain on cytologic preparations in cases with extensive tumor sclerosis.

Given the high incidence of malignant transformation of persistent udder papillomas in goats, wide surgical excision of these growths is the treatment of choice. Metastasis of squamous cell carcinoma to local lymph nodes can occur, but early and wide resection of squamous cell carcinoma could be curative.

MAMMARY GLAND

Tumors of the mammary gland are uncommon in farm animals. In cattle, fibroma and fibrosarcoma of the teat occur in yearlings. Inflammatory polyps that mimic neoplasia occur in the teat canal of cattle of any age. Mammary glandular tumors occur in cows 3 years of age or older and are most often adenocarcinoma or carcinoma. In contrast, adenomas are the most common mammary neoplasia in sheep and occur in adults. Mammary gland proliferative lesions in the goat include adenocarcinoma, cystic hyperplasia (fibrocystic change), and fibroepithelial hyperplasia. Nubian goats may be predisposed to fibroepithelial hyperplasia, which occurs in young goats, often less than 1 year of age. Mammary tumors are very rare in older sows, and reported cases have been carcinomas.

Teat fibroma and fibrosarcoma are smooth firm nodules covered by intact skin that occur at the base of the teat. Intramammary tumors and hyperplastic lesions cause firm localized to diffuse areas of mammary gland that may or may not result in overall enlargement of the affected gland. Mastitis and fistulation can occur secondary to malignant tumors. Milk production in nonpregnant animals and mastitis can be seen in goats with fibroepithelial hyperplasia.

Teat fibroma and fibrosarcoma are localized lesions consisting of proliferating fibroblasts with admixed collagen and variable mitotic activity. Adenomas are localized tumors formed by relatively well-differentiated and orderly epithelial cells forming glands. Adenocarcinoma and carcinoma are invasive tumors that can involve a large portion of the gland, and are composed of pleomorphic neoplastic epithelial cells that form glands or sheets of cells with a variable amount of collagenous stroma. Pleomorphic and atypical epithelial cells can be seen on cytologic preparations. Cystic hyperplasia in goats, also called *fibrocystic change*, consists of localized zones of dilated mammary ducts lined by epithelial cells lacking features of neoplasia. Fibroepithelial hyperplasia of goats consists of proliferation of ductal elements in a prominent loose to dense stroma and is similar to the mammary fibroepithelial hyperplasia seen in young female cats.

Surgical excision of teat fibromas and fibrosarcomas is apparently curative. Surgical excision of hyperplastic lesions and adenomas, which may necessitate removal of the entire affected gland, is also curative. Careful evaluation of cows with mammary neoplasia before surgery is warranted because metastasis of adenocarcinoma and carcinoma to local lymph nodes, internal organs, and to the peritoneum is common. Metastasis of mammary carcinoma in the goat has also been reported.

Tumors of the Female Genital Tract

Tumors of the female genital tract of farm animals are quite common and are probably second only to skin tumors in incidence. Various benign and malignant tumors occur. Although few clinical reports of surgical excision of genital tract tumors were found, the behavior of many of these tumors suggests that ovariectomy or hysterectomy could be curative.

TUMORS OF THE VULVA

Vulvar papillomas and fibropapillomas occur in cattle as a sexually transmitted papillomavirus disease. Squamous cell carcinoma of the vulva occurs in older cattle, sheep, and goats and may occur *de novo* or as the result of malignant transformation of viral papilloma. Poor pigmentation of vulvar skin and high solar exposure are predisposing factors. Smooth muscle tumors (leiomyoma and leiomyosarcoma) occur in the vulva of cattle. Ectopic mammary tissue in the vulva of goats will cause swelling during lactation and can be mistaken for neoplasia.

Papillomas and fibropapillomas are multinodular to multilobular tumors typically with a broad base of attachment and no evidence of invasion. Large tumors can be ulcerated. Squamous cell carcinoma is an invasive, ulcerated, spreading lesion of the vulvar skin. Ectopic mammary tissue in goats results in bilaterally symmetric nonulcerated vulvar swelling that occurs at parturition. Histologic evaluation will differentiate the relatively orderly epithelial proliferation, often with an associated fibrous component, of papilloma and fibropapilloma from the disorganized, pleomorphic, and invasive squamous epithelium of squamous cell carcinoma. Cytologic diagnosis of squamous cell carcinoma is possible, although frequent secondary infection and sclerosis can make interpretation of cytologic preparations difficult. Aspiration of ectopic mammary tissue in goats reveals milk and fat globules.

Papillomas and fibropapillomas often undergo spontaneous regression. Surgical excision or debulking may be desirable when tumors are large and/or ulcerated. Metastasis of vulvar squamous cell carcinoma to regional lymph nodes and lung is possible. Vulvar squamous cell carcinoma is also often a multicentric tumor, thus making wide surgical excision of this tumor difficult. The swelling of ectopic mammary tissue regresses spontaneously following lactation.

TUMORS OF THE VAGINA AND CERVIX

Smooth muscle tumors are the most common tumors of the vagina and cervix of farm animals and occur in adult cattle, goats and pigs. These tumors are rare in sheep. In goats, smooth muscle tumors may be multiple, especially in aged goats (greater than 10 years of age). Saanen goats may be predisposed to development of multiple genital smooth muscle tumors. Papilloma, fibropapilloma, and lymphoma can also involve the vagina and cervix, especially in cattle. Fibroma also occurs in the vagina of pigs.

Smooth muscle tumors and fibromas most often occur as nonulcerated nodular masses within the wall of the vagina or cervix. Large tumors of any type and leiomyosarcoma can become ulcerated and cause bleeding. Goats with multiple smooth muscle tumors often present with vulvar bleeding, recurrent pseudopregnancy, and spontaneous expulsion of uterine fluid ("cloud burst"). Straining, anorexia, depression, and weight loss can also be seen. Histologic evaluation is necessary to distinguish tumor types and to distinguish benign from malignant smooth muscle tumors. Genital papillomas and fibropapillomas have histologic features identical to those at other sites. Smooth muscle tumors consist of interlacing bundles of elongate cells. Leiomyoma consists of well-differentiated and noninvasive cells that resemble normal smooth muscle. Mitoses are not usually seen. Leiomyosarcoma is characterized by mildly to markedly pleomorphic spindle cells with variable mitotic activity and evidence of local invasion.

Surgical excision of papillomas, fibropapillomas and fibromas is possible and can be curative, although viral-induced lesions may recur. Isolated leiomyoma or leiomyosarcoma can also be surgically excised, although recurrence of leiomyosarcoma caused by local invasion is common. Peritoneal metastasis of leiomyosarcoma is also possible. Surgical removal is not usually possible in goats with multiple genital smooth muscle tumors, but biopsy can confirm the smooth muscle nature of these growths. Interestingly, this syndrome in goats is associated with ovarian cysts and is likely to be hormonally related. In one case, removal of the ovaries resulted in resolution of the vaginal tumors, and ovariectomy should be considered in goats with multiple genital smooth muscle tumors.

TUMORS OF THE UTERUS

Primary uterine tumors in farm animals include smooth muscle tumors (leiomyoma and leiomyosarcoma), epithelial tumors (adenoma and adenocarcinoma), and mixed tumors (carcinosarcoma). The uterus is also a common site of infiltration in cattle with multicentric lymphoma caused by BLV infection. Uterine smooth muscle tumors are most commonly reported in cattle but also occur in sheep, pigs, and goats. Endometrial adenocarcinoma is most common in the cow and is rare in sheep, goats, and pigs. Benign epithelial tumors of the uterus (adenomas) are very rare, and only one report of adenoma of the uterus occurring in a pig was found. Endometrial carcinosarcoma has been reported in an aged pig.

Clinical signs in animals with uterine tumors may be inapparent, even when tumors have achieved an extremely large size. Uterine masses are palpable during rectal examination of cattle. In other species, tumors may not be detected until systemic signs of anorexia and cachexia are apparent. Large uterine tumors in pigs can result in visible distension of the abdominal wall.

Leiomyoma is a smooth-surfaced, discrete mass within the uterine wall that closely resembles normal smooth muscle in appearance. Leiomyosarcoma is invasive and often contains areas of necrosis and hemorrhage. Uterine adenocarcinoma in cattle occurs most often in the horns and less commonly in the body of the uterus. Uterine adenocarcinoma arises within the uterine wall and does not generally extend to the mucosal or serosal surface. Diffuse thickening of the uterine wall as a result of adenocarcinoma can mimic pregnancy. Adenocarcinoma is sclerotic and can cause annular constriction of the uterus. Lymphoma causes diffuse thickening of the uterine wall by characteristic soft to slightly firm tan tissue with minimal to no sclerosis and no evidence of constriction (Figure 3-13).

Cytologic evaluation can help to distinguish smooth muscle tumors from epithelial and lymphoid neoplasia. Histopathologic evaluation is necessary to distinguish benign and malignant smooth muscle tumors; cellular pleomorphism, mitotic activity, and evidence of invasion indicate malignancy. Adenocarcinoma forms nests and

glands composed of pleomorphic neoplastic epithelial cells. Carcinosarcoma is characterized by neoplastic proliferation of both epithelial and mesenchymal elements. Lymphoma is characterized by invasive sheets of neoplastic lymphocytes that obliterate normal architecture.

Leiomyoma is a benign neoplasm that could be cured by hysterectomy. Leiomyosarcoma in early stages might also be cured by surgical excision; however, widespread metastases within the abdominal cavity are possible. Uterine adenocarcinoma typically metastasizes widely to lungs as well as abdominal organs, and surgical excision is not likely to be curative. Similarly, metastasis of carcinosarcoma to thoracic and abdominal viscera is likely. Cows with uterine lymphoma will also have lymphoid neoplasia within other organs.

TUMORS OF THE ACCESSORY SEX GLANDS

Tumors of accessory sex glands are very rare in all animals. An adenocarcinoma of the major vestibular gland (Bartholin's gland) has been reported in a 9-year-old Japanese Brown cow. Clinical signs were of persistent vulvovaginitis and hemorrhage. A large solitary invasive mass was found in the vestibule near the urethral opening. Histologic evaluation after slaughter revealed invasive, pleomorphic neoplastic epithelial cells that formed irregular tubules and glands with marked associated fibrous stroma and inflammation. Metastasis was not found; therefore treatment by surgical excision of this type of tumor may be possible.

TUMORS OF THE OVARY

Ovarian neoplasms are uncommon in farm animals. Granulosa cell/stromal tumors are most common in cattle and have been reported in heifers. Granulosa cell/stromal tumors occur much less commonly in pigs and sheep. Other ovarian tumors typically occur only in older animals. Adenoma, adenocarcinoma, and dysgerminoma occur rarely in cattle and pigs. Vasoproliferative lesions, classified as hamartoma, hemangioma, or hemangiosarcoma, occur most commonly in sows and are less common in cows. Ovarian teratoma is a rare neoplasm of cattle and sheep. Ovarian infiltration by lymphoma in cows with BLV infection can also occur. No reports of ovarian neoplasia in goats were found.

Granulosa cell/stromal tumors of cattle can result in signs of nymphomania. Clinical signs of masculine behavior are less common. Lactation can occur in virgin heifers with ovarian granulosa cell/stromal tumor. Ovarian tumors of all types in cattle typically result in palpable enlargement of the affected ovary on rectal examination. Ovarian tumors in sheep and pigs have most often been described in surveys of animals examined at slaughter, and no clinical information is available.

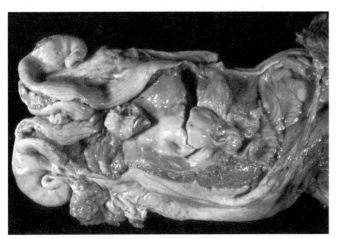

Figure 3-13 Localized thickening of the uterus of an adult cow by pale tissue typical of lymphoma.

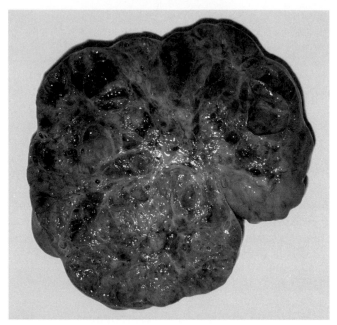

Figure 3-14   Granulosa cell/stromal tumor of the ovary of a cow.

(Courtesy of Dr. Barry Cooper.)

It is possible that affected animals were culled because of poor reproductive performance.

Gross examination reveals enlargement of one or both ovaries. Bilateral involvement is common in sows with vasoproliferative lesions. Adenoma, adenocarcinoma, and dysgerminoma often present as solid tissue tumors. Granulosa/stromal tumors often have multiple cystic spaces, which can be hemorrhagic, admixed with solid tissue (Figure 3-14). Teratomas contain multiple tissue types—including hair, bone, cartilage, and teeth—and a vascular nature is exhibited by the various vasoproliferative lesions. Histologic examination will distinguish the glandular pattern of adenoma and adenocarcinoma, the sheets of germs cells typical of dysgerminoma, the nests of plump granulosa cells often admixed with stromal cells typical of granulosa/stromal cell tumors, the multiplicity of tissue types in teratoma, and the vascular channels typical of vasoproliferative lesions.

Metastasis of ovarian neoplasia in farm animals is rare. Surgical excision of the affected ovary should be curative in most cases.

Tumors of the Male Genital Tract

Tumors involving the male genital tract occur in all farm animal species. Penile and preputial papillomas and fibropapillomas are most common. Various testicular tumors occur but are uncommon. Sperm granulomas, especially in polled cattle and goats, can mimic testicular

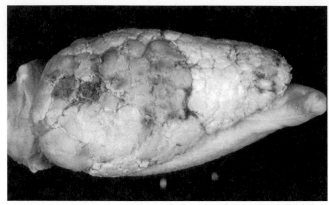

Figure 3-15   Fibropapilloma forming a cylindrical mass on the penis of a bull.

(Courtesy of Dr. Stan Snyder.)

neoplasia. A localized swelling within the testis or epididymis of cattle, sheep, or goats is more likely to be a sperm granuloma than a testicular tumor.

TUMORS OF THE PENIS, PREPUCE, AND SCROTUM

Papilloma and fibropapilloma as the result of papillomavirus involving the penis and/or prepuce are common in bulls 1 to 2 years of age and have also been seen in mature boars. A bovine tubular adenoma involving the prepuce has been reported. Mesothelioma is relatively common in the scrotum of adult bulls.

Papillomas and fibropapillomas of the penis can cause bleeding associated with breeding, and because of pain, affected bulls are often reluctant to breed. Large tumors can interfere with retraction of the penis. Tumors in the area of the urethral opening will cause dysuria. Tumors are single or multiple and most often appear as multinodular to multilobular masses with a broad base of attachment. These tumors in cattle can also be cylindrical and surround the penis (Figure 3-15). Fibrous proliferation is typical of genital tumors in cattle, whereas epithelial proliferation is characteristic of genital tumors in boars. Tubular adenoma occurs as a circumscribed tumor composed of well-differentiated glands. Mesothelioma presents as diffuse scrotal swelling with multiple soft granulomatous—appearing growths in the vaginal tunics. Scrotal mesothelioma in bulls can be unilateral or bilateral. Variable cell patterns are seen on histopathologic evaluation, and differentiating reactive from neoplastic mesothelium in cytologic and histopathologic preparations can be difficult.

Viral papillomas and fibropapillomas regress spontaneously. Surgical removal or debulking of larger tumors can be achieved, although tumors may recur in young bulls. Surgical excision of genital fibropapilloma in older bulls is often curative. Surgical excision of the testis and associated tunics of bulls with unilateral mesothelioma can be curative. Internal metastasis of mesothelioma to the abdominal and/or thoracic cavities is, however, also possible, and the prognosis for bulls with bilateral scrotal mesothelioma is poor. Surgical excision of adenoma would be curative.

TUMORS OF THE TESTIS

Various testicular tumors occur in older farm animals, although the incidence is low. Sertoli cell tumor, interstitial cell tumor, and teratoma occur in bulls. Shorthorn cattle may be predisposed to development of Sertoli cell tumors. Seminoma, rete testis tumors, and leiomyoma of the testis occur in rams. Teratomas and interstitial cell tumors are rare in boars, and no reports of testicular tumors in buck goats were found.

Testicular tumors cause palpable nodules or overall enlargement of the affected testis. Large tumors or Sertoli cell tumor with estrogen production can be associated with poor sperm production as a result of atrophy of testicular cords. Testicular tumors vary in gross appearance. Solid pale tan tumor tissue is typical of Sertoli cell, seminoma, and rete testis tumors. Sertoli and rete testis tumors are often associated with fibrous stroma. Interstitial cell tumor and leiomyoma are typically soft pink to red tumors that often contain areas of hemorrhage. Teratomas vary in appearance depending on the tissue types present. Hair, teeth, bone, and cartilage can be found in well-differentiated testicular teratomas. Histologic evaluation will differentiate the sheets of germ cells characteristic of seminoma, the sheets and nests of plump eosinophilic cells typical of interstitial cell tumor, the cords of often vacuolated columnar cells in fibrous stroma seen in Sertoli cell tumors, the glandular pattern of rete testis tumors, and the mixture of differentiated epithelial and mesenchymal tissue indicative of teratoma.

The majority of testicular tumors in farm animals are benign and cured by surgical removal of the affected testis. Seminoma can be invasive in sheep, although no reports of metastasis were found.

Tumors of the Kidney and Urinary Bladder

Tumors involving kidney or urinary bladder occur most often in pigs, cattle, and sheep. Renal cell tumors (adenomas and adenocarcinomas) and lymphoma involving the kidney occur most often in cattle and are much less common in sheep and pigs. Nephroblastoma occurs most often in pigs, less commonly in cattle, and rarely in sheep. Urinary bladder tumors—including papillomas, adenomas, and vascular tumors—occur most often in cattle and sheep, especially those grazing on bracken fern. Tumors that involve the kidneys or urinary bladder are very rare in goats.

KIDNEY

Renal cell tumors are found most often in adult to aged cattle and are described most often in females. Tumors can be single to multiple and can involve one or both kidneys. Lymphoma in cattle can involve one or both kidneys. Nephroblastoma (embryonal nephroma) occurs most often in pigs and is also the most common neoplasm encountered in this species. Nephroblastoma is rare in cattle and sheep. Nephroblastoma is a tumor of young animals seen most often in animals less than 1 year of age, and it can be seen in fetal animals. Renal tumors have not been described in goats.

Renal cell tumors in cattle have been found at necropsy, and *ante mortem* clinical signs have not been described. Clinical signs of renal lymphoma are variable and include cachexia and peripheral lymphadenopathy. The signs may or may not indicate renal dysfunction. Enlargement of one or both kidneys palpable on rectal examination is typical of renal lymphoma. Nephroblastoma rarely results in clinical signs of renal dysfunction, although abdominal distention caused by large tumors is possible.

Renal cell adenomas and adenocarcinomas are firm, irregular, yellow-orange, tan, or brown well-circumscribed cortical tumors that often protrude on the capsular surface and can also extend into the renal pelvis. Histologic features are similar for adenomas and adenocarcinomas, and size is not a good criterion for malignancy as even small (less than 2-3 cm in diameter) tumors have exhibited metastatic behavior. A variety of patterns from solid to papillary is seen, and a variant composed of renal cells with prominent clear cytoplasm (clear cells) occurs in cattle. Lymphoma results in locally extensive to diffuse enlargement and thickening of affected kidney by pale tan tissue. Histologic and cytologic preparations reveal sheets of neoplastic lymphocytes with marked infiltration and architectural effacement in tissue sections. Nephroblastoma is a firm, nodular, often multilobulated tumor that typically arises in the cortex of one pole of the kidney. Nephroblastoma can be quite large and can cause massive enlargement of the affected kidney (Figure 3-16). The tumor tissue is firm and pale and often contains cystic and necrotic zones. Foci of bone and cartilage are also possible. Nephroblastoma has a unique histologic pattern of admixed embryonal epithelial and mesenchymal elements.

Renal cell tumors can be multicentric within the kidneys, but extrarenal metastasis is uncommon. When

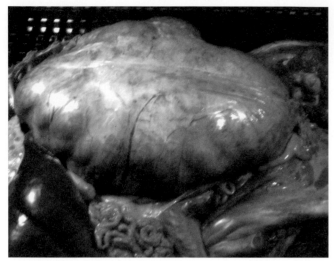

Figure 3-16   Massive enlargement of the kidney in a young pig with nephroblastoma.

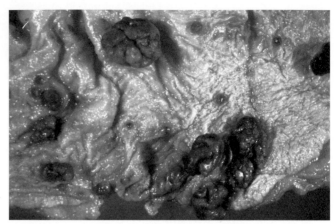

Figure 3-17   Multiple hemorrhagic tumors of the urinary bladder mucosa in a cow with enzootic hematuria.

(Courtesy of Dr. Stan Snyder.)

present, metastasis of renal cell tumors is most often to peritoneum and abdominal lymph nodes. If metastasis is not evident, surgery to remove the affected kidney would likely be curative. Lymphoma involving kidney occurs in cattle in association with multicentric lymphoid neoplasia caused by BLV infection, and surgical intervention would not alter the progressive course of this disease. Nephroblastoma of swine can achieve an extremely large size, but metastasis is rare. Therefore surgical excision of the affected kidney would likely be curative.

URINARY BLADDER

Tumors of the urinary bladder are most common in cattle and sheep. Enzootic hematuria, in which multiple animals are affected with a variety of urinary bladder tumors, occurs in areas where cattle and sheep have access to bracken fern. This disorder also occurs in areas with no bracken fern; therefore the exact etiology of this syndrome remains obscure. Types of tumors that occur in the urinary bladder include transitional cell papillomas, adenomas, carcinomas, and vascular tumors (hemangioma and hemangiosarcoma). Urinary bladder tumors are rare in goats and pigs. The most common clinical sign of tumors within the urinary bladder in all species is hematuria.

Tumors appear as single to multiple polypoid masses within the mucosa of the bladder. Papillomas and adenomas form noninvasive solitary masses, whereas carcinomas are invasive. A hemorrhagic appearance is typical of vascular tumors (Figure 3-17). Histologic evaluation will differentiate epithelial from endothelial tumors, and the degree of cellular pleomorphism, mitotic activity and tumor invasion will differentiate benign from malignant tumors. Cytologic evaluation of urine sediment can help to differentiate reactive from neoplastic processes within the urinary bladder, but differentiating reactive transitional cells from neoplastic transitional cells can be difficult. Moreover, neoplastic endothelial cells are rarely seen in urine.

Metastasis of urinary bladder tumors in farm animals is rare. Surgical excision of benign tumors should be curative. Most malignant tumors are in an advanced stage at the time of clinical diagnosis, thus making complete surgical excision difficult or impossible. Tumors caused by enzootic hematuria are generally multiple, and surgical excision is not an option.

Tumors of the Liver

Hepatocellular, biliary, and gall bladder tumors occur most commonly in cattle and sheep and are less common in goats and pigs. Malignant tumors are more common than benign tumors. Biliary and gall bladder tumors are most often found in older animals, whereas hepatocellular carcinoma occurs in cattle less than 3 years of age, in sheep less than 1 year of age, and in pigs less than 6 months of age. Hepatocellular carcinoma has been associated with carcinogens such as aflatoxin and nitrosamines, especially in pigs. In cattle, sheep, and goats, an association between liver fluke infestation and biliary carcinoma has been proposed but not proven. Lymphoma can involve the liver of cattle and goats with multicentric lymphoid neoplasia. Benign vascular lesions that may be hamartomatous rather than neoplastic occur in the liver of adult cattle as incidental findings. Cholangioma occurs in older pigs and nodular hyperplasia occurs in the liver of pigs of all ages.

Few clinical signs have been reported in farm animals with hepatic tumors. Progressive weight loss and

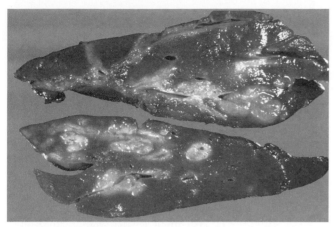

Figure 3-18 Pale zones with linear growth along biliary tracts characteristic of biliary carcinoma in the liver of a cow.

(Courtesy of Dr. Stan Snyder.)

abdominal effusion are possible. Tumors of the gall bladder and biliary tree can result in jaundice. Increased serum levels of liver enzymes and bilirubin are likely.

Hepatocellular and biliary adenomas are generally small and discrete, whereas carcinomas are often quite large at the time of diagnosis and can involve entire liver lobes. Hepatocellular carcinomas are composed of tissue that closely resembles normal hepatic parenchyma. Most hepatocellular tumors are confined to one liver lobe. Biliary tumors are often pale and firm because of the presence of connective tissue stroma and may be seen to follow the tracts of the biliary tree (Figure 3-18). Biliary carcinoma commonly involves multiple liver lobes, most likely because of intrahepatic metastasis. Lymphoma can be a diffuse or a multifocal tumor composed of pale tan, soft to slightly firm tissue. Vascular hamartomas in cattle can be single or multiple and are pale to red firm lesions that can be either depressed or pedunculated. Thrombi can be present within dilated vascular spaces.

Examination of histologic and cytologic preparations aids in the differentiation of hepatocellular from biliary tumors and of benign and malignant lesions and will identify neoplastic lymphocytes in cases of lymphoma. Hepatocellular tumors closely mimic normal hepatic parenchyma but lack portal zones and bile ducts, which differentiates them from hyperplastic nodules. Well-differentiated hepatocellular carcinoma can be difficult to distinguish from hepatocellular adenoma, although carcinoma is generally a larger and more extensive tumor than adenoma. Biliary adenomas are composed of well-differentiated biliary epithelium lining dilated spaces, whereas biliary carcinomas contain pleomorphic epithelial cells forming irregular ducts that are most often admixed in a dense fibrous stroma. Lymphoma is characterized by sheets of neoplastic lymphocytes effacing architecture. Vascular hamartomas consist of stromal and vascular proliferation often with prominent thick-walled arterioles.

Metastasis of biliary carcinoma is more common than is metastasis of hepatocellular carcinoma. Intrahepatic metastasis of biliary carcinoma often precedes spread to abdominal lymph nodes and lung. Lymphoma of the liver of cattle and goats will be part of a generalized neoplastic process. Surgical excision of biliary adenomas, hyperplastic nodules, and vascular hamartomas would be curative, although surgery would rarely be practical.

Tumors of the Spleen

Tumors of the spleen are rare in farm animals. Mast cell tumors in cattle and lymphoma in cattle and goats are most common. Tumors can cause diffuse splenic enlargement or form multifocal nodules throughout the splenic parenchyma. Cytologic and histologic examination will differentiate mast cell neoplasia from lymphoid neoplasia. Mast cell neoplasia confined to the spleen occurs in cattle, and splenectomy might be curative. Splenectomy in cases of lymphoma is not advised.

Tumors of the Abdominal Cavity

Abdominal tumors include mesothelioma, lymphoma, rhabdomyosarcoma, mast cell tumor, and mesenteric lipoma. Most tumors of the abdominal cavity occur in older cattle, although mesothelioma occurs in young as well as old cattle. Abdominal mesothelioma in bulls can occur as an extension of scrotal mesothelioma (see Tumors of the Male Genital Tract). Mesothelioma occurs rarely in sheep and pigs. Disseminated abdominal rhabdomyosarcoma, disseminated peritoneal mast cell tumors, and widespread abdominal lipomatosis occur in older cattle. Discrete focal mesenteric lipomas occur in adult cattle, sheep, and pigs.

Progressive weight loss accompanied by abdominal distention is the most common clinical sign of widespread abdominal neoplasia. Intraabdominal masses are often felt upon rectal examination. Cytologic evaluation of abdominal fluid most often reveals a modified transudate that may contain neoplastic lymphocytes or mast cells. Neoplastic mesothelial cells can also be seen, but the differentiation of reactive mesothelial cells from neoplastic mesothelium is often extremely difficult. Spread of abdominal mesothelioma to the thoracic cavity results in pleural effusion and can cause brisket edema and respiratory distress. Focal mesenteric lipoma is most often found as an incidental finding. Multiple mesenteric lipomas (lipomatosis) occur in older cattle and can result in signs of large intestinal obstruction.

Widespread soft to firm, nodular to infiltrative growths typify mesothelioma, lymphoma, and rhabdomyosarcoma. Mesothelioma is often a soft and granulomatous-appearing lesion of the peritoneum that can have a shaggy surface. Lymphoma is typically firmer, tan to white, and infiltrative into adjacent organs. Rhabdomyosarcoma, lymphoma, and mast cell tumors can appear similar on gross examination. Cytologic and histologic preparations will usually distinguish the sheets of neoplastic round cells typical of lymphoma, the granulated mast cells of mast cell tumor, the oval to spindle shaped cells of rhabdomyosarcoma, and the clusters and individual large round cells characteristic of mesothelial cells. Poorly differentiated tumors, however, may require stains for mast cell granules and/or immunohistochemistry for identification of the tumor cell type. Lipomas occur as focal nodular fatty masses within the mesentery or as multiple intraabdominal tumors (lipomatosis).

Abdominal lymphoma in cattle occurs as part of a more generalized neoplastic process associated with BLV infection. Abdominal mesothelioma and rhabdomyosarcoma metastasize widely within the abdominal cavity and can also spread to involve the thoracic cavity. A case of peritoneal mast cell neoplasia in a cow exhibited metastasis to lung and lymph nodes. Isolated mesenteric lipomas are benign lesions for which surgical excision is curative.

Tumors of Endocrine Glands

Endocrine tumors of farm animals include thyroid C-cell tumors, adrenal cortical and medullary tumors, and pancreatic islet cell tumors. In cattle, multiple endocrine tumors can occur in the same animal. In particular, C-cell tumors and islet cell tumors can be seen associated with pheochromocytoma. This concurrence of tumors in multiple endocrine glands has been compared to the syndromes of multiple endocrine neoplasias in humans. Adrenal cortical adenoma and pheochromocytoma occur in goats, but endocrine tumors are rarely reported in sheep or pigs.

Tumors of the thyroid (C-cell tumors, also called *ultimobranchial tumors*) are common in aged cattle of both sexes, although most reports are in aged dairy bulls. Both C-cell adenoma and C-cell carcinoma (medullary carcinoma) occur. Adrenal cortical tumors and pancreatic islet cell tumors occur in aged cattle. Sporadic reports of adrenal cortical and of adrenal medullary tumors in adult sheep and of adrenal cortical tumors in adult pigs exist. Adrenal cortical tumors occur in adult goats and may be more common in castrated male goats than in intact male goats.

Thyroid tumors in cattle can result in palpable enlargement of the thyroid gland. Thyroid tumors in aged bulls are often associated with degenerative changes in vertebrae and lameness, although the exact relationship between the thyroid C-cell tumors and the bony changes is not clear. Blood calcium levels in cattle with C-cell tumors are typically normal. Adrenal tumors in farm animals are most often incidental findings at necropsy, although cattle with pheochromocytoma excrete increased levels of catecholamines in urine. Pancreatic islet cell tumors in cattle can be found as an apparently incidental finding or are associated with recumbency ("downer cows").

Thyroid C-cell tumors form single to multiple firm, pale tan nodular masses within one or both lobes of the thyroid. Adenomas are smaller than carcinomas and average approximately 1 to 3 cm in diameter. Adrenal cortical adenomas are discrete, soft yellow to red nodular masses that often bulge from the adrenal surface. Pheochromocytoma causes overall enlargement of the adrenal gland and can become quite large and replace large portions of the affected gland. Pheochromocytomas are soft and dark tan to red. Pancreatic islet cell tumors occur as single to multiple, firm, pale creamy white to yellow nodular masses within the pancreas.

Cytologic and histologic evaluation of endocrine tumors reveals sheets of relatively homogeneous and bland round cells with a thin rim of clear to finely granular cytoplasm. Granules may be more obvious and have characteristic staining with argyrophilic silver stains, which distinguishes pheochromocytoma from adrenal cortical tumors. Immunocytochemical procedures to identify hormones and hormone-related compounds may be necessary to classify endocrine tumors. Mitoses and cellular pleomorphism can be inapparent, and distinguishing benign and malignant endocrine tumors on the basis of histologic and cytologic cell features is often difficult, if not impossible. Evidence of invasion is the best indication of malignancy in endocrine tumors.

Thyroid C-cell adenomas are localized tumors cured by surgical excision of the affected thyroid gland. C-cell carcinomas invade adjacent tissue, metastasize to local lymph nodes, and can spread to the lung. Metastasis of adrenal tumors has not been reported in farm animals. Pancreatic islet cell tumors in cattle are often malignant and exhibit multiple metastases throughout the abdominal cavity and also to lymph nodes within the thorax.

Tumors of Bone and Joint

Neoplasia of bones and joints is uncommon in farm animal species. Osteosarcoma, chondrosarcoma, and synovial cell sarcoma are primary tumors that can involve these tissues. Tumors that involve the bones of the jaw are discussed in Tumors of the Oral Cavity and Jaw. Bone tumors of nasal bones and sinuses are discussed in

Tumors of the Respiratory System. Lymphoma in cattle can involve multiple bones, but clinical signs are usually related to dysfunction of other organs.

Osteosarcoma occurs in older cattle and most commonly involves flat bones such as the skull at the base of the horn, the frontal bone, and the pelvis. Chondrosarcoma in cattle also occurs primarily in flat bones; most reported cases occur in the costosternal region and involving costal cartilage. Synovial sarcoma is rare and has been reported in a small number of cattle that were at least 3 years of age. In sheep, chondrosarcoma is more common than osteosarcoma. Chondrosarcoma in sheep most often affects flat bones such as the rib, scapula, and pelvis, but long bone chondrosarcoma also occurs. Chondrosarcoma can occur in sheep as young as 2 years of age. Chondrosarcoma of the costosternal region occurs rarely in goats, and bone and joint tumors of goats and pigs are extremely rare.

Long bone tumors and joint tumors result in lameness. Tumors involving the ribs or sternum may be mistaken for healing fractures. Tumors involving the pelvis can compress structures in the pelvic canal and interfere with parturition and defecation and can also cause signs of pelvic limb lameness.

Progressive swelling of affected bones and joints is typical. Radiographic findings of concurrent osteolysis and irregular mineralization can help to confirm the diagnosis of bone neoplasia, but differentiation of osteosarcoma from chondrosarcoma cannot be reliably achieved by radiographic evaluation. Synovial sarcoma results in increased soft tissue density within the joint and often lytic lesions within the adjacent bones.

Gross examination of bone tumors most often reveals expansion of the medullary cavity by tissue that may be soft, firm, bony, or cartilaginous and expansion and often disruption of the overlying cortex. Histologic evaluation reveals osteoblastic differentiation (osteosarcoma), chondrocytic differentiation (chondrosarcoma), or a mixture of these cell types (osteochondrosarcoma). *Ante mortem* diagnosis of bone neoplasia relies on evaluation of bone biopsies. Submission of multiple samples, including tissue from deep in the bone, is recommended because bone tumors are often associated with large areas of reactive bone and of necrosis. Evaluation of cytologic preparations for atypical osteoblasts, chondrocytes, or other neoplastic cell types can also be useful. Synovial tumors are characterized by marked and irregular proliferation of synovial tissue that may mimic synovitis or synovial hyperplasia but that can extend through the joint capsule into adjacent muscle following fascial planes. Histologic features include primarily a spindle cell component or an admixed spindle cell and epithelial cell population. Atypical cells indicative of neoplasia are seen in cytologic preparations and in biopsy samples.

Extensive local invasion and widespread metastasis of osteosarcoma and chondrosarcoma in farm animal species is often reported, which may reflect the advanced stage of the tumor at the time of diagnosis. Extrapolation from other species, however, would suggest that early detection and wide surgical excision might be curative. In sheep and goats, limb amputation could result in a viable animal and could be considered in cases of bone or joint neoplasia where internal metastases are not apparent. Too little information is available for synovial cell sarcoma in farm animals to be able to comment on behavior.

RECOMMENDED READINGS

Jubb KVF, Kennedy PC, Palmer N, editors: *Pathology of domestic animals,* ed 4, San Diego, 1993, Academic Press.

Kimberling CV: *Jensen and Swift's diseases of sheep,* ed 3, Philadelphia, 1988, Lea & Febiger.

McGavin MD, Carlton WW, Zachary JF, editors: *Thomson's special veterinary pathology,* ed 3, St Louis, 2001, Mosby.

Meuten DJ, editor: *Tumors in domestic animals,* ed 4, Ames, Iowa, 2002, Iowa State University Press.

Moulton JE, editor: *Tumors in domestic animals,* ed 3, Berkeley, 1990, University of California Press.

Radostits OM, Gay CC, Blood DC, Hinchcliff KW, editors: *Veterinary medicine,* ed 9, New York, 2000, WB Saunders.

Scott DW: *Large animal dermatology,* Philadelphia, 1988, W.B. Saunders.

Smith MC, Sherman DM: *Goat medicine,* Philadelphia, 1994, Lea & Febiger.

Straw BE, D'Allaire S, Mengeling WL, Taylor DJ, editors: *Diseases of swine,* ed 8, Ames, Iowa, 1999, Iowa State University Press.

Theilen GH, Madewelll BR: *Veterinary cancer medicine,* ed 2, Philadelphia, 1987, Lea & Febiger.

CHAPTER 4

SURGICAL CONSIDERATIONS

4.1—Preoperative Preparation

Susan L. Fubini and Ava M. Trent

Evaluation of the Patient

All animals that are surgical candidates should have a complete physical examination, including auscultation of the heart and lungs and an assessment of the surgical problem. For simple elective surgical procedures in young healthy animals, preoperative laboratory work is probably not necessary. Laboratory screening is of value for animals that undergo general anesthesia, those with a more complicated disorder, and those with significant potential hemodynamic complications associated with surgery (such as blood loss). Packed cell volume (PCV) and total protein (TP) are screening tests easily performed that may influence preanesthesia preparation and intraoperative response to blood loss. For cattle with complicated gastrointestinal disturbances, such as an abomasal volvulus, plasma electrolyte concentrations help determine appropriate replacement fluid therapy (see Chapter 5). A complete blood count would help identify animals affected with serious infectious processes and may influence preparation and the timing of surgery. If other systemic concerns about a farm animal, such as fatty liver syndrome in a cow, exist, specific tests such as a serum GGT can be run, or if finances permit, a large animal biochemical panel may be more appropriate.

Cattle that undergo elective surgical procedures under general anesthesia in lateral or dorsal recumbency should be fasted 24 to 48 hours before surgery to decrease the ruminal content and ruminal distension and risk of aspiration pneumonia. Furthermore, in ruminants subjected to general anesthesia, fasting is essential to improve venous return and ventilatory capacity (see Chapter 6).

Decision Making

The cost of surgery and perioperative care for farm animals usually requires that it make economic sense. This financial reality dictates good judgment in selecting preoperative preparation. If the surgical procedure is beyond the capabilities of the clinician or the available facilities, a referral should be considered. If this is impractical because of time, distance, or financial constraints and if the client understands the risk, it may be appropriate to attempt an unfamiliar procedure. Much can be gained through familiarity with the anatomy and through envisioning the operation step-by-step so that appropriate plans can be made. With farm animals, withdrawal times for meat and milk must be taken into consideration in the choice of pharmaceuticals.

With experience, clinicians develop a sense about which animals require intervention and what the likely outcome will be. This experience dictates recommendations to owners, choice of surgical approach, and procedures to be performed. However, one is inevitably humbled by finding the unexpected or a cow with a different disease than anticipated. If a problem arises or something does not work correctly during surgery, changing an aspect of the procedure (such as extending the incision, trying a different approach, performing an enterotomy, or asking for help from someone more experienced), rather than struggling for a long period of time, is ultimately best for that patient and the practitioner.

Patient Positioning

Determining the appropriate incision site is half the battle in gastrointestinal surgery in dairy cattle. Fortu-

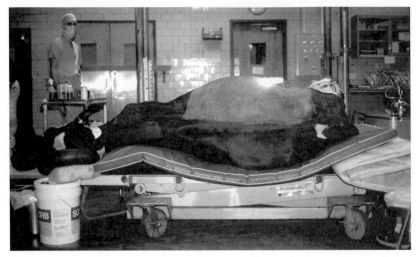

Figure 4.1-1   Cow in lateral recumbency under general anesthesia. Placing appropriate pads under the cow's shoulder and hip creates a cavity to support the distended rumen.

(Reproduced with permission from Smith DF: Bovine Intestinal Surgery: Part 1: *Mod Vet Pract* 65: 853-857, 1984, p 854—Fig 1).

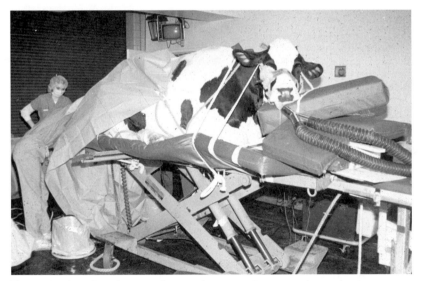

Figure 4.1-2   Cow in sternal recumbency under general anesthesia.

nately, the placid nature of the dairy cow permits many procedures to be done on a standing animal using a local anesthetic. For a more fractious animal, it may be possible to use small amounts of sedation, but this should be used with caution because it increases the risk that the animal will become recumbent. Lateral recumbency can be used for flank and inguinal approaches. Dorsal recumbency may be used for teat surgery, access to the cranial abdomen, and cesarean sections. Padding of bony prominences is indicated in recumbent procedures. For animals placed in left lateral recumbency, placing an inner tube or other pads under the shoulder and hip of a cow has been suggested as useful in making a so-called "sling" for the rumen (Figure 4.1-1). Rarely have we had to place animals in sternal recumbency, either for nasal or cervical surgery (Figure 4.1-2). Other acceptable padding includes air mattresses, water beds, foam pads, and inflatable surgery tables (Snell tables*).

---

*Snell, Wyke Farm, Sherborne, Dorset, UK DT9 6S2.

Preparation of the Surgery Site

Once the decision is made for the surgical approach, dirt and manure should be removed. Hair should be clipped and a generous area left free of hair and debris. Some advocate shaving the actual site of the skin incision, but this may increase chances of infection if the skin is inadvertently nicked. As a rule of thumb, a 25-cm hairless margin around the surgical site is recommended.

In thick-skinned animals, an initial prep with a clean, stiff brush may be helpful. This should be followed by repeated scrubs with a disinfectant solution. Scrub solutions typically contain povidone (polyvinylpyrrolidone)-iodine, 4% chlorhexidine gluconate, or 2% chlorhexidine diacetate. Povidone iodine and chlorhexidine products have a broad antimicrobial spectrum, including most bacteria, some fungi, and many viruses. Scrub solutions can be rinsed with water, saline, or 7% isopropyl alcohol. For long procedures (longer than 90 minutes), povidone iodine with an alcohol rinse, or chlorhexidine with a water or saline rinse is recommended. To aseptically prepare a skin incision, the planned incision site should be cleaned and followed by a circular motion moving from the center to the periphery. This should be repeated at least three times. Depending on the skin gross contamination, more cleansing may be indicated; the gauze should be checked for cleanliness at the completion of the scrub. Some clinicians don a sterile glove and use sterile gauze for the final preparation. This incision site should be draped if at all possible. Impervious drapes can be placed over cloth or paper drapes to help keep the incision dry and free of infection. If the surgery becomes contaminated (for example, if an enterotomy is performed), the area should be isolated with drapes or towels, and the surgeons should reglove after the procedure.

Preparation of the Surgeon

In a hospital setting, clean, comfortable cotton or cotton-blend clothing with use restricted to the operating room is ideal and helps reduce the number of environmental contaminants. Some type of clean head covering that confines hair has also been shown to reduce the incidence of surgical infections. Caps, hoods, and bouffant-style coverings are some options. Facial coverings other than masks protect the wound from droplets of saliva and nasal exudates but are not effective bacterial filters. When properly fitted, face masks direct airflow away from the surgical wound, which—theoretically—should cut down on wound infection. Studies have not supported this finding, but masks are still recommended. Shoe covers are fairly impractical in most farm animal surgery, although waterproof shoes add to the surgeon's comfort.

Surgical gowns are used for most lengthy procedures in a hospital environment. Lint-free gowns that are impervious to water and bacteria are most effective. Reusable gowns made of muslin or, more recently, of 270-count pima cotton, are somewhat resistant to water but not bacteria. Gowns treated with Quarpel, a flouro-chemical finish, combined with Pyridium or melamine hydrophobe, have a better barrier to water and bacteria and a pore size reduced to $10\,\mu m$. Gore-Tex fabric makes an even more durable bacteria-resistant gown.

Disposable gowns are made from olefin, which is regenerated cellulose, a petroleum by-product. Some gowns have extra layers of water repellent material in the sleeves to prevent constant dampness and subsequent capillary migration of skin flora, which lead to increased bacterial counts of surgical wounds. Advantages of disposable products are ease of handling and storage, and reduced bacterial contamination in the surgical environment compared to nondisposables. However, purchasing and disposing of disposable items is more expensive. Nondisposable gowns are more comfortable and less expensive but do need to be laundered and replaced on a regular basis.

Gloves should be worn for all surgical procedures. This helps avoid contamination from the residual flora on the surgeon's hands. Gloves also protect the surgeon from any allergens or contact dermatitis. Most gloves are made of latex and come in a single-use package in a wide variety of sizes. Hypoallergenic vinyl gloves are available for those with latex sensitivity. Magnesium silicate powder is preapplied to most gloves to make them easier to don; therefore gloves should be rinsed before handling tissues. Gloves commonly develop holes and should be checked often for defects. Double gloving is used if extensive draping is required or contamination of the surgeon's hands by sharp objects such as bony fragments and orthopedic implants is likely. Gloves can be applied with a closed or open gloving technique. Closed gloving techniques are preferred because the surgeon's skin will not make contact with the outside of the gown cuff. An open gloving is recommended to replace a glove during a procedure. Otherwise, the cuff of the gown that has been exposed to skin and perspiration will be pulled over "clean" hands. Cuffs of the surgeon's gown should be covered completely by gloves because the cuff material is not impervious to water penetration. Water often finds its way to the surgeon's hands regardless of the material chosen; therefore plastic safety sleeves and double gloving are often helpful during procedures in which the surgeon's hands and arms may be submerged. Although a gown is sterile when first applied, it should be remembered that only the front, above the waist, is considered sterile during the procedure.

Draping the Surgical Field

The purpose of drapes is to create and maintain a sterile field around the operative site. In stationary, recumbent animals, the surgical field is usually surrounded first by sterile towels held in place with penetrating towel clamps. Large cloth or disposable drapes are placed next. Impervious drapes are ideal if a lot of fluid or blood is expected or exteriorization of viscera is necessary.

If long enough, the tails of adult cows should be tied—usually to one hind leg—for standing procedures. Large disposable laparotomy cloths or disposable drapes are available.* They may be fenestrated, or an appropriate-sized hole can be made by the surgeon. They are usually used alone and secured in place with penetrating towel clamps. Although they are relatively expensive, they are a great help in allowing the surgeon to focus on the procedure without worrying about contamination from dirt, fecal material, or body fluids.

Prevention of Peritonitis and Surgical Infection

The surgeon must always be aware of their potential to promote or prevent peritonitis or other infections of the surgical site development during surgery in the cow. It is often possible is to reduce the risk of infection before contamination ever occurs or to intervene between the time contaminants are first introduced into the abdomen and the development of infection.

PRECONTAMINATION
The optimum time to intervene in the development of a surgical infection is before a known or anticipated episode of contamination. Careful planning of the procedure will minimize the period of contamination, ensure adequate restraint, and minimize the use of potential adjuvants to reduce the risk of infection. Prophylactic antibiotics should be considered in planning any clean-contaminated or contaminated procedure and clean procedures in patients with identified risk factors. Common patient risk factors include preexisting nonbacterial inflammatory peritonitis, malnutrition, circulatory shock, and remote or systemic infection. In the latter case, elective procedures should be delayed until

the preexisting infection can be treated and resolved. Similar steps should be considered when facilities, the animal's behavior, or its condition increase the risk of contamination (see Section 4.7). Field conditions often involve less than optimal restraint facilities, fractious animals, limited control of external sources of contamination, and conditions that might predispose to unexpected recumbency during standing procedures (hypocalcemia, exhaustion, extreme peritoneal tension), all of which increase morbidity.

Antibiotics should be administered just far enough before surgery to maintain high serum levels throughout the period of contamination. Intravenous (IV) administration of a single dose 15 minutes before surgery or intramuscular (IM) administration 60 minutes before surgery achieves this goal for most antibiotics. Parenteral, subcutaneous, and intraperitoneal routes are not recommended for prophylaxis because the time to peak levels is longer and less predictable and because peak levels are lower in comparison to IV and IM routes of administration. If intraoperative sample collection for culture is planned, some prophylactic effect can still be obtained by intravenously administering an appropriate antibiotic immediately after sample collection.

Prophylactic antibiotics should be selected with as specific a spectrum as possible, based on probable contaminants. This can be based on knowledge of common contaminants from planned surgical sites (e.g., anaerobes for rumenotomy), culture results from potential sites of leakage or preexisting infection (e.g., culture results from an umbilical abscess), or by predicting other common infectious agents. The ability of antibiotics to penetrate fibrin or function in the presence of necrotic debris or altered pH should not be a major concern in antibiotic selection during the precontamination or contamination stages. Antibiotic options are provided in Appendix 1.

CONTAMINATION
Preventive measures are similar to those described for the precontamination stage, with a few additions. Prophylactic antibiotics can still be of some benefit, but they should be given intravenously to achieve high serum and tissue levels as soon as possible. If a source of contamination first develops intraoperatively, rapid steps to minimize the amount and distribution of contamination are indicated. For example, in gastrointestinal surgery, gross contamination should be localized whenever possible by exteriorizing the site of leakage or isolating it with laparotomy sponges; physically removing all accessible contaminants; and avoiding palpation unless absolutely necessary so that contaminants are not physically transported from the site of leakage to other sites in the abdomen. If the site can be adequately exteriorized to

---

*Vet. Surgical Resources, Darling, MD, 21034.

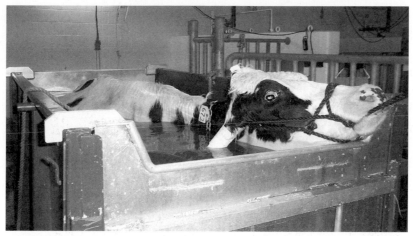

Figure 4.1-3   Cow in flotation tank.

allow external drainage, localized lavage with a sterile isotonic fluid can help remove contaminants. However, generalized lavage is more likely to distribute high concentrations of organisms to potentially clean areas and is only recommended if the site cannot be exteriorized or dissemination has already occurred. Adding antibiotics to the lavage fluid may be indicated even if appropriate systemic antibiotics have been administered.

Other important considerations in the after care of the surgical farm animal are supplying adequate hydration (see Chapter 5), keeping neonates warm, and providing adequate nutrition and oral electrolytes.

Down cattle need excellent footing that keeps them from slipping. They need to be supported by having food and water where it can be reached. Good padding in a heavily bedded stall or on soft dirt is ideal. If cattle remain down for prolonged periods of time it may be necessary to try to get them up with well-padded hip lifts. Alternatively, cattle can be "floated" in a commercial tub ("Aqua cow")* (Figure 4.1-3). This apparatus requires a fair amount of time, patience, and manpower. Regardless it has been successful in the right hands for recumbent cows that are amenable to therapy.

RECOMMENDED READINGS

St. Jean G: Decision making in bovine abdominal surgery, *Vet Clin NA, Food Animal Practice, Surgery of the Bovine Digestive Tract* 6: 335-354, 1990.

Stone WC: Preparation for surgery. In Auer JA, Stick JA, editors: *Equine surgery*, ed 2, Philadelphia, 1999, WB Saunders.

Turner AS, McIlwraith CW: Presurgical considerations. In Turner AS, McIlwraith CW: *Techniques in large animal surgery*, ed 2, Philadelphia, Lea & Febiger.

*New Brunswick, Canada
(http://www.gnb.ca/0389/1998/1998001e.html).

4.2—Perioperative Antimicrobials and Analgesics

Thomas J. Divers

The extra-label use of antimicrobials and analgesics is regulated under the Animal Medicinal Drug Use and Clarification Act of 1994 (AMDUCA) by the FDA Center for Veterinary Medicine. Penicillin and/or ceftiofur are the most commonly used perioperative antibiotics for cattle that undergo surgery without enterotomy. Each drug has its advantages and disadvantages: penicillin is more effective than ceftiofur against *Arcanobacterium pyogenes* and other bovine anaerobic pathogens. It should be used (alone or in combination with another compatible bacteriocidal drug) for surgery on anatomical locations that normally harbor anaerobic organisms (e.g., mouth, gastrointestinal tract, reproductive tract). Unfortunately, penicillin is not very effective against most gram-negative organisms, and the duration of withdrawal time for milk or meat is a disadvantage. At a dose of 27,000 IU/kg intramuscularly (~12,000 IU/lb IM—a 50-mL dose for a 1250 pound animal), the suggested withdrawal time for milk is 5 days and for meat 16 days; whereas for the generally clinically ineffective label dose of 7000 IU/kg, the respective withdrawal times are 2 and 5 days. Ceftiofur sodium (Naxcel), when used at the label dosage, has the advantage of no withdrawal time for meat or milk; ceftiofur hydrochloride (Excenel) has only a 2-day meat withdrawal and no milk withdrawal time.

If an enterotomy is performed, broad-spectrum coverage may be required. A therapy that combines penicillin and ceftiofur (both at 2 to 3 times label dosage) often is used. In a hospital setting, intravenously (IV) administered penicillin salts (22,000 units/kg) are sometimes substituted for procaine penicillin to achieve higher tissue concentrations, but more frequent administration (q6h) is required. If a venous catheter is used for penicillin salt administration, the water-soluble form of ceftiofur can also be given by this route. Ceftiofur IV administration causes less tissue irritation and discomfort with high peak serum and tissue levels of the parent drug. Using the water soluble form of ceftiofur IV is acceptable because it achieves plasma and tissue levels of the parent drug; and its metabolite, desfuroylceftiofur, exceeds the MIC of many gram-negative organisms of veterinary importance, as does its IM or subcutaneous (SQ) use. The SQ administration has the advantage of preserving beef quality because less muscle irritation occurs in comparison to that associated with an IM injection. Another option is oxytetracycline use, a broad-spectrum antibiotic that is moderately effective against gram-positive and gram-negative aerobic and anaerobic organisms. It is occasionally used at an extra-label frequency (6.6 to 11 mg/kg q12 h) to maintain higher tissue levels. Tetracycline is more lipid-soluble than either penicillin or ceftiofur; therefore higher tissue concentrations would be expected. Tetracycline disadvantages are its bacteriostatic activity and potential for causing renal failure when administered at high daily dosages and/or to dehydrated animals. At present, Liquamycin LA-200 is the only form of oxytetracycline with a label that allows use in lactating dairy cattle. Used at the label dose (6.6 to 11 mg/kg IV, SQ, or IM q 24 hr), the drug has a 28-day meat withdrawal and 4-day milk withdrawal.

All perioperative antibiotics should be administered only 1 to 2 hours before surgery so that the highest concentration of drugs is present when tissue is being incised and handled and when clots/fibrin are forming. If the surgery is uncomplicated (e.g., a routine laparotomy), many surgeons do not use antibiotics. If antibiotics are used, it is imprudent to use them for a shorter duration than the label recommendation. Most cattle antibiotics are labeled for 3 days minimum use. More complicated surgeries (e.g., enterotomy, internal fixation) require continuous treatment for at least 5 days. If infection is discovered at the time of or after surgery, treatment should be continued for longer periods. When bacterial infection is suspected before surgery, the decision to withhold preoperative antibiotics until a culture sample can be obtained should be based upon the location and predicted benefit of culturing the infected site. For most abdominal surgeries with preexisting infection (e.g., reticular or umbilical abscess), preoperative antibiotics are recommended because offending organisms are predictable, cultures are generally not taken, and some risk

of spreading the infection at the time of surgery exists. Conversely, antibiotics are generally withheld for orthopedic surgery that involves presumably infected bone until a culture sample can be obtained. If an offending organism's sensitivity is known from samples obtained before surgery, antimicrobial selection should be based upon the organism's sensitivity, predicted drug(s) tissue levels, confidence in drug safety and cost, and FDA approval of extra-label use.

Florifenicol (nonlactating cows), enrofloxacin (beef cattle with respiratory disease only), and tetracyclines are occasionally used as perioperative antibiotics. Aminoglycosides combined with penicillin, ampicillin, or Ticarcillin/clavulanate are rarely used in calves—and then only with strict adherence to extra label use (Table 4.2-1). Antibiotics prohibited under all circumstances in food animals are given in Box 4.2-1.

Perioperative Analgesics

Perioperative analgesics are indicated in most surgical procedures to temper the initial inflammatory response and decrease swelling as well as to improve the appetite and general well-being of the patient. In cattle with routine, relatively nontraumatic surgery (e.g., omentopexy), perioperative analgesics commonly are not used

---

TABLE 4.2-1

Combination Use of Antimicrobial Drugs in Farm Animal Surgery[a,b]

NONANTAGONISTIC	ANTAGONISTIC
Penicillin and aminoglycoside	Penicillin and tetracycline
Ampicillin and aminoglycoside	
Amoxicillin and aminoglycoside	
Cephalosporin and aminoglycoside	
Erythromycin and rifampin*	
Trimethoprim and sulfonamide (TMP/S)*	
TMP/S* and rifampin*	
Sulfonamide and tetracycline	
Lincomycin and spectinomycin	
Enrofloxacin[†]	

*To be used in calves only.
[†]Beef cattle for respiratory complications only.
[a]The American Association of Bovine Practitioners, in being cognizant of food safety issues and concerns, encourages its members to refrain from the intramuscular, subcutaneous, or intravenous extra-label use of the aminoglycoside class of antibiotics in bovines (Approved by the Board of Directors, December 1994).
[b]Until further scientific information becomes available, aminoglycoside antibiotics should not be used in cattle except as specifically approved by the FDA (Approved by the American Veterinary Medical Association House of Delegates, 1998).

BOX 4.2-1

ANTIMICROBIAL DRUGS PROHIBITED FOR USE IN FOOD ANIMALS

1. Chloramphenicol
2. Nitrofurans (including topical—e.g., nitrofurazone)
3. Most sulfonamides in lactating dairy cows (e.g., sulfamethazine)
4. Fluoroquinolones in dairy cows or calves (note: enrofloxacin, Baytril 100, is legal only for use in the therapy of beef cattle respiratory disease)
5. Nitromidazoles (e.g. metronidazole)
6. Glycopeptides (e.g. vancomycin, avoparcin)

simply because of cost and loss of product value as a result of milk withholding. This is particularly true if cattle are being treated perioperatively with ceftiofur, which has no withholding time. The most commonly used antiinflammatory drug is flunixin meglumine (1.1 mg/kg IV or IM). Flunixin is a cyclooxygenase inhibitor that provides excellent analgesia, including visceral analgesia, and is the only FDA-approved non-steroidal antiinflammatory drug for cattle—albeit only for beef cattle and only IV. It may be indicated during the time of routine (one or more dosages) bovine surgery and in the immediate postoperative period when withholding times for milk and meat are not a major issue (when used only preoperatively at label dose, it incurs 10 days of meat withholding and 3 days of milk withholding).

Phenylbutazone (PBZ) and aspirin are other antiinflammatory analgesics that historically have been used in food animals. Given that detection of PBZ at any level in food animals is considered illegal (milk and meat withdrawal are recommended at 10 and 45 days, respectively) and given the potential adverse reactions in human consumers, the Food Animal Residue Avoidance Databank (FARAD) strongly discourages PBZ use in any food animal. FARAD further discourages aspirin use in food animals for the following reasons: 1) no FDA approval for use in food animals; 2) flunixin is an available alternative; and 3) it has questionable efficacy (administered orally, the drug reaches baseline serum concentrations in 12 to 24 hours).

Additional analgesics that may be used are lidocaine, alpha-agonists, and butorphanol. Lidocaine is mostly used either for epidural administration to provide analgesia to the pelvic area during and after perineal or rectal surgery or as intravenous anesthesia (with a tourniquet) during surgery on a distal limb (15 to 30 ml lidocaine).

Lidocaine is most commonly used as a local analgesic for cutting skin to prevent an animal from becoming fractious.

Xylazine epidurals (0.05 mg/kg) or Medetomidine 5 to 15 µg/kg may provide slightly better analgesic effects than lidocaine. Xylazine 0.03 mg/kg can be combined with lidocaine (0.2 mg/kg) for both fast-acting and long-lasting (4 to 5 hours) analgesia. Butorphanol may also be used intramuscularly or intravenously (0.1 mg/kg) for severe pain that cannot be adequately diminished with NSAID therapy. For information regarding the use of nonapproved antibiotics and analgesics, the reader is encouraged to consult Food Animal Residue Avoidance Data Bank at www.farad.org.

RECOMMENDED READINGS

Brown SA, Robb EJ: Plasma disposition of ceftiofur and metabolites after intravenous and intramuscular administration of ceftiofur sodium to calves of various ages, *The Bovine Proceedings* 27: 206-207, 1995.

Extra-label drug use in animals: final rule. *Fed Reg* 1996; 61: 57732-57746.

Gingerich AG et al: Pharmacokinetics and dosage of aspirin in cattle. *J Am Vet Med Assoc* 167: 945-948, 1975.

Okker H et al: Pharmacokinetics of ceftiofur in plasma and uterine secretions and tissues after subcutaneous postpartum administration in lactating dairy cows, *J Vet Pharmacol Therap* 25: 33-38, 2002.

Payne, MA: Extra-label drug use and withdrawal times in dairy cattle, *Comp Cont Educ Pract Vet* 13: 1341-1351, 1991.

Payne M: Antiinflammatory therapy in dairy cattle: therapeutic and regulatory considerations, *Calif Vet* March 10-12, 2001.

Riviere JE et al: Primer on estimating withdrawal times after extra-label drug use, *J Am Vet Med Assoc* 213: 966-968, 1998.

Salmon SA et al: In vitro activity of ceftiofur and its primary metabolite, desfuroylceftiofur, against organisms of veterinary importance, *J Vet Diag Invest* 8: 332-336, 1996.

4.3—Facilities and Restraining Devices

Richard Wheeler

Introduction

When working with livestock, one faces inherent risks to the safety of the animal and handler. Livestock, by their sheer size, are a threat to human safety. Fearful or aggressive animals with horns are exponentially more dangerous and can inflict significant injury—or even death. Bulls are always dangerous and unpredictable and should never be trusted. Dairy bulls, because of their extensive human contact, lack a natural fear of humans and may be overtly aggressive. Beef bulls generally react out of fear toward humans. The protective, maternal instinct of a cow with a calf makes them significantly more dangerous then a single cow. Because beef cows usually are not intensively handled, they are more dangerous than dairy cows. It has been suggested that the position of the hair whorl between a cow's eyes correlates with the degree of agitation the cow demonstrates under restraint. Animals with whorls located high on the forehead, above the level of the eyes, were found to be more aggressive under restraint (high whorls, hot-headed) (Grandin, 1995).

Although small ruminants (sheep, goats, and calves) can inflict injury to their handlers, they are more likely to injure themselves when struggling against restraining devices or overly aggressive handlers. Sheep and goats have a strong herd instinct and become stressed when separated from herd mates. Stress adversely effects wound healing as well as general health, growth, and production. In pigs, stress has been associated with sudden death.

Animal Behavior

Consideration of the animals' natural instincts will enable a handler to humanely and safely move and restrain livestock. Livestock are prey animals whose primary defense mechanism is sight and flight. They have evolved wide-set eyes that afford them extensive peripheral vision in surveillance of predators. With an angle of vision approaching 300 degrees, their only blind spot is directly behind them. To avoid startling an animal when approaching it, the handler should remain within its line of sight. Startling an animal could elicit struggling, provoke the animal to kick, or incite a stampede.

Panoramic vision provides prey animals a wide angle of vision but sacrifices depth perception. This is why cattle commonly balk at shadows, are reluctant to step across different colored floors, and closely inspect objects in their paths. Handlers should be patient. They should allow the animal to assess the danger of a situation or novel object before forcing it to enter a foreign environment or head gate.

Animals naturally maintain a safe distance between themselves and potential predators. This distance is the flight zone. If the flight zone is invaded, the animal will move away from the invader to reestablish an adequate safe distance. In relation to people, this distance is influenced by the amount of contact the animal has had with humans. Dairy cattle, which are handled daily, may have practically no flight zone and can be readily approached. Alternatively, beef cattle, which often have greater fear because of limited human contact, may require several meters of space. Sheep and goats commonly move as a herd, and the comfort level of the first animal establishes the flight zone for the herd.

Knots

Ropes are invaluable assets in animal restraint. However, a rope is only as good as the knot that is tied. There is a unique knot, with a particular advantage, for practically any situation imaginable. However, every animal handler should be proficient with the three knots covered in the following discussion.

SQUARE KNOT
The square knot joins two rope ends. Joining the ends of a single rope forms a loop that allows the rope to be tied to a fixed object. Alternatively, the ends of two separate ropes can be joined to form one long rope. Once tightened, a properly tied square knot will not slip under tension. A common error is to tie a "granny knot" that slips when tension is applied (Figure 4.3-1).

QUICK-RELEASE SLIP KNOT
The quick-release slip knot and its modifications (see Tail Ties) secure the rope but allow it to be easily untied. For example, the free end of a halter may be tied to a post to restrain an animal's head. When properly tied, the bow end of the knot is entirely surrounded by rope; if the bow lies against the object to which it is tied, it is not secure and will loosen as the animal struggles. Because it is a slipknot, there will always be a little play in the rope as it slips down to its anchor; tying the knot as close to the anchor as possible is important (Figure 4.3-2).

BOWLINE KNOT
The bowline knot creates a permanent loop that will not tighten. It is useful to place around an animal's body, neck, or limb because it will not cinch down and compromise respiration or circulation (Figure 4.3-3).

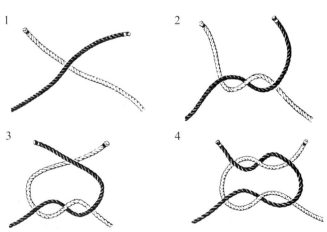

Figure 4.3-1   Square knot.

(Adapted from Leahy JR, Barrow P: *Restraint of animals*, ed 2, Ithaca, 1953, self-published.)

Restraint of Cattle

MOVING CATTLE

One should take advantage of ruminants' flight instinct when moving a single animal or a herd. The flight zone is entered slowly, steadily, and silently so the animal is not spooked. The rate at which the animal moves depends on how deeply and rapidly the flight zone is penetrated. If an animal gets too anxious or moves too quickly, the handler should back away and allow the animal to relax. Excited cattle are impossible to control

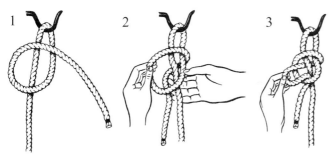

Figure 4.3-2   Quick-release knot.

(Adapted from Leahy JR, Barrow P: *Restraint of animals,* ed 2, Ithaca, 1953, self-published.)

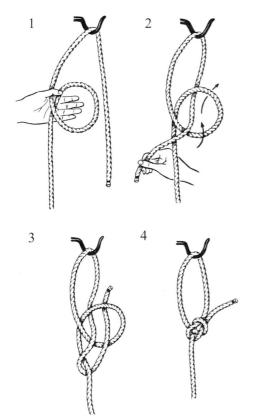

Figure 4.3-3   Bowline knot.

(Adapted from Leahy JR, Barrow P: *Restraint of animals,* ed 2, Ithaca, 1953, self-published.)

and are more likely to be injured or injure a person. Cattle should be moved no faster than a walk.

The spatial relationship between the handler and the animal's body dictates the direction the animal will move when approached. The animal's shoulder is the point of balance. If approached caudal to the shoulder, the animal will move forward; if approached cranial to the shoulder, the animal will generally move backward.

Getting a Cow to Stand

Most recumbent animals will stand as the handler enters the flight zone. However, dairy cows are so intensively managed that physical contact may be necessary to incite them to rise. Before a recumbent animal is prompted to stand, the animal should be evaluated to ascertain whether it is physically capable of standing. To encourage an animal to stand, a gentle kick on the caudal thigh with the inside of one's foot is often sufficient. If more substantial prompting is necessary, a pen, key, or other blunt object can be used to tap on the animal's spine. If the animal remains recumbent, the operator should stand at its back, buckle its knees into its ribs and simultaneously slap its chest on the contralateral side. If all else fails and it is certain the animal is physically able to stand, the electric cattle prod may be used as a last resort. Occasionally the animal can be intimidated to stand without being shocked. The humming noise made by activating the prod, or touching the uncharged nodes of the prod to the animal may prompt it to rise.

Moving Animals by Halter

A halter-broken cow may follow the handler when the lead is pulled. However, a novice to the halter will resist being pulled. Often the animal will move forward more willingly if the handler steps to the animal's side, caudal to the shoulder and behind the point of balance, while maintaining control of the lead. The animal's natural tendency is to move forward. The drawback is that the handler's position is deep in the animal's flight zone; therefore it may try to charge forward because it perceives that no one is there any longer. To maintain control, the handler pulls down the animal's head caudally toward its shoulder to force it to turn. If the animal gets out of control, the ropes should be released. Safety should not be compromised in a vain attempt to halt a stampeding animal.

If an animal is reluctant to proceed, the handler should make sure advancement is not impeded and no one is standing in the animal's path or line of vision. When encouragement is required, one should again start with the least noxious prodding necessary to stimulate the animal to move—a slap on the rump or a prod along the backbone with a blunt object. Although the discomfort from a tail twist is often effective, it holds potential for breaking a coccygeal vertebra. The electric prod should be used only as a last resort. Shouting should be discouraged because it increases confusion, stress levels, and impatience.

Moving Animals through Chutes

Using flight zone works well to move a single animal or group of animals through a chute. The handler walks alongside the chute in the *opposite* direction the cattle should move. Because the flight zone is deeply penetrated, the animals will move forward as the handler passes their point of balance. After the line of animals begins to move, the handler walks outside the flight zone back to the lead animal and penetrates the zone again to walk alongside the animals. Repeating this pattern causes the cow or group of cows to keep moving forward.

When moving cattle, one must eliminate as many distractions as possible. Chutes should be constructed in a curved pattern to facilitate uninterrupted forward movement. Cows will be leery of abrupt corners. The chute should terminate in a well-lit space because the animals will be reluctant to enter a great, dark abyss. Solid-sided chutes limit the animals' distraction, so they will move forward more readily. People should stay out of sight as much as possible. Objects that could distract or frighten the animals should not be left in or on the chutes.

HEAD RESTRAINT
Halters

Properly used halters provide excellent control of an animal's head. The halter should be placed with the nosepiece over the top of the animal's nose half way between the eyes and nostrils to prevent airway obstruction or trauma to the eyes. The lead rope should run below the jaw. Putting the halter on upside down with the lead rope running behind the ears or over the nose is a common mistake. An improperly fitted halter severely compromises control of the animal's head and is prone to slip off.

Nose Tongs

A nose tong is a pincer-type device with blunt bulbous ends that are inserted into each nostril to apply pressure to the nasal septum. The discomfort deters movement. Nose tongs should only be used in conjunction with another form of head restraint such as a halter or head gate. Tension must be maintained on the nose tongs, but they should never be tied to a fixed object. If nose tongs are not available, the nasal septum can be grasped between the thumb and middle finger.

A nose ring is a variation of the nose tong that is used on bulls. It is permanently inserted through the nasal septum. Again, excessive pressure can rip through the cartilage, so a halter should always be used in addition to the bull's nose ring.

Head Gates

Head gates are a necessity in working with large animals. Even the smallest cattle operation should be equipped with some type of head gate to provide ease in handling, restraint, and safety. Assorted head gates—ranging from homemade vertical wooden plank devices, dairy stanchions, and self-locking feeders to custom-made head gates—exist. Head gates constructed with curved bars reduce vertical head and neck movement but may increase asphyxiation potential from a blocked trachea or the carotid arteries if the animal lies down. Straight bars are less likely to result in asphyxiation, but they do not restrict vertical head movement.

Single file chutes provide an advantage in directing cattle into head gates while restricting sideways movement of the animal. Squeeze chutes are commercially manufactured with compressible side walls that apply pressure against the animal, creating a calming effect and supporting the animal if it attempts to lie down. Chutes are invaluable assets for controlling livestock, but they limit access to the animal and create a potential for operator injuries between the animal and chute. Also, spring-loaded levers and moving parts can cause severe injury to handlers.

KICKING

A major consideration for personal safety is the animal's ability to kick. Cows are very deft kickers and are notorious for kicking to the side—"cow kicking." They also kick forward surprisingly well, and can extend the leg as far cranial and dorsal as the shoulder. Cows are also very proficient at kicking straight backward. They may even "mule kick" with both hind feet at the same time. The safest place to stand when working at the hind end of a cow is immediately adjacent to the animal's body, so that the cow pushes the handler away rather then delivering a harmful blow at the snap of the kick. When working cranial to the hind legs, the operator should stay out of reach of a forward kick by standing level with the animal's shoulder at arm's length.

Hobbles

Hobbles may be used to tie the hind feet together to deter cattle from kicking. Commercial hobbles are available, but effective restraints can easily be fashioned out of rope.

Flanking

A manual method to deter an animal from kicking is called "flanking." The fold of skin in the flank is lifted, and the handler places a thigh against the animal's stifle. This provides mechanical resistance that interferes with the animal's ability to kick. A mechanical device working under the same premises lifts against the flank and attaches over the back beneath the lumbar vertebral processes.

Tailing

Tailing discourages kicking by causing discomfort and distracting the animal's attention. To tail an animal, the tail's base is grasped and lifted directly over the animal's back. Coccygeal vertebrae may fracture if too much force is exerted.

TAIL TIES

A swishing tail can be a source of frustration and potential for injury. It may contaminate a previously cleaned site, catch the handler in the eye, or otherwise be an annoyance. Tying the animal's tail out of the way is imperative for many surgical techniques and handler safety when he or she works near the back of the animal.

A secure tail-tie can be made using baling twine, rolled gauze, bandaging tape, or a light rope. One end of the rope is placed over the animal's tail below the last coccygeal vertebra. The switch (long hair at the end of the tail) is folded over the rope. The short end of the rope is run completely around the tail, made into a bow, and tucked underneath the loop that encircles the tail. This modified quick-release knot is tightened by pulling on the long end of the rope, which is then tied to a leg or around the neck. The tail should not be tied to a fixed object in case the animal escapes or falls down.

A proper tail tie will not loosen as the tail moves. Incorporating the switch into the tie prevents the rope from sliding off the end of the tail. If the tail has been docked or the switch cut short, the tail tie must be modified. A modified quick-release knot is tied at the tail's base with two or three half hitches made distally, creating an effective "Chinese finger trap" that prevents the rope from slipping off the bobbed tail. The free end of the rope is secured to the leg or neck as previously described.

SURGICAL POSITION
Surgical Tables

Surgical or tilt tables are convenient and effective for positioning animals for surgery or other procedures that require maximal restraint. Numerous variations are available, but the common theme uses belly bands or squeeze panels and leg wraps to secure the animal to the table. The table is then mechanically or hydraulically tilted until the animal is in lateral or dorsal recumbency. Tilt tables are convenient and offer excellent restraint but may be financially unfeasible unless a large number of surgeries are done to compensate the expense.

Casting

An animal may very effectively be maintained in lateral or dorsal recumbency by casting and rope restraint if no surgery table is available. The major disadvantage is that surgical procedures must be done at or near ground level, which may be inconvenient, uncomfortable, and exhausting, plus make it harder to maintain aseptic technique.

Casting is a technique used to force an animal to lie down (Figure 4.3-4). A loop of rope is placed around the animal's neck with a bowline knot or a quick-release honda. Some people prefer to run the loop over the neck and between the front legs to prevent undue pressure on the trachea. Two half hitches are placed over the back so that the knots lie against the animal's spine when tightened. The first half hitch is behind the shoulder, and the second is in the flank, cranial to the udder or caudal to the penis. With the head secured, the rope is pulled with steady pressure until the animal lies down. The rope is tied with a quick-release knot cranial to the second half hitch to maintain rope pressure and keep the animal recumbent. The front and hind legs are bound together with hobbles or ropes. The legs are extended and tied to sturdy supports to secure the animal. Alternatively, for a quick procedure, the hind legs can be tucked under the second half hitch. The animal can be balanced against a wall, between bales of straw, or supported manually if dorsal recumbency is required.

FOOT RESTRAINT
Hind Feet

Hind feet commonly are raised to treat claws, manage leg wounds, or increase exposure to the udder and teats. The method described here is versatile and practical (Figure 4.3-5). One end of a rope is secured around the

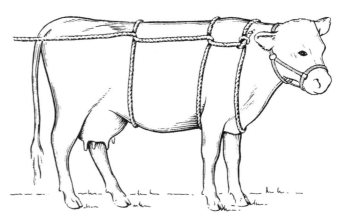

Figure 4.3-4   Position of the rope for casting a cow.

(From Leahy JR, Barrow P: *Restraint of animals*, ed 2, Ithaca, 1953, self-published.)

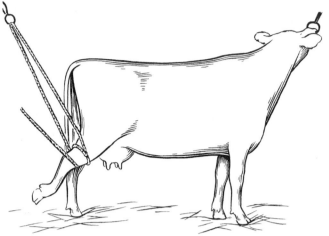

Figure 4.3-5   Position of a rope and beam hook used to lift a hind foot.

(Adapted from Leahy JR, Barrow P: *Restraint of animals,* ed 2, Ithaca, 1953, self-published.)

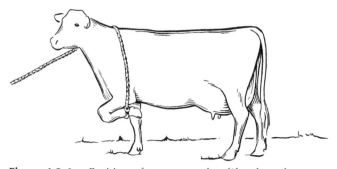

Figure 4.3-6   Position of a rope used to lift a front foot.

(From Leahy JR, Barrow P: *Restraint of animals,* ed 2, Ithaca, 1953, self-published.).

hind leg, dorsal to the hock, with a noose or quick-release honda. The free end of the rope is passed through a beam hook that is suspended from the ceiling. Coming from behind the cow, the rope is passed between the udder and hock, around the lateral aspect of the hock, and back through the beam hook. Pulling down on the free end of the rope, the pulley system created will elevate the hind leg as it bends at the stifle and hock. The free end of the rope is fastened by tying a quick-release knot around the rope itself close to the beam hook or by tying to the stanchion or another fixed object.

Front Feet

Raising the front feet is not as convenient as raising the back feet. The forelimb of an amenable cow can be raised manually. The handler's shoulder is placed at the crux of the cow's elbow. The dewclaws are grasped with one hand and the dorsum of the foot with the other. The handler presses his body into the cow's shoulder to displace its weight to the contralateral foot and simultaneously lifts the dewclaws and hoof, thus forcing the leg to bend at the carpus. Once flexed, the carpus and lower leg can be rested on a straw bale while the foot work is done.

Alternatively, a rope method can be used to elevate the front feet. A rope is placed around the leg, dorsal to the fetlock, and passed over a ceiling beam hook. The foot is raised and bent at the carpus. A second rope can be used to pull the foot laterally away from the animal's body to facilitate access to the foot. Both ropes should be secured with quick release knots for ease in untying.

A third option uses one rope tied above the fetlock, run over the back of the animal, and secured (Figure 4.3-6).

Restraint of Small Ruminants

MOVING SMALL RUMINANTS

When moving small ruminants (sheep, goats, or calves), one should use the same approach as for moving cattle. The natural flight instincts and points of balance are used. Sheep and goats are very flock-oriented. Whenever possible, the animals should remain with the flock. If a single animal must be removed, it may be necessary to forcibly move the animal. Pulling or pushing is not without risk. Undue force on the cervical vertebrae, strain on the joints of the animal's legs, or excessive wear on the hooves are potential problems with forcing an animal to move. Carrying the animal may be necessary. If the animal is too large or unruly to carry, it should be loaded onto a cart or wagon. Prudent use of sedation is advisable (see Chapter 6). Hand-raised animals may be coerced with small amounts of sweet feed or their favorite treats.

To catch an elusive small ruminant, one should first attempt to corner the animal against a wall or fence. The animal is restrained by holding it around the neck and over the rump or by reaching across its back and grasping the fold of skin in the flank. Horns serve as a convenient handhold but should be used with caution to avoid breaking them. Grabbing the wool can damage the fleece of a production animal and may cause trauma to the integument. Restraining the animal by a leg is also inadvisable because the ensuing struggle could injure the animal or handler.

HEAD RESTRAINT

As with cattle, control of the head is essential in controlling the animal. Ironically, horns, which evolved for sexual prowess and defense, serve as a convenient hand-hold for restraint. If the animal lacks horns, a halter is necessary. For many procedures, including jugular venipuncture, ophthalmologic examination, or early dehorning, sufficient head restraint can be maintained by straddling the animal's neck. The animal's head is turned caudally around the handler's leg and held between the handler's elbow and thigh.

SURGICAL POSITIONING

The appropriate use of chemical restraint and ropes allows small ruminants to be securely restrained in proper surgical position. With the exception of some approaches to the head, few procedures are done with the animal standing. Sheep are generally amenable to minor operations without sedation or general anesthesia if appropriate local or regional anesthesia is used. Sheep generally tolerate being restrained on their rumps or in dorsal recumbency. To force a sheep onto its rump, the handler stands alongside the animal with one hand under its jaw and the other over its back. With one swift movement, the sheep's head is turned toward its back, away from the handler, so that it faces its rump. Simultaneously, the animal's rump is pivoted around the handler's leg or lifted by the fold of skin in the flank. Once the animal is sitting, it can be held in this position, propped against the handler's legs or reclining in a sheep cradle. Alternatively, the animal can be lowered into lateral recumbency and held down bodily with pressure on its neck, or secured properly with ropes. Sheep placed in dorsal recumbency are quite content to lie in a V-shaped trough.

Unfortunately, calves and goats are not so willing to be constrained. To place a goat or calf in lateral recumbency, the handler reaches over the animal's back; one hand grasps the intended dependent foreleg, and the other hand grasps the fold of skin in the flank. The flank is lifted while the front leg is pulled out from under the animal, and it is lowered to the ground. If sufficient manpower is available, animals can be adequately held in position for minor procedures. Appropriate sedation is recommended for procedures of longer duration or if the animal is struggling excessively.

Restraint of Swine

MOVING SWINE

Hand-raised animals may voluntarily follow a handler offering food treats. Otherwise, the pig may be driven from behind to the intended destination. When driving unpredictable or aggressive animals, a portable, solid barrier (such as a slab of wood or a door) is used to provide a safe partition between the pig and handler.

When working with individual swine, the handler stands at the animal's shoulder. Aggressive or frightened animals may attempt to bite. However, their bulk and short necks make it impossible for them to turn their heads back without also turning their bodies, thus making the handler safe if positioned by the shoulder.

HEAD RESTRAINT—*SNARE*

A snare can be fashioned from a rope or wire noose. The loop is passed over the upper jaw and behind the tusks. When the snare is tightened, the pig will pull backward to resist. A metal pipe threaded over the standing end of the noose will provide additional control of the head and prevent the animal from moving forward. The pig can be held in place for minor procedures or as chemical restraint is administered.

SURGICAL POSITIONING
Body Restraint

Pigs are very vocal and will loudly protest any kind of restraint. Very small or well-socialized pigs may be managed with body restraint. Suspending a neonate by its back legs with its head downward sufficiently immobilizes it for early castration, ear docking, and clipping needle teeth. For more extensive procedures anesthesia is recommended.

Crate

Sows, and occasionally boars, in intensively managed herds are permanently housed in crates. Such confinement is often very conducive to veterinary examination and certain surgical procedures.

Barrier

Swine housed in pens individually, or in small groups, can be pinned against the pen wall with a slab of wood. The animal may still be able to move forward or backward; additional assistance may be necessary to keep the animal confined.

RECOMMENDED READINGS

Grandin T: Behavioural principles of handling cattle and other grazing animals under extensive conditions. In Grandin T *Livestock handling and transport*, ed 2, New York, 2000, CABI Pub.

Grandin T et al: Cattle with hair whorl patterns above the eyes are more behaviorally agitated during restraint, *App An Behav Sci* 46:117-123, 1995.

Leahy JR, Barrow P: *Restraint of animals,* ed 2, Ithaca, 1953, Cornell Campus Store, Inc.

4.4—Surgical Considerations

Jerry R. Roberson

This chapter deals with selected surgical instruments, suture patterns, equipment, and surgical procedures that are unique to farm animal patients.

Surgical Instruments

TROCARS

Trocars can be lifesaving devices, especially for cases of severe bloat. Several different types are available. Most older models have a stainless steel shaft with a handle made of wood, plastic, or stainless steel (Figure 4.4-1). Some of these older models (which work quite well) also come with a cannula that can be sutured in place. In extreme emergencies, trocars with stainless steel shafts may be driven directly into the bloated rumen without making a skin incision. The corkscrew trocar (Figure 4.4-2) is a self-retaining, screw-in type. The action of

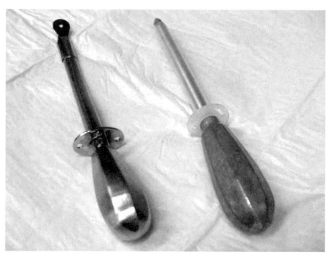

Figure 4.4-1   Stainless steel trocar.

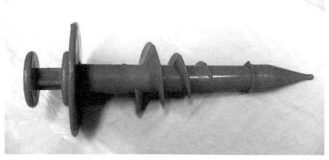

Figure 4.4-2   Corkscrew plastic trocar.

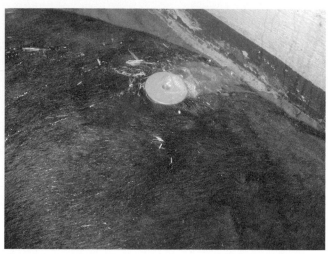

Figure 4.4-3   Dorsal view of the left paralumbar fossa in a heifer; this view shows the placement of the corkscrew trocar. Note frothy discharges. Trocars are quite effective in relieving free-gas bloats but may become plugged and ineffective against frothy bloats.

"screwing in" should bring the rumen tight against the peritoneum (Figure 4.4-3), thereby decreasing the chance of peritonitis. The corkscrew trocar requires a skin incision, so it can be inserted through the muscle and fascial layers. Leakage and peritonitis can be caused if the rumen is not pulled tight against the body wall in small calves. If the trocar fllange is not notably tight against the skin, Kerlix or rolled gauze can be placed under the fllange as a spacer for pulling the rumen against the body wall. Trocars can be maintained in place until the bloat is relieved, but peritonitis may occur with any trocar use; thus antimicrobials should always be considered.

OBSTETRIC WIRE AND HANDLES

Two types of obstetric wires exist: obstetric (OB) wire with handles (Figure 4.4-4A) and Gigli wires with handles (Figure 4.4-4B). Both types of wires are effective cutting tools. The difference in the weave can be seen in Figure 4.4-4. Several varieties of handles are available. An OB saw wire tends to be the most commonly used. Although originally developed for fetotomy use, both types of wires have several other uses such as dehorning, digit amputation, rib resection, and cast removal.

SPECIALIZED DEHORNING EQUIPMENT

The instrument in Figure 4.4-5 is designed to reduce hemorrhage associated with dehorning. The rubber-coated ends of the high tensile stainless steel apply pressure to the corneal artery. This instrument is especially useful during cosmetic dehorning.

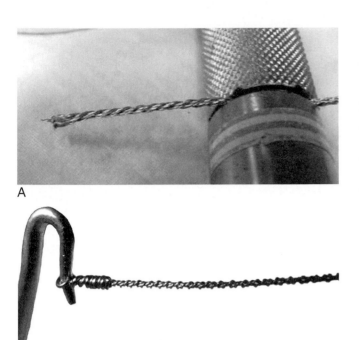

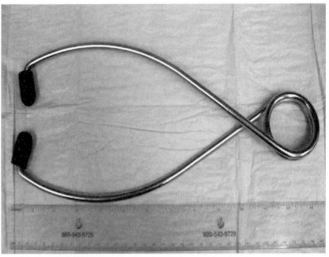

Figure 4.4-5 Specialized dehorning equipment used to decrease postoperative hemorrhage.

CASTRATING EQUIPMENT

The *Newberry* castrating knife allows the scrotal skin to be split without danger of other tissues being cut (Figure 4.4-6, *A*). Some producers do not prefer this method because, once it is healed, the scrotum may fill with fat

Figure 4.4-4 *A,* Close-up view of obstetric wire. *B,* Gigli wires with their respective handles.

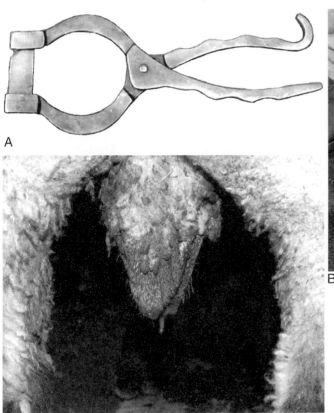

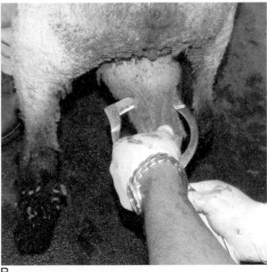

Figure 4.4-6 *A,* Newberry knife. *B,* The scrotum is grasped with the Newberry knife. *C,* Photographs taken show the scrotal flaps after the testes were removed.

so the animal may appear to be intact. More than one half of the scrotal length is grasped with the Newberry knife (Figure 4.4-6B). Pulling down and back with the Newberry knife splits the scrotum into fore and rear halves, thus allowing easy access to the testes and ample drainage (Figure 4.4-6C).

The *emasculatome* (Figure 4.4-7 and Figure 4.4-8) comes in a couple of sizes and is a bloodless form of castration. Each spermatic cord is crushed separately. Emasculatomes may also be used to remove warts and damaged or necrotic teats. The crushing effect may help control hemorrhage. Emasculators crush and cut

and are typically used on one spermatic cord at a time. They are usually left attached to the cut end of the spermatic cord for a few seconds up to a couple of minutes to enhance hemostasis. Emasculators should be applied to the spermatic cord without any cord tension; otherwise the cord may retract into the surgery site without any crushing effect (thus excessive hemorrhage may result). Key to using this piece of equipment is an adequate amount of spermatic cord proximal to the testis and placing the emasculator nut toward the testis ("nut-to-nut") (Figure 4.4-9). This places the crushing edge on the proximal end of the severed spermatic cord.

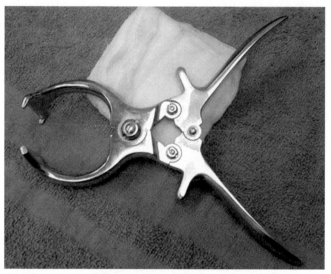

Figure 4.4-7   Single action (crushing) emasculatome.

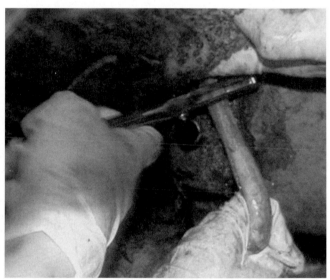

Figure 4.4-9   Placement of dual-action emasculatome on spermatic cord. Note the position of the nut in relation to the testis.

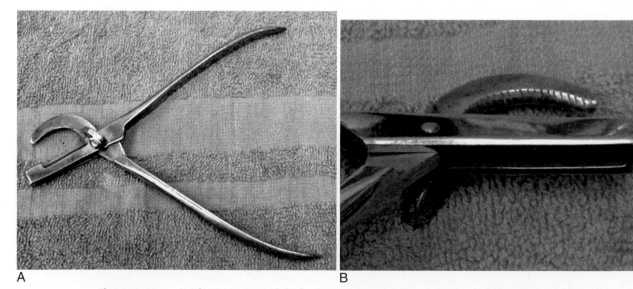

A   B

Figure 4.4-8   *A,* Close-up view of dual-action emasculatome showing cutting and, *B,* crushing surfaces.

Elastrators (Figure 12.1.1-10) have been used for several years to castrate neonatal male animals and dock lamb tails. Lately, this tool has been used to dock tails of dairy cattle. The critical step in using the elastrator is to make sure both testes are below the rubber band (Figure 4.4-10). This form of castration may be inadequate and potentially fatal when used to castrate older stock. In older stock with larger testes, the band is not strong enough to shut off the blood supply and may predispose to tetanus.

EZE-Bander and *Callicrate bander* have been developed to allow bloodless castration in practically any age male, including large bulls. Both methods rely on extremely tight elastic tubing to block the blood supply to the scrotum and testes. Both methods appear to be quite effective; however, tetanus prevention should be considered. The EZE-Bander is demonstrated in Figure 4.4-11A. The tubing is placed around the base of the scrotum (Figure 4.4-11B). Each end of the tubing is then hand-tightened (Figure 4.4-11C). A clamp is

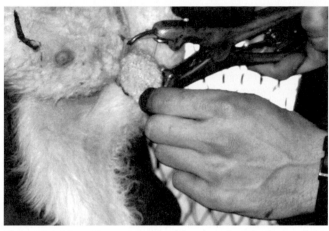

Figure 4.4-10   Placement of rubber band at the base of the scrotum.

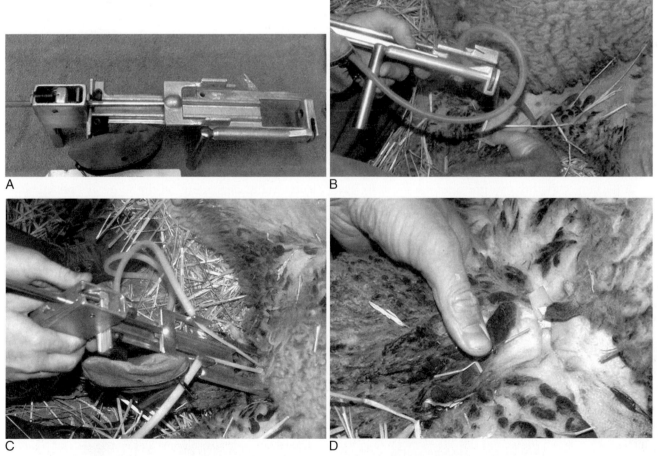

Figure 4.4-11   *A,* EZE-Bander. *B,* The tubing is placed around the base of the scrotum. *C,* Each end of the tubing is then tightened. *D,* After the tubing is cut free, the tightness of the band should be checked.

placed to keep the tubing tightly connected around the base of the scrotum and crimped into place. The tubing is then cut free. The band should be checked for tightness (Figure 4.4-11D).

The *Henderson castrating tool* (Figure 4.4-12) was also developed for larger more mature males. After the scrotum is opened by a preferred method, the tool is attached to the spermatic cord. An electric drill is placed on the handle of the tool and rotated. This twisting is reportedly very efficient in preventing excessive hemorrhage, even in large mature bulls.

S-CURVED NEEDLE
The S-curved needle (Figure 4.4-13A) has become a mainstay of bovine skin suturing, primarily because of the bovine's tough thick skin. Figure 4.4-13B shows how the needle should be held.

Suture Patterns

UTRECHT PATTERN
The Utrecht pattern is probably the most popular method of closing the uterus after a cesarean section. Although two-layer closures are sometimes used, the Utrecht pattern can maintain a tight seal with a one-layer closure. To begin the pattern, the first stitch is applied about 3 cm dorsal to the apex of the uterine incision and is angled up and out (Figure 4.4-14A and B). The needle is then inserted inward and downward so that the two ends are in close proximity. Tying the suture at this point should make a buried knot, thereby decreasing the chance of adhesions. The pattern is then continued using oblique bites that enter 2 cm from the cut edge and exit 0.5 cm from the cut edge without penetrating the lumen. It is important to pull the suture tight, so there are no

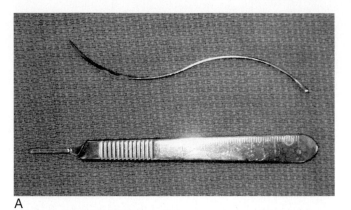

A

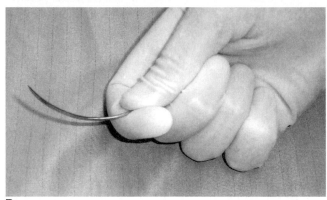

B

Figure 4.4-13   *A,* S-shaped needle. *B,* Hand positioned on needle.

gaps and the suture is minimally exposed. To end the Utrecht pattern, the needle first enters near the caudal apex of the incision and exits at an angle to the left (or to the right, depending on the surgeon's preference) as shown in Figure 4.4-14C. A loop of suture sufficient for tying needs to remain (Figure 4.4-14D). The needle's last entrance slants backward toward the distal apex of the incision and exits near the suture loop (Figure 4.4-14D). The Utrecht pattern should result in little suture exposure, including the initial and ending ligatures, as shown in Figure 4.4-14E.

TOGGLES
The practice of toggling left-displaced abomasums can be a time-saving, efficient, effective surgery for many cases. The concept was initially developed for less valuable dairy cows, but with experience and proper case selection, one can use it successfully on cows of any value. An excellent website has been developed (www.ldatogglesuture.com) The toggle kit includes a trocar, cannula, handle, and two T-shaped toggles (Figure 4.4-15A). Proper manipulation of the toggle and trocar is shown in Figure 4.4-15B-E.

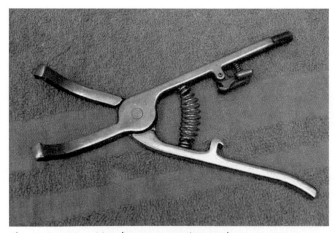

Figure 4.4-12   Henderson castrating tool.

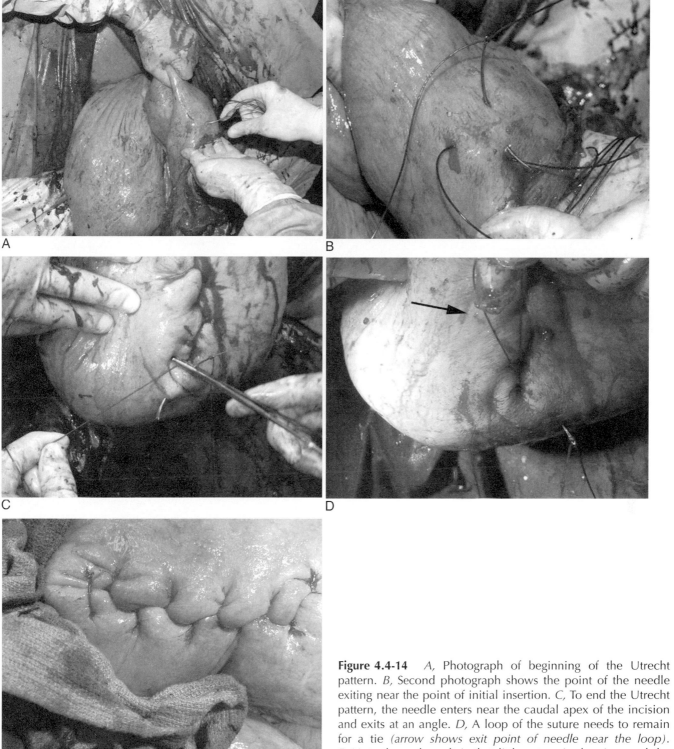

Figure 4.4-14 *A,* Photograph of beginning of the Utrecht pattern. *B,* Second photograph shows the point of the needle exiting near the point of initial insertion. *C,* To end the Utrecht pattern, the needle enters near the caudal apex of the incision and exits at an angle. *D,* A loop of the suture needs to remain for a tie *(arrow shows exit point of needle near the loop)*. *E,* Note the end result is that little suture is showing, and the knot is buried.

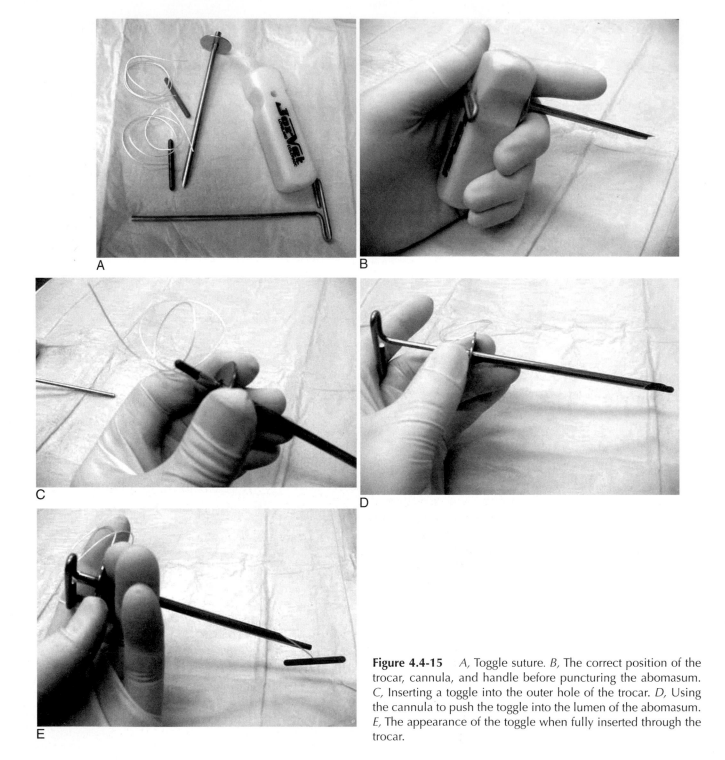

Figure 4.4-15   *A,* Toggle suture. *B,* The correct position of the trocar, cannula, and handle before puncturing the abomasum. *C,* Inserting a toggle into the outer hole of the trocar. *D,* Using the cannula to push the toggle into the lumen of the abomasum. *E,* The appearance of the toggle when fully inserted through the trocar.

FORD INTERLOCKING SUTURE PATTERN

The Ford interlocking suture pattern is probably the most common suture pattern used in bovine skin. A simple surgeon's knot is used to start the pattern. Figure 4.4-16A and B, shows the S-curved needle position and the suture position that results in the pattern "locking" on itself. Figure 4.4-16C shows the resulting pattern. The last stitch is completed by first inserting the needle in the opposite side that had been used previously. The tail of the suture is maintained on the side where the needle was inserted, and the loop of suture on the other side of the incision is tied to the tail (the single tail and loop can be seen in the second photo

Figure 4.4-16B). If any chance of the incision being contaminated exists, many surgeons close the remainder of the ventral skin incision with two to three simple interrupted stitches.

BÜHNER TAPE

Bühner tape (Figure 4.4-17A and B) is a very strong synthetic suture that can be used for rectal, vaginal, cervical, or uterine prolapses. Figure 4.4-17C shows the suture placed in a purse-string fashion to secure a rectal prolapse in a ewe lamb. Some veterinarians prefer to place the knot in a location such as dorsal placement shown in Figure 4.4-17C where it is least likely to be

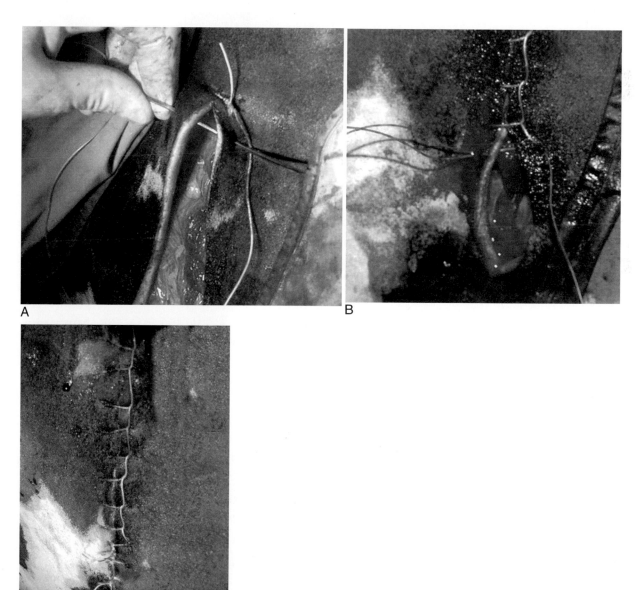

Figure 4.4-16 *A,* Start of Ford interlocking pattern. *B,* Ford interlocking pattern developing with, *C,* showing end result.

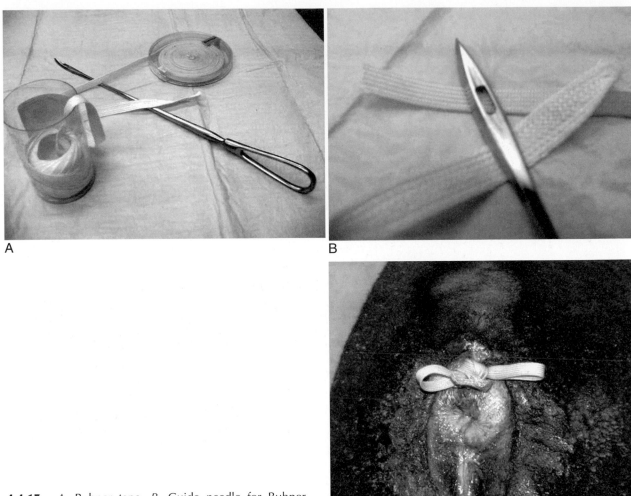

Figure 4.4-17   *A,* Buhner tape. *B,* Guide needle for Buhner tape. *C,* Rectal prolapse with a Buhner tape in place.

soiled. The Buhner stitch is typically tied in a shoestring fashion, which should allow easy adjustment and removal by the producer. Umbilical tape, which is not as strong as Buhner tape, may be supplied in cotton or polyester forms.

JOHNSON BUTTON

The Johnson button is used as an alternative to the Buhner stitch for vaginal prolapse repair. The major advantage of the Johnson button is the cow may undergo an unassisted parturition. The Johnson button may or may not be helpful in cases of cervical prolapse but is ineffective in cases of uterine prolapse. The Johnson button kit consists of two plastic "buttons"—a 6-inch plastic trocar, a 7-inch stainless steel pin, and a Cotter pin (Figure 4.4-18A). The large button with the trocar and pin (Figure 4.4-18B) are placed within the vagina and inserted through the sacrosciatic ligament, muscle, and skin. Care must be taken to avoid the

internal iliac artery. A scalpel incision must be placed in the skin to allow the plastic trocar to pass through. After the trocar is in place, the pin is removed, and the smaller button is placed over the trocar adjacent to the skin (Figure 4.4-18C). The Cotter pin is then inserted through holes in the trocar, and the excess trocar is removed. The area between the buttons would encompass everything between the vaginal mucosa and external skin.

Miscellaneous Procedures and Techniques

SURGICAL TIPS

Although numerous advances in castration equipment have been made, many practitioners still prefer to remove the lower half of the scrotum with a scalpel or castrating knife. The chance of cutting a finger, thumb, or the

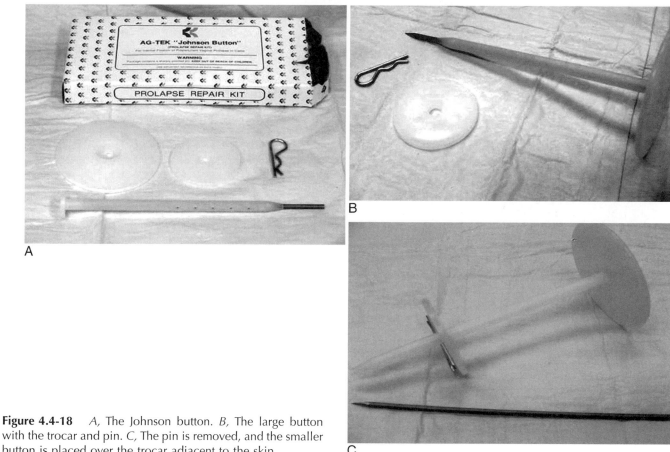

Figure 4.4-18 *A,* The Johnson button. *B,* The large button with the trocar and pin. *C,* The pin is removed, and the smaller button is placed over the trocar adjacent to the skin.

calf is greater with this method than with the others described. To decrease the chance of cutting something other than the scrotum, one can use towel forceps, as demonstrated in Figure 4.4-19. When drapes are used for surgery, two to three towel clamps placed directly along the spine will keep the drapes in place (Figure 4.4-20), and the cow is unlikely to kick when they are applied in this location.

RECTAL PROLAPSE RINGS

Rectal prolapse rings come in many sizes; most have a waist for anchoring the prolapsed rectum to the ring (Figure 4.4-21A). The emasculator and emasculator band can be used to secure the prolapsed rectum to the ring in smaller livestock. The EZE-Bander or Callicrate bander could be used with larger livestock. The following series of figures show the use of a prolapse ring in a 50-pound pig with a rectal prolapse. Figure 4.4-21B shows a typical rectal prolapse. Figure 4.4-21C shows the ring in the proper position. Figure 4.4-21D was taken the third day after the ring with the elastrator band was placed. Figure 4.4-21E shows the absence of

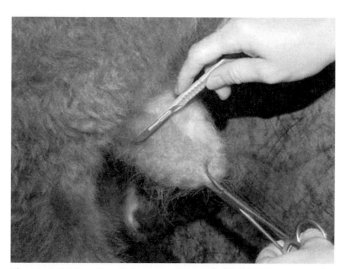

Figure 4.4-19 Special uses of towel forceps to tense the scrotum.

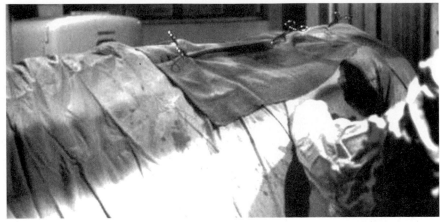

Figure 4.4-20   Uses of towel forceps to hold surgical drape on dorsal midline.

the ring and prolapsed rectum on day 5. The pig was separated from other pigs during this process to prevent cannibalism.

DRENCHING TOOLS

The McGrath pump is a simple device for administering fluids to the bovine. The pump has nose tongs that allow the hose portion to stay in place while the administrator pumps the fluid (Figure 4.4-22). The fluid should be pumped in slowly because too-rapid administration may result in aspiration and possibly even drowning.

WART REMOVAL

The following figures show a simple method to remove warts. Large curved hemostats are the preferred tool. The curved portion of the hemostat is pushed down around the base of the wart (Figure 4.4-23A). The jaws of the hemostat are then squeezed together firmly (Figure 4.4-23B), and the wart can be removed (Figure 4.4-23C) with one quick tug.

CANCER EYE EQUIPMENT

The three primary methods of treating eye cancer in cattle are eye enucleation, hyperthermia, and cryosurgery. Eye enucleation is described in Chapter 13. Hyperthermia treatment consists of a two-pronged probe that heats the tissues (cancerous or precancerous tissues) between the probes (Figure 4.4-24A). Figure 4.4-24B shows an example of a liquid nitrogen applicator/container that is used for cryosurgery.

APPLICATION OF BLOCKS
FOR BOVINE CLAWS

Because cattle have two claws per foot, applying a wooden or plastic block or shoe on the "good" claw

provides some pain relief and allows quicker healing of the affected claw. Figure 4.4-25A shows the supplies needed to apply a wooden block. Figure 4.4-25B shows a wooden block that has been worn for a couple of weeks. The affected claw shows healthy granulation tissue. Figure 4.4-25C shows the materials needed to apply a plastic type block. There are two shoe sizes. The shoe is attached with a fast-curing acrylic resin.

Surgical Equipment Unique to Farm Animal Practice

HIP LIFTERS

Historically, hip lifters (Figure 4.4-26A) were used to elevate a down animal and keep the animal up for an extended period of time. Although this treatment method may have been successful in some cases, the afflicted animal often would not benefit from this method and would sustain muscular damage around the tuber coxae. Hip lifters used by producers may not have the additional padding evident in Figure 4.4-26B. However, hip lifters can be used for diagnostic purposes. Completing a good physical exam on a down animal is difficult. The use of hip lifters allows a better physical examination and helps establish if the down animal can support its own weight.

CATTLE TRANSPORTER

The cattle transporter (Figure 4.4-27) allows a potentially fractious large animal patient to be transported to various areas of the large animal hospital, such as surgical suites or radiology, relatively easily.

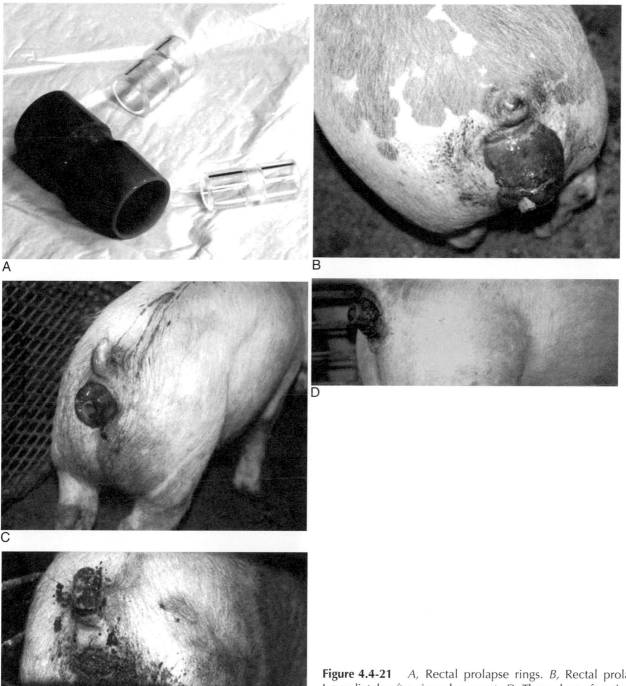

Figure 4.4-21 *A,* Rectal prolapse rings. *B,* Rectal prolapse. *C,* Immediately after ring placement. *D,* Three days after ring placement. *E,* Five days after ring placement.

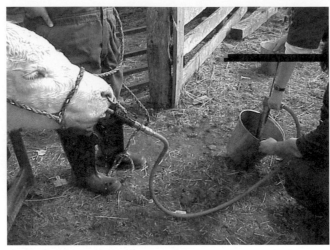

Figure 4.4-22   McGrath pump.

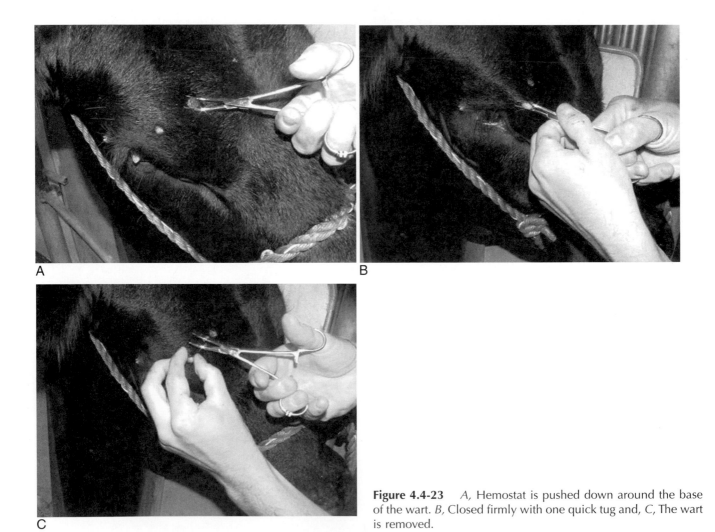

A

B

C

Figure 4.4-23   *A,* Hemostat is pushed down around the base of the wart. *B,* Closed firmly with one quick tug and, *C,* The wart is removed.

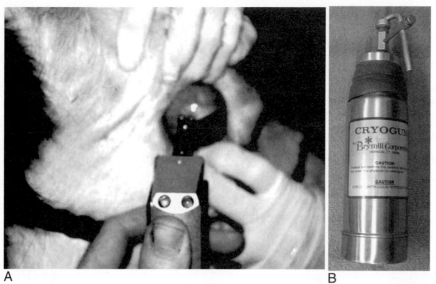

Figure 4.4-24   *A,* Hyperthermia treatment. *B,* Liquid nitrogen applicator/container.

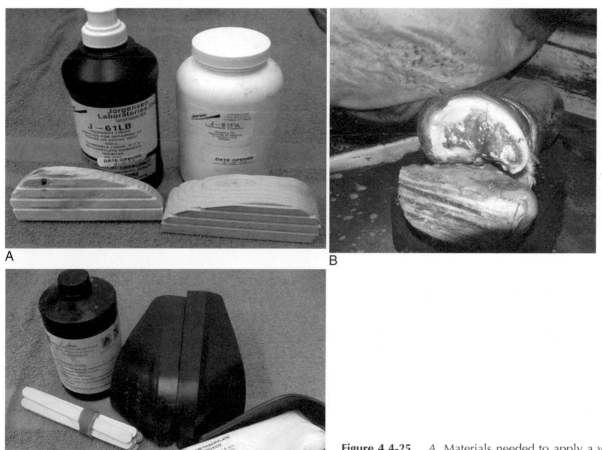

Figure 4.4-25   *A,* Materials needed to apply a wooden block (two different thicknesses are shown). *B,* Wooden block on unaffected claw provides affected claw protection from weight bearing and improves healing, as evidenced by healthy granulation tissue on the affected claw. *C,* Materials needed to apply a plastic-type block (two different sizes are shown).

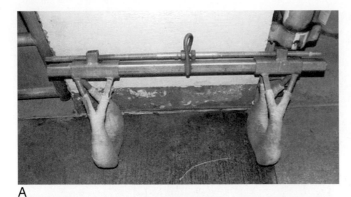

A

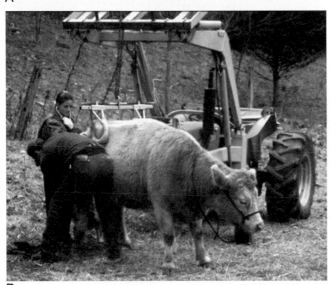

B

Figure 4.4-26   *A,* Hip lifters. *B,* Down animal being elevated.

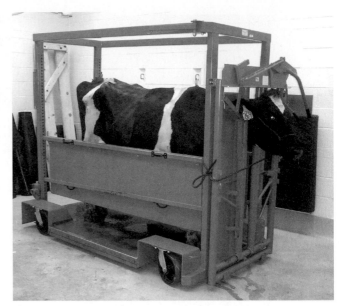

Figure 4.4-27   Cattle transporter.

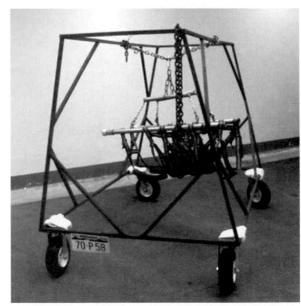

Figure 4.4-28   Walker with a sling for small ruminants.

THE WALKER

Figure 4.4-28 shows a a custom-designed walker with a sling used primarily for small ruminants. It is lightweight and easy to move.

TILT TABLE

Numerous styles of tilt tables are available. The selection of a tilt table should be based on ease of use and maximum size of the animal to be tilted. Although two or more people are ideal for placing an animal on a tilt table, some simple, portable, hydraulic tilt tables can be managed successfully and safely by a single person. Many tilt tables use broad bands (Figure 4.4-29C) to support the animal during the tilting. The tilt table pictured in Figure 4.4-29A is a hydraulic chute that supports the animal by squeezing it during tilting. All tilt tables have some method for securing all four legs. This chute can be rotated up to 360 degrees to permit the animal to be placed on either side or in dorsal recumbency for midline or paramedian surgery (Figure 4.4-29B). The table in Figure 4.4-29C is more dangerous to use and cannot

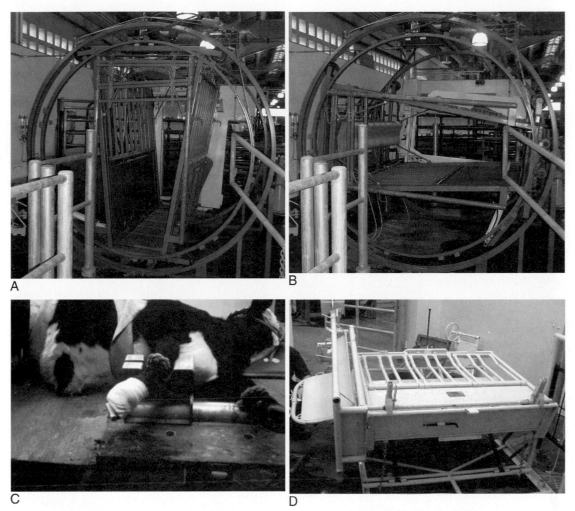

Figure 4.4-29 *A,* Tilt table with hydraulic chute. *B,* Tilt table with hydraulic chute rotated 90 degrees. *C,* Two-person tilt table. *D,* Tilt tables for small ruminants and young cattle.

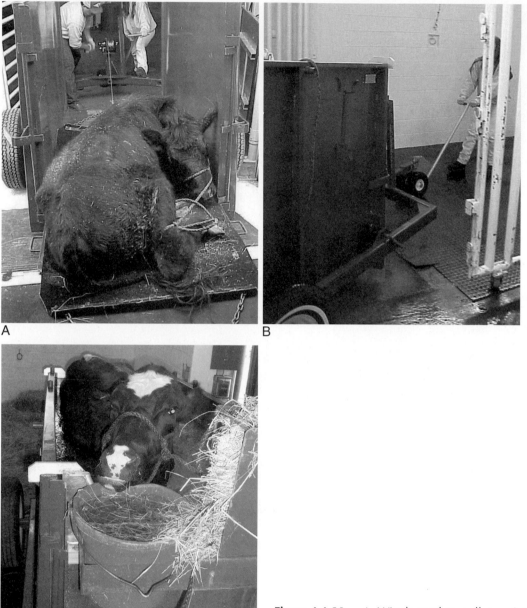

A

B

C

Figure 4.4-30   *A,* Winch used to pull cow into flotation tank. *B,* Wheel attachment to move floatation device. *C,* Cow in flotation tank. Note that feed and water can be offered.

be managed by a single person. The upper legs are secured after placing supports in place under the legs. Tilt tables have also been developed for small ruminants and young cattle (Figure 4.4-29D).

FLOATATION SYSTEMS

Whereas hip lifters may result in additional musculoskeletal damage, floatation tanks provide a much less harmful system to elevate down animals. Cows have been floated daily for greater than 14 hours. During floatation, muscle damage is prevented, and physical therapy can be performed. Figure 4.4-30A shows a winch being used to pull a down cow into the tank. Figure 4.4-30B shows a small wheel attachment that makes moving the tank with the cow easy. Figure 4.4-30C shows a cow standing in the floatation tank. These floatation tanks were developed in Europe and have gained worldwide acceptance.

4.5—Approaches to the Bovine Abdomen

J. Brett Woodie

Anatomy

The conformation of the bovine abdomen varies with age, weight, and physiologic condition. Normally it is bilaterally symmetric. The extent of the abdominal cavity is not readily apparent because a large portion is contained within the rib cage. The abdominal cavity is bounded cranially by the diaphragm, caudally by the pelvic inlet, dorsally by the lumbar vertebrae and epaxial musculature, laterally and ventrally by the abdominal musculature. The abdominal wall musculature is made of broad expansive sheets that attach by means of aponeuroses-forming connective tissue structures such as the linea alba and prepubic tendon. The abdominal muscles have many functions such as containing abdominal viscera, assisting respiration, stabilizing the pelvis, and flexing the vertebral column. The abdominal musculature also permits generation of an abdominal press necessary for defecation, micturition, and parturition. The abdominal wall is elastic in nature, thus allowing it to adjust to varying volumes.

The skin is thickest over the flank of the cow and becomes thinner over the ventral portion of the abdomen. The most prominent feature of the bovine flank is the paralumbar fossa. The paralumbar fossa is outlined by the transverse processes of the lumbar vertebrae, internal abdominal oblique muscle, and the thirteenth rib (Figure 4.5-1). Abdominal muscles and their aponeuroses form the main fibromuscular support of the ventral and lateral walls of the abdomen. The four pairs

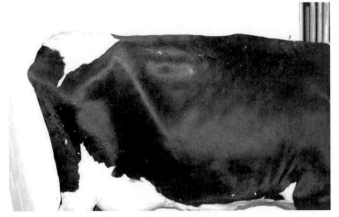

Figure 4.5-1   Right paralumbar fossa.

of muscles involved in the makeup of the abdominal wall are the external abdominal oblique, internal abdominal oblique, transversus abdominis, and the rectus abdominis. The most important nerves of the flank are the last thoracic, first lumbar, and second lumbar nerves. The caudal intercostal nerves innervate the floor of the abdomen ventral to the costal arch. Knowledge of these nerves is important in providing local anesthesia as part of performing a laparotomy. The ventral portion of the abdominal wall receives its blood supply from the cranial and caudal epigastric arteries, branches of the internal thoracic and external pudendal arteries. The flanks receive their blood supply from parietal branches of the aorta, the most important of which, from a surgical point of view, is the deep circumflex iliac artery.

The most extensive and superficial muscle of the flank is the external abdominal oblique muscle (EAO). The fibers of this muscle course in a caudoventral direction. However, in the area of the paralumbar fossa the fibers are seen in a more horizontal direction. This muscle terminates in an extensive aponeurosis near the lateral border of the rectus abdominis muscle. The EAO originates on the lateral aspect of the thorax from the fourth or fifth rib. It inserts on the tuber coxae, prepubic tendon, and linea alba by means of aponeurotic tissue. The aponeurosis of the EAO blends with the aponeurosis of the internal abdominal oblique muscle to form the external sheath of the rectus abdominis muscle.

The internal abdominal oblique muscle (IAO) is immediately under the EAO. This muscle is well developed and occupies the entire flank region from the tuber coxae to the last rib. The IOA originates from the tuber coxae, lumbar transverse processes, and the thoracolumbar fascia. Its fibers are directed cranioventrally. The fibers of the IAO insert on the costal cartilages or via an aponeurosis that fuses with that of the external abdominal oblique, which forms the external sheath of the rectus abdominis, which inserts on the linea alba.

The transversus abdominus muscle (TA) forms the deepest layer of the abdominal wall musculature. It is the least extensive and thinnest. The TA arises from the transverse processes of the lumbar vertebrae and the medial aspect of the last ribs. It forms an aponeurosis at the lateral edge of the rectus abdominis muscle, becomes the inner sheath of the rectus abdominis, and ultimately inserts on the linea alba. The fibers run transversely at right angles to those of the rectus abdominis muscle. The transversus abdominis is covered on the inside by the transverse fascia and peritoneum.

The rectus abdominis muscle (RA) is confined to the ventral aspect of the abdomen and travels on either side of the linea alba. It originates from the costal cartilages of the ribs and sternum and inserts on the cranial pubic ligament. The fibers of the RA are oriented in a sagittal direction. The rectus abdominis muscle lies within an aponeurotic sheath that is formed by the aponeuroses of the EAO, IAO, and TA.

The linea alba is formed from the aponeuroses of the EAO, IAO, and TA. The linea alba extends from the xiphoid process and inserts on the prepubic tendon. It consists of dense connective tissue composed of sheets of collagen bundles and fibroblasts. The fibers of each sheet cross between each other, which adds to its mechanical strength. The thickness and width vary depending on the location relative to the umbilicus. The linea is much thicker and wider at the level of the umbilicus. It becomes thinner and narrower as it courses cranially.

Approaches to the Abdomen

When deciding on an approach to the bovine abdomen, the surgeon must consider the large size of the abdominal cavity and viscera and the fact that the viscera has mesenteric and omental attachments that limit mobility.

Some portions of the intestinal tract can be exteriorized; some only palpated, and other portions are inaccessible (Figure 4.5-2). The surgeon must also consider the disease process when choosing an approach so that the organ(s) of interest can be accessed. Thus a careful diagnostic work-up before surgery is imperative. Other factors such as value of the animal, available facilities, temperament of the patient, and experience of the surgical team all influence the chosen approach.

Most abdominal surgeries can be performed as a standing procedure in the adult bovine patient by using local or regional anesthesia. Use of sedation or tranquilizers when performing standing surgery is not advisable because the cow might lie down during the procedure. However, in some instances general anesthesia or recumbency, sedation, and a local anesthetic are appropriate. For example, for exploration of the small intestine in a valuable cow that is uncomfortable and reluctant to stand, a recumbent approach is indicated. Use of perioperative antimicrobials and/or antiinflammatories is at the discretion of the surgeon.

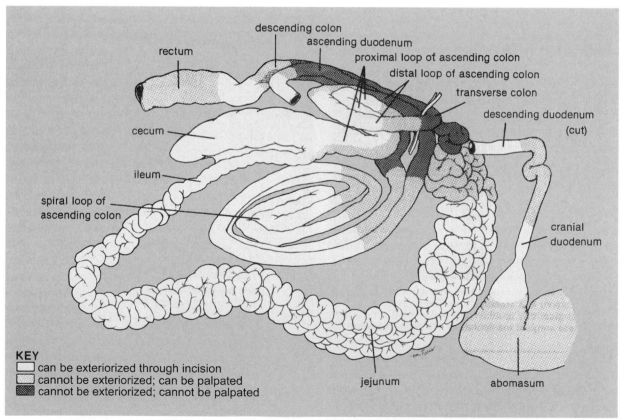

Figure 4.5-2   Schematic representation of the portions of the intestinal tract that can be exteriorized, some only palpated, and other portions that are inaccessible.

(Reproduced with permission from Smith DF: Bovine Intestinal Surgery: Part 1. *Mod Vet Pract* 65: 853-857, 1984, p 855, Fig 2).

LEFT PARALUMBAR FOSSA CELIOTOMY

This approach can be used to gain access to the rumen, reticulum, spleen, diaphragm, reproductive tract, bladder, left kidney, and the abomasum in the case of a left-displaced abomasum. The cow should be restrained in stocks, a head gate, or a mobile restraining chute such as the Ohio Bovine Transporter (Figure 4.5-3). Securing the cow's tail so that it does not contaminate the surgical field during prepping or surgery is advisable. The left flank should be clipped and aseptically prepared, and local or regional anesthesia should be used to desensitize the surgical area. Sterile draping should follow.

The location for the skin incision is typically centered over the paralumbar fossa. The location can vary somewhat depending on the disease process. The skin incision is begun 6 to 8 cm ventral to the transverse processes of the lumbar vertebrae and 4 to 6 cm caudal to the last rib. The incision is made in a dorsoventral direction for a length of 20 to 25 cm. In the case of a cesarean section, the incision can be started more caudal in the paralumbar fossa, lower in the flank, and will need to be longer in length (Figure 4.5-4). Once the skin and subcutaneous tissue have been incised, the external abdominal oblique muscle will be visible. Hemostasis is maintained by using hemostats and ligatures if necessary. All instruments and sponges should be moved off the surgical field before entry into the abdomen.

The external abdominal oblique muscle is incised in the same direction and for the same distance as the skin incision. The fibers of the internal abdominal oblique are now visible. This muscle layer is incised in the same manner as the external abdominal oblique. Because of the muscle fibers' direction, a tendency exists to incise the internal abdominal oblique muscle layer too far forward in the incision. The operator should strive to stay in the middle of the incision. The transversus abdominis muscle is encountered next. To prevent damage to underlying viscera upon entering the abdomen, it is helpful to "tent" the transversus abdominus by using thumb forceps and to incise the muscle and peritoneum the length of the incision by using Mayo scissors.

A sterile impervious sleeve should be used to palpate the abdominal cavity. A systematic approach should be used when exploring the abdomen. Because inflammatory conditions are more likely to be in the cranial abdomen, the caudal abdomen is usually explored first. The reproductive tract, bladder, ureters, lymph nodes, and inguinal rings should be palpated. The left kidney is large and covered by fat. It is easily palpable in the left caudal abdomen almost on midline, adjacent to the descending colon.

On the left side of the cranial abdomen the rumen, the spleen, reticulum, and diaphragm should be palpated. The presence of adhesions or abscesses in the area of the reticulum and diaphragm should be ascertained. The surgeon can palpate portions of the right side of the abdominal cavity by going behind the rumen and forward. The quality of the right-sided exploratory from the left side will depend on the size of the rumen and the cow's body size. A more thorough and informative exploratory of the right side of the abdomen can be done from the right side.

Closure of the flank laparotomy incision is done in four layers. The peritoneum and transversus abdominis are closed together with an absorbable suture (#2 in size)

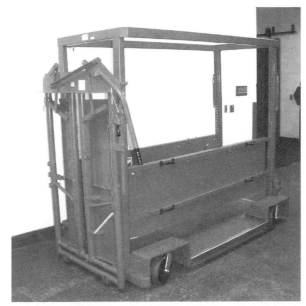

Figure 4.5-3 The Ohio Cattle Transporter.
(Bud Corporation, Columbus, Ohio).

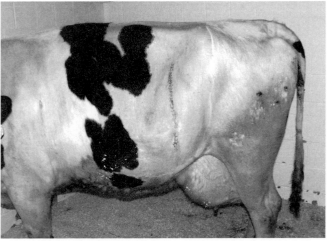

Figure 4.5-4 Left paralumbar fossa incision (cesarean section).

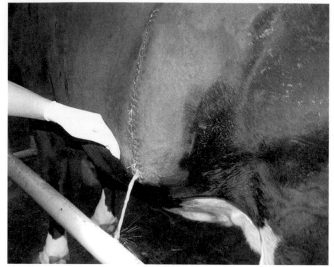

Figure 4.5-5   Drainage from an incisional infection.
(Courtesy of Dr. Chris Beinlich, Cornell University).

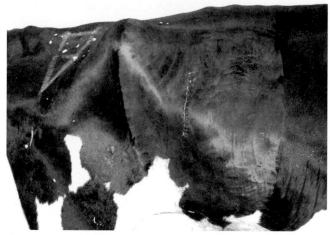

Figure 4.5-6   Right paralumbar fossa incision.

in a simple continuous pattern. The internal abdominal oblique and external abdominal oblique muscles are closed separately with an absorbable suture (#2 in size) in a simple continuous pattern. Between each layer of the closure, lavaging the muscles with sterile saline is advisable. The skin is closed with a nonabsorbable suture (#1 in size), a Ford interlocking pattern, and three simple interrupted sutures at the ventralmost aspect of the incision. The simple interrupted sutures can be removed to facilitate drainage should an incisional infection develop (Figure 4.5-5).

RIGHT PARALUMBAR FOSSA CELIOTOMY

This right paralumbar fossa approach can be used to gain access to the pyloric part of the abomasum, the majority of the small and large intestines, the reproductive tract, bladder, and kidneys. The restraint, preparation, and approach are the same as described in the left paralumbar approach. If a pyloropexy is anticipated, the initial incision is made closer to the last rib in a more ventral location as described for the left paralumbar fossa celiotomy (Figure 4.5-6).

A systematic approach to the abdominal exploratory is necessary. Again, exploration of the caudal abdomen first is recommended. This includes the reproductive tract, urinary bladder, left kidney, and descending colon. Cows typically urinate when the bladder is palpated.

In the cranial abdomen, the reticulum and diaphragm should be palpated for the presence of adhesions or abscesses. The omasum is identified caudal and medial to the reticulum. It should be filled with firm ingesta. The liver should be checked for rounded edges or irregularities. It is normal for the edges of the right lobe of the liver to be more rounded than the left lobe. The gall-

bladder is often enlarged in cattle that are anorectic. The position of the abomasum should be along the right body wall. The fundus and body of the abomasum normally contain fluid consistency ingesta. Ingesta in the pyloric portion is typically more dry and doughy. The pylorus is palpable as a firm structure at the level of the costochondral junction of the ninth and tenth ribs. Normally it can be exteriorized along with 6 to 8 cm of distal abomasum. The cranial portion of the duodenum leaves the pylorus and courses toward the liver. This portion of the duodenum is covered by the superficial sheet of the greater omentum. The cranial part of the duodenum in a fat cow may be totally obscured by fat. The descending duodenum can be seen just deep to the abdominal incision, running horizontally across the abdomen. The right kidney is dorsal to the cranial portion of the descending duodenum underneath the last two ribs.

To examine the intestinal tract distal to the abomasum, the omental sling is pulled forward; the surgeon palpates the viscera, most of which is contained in the supraomental recess. The apex of the cecum is exteriorized after identifying it as a blind sac of intestine 4 to 8 cm in diameter and located near the pelvic inlet. In some cows, the apex normally is rotated in a ventral direction. The ileocecocolic junction and proximal colon can be exposed when the greater omentum is moved cranially. Once the cecum is exteriorized and rotated cranially (180 degrees), the spiral colon can be examined. The distal flange of the small intestine is examined by tracing the ileum orad. The distal flange should be replaced in the abdomen, and the surgeon should palpate the small intestine proximally to the duodenojejunal junction. If an abnormality is felt or suspected, that portion of the small intestine can be exteriorized and examined. The descending colon and rectum should be palpated. The surgeon can examine the left side of the abdomen by advancing their arm caudal to the omental sling and dorsal to the rumen. The spleen can be palpated in the upper left quadrant of the abdomen.

Factors that affect the surgeon's ability to examine the gastrointestinal tract include size of the animal, fat content, distention of a viscus, stage of pregnancy, and the length of the surgeon's arms.

Closure of the right flank celiotomy incision is the same as described for the left paralumbar fossa approach.

RIGHT PARAMEDIAN CELIOTOMY

Access to the cranial abdomen is achieved with this approach. It is used primarily for correction of displacement of the abomasum, abomasal volvulus, or access to the reticulum. Rarely, a caudal paramedian celiotomy is used in a bull to access the urinary bladder. The incision is located 4 to 6 cm lateral to ventral midline and 6 to 8 cm caudal to the xiphoid (Figure 4.5-7). The length of the incision is approximately 15 to 20 cm. The cow should be positioned and restrained in dorsal recumbency (Figure 4.5-8). The area from the xiphoid to caudal to the umbilicus is clipped and aseptically prepared, and local anesthesia is used to desensitize the surgical field. A sterile drape is placed and secured over the incision site. The skin and subcutaneous tissues are incised. Branches of the subcutaneous abdominal vein often need to be ligated to provide hemostasis. Often the caudal portion of the pectoral muscle is encountered at the rostral aspect of this approach. This muscle is divided to expose the external sheath of the rectus abdominis muscles. The external sheath is incised sharply for the length of the incision. The rectus abdominis muscle is exposed and incised along its fibers with a combination

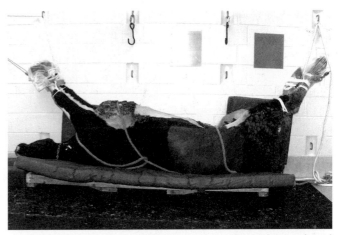

Figure 4.5-8 Cow positioned and restrained in dorsal recumbency (using sedation and casting rope).

of sharp and blunt dissection. Thumb forceps are used to tent the internal sheath of the rectus abdominis muscle and Mayo scissors are used to incise this layer. Once the incision has entered the abdominal cavity, the surgeon can use his or her fingers to protect underlying viscera while extending the incision.

An impervious sleeve is used for the abdominal exploratory. The abomasum is usually positioned under the incision unless it is displaced or the rumen is gas distended. The rumen and abomasum are identified and gas decompressed if necessary. This can help the ventilatory capacity of the cow and provide more room for surgical manipulations. The liver is palpable on the right side of the abdomen, the spleen on the left. The diaphragm is swept to check that it is intact. The omasum is present lateral to the abomasum and typically has firm ingesta. The abomasum is exteriorized with gauze sponges and the greater curvature followed from the pylorus to the reticulum (Figure 4.5-9). Access to the remainder of the intestinal tract is very limited, and another approach should be chosen if other abdominal organs need to be examined.

The peritoneum and internal sheath of the rectus abdominis muscle are closed together. If an abomasopexy is to be performed, the seromuscular layer of the abomasum is included in this layer closure. The suture material used for this layer can be a nonabsorbable or absorbable material (#2 or #3 in size), depending on surgeon's preference (see Chapter 10.4). The rectus abdominis muscle is closed with an absorbable suture material (#2 in size) in a simple continuous or interrupted pattern. The external sheath of the rectus abdominis muscle is the holding layer of the closure. Closure of this layer is accomplished by using an absorbable suture material (#2 in size) in a simple continuous or interrupted pattern. Closure of the skin is performed by using a nonabsorbable suture material (#1 in size) in a Ford interlocking pattern (Figure 4.5-10).

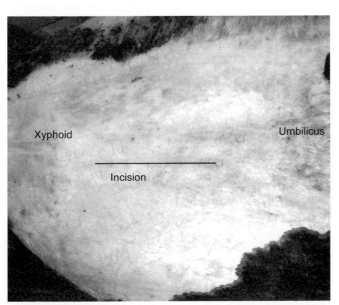

Xyphoid

Umbilicus

Incision

Figure 4.5-7 Diagram that shows the location of a right paramedian incision.

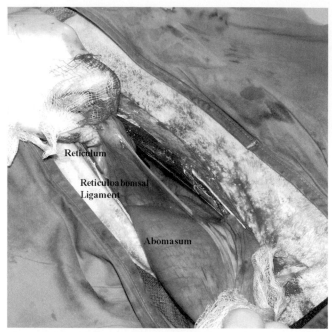

Figure 4.5-9   Exposure of the abomasum, reticuloabomasal ligament, and reticulum through a right paramedian incision.

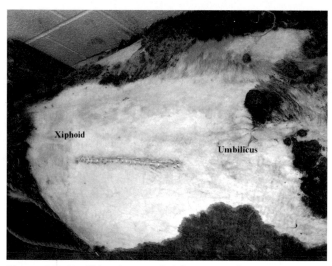

Figure 4.5-10   Skin closure of right paramedian incision.

VENTROLATERAL CELIOTOMY

This approach is especially useful in accessing the uterus for a hysterotomy in the case of an emphysematous fetus. Postpartum uterine lacerations can be accessed and sutured with this approach. The incision is made laterally to the subcutaneous abdominal vein (milk vein) and extends caudally curving dorsally staying lateral to the attachment of the udder. The length of the incision depends on the amount of exposure needed. The subcutaneous abdominal vein should be marked with sutures before positioning the cow in lateral recumbency. This

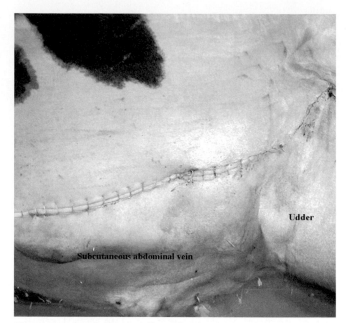

Figure 4.5-11   Left ventrolateral celiotomy incision.

is necessary to avoid lacerating the vein during the approach because its location will not be as obvious when the cow is recumbent. The cow is restrained in lateral recumbency with the upper hind limb abducted and secured so the inguinal area and base of the udder are accessible. The area from the xiphoid cartilage to the inguinal region should be clipped and aseptically prepared. Local anesthesia should be used to desensitize the region, and the surgical site should be draped for aseptic surgery. The skin incision is made and the subcutaneous tissues are divided to expose the external sheath of the rectus abdominis muscle. This layer is sharply incised, thereby exposing the rectus abdominis muscle, which is opened along its length by splitting muscle fibers with a combination of sharp and blunt dissection. Extreme caution should be used when entering the abdominal cavity. The gravid uterus is usually beneath the peritoneum. The internal sheath of the rectus abdominis muscle is elevated by using thumb forceps and then incised by using Mayo scissors. The surgeon's fingers work best to protect underlying viscera when opening this final layer. The incision can be lengthened cranially or caudally to provide the necessary exposure. This approach provides excellent exposure to the uterus at the expense of a time-consuming and difficult body-wall closure. The caudal aspect of the incision will not have as many layers as the cranial portion of the incision because caudally the abdominal muscles are largely aponeurotic. The layers at the cranial aspect of the incision will include the peritoneum, rectus abdominis muscle, and internal and external sheaths of the rectus abdominis muscle. The external sheath of the rectus abdominis muscle is the holding layer for closing this incision. The surgeon can close the internal sheath of the rectus abdominis muscle with an absorbable suture (#2 in size) in a simple continuous pattern. However, this layer often does not hold sutures well; therefore the suture can tear through the tissues. One can choose not to close this layer and begin by closing the rectus abdominis muscle with an absorbable suture material (#2 in size) in a continuous or interrupted pattern. The external sheath of the rectus abdominis muscle is closed by using an absorbable suture material (#2 or #3 in size) in an interrupted or simple continuous pattern. This fascial layer is the most critical for providing body wall support. Tension-relieving suture patterns such as near-far-far-near can be used if necessary. Finally, the skin is closed with a nonabsorbable suture material (#1 in size) in a Ford interlocking pattern. Lavage of the soft tissue between closure layers is advisable. Seroma and peri-incisional edema are very common with this approach.

VENTRAL MIDLINE CELIOTOMY

Ventral midline celiotomy can be used for cesarean section. In cattle that have very large and branching subcutaneous abdominal veins the surgeon can avoid them by using this approach. The linea alba is composed of dense fibrous tissue that provides a secure closure and makes enlarging the incision, if necessary, easy. The cow is restrained in dorsal recumbency, and the ventral abdomen from the umbilicus to the udder and extending to the folds of the flank is clipped, aseptically prepared, and draped for surgery. Local anesthesia is used to desensitize the area. The skin incision is started at the umbilicus and extended caudally. The incision is continued through the subcutaneous tissue to the level of the linea alba. A small incision made through the linea alba and peritoneum, while carefully avoiding underlying viscera, provides access to the abdomen. In some instances substantial retroperitoneal fat must be dissected before the peritoneum can be seen. The surgeon can use a finger to determine whether adhesions are present at the entry incision. The incision through the linea alba is continued caudally. The surgeon can use an instrument such as a thumb forceps to protect underlying viscera as the incision is extended. A sterile impervious sleeve should be used for exploration. When using a ventral midline celiotomy for cesarean section, some operators advocate tilting the cow 45 to 60 degrees to facilitate delivery of the calf. This approach may be especially useful for fractious beef cattle.

Closure of the incision should be in three layers. The linea alba is closed with #2 or #3 absorbable suture material in a simple continuous pattern or an interrupted pattern. The subcutaneous layer is closed using #0 absorbable suture material in a continuous pattern. The skin is closed using #1 nonabsorbable suture in a Ford interlocking pattern.

RIGHT PARACOSTAL APPROACH

This approach provides access to the abdomen through the low flank. It can be used to gain access to the abomasum in adult cattle and calves. Because of the smaller and more mobile gastrointestinal tract in calves a more thorough exploratory can be performed in comparison to that for adult cattle. The animal is placed in left lateral recumbency under general anesthesia. The area is clipped, prepped, and draped in routine fashion. The skin incision is made parallel and 5 to 10 cm (adult) caudal to the last rib. The length of the incision will vary depending on the surgical exposure needed. After the skin and subcutaneous tissues are incised the aponeurosis of the external abdominal oblique is exposed and incised in the direction of the skin incision. The muscular portion of the internal abdominal oblique may be encountered dorsally and the aponeurotic portion ventrally. This depends on the location of the incision. Once the internal abdominal oblique muscle/aponeurosis is incised in the direction of the skin incision the transversus abdominis should be tented with thumb forceps and incised with Mayo scissors. Access to the abdomen in completed by incising the peritoneum and transversus abdominis together.

Closure of the incision is accomplished by suturing the transversus abdominis and peritoneum as the first layer with an absorbable suture material. The suture size will depend on the size of the animal. The subsequent muscle/aponeurotic layers should be closed separately with an absorbable suture material of appropriate size. The skin is closed using a nonabsorbable suture material in a Ford interlocking pattern. The closure of the aponeurosis of the external abdominal oblique muscle is the strongest layer of this closure.

LEFT OBLIQUE CELIOTOMY

A left oblique celiotomy has been recommended for cows requiring cesarean section (Figure 12.2.2-6, A and B). The skin incision starts 10 cm ventral to the transverse processes of the lumbar vertebrae and angles forward to finish at the level of the costochondral junction. The abdominal oblique muscles are sharply incised in the same direction. The transversus and peritoneum are tented as for the other approaches and are incised with scissors.

It has been suggested that this approach extends further cranial and ventral than the classical flank approaches, thus permitting superior manipulation and exteriorization of the uterus. In 18 standing cows, closure of the abdomen was easily accomplished. Three cows developed incisional complications, and persistent anesthesia of the body wall was noted.

RECOMMENDED READINGS

Campbell ME, Fubini SL: Indications and surgical approaches for cesarean section in cattle, *Compend Contin Educ Pract Vet* 12: 285-291, 1990.

Dyce KM, Sack WO, Wensing CJG: The abdomen of the ruminants In *Textbook of veterinary anatomy*, Philadelphia, 1987, WB Saunders.

Parish SM, Tyler JW, Ginsky JV: Left oblique celiotomoy for cesarean section inn standing cows, *J Am Vet Med Assoc* 15: 207(6): 751-2.

Smith DF: Bovine intestinal surgery: part 1, *Mod Vet Pract* 65: 705-710, 1984.

Smith DF: Bovine Intestinal surgery: part 2, *Mod Vet Pract* 65: 853-857, 1984.

Turner AS, McIlwraith CW: Flank laparotomy and abdominal exploration, *Techniques in large animal surgery*, ed 2, Philadelphia, 1989, Lea & Febiger.

Turner AS, McIlwraith CW: Right flank omentopexy, *Techniques in large animal surgery*, ed 2, Philadelphia, 1989, Lea & Febiger.Turner AS, McIlwraith CW: Ventral paramedian abomasopexy. *Techniques in large animal surgery*, ed 2, Philadelphia, 1989, Lea & Febiger.

4.6—Laparoscopy

David E. Anderson

Laparoscopy has been used in ruminants primarily to evaluate reproductive structures and for artificial insemination. More recently, minimally invasive viewing of abdominal structures has been recognized to have many applications in diagnostic and therapeutic procedures. Laparoscopy has also been used to guide serial renal biopsies in cattle. A technique that uses a paralumbar fossa approach and a rigid laparoscope to view the uterus and ovaries of cattle has been described. Recently, laparoscopic abomasopexy has been performed in cattle affected with left displacement of the abomasum (see Chapter 10.4-1).

Appropriate treatment selection is vital for managing gastrointestinal tract disease. Differentiating between medical and surgical conditions requires certain diagnostic techniques. Physical examination alone is often sufficient; however, other ancillary evaluations can yield more specific diagnoses. Abdominocentesis in cattle is often unrewarding because of the low volume of peritoneal fluid usually present. Failure to obtain peritoneal fluid by abdominocentesis does not preclude the existence of abdominal lesions. When a diagnosis cannot be obtained with standard techniques, laparoscopy may provide a safe, efficient, less-invasive procedure than an exploratory celiotomy can.

Surgical Techniques

In a 1984 study, a flexible colonoscope was used to examine the abdominal cavity of cattle through the right or left paralumbar fossa. Disadvantages included a 10-cm incision through the skin and abdominal musculature, difficulty controlling the colonoscope because of its flexible end, and requirement of a second operator's guidance through rectal palpation. This technique was accurate for diagnosing traumatic reticuloperitonitis from the left side of the cow; but the investigators were unable to observe left abomasal displacement in 10 cows from the right side of the abdomen. In this study, use of the colonoscope for laparoscopy was considered less stressful and more innocuous than an exploratory celiotomy based on serial hematologic results and clinical observation. However the authors acknowledged that trocar placement of the laparoscope would be superior and that the technique needed modification.

More recent laparoscopies have feed and water withheld for 24 hours before the procedure. Standing laparoscopy is performed with the cows under light sedation (acepromazine maleate, 0.03 mg/kg of body weight, IM). Xylazine hydrochloride (0.05 mg/Kg, IM) is administered before ventral midline or paramedian laparoscopy. A 32-cm or preferably 54-cm rigid laparoscope with direct viewing lens has been used to view the abdomen and viscera. The 32-cm length laparoscope presents some difficulty for viewing the caudal abdomen. An angled viewing lens may be beneficial in a few cases.

Laparoscopy through the right or left paralumbar fossa is performed with the cow sedated standing in a chute (Figure 4.6-1). The cow is prepared for aseptic surgery, and a 2 cm incision is made through the skin and abdominal musculature after infiltration with 2% lidocaine hydrochloride (5 ml, SC/IM). The view port incision (10 mm) is made 8 cm ventral to the tip of the transverse process of the third lumbar vertebra and 5 cm

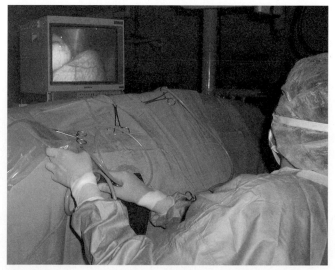

Figure 4.6-1   Standing right flank laparoscopy in a cow.

(Courtesy of Dr. Andre Desrochers, University of Montreal)

caudal to the caudal aspect of the last rib. The laparoscope is introduced by inserting a cannula with trocar and insufflating the abdominal cavity with carbon dioxide gas. Room air may be used to insufflate the abdomen, but an inline filtration system should be used to avoid introducing aerosolized contaminants into the abdomen. The abdominal cavity is insufflated as needed to view the abdominal viscera without exceeding 20 mm Hg (30 cm water) intraabdominal pressure. Thorough examination is completed by initially directing the laparoscope caudally for left-flank laparoscopy or cranially for right-flank laparoscopy. This avoids trauma to the rumen or spleen and prevents introduction of the scope into the omentum or omental bursa, respectively. The scope is then moved counterclockwise to examine the remaining portions of the abdomen. After each laparoscopy is completed, the abdomen is passively deflated through the laparoscopic cannula, and the skin is closed with two simple interrupted sutures.

Cranioventral midline laparoscopy is performed with the cow in dorsal recumbency, whereas paramedian laparoscopy is done with the cow in dorsal recumbency positioned at a 45- to 60-degree angle to the ground (Figure 4.6-2). The site is aseptically prepared, and local anesthesia is induced. A 2-cm incision is made through the skin, subcutaneous tissues, and linea alba or rectus abdominis 10 cm caudal to the xiphoid process. For a laparoscopic abomasopexy, the viewing port is placed caudal to the umbilicus on the right paramedian aspect of the abdomen to decrease the chance of perforating the gas-distended abomasum. To examine the cranioventral abdomen, the laparoscope is moved in a counterclockwise circle starting at the central portion of the diaphragm. The cannula is also introduced caudally for this procedure to avoid the abomasum.

RIGHT PARALUMBAR FOSSA LAPAROSCOPY

Right paralumbar fossa laparoscopy can be used to view a variety of viscera (Table 4.6-1). Cranially, the descending duodenum, (Figure 4.6-3) caudate and right lobes

TABLE 4.6-1			
Observation of Abdominal Viscera from Right and Left Paralumbar Fossa and Cranioventral Midline Laparoscopy			
VISCERA	RIGHT PLF	LEFT PLF	CVML
Diaphragm	Yes	Yes	Yes
Rumen	Yes	Yes	Yes
Reticulum	No	No	Yes
Abomasum	No	No	Yes
Pylorus	No	No	Yes
Duodenum	Yes	No	No
Pancreas	Yes	No	No
Small intestine	Yes	Yes	No
Cecum	Yes	No	No
Spiral colon	No	No	No
Descending colon	Yes	No	No
Right kidney	Yes	No	No
Left kidney	No	Yes	No
Urinary bladder	Yes	Yes	No
Liver:			
Right and caudate lobes	Yes	No	No
Left lobe	No	No	Yes
Spleen	No	Yes	Yes
Right ovary	Yes	No	No
Left ovary	Yes	No	No
Uterus	Yes	No	No

*CVML = cranioventral midline laparoscopy. PLF = paralumbar fossa laparoscopy.

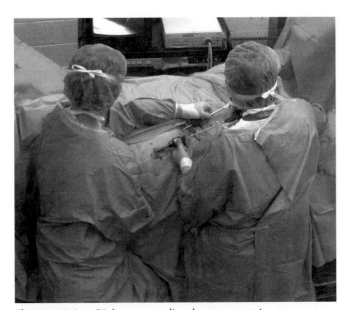

Figure 4.6-2   Right paramedian laparoscopy in a cow.

(Courtesy of Dr. Andre Desrochers, University of Montreal)

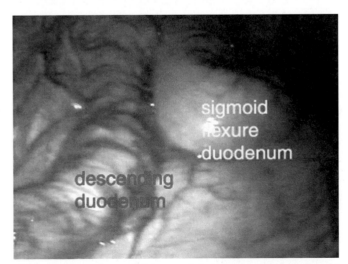

Figure 4.6-3   View of right cranial abdomen through a right paralumbar fossa laparoscopy.

(Courtesy of Dr. Andre Desrochers, University of Montreal)

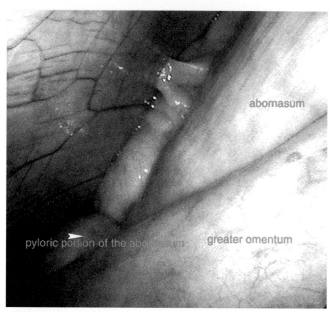

abomasum

pyloric portion of the abomasum

greater omentum

Figure 4.6-4   RDA view from right paramedian laparoscopy in a cow.

(Courtesy of Dr. Andre Desrochers, University of Montreal).

of the liver, and right kidney are viewed. The costal and lateral parts of the right crus and central tendinous portions of the diaphragm are evident. The descending duodenum is identified by the attachments of the mesoduodenum dorsally and the greater omentum ventrally (see Figure 4.6-3). In cases of RDA, the abomasum can be recognized by it smooth distended surface (Figure 4.6-4). Multiple peristaltic movements are evident during laparoscopy. The laparoscope can be easily manipulated around the caudate and right lobes of the liver. The cystic duct or gallbladder usually is not visible. The right kidney is identified as a focal blue-grey region protruding from the surface of the parietal peritoneum in the cranial dorsal abdomen but caudal to the liver attachment to the dorsal abdominal wall. The body and right lobe of the pancreas can be identified by the typical tan-to-pale pink color of the tissue with a granular-appearing surface that is located in the mesoduodenum ventral to the right kidney, caudal to the caudate lobe of the liver, and dorsal to the proximal portion of the descending duodenum.

The laparoscope is advanced through a caudal space created by the free edge of the greater omentum and cranial border of the broad ligament to view the female urogenital tract and caudal abdomen. The ovarian artery and vein are identified as tortuous vessels coursing ventrally on the free edge of the broad ligament. The right ovary is identified by following the ovarian artery and vein from the broad ligament. The descending colon is observed along the dorsal midline within the mesocolon.

The nongravid uterus can be seen lying over the abdominal margin of the pubis in the caudal portion of the abdominal cavity. Smooth serosal surfaces, vascular arcades emanating from the mesenteric border, and free mobility with peristaltic movements differentiates the small intestine from other segments of the intestinal tract. The cecum is identified as a variably dilated viscus. Its diameter is larger than the small intestine's, and it has multiple branching vessels and segmental motility. Intestine segments connected by a short mesentery and a lack of prominent vascular arcades (as seen in the small intestine) identify the spiral colon. The urinary bladder is visualized as a distended viscus with prominent vessels. The caudomedial aspect of the dorsal sac of the rumen may be observed. With some difficulty, the cranial root of the mesentery is viewed. Alternatively, the laparoscope may be introduced into the omental recess by inserting it directly through the omental curtain.

LEFT PARALUMBAR FOSSA LAPAROSCOPY
When the laparoscope is inserted into the left paralumbar fossa, it can be directed cranially to view the dorsal sac of the rumen and the spleen. The rumen is large and occupies most of the paralumbar fossa (Figure 10.4-5, *B*). The spleen is dark blue-grey, with an irregular surface marked by white lines in the splenic capsule. The laparoscope is manipulated between the spleen and rumen to view the costal part and central tendinous portion of the diaphragm. The reticulum cannot be observed, but fibrinous adhesions are found along the cranial and ventral aspects of the lateral rumen wall in cases of traumatic reticulitis. The dorsal sac and caudodorsal blind sac of the rumen are visible caudally. The left kidney, seen medial to the rumen in the middorsal portion of the abdomen, has an appearance similar to the right kidney. Portions of the small intestinal tract are identified caudomedial to the rumen.

CRANIOVENTRAL MIDLINE LAPAROSCOPY
The cannula and trocar are directed perpendicular to the parietal peritoneum to enter the abdominal cavity, and the cannula is advanced caudally and dorsally. Cranially, the sternal part and tendinous center of the diaphragm are visualized. To the right of midline, the body of the abomasum is recognized by its smooth serosal surface without overlying omentum and large fundus tapering caudally into its pyloric part. The left lobe of the liver is visible on the right side of midline (Figure 4.6-5). Distention of the abomasum, reticulum, or both, can obscure the liver from view. The omasum is obscured by the greater omentum. The reticulum is difficult to distinguish from the adjacent rumen unless it is distended with gas. When the reticulum is distended with gas, it has an irregular serosal surface with multiple indentations

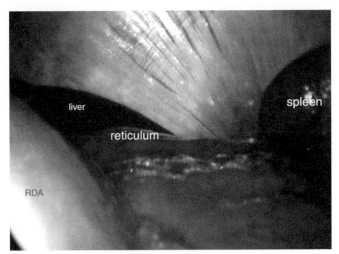

Figure 4.6-5 Cranial abdomen of a cow with a LDA showing relative position of the liver, reticulum, spleen and abomasum. Note that with cow in dorsal recumbency, the abomasum returns to the right (RDA).

(Courtesy of Dr. Andre Desrochers, University of Montreal).

similar to the honeycombed interior. The distal portion of the spleen that is not attached to the rumen can be identified. The caudal portion of the abdominal cavity is obscured by the greater omentum. Inadvertent entry into the omental bursa can be recognized when the immense ventral aspect of the rumen (normally obscured by the omentum) is observed without being able to view the abomasum.

Laparoscopic Abomasopexy

Laparoscopic abomasopexy has been described as a two-step procedure. The author has developed a one-step procedure as a time- and labor-efficient alternative. Laparoscopic abomasopexy is a more specific method for toggle-pin abomasopexy in cattle with a left displaced abomasum. This technique allows the abomasum to be viewed directly so that a toggle-pin suture can be accurately placed. This technique should not be used in cattle with a right displaced abomasum or suspected of having abomasal adhesions. However, laparoscopy can be used to definitively determine if abomasal adhesions are present and to select the best surgical approach to treat the adhesions.

TWO-STEP LAPAROSCOPIC ABOMASOPEXY

Two-step laparoscopic abomasopexy is discussed in Chapter 10.4. The first step involves left paralumbar fossa laparoscopy to identify the abomasum, integrity of the abomasal wall, and to introduce a toggle-pin suture implant (Figure 10.4-5, *B*). The viewing portal should be placed caudally in the left paralumbar fossae to avoid

accidental penetration of the abomasum (Figure 10.4-5, *A*). A long, laparoscopically-guided cannula is used to penetrate the abomasum. After penetrating the abomasum, a toggle pin is inserted into the lumen of the abomasum and is followed by deflation of abomasal gas. The instruments are removed, and the incisions are closed after the abomasum has been decompressed. The cow is then placed on the right side and rolled into dorsal recumbency. A viewing portal is placed in the right paramedian abdomen slightly caudal to the umbilicus. An instrument portal is placed 10 to 15 cm caudal to the xiphoid cartilage in the right paramedian abdomen with laparoscopic guidance. A grasping forceps is used to retrieve the toggle-pin suture, and this suture is tied over a roll of gauze padding (Figure 10.4-6). The laparoscope is removed after the insufflated gas is evacuated from the abdomen.

ONE-STEP PROCEDURES

The cow is placed on the right side and rolled into dorsal recumbency. The cow is then maneuvered into left dorsal recumbency (45 to 60 degree angle to the ground). A viewing portal is placed in the right paramedian abdomen slightly caudal to the umbilicus. An instrument portal is placed 10 to 15 cm caudal to the xiphoid cartilage in the right paramedian abdomen by using laparoscopic guidance (see Figure 4.6-2). A long cannula is used to penetrate the abomasum. After the abomasum is penetrated, a toggle pin is inserted into the lumen of the abomasum and is followed by deflation of abomasal gas. The instruments are removed, and the incisions are closed after the abomasum has been decompressed. The toggle-pin suture remains outside of the abdomen throughout the procedure, and this suture is tied over a roll of gauze padding.

Alternatively, Desrochers reported that a sutured-abomasopexy can be performed under laparoscopic control (Figure 4.6-6) and result in excellent postoperative adhesions (Figure 4.6-7). After placement of the laparoscope as described above (some abdominal inflation may be needed), the abomasum is decompressed with a long needle placed through the abdominal wall. A 10-mm instrument port is placed to the right of the ventral midline in the cranial abdomen near the xiphoid process. A Babcock laparoscopic forceps is inserted into the abdomen, and the fundus of the abomasum is grasped near the intended "pexy" site. A second instrument portal (5 mm) is made on the right side of the umbilicus, and a laparoscopic needle driver is inserted. Four small incisions (5 mm in length) 2 cm apart are made through the skin only, at the intended "pexy" site—2 cm to the right and 15 cm caudal to the xiphoid process and parallel to the ventral midline. A USP 2 polydioxanone suture is passed with a straightened swaged-

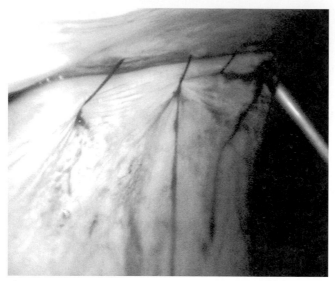

Figure 4.6-6 Sutured-abomasopexy under laparoscopic guidance.

(Courtesy of Dr. Andre Desrochers, University of Montreal)

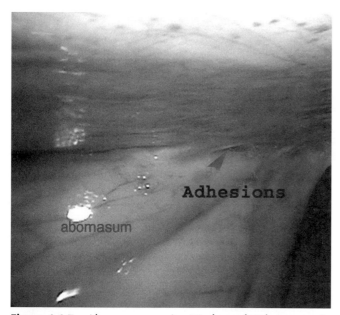

Figure 4.6-7 Abomasopexy site 60 days after laparoscopic abomasopexy.

(Courtesy of Dr. Andre Desrochers, University of Montreal)

on needle through the previously made skin incision. The needle is grasped in the abdomen with the needle driver and passed through the abomasum held by the Babcock forceps approximately 2 to 3 cm from the attachment of the greater omentum on the abomasum. The needle is then pulled through the abomasal wall and driven back through the abdominal wall at the first inci-

sion site. The procedure is repeated at the other three incision sites. The sutures are tightened (see Figure 4.6-6); all instruments are removed; and the abdomen is deflated. The skin incisions are closed with absorbable sutures.

Conclusion

Laparoscopy of the abdomen provides a safe alternative to exploratory celiotomy in cattle, but access to many portions of the abdomen is limited or impossible. In six cattle that had trial abdominal laparoscopy, no apparent adverse effects occurred; the cows had no changes in physical exam, CBC, serum biochemical profile, or peritoneal fluid assessment. Serial laparoscopy does not appear to increase the risk of intraabdominal complications or adversely affect pregnancy and may provide a means for obtaining repeat diagnostic samples with better precision. Performing laparoscopy in an animal with gastrointestinal distention greatly increases the likelihood of visceral trauma; therefore the animal should be carefully prepared. The laparoscope must have sufficient length to maneuver into the caudal portion of the abdominal cavity. Insufficient length may prevent observation of portions of the abdomen.

RECOMMENDED READINGS

Anderson DE, Gaughan EM, St-Jean G: Normal laparoscopic anatomy of the bovine abdomen, *Am J Vet Res* 54: 1170-1176, 1993.

Blood DC, Radostitis OM, Henderson JA: Diseases of the alimentary tract I. In *Veterinary medicine*, ed 6, London 1983, Balliere Tindall.

Hulet CV, Foote WC: A rapid technique for observing the reproductive tract of living ewes, *J Anim Sci* 27: 142-145, 1968.

Janowitz H: Laparoscopic reposition and fixation of the left displaced abomasum in cattle, *Tierarztl Prax* 26: 308-313, 1998.

Lambert RD, Bernard C, Rioux JE et al: Endoscopy in cattle by the paralumbar route: technique for ovarian examination and follicular aspiration, *Theriogenology* 20: 149-161, 1983.

Maxwell DP, Kraemer DC: Laparoscopy in cattle. In Harrison RM, Wildt DE, editors: *Animal laparoscopy*, Baltimore, 1980, Williams and Wilkins.

Megale, Fincher MG, McEntee K: Peritoneoscopy in the cow: visualization of the ovaries, oviducts, and uterine horns, *Cornell Vet* 46: 109-121, 1956.

Miller SJ: Artificial breeding techniques in sheep. In Morrow DA, editor: *Current therapy in theriogenology*, Philadelphia, 1986, WB Saunders.

Naoi M, Kokue E, Takahashi Y et al: Laparoscopic-assisted serial biopsy of the bovine kidney, *Am J Vet Res* 46: 699-702, 1985.

Snyder DA, Dukelow WR: Laparoscopic studies of ovulation, pregnancy diagnosis, and follicle aspiration in sheep, *Theriogenology* 2: 143-148, 1974.

Wass WM, Thompson JR, Moss EW, et al: Diseases of the ruminant forestomach. In Howard JL, editor: *Current veterinary therapy 2 (food animal practice)*, Philadelphia, 1986, WB Saunders.

Wilson AD, Ferguson JG: Use of a flexible fiberoptic laparoscope as a diagnostic aid in cattle, *Can Vet J* 25: 229-234, 1984.

4.7—Herd Health Considerations for Treating Food Animal Surgical Patients in the Veterinary Hospital Setting

Susan M. Stehman

Introduction

Individual food animals presented to a Veterinary Hospital for surgical procedures are typically members of a larger operation or food animal production system. Animals may be presented from a variety of types of operations, including registered high genetic breeding farms, commercial production farms, or farms that specialize in niche markets such as organic or transgenic production. Each type of production unit operates under different management systems and standards of production. Livestock producers are increasingly being asked to document on-farm processes, including biosecurity; herd health programs; and vaccine and antimicrobial usage to meet animal health, welfare, food safety, and quality standards set by regulators and marketing groups. These trends in food animal production agriculture need to be taken into consideration when treating individual food animals that will be returning to a farm or that may enter the market system. The objective of this chapter is to provide the reader with a broad overview of the livestock industry trends and challenges faced by producers and veterinarians who treat food animals in a referral hospital setting.

Trends in Food Animal Production— Commercial Operations

The structure of the livestock production units is changing. Commercial livestock operations are increasing in size, with trends toward larger intensively managed farms with high densities of livestock. The swine industry tends toward closed, vertically integrated systems with an emphasis on biosecurity and quality assurance procedures. The ruminant livestock industries are typically more open systems. Large cattle farms, especially dairy operations, often require purchase of replacement animals and feed from external sources to meet ex-

pansion goals. The potential risks for introducing and transmitting infectious diseases increase in large, open, high-density operations. Bovine leukosis, bovine virus diarrhea, contagious mastitis, salmonella infection, and Johne's Disease have become common endemic infections in our dairy herds. Introduction of contagious respiratory, intramammary, reproductive, gastrointestinal, and foot infections can have immediate and long-term implications for the health and productivity of a herd. Salmonella, Johne's Disease, bovine virus diarrhea, and contagious mastitis (dairy cattle) are of particular concern to the cattle industry. *Corynebacterium pseudotuberculosis*, contagious foot rot, anthelmintic-resistant parasites, scrapie, and ovine and caprine lentiviruses (OPPV and CAEV) are biosecurity concerns to small ruminant producers. Increasingly, producers are adopting biosecurity programs to limit the introduction and spread of these infections in their herds.

Livestock producers are also being challenged to respond to public health concerns about zoonotic agents that can be present on farms with and without causing animal health problems. Such agents can be exported into the food chain by carrier animals and environmental contamination of water and vegetable crops from land application of livestock manure. Examples include *Listeria* spp., *Campylobacter* spp., *Salmonella* spp., *E. coli* O157:H7, *Cryptosporidium parvum* and *Giardia* spp. Antimicrobial resistance and the potential of spreading resistant microbes through the food chain are also public health concerns. In addition to addressing microbial hazards, food animal producers are required to prevent chemical contamination of milk and meat.

Prevention of chemical contamination by pesticides, animal health products—including vaccines, antimicrobial, reproductive, and antiinflammatory drugs and toxicants that could adulterate meat and milk products—is required of meat and milk products that enter the food system. Treatment records must be kept to show identification of the animal treated, type of medication, dose, and amount injected per site, with a clear indication of meat and milk withholding times. Record-keeping is especially important if extra-label drugs are used.

Increasingly, product quality is required for premiums and even access to certain markets. Market Quality Assurance Programs have been developed for the beef, sheep, and pork industries to prevent quality defects associated with injection practices. Injection practices can result in injection-site lesions and abscesses that cause carcass quality defects. Injections given to calves can cause detectable lesions at slaughter and affect beef tenderness up to a year after administration. Muscle tissues respond to injections with increased amounts of connective tissue and fatty deposits. Meat tenderness is affected at the core of the lesion and up to several inches from the center of the injection site. To enhance meat quality and minimize injection site reactions, the following general recommendations are suggested:

- Use vaccines and drugs labeled for subcutaneous use whenever possible. Each commodity group may have specific designated injection site recommendations.
- Eliminate intramuscular injections in the loin and hind leg to protect these higher-priced cuts. The preferred sites for intramuscular injection include the large muscle masses of the shoulder and neck. Highly irritating intramuscular injections should be avoided in the neck near the spinal column.
- Use single-use needles to prevent spread of blood-borne infections such as bovine leukosis virus and anaplasmosis. Use the smallest diameter needle necessary for the product used.
- Limit amount per injection site.

Niche Markets

In a smaller segment of the livestock industry, producers are pursuing niche markets that require more stringent health and production standards. Access to global markets for replacement cattle, semen, and embryos requires a focus on control and elimination of livestock infections often considered endemic in commercial operations. Examples include Office International des Epizooties (OIE) List B and C diseases. Some of these diseases are addressed in national and regional disease status programs administered by the federal government and include regulatory and voluntary disease status programs. Diseases such as tuberculosis and brucellosis are addressed in federal regulatory programs. Blue tongue virus infection is addressed on a regional disease status level with some regions free and some endemically infected. Voluntary herd status programs such as the USDA Voluntary Bovine Johne's Disease Control Program (VBJDCP) are implemented at the herd level by using state guidelines that meet minimum requirements as outlined in federal program standards (Uniform Program Standards VBJDCP APHIS 91-45-014). Herd status for other endemic infections, such as bovine leukosis, infectious bovine rhinotracheitis virus, ovine progressive pneumonia virus, and caprine arthritis encephalitis virus are not defined by national program standards, but herds may elect to control or eliminate these diseases to meet requirements for export markets. Production units such as bull studs and registered herds that sell germplasm, embryos, and seed stock are required to meet international health standards for export. Because the health status of an individual animal from a herd is difficult to verify, the trend toward requirements for health certification of the herd will increase.

The above trends and the publicity and costs of losses incurred by the 2001 foot-and-mouth disease outbreak in England have increased awareness about biosecurity and preventive herd-health programs within the livestock industries in North America. On-farm quality or health assurance programs for livestock based on the Hazard Analysis Critical Control Point (HACCP) system, the Total Quality Management System, or modifications of these systems are being used to address herd health management as well as product quality on farms. Herds identify and prioritize risks important to their operation and establish management practices to mitigate or eliminate these risks within their operation. Risks of chemical and biological contamination from external sources that could be introduced to the farm as well as on-farm risks are typically addressed in farm health management plans. Broad interventions—sometimes called *Best Management Practices* or *good farming practices*—are implemented to address general risk conditions common to multiple infectious agents and contaminants. More specific management practices or critical control point interventions are implanted to address specific risks posed by a certain agent or contaminant on a particular premise. Biosecurity and biocontainment of respiratory, reproductive, intramammary and gastrointestinal diseases of the neonatal and adult cattle have been covered in detail elsewhere (Dargatzel, 2002). Examples of general and specific management practices—as well as the process of hazard identification, exposure assessment, risk management and monitoring—are also covered.

Although participation in nonregulatory programs may be voluntary, some producers choose to meet higher standards that require third-party certification and monitoring. Some of the disease-specific and more general best management practices being used on farms are becoming part of an expected standard of care. Veterinarians in hospitals that primarily handle individual patients need to be aware of these industry trends and expectations. The potential for exposure to traditional nosocomial infections and an expanding range of other infectious diseases, selection of injection sites appropriate for food animal use, and the potential for chemical residues must be taken into account when one treats individual livestock within a hospital setting.

Challenges within the Veterinary Hospital or Clinic

Hospitalization of livestock presents biosecurity risks both to the hospital environment and—upon return—to the farm of origin. The potential exists for patients to be exposed to other animals, either directly or indirectly, from herds of different health status and to different species. Many hospitals/clinics have isolation facilities and protocols designed to manage transmission from highly infectious patients. However, the facility's design and operational procedures for flow of work, traffic, and equipment and personnel hygiene may or may not address biosecurity risks to animals with different levels of susceptibility to exposure within a hospital setting. When producers present livestock for surgery, expected standards of care used in farm health management programs may not be communicated to hospital personnel when livestock are delivered or may not be communicated within the hospital as cases are handled by multiple individuals or services. Awareness of the expected standards for health programs provides hospital staff with the opportunity for discussion of risks presented by hospitalization. Clients can then make informed decisions about risks to an animal's or herd's heath status that might arise from the biosecurity challenges presented by hospitalization or risks to marketability that might arise from a procedure. Furthermore, training in risk evaluation, communication, and biosecurity promote skills in disease prevention that not only address nosocomial infections that affect the patient but also reduce risks to public health for clients and for the hospital staff, should zoonotic agents be present.

A risk identification, assessment (likelihood and magnitude), management, and communication approach similar to that being used in livestock and food production systems can and has been applied to veterinary hospitals to address infection control (P Morley 2002). Key points will be outlined in the following discussion.

Veterinarians and hospitals have their own standards of care to reduce risks of disease transmission from a variety of agents. General recommendations for breaking transmission cycles within a facility include the following:

1. Minimizing direct transmission by segregation or quarantine of animals with known or suspected contagious infections and animals at high risk of acquiring infections
2. Limiting human contact with high-risk patients, especially if the infection is highly contagious, has zoonotic potential (rabies, salmonella, etc.) or if the patient is particularly susceptible to infection
3. Hygiene of personnel, equipment, and other fomites (banked blood, colostrum) and the environment need to be adequate to minimize indirect transmission.

The effectiveness of standard operating procedures in infection control cannot be measured without monitoring and surveillance. Both patient monitoring and procedural monitoring are important to identify the potential for transmission of infectious agents within the hospital environment. To give one example, foot baths were routinely used in one facility to control salmonella infection. The foot baths were kept clean and filled daily with a broad-acting disinfectant. In the middle of a salmonella outbreak, the epidemic strain of salmonella was isolated from a foot bath that from all appearances should have been an effective control point that restricted spread from contaminated footwear to the rest of the facility. Without monitoring, the assumption would have been made that risks of spread by footwear had been addressed, and an important risk contributing to the outbreak would have been missed.

Although general hygiene procedures will help reduce risks from multiple agents, a systematic approach may be needed to address risks for transmission of specific agents or to enhance general operating procedures should monitoring identify risks. The process to address biosecurity risks and interventions can be used across facilities; however, each facility or practice will need to tailor the program to its own client base, facilities constraints, and resources and level of risk aversion. The general risk evaluation process to determine the need for a specific program follows (adapted from Morley, 2002):

1. Identify the infectious agents that may be of concern to the clients and to the operations of the facilities including zoonotic agents.
2. Prioritize the infections based on the risk posed. The level of risk or hazard will depend on the likelihood and magnitude of exposure, characteristics of the agent (infectious dose, virulence, environmental persistence, etc.), characteristics of the patient population (immune or susceptible), value of the patient, zoonotic potential, and the potential for liability.
3. Assess management practices currently in place to address introduction and spread of the identified hazards. Also, procedures that might increase risk of transmission not only to an individual patient but also to other patients within the facility are identified. Facility design, traffic, flow of work, and hygiene are taken into consideration in steps 2 and 3. Are the precautions in place understood by and routinely followed by staff (i.e., has the management plan been communicated to all levels of the staff, suppliers, and clients?).
4. Do the current operating procedures effectively protect against the risks identified to the clients and to the hospital?

If gaps in protection are identified and deemed important to the operations of the hospital and to the clients served, a more systematic approach should be considered.

A risk-analysis approach has been used by a number of authors to describe specific and general management practices to minimize risks for specific agents of concern to cattle producers (see Recommended Readings). The application of the Hazard Analysis Critical Control Point process to develop a tailored veterinary hospital biosecurity plan is discussed in detail by Morley, 2002. The reader is referred to these references for more details.

Summary

Veterinarians in referral hospitals that primarily handle individual food animal patients need to be aware of industry trends in livestock production systems, including increased attention to farm biosecurity and product quality assurance programs. Trends in food animal production agriculture need to be taken into consideration when one treats individual food animals that will return to a farm or that may enter the market system. Industry trends toward larger farms and niche markets present patients with both an increased risk of shedding organisms and an increased risk of susceptibility to the veterinary referral hospital. The potential for exposure to nosocomial infections and an expanding range of other infectious diseases of importance to herd productivity or export markets, selection of injection sites appropriate for food animal use, and the potential for chemical residues must be taken into account in the treatment of individual livestock within a hospital setting. A risk assessment, management, and communication process similar to those being used on farms can be applied to hospitals to optimize infection control.

RECOMMENDED READINGS

Callan RJ, Garry FB: Biosecurity and bovine respiratory disease. In Dargatz DA, ed: *Veterinary Clinics of North America Food Animal Practice* 18: 57-78, 2002.

Dargatz DA, Garry FB, Traub-Dargatz JL: An introduction to biosecurity of cattle operations. In Dargatz DA, ed: *Veterinary Clinics of North America Food Animal Practice* 18: 1-7, 2002.

Dinsmore RP: Biosecurity for reproductive diseases. In Dargatz DA, ed: *Veterinary Clinics of North America Food Animal Practice* 18: 79-98, 2002.

England JJ: Animal health emergency diseases. In Dargatz DA, editor: *The Veterinary Clinics of North America Food Animal Practice* 18: 373-572, 2002.

Faust MA, Kinsel ML et al: Characterizing biosecurity, health, and culling during dairy herd expansions, *J Dairy Sci* 84: 955-965, 2001.

Konkle DM, Nelson KM et al: Nosocomial transmission of Cryptosporidium in a veterinary hospital, *J Vet Intern Med* 11: 340-343, 1997.

Moore C: Biosecurity and minimum disease herds. In Tubbs RC, Leman AD, eds: *Vet Clin N Am Food Anim Pract* 8: 461-474, 1992.

Morley PS: Biosecurity of veterinary practice. In Dargatz DA, ed: *Vet Clin North Am Food Anim Pract* 18: 133-155, 2002.

Noordhuizen JP, Welpelo HJ: Sustainable improvement of animal health care by systematic quality risk management according to the HACCP concept, *Vet Q* 18: 121-126, 1996.

Noordhuizen JP, Wentink GH: Developments in veterinary herd health programs on dairy farms: a review, *Vet Q* 23: 162-169, 2001.

Oliveira MR, Batista CR et al: Application of Hazard Analysis Critical Control Points system to enteral tube feeding in hospital, *J Hum Nutr Diet* 14: 397-403, 2001.

Sanderson MW, Gnad DP: Biosecurity for reproductive diseases. In Dargatz DA, ed: *Vet Clin North Am Food Anim Pract* 18: 115-132, 2002.

Wells SJ, Fedorka-Cray PJ et al: Fecal shedding of *Salmonella* spp. by dairy cows on farm and at cull cow markets, *J Food Prot* 64: 3-11, 2001.

Wells SJ: Biosecurity on dairy operations: hazards and risks, *J Dairy Sci* 83: 2380-2386, 2000.

Wells SJ, Dee S, Godden S: Biosecurity for gastrointestinal diseases of adult dairy cattle. In Dargatz DA, ed: *Vet Clin North Am Food Anim Pract* 18: 35-56, 2002.

Weese JS, Staempfli HR et al: Isolation of environmental *Clostridium difficile* from a veterinary teaching hospital, *J Vet Diagn Invest* 12: 449-452, 2000.

LINKS AND PUBLICATIONS

Office International des Epizooties (OIE) International Animal Health Code athttp://www.oie.int/eng/normes/en_mcode.htm

The Sheep Safety and Quality Assurance Program http://www.colostate.edu/programs/SSQA/

USDA Uniform Program Standards for the Voluntary Bovine Johne's Disease Control Program APHIS 91-45-014.

CHAPTER 5

FLUID THERAPY

Allen J. Roussel

Patients who undergo surgery often require rehydration and electrolyte therapy, particularly in cases of surgery of the gastrointestinal tract. Dehydration and shock are the most important indications for rehydration therapy, especially intravenous therapy. Failure to institute appropriate fluid therapy can result in case failure, regardless of surgical expertise.

Estimating Rehydration Needs

Constable and coworkers showed that the time required for cervical skin to return to its normal position after tenting and the degree of eyeball recession in dehydrated preruminant calves are reasonably accurate methods to determine the state of hydration for calves. Table 5-1, based on this work, is a guide for estimating dehydration. Rehydration by intravenous fluid administration is recommended once dehydration reaches 8%. When skin pinched on the neck takes 6 seconds to return to normal and an eyeball is recessed 4mm, it indicates the 8% dehydration point has been reached. Similar quantitative studies of the relationship between clinical signs and degree of dehydration for mature ruminants have not been undertaken. In the absence of data to suggest otherwise, the values for estimating dehydration in calves by using skin tent is probably a reasonable guide for mature cattle. However, emaciation can cause eyeball recession and loss of skin turgor, thus making these tests more difficult to interpret in cattle that have recently lost substantial weight. The body weight of mature ruminants can change dramatically based on the amount of ingesta and water in the rumen; therefore estimates of percent dehydration measured as a percent of body weight are probably not very accurate. Therefore from a clinical standpoint, we predict that a cow that is 10% dehydrated will have a normal or near-normal hydration status if 10% of her body weight in fluids is restored. She may still be well under her "normal" body weight because of lack of rumen fill. On the other hand, a cow with forestomach distension from vagal indigestion or carbohydrate engorgement may gain weight from fluid sequestered in the third space compartment (inside the rumen) during the disease process but lose significant extra-cellular body water. Even if we could predict the hydration status of a ruminant patient with certainty, factors other than hydration must still be considered in planning and executing the rehydration process. At times an experienced veterinarian can or must break the 8% rule. Sometimes cattle with severe dehydration and normal gastrointestinal function will recover uneventfully with only oral or intraruminal rehydration or with a combination of intraruminal rehydration and a small amount of fluids administered intravenously. In these cases, breaking the rule saves substantial time and expense. However, endotoxemic or hypovolemic cattle or those in shock—with only mild or moderate dehydration—should receive intravenous fluids. Acute strangulating gastrointestinal disease and acute mastitis are examples of conditions that result in this situation. Rapidly correcting or preventing shock is particularly important if a standing surgical procedure is planned. Finally, patients with fatty liver, chronic or refractory ketosis, and pregnancy toxemia may benefit from intravenous glucose therapy regardless of hydration status.

A flow rate of less than 80ml/kg/hr has been recommended for calves because of studies of central venous pressure in clinically dehydrated calves. Similar studies have not been performed to determine the maximum

TABLE 5-1

Guide for Estimating Dehydration of Calves

% DEHYDRATION	0	2	4	6	8	10	12	14
Eyeball recession (mm)	0	1	2	3	4	6	7	8
Skin tent duration (seconds)	2	3	4	5	6	7	8	9

safe flow rate in mature cattle or small ruminants. However, significant elevation in central venous pressure occurred when approximately 40 ml/kg/hr of an isotonic crystalloid was administered intravenously to dehydrated cattle with experimentally induced intestinal obstruction, even though no clinical signs were observed. Although this is a much slower flow rate than the maximal flow rate recommended for calves (80 ml/kg/hr) and dogs (90 ml/kg/hr), a 20 L/hr total flow rate for an average dairy cow is a volume difficult to achieve with a single 14-gauge intravenous catheter. Therefore in most situations, intravenous fluids can be administered to mature cattle through a 14-gauge catheter as quickly as they will flow. Exceptions include cattle with heart disease, oliguric renal failure, and hypoproteinemia and those in recumbency.

A significant energy penalty is incurred if fluids are intravenously administered cold and must be warmed by the patient, especially neonates. Commercially prepared solutions ideally should be used. However, optimal solutions for many ruminant conditions are not readily available in some countries. In those cases, sterilizing locally prepared fluids is recommended. All of the usual components of solutions for cattle can be heat-sterilized, except sodium bicarbonate, which must be filtered. Alternatively, sterile distilled water and reagent grade salts can be used to formulate solutions. Contamination should be carefully avoided during and after preparation, and solutions should be used immediately after preparation. Bacteria can be eliminated by autoclaving, but heat-stable endotoxins and pyrogens may be present in rural and municipal tap water. Therefore the use of pyrogen-free water is important.

Choice of Solution

Ideally, a rehydration solution is formulated after determining the individual patient's needs by laboratory evaluation. However, this is usually not practical or necessary. In general, ruminants, especially cattle, have rather consistent acid-base and electrolyte abnormalities associated with particular diseases, especially surgical diseases. The following data illustrate that alkalizing solutions are not indicated in most sick cattle, especially those with surgical diseases.

In a study of over 500 cattle older than 1 month of age, blood gas and electrolyte determinations were made from patient venous blood samples. Dehydrated cattle were about twice as likely to have metabolic alkalosis as metabolic acidosis. If cattle with 3 diseases that are easily recognized (pneumonia, carbohydrate engorgement, and diarrhea) were excluded, only 16% of dehydrated cattle had metabolic acidosis. About 20% of the dehydrated cattle were hyponatremic or hypokalemic, whereas over 40% were hypochloremic. In another study of 350 sick cattle, approximately 60% had pH values within the reference range. However, many had compensated acidosis or alkalosis. About 53% had abnormally elevated concentrations of HCO_3^-, whereas about 10% had decreased HCO_3^- concentrations. The only conditions of mature cattle in which metabolic acidosis was more common than metabolic alkalosis were carbohydrate engorgement, urinary tract disease, small intestine strangulation/obstruction (torsion of the root of the mesentery, intussusception, etc.), and enteritis/diarrhea. Cattle with abomasal displacement or volvulus, vagal indigestion, cecal displacement, or torsion and (in our study and experience) intussusception are usually alkalotic.

FLUID THERAPY IN CATTLE WITH METABOLIC ACIDOSIS

Although relatively few in number, those conditions in cattle that are consistently associated with acidosis in ruminants are important to remember. Acidosis is the norm for calves with diarrhea and dehydration but not for other sick calves such as those requiring surgery for umbilical masses, fractured limbs, or gastrointestinal diseases. Calves with abomasal and intestinal surgical diseases are similar to mature cattle in their metabolic abnormalities. The most consistent causes of acidosis in cattle older than 1 month of age include carbohydrate engorgement and choke or dysphagia. Carbohydrate engorgement is the only condition that usually causes acidosis and may also require surgery. Carbohydrate engorgement results in systemic acidosis because large amounts of volatile fatty acids and lactic acid are produced by bacterial fermentation. Both D- and L-lactic acid are produced, but only the L isomer is efficiently metabolized by mammalian tissues. Choke or other causes of salivary loss also cause acidosis, because ruminant saliva is rich in bicarbonate. Diarrhea, fatty liver disease, severe ketosis, and urinary tract disease are relatively common diseases that have the potential to cause serious acidosis. In the author's experience, cattle and small ruminants with urethral obstruction or uroperitoneum are unpredictable in their acid-base and electrolyte status. Some diseases usually associated with alkalosis may be accompanied by acidosis in their later stages. These include abomasal volvulus, intussusception, and torsion of the mesenteric root.

ALKALIZING SOLUTIONS

Bicarbonate or metabolizable bases in alkalizing solutions results in a hydrogen ion being consumed. This means the strong ion difference is increased. Lactate, acetate, gluconate, and citrate are some of the metabolizable bases commonly used to treat acidosis. Research has shown that simply restoring extracellular fluid volume is insufficient to rapidly correct acidosis in calves with naturally occurring diarrhea. Sodium bicarbonate is the most economical and readily available alkalinizing agent. However, it cannot be heat-sterilized and forms an insoluble compound if used in solutions that contain calcium.

Alternative alkalinizing agents offer advantages and disadvantages. Lactate is probably the most widely used alkalinizing agent in veterinary medicine in the United States. Commercial preparations of lactated Ringer's solution contain racemic mixtures of D- and L-lactate. Only the L-isomer is metabolized efficiently, whereas most of the D-isomer is excreted unchanged in the urine. Therefore the racemic mixture has only about half the alkalinizing potential of an equimolar amount of the L-isomer. Unlike lactate, acetate is metabolized by peripheral tissues (not just the liver), has no significant endogenous source, and has no unmetabolized isomer. Citrate is used in some oral rehydration solution (ORS) products, but its calcium-chelating properties preclude its inclusion in solutions for intravenous administration. Gluconate, an alkalinizing agent used in combination with acetate in commercially prepared solutions for intravenous administration to humans, dogs, and horses, is ineffective as an alkalinizing agent in calves. Widespread dire warnings in the veterinary and medical literature about the dangers of rapid administration of sodium bicarbonate solution appear to be based on scant evidence and unfounded in cattle practice. Much anecdotal experience and a recent research report suggest that rapid correction of acidosis in cattle is usually without the complication of CSF acidosis.

CALCULATING BASE DEFICIT

Total base replacement needs for mature cattle is calculated by the following formula:

$$BD \times 0.3 \times BW = \text{Base required}$$

BD is base deficit in mEq/L; 0.3 is a conversion factor for extracellular water or the "bicarbonate space;" and BW is body weight in kilograms (which is equivalent to liters of water). The base required is expressed as total mEq of base. Because a larger percent of body weight in neonates is extracellular water than in mature cattle, a 0.6 conversion factor is used for calves instead of 0.3.

When the acid-base status cannot be measured but acidosis is suspected based on the diagnosis, the veterinarian can correct for a base deficit of 10 mEq/L without substantial risk. Calculating the total base deficit in a 500-kg cow yields the following:

$$10\,\text{mEq/L} \times 0.3 \times 500\,\text{kg} = 1500\,\text{mEq}$$

When sodium bicarbonate is the chosen alkalizing agent, one divides the total milliequivalents derived in the formula above by 12, the approximate number of milliequivalents of HCO_3^- contained in 1 g of sodium bicarbonate, to arrive at 125 g, the calculated replacement needs. Because approximately 13 g of sodium bicarbonate dissolved in enough water to make 1 L of solution is isotonic, it would require just under 10 L of isotonic (1.3%) sodium bicarbonate solution to correct a BD of 10 mEq/L in this cow. Therefore about 10 L of isotonic sodium bicarbonate solution, or 125 g of sodium bicarbonate, is needed empirically to treat moderate acidosis in an average-sized cow.

ELECTROLYTE NEEDS

Although acidosis is often accompanied by hyperkalemia, potassium moves from the intracellular to the extracellular compartment during acidosis, and much is excreted in the urine; therefore a total body potassium deficit may exist. Serious hypokalemia may result when potassium moves from the extracellular to the intracellular compartment while acidosis is being corrected. For this reason, potassium should be included in alkalizing fluids or should follow immediately after correction of acidosis. A moderate concentration of 10 mEq of K^+/L is safe for hyperkalemic acidotic cattle, even at the 20 L/h rate, if it is administered simultaneously with bicarbonate. If possible, additional potassium should be supplied orally or intravenously after the acidosis is corrected.

Some cattle with acidosis, especially those with carbohydrate engorgement, are hypocalcemic. Because acidosis causes a relative increase in ionized calcium, clinical signs of hypocalcemia may not appear until the acidosis is corrected. Because all patients, especially those with acidosis, that receive intravenous calcium therapy may develop potentially fatal cardiotoxicity, they should be monitored very closely. Subcutaneous or oral administration is certainly safer than intravenous administration.

SUMMARY

In summary, neonatal diarrhetic ruminants commonly suffer from metabolic acidosis. Clinically important is the fact that metabolic acidosis is not common in mature ruminants except in those with specific diseases. Calves—and perhaps other ruminants—should receive alkalinizing therapy when they have moderate or severe acidosis. Bicarbonate is the most efficient alkalinizing agent, but lactate and acetate are also effective.

Fluid Therapy in Cattle Without Metabolic Acidosis

Alkalosis is treated by providing extracellular anions in relative excess to cations. The strong ion difference theory explains how this works. In practice, this is accomplished with chloride-rich, potassium-rich solutions. Given adequate circulatory volume and plasma electrolytes, the kidneys can usually correct the alkalosis. Numerous surgical and nonsurgical conditions can result in significant metabolic alkalosis, including vagal indigestion, abomasal displacement or volvulus, traumatic reticulitis, abomasal ulcer disease, peritonitis, renal disease, and almost any condition that results in anorexia and gastrointestinal stasis. Hypochloridemia and hypokalemia often accompany metabolic alkalosis in cattle. For efficient renal correction of metabolic alkalosis and prevention of recurrence, replacing sodium, chloride, and potassium, as well as extracellular fluid volume, is necessary.

NONALKALIZING SOLUTIONS

For large volume replacement, isotonic or nearly isotonic solutions are used. Sodium chloride (0.9%) solution or Ringer's solution (*not* lactated Ringer's) is a good base solution. Potassium chloride should be added to either solution at a rate of 20-40 mEq/L. For ease of calculation, one can remember that 1 g of potassium chloride contains about 14 mEq of potassium ion. Therefore 2 g of potassium chloride/L yields 28 mEq/L, a reasonable concentration for most cattle without acidosis. Oral potassium supplementation should be provided as well because safely administering adequate intravenous potassium replacement is often difficult. Surgical diseases, such as abomasal displacement or volvulus, often occur in dairy cattle in early lactation and risk for metabolic disease such as ketosis or hypocalcemia is great. Therefore including glucose and/or calcium in intravenously administered solutions is often desirable.

A 5% glucose solution can be administered at a slow intravenous rate for several days. It is usually preferable to infuse 2.5% to 5% glucose in 0.45% to 0.9% sodium chloride or other electrolyte solution. The veterinarian should base his or her decision on the relative energy, electrolyte, and fluid volume needs of the patient. Using hypertonic solutions of 550 mOsm/L or less has not caused adverse clinical effects in our hospital when elec-

---

trolytes contribute 350 mOsm/L or less of the total osmolality with glucose contributing to the balance. Urine glucose is monitored so that the flow rate can be adjusted to minimize glucosuria. A minidrip administration set can be used to administer 50% glucose as an alternative to large volume isotonic glucose therapy.

Calcium may be added to solutions for intravenous administration. Ringer's solution contains 5 mEq of calcium/L. Not only is calcium necessary for skeletal muscle contraction and neuronal function and as an intracellular messenger for countless cellular functions; it is also necessary for gastrointestinal smooth muscle function. Calcium homeostasis is precariously balanced in postpartum dairy cattle and is particularly important in cattle that require surgery for gastrointestinal disease. Consequently, inclusion of calcium is recommended in all fluids administered intravenously to lactating dairy cows unless calcium supplementation has been administered within the previous 12 hours. As a rule of thumb, 500 ml of a commercial calcium borogluconate solution may be added to 20 L of solution for intravenous administration. Alternatively, 10 g of calcium chloride may be substituted.

A solution has been formulated and administered in our hospital by the intraruminal and intravenous routes (Box 5-1). It is prepared by adding reagent-grade electrolytes to filtered, deionized water for intravenous administration or feed-grade electrolytes to tap water for intraruminal administration. This solution is superior to calf ORS, which usually contains unneeded alkalizing agents and glucose and is rapidly metabolized by ruminal microbes. Calf ORS is also relatively expensive in comparison to alternative homemade solutions.

HYPERTONIC SALINE SOLUTION

The merit of hypertonic saline solution combined with intraruminal water or rehydration solution has been documented and offers another option for rehydration. The usual dose is 4 to 5 ml of hypertonic saline (2400 mOs/L) solution/kg BW administered intravenously over 5 minutes and 20 liters of water administered orally. Water should be pumped into the rumen of cattle treated with hypertonic saline if they do not drink when allowed access to water. If electrolytes other than sodium and chloride are required, they should be added to the oral fluids. To the author's knowledge, no clinical studies to determine the efficacy of hypertonic saline compared to isotonic solutions have been undertaken.

SUMMARY

In summary, replacement electrolyte solutions for intravenous administration to cows with normal acid-base status or metabolic alkalosis should contain approximately 300-500 mOsm/L. The solution should contain sodium (135-155 mEq/L), chloride (150-170 mEq/L), and potassium (10-20 mEq/L). Lesser concentrations of electrolytes may be included if glucose is added to the solution. In dairy cows, calcium borogluconate (5-8 g/L) or calcium chloride (0.5 g/L) should be added. Cattle with ketosis, fatty liver, or negative energy balance may benefit by adding 10 to 50 g/L glucose. Hypertonic saline (2400 mOs/L) solution administered at a dose of 4 to 5 ml/kg BW intravenously and accompanied by intraruminal fluid is an alternative to large-volume intravenous isotonic fluid therapy.

Equipment and Techniques

Although intravenous administration is sometimes essential, the time and supply costs for complete rehydration of mature cattle with isotonic electrolyte solution is great. Fortunately, the rumen provides a large reservoir that may allow reduction of the cost and time for administrating large volumes of fluids. In many cases, a combination of intravenous and intraruminal administration provides the optimal cost-benefit balance

INTRARUMINAL ADMINISTRATION

Intraruminal administration may be accomplished by using a Frick speculum and orogastric tube, a nasogastric tube, or a specially designed cattle pump system with a self-retraining flexible esophageal probe.* Nasogastric intubation is probably the least stressful technique in mature cattle, although it requires a bit more finesse and a smaller tube than orogastric intubation requires. The pump system is the quickest and most efficient technique, but it is also the method most likely to lead to complications if care is not taken. The oral pump system flow rate must be moderated in some cattle, especially very sick ones, to avoid regurgitation and aspiration. In hospital pens or veterinary clinics, gravity flow devices can be constructed to facilitate oral fluid administration.

---

*Magrath Cattle Pump System (Magrath Manufacturing Co, McCook, NE)

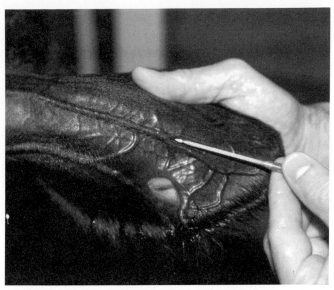

Figure 5-1 Proper site to place auricular vein catheter in the ear of a cow. Note: to avoid a kink, the vein is entered distally so the tip is at least 3 cm from the base of the ear when the entire catheter is inserted.

INTRAVENOUS ADMINISTRATION

The jugular vein is most commonly used for intravenous administration in adult cattle and is also the most useful for administering large volumes very rapidly. However, the auricular vein is quite satisfactory for longer-term administration (Figure 5-1). It provides easy accessibility and seemingly tends to have less catheter failure (accidental removal, kinking, or clotting). Besides fluids, other medications can also be easily administered via an auricular vein catheter. A 14-gauge catheter can usually be inserted in an auricular vein of a mature cow. Flow rates greater than 7.5 L/hr have been achieved with a 14-gauge catheter in the auricular vein. Auricular vein catheters have been maintained for more than 96 hours with heparinized saline flushed just twice daily.

RECOMMENDED READINGS

Constable PD et al: Use of hypertonic saline-dextran solution to resuscitate hypovolemic calves with diarrhea, *Am J Vet Res* 57: 97-104, 1996.

Roeder BL: Acute effects of intravenously administered hypertonic saline solution on transruminal rehydration in dairy cows, *Am J Vet Res* 58: 549-554, 1997.

Roussel AJ, Constable PD: Fluid and electrolyte therapy, *Veterinary Clinics of North America, Food Animal Practice* 15:3, 447-68, 1999.

Roussel AJ et al: Catheterization of the auricular vein of cattle, *J Am Vet Med Assoc* 208: 905-907, 1996.

Roussel AJ et al: Alterations in acid-base balance and serum electrolyte concentration in cattle: 632 cases (1984-1994), *J Am Vet Med Assoc* 212: 1769-1775, 1998.

CHAPTER 6

FARM ANIMAL ANESTHESIA

Jennifer M. Ivany, William W. Muir

Sedation of Farm Animals

Xylazine, acepromazine, diazepam, pentobarbital, butor-phanol, and chloral hydrate are used as preanesthetic medications and sedatives in farm animals (Table 6-1). Xylazine and detomidine are alpha-2 agonists that act on the central nervous system alpha-2 adrenoreceptors to cause sedation, analgesia, and muscle relaxation. Higher doses of xylazine and detomidine induce recumbency and profound CNS and respiratory depression. The amount of drug required to produce sedation depends on an animal's temperament and excitement at the time of administration. Excited animals cannot be sedated with standard drug dosages. In general, a xylazine dose one-tenth that needed to sedate horses is required to sedate cattle. A low concentration of xylazine (20 mg/mL vs. 100 mg/mL) is recommended to avoid over-dosage because of farm animals' sensitivity to the drug. Intravenous or intramuscular doses of xylazine (0.015 to 0.025 mg/kg) will sedate cattle without inducing re-cumbency. Higher doses of xylazine (0.1 to 0.2 mg/kg) induce recumbency and light anesthesia. Sedation is a common side effect after epidural administration of xylazine (see Local Anesthetic Techniques).

Sheep and goats are more sensitive than cattle to xylazine's sedative effects. A low concentration of xylazine (20 mg/mL vs. 100 mg/mL) is recommended to avoid overdosage because of farm animals' sensitivity to the drug. Respiratory depression, hypotension, brady-cardia, hyperglycemia, hypoinsulinemia, and increased urine production are side effects of xylazine. Anecdotal reports of pulmonary edema and cardiovascular instabil-ity in small ruminants exist. Pulmonary edema is most likely precipitated by hypoventilation and alveolar hypoxia. Reports of an oxytocin-like effect from xylazine in near-term pregnant cows suggest that it should be used with care during pregnancy. Detomidine appears to have less of an oxytocin-like effect than does xylazine.

Xylazine sedation, analgesia, cardiopulmonary depres-sion, and muscle relaxation are reversible (see Table 6-1). Tolazoline and yohimbine often are used to reverse sedation and cardiopulmonary depression. Tolazoline seems to have a faster onset of action than yohimbine. Adverse side effects include hypertension and cardiac arrhythmias. The recommended dose for yohimbine is 0.12 mg/kg IV in cattle, with higher doses required for small ruminants (up to 1 mg/kg IV). The recommended dose of tolazoline for ruminants is 0.5 to 2.0 mg/kg IV, and fewer instances of adverse effects occur than with yohimbine.

Xylazine (0.5 to 3 mg/kg IM) can be used alone for sedation in swine but is usually combined with other drugs, such as ketamine (2-5 mg/kg IV or 5-10 mg/kg IM) or Telazol (1-3 mg/kg IV or 2-5 mg/kg IM). It can induce vomiting and cardiopulmonary depression, espe-cially at high doses.

Acepromazine is a phenothiazine tranquilizer com-monly used in horses but infrequently in cattle because of its long duration of action and withdrawal times. The acepromazine dose for cattle is 0.03 to 0.05 mg/kg IV; for sheep and goats it is 0.05 to 0.1 mg/kg IV. Intra-muscular injection is extremely painful, and absorption is variable. Injection into the tail vein should be avoided because accidental intraarterial injection can cause sloughing of the tail as a result of arterial vasospasm and ischemic necrosis. Acepromazine may also increase the risk of phimosis in breeding males and predisposes adult cattle to regurgitation during anesthesia. In swine,

TABLE 6-1

Range of Drug Dosages Used to Sedate and Tranquilize Ruminants and Swine (mg/kg)*

DRUG	CATTLE		CALVES		SHEEP		GOATS		SWINE	
	IV	IM	IV	IM	IV	IM	IV	IM	IV	IM
Acepromazine	0.03-0.05	0.05-0.1	0.03-0.05	0.05-0.1	0.03-0.05	0.05-0.1	0.03-0.05	0.05-0.1	0.03-0.05	0.05-0.1
Diazepam	0.2-0.5	0.5-1.0	0.2-0.5	0.5-1.0	0.2-0.5	0.5-1.0	0.2-0.5	0.5-1.0	0.1-0.2	0.5-1.0
Alpha-2 Agonists										
Xylazine	0.02-0.1	0.02-0.5	0.02-0.1	0.1-0.2	0.02-0.1	0.1-0.3	0.02-0.1	0.1-0.3	0.5-2.0	1.0-4.0
Detomidine	0.01-0.02	0.02-0.05	0.01-0.02	0.03-0.05	0.01-0.02	0.02-0.05	0.01-0.02	0.02-0.05	0.02-0.04	0.04-0.08
Medetomidine		0.02-0.05		0.02-0.05		0.01-0.03		0.01-0.03		0.04-0.08
Alpha-2 Antagonists[†]										
Yohimbine	0.1-0.2		0.1-0.2		0.1-0.5		0.1-0.2		0.1-0.2	
Tolazoline	1.0-2.0		1.0-2.0		1.0-2.0		1.0-2.0		1.0-2.0	
Atipamezole	0.02-0.05		0.02-0.05		0.02-0.05		0.02-0.05			

*Atropine, 0.05-0.1 mg/kg IV, and glycopyrrolate, 0.005-0.01 mg/kg IV, can be used to treat vagal-induced bradycardia but are only partially effective in reducing salivary secretions, which become more viscous and more difficult to remove from the airway, thus predisposing to airway obstruction.
[†]Doxapram 0.5-1.0 mg/kg is partially effective in stimulating respiration and reversing sedation produced by alpha-2 agonists.

acepromazine helps reduce the risk of hyperthermia and porcine stress syndrome. The dose of acepromazine to tranquilize swine is 0.5 mg/kg IM.

Diazepam (0.25 to 0.5 mg/kg IV) can be used to provide brief sedation in small ruminants. Low doses of pentobarbital (2 mg/kg IV) can also be used in cattle to produce sedation, but large doses should be avoided because of the risk of ataxia and delirium. Sedation is moderate and lasts 30 to 60 minutes. Butorphanol provides sedation and analgesia in ruminants at doses ranging from 0.05 to 0.5 mg/kg IM or 0.05 to 0.2 mg/kg IV. Side effects include ataxia, agitation, vocalization, and stimulation of appetite. Although rarely used, chloral hydrate produces long-acting sedation to hypnosis in farm animals. It has also been used to treat tetanus because its effects are long-lasting. Dosages range from 40 to 60 mg/kg IV and up to 0.5 mg/kg orally (50 g in 1 L warm water). In swine, 0.25 mg/kg chloral hydrate can be given orally to induce sedation.

Local and Regional Anesthetic Techniques

The use of local or regional anesthetic techniques in farm animals is preferred over general anesthetic techniques because of ease of administration, minimal equipment requirements, low cost, and reduced incidence of complications. Many surgical techniques, such as an abdominal exploratory, cesarean section, umbilical surgery, dehorning, enucleation, perineal surgery, or castration, can be performed with local or regional techniques. General anesthesia is reserved for more complicated surgeries or extremely painful procedures. Unlike general anesthetic procedures, holding the patient off feed is usually unnecessary. However, in some instances it may be useful to decrease the bulk of the rumen to allow better visualization and manipulation of abdominal viscera for procedures such as ovariectomy. Lidocaine hydrochloride is the most commonly used drug in farm animal practice for local and regional anesthesia. It has an analgesic duration of 90 to 180 minutes, and less than 100 mL of a 2% solution is usually sufficient, even for a large bovine. Other local anesthetics, including bupivacaine, mepivacaine, and procaine have been used, but they are all more costly and potentially more toxic—and therefore less popular than lidocaine. None of the local anesthetics is approved for use in farm animals in the United States; therefore clients must be advised of appropriate withdrawal times (see Table 6-5).

Other drugs have been administered with lidocaine to prolong its local anesthetic effects. Epinephrine at concentrations of 5 to 20 µg/mL has been suggested to prolong local anesthesia and possibly reduce toxicity by causing vasoconstriction. However, this also increases the risk of tissue necrosis, especially at skin edges or in thin-skinned animals. Lidocaine with epinephrine should not be used for epidural administration. Hyaluronidase has been added to shorten onset time and improve anesthetic dissipation into adjacent tissues, thereby reducing the amount of lidocaine required. This is most commonly done for ocular nerve blocks.

ANESTHESIA FOR ABDOMINAL SURGERY

Regional anesthesia in the bovine is most commonly used to access the abdominal cavity. This can be accomplished by a proximal paravertebral nerve block, distal paravertebral nerve block, infiltration anesthesia,

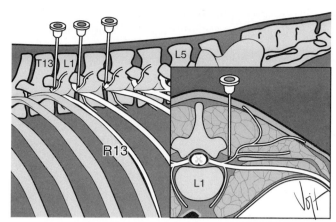

Figure 6-1 Proximal paravertebral nerve block. Note that the needles are placed just cranially to the transverse processes and less than 2.5 cm from midline.

(From Muir WW, Hubbell JAE, Skarda RT, Bednarski R: *Handbook of veterinary anesthesia*, ed 3, St Louis, 2000, Mosby.)

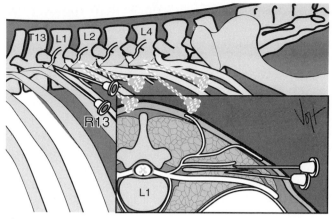

Figure 6-2 Distal paravertebral nerve block. Note that the needles are placed just above and below each transverse process, and lidocaine is infiltrated in a fan pattern.

(From Muir WW, Hubbell JAE, Skarda RT, Bednarski R: *Handbook of veterinary anesthesia*, ed 3, St Louis, 2000, Mosby.)

segmental epidural anesthesia, and (in smaller animals) high epidural anesthesia. All provide anesthesia of the flank region for abomasal displacements, rumenotomy, cesarean section, or intestinal surgery.

PROXIMAL PARAVERTEBRAL ANESTHESIA (FARQUHARSON, HALL, OR CAMBRIDGE TECHNIQUE)

Proximal paravertebral anesthesia provides excellent anesthesia of the entire flank region through blockade of the last thoracic (T13) and first two lumbar (L1 and L2) spinal nerves. The nerves are approached from the dorsal aspect of the transverse processes of the lumbar vertebrae. The ends of the transverse processes are palpated, starting caudally just in front of the tuber coxa with L5 and working cranially to the often very small, shorter, and harder-to-palpate L1. A 14-gauge, 1-inch needle is placed as a trocar 1 to 2 cm off dorsal midline, in line with the cranial aspect of the transverse process of L1 (Figure 6-1). A 5-inch, 18-gauge needle is then used to perform the nerve block through this trocar. The needle is passed ventrally until the transverse process is encountered (5 to 7 cm deep). The needle is then walked off the cranial edge of the process and passed ventrally to penetrate the transverse ligament and fascia. After penetration of the fascia, usually palpable as a "pop," 10 to 15 mL of 2% lidocaine is injected. The needle is then withdrawn 1 to 2 cm so that the tip of the needle is above the fascia, where an additional 10 to 15 mL of lidocaine is injected. The authors recommend injecting an additional 2 to 3 mL of lidocaine as the needle is slowly withdrawn through the epaxial musculature to desensitize branches of the spinal nerves. Advantages of this

technique include minimal amount of anesthetic required, a relatively large area of desensitization, no lidocaine in the incision site, and rapid onset of local anesthesia. Disadvantages of this technique include difficulty in finding landmarks in fat cattle, scoliosis and moderate ataxia, and risk of penetrating major blood vessels or the spinal canal.

DISTAL PARAVERTEBRAL ANESTHESIA (MAGDA, CAKALA, OR CORNELL TECHNIQUE)

Distal paravertebral anesthesia provides excellent anesthesia of the entire flank region of the cow through blockade of T13, L1 and L2 at the tips of the transverse processes of the lumbar vertebrae. Injections are made with an 18-gauge, 1.5-inch needle inserted parallel to the tips of the processes of L1, L2, and L4 (Figure 6-2). Ten to 20 mL of 2% lidocaine is infiltrated in a fan-shaped area dorsal to the tip of the process, after which time the needle is withdrawn until it can be redirected ventral to the process and infiltration repeated with 10 to 20 mL of lidocaine. Advantages of this technique include lack of scoliosis and ataxia, reduced risk of penetrating large blood vessels or nerves, and the use of common-sized needles. Disadvantages include the increased amount of lidocaine required, variable position of nerves leading to incomplete or inadequate anesthesia, and difficulty in locating the transverse processes in fat cows.

INFILTRATION ANESTHESIA

Infiltration of lidocaine at or around the incision site can provide adequate analgesia for most minor surgical procedures. Infiltration anesthesia is usually performed by using a line block or an inverted-L or -7 pattern. The line block is performed by making multiple subcutaneous (1 cm deep) and deep (2-7 cm deep) injections of 1 to 2 mL of 2% lidocaine along a proposed incision line. Up to 100 mL of 2% lidocaine may be required in cattle, depending on the required incision size and thickness of the body wall. Small amounts of lidocaine are used for line blocks in small ruminants, especially goats, because of their sensitivity to the drug. When possible, lidocaine should be diluted to a 1% solution with equal parts of sterile saline before injection in small ruminants. Potential disadvantages of this technique include delayed healing as a result of lidocaine in the incision site, incomplete anesthesia of the deeper layers, increased amounts of lidocaine required, length of time required to perform the block, risk of toxicity, potential for sloughing of skin (especially if epinephrine is added to the lidocaine), and inability to extend the incision during surgery without additional lidocaine infiltration.

An inverted-L or -7 pattern is used for flank laparotomy and is performed by first injecting lidocaine along the last rib and then horizontally just ventral to the transverse processes. The technique is similar to the line block, with multiple subcutaneous injections (1 cm deep) and deeper muscle injections (2 to 7 cm deep). The disadvantages are the same as for the line block, except lidocaine is not in the incision site and therefore should not interfere with healing.

SEGMENTAL EPIDURAL ANESTHESIA (ARTHUR TECHNIQUE)

Segmental epidural anesthesia can be performed for flank incisions. This is the most technically challenging spinal nerve block to perform. The local anesthetic is injected into the epidural space between L1 and L2 or between T13 and L1. A 14-gauge, 1-inch needle is placed similar to proximal paravertebral anesthesia at the cranial edge of the transverse processes of L2. An 18-gauge, 5-inch spinal needle with stylet is placed and advanced slightly cranially and ventrally between the transverse processes into the interosseous canal until a sudden change in resistance is palpated. At this point, the stylet is withdrawn and needle placement confirmed by using minimal resistance to injection or by filling the needle hub with lidocaine and advancing slowly until the lidocaine is sucked into the epidural space. If the location is correct, 8 to 10 mL lidocaine is slowly injected to provide anesthesia in an average adult bovine. If the dura is penetrated so that CSF can be aspirated from the needle, subarachnoid anesthesia should be performed, or the needle should be withdrawn 1 to 2 cm before injection. The amount of lidocaine should be reduced if subarachnoid anesthesia is performed.

Advantages of this technique include minimal desensitization of the hind limbs, good regional anesthesia of

the flank, only one injection required, and minimal lidocaine required. Disadvantages include technical difficulty, risk of trauma to the spinal cord or bleeding in the epidural space, and abnormal migration of lidocaine cranially or caudally causing respiratory difficulty (rare) or pelvic limb paresis.

ANESTHESIA FOR PERINEAL SURGERY

Anesthesia of the perineal region may be required for surgeries of areas such as the tail, vagina, vulva, anus, rectum, caudal prepuce, or scrotum; for repair of a prolapsed rectum or vagina; difficult parturition; fetal manipulation during dystocia; or perineal urethrostomy. Perineal anesthesia is also useful to control tenesmus and uterine contractions. Anesthesia of the perineal region is obtained by epidural anesthesia and is performed at the sacrococcygeal region ("caudal" or "low" epidural) or the lumbosacral region ("high" epidural).

CAUDAL EPIDURAL ANESTHESIA

The caudal epidural is commonly performed in all farm animals. It is technically easy to perform and requires no special equipment. The location is the sacrococcygeal (S5-Cx1) or first coccygeal (Cx1-Cx2) space. The S5-Cx1 interspace is caudal to the spinal cord, and only the coccygeal nerves are present. The correct location is palpated by moving the tail up and down with one hand while palpating the dorsal spinous processes of the sacrum and coccygeal vertebrae with the other hand. The most proximal moving intervertebral space is the location for drug injection (Figure 6-3). The sacrococcygeal space is generally ossified in older animals, especially in cows. The intercoccygeal space is larger in most cows,

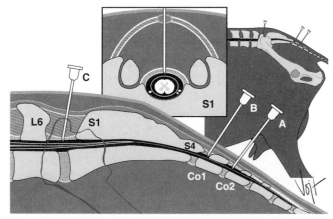

Figure 6-3 Locations for cranial and caudal epidural in a goat. The locations are similar for the cow and sheep. The sacrococcygeal location is usually ossified in the adult cow.

(From Muir WW, Hubbell JAE, Skarda RT, Bednarski R: *Handbook of veterinary anesthesia*, ed 3, St Louis, 2000, Mosby.)

thus making penetration of this interspace easier. An 18-gauge, 1.5-inch needle is used to penetrate the space directly on the dorsal midline in an adult cow. The needle is directed slightly cranially with the bevel in a lateral or cranial orientation to the animal. The needle is advanced until a "pop" is felt (usually 2 to 4 cm deep), thus indicating entrance into the epidural space. If the ventral floor is encountered, the needle is withdrawn slightly (1 cm) into the epidural space. The bevel is rotated cranially, and its position is checked by placing a few drops of lidocaine into the needle hub and waiting until the lidocaine is aspirated into the epidural space. Injection should be easy and without resistance. If previous epidurals have been performed or attempted, there may be no negative pressure to aspirate the lidocaine from the needle hub. Injection of 1 mL lidocaine per 100 kg body weight is recommended in adult cattle. This approximates 5 to 6 mL for an average adult cow. Larger doses may paralyze the spinal nerves to the hind limbs of smaller cattle, thus causing recumbency. Time to onset is usually 10 to 20 minutes, with a 30- to 150-minute duration range.

Xylazine alone or added to the lidocaine epidural has been reported to provide a longer duration of local anesthesia. Xylazine at 0.03 mg/kg diluted with lidocaine to a 5 mL volume for an adult cow can provide anesthesia of the entire perineal region, including the udder and flank. Onset of action is within 3 to 4 minutes, and duration is approximately 100 minutes. Ataxia and sedation will occur with this method, and some animals may become recumbent. The sedation provides an added benefit for agitated or fractious cattle. If animals are excited when the epidural is administered, higher xylazine doses may be required for sedation.

Xylazine (0.05 mg/kg) diluted to 5 mL in sterile water provides longer duration (up to 3 hours) of epidural anesthesia. Sedation also occurs with this method, which can be antagonized by administering intravenous tolazoline (0.3 mg/kg) without decreasing the anesthesia.

Caudal epidural anesthesia in small ruminants is performed by administering no more than 1 mL 2% lidocaine per 50 kg at the sacrococcygeal or first coccygeal space with an 18- or 20-gauge needle (see Figure 6-3).

CRANIAL EPIDURAL ANESTHESIA

Cranial epidural anesthesia ("high" epidural) can be performed for procedures as far cranial as the diaphragm, depending on the amount of local anesthetic used. A similar amount of anesthesia can also be obtained by administering larger volumes of lidocaine at the sacrococcygeal space (S5-Cx1) or the first coccygeal space (Cx1-Cx2), but ataxia and recumbency usually occur. The injection location is at the lumbosacral space (L6-S1). This L6-S1 space is palpable as a depression in the

spinal column just caudal to a line drawn between the wings of the ilium (see Figure 6-3). The block is performed with a 3- to 5-inch 18-gauge needle. Similar to the caudal epidural, the needle is advanced through the skin and musculature to a depth of approximately 10 cm, where a sudden decrease in resistance should be felt. Testing of the location and injection are similar to the caudal epidural. The dosage of lidocaine is approximately 0.5-1 mL of 2% lidocaine per 4.5 kg body weight for cattle. At either of the lower epidural locations, 40 to 150 mL (average 80 mL) may be required for adult cattle and 5 to 25 mL (average 15 mL) in calves. The volume of lidocaine injected is determined by the animal's response to the injection and the desensitization area size required by the procedure. The position of the animal affects local anesthetic distribution. Elevation of the head confines local anesthetic to the caudal region of the epidural space, whereas elevation of the hindquarters (not recommended) causes cranial migration of the anesthetic. Lateral recumbency provides lateral anesthesia, whereas dorsal recumbency provides bilateral distribution of the anesthesia. Care should be taken with high-volume infusions because improper positioning of the animal (elevated hindquarters) may lead to respiratory paralysis and death. Slow injection produces a smaller area of desensitization than does rapid injection. Cattle that are recovering from a "high" epidural should have excellent footing with their hind legs "hobbled" to prevent abduction of the hind limbs and damage to the inner thigh musculature.

The lumbosacral space is the only easily accessed epidural space in swine; therefore this site is preferred for administering a local anesthetic. The injection site is located in a similar place to that in ruminants, as a depression in the spinous processes between the wings of the ilium (Figure 6-4). Injection is made with an 18 or 20-gauge 3- to 7-inch needle. A 14-gauge, 1-inch needle may be used as a trocar. The dose for swine is the same as that for cattle (0.5-1 mL of 2% lidocaine per 4.5 kg body weight). Evidence suggests that a smaller dose may also work (1 mL per 7.5 kg, plus 1 mL for every 10-kg increase over 50 kg). Epidural xylazine has been examined in swine by using 2 mg/kg in 5 mL saline. This produced effective immobilization and analgesia for 120 minutes after administration. In sows, 1 mg/kg xylazine in 10 mL lidocaine produced anesthesia and analgesia of the hindquarters.

ANESTHESIA FOR PROCEDURES INVOLVING THE HEAD

Dehorning and ocular surgery are the two most common reasons for providing local anesthesia of the head in farm animals. Local anesthetic procedures are easily performed in standing animals in conjunction with adequate

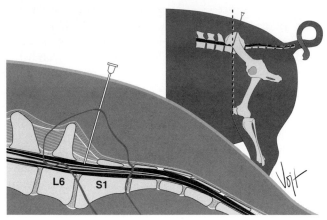

Figure 6-4   Cranial epidural in swine. Note the large amount of soft tissue overlying the lumbosacral space in the pig, necessitating the use of a long needle.

(From Muir WW, Hubbell JAE, Skarda RT, Bednarski R: *Handbook of veterinary anesthesia*, ed 3, St Louis, 2000, Mosby.)

head restraint. Occasionally, anesthesia of other areas of the head, such as the nose, lips, and face is required.

ANESTHESIA OF THE EYE

Topical anesthetics such as proparacaine hydrochloride desensitize the cornea, which relieves corneal irritation and facilitates corneal procedures. Proparacaine is approved for use in farm animals in the United States. If more invasive procedures are necessary, local anesthesia can be performed by using desensitization of the auriculopalpebral branch of the facial nerve, four-point retrobulbar injection, or a Peterson eye block.

The auriculopalpebral nerve is occasionally palpable along the zygomatic arch, rostral to the base of the auricular muscles. Infiltration of 5 to 15 mL of 2% lidocaine in this region will desensitize the nerve, thus causing akinesia (but not analgesia) of the eyelids. If necessary, the eyelids themselves can be infiltrated with 10 mL of 2% lidocaine approximately 1 cm from the edges of the dorsal and ventral lids.

The four-point retrobulbar injection will desensitize all the ocular muscles and the optic nerve. Injections are made using a 3- to 4-inch 18-gauge needle with a large curve in it. The eyelids are penetrated at the medial and lateral canthus and at the dorsal and ventral orbital rims. The needle is inserted at the medial and lateral canthus while using the finger to reflect the globe away from the needle. The needle is advanced through the conjunctiva in a curve medially to the orbital apex (7 to 10 cm). The needle is aspirated to ensure that it is not placed within the optic nerve or meninges, and a total of 15 mL of 2% lidocaine, divided between the four sites, is slowly injected as the needle is withdrawn from the orbit.

Disadvantages of this procedure include possible damage to the globe, intraneural or meningeal injection (rare but causes death), retrobulbar hemorrhage, or damage to the optic nerve. Obviously, some of these are not important if anesthesia is used for enucleation.

The Peterson eye block is performed by using a straight, or only slightly curved, 3- to 4-inch, 18-gauge needle. The needle is inserted into the most rostral aspect of the notch formed by the supraorbital process and zygomatic arch. It is advanced medially until the coronoid process of the mandible is encountered. The needle is then walked rostrally until it passes medial to the coronoid process and reaches the solid bony plate in the region of the foramen orbitorotundum. At this point, 15 mL of 2% lidocaine is slowly injected after aspirating to ensure the meninges or maxillary artery has not been penetrated. When the needle reaches the correct position, the globe is often seen to move with needle pressure. After injection, the entire globe and its associated muscles are desensitized, thus allowing proptosis of the globe. The eyelids must be desensitized separately with an auriculopalpebral block. The Peterson eye block is technically difficult to perform but has a lower risk of hemorrhage, penetration of the globe, damage to the optic nerve, or injection into the meninges.

ANESTHESIA OF THE HORNS

Anesthesia of the base of the horn for dehorning or disbudding requires anesthesia of the cornual nerve, a branch of the zygomaticotemporal nerve, which is part of the trigeminal nerve. This nerve is often palpable along the ventrolateral aspect of the frontal ridge, halfway between the lateral canthus of the eye and the base of the horn (Figure 6-5). Anesthesia is performed by using a 20-gauge, 1- or 1.5-inch needle inserted just under the frontal ridge. Five to 10 mL of 2% lidocaine is infiltrated in a fan pattern to desensitize the nerve. The nerve lies deeper (1 cm) in older animals than in young animals. Older animals will also require hemicircumferential infiltration of the caudal aspect of the horn base to anesthetize cutaneous branches of the second cervical spinal nerve.

Goats have different innervation of the horn base region. In addition to the cornual nerve, branches of the infratrochlear nerve extend to the horn base (see Figure 6-5). In adult goats, the cornual branch of the zygomaticotemporal nerve is desensitized with a 22-gauge, 1-inch needle and 2 to 3 mL of lidocaine at a location halfway between the lateral canthus of the eye and the lateral horn base, as close as possible to the ridge of the supraorbital process. The infratrochlear branches are desensitized by injecting 2 to 3 mL of lidocaine halfway between the medial canthus of the eye and the medial horn base dorsal and parallel to the dorsomedial margin

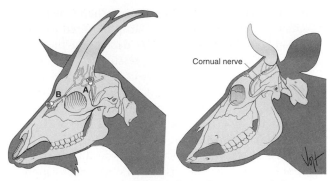

Figure 6-5 Cornual nerve block in the cow and the goat. Note the additional location for infiltration in the goat.

(From Muir WW, Hubbell JAE, Skarda RT, ;Bednarski R: *Handbook of veterinary anesthesia*, ed 3, St Louis, 2000, Mosby.)

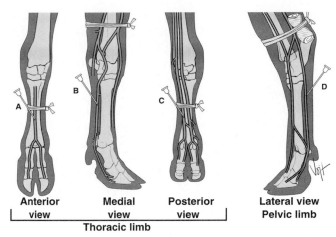

Figure 6-6 Intravenous regional anesthesia of the distal limb in the bovine. The suggested sites are only for reference; any visible or palpable vessel may be used.

(From Muir WW, Hubbell JAE, Skarda RT, Bednarski R: *Handbook of veterinary anesthesia*, ed 3, St Louis, 2000, Mosby.)

of the orbit. This infiltration should be performed as a line block because the nerve is branched. It is important to use as small an amount of lidocaine (maximum dose of 10 mg/kg) as possible in goats because of their extreme sensitivity to lidocaine toxicity. When disbudding kids younger than 14 days of age, one can divide 1 mL of 2% lidocaine between the four sites to desensitize the horn bud. Young kids should also be sedated with xylazine (up to 0.05 mg/kg IV) to minimize movement and vocalization during the procedure.

ANESTHESIA OF THE UDDER

Anesthesia of the udder can be achieved by performing a high or low caudal epidural or sometimes paravertebral nerve block. These techniques are not as easy to perform nor as safe as direct local infiltration of the teats. Placement of an elastic band around the base of the teat will hold the lidocaine in the teat for the duration of the teat surgery. Five to 10 mL of 2% lidocaine injected into the teat cistern provides anesthesia of the interior of the teat only. A ring block is performed around the base of the teat with 5 mL of 2% lidocaine for procedures that involve the external teat surface, such as laceration repair. Alternatively, 2.5 mL of 2% lidocaine can be injected into a teat vessel just below an elastic band tourniquet. All techniques provide adequate anesthesia for most procedures that involve the teats and can be performed in standing cows. The anesthetic is released into the circulation when the rubber band tourniquet is removed.

ANESTHESIA OF THE FOOT

Anesthesia of the foot may be required for debridement of severe foot abscesses, corn removal, digit amputation, or laceration repair. Anesthesia can be accomplished by performing a ring block of the limb above the surgical site; however, this provides only minimal anesthesia and is often incomplete in its distribution. For interdigital

surgery, such as corn removal, adequate anesthesia can be provided by injecting 5 to 10 mL of 2% lidocaine deeply (5 cm) approximately 2 to 3 cm proximal to the interdigital space.

The Bier block (intravenous regional anesthesia that produces effective regional limb anesthesia) requires placing a tourniquet and injecting lidocaine into the distal limb veins. Regional anesthesia is produced for as long as the tourniquet is in place. The tourniquet is placed in the midmetacarpus or metatarsus for foot surgery, and up to 30 mL of 2% lidocaine is injected into one of the following: dorsal metacarpal (metatarsal) vein, palmar (plantar) digital vein, dorsal digital vein, or lateral saphenous vein with a 20- or 22-gauge butterfly catheter (Figure 6-6). The particular vein that is used is immaterial as long as it is easily accessed. Advantages of intravenous regional anesthesia include complete anesthesia of the foot, reduced bleeding, only one injection required, a smaller amount of lidocaine required, and rapid onset of anesthesia. Disadvantages include the need for knowledge of vessel anatomy in the foot, and failure of the nerve block despite accurate penetration of the vessel. The tourniquet should be released slowly to prevent signs of lidocaine toxicity from rapid release of the lidocaine into the systemic circulation. A tourniquet can be safely left in place for up to 90 minutes without loosening.

General Anesthesia in Farm Animals

PREANESTHETIC PREPARATION

Several factors must be considered before producing anesthesia. First, feed should be withheld, if necessary, to reduce the risk of aspiration and bloating during anesthesia. The forestomach of adult cattle can hold a large quantity of feed, and fasting for at least 18 to 24 hours is recommended. Small ruminants and young ruminating cattle require slightly less fasting time; 12 hours is usually sufficient. Non-ruminant calves require minimal if any feed withholding because they are essentially monogastrics. Skipping a milk feeding is usually sufficient. Water should be withheld from adult cattle for at least 6 to 8 hours but does not need to be withheld from small ruminants and young cattle. Emergencies preclude feed restriction, but attempts should be made to decompress the rumen (Kingman tube) if the animal is thought to be at high risk for developing bloat or aspiration pneumonia. Feed restriction has the added benefit or reducing abdominal filling, thereby facilitating abdominal surgery and reducing abdominal pressure on the lungs during anesthesia. Feed restriction is known to increase vagal tone in adult cattle, thus producing bradycardia and increasing ruminal motility, which paradoxically increases the risk of regurgitation. Regardless, the benefits of feed restriction outweigh relatively rare potential problems.

A complete physical examination should be performed within 2 hours of inducing anesthesia. Evidence of respiratory or cardiovascular disease should delay anesthesia until the problem is resolved or a more diagnostic procedure (radiographs, echocardiogram) can be performed. If disease is present in an emergency situation, appropriate medical support should be available. Preanesthetic hemogram (complete blood count, serum chemistry profile) is ideal for assessing the animal's general health and organ function. A packed cell volume (PCV) and total protein are the minimum requirements prior to inducing general anesthesia. Additional blood chemical tests (pH, blood gases [PO_2, PCO_2], electrolytes) may be required in sick, debilitated or depressed animals. Correction of life-threatening abnormalities (e.g., hypovolemia, hyperkalemia) should occur prior to anesthesia.

INDUCTION OF ANESTHESIA

Induction of general anesthesia should only be attempted in animals that have received a physical examination and are properly restrained and sedated. Animals that are not properly restrained pose a physical threat to their attendants and can produce considerable damage to themselves and their environment if they react adversely to physical manipulation or anesthetic drug administration. Ideally, all animals should receive preanesthetic medication before being administered drugs to produce general anesthesia (see Sedation). This is important in fractious or dangerous animals and in sick or debilitated animals (e.g., obstructed urethra in a

goat). The administration of preanesthetic medication typically reduces the amount of drug required to induce and maintain anesthesia, thereby decreasing the potential for drug overdose and drug related adverse effects.

Induction of general anesthesia in cattle, sheep, and goats is easily produced in sedated or calm animals by intravenous administration of combinations of muscle relaxants and dissociative anesthetics (Table 6-2). Most commonly, 1 g of ketamine is added to a 1 liter bag or bottle of a 5% guaifenesin solution ("double drip"), and this combination is administered IV to effect (approximately 0.5-1.0 ml/kg). It is important not to use more concentrated solutions (>5%) of guaifenesin in cattle, sheep, or goats because it could cause significant hemolysis. Xylazine (25-50 mg) can be added to this cocktail to produce a final solution of 1 g ketamine and 25 to 50 mg of xylazine in a 1 liter bag of 5% guaifenesin ("triple drip"). This is a different formulation than that

TABLE 6-2

Intravenous Anesthesia Drug Dosages Used in Ruminants and Swine (mg/kg)*

DRUG	CATTLE	SHEEP	GOAT	SWINE
Thiopental	3-6	2-4	2-4	3-6
Propofol	2-4	2-4	2-4	2-6
Ketamine	2-4	2-4	1-3	2-4
Telazol	2-4	2-4	2-5	2-5
Guaifenesin[†]	20-50	20-50	20-50	
Thiopental	2-4	2-4	2-4	
Guaifenesin[†]	20-40		20-40	
Ketamine	0.3-0.5		0.3-0.5	
Xylazine[‡]	0.04	0.04	0.02	0.5-1.0
Ketamine	1-2	1-2	1-3	2-4
Xylazine	0.05	0.05	0.04	0.5-1.0
Telazol	1-3	1-3	1-3	1-3
Diazepam[§]	0.2	0.2	0.2	0.4
Ketamine	2-4	2-4	2-4	2-5

Xylazine	25 mg	[ruminants] approximately 0.5-	
Guaifenesin[†]	500 ml 5%	1.0 ml/kg to effect for	
Ketamine	500 mg	induction	
Telazol	500 mg	and 0.5-2 ml/kg/hr by infusion	
Ketamine	250 (2.5 ml)	1 ml/25-50 kg required, depend-	
Xylazine	250 mg	ing upon the depth of	
	(2 ml of	anesthesia	
	100 mg/ml)		

Be prepared for respiratory depression, apnea, and regurgitation that may occur in ruminants.
*Use after preanesthetic medication.
[†]Use dilute solutions (<6%) of gauifenesin in cattle, sheep, and goats.
[‡]Xylazine, 0.05 mg/lb IV, can be used to dehorn goats.
[§]Midazolam, 0.1-0.3 mg/lb IV, can be used in diazepam drug combinations.

commonly used in horses because of ruminant sensitivity to xylazine. If both formulations commonly are used by the practitioner, careful labeling is required to avoid xylazine overdose in ruminants. Triple drip is administered to animals that are more fractious or alert or have not responded adequately to preanesthetic medication. Double drip or triple drip is administered by using a standard solution administration set and produces a slow, controlled, and uneventful induction to recumbency in most animals. The bag of triple drip may be placed in an inflatable pressure sleeve and administered under pressure to hasten induction because the duration of induction to anesthesia may take as long as 5 to 10 minutes with the simple gravity technique. Care must be taken not to inadvertently administer too much of the drug cocktail (>1 ml/kg) if the latter technique is used because it may result in respiratory depression and hypotension. Furthermore, administering double or triple drip under pressure from a glass bottle or plastic container is not recommended; air may be inadvertently pumped into the venous circulation producing a pulmonary air embolus.

Smaller cattle (<200 kg), goats, sheep, and calves are generally less fractious and easier to restrain and are induced to general anesthesia by the intravenous bolus administration of various drug cocktails (see Table 6-1). The 50:50 combination of diazepam and ketamine (Ket-Val) mixed in the same syringe and administered IV at a dosage of 1 ml/15 to 20 kg generally produces rapid (1- to 2-minute) induction to anesthesia without incident. Alternatively, 1 ml/20 kg IV, of Telazol® can be administered to induce general anesthesia. Either drug cocktail (Ket-Val or Telazol®) can be administered IM at approximately twice the IV dose to produce calming to profound sedation in animals that are difficult to restrain and fractious. Small dosages of propofol (2-4 mg/kg to effect) can be used to provide additional relaxation to facilitate endotracheal intubation and induction to an inhalant anesthetic. Small ruminants that are easily restrained or are very young (days-weeks) can be mask induced to general anesthesia with halothane, isoflurane, or sevoflurane. All three inhalant drugs produce relatively rapid induction to anesthesia; sevoflurane is the fastest and most controllable but also the most expensive. An appropriately sized mask, fashioned from an empty water or detergent bottle, is connected to the Y-piece of the anesthetic hoses and slowly and gently placed over the animal's muzzle. Oxygen (3-5 L/min) should be allowed to flow for 1 to 2 minutes before gradually introducing the inhalant anesthetic (Table 6-3). Once the animal begins to show signs of anesthesia (weakness, ataxia) the anesthetic concentration should be increased to maintenance levels and maintained for the duration of the surgery or until the animal can be intubated. Although not preferred, the initial inhalant anesthetic concentra-

TABLE 6-3			
Important Characteristics of Inhalant Anesthetics in Ruminants* and Swine			
PROPERTY/ CONCENTRATION	HALOTHANE	ISOFLURANE	SEVOFLURANE
Boiling point (°C)	50	49	59
Vapor pressure (mmHg): 20°C (68°F)	243	240	160
mL vapor/mL liquid, 20°C (68°F)	227	194.7	182.7
Preservative	Present	None	None
Stability[†] in			
Soda lime	Decomposes	Stable	Decomposes?
UV light	Decomposes	Stable	Stable?
Maintenance concentration (%)	**1-2**	**1.5-2.5**	**3-4**

*Nitrous oxide (N20) is not recommended in adult cattle, sheep, and goats. It can be used in swine at 40% to 60% of the inspired concentration.
[†]All inhalant anesthetics should be scavenged.

tion may have to be increased to above maintenance concentrations in animals that are difficult to restrain and/or object to the placement of the mask. If this is done, the animal should be closely monitored for signs of respiratory depression or hypotension and immediately checked for cardiovascular depression once recumbency has been produced.

Anesthesia in swine is similar to that in small ruminants. Intravenous bolus, IM, and inhalant anesthetic techniques are used (see Table 6-1). The combination of Telazol®, ketamine, and xylazine (TKX) can be administered to produce induction of general anesthesia or for short periods of anesthesia (5-10 minutes). This combination, created by adding 4 ml of ketamine (100 mg/ml) and 1 ml of xylazine (100 mg/ml) to a 5 ml bottle of Telazol® and administering 1 ml/ 20 to 40 kg IM, produces variable degrees of sedation to anesthesia lasting for 10 to 30 minutes. The degree of sedation and depth of anesthesia depend on the dose administered and the site of drug administration, which determines the rate of drug absorption into the systemic circulation. Intramuscular injections should be performed along the back or in the shoulder area in swine. Gluteal or "ham" drug injections are not recommended because of the potential for the development of muscle inflammation and fibrosis. Small swine or heavily sedated swine can be masked induced to general anesthesia with either isoflurane or sevoflurane. Halothane is not used because of its tendency to induce malignant hyperthermia in susceptible pigs. Sevoflurane produces more rapid and controlled anesthesia, as previously discussed, and, like isoflurane, is not known to produce hyperthermia. However, it is considerably more expensive. The techniques used to induce general anesthesia by mask induction in swine are identical to those for small ruminants.

Once recumbent, adult farm animals (>100 kg) should be placed on thick foam pads or inner tubes to minimize muscle and nerve trauma and the development of myositic or nerve palsy, respectively. The front forelimb on the down side should be pulled as far forward as possible in animals placed in lateral recumbency. The shoulder should be well padded, and the head should be positioned so that it is lower than the shoulder when the animal is placed in lateral recumbency. An esophageal tube should be placed after the endotracheal tube and inflation of the endotracheal tube cuff to prevent the accumulation of regurgitated material in the pharynx and mouth in adult ruminants that are regurgitating in order.

ENDOTRACHEAL INTUBATION

Endotracheal intubation is performed digitally in adult cattle. A speculum is placed in the animal's mouth, and the jaws are separated as far as possible (18-inch Wisconsin laryngoscope blade,* Model number 04408). Care should be taken not to injure the tongue while positioning and opening the mouth. All jewelry should be removed from the hands or wrists. The left or right hand is placed into the animal's mouth until the epiglottis can be palpated. The other hand is used to insert an appropriately sized (generally determined by palpation of the trachea, 18-30 mm ID) cuffed endotracheal tube[†] into the animal's mouth under the first hand and using the first hand to guide it into the trachea. The hand, arm, and endotracheal tube should be thoroughly lubricated with the animal's saliva or a lubricant jelly (KY gel) before inserting them into the animal's mouth. The endotracheal tube should be advanced into the trachea to about the middle of the neck. Care should be taken not to advance the tube too far because this could result in endobronchial intubation and hypoxemia. The endotracheal tube should be secured at all times; because once it is in placed in the trachea, the animal usually coughs and could displace the tube. The endotracheal tube can be secured to the animal's muzzle with gauze bandage or tape to prevent it from becoming dislodged during the operative procedure. Once it is positioned, the endotracheal tube is connected to the Y-piece of the anesthetic machine hoses. The rebreathing bag on the anesthetic machine should be slowly squeezed while the endotracheal tube cuff is inflated (approximately 50-70 ml in adult cattle) until air can no longer be heard coming from the mouth. Overinflation of the

endotracheal tube cuff can result in obstruction of airflow; increased work of breathing; and respiratory distress, including pulmonary edema. A second tube should be placed into the animal's esophagus in larger cattle or in cattle that are regurgitating to control the regurgitation and prevent material from accumulating in the posterior pharynx. Positioning the animal so that the shoulder is padded and situated higher than the head and rumen when the animal is in lateral recumbency is believed to limit regurgitation and facilitate the flow of saliva out of the mouth. Positioning the animal with the head lower than the body (head down) when the animal is on its back is not recommended because the weight of the rumen and abdominal contents could severely restrict lung inflation. Finally, the tube should be removed with the cuff still inflated or partially inflated and only after the animal has begun to swallow. These latter techniques are performed to minimize the chance for aspiration of rumen contents or excessive quantities of saliva.

Several techniques have been developed for endotracheal intubation in small ruminants and swine, each with their own proponents and supposed advantages. The technique described here ensures tracheal intubation and is universally applicable to all small ruminants and swine. Anatomical differences, particularly in swine, make it extremely difficult to perform endotracheal intubation in small ruminants and swine without the use of a speculum, laryngoscope, and endotracheal tube stylet. The pharynx and larynx of small ruminants and swine are not normally visible without the aid of a speculum and laryngoscope. The animal should be positioned on its sternum, and the head should be elevated and extended straight up at a right angle to the body. The laryngoscope is advanced into the mouth until the larynx is observed and its tip is then used to hold down the epiglottis, visualizing the opening to the trachea (Figure 6-7). A 1-meter plastic or metal dowel (stylet) is placed through and should extend approximately 20 cm beyond the end of an appropriately sized (generally determined by palpation of the trachea), lubricated (KY gel), cuffed endotracheal tube (6-12 mm ID; Figure 6-8). The stylet is then placed into the mouth and visually guided through the larynx. It advances about 5 to 10 cm into the trachea, depending upon the size of the animal. The endotracheal tube is then slowly advanced over the stylet. It is rotating slowly as it approaches and passes the larynx. Care should be taken not to move the stylet once it has been positioned in the trachea to avoid unnecessary trauma and inadvertent puncture of the larynx or trachea. Once the endotracheal tube is positioned in the trachea, the stylet is removed and the endotracheal tube cuff inflated (until no air exits the mouth). It is secured to the animal's head or muzzle and connected to the Y-piece of the rebreathing hoses on the anesthetic machine.

---

*AM Bickford Co.; Wales Center, NY
[†]Bivona Inc.; Gary, IN

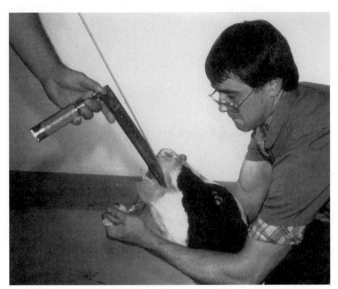

Figure 6-7 Endotracheal intubation in a calf. Note that the head and neck are extended perpendicular to the body. A long (18″) laryngoscope blade can be used to visualize the larynx and deflect the epiglottis ventrally to provide a clear view of the opening to the trachea.

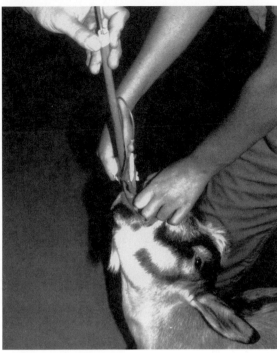

Figure 6-8 Endotracheal intubation in a goat. Note that the head and neck are extended perpendicularly to the body and that a stylet is used to stiffen the endotracheal tube for placement through the larynx into the trachea.

The animal should be administered one or two breaths of oxygen and monitored for adequate respiratory rate and volume.

Adult cattle, small ruminants, and swine are allowed to breathe spontaneously unless there are signs of respiratory depression (low rate or volume), hypoxemia (cyanosis) or respiratory distress. Ventilators are useful for longer (>1hour) procedures; otherwise respiration can be supported by manual inflation of the lungs (Ambu bag, rebreathing bag) with the animal breathing 6 to 10 times per minute to an inspiratory pressure of 20 to 30 cm H_2O.

MAINTENANCE OF ANESTHESIA

Anesthesia in cattle and small ruminants can be maintained by infusing ketamine and guaifenesin (double drip) or by administering an inhalant anesthetic (see Tables 6-2 and 6-3). The intravenous administration of double drip to effect (approx. 0.2-0.5 ml/kg/hr) will produce satisfactory anesthesia that can be maintained for several hours or longer in combination with local (line) or regional anesthesia (see Regional and Local anesthesia). The infusion of a triple drip (alpha-2 agonist, guaifenesin, ketamine) is not recommended for maintaining general anesthesia in ruminants because of its potential for producing excessive respiratory depression and bradycardia. Anesthesia in swine can be maintained by repeated injections of TKX or administration of inhalant anesthetics (see Tables 6-2 and 6-3).

Inhalant gases (nitrous oxide) and anesthesia with controlled ventilation (when possible) are recommended for complicated surgical procedures lasting more than 1 hour. The administration of nitrous oxide (N_2O) is not recommended in ruminants because of its potential for producing bloat and diffusion hypoxia. Nitrous oxide is relatively insoluble in the blood in comparison to oxygen and inhalant anesthetics and diffuses rapidly into gas-filled compartments such as the rumen. Nitrous oxide can be used safely in swine and young ruminants (<3-4 months) before the rumen becomes active. Inspired concentrations should not exceed 70% of the total inspired gas flow and generally range from 50% to 70% (e.g., 50% N_2O + 50% O_2).

Halothane (1%-2%),* isoflurane (1.5-3.0%),* and sevoflurane (2.5-4.0%)* in oxygen (20-50 ml/kg) can be safely used in cattle, sheep, and goats, and isoflurane and sevoflurane are suitable and safe in swine because they are not likely to cause malignant hyperthermia (Figure 6-9). All three drugs possess different physical-chemical properties, thus resulting in clinically relevant differences in their anesthetic characteristics (see Table 6-2). Halothane is the least expensive inhalant anesthetic

---

*Mallard Medical Inc.; Irvine, CA

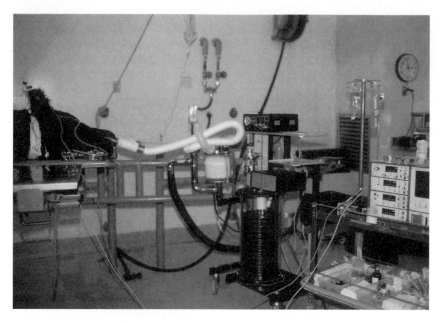

Figure 6-9   Inhalation anesthesia in large ruminants can be facilitated by using a large animal breathing circuit that permits spontaneous or controlled ventilation.

but is noted for its comparative potential to produce cardiovascular depression, sensitize the myocardium to catecholamine-induced arrhythmias, and produce hyperthermia in swine. Sevoflurane is more controllable than halothane or isoflurane and produces the fastest induction to and recovery from anesthesia. Its cardiorespiratory effects are similar to isoflurane. All three drugs can produce significant respiratory and cardiovascular depression if the patient is not closely monitored during anesthesia. Eye signs are a reasonable method of monitoring anesthetic depth during inhalant anesthesia: eyeballs rotated ventrally and medially and/or nystagmus suggest a light plane of anesthesia. Eyeballs minimally rotated medially or located centrally with normal pupil size suggest a surgical plane of anesthesia. Eyeballs centrally located with a dilated pupil suggest a deep plane of anesthesia or excessive anesthesia. Animals occasionally will become light during the maintenance phase of anesthesia and require a transient increase in the rate of infusion of double drip or an increase in the inhalant anesthetic vaporizer setting. Alternatively, a low intravenous dose of Ket-Val (1 ml/200 kg) or thiopental (0.25-0.5 mg/kg) can be administered to restore an appropriate anesthetic depth.

PERIOPERATIVE AND OPERATIVE CONSIDERATIONS

The perioperative and operative considerations in cattle, sheep, goats, and swine are similar to those in other species and emphasize appropriate time and method of extubation (patient swallowing, cuff inflated, sternal position if possible), pain management, fluid therapy, patient monitoring, and anticipation of common anesthetic-associated species-specific mishaps.

Pain management is an important consideration in any animal subjected to surgery. Attempts should be made to categorize the intensity (mild, moderate, severe) of pain the animal is likely to suffer (based on the extent and type of surgery) before surgery. Analgesics should be prescribed based upon the presumed severity of pain and administered several hours before inducing anesthesia (preemptive analgesia)—intraoperatively and postoperatively, if necessary. Nonsteroidal analgesic drugs (NSAIDs) can be administered for mild pain, alpha-2 agonists or opioids for moderate pain, and opioids in combination with local anesthetic procedures for severe pain (Table 6-4). The appropriate preemptive use of analgesic drugs reduces stress and the need for increased dosages of injectable or inhaled anesthetics, thereby reducing the risk of anesthesia. Opioids can be administered intraoperatively or postoperatively to treat breakthrough pain. Lidocaine can be added to the intravenous fluids and administered by infusion (25-50 µg/kg/min) to treat pain and reduce the anesthetic requirements. Drug withdrawal times must be considered depending upon the circumstances, and clinicians must adhere strictly to them (Table 6-5).

All patients to be anesthetized should have an intravenous catheter placed in a peripheral vein for rapid IV access and administration of fluids and drugs. Fluid

TABLE 6-4

Analgesic Drugs Used to Treat Pain in Ruminants and Swine (mg/kg)

DRUG	CATTLE	SHEEP/GOAT	SWINE
Aspirin	100 PO q12h	100 PO q12h	10 PO q4h
Phenylbutazone	NA	10 PO	NA
Flunixin meglumine	1.0 IM	1.0 IM	1.0 IM
Butorphanol	0.005 IM	0.005 IM	0.1 IM
Buprenorphine	NA	0.005 IM q12h	0.005-0.01 IM q12h
Meperidine	2.0 IM	0.5 IM	2.0 IM q4h
Morphine	NR	≤10 mg IM total dose	0.2 IM
Oxymorphone	0.005 IM	0.005 IM	0.02 IM
Xylazine	0.1 IM	0.05-0.1 IM	1.0 IM

NA, not available.
NR, not recommended.

therapy is rarely indicated or needed for surgical procedures that last less than 1 hour, during which little or no blood is lost. However, longer procedures require fluid therapy to replace insensible losses, counteract the hypotensive effects of anesthetic drugs and ensure appropriate tissue perfusion. Standard fluid administration rates of 10 ml/kg/hour of a balanced electrolyte solution (lactated or acetated ringers) can be safely administered to most patients but should not exceed a total volume of more than 20 ml/kg unless there has been significant blood loss (>20 ml/kg). Patients should receive 3 mL of a balanced electrolyte solution for every 1 mL of blood lost. Patients subjected to surgical procedures expected to result in significant blood loss (>20 ml/kg; 20% blood volume) should be administered a colloid (10 ml/kg; 1:1 for blood lost). Every attempt should be made to maintain the packed cell volume (PCV) greater than 20% (Hb >6 g/dL). A low PCV in conjunction with hypotension can result in tissue ischemia and hypoxia and thus lead to muscle weakness; prolonged recovery from anesthesia; and a variety of postoperative complications, including blood clotting abnormalities, seizures, diarrhea, renal failure, and death. Every attempt should be made to minimize blood loss in patients with a PCV less than 20%, and blood or blood substitutes (Oxyglobin;® 10-15 ml/kg) should be administered if the PCV falls below 15%. Blood substitutes are currently extremely expensive (approx. $1.00/ml), which makes their use impractical for all but selective procedures. Colloids are an excellent alternative to balanced electrolyte solutions when blood is not available and the administration of Oxyglobin® is impractical. Hetastarch,® a colloid, can be administered in quantities averaging no more than 10 to 20 ml/kg or in volumes equal to the amount of blood lost. Less potential to produce hypothermia and dilute plasma elements (PCV, TP, and serum electrolytes) exists because of the smaller volumes required in comparison

TABLE 6-5

Approximate Withdrawal Times for Anesthetic Drugs in Ruminants and Swine*

DRUG	WITHDRAWAL TIME		COMMENTS
	MEAT	MILK	
Diazepam	7 days	3 days	
Midazolam	7 days	3 days	
Xylazine	7 days	3 days	Withdrawal times established in Canada
Acepromazine	7 days	2 days	Withdrawal times established in Canada
Thiopental	4 days	2 days	Drug accumulation may occur in fat
Butorphanol	>3 days	>3 days	Believed to be rapidly eliminated
Morphine	>3 days	>3 days	Believed to be rapidly eliminated
Oxymorphone	>3 days	>3 days	Believed to be rapidly eliminated
Lidocaine	3 days	2 days	Rapidly eliminated in sheep
Mepivacaine	3 days	2 days	Rapidly eliminated in sheep
Ketamine	2 days	2 days	Short half-life in cattle (<1 hr) and swine (<3 hr)
Guaifenesin	>2 days	>2 days	Rapid elimination in ruminants
Inhalant Anesthetics†			
Halothane	>3 days	>3 days	
Isoflurane	>3 days	>3 days	
Sevoflurane	>3 days	>3 days	

*Modified from: Papich MG: Drug residue considerations for anesthetics and adjunctive drugs in food-producing animals. CR Swanson: *Vet Clin North Am: Food Animal Pract*, Philadelphia, 1996, WB Saunders.
†Rapid elimination in expired gases; temporary accumulation in fat.

to balanced electrolyte solutions. Colloids also help keep fluid within the vascular compartment, thereby limiting tissue edema.

The three most common mishaps encountered during or after anesthesia include hypoventilation, hypotension, and development of cardiac arrhythmias. All of these problems can be detected with appropriate portable monitoring equipment, including the use of portable pH* and blood gas,[†] ECG,[‡] and blood pressure[§] analyzers. This type of equipment should be available and routinely employed in all but the shortest surgical procedures. Hypoventilation can be detected by an increase in the arterial concentration of carbon dioxide ($PaCO_2$ >60 mm Hg) and should be treated by assisted or controlled ventilation (Ambu bag; anesthetic machine) until adequate breathing resumes. The administration of respiratory stimulants (doxapram HCl 1-5 mg/kg IV), although not routinely recommended, may be helpful in patients suffering from anesthetic-induced respiratory depression or that have received an alpha-2 agonist (xylazine, medetomidine).

Bradycardia and cardiac rhythm disturbances should be treated with anticholinergics (atropine, glycopyrrolate) (see Table 6-1) and antiarrhythmic drugs, respectively. Atrial and ventricular premature depolarizations and atrial fibrillation are the most common cardiac arrhythmias in ruminants after sinus bradycardia and tachycardia. Ventricular arrhythmias are treated with lidocaine (0.5-1.0 ml/kg IV), whereas atrial fibrillation can be treated with quinidine (0.2-0.5 mg/kg IV). Cardiac arrhythmias are uncommon in swine but are treated similarly to those in ruminants. Most cardiac arrhythmias in ruminants and swine do not require therapy and resolve shortly after anesthesia is terminated. Short periods (<5 minutes) of mild hypotension (mean arterial blood pressure <60 mm Hg) are generally inconsequential, but more severe hypotension (<40 mm Hg) for longer periods can result in dementia, prolonged difficult recovery from anesthesia, seizures, hypothermia, shock, and death. Mean arterial blood pressure should be maintained above 70 mm Hg. Fluid therapy in combination with the judicious use of pressors (ephedrine, 0.1-0.25 mg/kg IV) when needed will help maintain arterial blood pressure within acceptable limits. Either dopamine or dobutamine (0.05-2.0 µg/kg/min) can be administered by infusion during more involved and prolonged surgical procedures to help maintain arterial blood pressure and tissue blood flow (cardiac output). Epinephrine (0.1 ml/10 kg of 1:1000 solution) should

be administered to any patient that develops bradycardia and weak pulse or pulselessness.

The key to safe anesthesia is familiarity with a select group of anesthetic drugs, knowing what can go wrong, and having appropriate therapies available to treat these problems when/if they occur.

AMDUCA Regulations and Anesthetic Drug Concerns

Very few anesthetic drugs have been approved for use in food-producing animals. Therefore almost all anesthetic drugs are used in an extra-label manner, and withdrawal times for meat and milk are not available or approved. Fortunately, the Food and Drug Administration (FDA) approved extra-label drug use in farm animals under the Animal Medicinal Drug Use Clarification Act (AMDUCA) in 1994. This act allows veterinarians to use drugs in an extra-label manner provided a valid veterinarian-client-patient relationship (VCPR) exists. The valid VCPR is defined as the following:

1. The veterinarian has assumed responsibility for making clinical judgments regarding the health of the animal(s) and the need for medical treatment, and the client has agreed to follow the veterinarian's instruction.
2. The veterinarian has sufficient knowledge of the animal(s) to initiate at least a general or preliminary diagnosis of the medical condition of the animal(s). This means that the veterinarian has recently seen and is personally acquainted with the keeping and care of the animal(s) by virtue of an examination of the animal(s) or by medically appropriate and timely visits to the premises where the animal(s) are kept.
3. The veterinarian is readily available for follow-up evaluation in the event of adverse reactions or failure of the treatment regimen.

Use of drugs in an extra-label manner without fulfillment of the above requirements is a violation of the AMDUCA regulations and is considered illegal by the FDA.

Fortunately, reported residues from anesthetic drugs are rare. This may be caused in part by the rapid metabolism of most anesthetic drugs, administration by ventilation or intravenously, which speeds metabolism and elimination, low doses of anesthetic drugs, use of local anesthetics in the majority of cases, and minimal surveillance for anesthetic drugs in residue testing. Unlike many antibiotics made available to producers, anesthetic drugs

---

*I-Stat,® I-Stat Corp.; Princeton, NJ
[†]IRMA,® Diametrics Medical Inc.; St Paul, MN
[‡]Heska,® Prospect Parkway; Fort Collins, CO
[§]Datascope® Corp.; Paramus, NJ

are used directly by veterinarians so that the possibility of uninformed use is reduced.

Very few anesthetic drugs are approved for use in farm animals in the United States. Those known to the authors include azaperone, lidocaine, methoxyflurane, pentobarbital, and thiamylal. Xylazine is approved for use in cattle in Canada and the United Kingdom, and acepromazine is also approved for use in cattle in Canada. The approved drugs either have withdrawal times on the label, or no withdrawal times are established. Some drugs were approved by the FDA long before concerns about drug residues were commonplace. The remaining anesthetic drugs used in farm animal anesthesia are used in an extra-label manner. Some are approved for use in other animal species, whereas others are approved only for use in humans. The veterinarian is responsible for recommending adequate withdrawal times to protect humans from drug residues in meat or milk and to protect the producer from penalties caused by drug residues (see Table 6-5).

Withdrawal times for extra-label drug use can be calculated from the drug half-life and pharmacokinetic data. Drug withdrawal times are usually based on the principle of ten plasma half-lives. This provides an estimate of the amount of time it takes 99.9% of the drug to be eliminated from the plasma. This principle does not take into account the possibility of drug concentration in tissues such as liver or kidney. Fortunately, anesthetic drugs are not known to concentrate in certain tissues, so the principle of ten half lives is accurate. Compensation must be made for animals with diseases that may affect drug clearance (liver disease, renal disease, respiratory compromise). Most anesthetic drugs have very short half-lives, so waiting 96 to 120 hours is usually enough to allow most drugs to clear from the body of healthy animals.

A very useful source of information about withdrawal times is the Food Animal Residue Avoidance Databank (FARAD). This computerized database is supported by the government and provides information about residue tolerances, pharmacokinetics, and recommended withdrawal times. FARAD can be reached through their website at www.farad.org, by telephone at 888-USFARAD, or by phone at (919) 829-4431 or (916) 752-7507.

RECOMMENDED READINGS

Arthur GH: Some notes on a preliminary trial of segmental epidural anesthesia of cattle, *Vet Rec* 68: 254-256, 1956.

Baker JS: Dehorning goats, *Bovine Pract* 2: 33-39, 1981.

Bednarski RM, McGuirk SM: Bradycardia associated with fasting in cattle (Abstract), *Vet Surg* 15: 458, 1986.

Benson GJ, Thurmon JC: Anesthesia of swine under field conditions, *J Am Vet Med Assoc* 174: 594-596, 1979.

Bhokre AP, Deshpande KS: Experimental study on effect of hyaluronidase in pudic nerve block in bovines, *Indian Vet J* 56: 872-874, 1979.

Bogan JA, Weaver AD: Lidocaine concentrations associated with intravenous regional anesthesia of the distal limb of cattle, *Am J Vet Res* 39: 1672-1673, 1978.

Booth NH: Anesthesia in the pig, *Fed Proc* 28: 1547-1552, 1969.

Bristol D: Teat and udder surgery in dairy cattle, part I, *Compend Cont Educ Pract Vet* 11: 868-872, 1989.

Brock KA, Heard DJ: Field anesthesia techniques in small ruminants, part I: local analgesia, *Compend Cont Educ Pract Vet* 7: S417-S425, 1985.

Brody MD: Congress entrusts veterinarians with discretionary extra-label use, *J Am Vet Med Assoc* 205: 1366-1370, 1994.

Browne TG: The technique of nerve-blocking for dehorning cattle, *Vet Rec* 50: 1336-1337, 1938.

Butler WF: Innervation of the horn region in domestic ruminants, *Vet Rec* 80: 490-492, 1967.

Cakala S: A technique for the paravertebral lumbar block in cattle, *Cornell Vet* 51: 64-67, 1961.

Caron JP, LeBlanc PH: Caudal epidural analgesia in cattle using xylazine, *Can J Vet Res* 53: 486-489, 1989.

Caron JP, LeBlanc PH: Epidural analgesia in cattle using xylazine (abstract), *Proc Am Coll Vet Anesth*, San Francisco, 1988.

Elmore RG: Food-animal regional anesthesia, bovine blocks: epidural, *Vet Med Small Anim Clin* 75: 1017-1029, 1980.

Elmore RG: Food-animal regional anesthesia, bovine blocks: intravenous limb block, *Vet Med Small Anim Clin* 75: 1835-1834, 1980.

Elmore RG: Food-animal regional anesthesia; porcine blocks: lumbosacral (epidural), *Vet Med Small Anim Clin* 76: 387-388, 1981.

Estill CT: Intravenous local analgesia of the bovine lower leg, *Vet Med Small Anim Clin* 72: 1499-1502, 1977.

Farquharson J: Paravertebral lumbar anesthesia in the bovine species, *J Am Vet Med Assoc* 97: 54-57, 1940.

Framstad T, Austad R, Knaevelsrud T: Epidural anesthesia of sows: techniques and dosage for obstetric procedures, *Norsk Veterinaertidsskrift* 102: 363-369, 1990.

Getty R: Epidural anesthesia in the hog—its technique and application, *Am Vet Med Assoc Sci Proc 100th Annu Mtg*, New York, 1966.

Gray PR: Anesthesia in goats and sheep, II: general anesthesia, *Compend Cont Educ Pract Vet* 8: S127-S135, 1986.

Gray PR, McDonell WN: Anesthesia in goats and sheep, part I: local analgesia. *Compend Cont Educ Pract Vet* 8: S33-S38, 1986.

Hall LW: Local analgesia. In Hall LW: *Wright's veterinary anesthesia and analgesia*, ed 7, London, 1971, Bailliere Tindall.

Hare WCD: A regional method for the complete anaesthetization and immobilization of the bovine eye and its associated structures, *Can J Comp Med* 21: 228-234, 1957.

Harris T: Caudal epidural anaesthesia in the ewe, *In Practice* 13: 234-235, 1991.

Heavner JE, Teske RH: Legal implications of the extra-label use of drugs in food animals, *Vet Clin North Amer Food Anim Pract* 2: 517-525, 1986.

Hopcroft SC: Technique of epidural anaesthesia in experimental sheep, *Aust Vet J* 43: 213-214, 1967.

Hopkins TJ: The clinical pharmacology of xylazine in cattle, *Aust Vet J* 48: 109-112, 1972.

Hull BL: Personal communication. August 1, 2001.

Knight AP: Intravenous regional anaesthesia of the bovine foot, *Bovine Pract* 1: 11-15, 1980.

Ko JCH, Althouse GC, Hopkins SM et al: Effects of epidural administration of xylazine or lidocaine on bovine uterine motility and perineal analgesia, *Theriogenology* 32: 779-786, 1989.

Ko JCH, Thurmon JC, Benson JG et al: A new drug combination for use in porcine cesarean section, *Vet Med Food Anim Pract* May: 466-472, 1993.

Ko JCH, Thurmon JC, Benson JG et al: Evaluation of analgesia produced by epidural injection of detomidine and xylazine in swine, *J Vet Anesth* 19: 56-60, 1992.

Johnson R, Lopez MJ, Hendrickson DA, Kruse-Elliott KT: Cephalad distribution of three differing volumes of new methylene blue injected into the epidural space in adult goats, *Vet Surg* 25: 448-451, 1996.

LeBlanc MM, Hubbell JAE, Smith HC: The effect of xylazine hydrochloride on intrauterine pressure in the cow and the mare, *Proc Annu Mtg Soc Theriogenol*, Denver, 1984.

Link RP, Smith JC: Comparison of some local anaesthetics in cattle, *J Am Vet Med Assoc* 129: 306-309, 1956.

Lopez MJ, Johnson R, Hendrickson DA, Kruse-Elliott KT: Craniad migration of differing doses of new methylene blue injected into the epidural space after death of calves and juvenile pigs, *Am J Vet Res* 58: 786-790, 1997.

Modransky P, Welker B: Management of teat lacerations and fistulae, *Vet Med* 88: 995-1000, 1993.

Moore DC: An evaluation of hyaluronidase in local and nerve block analgesia: a review of 519 cases, *Anesthesiology* 11: 470-484, 1950.

Morishima HO, Pederson H, Finster M et al: Toxicity of lidocaine in adult, newborn, and fetal sheep, *Anesthesiology* 55: 57-60, 1981.

Muir WW, Hubbell JAE, Skarda RT, Bednarski R: Local anesthesia in cattle, sheep, goats, and pigs. In Muir WW: *Handbook of veterinary anesthesia*, ed 3, St Louis, 2000, Mosby.

Nelson DR, RS Ott, GJ Benson et al: Spinal analgesia and sedation of goats with lignocaine and xylazine, *Vet Rec* 105: 278-280, 1979.

Nicoll JMV, Treuren B, Acharya PA et al: Retrobulbar anesthesia: the role of hyaluronidase, *Anesth Analg* 65: 1324-1328, 1986.

Papich MG: Drug residue considerations for anesthetics and adjunctive drugs in food-producing animals, *Vet Clin North Amer Food Anim Pract* 12: 693-706, 1996.

Peterson DR: Nerve block of the eye and associated structures, *J Am Vet Med Assoc* 118: 145-148, 1951.

Powell JD, Denhart JW, Lloyd WE: Effectiveness of tolazoline in reversing xylazine-induced sedation in calves, *J Am Vet Med Assoc* 212: 90-92, 1998.

Prentice DE, Wyn-Jones G, Jones RS et al: Intravenous regional anaesthesia of the bovine foot, *Vet Rec* 94: 293-295, 1974.

Riviere JE: Pharmacologic principles of residue avoidance for veterinary practitioners, *J Am Vet Med Assoc* 198: 809-816, 1991.

St Jean G, Skarda RT, Muir WW et al: Caudal epidural analgesia induced by xylazine administration in cows, *Am J Vet Res* 51: 1232-1236, 1990.

Scarratt WK, Troutt HF: Iatrogenic lidocaine toxicosis in ewes, *J Am Vet Med Assoc* 188: 184-185, 1986.

Scott PR: Extradural analgesia for field surgery in sheep, *Compend Cont Educ Pract Vet* 22: S68-S75, 2000.

Skarda RT: Techniques of local analgesia in ruminants and swine, *Vet Clin North Amer Food Anim Pract* 2: 621-663, 1986.

Skarda RT: Local and regional anesthesia in ruminants and swine, *Vet Clin North Amer Food Anim Pract* 12: 579-626, 1996.

Skarda RT: Local and regional anesthetic techniques: ruminants and swine. In Lumb WV, Jones EW: *Veterinary Anesthesia*, ed 3, Baltimore, 1996, Williams & Wilkins.

Skarda RT, Muir WW: Segmental lumbar epidural analgesia in cattle, *Am J Vet Res* 40: 52-57, 1979.

Skarda RT, St Jean G, Muir WW et al: Influence of tolazoline on caudal epidural administration of xylazine in cattle, *Am J Vet Res* 51: 556-560, 1990.

Spaulding CE: Procedures for dehorning the dairy goat, *Vet Med Small Anim Clin* 72: 228-230, 1977.

Strade A: Epidural anaesthesia in young pigs: dosage in relation to the length of the vertebral column, *Acta Vet Scand* 9: 41-49, 1968.

Symonds HW, CB Mallison: The effect of xylazine and xylazine followed by insulin on blood glucose and insulin in the dairy cow, *Vet Rec* 102: 27-29, 1978.

Symonds HW: The effect of xylazine upon hepatic glucose production and blood flow rate in the lactating dairy cow, *Vet Rec* 99: 234-236, 1976.

Thurmon JC, Lin HC, Tranquilli WJ et al: A comparison of yohimbine and tolazoline as antagonist xylazine sedation in calves (Abstract), *Vet Surg* 18: 170-171, 1989.

Thurmon JC, Nelson DR, Hartsfield SM, Rumore CA: Effects of xylazine hydrochloride on urine in cattle, *Aust Vet J* 54: 178-180, 1978.

Thurmon JC, Sarr R, Denhart JW: Xylazine sedation antagonized with tolazoline, *Compend Cont Educ Pract Vet* 21: S11-S20, 1999.

Uggla A, Lindqvist Å: Acute pulmonary oedema as adverse reaction to the use of xylazine in sheep, *Vet Rec* 113: 42, 1983.

Valverde A, Doherty TJ, Dyson D, Valliant AE: Evaluation of pentobarbital as a drug for standing sedation in cattle, *Vet Surg* 18: 235-238, 1989.

Waterman AE, Livingston A: Analgesic activity and respiratory effects of butorphanol in sheep, *Res Vet Sci* 51: 19-23, 1991.

Watson D: Hyaluronidase, *Br J Anaesth* 71: 422-425, 1993.

Wheat JD: New landmark for cornual nerve block, *Vet Med* 45: 29-30, 1950.

CHAPTER 7

POSTOPERATIVE MANAGEMENT

Allen J. Roussel

Little has been written about proper postoperative nutritional management of the ruminant patient, even though all successful veterinary surgeons recognize its importance. In the absence of data from controlled clinical trials, this chapter attempts to record contemporary recommendations for postoperative feeding and nutritional support and is based largely upon the author's opinions and experiences. Nevertheless, the recommendations made consider the physiology and pathophysiology of the relevant animal species and their clinical syndromes. The focus is on strategies for returning the gastrointestinal tract to normal function in the immediate postoperative period with less attention on specific long-term nutritional needs of the patient. More attention must be given to the nutritional needs of neonates and debilitated patients immediately after surgery, including partial and total parenteral nutrition. The nutritional support of these critical care patients is beyond the scope of this chapter.

Evaluation of Gastrointestinal Function

Evaluation of the gastrointestinal tract, especially the forestomachs and abomasum, is fundamental to postoperative evaluation of a ruminate patient. During the immediate postoperative period, the most important gastrointestinal tract features to monitor are gastrointestinal fill, motility, and microflora.

GASTROINTESTINAL FILL

In most surgical cases, the forestomachs are less full than normal because of anorexia or intentional preoperative fasting. Notable exceptions include vagal indigestion, carbohydrate engorgement, and obstructive diseases of the gastrointestinal tract. As appetite returns postoperatively, the rumenoreticulum and eventually the entire tract regain the appropriate fill. Gastrointestinal fill can best be evaluated by observing the abdominal contour facing the animal's rear, combined with rectal palpation in cattle or transabdominal palpation and ultrasound examination in small ruminants. Extensive discussion of evaluation of abdominal distension can be found elsewhere. The most important abnormal contours of postoperative patients include the following: 1) dorsal and ventral distension on the left with ventral distension on the right; 2) prominent dorsal distension on the left with ventral distension on the right; and 3) bilateral ventral distension.

Dorsal and Ventral Distension on the Left with Ventral Distension on the Right

Dorsal and ventral distension on the left with ventral distension on the right indicates rumenoreticular distension—with or without abomasal distension—that is often, but not exclusively, caused by vagal indigestion. Rectal palpation of a full rumen confirms the assessment. Deep palpation of the right ventral flank is recommended to determine whether the abomasum is involved, but experience indicates a distended ventral sac of the rumen can also be palpated in that area. Sonographic examination and visualization of an enlarged fluid-filled abomasum confirms abomasal distension. Evaluating plasma electrolyte values is often necessary to determine whether the abomasum is functioning properly. Hypochloridemia and alkalosis indicate abomasal outflow failure, but postoperative intravenous fluid therapy may obfuscate interpretation of this important preoperative test in the postoperative period.

Prominent Dorsal Distension on the Left with Ventral Distension on the Right

Prominent dorsal distension on the left with ventral distension on the right usually indicates the same functional failures as the first abdominal contour, with the additional problem of free gas bloat or eructation failure. This can be confirmed by rectal palpation and passing an orogastric tube. Periruminal abscess and acites are two uncommon causes of this contour that must be differentiated from vagal indigestion. A periruminal abscess may occupy the left paralumbar fossa, thus giving the external appearance of bloat. Often, the diagnosis is missed or delayed because the history includes bloating in the past, which tends to lead the examiner to assume the distention continues to be caused by ruminal typany. There may also be a history of bloat treated with needle trocarization or intraruminal injection of antisurfactant products or by rumenotomy. Through the paralumbar fossa, the structure may even feel like a gas-filled rumen because of gas in the abscess. However, upon rectal examination, the examiner is unable to pass a hand between the rumen and left abdominal wall, and the abscess usually feels firmer than a rumen. Sonographic examination per rectum or transabdominally is useful, and centesis of the mass is confirmatory. In ascites secondary to uroperitoneum or peritonitis, the large amount of peritoneal fluid can push a rather small gas-filled rumen into the left paralumbar fossa and give the external appearance of rumen distension with bloat. Rectal palpation and abdominal sonography or centesis is confirmatory.

Bilateral Ventral Distention

Bilateral ventral distention usually indicates free abdominal fluid such as that accompanying uroperitoneum or diffuse peritonitis. It is similar to the second shape but without the dorsal distension and yields a more symmetrical shape. Sonography can differentiate abdominal fluid from intestinal ileus, another possible cause of this contour. Abdominocentesis will allow characterization of the fluid and definitive diagnosis.

The relationships between ruminal fill and feed intake and ruminal fill and fecal production are important to consider. If the rumenoreticulum fills rapidly with dehydration present or commensurate fecal production absent during the postoperative period, there is most likely a dysfunction of the forestomachs or abomasum. As mentioned previously, plasma electrolytes are often useful in assessing abomasal outflow, which may indicate abnormal abomasal motility, intestinal hypomotility, or obstruction. Other means of indirectly assessing abomasal and intestinal motility are auscultation, rectal palpation, and ultrasonography. The absence of gut sounds is a more reliable sign than the presence of sounds. The presence of sounds emanating from one area of the gastrointestinal tract does not mean that the other areas of the tract are moving, nor does it prove that the area producing sounds is functioning properly. However, the total absence of gut sounds can be a foreboding sign. Rectal palpation of the intestines does not detect motility, but fluid-filled intestines indicate functional or physical obstruction of the intestinal tract.

GASTROINTESTINAL MOTILITY

As defined in human medicine, postoperative ileus is abnormal motility of the gastrointestinal tract that follows almost every major surgical procedure, especially abdominal surgery. A postoperative paralytic ileus is a pathologic ileus that occurs after some surgical procedures and causes clinical signs and serious complications. In cattle, the rumen usually continues to contract during standing surgery; postoperative ruminal paralytic ileus is not usually a problem unless ruminal stasis was present prior to surgery. However, other parts of the ruminant GI tract are susceptible to ileus. No studies have been performed to define the duration of postoperative ileus in the different parts of the gastrointestinal tract of ruminants. In most species, the small intestine recovers within the first 24 hours and is followed closely by the stomach. The large intestine is the last region to recover. Understanding that gastrointestinal motility dysfunction always follows surgery and recognizing when expected "postoperative ileus" turns into pathologic and serious "postoperative paralytic ileus" is important.

Evaluation of gastrointestinal motility involves auscultation and palpation. Intestinal and abomasal sounds can be ausculted on the right side and ventrum, respectively. Rumenoreticular motility can be assessed by auscultation or by placing a fist in the left paralumbar fossa to feel the contractions. When evaluating ruminal contractions, one should note both the frequency and strength of contractions. The author prefers palpation to auscultation for initial assessment of ruminal motility. The normal rumen contracts about 2 to 3 times every 2 minutes. More complete evaluation of the rumen can be accomplished by combining auscultation and palpation through the left paralumbar fossa as well as rectally. In addition to frequency and strength of contractions, the physical character of the ruminal contents can be appreciated. A sutured surgical incision in the left paralumbar fossa, often present in postsurgical patients, may complicate the execution of auscultation and palpation in this area. The rumen has two contractile cycles that are called *primary* and *secondary*. The primary cycle is associated with mixing ingesta, while the secondary is associated with eructation. The primary cycle stratifies ingesta so the firm fibrous material floats in a mat on top of ruminal liquid. Small particles exit the rumen while larger ones are retained. Plant fibers more than 0.5 cm long in the feces indicate abnormal ruminal contractile activity. The primary cycle is under vagal parasympathetic control. Factors that stimulate contractions include feeding, low environmental temperature, and a slight distension sufficient to stimulate low threshold receptors in the rumen. The low threshold receptors can sometimes be exploited by pumping water and gruel into an empty rumen until mild distension is achieved. This helps stimulate ruminal contractions in anorectic ruminants. Factors that depress ruminal contractile activity include depression, fever, pain, endotoxin, volatile fatty acids, and abdominal distension sufficient to stimulate high threshold receptors. Ruminal motility can sometimes be improved by physically or pharmacologically reversing one or more of these inhibitory factors. Because these stimuli and suppressors of ruminal activity are mediated through the vagus nerve, an intact vagus is required for them to have an effect. Hypocalcemia reduces ruminal contractility by reducing the contractility of smooth muscle fibers irrespective of neural input.

Secondary ruminal contractions result in eructation of ruminal gas. They occur about every 2 minutes and are independent of the primary cycle contractions. Secondary contractions are stimulated by moderate distension and inhibited by severe distension. The secondary cycle can most easily be recognized by the occurrence of an eructation coincident with a contraction. Rumination is a specialized form of secondary contraction stimulated by coarse material in the reticulum and rumen. Rumination may actually be a source of pleasure for ruminants. Subjectively, the occurrence of rumination is a positive prognostic sign in the postoperative patient and is always a welcome sight in the eyes of this author.

The motility of the remainder of the ruminant gastrointestinal tract is similar to the nonruminant. The vagus nerve plays a significant role in controlling abomasal motility, but the intestinal tract is controlled principally by locally-produced substances and the enteric nervous system. In diseased animals, external factors such as electrolyte imbalances, inflammation, and endotoxemia can affect intestinal motility. In contrast to the simple and direct techniques for assessing ruminal motility, techniques for assessing abomasal and intestinal motility are indirect and not completely reliable. Auscultation, as described above, is perhaps most useful to confirm ileus through the absence of sound but is less reliable for confirming normal motility through the presence of sound. Ultrasound is being used in many species and holds promise for ruminants as well. Plasma electrolyte concentrations, especially chloride and bicarbonate ion, can be useful in determining functional or physical obstruction of the gastrointestinal tract. Severe hypochloridemia and alkalosis is usually associated with abomasal outflow problems, or obstruction or dysmotility of the orad small intestine. Less profound electrolyte abnormalities are observed in obstruction of the aborad small intestine and cecum.

RUMINAL MICROBES

The ruminant forestomachs are a physiologic and biologic wonder, a marvelous example of symbiosis. In the mature cow, the rumen and reticulum represent 64% of the total stomach capacity, whereas the abomasum makes up only 11%. During the transition from preruminant to ruminant, the stomach changes in form, function, and fauna. The rumen and reticulum become a fermentation vat containing between 10^5 and 10^{12} bacteria/ml. The vast majority of ruminant microbes of animals on a forage diet are gram-negative anaerobic bacteria. The proportion of gram-positive organisms increases as the amount of grain in the diet increases. The ruminant's ability to use poor quality roughage, inadequate to sustain nonruminant animals, is facilitated by the bacteria in the rumen. Although bacteria are more important for digestive function, the ruminal protozoa are easier to assess diagnostically, and they provide a reasonable index of ruminal health. Therefore a substantial proportion of the ruminal microbe examination focuses on the protozoal population. For clinical purposes, the ciliate protozoa can be divided into 2 morphologic types: holotrichs and entodiniomorphs. Holotrichs have cilia surrounding their one-celled bodies, whereas entodiniomorphs have cilia at one end (Figure 7.1-1).

Ruminal Fluid Analysis

Indications for clinical evaluation of ruminal microflora include suspicion of ruminal acidosis (e.g., carbohydrate engorgement), vagal indigestion, abomasal emptying defect of sheep, and rumen atony. Sometimes the analysis precedes surgery, but correction of the problem occurs during the postoperative period. A weighted stomach tube or a needle and syringe can be used to collect ruminal fluid for analysis. When a weighted collection tube is used, it is simply passed into the rumen, pushed back and forth to sink the tube, and aspirated. The first 100 ml or so is discarded to reduce salivary contamination. Aspirating transabdominally through the left

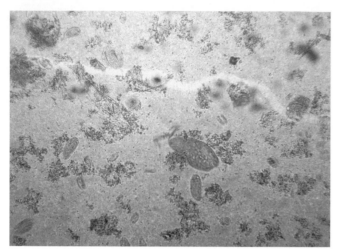

Figure 7.1-1 The microscopic appearance of ruminal fluid from a healthy cow. Notice the variety of sizes and shapes of the protozoa, which indicates healthy rumen microflora.

flank by using a 16- to 18-gauge, 5-inch needle also helps eliminate salivary contamination.

A relatively simple analysis is sufficient for clinical evaluation of most presurgical and postsurgical cases. Color, odor, and smell should be evaluated immediately. Normal color is gray-green to green to brownish-yellow, depending on the diet. Milky gray or yellow fluid is associated with CHO engorgement. The pH of rumen fluid ranges from 5.5 to 7.0 in healthy cattle on a balanced ration. A pH paper with half-unit sensitivity is sufficient to diagnose ruminal acidosis or alkalosis of a single clinical case. A hand-held pH meter is required for adequate sensitivity at herd-level diagnosis of mild chronic acidosis. Cattle on high carbohydrate diets have lower pH values than those on roughage diets. Acid pH less than 5.5 in an anorectic ruminant indicates ruminal acidosis. Ruminal pH greater than 7.0 indicates ruminal alkalosis. Simple ruminal inactivity, or anorexia, results in ruminal alkalosis. Cattle with abomasal reflux may have an unusually low pH for an animal that has been off of feed for several days (e.g., 6.5 in comparison to an expected value of 8.0). This is because the abomasal acid has refluxed or been "vomited" into the rumen.

A very simple function test, the methylene blue reduction (MBR) time, can be performed rapidly without special equipment. The MRB test measures metabolic activity of the ruminal flora by indicating the relative redox potential of the rumen. One part of 0.03% methylene blue is added to 20 parts of strained ruminal fluid in a glass blood collection tube and is incubated at 37°C. A second tube of ruminal fluid serves as a control. Clearing of the dye in 5 to 6 minutes indicates active ruminal microbes. Delayed clearing indicates diminished anaerobic bacterial activity. In some cases, measurement of

ruminal chloride is indicated. Ruminal chloride can be measured by standard electrolyte analyzers if the sample is filtered. It is elevated (>30 meq/L) in abomasal impaction and some other obstructive diseases in cattle and abomasal emptying defect in sheep.

Direct microscopic examination of fresh ruminal fluid on a slide is a quick and useful way to assess the health of the ruminal microflora. Abundant, live, active protozoa of various sizes and shapes will be present in cattle with a normal rumen (see Figure 7.1-1). Very large entodiniomorphs are the most fragile species; their presence suggests a healthy rumen. For further evaluation of the microflora, a drop of Lugol's iodine can be added to a few drops of fresh rumen fluid. Lugol's iodine kills the protozoa and stains carbohydrate in protozoa and bacteria. If the protozoa are depleted of carbohydrate, this indicates a depletion of carbohydrate in the rumen. Transfaunation of such an animal without concomitant force-feeding is likely to be ineffective because the newly introduced fauna will not have the substrate to allow them to multiply. Gram staining of the ruminal bacterial population, except in carbohydrate engorgement, has not been diagnostically useful in the author's experience. If gram staining is performed on ruminal contents, one should expect to see primarily gram-negative organisms of a size and shape quite different from those encountered elsewhere in veterinary medicine. In CHO engorgement, chains of the gram-positive cocci *Strep bovis* proliferate first; then the large gram-positive rods of *Lactobacillus* sp become the predominant bacterial type.

Transfaunation

Transfaunation of an inactive rumen can be accomplished by providing ruminal fluid from a healthy ruminant of the same species. Cross-species transfaunation may be of some benefit as some species of ciliates are common to different ruminants. Ruminal contents may be obtained at a slaughterhouse or from another animal that has been fitted with a ruminal cannula. Ruminal fluid collection devices, like the one described by Geishauser, also can be used. The potential to transmit certain diseases exists; therefore a tested donor or a herd mate of the patient is desirable. The author is not aware of studies that have demonstrated the minimum effective dose of ruminal fluid to restore functional microflora to a rumen of a diseased animal rapidly. At our hospital, the usual amount administered is 4 liters. Figure 7.1-2 shows a collection device made from PVC pipe. It is a meter long, 5 cm in diameter and capped at one end. Beginning about 35 cm from the capped end and extending to the cap are hundreds of 2- to 3-mm holes drilled through the wall. The capped end is inserted into the ventral sac of the rumen through the rumen cannula,

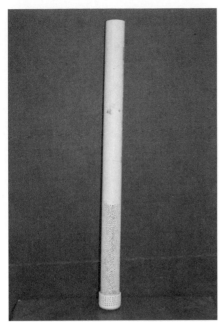

Figure 7.1-2 Device for collecting large quantities of rumen fluid from a cannulated cow.

and a small stomach tube is used to siphon ruminal fluid out of the pipe. This device obviates the need for the messy process of straining the fluid after collection.

Postoperative Feeding

NEONATES

At birth, preruminant animals are physiologically similar to nonruminants. The abomasum represents over half of the total stomach capacity, and the esophageal groove allows the nursing preruminant to function as a simple-stomached animal. Groove closure is a vago-vagal reflex mediated by receptors in the mouth and pharynx. In normal suckling animals, virtually all milk is channeled directly into the abomasum. During the first several days of life, if milk or other liquid is placed directly into the rumen by esophageal or intraruminal intubation, the liquid is rather quickly emptied into the abomasum. Later in the calf's life, however, the efficiency and completeness of emptying of fluid introduced directly into the rumen is reduced, and fermentation and ruminal acidosis can occur if milk remains in the rumen. Therefore every attempt should be made to encourage young ruminants to suckle milk rather than to force-feed them by intubation. Intubation with electrolyte solution does not pose the same threat to the ruminal environment as milk. When a calf is reluctant to voluntarily consume milk, providing fluids, electrolytes, and energy (in the form of glucose) by intravenous infusion or intraruminal intubation and refraining from administering intraruminal milk

as long as possible without compromising the health of the calf (up to 48 hours) is probably better. When an anorectic calf is relatively bright, alert, and not emaciated, the author prefers to maintain hydration with intravenous fluids and moderate amounts of intraruminal oral rehydration solution and allow the calf to become hungry. This often results in spontaneous nursing within 24 hours. On the other hand, when the caregiver is overly concerned about providing enteral nutrition to a calf and frequently intubates it with milk, the calf is less likely to nurse on its own, thus further delaying voluntary nursing.

Unlike foals, neonatal ruminants do not normally nurse frequently during the day. However, after surgery of the gastrointestinal tract, offering four or more small feedings per day is probably best for a few days. It is difficult to make hard recommendations concerning the amount to feed. In neonatal calves, milk equalling nearly 10% of the calf's body weight is required for maintenance alone, but after gastrointestinal surgery such as correction of abomasal volvulus, the amount fed for 1 to 2 days should be less than the usual ration. Ideally, intravenous fluid therapy should be continued for 24 to 48 hours postoperatively while milk (and dry foodstuffs if the calf had been consuming them before surgery) is reintroduced gradually. A conservative and easy guideline to follow is to feed one-fourth, one-half, three-fourths, and full ration on the four consecutive days after surgery, provided it is tolerated. In nursing beef calves, lambs, and kids, the amount of milk available to the patient can be limited by milking the dam one or more times daily and discarding the milk. Calves under 3 weeks of age should receive whole milk or milk replacer that contains only milk-derived protein. The milk replacer should contain at least 22% protein and 15% fat on a dry matter basis. Lambs and kids should receive only milk replacer designed for their species. In a hospital situation, whole retail milk is a reasonable feed for calves. Waste milk, especially from animals from a different farm, should be avoided because it may transmit *Mycobacterium avium* ssp. *paratuberculosis*, bovine leukemia virus, CAE virus, mycoplasma, salmonellae, or other pathogens. Some veterinarians feed lamb milk replacer to calves as a convalescent diet because it contains higher concentrations of fat and protein than cow's milk does.

MATURE RUMINANTS

Postoperative feeding strategies should be aimed at providing adequate nutrition for healing the surgical wound and any other tissue damage as well as maintaining body systems, restoring or maintaining functional microflora in the forestomachs, and returning the animal to production as soon as possible, especially in dairy cows. At the same time, consideration must be given to 1) the possibility that anorexia before surgery may have rendered the rumen unprepared for a typical high production grain-rich diet; and 2) the time for recovery of the compromised gut in cases of diseases that involve the GI tract. In cases such as intussusception and abomasal volvulus, in which ileus is likely to be a problem, small amounts of hay (1 kilogram) and grain (1/2 kilogram) 2 to 3 times daily should be fed for a few days. The amount can be increased gradually if abdominal distension is absent and feces is being passed. For other procedures, beginning with half rations and working up to a full ration in 3 to 5 days is usually done without complication.

In anorectic cattle, force-feeding is often beneficial. Although many "recipes" for force-fed rations exist, the base ration is usually a pelleted feed or alfalfa meal soaked in water to create a slurry. In areas where it can be purchased, hominy grits works well to provide energy because it flows through a tube easily. It is best to use a pellet without large pieces of grain; otherwise the slurry will plug the stomach pump. About 1 kg of feed in 12 L of water usually yields a slurry with the right consistency. We use a complete horse feed or one of the equine geriatric diets. A hand bilge pump or cattle pump system* with a self-restraining flexible esophageal tube works well. It is important to keep stirring the slurry during pumping to prevent it from settling and plugging the pump. Depending on the class of animal (lactating dairy cow versus wether goat) and its metabolic status, other ingredients such as yeast, electrolytes, propylene glycol, and calcium may be added. When the ruminal microflora are compromised, there may not be adequate, or at least optimal, production of B vitamins for the animal. Therefore injectable B vitamins are warranted in anorectic ruminants.

Postoperative ileus, as described previously, may complicate recovery following surgery. The most prominent clinical sign of postoperative ileus, irrespective of the location of the problem, is often ruminal distension. The use of motility modifiers to treat postoperative ileus in cattle is the subject of a different section in this book. From a postoperative nutritional and medical management perspective, a simple rule to follow is to cease enteral feeding at the first sign of ruminal distention. Remove excess ruminal contents if necessary with a large-bore stomach tube and provide fluid, electrolyte, and energy by the parenteral route described in Chapter 5, Fluid Therapy.

The author believes when attempting to coax anorectic animals to eat, one must offer small amounts of a variety of foodstuffs. Predicting which type of foodstuff the animal will consume first is difficult, but it is not always the feed to which they are accustomed. By putting small piles of a dry feed like cracked corn or oats, a pelleted feed, and a coarse sweet feed in the trough, one offers the animal choices and enhances the chance of finding a foodstuff the animal will eat. The author's opinion is that finicky cattle eat best when just a small amount of feed is available. Perhaps this is simply because when excess feed is available, consumption of small amounts cannot be detected. At any rate, this method appears to enhance consumption and certainly facilitates quantifying what is being consumed.

7.1.3—Motility Modifiers

Adrian Steiner and Peter C. Rakestraw

Physiological gastrointestinal (GI) motility patterns, regulation of GI motility, pathological motility patterns during GI disease, and pharmacological modification of GI motility are extremely complex and far from being fully understood. The GI problems in cattle that potentially benefit from pharmacological motility modification include intestinal obstruction, cecal dilatation/-dislocation (CDD), and displacement of the abomasum (DA); displacement of the abomasum to the left (LDA) being by far the economically most important of these diseases. As a prerequisite for understanding and correct interpreting of scientific publications and results in the field of motility modifiers, the reader needs to be familiar with the basic concepts of motility monitoring, physiological and pathological motility patterns, and motility regulation.

Motility Registration

Techniques for registration of GI motility in vivo include direct visualization, indirect visualization—using radiography, ultrasonography, or nuclear scintigraphy—acetaminophen absorption test, transit of nonabsorbable microspheres, intraluminal and intramural pressure measurements, and analysis of myoelectric activity (Figure 7.1.3-1). Most of the recent motility studies in cattle are based on registration and analysis of myoelectric activity.

Physiological Gastrointestinal Motility

Myoelectric signals of the digestive tract in cattle follow the same basic patterns as in other species. They are characterized by slow waves (electric control activity) and superimposed spike bursts (electric response activity).

---

*Magrath Cattle Pump System (Magrath Manufacturing Co, McCook, NE)

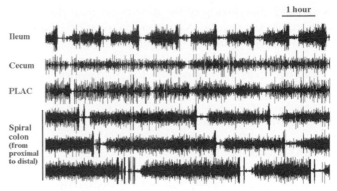

Figure 7.1.3-3 Myoelectric activity of the ileum, cecum, proximal loop of the ascending colon and spiral colon of a healthy adult cow, recorded over 9-hours.

(Courtesy of Dr. Mireille Meylan.)

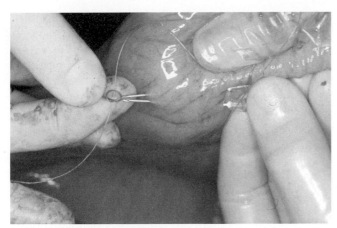

Figure 7.1.3-1 Implantation of retrievable bipolar electrodes in the cecum of an adult cow for registration of myoelectric activity.

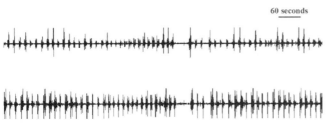

Figure 7.1.3-2 Myoelectric activity of the pyloric antrum of a healthy adult cow.

(Courtesy of Dr. Mireille Meylan.)

Slow waves are spontaneous, regular oscillations of the smooth muscle cell membrane potential, which remains below the depolarization threshold. If the depolarization threshold is exceeded, a maximum of one spike burst can be superimposed on one slow wave. Thus the maximal frequency of spike bursts is determined by the frequency of slow waves. Spiking activity is directly correlated with smooth muscle contractions (i.e., mechanical activity) and propulsion of gut contents is correlated with propagated smooth muscle contractions. Therefore recording of myoelectric activity of the gut wall may be used as a technique for characterization of gastrointestinal motility.

ABOMASUM

Myoelectric activity of the abomasal antrum is characterized by slow waves, regularly occurring at a mean frequency of 3.3 per minute. Eighty-two percent of the slow waves are superimposed by spikes (Figure 7.1.3-2). Almost half of the antral spikes are propagated to the proximal duodenum. This most likely represents abomasal emptying. Further coordination between antral and small intestinal motility exists. It is characterized by

a reduction of the frequency of slow waves and spike bursts in the abomasal antrum immediately after phase III of the migrating myoelectric complex (MMC) occurs in the duodenum. (See next section on the small intestine.)

SMALL INTESTINE

Motility of the small intestine is well organized and consists of a 30- to 90-minute regularly recurring, aborally propagated pattern of myoelectric activity, termed MMC. The MMC is initiated in the duodenum and consists of three phases. Phase I is characterized by less than 10% of the slow waves being superimposed by spikes. It immediately follows phase III and is immediately followed by phase II. Phase II is usually the longest of the three phases. It is the phase of irregular spiking activity, with more than 10% but less than 100% of the slow waves superimposed by spikes. Intense mixing of gut contents takes place during phase II. The last few minutes of phase II are thought to be responsible for propulsion of intestinal contents. Phase III is the phase of regular spiking activity with 100% of the slow waves being superimposed by spikes (Figure 7.1.3-3). The role attributed to phase III is to clean the lumen from debris and residual content, and to prevent retrograde flow of intestinal contents ("housekeeping" function). In ruminants, feeding does not interrupt the MMC. Propagation velocity of phase III ranges from 30 cm per minute in the duodenum to less than 10 cm per minute in the ileum.

CECUM AND PROXIMAL LOOP OF THE ASCENDING COLON (PLAC)

Cyclical activity and propagated spike sequences are also found in the cecum and PLAC. Occurrence of hyperactivity in the cecum is coordinated with phase III of each MMC in the ileum. Hyperactivity in the cecum may be responsible for mixing of the new bolus with the stored contents in the cecum. Nonpropagated spikes and spike sequences propagated in both directions are responsible for mixing of intestinal contents. Aborally propagated spike sequences are responsible for propagation of contents from the cecum to the PLAC. Regular emptying of the PLAC is well coordinated with the myoelectric motility pattern of the spiral colon.

SPIRAL COLON

Myoelectric activity of the spiral colon is characterized by a regularly recurring, aborally propagated pattern, termed bovine colonic migrating myoelectric complex (bcMMC). The bcMMC lasts about 3 hours and consists of four phases. More than 90% of the bcMMCs are propagated throughout the entire spiral colon. Similar to the MMC in the small intestine, phase II is by far the longest phase. The last few minutes of phase II are thought to be responsible for aboard propulsion of intestinal contents in the bovine spiral colon. The "housekeeping" function is attributed to phase III with its regular and intense spikes of long duration (see Figure 7.1.3-3). Function of phase IV is not clear.

Pathological Motility Patterns

INTESTINAL OBSTRUCTION

Myoelectric activity patterns occurring during small intestinal obstruction are characterized by the disorganization of the MMC in the segment oral to an obstruction. The MMC is replaced by rapidly migrating, prolonged, high amplitude spikes that sometimes occur in clusters. This characteristic pattern is termed colic motor complex (CMC). The pattern occurring aboral to an obstruction is not consistent and depends on the species affected and the degree of luminal occlusion. Myoelectric activity of the PLAC during obstruction of the proximal part of the spiral colon is similarly characterized by increased spike duration, increased number of spikes propagated towards the obstruction site, and increased velocity of spike propagation. In analogy to small intestinal obstruction, this pattern was termed colonic CMC. The CMCs may represent an effort of the intestine to overcome the obstruction to reestablish the continuity of digesta passage.

CECAL DILATATION/DISLOCATION

Atony, or hypotony, affecting the cecum and the PLAC, were postulated to trigger CDD. However, during the past three decades, scientists were not able to confirm this hypothesis. Attempts of scientific induction of CDD were not successful, and an accepted disease model for CDD has never been established. In cases of delayed

recovery and/or recurrence after surgical evacuation of spontaneous CDD, a pattern of myoelectric activity in the cecum and PLAC similar to the CMC was found. It was suggested that atony and/or hypotony of the cecum were not the cause of recurrence of CDD. An alternative hypothesis offered was that an obstruction of the spiral colon might be responsible for recurrence of CDD after surgical correction of spontaneous CDD.

DISPLACEMENT OF THE ABOMASUM

In the early seventies, abomasal atony has been postulated to precede distention and displacement of the abomasum. Since then, scientists were not able to confirm this hypothesis. In a more recent study, extended periods of atony preceding LDA were not found. However, during periods of left displacement as compared to periods of normal abomasal position, significant decrease of the number of spike bursts was found in the abomasal corpus and pyloric antrum. Therefore significant decrease of myoelectric activity was found during rather than immediately before DA. Smooth muscle preparations collected from displaced abomasa as compared to nondisplaced abomasa showed an increase in nitric oxide mediated inhibition and a decrease in sensitivity to acetylcholine-mediated excitation. This suggests a malfunction at the level of the intrinsic nervous system and/or abomasal smooth muscle cells. Whether this is a preexisting condition predisposing the animal to DA or a result of the displacement has yet to be determined.

Prokinetics in Ruminants

Numerous causes of hypodynamic gastrointestinal motility disorders have been demonstrated in various species. These include electrolyte imbalances, such as hypocalcemia, shock, inflammation, endotoxemia, and intestinal ischemia. Although the effects of these pathological conditions may not have been evaluated specifically in ruminants, there are enough similarities between species to suggest these abnormalities will also adversely affect motility in ruminants. Treatment plans to correct impaired gastrointestinal motility should initially evaluate and correct these problems if they exist. Prokinetic drugs will have little therapeutic effect in ruminants with ischemic bowel, hypocalcemia or a mechanical obstruction.

The primary areas of the ruminant digestive tract that have been studied in relation to the use of prokinetics to treat hypomotility disorders are the abomasum, small intestine, cecum, and proximal ascending colon. Although recent literature has not been able to support the thought that abomasal atony and/or delayed abomasal emptying predispose ruminants to abomasal displacement, it is possible that drugs which alter the pattern of contractile activity may be beneficial in treating these disorders in some instances. Paralytic ileus involving the small intestine, as well as the large intestine, can occur after any abdominal insult, such as impaction or volvulus, resulting in traumatized/inflamed intestine. Prokinetics may act by stimulating contractile activity directly, or by attenuating the inflammatory process and resulting motility depression. Motility dysfunction of the cecum and proximal loop of the ascending colon are thought to predispose to cecal dilatation/volvulus. Drugs that promote normal motility patterns in these areas may have efficacy in the medical treatment of cecal dilation.

The following is a list of prokinetic drugs that may be beneficial in treating certain gastrointestinal conditions in the ruminant. Unfortunately, there are few studies which have evaluated these drugs in a clinical setting in the ruminant.

BETHANECHOL

Bethanechol hydrochloride is a direct-acting parasympathetic agonist that stimulates acetylcholine receptors on the gastrointestinal (GI) smooth muscle, increasing contractile activity. There is some preliminary support showing that bethanechol may improve small intestinal motility in the ruminant. Bethanechol (0.07 mg/kg SC) increased the duodenal spike rate (associated with contractile activity) for the first hour after administration in normal yearling cattle. However, a combination of bethanechol (0.07 mg/kg SC) and metoclopramide (0.1 mg/kg SC) significantly improved propagating spike activity, which is more likely to indicate propulsive motility in the duodenum. In the large bowel, bethanechol (0.07 mg/kg SC) has been shown to increase the number of cecocolic spikes, the duration of cecocolic spiking activity and the number of propagated spikes in normal cows. Although the underlying cause of CDD is not known, these results indicate that bethanechol at this dosage may be a suitable medical or postoperative treatment for cecal dilatation in cattle in which hypomotility of the cecum and proximal loop of the ascending colon are present. It should be kept in mind in evaluating the results of the above studies that these were performed in normal animals. Extrapolation to pathological states may not always be valid.

NEOSTIGMINE

Neostigmine methylsulfate is a cholinesterase inhibitor that prolongs the activity of acetylcholine by retarding it's breakdown at the synaptic junction. The effect of neostigmine (0.02 mg/kg, SC) on myoelectric activity of the ileocecocolic area in normal cows was mainly to increase the number of cecocolic spikes. However, neostigmine increased the ratio of orally to aborally propagated spike sequences suggesting that neostigmine may promote retrograde versus antegrade propagation of GI motility. Consequently, based on studies in normal cows, bethanechol may be a more suitable drug to treat cecal dilatation in cattle in which hypomotility of the cecum and proximal ascending colon are thought to contribute to the pathological process.

Another report describes the use of neostigmine administered as a continuous drip (87.5 mg/10 l of NaCl administered at 2 drops/sec) to treat cattle with cecal dilatation. Bradycardia and restlessness were commonly seen side effects necessitating careful monitoring of the animal. To date, there is little more information on the use of neostigmine in ruminants.

METOCLOPRAMIDE

Metoclopramide acts to stimulate progressive motility by antagonizing the inhibitory neurotransmitter dopamine, augmenting the release of acetylcholine, and acting through both inhibitory and excitatory serotonergic receptors. It has been suggested that metoclopramide improves antroduodenal coordination and consequently is an effective prokinetic to treat delayed gastric emptying in different species. Metoclopramide (0.1 mg/kg SC), used together with bethanechol (0.07 mg/kg SC), was more effective than either medication used alone in increased propagated spike activity in the abomasum and duodenum in normal cattle. Metoclopramide was not effective in improving myoelectric activity in the cecum and proximal ascending colon. Administered at a higher dose (0.5 mg/kg IM) in another study, metoclopramide transiently increased electrical activity of the proximal duodenum in goats. These results support the observation that this drug may be more suitable for proximal motility disorders, such as rumen and abomasal emptying problems, as well as small intestinal hypomotility disorders. This is in agreement with findings in other species where metoclopramide is primarily used to treat gastric and small intestinal motility disorders. Metoclopramide has been used in the treatment of abomasal emptying defects in sheep and vagal indigestion in cattle. The recommended dose in ruminants is 0.1 to 0.5 mg/kg SC or IM. Hypotension has been reported to occur after intravenous use. Reported side effects are restlessness, excitement, and somnolence.

ERYTHROMYCIN

Erythromycin is a macrolide antibiotic with recognized gastrointestinal side effects. When administered at subtherapeutic antimicrobial levels, erythromycin has been shown to stimulate gastric emptying, antroduodenal coordination, increased contractile activity in the small intestine and increased cecal emptying in nonruminant species. Erythromycin is a motilin agonist that stimulates motilin receptors on the gastrointestinal smooth muscle. It also stimulates the release of acetylcholine. Since erythromycin appears to stimulate motility throughout the GI tract in other species, its use may be indicated for rumen, abomasum, and small and large intestine hypomotility disorders. The dose used to treat postoperative ileus in horses is 1.0 mg/kg in 1 L of saline infused over 60 minutes, every 6 hours. Abdominal pain is the most commonly reported side effect seen with this drug. There have also been occasional reports of diarrhea even though it is administered at a level that should not cause antibiotic induced diarrhea.

LIDOCAINE

Inhibitory reflexes that are confined to the gut as well as involving the prevertebral ganglia and spinal cord are involved in the pathogenesis of certain motility disturbances. These become important after abdominal surgery where the original GI insult, as well as the bowel manipulations during surgical correction, causes an inflammatory response. Endotoxemia associated with enteritis/colitis will also activate these inhibitory reflexes. Intravenous lidocaine can promote motility by reducing the level of circulating catecholamines, blocking the inhibitory reflexes and decreasing the production of inflammatory mediators in the bowel wall, many of which are inhibitory. Some work has shown that normal small intestine and colon is under a basal inhibitory neural tone. Addition of lidocaine blocks this inhibitory tone and has been shown to increase contractile activity. For this reason lidocaine may also be beneficial in motility disorders which lack an inflammatory component. There is no research in the ruminant using this drug, but in the horse, the recommended protocol is an initial bolus of 1.3 mg/kg IV administered slowly over 5 minutes followed by 0.05 mg/kg/min in saline or LRS over 24 hours.

Certain drugs should be avoided or used with caution when treating a ruminant with hypomotility problems. The adrenergic agonists have been shown to depress gastrointestinal motility in many species. In cattle xylazine increased the duration of inactivity of the ileocecolic area. In horses detomidine has been shown to depress intestinal motility for a longer period than xylazine. In general opioids inhibit progressive motility. In calves the opioid agonist/antagonist butorphanol has been shown to inhibit ruminoreticular contractions for up to 40 minutes. Consequently, opioids should also be used with caution in ruminants with motility disorders.

RECOMMENDED READINGS

Braun U, Steiner A, Bearth G. Therapy and clinical progress of cattle with dilatation and torsion of the caecum. *Vet Rec* Oct: 430-433, 1989.

Brikas P: Motor-modifying properties of 5-HT₃ and 5-HT₄ receptor agonists on ovine abomasum. *J Vet Med A* 41: 150-158, 1994.

Constable PD et al: The reticulorumen: normal and abnormal motor function, part I: primary contraction cycle, *Compend Cont Ed Pract Vet* 12: 1008-1014, 1990.

Divers TJ et al: Parenteral nutrition in cattle, *Bovine Practitioner* 22: 56-57, 1987.

Doherty T et al: Acetaminophen as a marker of gastric emptying in ponies. *Equine Vet J* 30: 349-351, 1998.

Garry F: Diagnosing and treating indigestion caused by fermentative disorders, *Veterinary Medicine* 85: 660-670, 1990.

Geishauser T et al: Identification of motility disorders associated with displaced abomasum in dairy cows. *Neurogastroenterol and Motility* 10: 395-401, 1998.

Guard C, Schwark W, Kelton D, et al. Effects of metaclopramide, clenbuterol, and butorphanol on ruminoreticular motility of calves. *Cornell Vet* 78: 89-98, 1988.

Huhn JC, Nelson. The quantitative effect of metoclopramide on abomasal and duodenal myoelectric activity in goats. *J Vet Med Assoc* 44: 361-371, 1997.

Kopcha M: Myoelectrical and myomechanical response of the pyloric antrum in sheep to metoclopramide. *Proc ACVIM Meeting*, 1988. pp 733.

Lohmann KL et al: Comparison of nuclear scintigraphy and acetaminophen absorption as a means of studying gastric emptying in horses. *Am J Vet Res* 61: 310-315, 2000.

Madison JB and Troutt HF: Effects of hypocalcaemia on abomasal motility. *Res Vet Sci* 44: 264-266, 1988.

Malone ED, Turner TA, Wilson JH. Intravenous lidocaine for the treatment of equine ileus. *J Vet Intern Med* 13: 229, 1999.

Meylan M et al: Myoelectric activity of the sprial colon in dairy cows. *Am J Vet Res*. In press, 2001.

Nappert G and Lattimer JC: Comparison of abomasal emptying in neonatal calves with a nuclear scintigraphic procedure. *Can J Vet Res* 65: 50-54, 2001.

Nelson DR et al: Electromyography of the reticulum, abomasum and duodenum in dairy cows with left displacement of the abomasum. *J Vet Med A* 42: 325-337, 1995.

Nicholson T et al: Radionuclide imaging of abomasal emptying in sheep. *Res Vet Sci* 62: 26-29, 1997.

Nieto J et al: In vitro effects of 5-HT and cisapride on the circular smooth muscle of the jejunum of horses. *Am J Vet Res* 61: 1561-1565, 2000.

Plaza MA et al: Effect of motilin and somatostatin on the myoelectrical abomasal and duodenal activity in sheep. *J Gastrointest Mot* 4: 236, 1992.

Plaza MA et al: Effect of motilin, somatostatin and bombesin on gastroduodenal myoelectric activity in sheep. *Life Sci* 58: 1413-1423, 1996.

Roussel AJ, Brumbaugh GW, Waldron RC, et al. Abomasal and duodenal motility in yearling cattle after administration of prokinetic drugs. *Am J Vet Res* 55: 111-115, 1994.

Steiner A, Roussel AJ, Ellis WC: Colic motor complex of the cecum and proximal loop of the ascending colon in an experimental cow with large intestinal obstruction. *Zentralbl Veterinarmed A* 41: 53-61,1994.

Steiner A et al: Myoelectric activity of the cecum and proximal loop of the ascending colon in cows. *Am J Vet Res* 55: 1037-1043, 1994.

Steiner A et al: Effect of xylazine, cisapride and naloxone on myoelectric activity of ileo-ceco-colic area in cows. *Am J Vet Res* 56: 623-628, 1995.

Steiner A, Roussel AJ, Martig J: Effect of bethanechol, neostigmine, metoclopramide, and propranolol on myoelectric activity of the ileocecal area in cows. *Am J Vet Res* 56: 1081-1086, 1995.

Stocker S et al: Myoelectric activity of the cecum and proximal loop of the ascending colon in cows after spontaneous cecal dilatation/dislocation. *Am J Vet Res* 58: 961-968,1997.

Svendsen P: Abomasal displacement in cattle. *Nord Vet Med* 22: 571-577, 1970.

Svendsen P, Kristensen B. Cecal dilatation in cattle. An experimental study of the etiology. *Nord Vet Med* 22: 578-583, 1970.

Taniyama K et al: Functions of peripheral 5-hydroxytryptamine receptors, especially 5-HT$_4$ receptor, in gastrointestinal motility. *J Gastroenterol* 35: 575-582, 2000.

CHAPTER 8

SURGERY OF THE BOVINE INTEGUMENTARY SYSTEM

8.1—Wounds

Richard Wheeler

Wound Healing

Wound healing is a complex orchestration of cellular and biochemical processes intricately balanced to achieve healing without potentiating further tissue damage or causing uncontrolled tissue proliferation. The cells that mediate wound healing include platelets, macrophages, neutrophils, epithelial cells, lymphocytes, fibroblasts, and endothelial cells. These cells interact, grow, divide, and migrate as directed by chemotactic agents, growth factors, and cytokines. The process of wound healing is a continuum of overlapping events described here as four stages: inflammation, debridement, repair, and maturation.

INFLAMMATION

Inflammation is the body's attempt to arrest fluid loss, prevent infection, and initiate healing. When tissue damage compromises vascular integrity, platelet aggregation and the clotting cascade stop blood loss by forming a fibrin clot. Local cells simultaneously release catecholamines, histamine, cytokines, and prostaglandins. These inflammatory mediators initially induce vasoconstriction to contribute to hemostasis. Once hemorrhage is controlled, these inflammatory factors increase vascular permeability and induce diapedesis of phagocytic cells into the wound, resulting in the classic signs of heat and swelling.

The inflammatory response is a critical and necessary stage of wound healing. It prevents systemic complications by controlling hemorrhage and initiating local immune reactions to prevent systemic infection. Because the vascular changes and cellular responses elicited by inflammatory mediators are characterized by heat, redness, swelling, and pain, a clinician's first response is to eliminate inflammation with antiinflammatory drugs. Controlling the negative effects of inflammation is beneficial to the patient, provided cellular and chemotactic function necessary for wound healing is unimpaired. However, elimination of the entire inflammatory response will prolong wound healing.

DEBRIDEMENT

Ultimately, the fibrin clot formed during the inflammatory phase organizes, dries, and becomes a scab. The scab protects the underlying tissue from recurrent injury and maintains a moist environment for phagocytic cells and fibroblasts. It maintains a hypoxic and acidic environment that inhibits bacterial growth and stimulates fibroblast proliferation. In addition, the scab provides scaffolding for the second stage of wound healing, debridement. The platelets and fibrin that comprise the scab form a network of proteins and chemotactic factors that attract neutrophils and macrophages into the wounded area. The neutrophils and macrophages remove necrotic debris, foreign matter, and bacteria.

REPAIR
Fibroplasia

Soon after injury, fibroblasts move out of the connective tissue adjacent to the wound and migrate across the protein lattice formed by the clot. Fibroblasts replace damaged dermis with ground substance and collagen. This collagen forms scar tissue that is structurally altered and functionally inferior to the original dermis.

Granulation

Granulation tissue is highly vascular connective tissue that functions to nourish the epithelial cells, fibroblasts, and macrophages. By the process of angiogenesis, endothelial cells migrate and anastomose to revascularize the wounded tissue. The mechanisms that control endothelial cell and fibroblast proliferation in the formation of granulation tissue are ill-defined but include a plethora of growth factors produced by platelets, macrophages, fibroblasts, and endothelial cells. Hypoxia also seems to play an important role.

Epithelialization

After injury, the epithelial layer is capable of regenerating. Epithelial cells at the wound margin proliferate and migrate over the granulation tissue toward the center of the wound. Epithelialization is complete when apposing margins meet. Contact inhibition prevents further epithelial cell division.

Contraction

Wound contraction is the centripetal closure of the total wound area. The full thickness of skin is pulled together. Wound contraction reduces the defect so less scar tissue and epithelialization occurs. For contraction to proceed, select fibroblasts differentiate into myofibroblasts that are capable of contracting to pull the wound margins together. Contraction stops when the wound margins are apposed or when tension across the wound exceeds the potential strength of myofibril contraction.

MATURATION

Remodeling of the collagen scar tissue occurs over the next several months. The collagen matrix initially produced by the fibroblasts is converted from Type III collagen to Type I collagen. Reorganization and structural cross-linkage develops between the collagen fibers increasing tensile strength of the scar.

FACTORS THAT AFFECT WOUND HEALING

The process of wound healing strives toward completion, but numerous factors affect the body's ability to repair itself.

Foreign Bodies/Contamination

Foreign matter and organic debris pose a physical barrier to wound healing. They are also infection-potentiating factors, the presence of organic debris reduces the minimum concentration of bacteria necessary to cause infection.

Necrotic Tissue

Presence of necrotic debris prevents formation of granulation tissue and provides a substrate for bacterial growth.

Infection

Open wounds expose the fibrin clot to the environment. Pathogenic or opportunistic bacteria take advantage of the same binding sites and scaffolding used by neutrophils and fibroblast to adhere to the wound. Some bacteria produce toxins that increase tissue damage and further the ability of bacteria to colonize and infect the tissue. Wounds with significant tissue damage and decreased perfusion, such as blunt trauma injuries, are at increased risk of infection because the devitalized tissue provides an optimal environment for bacterial proliferation and growth.

Movement

Wounds located over joints or tendons are subject to excessive motion, which delays wound healing. Tension against the wound and recurrent irritation may cause chronic inflammation and exuberant granulation tissue development.

pH

A slightly acid environment has been shown to enhance wound healing. This may be the result of enhanced oxygen release from hemoglobin in acidic environments. The acidic environment may also inhibit bacterial growth. However, too low a pH causes cell damage and delayed healing.

Blood Supply

An adequate blood supply is essential for wound healing. Blood delivers nutrients, oxygen, neutrophils, and macrophages and removes cellular wastes.

Temperature

Wounds heal faster at higher temperatures, possibly because secondary vasodilation increases perfusion. Body temperature of the distal limbs is generally slightly lower then core body temperature and may contribute to delayed wound healing and exuberant growth of granulation tissue in these locations.

Oxygen Tension

The presence of oxygen is necessary to meet the aerobic demands of metabolically active cells involved in healing. However, some degree of hypoxia stimulates wound healing. Low oxygen tension stimulates longevity and multiplication of fibroblasts. Hypoxia also induces the secretion of growth factor and angiogenic substances.

Nutrition

Poor nutrition can result in compromised immune function and deficiency in vitamins and building blocks necessary for protein synthesis and wound healing.

Wound Management

Veterinary care requires adequate assessment of the whole animal and appropriate triage when treating tissue injuries. The factors that affect wound healing must be considered when one is deciding on the most practical and effective treatment.

ANESTHESIA

Appropriate restraint; sedation; and local, regional, or general anesthesia are essential to effectively examine and manage any wound. Local anesthetics can delay wound healing. Lidocaine is acidic and can cause cell damage when injected at the site of injury. To prevent inhibition of wound healing caused by local anesthetic agents, regional anesthesia should be used whenever possible. When local anesthesia is unavoidable, injections should be made through the wound and under the skin. In this way, the needle does not penetrate the skin; pain receptors are avoided; and the anesthetic can be deposited a needle's length away from the wound margin.

WOUND CLOSURE

The decision to leave a wound open or to suture the skin closed is based on the span of time since injury occurred, mechanical cause of the laceration, degree of contamination, and location of the wound.

Second Intention Closure

Second intention closure relies on the wound's natural ability to contract and epithelialize. It is applicable to wounds that are heavily contaminated, have excessive soft tissue damage (contusions), dead space, or extensive tissue loss that prevents closure of the defect. Second intention healing provides maximum drainage and is optimal for deep, penetrating wounds. Wounds healing by second intention require greater time to heal and may be unsightly and disturbing to the owner, but the final result is often a surprising, aesthetically acceptable return to function.

Once the decision has been made to allow a wound to heal by second intention, the wound is cleaned and debrided. Topical treatments may be used, and a bandage is applied. Petroleum jelly applied to the skin ventral to the wound helps prevent serum scald. If the injury lies over a highly mobile location on a limb, immobilizing the area with a splint or cast may be necessary.

If tissue contraction is insufficient to close the wound, the final result is epithelialization. Epithelial cells extend across the lesion but are structurally weaker and more prone to recurrent injury than full thickness skin is. If extensive epithelialization results, reconstructive surgery or grafting may be necessary.

Primary Wound Closure

With primary wound closure, the defect is closed by apposing and suturing skin edges. The best example is closure of a surgical incision. Primary wound closure provides the greatest rate of healing and the most normal return to function. It is the ideal route of healing because it results in the most physiologically normal tissue and the least amount of scarification. It should be used when the wound is very recent or the result of sharp incision with minimum contamination or soft tissue damage.

If necessary, the wound should be lavaged and debrided. Then the wound edges are apposed and sutured. To minimize the inflammatory reaction, nonreactive suture material and the minimum number of sutures necessary to close the defect are used. A bandage or cast may be applied over the closed wound to minimize contamination and restrict motion.

When excessive dead space remains, a drain should be placed alongside the suture line to facilitate drainage; it should not be directly beneath the sutured wound edge. Drains should be sutured proximally and distally and exit the skin through incisions separate from the sutured wound. Where the drain is exposed, it should be protected by a sterile bandage or stent; otherwise it may wick bacteria and contaminants into the wound. Drains should remain in place for 24 to 48 hours or until drainage ceases.

With primary wound closure, drainage is reduced, and contamination trapped in the wound site could cause abscessation. Also, excessive tension across the wound can cause pressure necrosis, suture failure, or can interrupt circulation and inhibit wound healing. If necessary, tension-relieving sutures can be placed initially and can

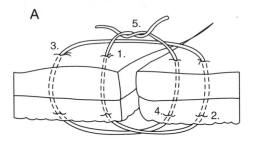

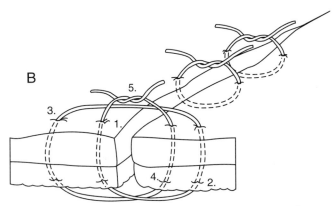

Figure 8.1-1 Primary wound closure using tension-relieving sutures placed at regular intervals to appose wound edges. *A,* Placement of a near-far-far-near tension-relieving suture, with *1-4* indicating order the bites are placed and *5* indicating the knot. *B,* Two simple interrupted sutures placed next to a near-far-far-near tension-relieving suture.

be followed by simple interrupted sutures placed between the tension-relieving bites (Figure 8.1-1). Interrupted near-far-far-near tension-relieving sutures placed at regular intervals along the incision starting in the center work well to bring skin edges into apposition. For wounds under a lot of tension, using penetrating towel clamps to help align tissues may be necessary. Rubber stents or "quills" placed on the tension sutures help prevent tissue necrosis under the suture material. After 3 to 4 days, the tension sutures are removed, and the simple interrupted sutures are left for 10 to 14 days.

Delayed Primary or Secondary Closure
These approaches to wound closure should be applied to wounds that did not receive immediate attention, had topical therapies that should not be closed into the wound applied, or are moderately contaminated.

Delayed primary closure makes use of lavage and manual debridement to clean a contaminated wound before it is closed. The wound is sutured several days after the injury but before granulation tissue develops.

Secondary closure allows a healthy bed of granulation tissue to develop before the wound is sutured. Excessive granulation tissue is sharply excised and the skin edges apposed over the granulation tissue.

These methods are particularly applicable to wounds of the distal limb that have degloving injuries or tissue flaps. When the viability of a tissue flap is uncertain, the skin is temporarily tacked down with a minimal number of sutures. This protects the skin flap and the underlying tissue from further damage, contamination, and desiccation. In 24 to 48 hours, the skin flap can be assessed. Viable tissue will be warm and pliable and will have good blood flow. The nonviable tissue is sharply debrided and the wound closed.

WOUND LAVAGE
Regardless of which closure technique is selected, removal of organic debris, necrotic tissue, and bacteria is essential. Lavage effectively removes contamination and decreases the inflammatory and debridement phases. To overcome the adhesive ability of bacteria and debris, irrigation fluid must be delivered at a minimum pressure of 8 psi. Forcing the irrigation solution through an 18-gauge needle attached to a 60-cc syringe effectively attains this pressure. Pressure in excess of 15 psi increases the potential to separate facial planes and drive bacteria and contaminants deeper into the tissue.

Warm irrigation increases the circulation to the injured area, delivering vital nutrients and removing wastes. Ideally, lavage fluids should be 45° C. Fluids that exceed 60° C will cause tissue damage and delayed healing.

To prevent osmotic damage to healing tissues and cells, lavage solution should be isotonic. Lactated Ringer's solution or isotonic saline is ideal. Antiseptics added to the irrigation solution enhance the lavage by combining antisepsis with the physical removal of contaminants. The antiseptic agent used must be bactericidal but should not inhibit neutrophils, macrophages, or fibroblasts.

Povidone Iodine
At a 0.1% concentration (10 cc of 10% stock solution in 1 liter of saline), povidone iodine is antibacterial and does not interfere with healing. At concentrations less than 0.1%, povidone iodine has a stimulatory effect on neutrophils but minimal bactericidal effect. At higher concentrations, povidone iodine is toxic to fibroblasts. Povidone iodine is inactivated by organic debris and has little residual effect.

Chlorhexidine Diacetate
Chlorhexidine solution at a 0.05% dilution (25 cc of 2% stock solution in 1 liter saline) has antibacterial effects without inhibiting wound healing, Chlorhexidine diacetate has a longer residual effect than povidone iodine

and has shown greater efficacy in the presence of organic debris.

Hydrogen Peroxide

Despite its impressive foaming action, hydrogen peroxide has not shown effective bactericidal activity and is cytotoxic at concentrations greater than 10%. However, hydrogen peroxide maintains sporicidal activity and may be indicated for treatment of potential spore-forming bacterial infections.

MANUAL DEBRIDEMENT

In conjunction with lavage, manual debridement of devitalized tissue allows tissue healing to proceed. Sharp excision using a scalpel blade creates less tissue damage and is preferred to scraping the tissue with a scalpel blade or abrasively scrubbing with gauze.

BANDAGING

When properly applied, bandages promote wound healing by limiting inflammation, assisting debridement, preventing desiccation, maintaining a slightly hypoxic and acidic environment, increasing local temperature, preventing contamination, and limiting motion.

Adherent Bandages

Adherent bandages are used during the inflammatory and debridement phases of wound healing. Mesh gauze is used as the contact layer and may be alternated "wet-to-dry" with each bandage change. Necrotic tissue and debris adhere to the gauze and are removed when the bandage is changed. Once granulation tissue develops debridement is no longer necessary, and adherent bandages are no longer used.

Semiocclusive, Nonadherent Bandages

Semiocclusive, nonadhesive bandages are used once granulation tissue has developed. Being semiocclusive, the bandage maintains hydration of the wound but retains some absorbency to prevent exudate buildup. The contact layer should be nonadhesive material. Numerous nonadhesive pads are available commercially. They can also be made by coating gauze with triple antibiotic ointment, povidone-iodine ointment, or other topical ointments to prevent gauze adhesion to the wound.

Amnion has been used as a semiocclusive, nonadherent wound dressing. Qualitative assessment of wound healing indicates amnion increases wound healing and diminishes the amount of exuberant granulation tissue on wounds of the distal limb. The exact mechanism by which amnion potentiates wound healing is unknown. Because it clings tightly to the wound margin without adhering to developing granulation or epithelial tissue,

amnion may simply be acting mechanically to prevent bacterial contamination. It is possibly less abrasive than synthetic pads and causes less irritation. The natural, low immunogenicity of amnion may induce less immune reaction when it contacts the wound surface.

Amnion can be stored for up 6 months at 4° C in a 0.05% chlorhexidine diacetate solution in water. The benefits and availability of amnion make it an affordable alternative to nonadherent pads.

Occlusive Bandages

Occlusive bandages prevent absorption of exudates and impede gas exchange across the wound surface. They are used extensively in human medicine but are of limited value in veterinary medicine. They have been shown to inhibit wound healing and promote excessive granulation in horses.

TOPICAL MEDICATIONS

Topical medications are commonly applied to wounds to enhance wound healing, decrease further contamination, or repel insects. When choosing a topical therapy, one must select a treatment that will not inhibit healing.

Aloe Vera Extract

Aloe vera extract has been shown to have both antibiotic and antiinflammatory properties. In combination with allantoin, aloe vera extract has been shown to increase the rate of wound healing.

Triple Antibiotic Ointment

Triple antibiotic ointment of bacitracin zinc, neomycin sulfate, and polymixin B sulfate has been shown to increase reepithelialization by 25%.

Silver Sulfadiazine

Silver sulfadiazine is commonly used in human medicine to treat burn victims and promote wound healing.

Nitrofurazone

Nitrofurazone (a potential carcinogen) use in food animals is strictly prohibited by the Food and Drug Administration. Even topical administration has resulted in systemic detection of drug residue.

Povidone Iodine Ointment

Application of povidone iodine ointment decreases bacterial concentrations and infection rates, but it may also decrease tensile strength of the wound.

Petroleum

Although commonly used in nonadherent bandages, petroleum has no apparent antibacterial properties and decreases the rate of wound contraction.

Topical Antibiotic

Application of topical antibiotics such as penicillin to a wound or incision decreases infection rate and does not suppress wound healing.

SYSTEMIC MEDICATION
Tetanus Toxoid

Tetanus prophylaxis boosters should be administered to animals with significant tissue damage or penetrating wounds at risk of anaerobic bacterial growth. Tetanus vaccines should be used in accordance with manufacturers' directions and species specificity. If the animal has not been vaccinated before injury, tetanus antitoxin may be administered. However, anaphylactic reactions or acute hepatic disease (Theiler's Disease in horses) are potential side effects to antitoxin.

SYSTEMIC ANTIBIOTICS

The use of systemic antibiotics is a topic of great debate. Indiscriminate use may propagate antibiotic resistance or upset the commensal flora of the skin or gastrointestinal tract. However, if the likelihood of systemic infection is high, such as with a penetrating wound or involvement of synovial structures, implementing systemic antibiotic therapy is certainly advisable.

VITAMIN SUPPLEMENTATION

Vitamins A, C, and E are crucial cofactors in wound healing. During inflammation and debridement, they are potent antiinflammatories and antioxidants that stabilize cell membranes and neutralize free radicals. They are also associated with growth and differentiation of epithelial cells and stabilization of collagen.

However, vitamin supplementation does not enhance wound healing unless a deficiency exists. Because Vitamins A, C, and E are natural component of green plants, it is very rare for ruminants to be deficient, unless the animal is severely malnourished. Therefore vitamin supplementation in well-nourished animals is unnecessary.

MYIASIS

The invasion of flesh wounds by fly larva can occur within 24 hours. Opportunistic species of maggots preferentially feed on necrotic tissue and may serve a reasonable benefit by facilitating debridement. However, these larvae may inadvertently damage the healthy tissue at the wound margins. Obligatory parasites, such as the larva of *Cochliomyia hominivorax* (New World screwworm), aggressively tunnel into the healthy subcutaneous tissue and exacerbate tissue damage. *C. hominivorax* infestations must be reported to state and federal authorities. Effective control against myiasis requires keeping the wound clean and dry, removing matted hair, and using topical insecticides or repellants. Recently, systemic larvicides have shown potential benefits in controlling myiasis.

Ivermectin has been shown to be larvicidal to many common barnyard fly larva, including *Musca domestica* (House fly), *Musca autumnalis* (Face fly), *Stomoxys calcitrans* (Stable fly), and *Haematobia irritans* (Horn fly). It has also been shown to directly prevent or eliminate subcutaneous infestations of *Chrysomyia bezziana* (Old World screw worm), *Cochliomyia hominivorax* (New World screw worm), and *Lucilia cuprina* (sheep blow fly) at a dose of 0.2 mg/kg . Infestation with screwworm larva was also effectively eliminated with Doramectin. Other studies have not shown ivermectin as having the same efficacy to reduce larval infestations and the potential for drug resistance to develop exists.

At a dose of 0.2 mg/kg, ivermectin did not affect the rate of larval infestation in goats. Empirical use of ivermectin in goats suggests a dose twice that labeled for cattle is necessary to attain the same effect. Ivermectin has not been approved for use in goats, and its administration must be deemed extralabel.

EXUBERANT GRANULATION TISSUE (PROUD FLESH)

Although exuberant granulation tissue is considerably more common in horses, excessive granulation tissue growth does occur on distal limb injuries of food animal species. The development of exuberant granulation tissue may be caused by several contributing factors associated with the anatomy and function of the distal limb: low oxygen tension and blood flow, high motion areas, chronic contamination, excess tension on the skin, a difference in concentration of growth factors, and a lower body temperature.

The most affective management of exuberant granulation tissue is prevention. Applying a bandaging or cast helps prevent development of exuberant granulation tissue by decreasing movement, applying pressure, maintaining a warm, moist environment, and increasing the rate of wound healing. The use of amnion as the contact layer in bandages may also impede excessive granulation and speed healing. Corticosteroids may be applied topically to granulation tissue to inhibit production. However, corticosteroids must be reserved until a healthy bed of granulation tissue has developed, because they inhibit macrophages and neutrophils and delay wound healing.

Caustic substances are commonly used to reduce granulation tissue once it has developed. However, they may also suppress epithelialization. When it is necessary to remove granulation tissue, sharp excision and proper management is preferable to caustic substances.

ALTERNATIVE MEDICINE

Integrative medical modalities to enhance wound repair include ultrasound, acupuncture, and phototherapy with lasers. These modalities decrease the inflammatory phase and promote the proliferative phase of healing. The proposed mechanism involves stimulation of cell membrane permeability and the release of growth factors and cytokines. The efficacy, feasibility, practicality, and potential use of these modalities are yet to be realized or proven.

MONITORING WOUND HEALING

The progress of wound healing should be monitored to ascertain whether treatment modalities are effective and nondetrimental to wound healing. The most noninvasive technique to assess the wound is an evaluation of color and size and the presence of discharge or blood. However, deep structural changes cannot be monitored visually. Under certain circumstances ultrasound examination may benefit assessment of deep, healing wounds. If a possibility of bony involvement or draining tract development exists, radiographs of the area should be pursued. Contrast radiography may also be useful in the delineation of a foreign body or sequestrum. If body cavity involvement is a risk, radiographs and abdominocentesis or thoracocentesis may be indicated.

Skin Grafts

Susan L. Fubini

Skin graft reconstructive surgery is rarely used in cattle. However, at times, wounds are amenable to skin grafts, especially areas such as the distal limbs and back that have very little loose skin (Figure 8.1-2). Grafts can be performed on fresh wounds or after granulation tissue development by using a delayed technique. Pedicle flaps are a type of graft in which a portion of skin and subcutaneous tissues are transferred to preserve a neurovascular pedicle. Unlike flaps, free skin grafts are devoid of all vascular and neural connections and rely on the recipient site for survival.

A free graft called an *island graft* is the most practical graft to perform on cattle. Island grafts are portions of skin substantially smaller than the recipient site that can be applied in several ways known as pinch, punch, stamp, and tunnel grafts. Skin conditions have to be favorable for attachment and revascularization to have the graft "take" successfully. The recipient bed must provide an environment conducive to graft survival. A bed of healthy granulation tissue gives the best results.

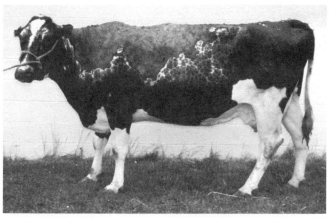

Figure 8.1-2   An adult dairy cow that survived a barn fire with a large granulating wound along the back.

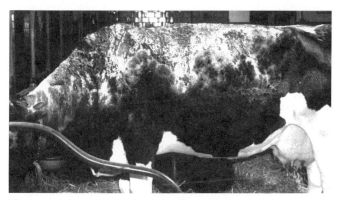

Figure 8.1-3   The adult dairy cow shown in Figure 8.1-2 three months after multiple pinch grafts.

ISLAND GRAFTS

Island grafts are small pieces of skin harvested and transferred to a healthy bed of granulation tissue. Unlike other more sophisticated graft techniques, the surgery can usually be done in the standing animal, is simple, and requires no special equipment. The limited amount of dermis and adnexa transferred means the cosmetic results will not be excellent. Hair growth is oriented in different directions and can have a "tufted" appearance with hairless skin between the plugs of hair. However, a functional result is achievable (Figure 8.1-3).

The technique involves harvesting small plugs of skin from the neck or ventral part of the abdomen and transferring them to a healthy granulation bed. To obtain the grafts, the donor and recipient sites are clipped and prepared for aseptic surgery. An inverted-L block is used to desensitize the donor site. Grafts are obtained by using either a punch biopsy instrument (punch graft) or by elevating a segment of skin with a hypodermic needle and using a scalpel blade to excise a small (approximately 3- to 5-mm) diameter portion of skin. The harvested skin grafts are placed on sterile gauze moistened with sterile saline. They are placed into the granulation bed by creating a "pocket" with a #15 scalpel blade. This works best if the pockets are oriented obliquely in the granulation tissues. The grafts are placed by using a hemostat or thumb forceps. It may be helpful to use a small gauge hypodermic needle to "tease" the graft into the pocket and then hold it in place with direct pressure for 10 to 20 seconds. The most distal grafts should be placed first so that the field is not obscured by blood. The grafts should be placed as close together as possible (3- to 5-mm intervals) because not all will survive. Upon completion of the process, the limb should be wrapped with a sterile, nonadherent bandage. Minimizing motion with a bandage, splint, or cast enhances graft survival. The donor site is left to heal by second intention.

The expected graft survival rate ranges from 50% to 75%. In 4 to 5 weeks, epithelialization should be evident, with some hair growth by 6 weeks.

Mammary Vein Hematoma

Cattle can sustain huge hematomas cranial to the udder, probably resulting from trauma to the subcutaneous abdominal vein. Possible mechanisms that cause the trauma include lacerations, getting up and down, or fighting other cattle. Regardless, the blood loss can be life-threatening, and swelling can be massive. Progressive enlargements of the swelling coupled with worsening anemia are poor prognostic indicators. The anemia is manifested by tachycardia, pale mucous membranes, and weakness.

Differential diagnoses include abscesses and seromas. An abscess is usually hot, painful, and rarely as large. Seromas also do not usually become so large or result in progressive anemia. Ultrasound can confirm the presence of a fluid-filled mass but is not necessary. An aspirate can be performed, but a substantial, and possibly catastrophic, risk of introducing infection exists.

A CBC and coagulation panel is indicated in valuable cows to rule out a bleeding disorder. If a major vein is severed and encountered right away (such as during a surgical approach), the vessel can be sutured with 4-0 monofilament absorbable suture. In more typical, chronic cases, supportive care is indicated. This consists of a blood transfusion, packed cell volume (PCV) ≤13%, belly bandage, confinement, excellent footing and bedding.

Stabilization of the hematoma's size and no further decreases in PCV are positive prognostic indicators. Over time, the swelling will resolve. Incising udder hematomas is contraindicated when no infection is present.

8.2—Dehorning/ Cornuectomy

Daryl Van Nydam and Charles W. Nydam

Historical Perspective

As a surgical procedure, dehorning is one of the oldest and most common procedures done on cattle. Notwithstanding illustrations of cows in many children's books or on craft items such as cow saltshakers or towels, most cattle in countries with a developed bovine industry are dehorned. Although horns are useful to cattle in the wild state, dehorned cattle are safer for handlers and other cattle. Animal welfare concerns are decreased because cattle with no horns, especially when confined in relatively small areas, do not have the opportunity to gouge and bruise one another, either accidentally or on purpose as individuals seek dominance. Effective January 2001, Australia has excluded horned cattle from transport in the export market in an attempt to improve cattle welfare and economic efforts. Carcass losses from bruising are significantly lessened by dehorning, as is damage to other areas, such as the eyes. The incidence of infected lacerations and loss of blood from wounds is also lessened by removing horns. The same effect has not been seen with tipped horns. Dehorning is primarily an elective procedure, except for in cattle with fractured horns or osteomyelitis.

Aside from some polled breeds (e.g., Polled Hereford and Polled Shorthorns), most beef and dairy cattle would have horns if they were not removed. Historically, some breeds, particularly Ayrshires, were prized for their horns, and much effort was put into training horns to shape for show purposes. Some beef breeds, such as Texas Longhorns and Scottish Highlands, still value horns. Pictures of the ideal dairy cow shortly after World War II showed horned animals. In northern climates, several cows 18 to 36 months old had their horns cut off on a cold winter day and were turned outdoors so the frigid air would help constrict spurting and dripping blood vessels to stem the bleeding. It is reputed some animals lost enough blood that they became weak but seldom died.

Cattle owners came to veterinarians for a procedure that could be done cleaner with less blood loss and fewer aftereffects. Veterinarians could provide analgesia and anesthesia as options. The horns were likely to be removed better and avoid regrowth of remnant horn tissue that might still allow infliction of trauma as well as be unsightly. For veterinarians in food animal practice the surgery is repetitive and not especially challenging. Over the years, dehorning gave the veterinarian a chance to get to know the farmer and his cattle operation better, thus providing an opportunity to talk about other bovine production and health matters. With the increase in large herds and development of newer and easier dehorning methods, the job has often been taken over by lay help. Even so, veterinarians instruct the lay help on effective dehorning. In addition, there will often be some that "got away," or there will be smaller or niche farmers, even hobbyists, who will want the veterinarian's attention for dehorning.

Anatomy

Horns begin as "buds" in the newborn when modified epithelium grows outward from the skin. Until 2 months of age, the horn bud is not attached to the skull. Under the bud, the continuing outgrowth of the cornual process of the frontal bone connects it to the skull after 2 months. The bone is covered by a blood-bearing corium that is covered by cornified epithelium. Initially, the frontal sinus does not extend into the horn, but at 4 to 6 months of age, the sinus opens into the horn and becomes larger as the horn grows with age. To keep a scur of horn from growing back after dehorning, a ring of skin tissue 1 to 1.5 cm around the base of the horn needs to be removed, because this is origin of the germinal epithelium where horn growth occurs. If this entire area is removed, the surrounding haired skin will replace the defect without producing a horn.

The horn blood supply is mainly from a branch of the superficial temporal artery, the cornual artery, which lies at the ventral side of the horn (Figure 8.2-1). It arises from behind the orbit, courses caudally along the temporal line, and branches into dorsal and ventral arteries just as it approaches the horn. A proper cut will expose these branches on the edge of the bone. Some smaller arteries may also be exposed on the dorsal side of the horn.

The cornual nerve, a branch of the zygomaticotemporal nerve, innervates the horn area. It courses caudally from the orbit under the bony ridge of the temporal line to the horn, where it divides into two or more branches. The nerve runs with the cornual artery and vein below the temporal line.

Restraint

Adequate restraint of the unwilling patient is crucial for rapid and efficient dehorning. Sufficient lighting facilitates the surgery. Young calves can be straddled and handheld. Ideally, a wooden stake, stanchion, or a head gate on a chute, along with a halter to secure the head

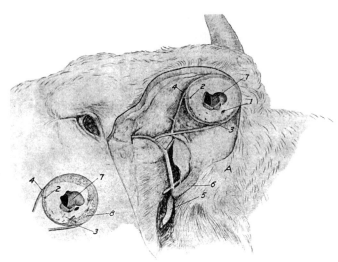

Figure 8.2-1 Schematic of mature bovine poll area and arteries of interest. A, head. 1, intraosseous ventral branch of cornual artery. 2, intraosseous dorsal branch of cornual artery. 3, ventral branch of cornual artery. 4, dorsal branch of cornual artery. 5, external carotid artery. 6, ear cartilage. 7, Frontal sinus. 8, Horn matrix.

(Reprinted from Williams WL: *Surgical and Obstetrical Operations*, ed 4, Ithaca, NY, 1919, William L. Williams.)

snugly against the side of the restraint with room to do so in either direction, should be available for larger animals. Nose leads can be used in place of, or in addition to, a halter on cows and bulls. In reality, animals to be dehorned are often presented in poorly illuminated and cramped areas and fastened loosely by a tie-rail or tether, all of which make restraint and subsequent dehorning more of an effort than one would wish. However, with practice one learns to improvise and cope to still do a satisfactory job.

Anesthesia

Anesthesia is one feature that veterinarians can add to dehorning. It increases the time needed, especially when calves loose in a pen have to be caught individually for anesthetic and dehorning. Some people debate the need for the extra time and handling trauma; they prefer the "brief grief" technique. This is particularly so for very young calves being dehorned by cautery. Nevertheless, United Kingdom law requires use of some form of analgesia when dehorning cattle, unless a caustic disbudding paste is used on animals younger than 7 days old. A study performed in Denmark on Holstein calves showed that the negative behavioral effects and rise in cortisol associated with dehorning were lessened by a cornual nerve block. Larger animals are more easily controlled, especially for hemostasis procedures, if local anesthesia is used.

In all cases, 2% (20 mg/ml) lidocaine can be given with an 18-gauge, 1- to 1.5-inch needle in quantities of 3 to 10 ml per side—needle size and volume depending on the size of animal. The injection site to block the cornual nerve is just under the shelf of the frontal crest/temporal line halfway between the orbit and base of the horn. Loss of sensation generally begins in 5 to 10 minutes. Occasionally, this technique fails to produce the intended anesthesia of the area. Reasons for this include: 1) variation in the nerve's relationship to the bony temporal line; 2) aberrant innervation of the area by other nerves (supraorbital and infratrochlear); 3) a long nerve of the frontal sinus; and 4) premature division of the cornual nerve (See Chapter 6 for more details).

Xylazine hydrochloride can be given to large or unruly patients, particularly if facilities for restraining the head are less than desirable, at a dose of 0.1 mg/kg intramuscularly or 0.05 mg/kg intravenously (some subjects may be refractory to this dose and require more). Fifty to 100 milligrams of xylazine can be added to a hundred-milliliter vial of 2% lidocaine; the resultant mix then is given as usual for dehorning anesthesia to better calm the animal. For example, if 100 milligrams of xylazine is added to 100 ml of lidocaine, the resulting mixture is a 1 mg/ml concentration. If the desired dose of xylazine is 0.1 mg/kg and one is dehorning a 60 kg calf, 6 mg of xylazine is indicated. Therefore administering 3 ml of the xylazine mixture to each side to be dehorned requires 6 mg. If xylazine is used, sedated animals should have adequate footing both during and after dehorning. One disadvantage to xylazine use is that some animals lie down and will not get back up for proper positioning. Another possible untoward effect is bloat if the animal becomes and remains recumbent too long. Furthermore, decreased blood pressure induced by xylazine at the time of dehorning may give a false sense of security about the level of hemostasis achieved. To reverse the effects of xylazine, tolazoline, an alpha-2 adrenergic antagonist, can be administered at a dose of 4.0 mg/kg (4 ml/100 kg). Onset of recovery usually becomes apparent within 5 minutes. Neither xylazine or tolazoline nor compounding of lidocaine with xylazine is approved for use in cattle at this time in the United States. Consult AMDUCA (Animal Medicinal Drug Use Clarification Act) for usage guidelines of extralabel use of drugs and the Food Animal Residue Avoidance Databank (FARAD) for withdrawal times (see Chapter 6, Farm Animal Anesthesia).

Methods

The main methods of dehorning cattle are chemical, thermal cautery, cutting, or genetic. The first two are done on younger calves and require no hemostasis. They also leave no sinus open to infection and can be done any time of year. With proper attention, small horns can also be removed in summer, but cutting horns during fly season, particularly when the frontal sinus is opened, is generally not recommended because of the greatly increased possibility of infection.

The various means of cutting horns also opens the possibility of transfer of bloodborne pathogens such as *Anaplasma, Babesia,* or bovine leukemia virus. Complete disinfection of the dehorner between animals would prevent this, but is not very practical in real field situations. This is another reason to dehorn young cattle by cautery. Dropping the dehorner in a bucket of disinfectant (chlorhexidine) between each use is of some value for diminishing infections transmitted by dehorning (DiGiacomo et al, 1985).

CHEMICAL DEHORNING

For chemical dehorning, a caustic paste of potassium, sodium, or calcium hydroxide is applied to the horn button (Figure 8.2-2). For best results, it is imperative the paste be applied as soon as the horn button can be felt (i.e., within 3 to 7 days of birth); otherwise all of the horn-germinating cells will not be destroyed, and regrowth will occur. It does cause some discomfort to the calf, which must be monitored to ensure that the paste does not gravitate toward its eyes if the calf starts rubbing the buttons or is out in the rain. A 1920 text oriented toward farmers, *The Practical Stock Doctor,* recommends an old technique of clipping the hair off the button to allow better paste contact and use of smaller amounts to lessen the chance of runoff.

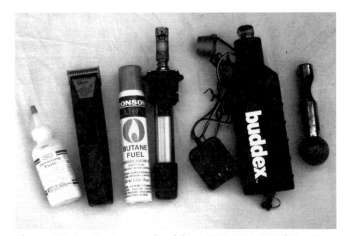

Figure 8.2-2 Equipment for dehorning younger calves. From left to right: dehorning paste, rechargeable clippers, butane fuel, Portasol dehorner, Buddex dehorner, Roberts dehorner.

THERMAL DEHORNING

Various means of thermal dehorning are available. In all cases, it is important to burn thoroughly enough to kill the germinal tissue surrounding the horn bud. This technique is restricted to calves small enough that the dehorner being used will fit entirely to the base of the horn button. It is helpful to clip the hair away first with scissors, a small clipper, or a rechargeable battery powered clipper (see Figure 8.2-2). With small calves, straddling the calf and holding the head firmly against the thigh may be sufficient restraint; otherwise a halter snugged to a firm object is desired.

Portable

Small butane-powered dehorners have become a favorite of many veterinarians and herdsmen (see Figure 8.2-2). They, like other thermal cautery devices, operate at 500° to 600° C. These portable dehorners do not need a cord, heat fast, and work quickly by cutting through the skin to the bone in 5 to 10 seconds, depending on the size of the calf. They can be used on calves about 7 days to 2 months old, which makes them useful for scheduled herd health visits. No risk of transferring bloodborne diseases exists, and they can be used year round. Petrie et al (1996) substantiate this in their report of a surge in cortisol 3 to 7 hours after scoop dehorning but not after thermal cautery. The authors' preference is to have herds accustomed to the thermal cautery dehorners because they seem to be the least traumatic yet offer excellent dehorning results.

Rechargeable battery-powered dehorners for 7-day to 2-month-old calves are available (see Figure 8.2-2). They need to be kept charged and occasionally discharged for recharging, and the power weakens between calves if used in too rapid fashion.

Sufficient pressure must be applied to the skull of small calves while burning with thermal dehorners, best done while twisting the dehorner back and forth. It must be done long enough to see a complete white rim of bone at the base of the burn effort to ensure the blood supply to the horn bud is completely cut.

Corded

Several different types of corded electric dehorners can also be found (Figure 8.2-3). Some are large enough to be used on older calves up to 8 months old, but more contact time is needed with more tissue damage and the smell of burning hair and skin. It is best to perform the procedure in young calves. Adequate time must be allowed for the dehorner heating element to get a cherry red color so it is hot enough to use. The dehorner *must* be applied firmly and long enough to get a copper-colored ring all around the base of the horn. With some smaller units, the heating element may not stay

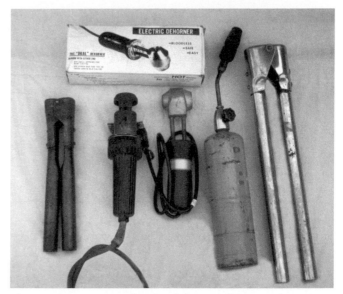

Figure 8.2-3   Instruments for dehorning bigger calves. From left to right: small Barnes, electric dehorner 1, electric dehorner 2, propane dehorner, large Barnes.

sufficiently hot to do a number of calves quickly, particularly if they are large. Dehorners attached to a small propane tank or via hose to a larger tank are heated and used in the same way.

Some owners or operators working in confined areas find the smell of burning hair and skin from this method objectionable. This can serve as a teachable moment when one is trying to convince a producer to more adequately ventilate a housing facility as the smell and smoke should clear out more quickly in a well-ventilated facility.

CUTTING DEHORNING

If young stock are missed at a young age or an owner prefers the final look of a gouge dehorning, then cutting the horns off is an option. Several cutting dehorner devices exist for this, including gouging forceps and a saw. The cutting operation is easier and cleaner if the instruments are kept sharp.

Tube Dehorner

A tube gouge or Roberts dehorner makes a circular cut when twisted over the base of a horn bud on young calves (see Figure 8.2-2). Then a twist upward scoops out the horn. Hemorrhage is minimal, and pressure can be applied to the opening to arrest the bleeding.

Scoop/Gouge Dehorner

Once horns have erupted, scoop dehorners, such as various-sized Barnes dehorners, can be used on calves from 3 months to a year or more, as long as the dehorner fits over the base of the horn enough to remove a one centimeter ring of skin (see Figure 8.2-3). By pushing down on the handles and forcing them apart, the sharp metal edges make an elliptical cut that removes the horn and exposes the cornual arteries. If conditions allow, one can tilt the head over to one side to cut the top horn and pull the head over in the opposite direction to cut the other horn; although both horns can usually be cut with the head tilted in just one direction by maneuvering the handles a little. The exposed cornual arteries and any available branches are grasped with hemostatic forceps and pulled out slowly in the same plane as the head until they snap. That way, the artery remnants are beneath the bone and under the skin where they can clot. One to four arteries may be seen spouting and can be pulled. Often doing the one main ventral artery is sufficient. A thermal cautery dehorner can be applied to the exposed bleeding area for hemostasis. The opening into the sinus can be left open, or a thin piece of gauze can be laid across it to help stem minor bleeding and cover the sinus opening to keep it clean.

Keystone

A large cutting instrument is the guillotine or Keystone-type dehorner, which has two opposing blades that cut the horn when brought together by two long handles (Figure 8.2-4). These are used on large heifers, cows, and smaller bulls. Room is needed to accommodate the handles. After the animal's head is secured, the blades are set far apart and pushed to the base of the topmost horn. The handles are pulled sharply together to cut the horn. If the horns are so large that the operator cannot close the handles easily, separating the handles slightly and rotating the blades a bit before pulling the handles together again can help complete the cut. Ideally, the head can be turned and the other side properly cut in like manner. Pulling the arteries achieves hemostasis if the cuts are done well. If the arteries cannot be pulled, a tourniquet around the base of the horns and across the poll will usually suffice. Baler twine, large rubber bands, canning jar rubbers, and cut pieces of inner tube have been used as tourniquet material. With twine, another piece of twine across the top of the poll drawing the circle tighter may be necessary. Caution the owner to remove the tourniquet in a few days, because it can keep drawing together and get hidden if ignored, creating a nonhealing wound until it is removed.

Electrically Powered

Various electrically powered dehorning saws or cutters are available for use on large horns when electricity is available (see Figure 8.2-4). They cut quickly, but some types can be left open; therefore an ear can be accidentally removed as well. Caution is required to protect the

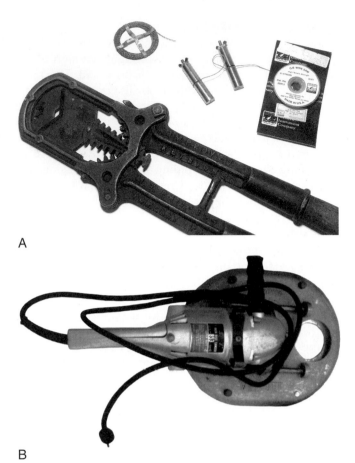

A

B

Figure 8.2-4 Instruments for dehorning mature cattle. *A*, From left to right: keystone, obstetrical wire, and handles. *B*, electric guillotine.

operator and patient. Hemostasis and covering is the same as for other cutting methods.

Obstetrical Wire and Others

Obstetrical wire can be used when a cutting device will not work for really large horns occasionally found on cows and bulls and horn regrowth that curves into the head (see Figure 8.2-4). As with other techniques, it is essential to include a 1.0 cm ring of haired skin with the horn when one makes the cut. Anesthesia is recommended for cutting with an OB wire because the technique is relatively slow. Handheld saws with a stiff back can also cut horns. Because of the horn dust produced and the jaggedness of the cut, hemorrhage may be less, especially from capillaries and small arteries. Any horn dust can fall into the open sinus and be an irritant. Again, hemostasis is via pulling arteries as described above. Occasionally, other cutting devices such as convex nippers or pruning shears can be used to remove horns.

GENETIC

Some beef breeds are now naturally polled and occasional individuals of any breed are polled as the result of an autosomal dominant gene. In fact, the Australian Model Code of Practice for the Welfare of Animals recommends breeding polled cattle where applicable. In the future, gene manipulation may offer an additional alternative to achieve hornless animals.

Although not in use yet except in extraordinary situations, cryosurgery and laser surgery may someday be added to the common ways of dehorning.

Cosmetic Dehorning

Cosmetic dehorning allows primary closure of the skin over the defect created by removing the horn and is occasionally done to create a more predictably desirable-looking head. It is employed in situations in which the following conditions apply: 1) less scarring is desirable; 2) a short healing time is necessary; and/or 3) a cutting dehorning procedure is to be performed on mature subjects during fly season. It is easiest to attain apposition of the skin if this procedure is performed in animals younger than 2 years old. Disadvantages of this procedure include the following: 1) it takes more time and is more expensive than the aforementioned techniques; and 2) greater care must be given to sterile technique because the potential for drainage is eliminated. Clients whose cattle have shown potential or high live market value often request this procedure. Generally, it involves cutting and reflecting skin around the horn base, removing the horn, undermining the skin, and suturing over the wound. Other texts offer additional instruction for the procedure (Hoffsis, 1995).

PREPARATION

Restraint for the procedure should be done as suggested previously, with a chute equipped with a head gate being the optimal alternative. To perform this operation, the veterinarian needs a sterile scalpel, hemostats, needle holder, #2 nonabsorbable suture, and obstetrical wire. A cornual nerve block should be performed as described previously, along with a ring block around the horn and intravenous administration of a 0.05 mg/kg xylazine dose through the tail vein. No complications are anticipated with 20 ml of 2% lidocaine per horn.

The hair should be clipped in a wide area around the horns and across the poll. The area should receive a standard surgical preparation.

TECHNIQUE

Elliptical incisions are made leaving no more than a 1 cm margin around the base of the horn beginning 5 to 7 cm dorsal to and ending 5 to 7 cm ventral to the base of the

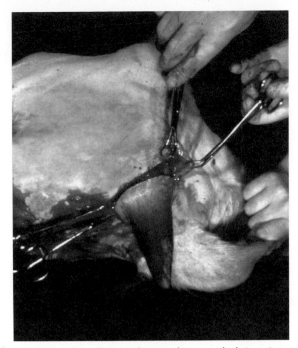

Figure 8.2-5 Skin dissected away from underlying tissues.

horn. The incisions are made with the blade resting on the underlying bone. The skin is sharply dissected from the underlying tissues in the ventral incision, and the veterinarian must be careful not to transect the auricular muscles of the area (Figure 8.2-5). The obstetrical wire is placed in the ventral incision against the frontal bone with the wire directed towards the poll and used to saw off the horn. It is essential the saw be seated properly at the very base of the horn. This should remove the germinal epithelium to prevent horn regrowth, adequately expose the cornual artery for pulling to provide hemostasis as described earlier, and allow apposition of the skin (Figure 8.2-6). The area is examined for loose bone chips and debris, and the site is lavaged with physiologic saline after adequate hemostasis has been achieved. The incised skin is undermined if necessary and brought into direct apposition by using #2 nonabsorbable sutures in a simple interrupted or mattress pattern. If there is a lot of tension on the wound, it may be helpful to put one tension-relieving suture in the middle of the wound. The sutures are removed in 2 to 3 weeks. The opposite horn is removed in like manner to achieve symmetry.

Complications and Aftercare

Hemorrhage is the most common possible complication. If a "bleeder" persists, the operator should check again for an artery to be pulled or ligated. A tourniquet can be applied. It has also been suggested that large

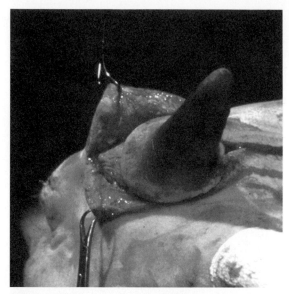

Figure 8.2-6   Exposure of area adjacent to horn.

quantities of sweet clover hay feed can have mold that interferes with hemostasis and should be investigated as a cause of uncontrolled bleeding. To give the clot a matrix on which to form, padding such as cotton can be pressed on the wound and left until it falls off. Blood-stop powders, mainly astringents, can be applied to the bleeding areas as well. Other powders that have been used include flour and corn starch. Dressings in the sinus should be avoided as they can be irritating and delay healing. In yesteryear, farmers applied cobwebs from the barn ceiling for the same purpose. With any form of dehorning, the seal that forms can be prematurely knocked off; occasionally exposing a bleeder that warrants attention. Cautery from a thermal-type dehorner can be used for hemostasis.

Infection is a serious complication, although it is rare with proper technique. Affected cattle are generally febrile, lethargic, inappetent, and may have a malodorous discharge from the site. The resultant acute sinusitis needs to be drained by opening the dehorning site, flushing it copiously with a disinfectant, and tipping the head to drain it on a daily basis until it dries up and drainage ceases. Occasionally, systemic antibiotics may be needed. Sometimes sinusitis may become chronic, which is best treated by trephination and lavage, administration of topical and systemic antibiotics, and analgesics. If drainage persists, osteomyelitis and bone sequestrum may be the cause of a chronic condition. Surgical curettage of the affected area is performed. These chronic sinus infections can be difficult, if not impossible, to clear up. For these reasons, the surgery should not be done in rainy, dusty conditions or during fly season. If dehorning occurs during fly season, appropriate fly control

measures should be instituted, particularly in screw worm–endemic areas. Maggot infestation is handled as in sinusitis.

Another complication of dehorning, especially with the large cutting instruments, is a fractured skull, which can generally be avoided by keeping guillotine blades sharp.

Ketoprofen and other NSAIDs (nonsteroidal anti-inflammatory drugs) have been tried as an aid to reduce stress. One trial that used oral ketoprofen before dehorning and at 2 and 7 hours after dehorning showed reduced levels of behavioral responses to pain compared to the control group (Faulkner and Weary, 2000). The administration of an oral medication three times per day along with xylazine, cornual nerve block, and ring block employed in this study may be difficult to implement given the typical management on United States dairy operations. Note that these drugs are not approved in the United States for this purpose in cattle, but they could be employed under AMDUCA and/or approved in the future.

8.3—Insertion of a Nose Ring

Robert O. Gilbert

Nose rings are commonly used to control bulls. They are inserted into the soft tissue of the nasal septum just cranial to the cartilaginous septum. For insertion the bull should be tightly restrained, so head movement is restricted as much as possible. Infiltration of local analgesia is not practical, but sedatives or systemic analgesics may be administered. Most nose rings have a sharp point designed to be forced through the septum. However, the size and shape of the (hinged and open) ring and the rough nature of the pointed end make controlling and accurately placing the ring extremely difficult. Instead, it is easier to use an appropriately-sized trocar and cannula to pierce the septum at the desired site, and then introduce the nose ring as the cannula is withdrawn. The ring is then snapped shut, screwed closed, and filed, if necessary, to ensure a completely smooth surface.

Although a nose ring is extremely useful in restraining bulls, it is often misused. The nose ring should not be used as the sole form of restraint. Ideally, a rope attached to a neck loop or halter serves as the primary form of restraint, with the nose ring rope used to get the bull's attention or provide additional restraint, if necessary. Constant tension on a nose ring eventually reduces the bull's sensitivity and may be counterproductive.

There is some debate about whether rigid poles or ropes are safer for handling bulls. Some feel there is a danger of a bull using a rigid pole as an instrument to injure the handler; whereas others feel that a rigid pole helps keep the bull at a safe distance from the handler. Ideally, ropes can be used and the handler kept safe by having appropriate facilities with specially designed walkways that allow separation of the handler and bull.

Occasionally, bulls may tear out their nose rings. This sometimes happens during handling; otherwise it may result from the ring being trapped on an immovable object. A nose laceration can be sutured to allow placement of a second ring. For this to be accomplished, the bull should be sedated and firmly restrained. Local analgesic is infiltrated into the area of the laceration. As large an area as possible is freshened on both sides of the laceration, and the anatomy restored by multiple simple interrupted sutures of absorbable material, taking care to restore as much nasal septum as possible. A ring may be inserted once healing is complete, usually in about a month.

RECOMMENDED READINGS

Anziani OS et al: Persistent activity of doramectin and ivermectin in the prevention of cutaneous myiasis in cattle experimentally infested with *Cochliomyia hominivorax*, *Vet Parasit* 87: 243-247, 2000.

Anziani OS, Loreficce C: Prevention of cutaneous myiasis caused by screw worm larva (*Cochliomyia hominivorax*) using Ivermectin, *J Vet Med series B* 40: 287-290, 1993.

DiGiacomo RF et al: Natural transmission of bovine leukemia virus in dairy calves by dehorning, *Can J Comp Med* 49: 340-343, 1985.

Farkas R et al: Efficacy of ivermectin and moxidectin injection against larvae of *Wohlfahrtia magnifica* (Diptera: Sarcophagidae) in sheep, *Parasitol Res* 82: 82-86, 1996.

Faulkner PM, Weary DM: Reducing pain after dehorning in dairy calves, *J Dairy Sci* 83: 2037-2041, 2000.

Goodrich LR et al: Comparison of equine amnion and a non-adherent wound dressing material for bandaging pinch-graft wounds in ponies, *Am J Vet Res* 61: 326-329, 2000.

Grondahl-Nielsen C et al: Behavioural, endocrine, and cardiac responses in young calves undergoing dehorning without and with use of sedation and analgesia, *Vet J* 158: 1-3, 1999.

Hoffsis G: Surgical (cosmetic) dehorning in cattle. In *The Veterinary Clinics of North America, Food Animal Practice*, Philadelphia, 1995, WB Saunders.

Howard RD et al: Evaluation of occlusive dressings for management of full-thickness excisional wounds on the distal portion of the limbs of horses, *Am J Vet Res* 54: 2150-2154, 1993.

Kashyap A et al: Effect of povidone iodine dermatologic ointment on wound healing, *Am Surg* 61: 486-491, 1995.

Knottenbelt DC: Equine wound management: are there significant differences in healing at different sites on the body? *Vet Derm* 8: 273-290, 1997.

Lee AH et al: Effects of chlorhexidine diacetate, povidone iodine, and polyhydroxydine on wound healing in dogs, *JAAHA* 24: 77-83, 1988.

Lee AH et al: The effects of petrolatum, polyethylene glycol, nitrofurazone, and a hydroactive dressing on open wound healing, *JAAHA* 22: 443-451, 1986.

Lingaraj HD et al: Histological and histochemical evaluation of bovine amnion and porcine skin as biological dressings in bovine wounds, *Ind J An Sci* 65: 849-852, 1995.

Lozier S et al: Effects of four preparations of 0.05% chlorhexidine diacetate on wound healing in dogs, *Vet Surg* 21: 107-112, 1992.

McMeekan CM et al: Effects of local anesthesia of 4 to 8 hours' duration on the acute cortisol response to scoop dehorning in calves, *Aust Vet J* 76(4): 281-285, 1998.

Miller JA et al: Larvicidal activity of Merck MK-933, an avermectin, against the horn fly, stable fly, face fly, and house fly, *J Econ Ent* 74: 608-611, 1981.

Petrie NJ et al: Cortisol responses of calves to two methods of disbudding used with or without local anesthetic, *NZ Vet J* 44: 9-14, 1996.

Rebhun WC: Diseases of the teats and udder. In Rebhun WC, editor: *Diseases of dairy cattle*, Philadelphia, 1995, Wilkins and Williams.

Shaw FD et al: The contribution of horned cattle to carcass bruising, *Vet Rec* 98: 255-257, 1976.

Southwood LL, Baxter GM: Instrument sterilization, skin preparation, and wound management, *Vet Clin N Am* 12: 173-194, 1996.

Stashak TS: *Equine wound management*, Philadelphia, 1991, Lea and Febiger.

Swaim SF: Advances in wound healing in small animal practice: current status and lines of development, *Vet Derm* 8: 235-242, 1997.

Turner AS, McIlwraith CW: Cosmetic dehorning. In Turner AS, McIlwraith CW: *Techniques in large animal surgery*, ed 2, Philadelphia, 1989, Lea & Febiger.

Ward JL, Rebhun WC: Chronic frontal sinusitis in dairy cattle: 12 cases (1978-1989), *J Am Vet Med Assoc* 201: 326-328, 1992.

Wohlt JE et al: Cortisol increases in plasma of Holstein heifer calves from handling and method of electrical dehorning, *J Dairy Sci* 77: 3725-3729, 1994.

Wythes JR et al: Effect of tipped horns on cattle bruising, *Vet Rec* 104: 390-392, 1979.

CHAPTER 9

SURGERY OF THE BOVINE RESPIRATORY AND CARDIOVASCULAR SYSTEMS

Earl M. Gaughan, Judy Provo-Klimek, Norm G. Ducharme

Need for surgical treatment for respiratory and cardiovascular disease in cattle is not common. However, several disorders are well documented and are most expediently addressed with surgical therapy. Although some of these disorders are congenital malformations, the majority are infectious in origin. Thorough physical examination can often determine an accurate diagnosis and the treatment most likely to be successful. Several ancillary diagnostic exercises can assist physical examination findings to further direct specific treatment selection. This chapter will focus on surgical considerations in the treatment of cardiovascular and respiratory diseases, but other factors such as cost, genetic potential, and other business considerations should be included in the decision-making process.

Diagnostics

PHYSICAL EXAMINATION

Clinical signs can often dictate the specific target of a physical examination. However, any thorough examination should evaluate the respiratory and cardiovascular systems. The focus of the exam should be on both the morphology of the relevant anatomical structures and evidence of physiological dysfunction of each of these systems.

When the animal is approached, indications of respiratory system dysfunction can be appreciated by noting respiratory characteristics such as rapid, shallow breaths, coughing and open-mouth breathing, which are all signs of impaired ventilation. Determination of respiratory rate is not as important as noting the pattern and ease of respiratory effort. Upper respiratory sounds can increase or be abnormal in cases of upper airway obstruction. In addition, other vital signs such as heart rate and body temperature are very important in assessing a patient. These can often help determine the likelihood of involvement of a septic process. Body condition and knowledge of the duration of the problem can help in determining potential success when considering surgical therapy.

The upper respiratory tract can be evaluated relatively readily via palpation, percussion, and auscultation. The nares of cattle should be moist and readily and regularly cleaned by the tongue; therefore the presence of even serous nasal discharge is abnormal. The openings of the nares do not flare or move as much as those of horses. Patency of the nares and nasopharynx can be readily accomplished by placing cupped hands in front of the nares and assessing the volume of air flow or, in cold climates, observing the condensed expired air. Inspiration is difficult to assess, but the relative volume of expired air can be readily determined. Symmetry of air flow may be the most important aspect of expiration to be determined at the nares. The nature of any fluid at the nares should be examined. Expired air should be evaluated for odors that may be indicative of an infectious and/or necrotic process. Any abnormal sounds associated with inspiration or expiration should also be noted. Audible whistles, gurgles, or other abnormal sounds can be indicative of upper airway compromise.

Facial symmetry should be assessed and any distortion may indicate underlying disease disrupting upper airway anatomy. Percussion of the nasal passages and paranasal sinuses can be performed with fingers or with a plexometer. Placing a stethoscope over the percussed region may help determine the presence of abnormal tissue or fluid presence in otherwise air-filled spaces. The sounds can be augmented by opening the mouth during percussion.

The ventral aspect of the head should be visually examined and palpated. The intermandibular space should be examined for swelling and painful response to palpation. Congenital malformation, trauma associated with bawling gun injury or foreign body penetration may result in a perilaryngeal mass that can compromise the upper respiratory tract at the pharynx, larynx and proximal trachea. These can be suspected by detection of proximal cervical swelling (see Figure 10-14). The cervical locations of palpable lymphatic tissues should be closely examined visually and by hand. The trachea should be auscultated with attention to airflow, or abnormal sounds indicating the presence of fluid. The trachea and tracheal region should be palpated. Subcutaneous crepitation should be noted. Tracheal sensitivity to pressure and the ease of eliciting a cough should also be determined.

The thoracic cavity should be evaluated by observing the overall condition of the patient as well as the basic movements of the thoracic wall during respiratory efforts. A decline in body score and abnormal respiratory movements can indicate a primary disease process in the thorax. Auscultation is important in evaluating the thorax. Careful attention and assessment of ventilation and lung sounds should be performed. This should include notation of the location or regionalization of abnormal findings. Abnormal lung sounds can indicate different pulmonary diseases, which may or may not need surgical therapy. Thoracic and cardiac surgical diseases are suspected by the absence of respiratory sounds or muffled normal sounds, which indicates a need for further diagnostic procedures. In conjunction with auscultation, percussion of the thoracic wall should be performed. A normal bovine thorax should have air-filled resonance throughout the thorax except for sites of closest cardiac association. Fingers or a plexometer used in a dorsal-to-ventral direction in the intercostal spaces can help detect loss of resonance associated with accumulated fluid or solid tissue in the pleural space. Notation of the interface between resonant and dull percussing regions can often indicate the relative level and severity of abnormal pleural fluids. This can also help when deciding if thoracocentesis will be of value.

Other physical manipulations can also assist when assessing the thorax of cattle. Hand pressure can be applied to the dorsal aspect of the spinous processes over the thorax or from the ventral aspect of the sternum. Observation while applying pressure can reveal a pain-avoidance response (grunt test), which can indicate an intrathoracic disorder that may require surgical treatment.

ENDOSCOPIC EXAMINATION

Endoscopy is a very useful tool for evaluating the upper respiratory tract. Endoscopy is certainly most familiar in equine practice, yet the same general techniques can be applied to cattle. Standing restraint is necessary and is likely best in a stanchion or substantial head catch. Although anatomy can be evaluated with any form of restraint, normal upper airway function can only be assessed in a nonsedated animal. Therefore physical restraint alone is encouraged. Nose tongs can help gain control of the head. If these are used, care should be taken not to occlude passage of an endoscope through the nares into the nasal passages. It is advised to evaluate each nasal passage, which requires passing the endoscope though the left and right sides. Anatomical variation from the more familiar equine upper airway includes the following:

1. Pharynx: a caudodorsally tapering nasal septum in the caudal one third of the nasal passage (Figure 9-1), visualization of both ethmoid turbinates from

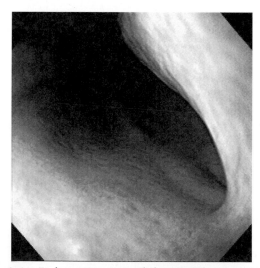

Figure 9-1 Endoscopic view of the nasopharynx; note the caudodorsally tapering nasal septum in the caudal third of the nasal passage.

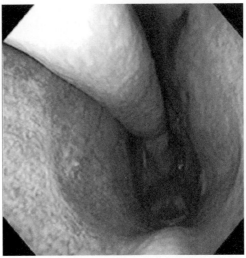

Figure 9-2   Endoscopic view of the nasopharynx: note the nasopharyngeal septum.

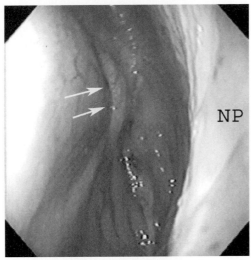

Figure 9-3   Endoscopic view of the nasopharynx: note the right nasopharyngeal opening of the auditory tubes (arrows) located dorsolateral to the nasopharyngeal (NP) septum.

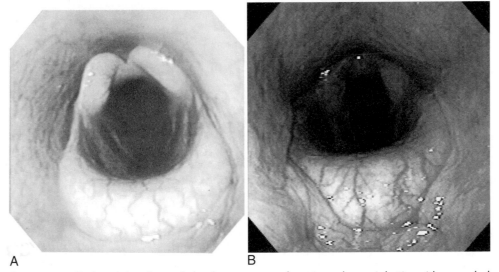

Figure 9-4   Endoscopic view of the larynx: note the triangular epiglottis with rounded borders and very prominent rounded corniculate processes of the arytenoid cartilages.

the same viewing side, a pharyngeal septum (Figure 9-2), location of the nasopharyngeal openings of the auditory tubes dorsolateral to the pharyngeal septum (cattle do not have guttural pouches) (Figure 9-3)

2. Larynx: a triangular epiglottis with rounded borders and very prominent corniculate processes of the arytenoid cartilages (Figure 9-4). Jersey cows have irregular, dark pigmentation of the mucosa of the pharyngeal and laryngeal structures (Figure 9-5). Finally, dorsal displacement of the soft palate is common after withdrawal of the endoscope from the trachea.

If sedation is deemed necessary to complete an endoscopic evaluation of an individual's upper airway, care should be exercised in choosing sedative agents. Xylazine can substantially alter the anatomic position of laryngeal structures and reduce response to stimuli. Therefore assessments of laryngeal function may be inaccurate. Acepromazine appears to result in much less interference with evaluation and may be preferable over xylazine if time and the animal's demeanor allow use of this agent.

IMAGING EXAMINATION

Ultrasonography can be a very helpful tool in evaluating the airway for disease. It should be recalled that sound

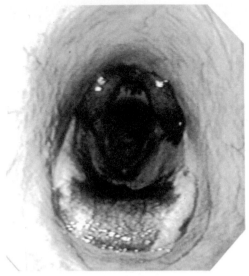

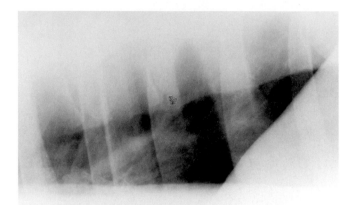

Figure 9-6   Pleural fluid accumulation in a cow with septic pleuritis.

(Courtesy of Dr. A. Yeager, Cornell University.)

Figure 9-5   Endoscopic view of the nasopharynx and larynx in a Jersey cow; note the irregular, dark pigmentation of the mucosa of the pharyngeal and laryngeal structures.

waves reflect from gas or air; therefore the aerated aspects of the respiratory tract cannot be satisfactorily imaged. However, a great deal of indirect information can be obtained with ultrasonography. Soft tissue facial distortion, peritracheal swelling, and pleural space fluid accumulation can be readily assessed. Ultrasonography is indicated anytime soft tissue or fluid-associated abnormalities are evaluated in and around the respiratory tract of cattle.

Radiography can also be critical in imaging the respiratory tract of cattle. The upper airway is best imaged with lateral and dorsoventral radiographic projections. However, various oblique views can certainly assist in defining mass lesions and lesions associated with fluid accumulation. With the increasing availability of three dimensional imaging, computed tomography (CT) and magnetic resonance imaging (MRI) can assist the clinician in completing diagnoses in cattle. However, animal size and economic considerations will likely limit the practicality of these imaging modalities. The lower airway can also be imaged with radiographs (Figure 9-6); however, animal size often interferes with the ability to identify abnormalities. It should be assumed that radiographic detail will be lost as body size increases. When one is considering the caudal thorax and cranial abdomen, positioning the bovine patient may be an important for successful radiographic assessment. Metallic foreign material that penetrates the reticulum and entering the thoracic cavity may be more easily identified radiographically with the patient in dorsal

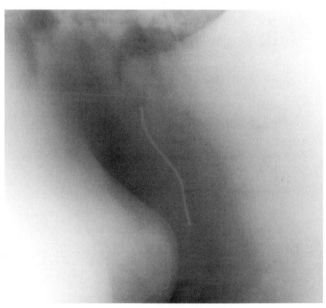

Figure 9-7   Radiograph of the caudal thorax and cranial abdomen in a mature cow with traumatic reticuloperitonitis and pericarditis. Note the metallic foreign body sticking out of the confines of the reticulum in the caudal thoracic area.

(Courtesy of Dr. N. Dykes, Cornell University.)

recumbency rather than standing (Figures 9-7 and 9-8). This allows for reduced tissue thickness and better detail of reticular and pericardial structures with the gas content displaced in the ventral aspect of the reticulum. Care should be exercised as some animals do not tolerate casting or the sedation needed for this position. Dorsal recumbency is not advised for very sick and/ or debilitated animals or animals with impaired ventilation.

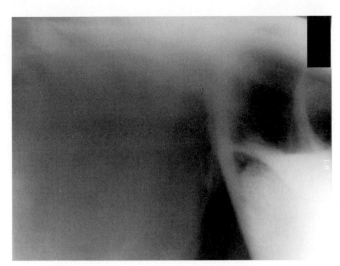

Figure 9-8 Radiograph of the cranial abdomen in a mature cow in dorsal recumbency: note the improved visibility of the reticulum in comparison to Figure 9-7.

(Courtesy of Dr. N. Dykes, Cornell University.)

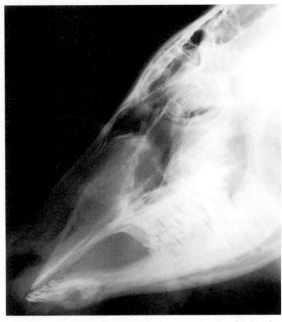

Figure 9-9 Lateral radiograph of a 7-month-old heifer calf with nasal conchae cysts. Note oblong opacity in the nasal cavity.

(Courtesy of Dr. N. Dykes, Cornell University.)

Upper Airway

NASAL OBSTRUCTION

Nasal obstruction in cattle, as in other animals, is typically marked by respiratory noise, which is readily localized to the upper airway. Unilateral obstruction can usually be detected with cupped hands near the nares to evaluate symmetry of expiration. Bilateral obstruction is accompanied by severe dyspnea and often with labored open-mouthed breathing. Disease entities most commonly associated with nasal obstruction include congenital malformation—such as conchal cyst (Figure 9-9) and choanal atresia—and acquired conditions, such as granulomas, polyps, and neoplasia (i.e., adenocarcinoma).

Physical and endoscopic examinations in combination with radiography can usually delineate the presence of a discrete mass lesion (see Figure 9-9). This is desirable when surgical treatment is considered, as a specific target helps in formulating a surgical plan. Some small and pedunculated nasal masses can be resected with transendoscopically-guided long instruments, wire loop (with or without cautery), or laser. Small masses may also be amenable to traditional trephination approaches and therefore can be removed in standing cattle. It is possible to resect membranous choanal atresia using a laser (Nd : Yag or diode) under video endoscopic guidance, but a well vascularized membrane can hemorrhage and obstruct vision of the surgery site.

Nasal flap elevation is typically necessary to reach larger masses in the nasal passage or bony choanal atresia of affected animals. Often nasal masses come to

veterinary attention after the size and potential invasiveness of the primary disease process indicates a need for general anesthesia and performance of a large facial flap procedure.

The typical preanesthetic preparations (including acceptable antibiotic and antiinflammatory therapies), induction and maintenance of general anesthesia are recommended (see Chapter 6). Orotracheal intubation is essential to allow surgical manipulation within the nasal cavity. Lateral recumbency with the affected nasal side uppermost is usually a satisfactory position for unilateral disease. On rare occasions, sternal recumbency is desirable to reach bilateral lesions from a single incisional approach. A flap should be designed to allow as complete exposure as possible without potentially damaging vital structures. It should be noted that many—if not most—facial flaps will enter the paranasal sinuses. This is especially true in the caudal region of the nasal passages. The maxillary and frontal sinuses are often the first cavity entered in an approach to the nasal cavity.

A curvilinear skin incision is made over the underlying bone and soft tissues that require elevation. Periosteum should be sharply incised, gently elevated, and moved from the line of incision into bone. An oscillating bone saw is ideal for this procedure; however, an osteotome and mallet can also be successful in producing a bone flap. The rostral, caudal, and axial aspects of the bone flap should be completely osteotomized. The dorsal and rostral aspects should be "notched" at the corners to allow the flap to be gently hinged away from the normal position. This generally produces good exposure to allow needed manipulations of diseased tissues in the nasal cavity. The nasal passages and paranasal sinuses are highly vascular regions, and extensive hemorrhage should be expected with aggressive manipulations. Hemostasis is difficult to obtain without direct packing of gauze into the affected airways. With unilateral surgical procedures, firm packing of the affected airway with continuous rolled gauze is very effective in controlling bleeding. In our experience, nasal bleeding is not as marked in cattle in comparison to horses. If bilateral disease is present, a tracheostomy should be placed. The gauze packing can be exited from the nares and secured to the skin. Alternatively, the packing can be exited from the lateral aspect of the incision. This usually requires removal of a corner of bone with a rongeur forceps or osteotome. The bone flap can be repositioned and manually pushed back to its normal position. Periosteum, subcutaneous tissues, and skin are then closed. The facial bone of the flap can be wired to the parent bone, but this is rarely necessary if the overlying soft tissues can be successfully closed.

Gauze packing should be left in place for 24 to 72 hours. The gauze can usually be readily pulled from the airway without chemical restraint. Some form of confinement housing is probably best for several days after surgery. During this time, continued antibiotic and anti-inflammatory therapy is usually indicated. Benign nasal polyps, foreign bodies, and infectious or allergic granulomas usually respond well to surgical removal and supportive medical management. Alternatively, some granulomatous masses can be treated or managed with repeated injection of formaldehyde (neutral buffered 10% formalin) (one should consult with your regulatory veterinarian, as this may vary between countries). Nasal neoplasia is often very difficult to completely excise; therefore surgery is, at best, palliative, and recurrence is common.

DISORDERS OF THE PARANASAL SINUSES

Disease of the paranasal sinuses is most commonly marked by discharge from the nares or a site of previous dehorning or fracture. The frontal or maxillary sinuses or both can be affected. The sinuses can be primarily affected—usually with infectious, congenital, or neoplastic disorders—or secondarily a disease process extension from a distant or near site. The most common cause of infectious sinusitis is extension of a septic complication after dehorning. Other causes of sinusitis are trauma, sinus cysts, and parasites. Sinus disease should be considered with unilateral or bilateral nasal discharge; facial

distortion; and signs of abnormal head posturing, which possibly indicates pain. Other clinical signs may include foul breath odor, dullness upon sinus percussion, fever, anorexia, depression, weight loss, or decreased production.

Diagnosis of paranasal sinus disease is based upon physical examination findings and imaging studies. On physical examination, bulging of the sinus and purulent exudates at the site of dehorning or nasal discharge are typical of sinusitis (Figure 9-10). Endoscopy may help rule out other sources of nasal discharge, but the best definition of sinus involvement is obtained with radiography. Lateral and dorsoventral radiographic projections will delineate abnormal soft tissue and fluid components within the airspace and walls of the sinuses (Figure 9-11, A and B). Occasionally, oblique projections may be necessary to more fully understand the extent of the disease process. Final etiologic diagnosis depends on microbial culture, cytology, and/or histology of the abnormal tissues within the affected sinus. This may be obtained from sinus centesis and aspiration after a small trephine hole is produced with a Steinmann pin (4 mm or 5/32 inch). *Actinomyces pyogenes* is commonly isolated after dehorning, and *Pasteurella multocida* is often associated with sinusitis unrelated to dehorning.

Refractory or chronic infectious sinusitis is best treated by open drainage and lavage of the affected sinus. This is most directly performed with 1 or 2 trephine holes positioned to allow drainage. The site of trephination for each sinus is indicated in Figure 9-12. This can

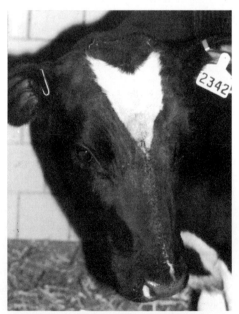

Figure 9-10 Young bull with sinusitis. Note purulent drainage at the right nostril.

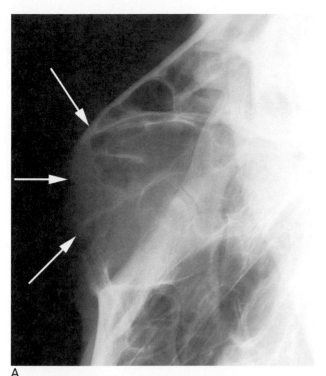

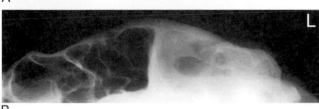

Figure 9-11   *A,* Right lateral radiograph of the frontal sinus in a 3-year-old Jersey cow. Note the fluid line in the left frontal sinus. *B,* Rostral to caudal radiograph view of the frontal sinuses. Note complete opacification of the left frontal sinus.

(Courtesy of Dr. Anthony P. Pease, Cornell University.)

be done with physical restraint and local anesthesia. Generally, the site of drainage is localized in the middle of the bulging frontal or maxillary bone. The frontal sinus is the most commonly affected sinus, and one needs to effectively drain the postorbital diverticulum. The drainage site is 4 cm caudal to the caudal edge of the orbit just above the temporal fossa (Figure 9-12A). The rostral site of the frontal sinus can be drained by trephining 2.5 cm from the midline on a line passing through the orbit center (Figure 9-12B). The turbinate part of the frontal sinus can be drained by trephining just caudal to the nasal bone divergence point, again 2.5 cm from midline (Figure 9-12C). The main part of the frontal sinus can also be trephined if it bulges (Figure 9-12D). A ³/₄-inch (19 mm) trephine is recommended. Addi-

tional trephine holes may be required, depending on individual needs. The maxillary sinus can be opened with a trephine hole immediately dorsal and caudal to the facial tubercle. It may be necessary to place this hole more dorsally in younger cattle to avoid the maxillary teeth. After trephination, large volume lavage with sterile fluid is often necessary to remove exudate and debris. Saline (0.9%), lactated Ringer's, or tap water with povidone iodine solution can work well. Occasionally, debridement will be required to completely remove inspissated material and necrotic tissue. This can be performed though the trephine holes or a more aggressive sinus flap. The technique is the same as described for the various approaches to the nasal passages. Flaps should be elevated toward midline with sufficient exposure to accomplish the necessary excision or debridement. General anesthesia is usually required when large flaps are considered. Complete curettage and aggressive lavage are easier to perform via a sinus flap. Voluminous hemorrhage is more likely after creation of a flap and aggressive intrasinus manipulation. Therefore packing the sinus with gauze may be required before flap closure. Creating portals for lavage and drainage is recommended before closing the flap. Removing one or two corners of the facial bone flap allows easy access for subsequent lavage. This is essential to resolve septic disease processes in conjunction with systemic and local antibiotic therapy.

In cattle with dental disease as the primary cause of sinus involvement, dental extraction is required. Often oral extraction of the affected tooth can be successful. Because the tooth root is shorter in cattle and the disease process is usually chronic, oral extraction is easier than it is for horses. The crown of the affected tooth is grasped with a forceps and rocked back and forth until it loosens and can be extracted. Postextraction drainage through the mouth with, or without, lavage usually resolves the problem. Alternatively, either a trephine hole over the affected tooth or a sinus flap can be effective in providing access for tooth repulsion. A general-purpose acrylic or special dental putty should be placed into the oral aspect of the dental alveolus to prevent oral contamination of the sinus. Plaster of Paris can be used for this purpose as well. The packing is an effective temporary barrier and is usually extruded (or removed) when sufficient granulation or fibrous tissue forms to occlude the mouth from the sinus. Treatment of the sinusitis with local lavage as described earlier is also required.

Cattle with infectious sinusitis appear to respond well to surgical treatment if it is performed prior to general debilitation and development of deteriorating secondary clinical signs. If a neoplastic disorder causes the sinusitis, treatment (surgical debridement of an affected sinus) is

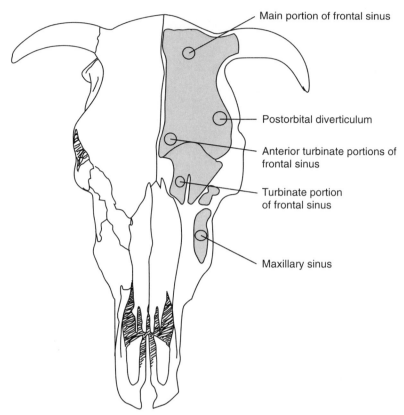

Figure 9-12   The circles indicate the site(s) of trephination for each sinus, and shaded areas are the frontal and maxillary sinuses.

palliative, but long-term prognosis is poor because complete excision is usually not possible.

DISORDERS OF THE NASOPHARYNX

Localized infectious disease is the most common disorder of the bovine pharynx. Trauma from puncture or laceration can be problematic and can also result in abscess, hematoma, or granuloma formation in the pharyngeal and retropharyngeal tissues (see Figure 10.1-4). Lymph node abscesses can also result from delivery of bacteria to lymphatic tissue in this region. Pharyngeal polyps and various neoplastic disorders have been reported in cattle but are rare. Finally, cleft palate is occasionally seen in cattle (see Figure 10.1-20). Most cleft palates are congenital, but injury during oral administration of medication can occasionally result in iatrogenic palate laceration. Animals with cleft palate typically present with nasal regurgitation of milk, water, and food material immediately after eating. They are likely to have secondary aspiration pneumonia, and signs of lower airway disease may be present.

Clinical signs associated with trauma to the pharynx can mimic those of other regions of the upper airway.

Nasal discharge with foul breath may be the mildest sign noted. The spectrum of clinical signs can progress to dyspnea and dysphagia, fever, and systemic fluid and electrolyte derangement. Diagnosis can usually be made from a thorough physical examination, which includes a speculum-assisted visual and manual oral examination. Endoscopy can also be helpful to inspect suspected lesion sites more closely. Ultrasound examination can reveal an abscess or thickened perilaryngeal tissue with edema or fluid/air around the larynx, which indicates cellulitis. Radiography can also delineate an abscess location and dimensions. Close attention should be given to the systemic repercussions of pharyngeal obstruction because respiratory and gastrointestinal malfunction (such as ruminal bloat) may initially require treatment before the primary pharyngeal lesion is addressed. For example, if an animal cannot swallow, marked dehydration and acidosis can occur associated with the loss of fluids and bicarbonate through the saliva.

Pharyngeal trauma that does not result in abscess formation rarely requires surgical treatment. Instead, systemic antibiotics, analgesics, and medical therapy (appropriate fluid and electrolyte supplementation) can often lead to resolution of lacerations, hematomas, and granulomas. However, if cervical cellulitis (see Section 10.1) and/or a pharyngeal abscess develops, surgical drainage is the most expedient means of returning to normal function (see Section 10.1 for management of cervical cellulitis secondary to oropharyngeal disease). An abscess can cause significant upper airway obstruction and requires immediate attention to prevent suffocation. Depending on the degree of airway compromise, a temporary tracheostomy may be needed before surgical intervention. Abscesses in—or very near—the pharyngeal wall can often be incised and drained into the pharyngeal cavity. Retropharyngeal and perilaryngeal abscesses are more common than abscesses directly in the pharyngeal wall. These abscesses usually result from trauma or esophageal rupture or develop in regional lymph nodes. As for pharyngeal abscesses, the diagnosis is usually based on clinical signs that can vary from local swelling to dyspnea, anorexia, excessive salivation, and dysphagia. Ultrasonography and radiography can help more accurately define the location, structure, and quantity of abscesses (see Figure 10.1-6, A). These imaging techniques can also confirm the presence of foreign material that requires removal. The treatment of retropharyngeal abscesses is also based on establishing good ventral drainage.

Drainage of both pharyngeal and retropharyngeal abscesses can be readily accomplished in standing cattle with physical or chemical restraint. Drainage can be obtained through the nasopharynx, oropharynx, or proximal cervical area. An incision adequate enough for complete drainage is important. Debridement and lavage may assist in completing drainage but may not be essential to a good outcome. The incision should be left open to heal by second intention.

This drainage is best accomplished with a carefully restrained, standing, and occasionally sedated animal after infiltrating the surgical site with local anesthesia. Sedation must be used with great caution because sedation relaxes the nasopharynx musculature, which can accentuate the degree of upper airway compromise. Nasopharynx drainage is done with endoscopic guidance by using either laser incision or cautery. Oropharynx drainage is performed, after placing an oral speculum, using a scalpel blade, guarded by hand, introduced into the mouth. The abscess can be incised and drained, either blindly or with endoscopic guidance. Ideally, incisions should be located ventrally and be large enough to allow continuous drainage. When possible, the abscess cavity should be explored digitally for blunt debridement of fibrinous and fibrous septa, which can interfere with complete decompression. After surgery, oral or pharyngeal lavage can be attempted, but the practicality and efficacy of this may be frustrating.

A large retropharyngeal abscess that extends near the skin surface in the cervical area may require a cervical approach for surgical decompression of the ventral pharyngeal and laryngeal regions. Because many perilaryngeal and pharyngeal structures (linguofacial vein and artery; parotid glands; facial, vagal, and pharyngeal branch of the vagal and hypoglossal nerves) are important, great care should be used during surgical exploration. Cellulitis or periabscess fibrosis can greatly diminish the ability to recognize these vital structures. The authors have found the following procedure minimizes the risk and morbidity associated with drainage of these abscesses. First, (preferably under ultrasonographic control) a 6-inch (15.24 cm), 14-gauge needle is placed into the abscess. A 2-cm skin incision is made adjacent to the lesion, and the needle is left in place. A curved Mayo scissors is advanced a few cm into the incision and the blades opened to bluntly to separate the tissue. This procedure is continued until the scissors penetrate the abscess, and the needle is loosened. The abscess cavity is then probed digitally, and if necessary, the tract is enlarged one to two more centimeters. A draining fistula should be enlarged conservatively where adjacent vital structures cannot be identified. Depending on the extent and location of the lesion, a midline incision, or a lateral incision below the linguofacial vein, is used to drain a pharyngeal abscess and reach a quicker resolution.

Finally, a pharyngotomy can be used to provide limited surgical access for addressing pharyngeal abscesses, polyps, or tumors. Most polyploid and neoplastic disorders of the pharynx will not be resolved by surgical resection. A caudal ventral midline skin incision can be made between the basihyoid bone and thyroid cartilage. The incision is extended toward the pharynx using a combination of sharp and blunt dissection to enter the ventral aspect of the oropharynx. As described under Transhyoid Pharyngotomy, the basihyoid bone can be transected with an osteotome to increase visibility of the oropharynx. The authors prefer to close the oropharyngeal mucosa with simple continuous sutures. If the basihyoid bone has been split, a number 2 or 5 stainless steel suture is used to stabilize the basihyoid bone. The sternothyrohyoid muscles are reapposed over the basihyoid bone only, and the remainder of the incision is left open to heal by second intention. If the pharyngeal and laryngeal aspects of the upper airway are still compromised to the point of dyspnea, a temporary tracheotomy may also be required.

Persistent dorsal displacement of the soft palate is an extremely rare cause of upper airway obstruction in farm animals. Unlike horses, dorsal displacement of the soft palate results in respiratory noise that is most evident on inspiration, although it is apparent on expiration as well. Diagnosis is suspected on the basis of upper respiratory noise and confirmed by endoscopy. If the upper airway obstruction is significant, strap muscle resection has been shown effective in relieving DDSP. The procedure can be done with the animal standing, head tied-up, and the middle cervical infiltrated with local anesthetic. Alternatively, general anesthesia can be used. After aseptic preparation of the area, a 10-cm ventral midline incision in the cranial cervical region is used to expose the sternohyoideus and sternothyroideus muscles at the ventral and ventrolateral aspects of the trachea. These muscles are elevated and transected, and a segment (10 cm) of each muscle is resected. The subcutaneous tissues and skin are closed separately. Normal husbandry and function as well as reduction of respiratory noise have been reported within 24 hours of surgery.

PALATOSCHISIS (CLEFT PALATE)

The etiology of cleft palate can be congenital or acquired. In utero, the left and right sides of the palate should fuse following descent of the tongue out of the nasal cavity. A delay in tongue descent is theorized to cause cleft palate in many species. Palate fusion normally starts at the rostral aspect of the palate and extends caudally. Therefore a hard palate cleft typically involves the soft palate. Congenital clefts can be caused by heritable factors seen in some breeds (such as Charolais) or associated with the ingestion of teratogenic substances by the dam during pregnancy. Piperidine alkaloids contained in various plants (Poison-hemlock [*Conium maculatum*] and *Nicotiana* spp., including *N. tabacum* and *N. glauca*) have been reported to cause cleft palate in goats, sheep, pigs, and cattle. These substances may reduce fetal movement, resulting in cleft palate (by decreased tongue movement) and multiple skeletal contractures. Iatrogenic cleft palate usually results from inappropriate or forceful delivery of oropharyngeal medication.

Cleft palate is most often associated with regurgitation of milk from the nose and complications from aspiration pneumonia. The diagnosis can be made by oral examination in cases in which the cleft extends into the hard palate (see Figure 10.1-20) and by endoscopy in all other cases. Because aspiration pneumonia is the main consequence of cleft palate, the lower airway status should be carefully evaluated. It follows that animals with recurrent pneumonia may need to have their palate evaluated. Because of cleft palate's association with orthopedic malformations, it is wise to closely evaluate any calf affected with congenital orthopedic abnormalities (specifically arthrogryposis) for other anomalies, such as cleft palate.

Most affected animals are removed from replacement considerations or herd additions. Euthanasia is the suggested appropriate treatment in cases where heritability is thought to cause the disease. The duration and degree of aspiration in cleft palate cases determines the optimal management of animals not intended for reproduction or with nonheritable congenital or acquired cleft palate. Small soft palate clefts that have minimal degrees of aspiration may be compatible with life with minimal or no impairment in growth or production. Larger cleft palates need to be repaired surgically as described in the following discussion.

The choice of surgical approach includes a) oral—using laparoscopic instruments; b) transhyoid pharyngotomy; and c) mandibular symphysiotomy. Sometimes a combination of these approaches is required. Factors that influence the choice of optimal approach include the size of the animal's head and length and location of the palate defect. Whenever possible, the least invasive approach should be used. The optimal time to repair a cleft palate is still unclear. The advantages of early intervention include minimizing the consequences of aspiration, ability to rely on a liquid-only diet, and absence of rumination in the postoperative period. However, the small surgical field makes the procedure more difficult, and the reduction in pharyngeal size associated with postoperative swelling can result in respiratory distress. The advantage in delaying repair 1 to 4 months is that the animal's larger size may make the surgical procedure easier. However, aspiration pneumonia may increase the anesthetic risks.

The transhyoid pharyngotomy approach is less invasive than a symphysiotomy and has minimal morbidity. The animal must be older for the approach to provide enough exposure for surgical repair. This is only indicated for soft palate cleft repair. A ventral midline incision from the rostral aspect of the basihyoid to the cricoid cartilage is made. The incision is extended with scissors between the thyroid cartilage and basihyoid bone until the pharyngeal mucosa is identified. Using an osteotome, the veterinarian splits the basihyoid into two equal halves. The oropharyngeal mucosa is incised through the length of the pharyngotomy. A Gelpi retractor is used to keep the pharyngotomy incision open, and an Army-Navy retractor is used to rostrally retract the base of the tongue underneath the split basihyoid bone. Closure of the pharyngotomy incision is obtained with a simple continuous pattern by using absorbable sutures (00) in the mucosa. The basihyoid bone is reapposed with a single steel suture. The sternohyoid muscles are reapposed with a simple continuous pattern of absorbable sutures (00) to cover the basihyoid bone. The rest of the incision is left open to heal by second intention.

Mandibular symphysectomy gives the best exposure and is required for repair attempts of all clefts extending to the hard palate. Affected calves should be fasted, supported intravenously with fluids and glucose, and placed under general anesthesia. A skin incision is made from the basihyoid bone extending rostrally to the mandibular symphysis just caudal to the lip attachments on the mandible. The incision is extended through the mylohyoid muscle. The incision does not have to extend rostrally through the lip. Instead, a transverse skin incision can be made by extending through the oral mucosa perpendicularly to the midline incision. The lip can then be placed orally by exposing the mandibular symphysis. This procedure spares the lip from being incised, which decreases the morbidity of this invasive procedure. The symphysis is separated with an osteotome. An abaxial plane of dissection is made approximately 1.5 cm axial to the mandible as follows: the tendon of insertion of the geniohyoid is incised 1 cm from its mandibular insertion. The genioglossus is separated, and the soft tissues are separated bluntly so the mandibular salivary glands, hypoglossal nerve, and tongue are axial to the plane of dissection. After incising the oral mucosa and widely separating the incised mandibular symphysis and soft tissues, the palate can be reasonably exposed.

The soft palate's ability to mobilize tissues to close the cleft should be evaluated. If there is not enough redundant tissue available to appose the palate margins without great tension, tissues must be elevated and advanced toward the midline. Most cleft palate repair attempts in which this step is necessary are likely to fail. If tissue can be apposed, the free edge should be incised, and closure should be completed in three layers (Figure 9-13). A 0-0 to 2-0 size absorbable suture material is recommended. The first layer reapposes the mucosa of the nasopharyngeal side with a simple continuous pattern. The second layer incorporates the stromal and mucosal tissues on the oropharyngeal side in an interrupted vertical or horizontal mattress pattern. The third layer is a simple continuous pattern of the everted mucosa on the oral side. In this third layer, knots on the oral side should be buried to reduce the tendency of the tongue to irritate the reconstructed palate. Hard-palate defects are repaired by first making an incision into the mucoperiosteum covering the hard palate. This incision is made parallel and approximately 2 cm abaxial to the defect. This incision should be carefully made to avoid the path of the palatine artery that runs parallel and approximately 0.5 to 1 cm axial to the cheek teeth. The mucoperiosteal flaps are elevated with a blunt periosteal elevator and slid axially. They are sutured together with no. 0 absorbable sutures in a horizontal mattress pattern.

Most cleft palate repair attempts are undertaken when the affected animal is nursing. The suckling response appears to complicate appropriate healing, and dehiscence is a common complication. Feeding by stomach tube may help reduce this tendency. However, incomplete repair and complete dehiscence are common after attempted surgical repairs of the cleft palate. In the

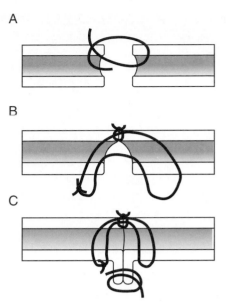

Figure 9-13   *A*, The first layer is reapposing the mucosa of the nasopharyngeal side with a simple continuous pattern. *B*, The second layer incorporates the stromal tissue and mucosa on the oropharyngeal side in an interrupted vertical or horizontal mattress pattern. *C*, The third layer is a simple continuous pattern of the everted mucosa on the oral side.

authors' experience, two or three revisions may be needed to complete the repair. This—and the possible heritability status—makes this procedure one to pursue only after careful consideration and counseling of the client/owner.

DISORDERS OF THE LARYNX

Surgical treatment of the larynx of cattle is not commonly indicated. Disorders that require surgical manipulation of the laryngeal cartilages (laryngeal hemiplegia, arytenoid chondritis, dorsal displacement of the soft palate, subepiglottic cyst) common to the horse are not encountered as commonly in cattle and rarely require surgical treatment because athletic soundness or noise reduction are not significant concerns for farm animals. Indications for surgery may include trauma by or lodging of a foreign body at the larynx, necrotic laryngitis with associated chondritis (Figure 9-14), and perilaryngeal abscesses.

The clinical signs associated with laryngeal disease in cattle depend on the location and severity of laryngeal obstruction. With increasing glottic obstruction, inspiratory noise and dyspnea appear. Occasionally, the throatlatch region may appear swollen secondary to abscess and/or cellulitis. Severe necrotizing disease can have systemic signs of debilitation in addition to the upper airway signs.

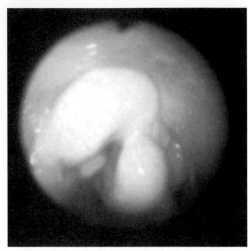

Figure 9-14   Arytenoid chondritis in a calf. Note left arytenoid cartilage on the midline with enlarged right arytenoid cartilage. There is a mass on the axial surface of the right arytenoid cartilage.

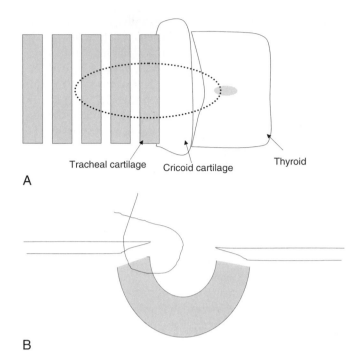

Tracheal cartilage   Cricoid cartilage   Thyroid

A

B

Figure 9-15   Schematic representation of surgical approach. *A,* Ventral view: dotted lines represent intended line of resection. *B,* Larynx view in cross-section at the level of the first tracheal cartilage: This skin incision is made at an angle, and the cartilage is cut to match this angle to facilitate closure.

Diagnosis of laryngeal disease can be presumed from physical examination findings and confirmed with endoscopy, ultrasonography, and radiography. Careful restraint is essential when animals are maintaining a marginal airway, as any additional stress may cause a respiratory crisis. Endoscopy is best performed with minimal physical and chemical restraint when possible. Ultrasonography can define soft tissue and fluid abnormalities and radiography can provide pertinent information in regard to airway dimensions and potential distortion of cartilaginous structures.

Laryngeal disease in cattle is often accompanied by lower airway disease secondary to aspiration complications. Therefore affected cattle often require systemic antibiotic and antiinflammatory therapy. Physical therapy directed toward reduction of perilaryngeal swelling (hydrotherapy) may also assist in the reduction of clinical signs.

Surgical therapy of the larynx can be performed with trans-endoscopic or trans-oral approaches in standing cattle. These approaches facilitate placement of wire and cautery loops, and use of laser instruments. These have been successful in removing foreign bodies, subepiglottic cysts, and laryngeal granulomas and allowing regional debridement.

Several incisional approaches to the larynx can also be used. Ventral laryngotomy can be performed after infiltration with local anesthesia but this is preferably done with the animal under general anesthesia. Cattle do not have a wide cricothyroid ligament that can be incised to provide good laryngeal visualization. Incising through the ventral midline of the thyroid, cricoid, and even cranial tracheal cartilages to provide adequate exposure for substantial debridement of diseased tissues is advisable. In addition, a pharyngotomy can allow access the rostral aspect of the larynx or pharynx where manipulation is required. Alternatively, a very cranial, ventral tracheotomy allows access to the caudal aspects of the laryngeal region. Regardless of the chosen approach, the incisional site should be left open to heal by second intention. A permanent tracheostomy should be considered for advanced laryngeal disease or situations where repeated access to the caudal aspect of the larynx may be required.

In the authors' experience, the most successful surgical treatment of necrotizing laryngitis with associated chondritis in cattle is the tracheolaryngostomy technique described by Gasthuys et al. Anesthesia is maintained with a tracheostomy distal to the surgical site. The calf is placed in dorsal recumbency with its head extended. After appropriate aseptic preparation of the ventral cervical area, an oval section of skin overlying the ventral aspect of the larynx and proximal tracheal ring is incised (Figure 9-15A). This skin incision is made at an angle (Figure 9-15B). The incision is extended toward the larynx by bluntly separating the sternohyoid muscles at the midline. The incision is sharply extended through the larynx by incising the cricothyroid membrane, cricoid cartilage, and first three tracheal rings. After a self-retaining retractor is placed and necrotic tissue is removed, the draining tract(s) are curetted, and the affected vocal cords and arytenoid cartilages removed as necessary. After a section of the cricoid and tracheal cartilages matching the skin incision is removed, the stoma is closed by reapposing the laryngeal and tracheal mucosa to the skin while incorporating the cartilage in the closure (Figure 9-15, B). Closure is obtained with simple interrupted sutures. The tracheostomy is maintained for 24 to 48 hours after surgery; afterwards the tracheostomy tube is removed if the created stoma is sufficient in size. Appropriate antibiotics are continued after surgery for 2 weeks, at which time the skin sutures are removed. The tracheostomy site will close a few months after surgery in a percentage of animals.

DISORDERS OF THE EXTRATHORACIC TRACHEA

Upper airway obstruction in cattle is the most common indication for surgical treatment of the trachea. An emergency tracheostomy can be lifesaving when indicated, and placement of an indwelling tracheostomy tube can provide an airway for prolonged upper airway surgery or an upper airway occlusion because of potential complications. Tracheostomy can be performed midtrachea in standing or recumbent cattle. If time and airway status allow, the ventral cervical site should be clipped, aseptically prepared, and infiltrated with local anesthetic. If this is not possible, all priorities should be directed at opening the tracheal airway. A 7-cm skin incision is made through the skin at a midcervical area, where the trachea is most easily palpated (junction of the middle and cranial thirds of the cervical trachea). The trachea can usually be grasped with one hand and a ventral midline skin incision performed. The musculature ventral to the trachea (sternohyoideus and sternothyroideus muscles) is paired and has a midline raphe. The ideal incision should part the musculature on the midline to expose the ventral aspect of the trachea. The incision is extended bluntly by separating the sternohyoid muscles with scissors. With a surgical blade, the membrane between two tracheal rings is incised parallel to the tracheal rings over approximately one third of its circumference. Care must be taken not to incise a cartilaginous ring. An indwelling tracheostomy tube can be inserted to maintain an open airway. Various designs of tracheostomy tubes are available. (A semilunar section of tracheal ring that encompasses no more than one third of the tracheal ring diameter can be cut if a tracheostomy tube cannot be inserted.) The tracheostomy tube is inserted and secured in place with one loop of suture on either side of the tracheostomy tube. Umbilical tapes are used to secure

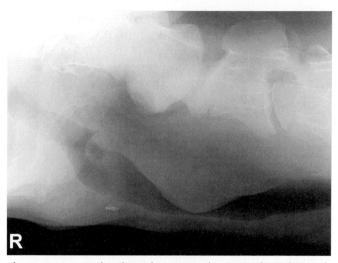

Figure 9-16   Right lateral proximal cervical radiograph showing soft tissue opacity confluent with the dorsal tracheal wall in a calf. This mass was an abscess. Note partial obstruction of the trachea. The abscess was drained through endoscopy, and the calf recovered.

(Courtesy of Dr. Anthony P. Pease, Cornell University.)

the tracheostomy tube to the loops of sutures placed in the skin.

After surgery, the tracheostomy tube should be removed and cleaned daily or more frequently if substantial volumes of exudate and debris accumulate in and around the tube's lumen. The tracheostomy site is cleaned, and all secretions removed during each cleaning. Petroleum jelly should be liberally applied ventrally to the tracheotomy site to prevent scalding by tracheal secretions. The tube is removed once the primary respiratory obstruction is resolved, and the tracheostomy site is allowed to granulate in. Second intention healing of the tracheotomy site can occasionally lead to formation of excessive amounts of granulation tissue and granulomas. This tissue can be large enough to partially occlude the tracheal airway; therefore careful monitoring of the tracheotomy site healing is suggested.

For unusual, chronic conditions when efforts are directed toward short-term salvage, or an upper airway obstruction cannot be resolved, a permanent tracheostomy is indicated to provide an adequate airway. The preferred site and procedure for permanent tracheostomy is the tracheolaryngostomy technique described earlier. If the trachea is obstructed distal to the proximal trachea (Figure 9-16) or a midcervical is desired, the following procedure is done. A more extensive exposure is required for a permanent tracheostomy as all local musculature, excessive skin, and portions of three to four tracheal rings are excised. A 10-cm skin incision is first made over the ventral aspect of the mid-trachea. After a section of strap muscles (sternothyroid and sternohyoid muscle) is removed, one-fourth to one-third of the tracheal circumference should be removed from each cartilage ring. The mucosa should be preserved and incised on the midline. Enough skin should be excised to prevent loose skin from occluding the tracheostomy site. The tracheal mucosa is sutured to the skin to produce the desired stoma. These sites should be expected to narrow markedly during the healing and contracture periods. It is not unusual to have a permanent tracheostomy site end up with 25 percent or less of the original stoma size.

External trauma to the trachea is rare. Typical clinical signs associated with a wound site involving the trachea include subcutaneous emphysema and dyspnea if the airway lumen is compromised or the thoracic inlet opened. The most likely treatment for affected cattle is to establish an open airway with either an indwelling tracheostomy tube or permanent tracheostomy if a normal tracheal lumen is not possible because of the extent of tissue damage. Systemic antibiotic and antiinflammatory therapy is also indicated. Tracheal stenosis and granuloma formation may result after penetrating trauma and management of the tracheostomy. Local excision of a mass or compromising tissue can be palliative of clinical signs. Total, circumferential resection of segments of trachea up to 3 to 5 rings can be successful. Careful apposition of the remaining trachea and suturing of the ring with interrupted patterns of monofilament suture material are suggested. Sutures should not enter the lumen. Intensive housing and feeding that discourages head and neck extension are indicated to reduce suture line tension. Some recurrence of luminal restriction is likely after complete repair.

Tracheal collapse is occasionally observed in calves. Inspiratory and expiratory dyspnea with open-mouthed breathing and poor body condition are common clinical signs. A "honking" noise is often associated with collapse within the thorax. A common association with tracheal collapse is cranial rib fractures. Most calves are clinically affected with airway compromise by 3 to 10 weeks of age after forced extraction at birth. Lateral radiographs often demonstrate substantial osseous callus at the first or second ribs, associated with the narrowed tracheal lumen. Some calves, treated without surgery, can be confined to a stall to reduce environmental pressures until slaughter. Generally, by the time this syndrome is recognized, the trachea damage requires surgical treatment to return a normal airway. Extraluminal tracheal prostheses can be successful in restoring an airway for about 30% of affected calves. The prostheses can be made from the polypropylene syringe barrels of either 35 or 60 ml

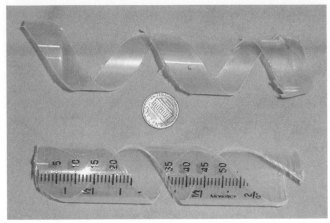

Figure 9-17   The prostheses can be made from 60-ml polypropylene syringe barrels or cases as follows: with a pruning shear, a spiral cut is made along the length pf the syringe case or barrel. A second spiral is made one cm parallel to the first cut. The section created is removed (top) leaving the prosthesis (bottom). The rough edges are sanded for a smooth finish. The desired length should approximate the length of 2 to 4 tracheal rings.

syringes (Figure 9-17). The desired length should approximate 2 to 4 tracheal rings. A length-wise slot should be created to allow the prosthesis to pass around the trachea, and predrilled holes around the circumference allow sutures to secure the device to the tracheal rings. More than one prosthesis may be necessary to open the airway, depending on the length of the defect.

To place a tracheal prosthesis, affected calves should be placed under general anesthesia in dorsal recumbency with the head and neck extended and forelimbs pulled caudally. A ventral midline incision is performed over the area of collapse. The ventral musculature is divided on midline and/or transected to expose the trachea. Large callused regions of affected ribs should be resected either with Gigli wire or rongeurs. The polypropylene rings can be placed around the affected aspects of the trachea and secured with 2-0 polypropylene sutures. Muscle, subcutaneous tissues, and skin are routinely closed.

The tracheal prosthesis may need to be removed 2 to 3 months after placement to allow unrestricted growth and more normal development. However, this procedure is often accompanied by complications that include collapse of tracheal segments that adjoin the prostheses and failure of affected cattle to thrive. Surgically treated calves have been observed to be smaller than similarly aged herd mates.

Lower Airway

DISORDERS OF THE LUNGS AND PLEURAL CAVITY

Cattle frequently experience pulmonary disease; however, surgical treatment of the lungs is not commonly indicated. Cattle have a propensity to develop pleuritis and pulmonary abscesses secondary to penetration of foreign objects from the reticulum. In addition, pleuritis may result from an extension of pneumonia, abscesses in the lungs or liver, or other penetrating trauma.

Pneumothorax can result from penetrating trauma or pulmonary disease. The typically complete mediastinum of cattle usually prevents life threatening consequences; however, correction of the pneumothorax is desirable to prevent further complications in the pulmonary tissues or pleural space. Wounds can be primarily closed if deeper tissue complications are not likely, or these wounds can be managed by second intention wound healing. A one-way valve allows evacuation of pleural/air from the pleural space and assists normal healing by allowing lung reinflation. If the purpose of a chest drain is to evacuate air, it should be placed dorsally in the caudal thoracic cavity. Fluid is best drained from a more cranial and ventral portal. Drains (24 to 28 French) should be introduced through the thoracic wall from a skin incision placed 1 to 2 cm caudal of a penetration site carefully placed at the caudal aspect of the chosen intercostal space. This will avoid intercostal neurovascular structures immediately caudal to each rib. A one-way valve or multiway stopcock can be used for effective air or fluid evacuation.

More aggressive approaches to the pleural space are indicated for advanced pleuritis and septic diseases that require lavage therapy of the pleural cavity. Large-bore chest tubes (26-32 French) can be placed in the pleural cavity with the affected animal standing by using local anesthesia at the tube placement site. Ultrasonographic guidance has been suggested to avoid trauma to major intrathoracic structures. The fifth and sixth intercostal spaces at the costochondral junction approximately level with the elbow are the most successful sites for tube placement. After skin incision, a chest tube with trocar can be pushed into the pleural space. Fluid will usually be apparent after the typical "pop" of pleural penetration and trocar removal. A single tube can be used for drainage and lavage. More than one tube may be used with difficult or refractory cases but often indicates a poor prognosis.

Thoracic exploration is indicated as a diagnostic procedure such as characterization (location, degree of adhesion) of thoracic abscesses by laparoscopy or even by the more invasive thoracotomy. Disease entities such as pulmonary abscesses and neoplasia may therapeutically benefit from surgical treatment.

ANESTHETIC CONSIDERATIONS

The thoracoscopy and thoracotomy surgical approaches can be performed in standing or recumbent cattle. Standing thoracic procedures (such as standing thoracoscopy and thoracotomy) result in unilateral pneumothorax that remains unilateral because cattle typically have an intact mediastinum that allows unventilated procedures. Despite the decreased ventilation associated with unilateral pneumothorax, standing thoracic procedures are still preferable because lateral recumbency results in poor ventilation of the down (usually normal) side. The mortality rate from general anesthesia is high if the disease process affects a significant portion of the up side lung.

The patient is placed in stocks without sedation because sedated cattle tend to lie down and sedation impairs ventilation. Local anesthetic is applied to the intercostal nerves of the rib to be resected, and 2 to 3 ribs cranial and caudal to the intended surgical site, or at two adjacent ribs if an intercostal approach is planned. Local linear infiltration of an anesthetic agent should also be performed at the intended surgical site. Preparation should be made for emergency ventilation in case the animal shows signs of distress. Typical preparation includes 100% oxygen available for nasal insufflation, endotracheal tube for emergency intubation, preparation of the midcervical area for an emergency tracheostomy, availability of positive pressure ventilation, an impervious material to seal the thoracotomy site, and gas suction to reverse a pneumothorax.

The greater control and analgesia offered by general anesthesia is recommended when extensive pleural debridement is required, because of the likelihood of creating potentially fatal bilateral pneumothorax. An individual animal's ability to tolerate general anesthesia is best determined by thorough physical examination, CBC, and blood gas analysis. If general anesthesia is selected, placing the animal in sternal recumbency to optimize ventilation is best. Positive pressure ventilation is a requirement.

SURGICAL CONSIDERATIONS

One must first consider the location of the lesion when deciding on the approach. Whenever possible, thoracic lesions need to be localized by a combination of ultrasound and thoracic radiographs. Lesions located in the cranial aspects of the thorax are very difficult to access surgically. The caudal lung lobes can be reached through a partial rib resection or intercostal approach from the seventh to ninth ribs. The size of the lesion and purpose of the surgery determine the surgical procedure: thoracotomy through an intercostal space allows limited manipulations but is sufficient for simple drainage, lavage, limited manual debridement of the pleural space, and marsupialization of an abscess adhered to the parietal pleura if postoperative access to the thorax is not required after surgery.

Aseptic site preparation is necessary in all cases. If an intercostal thoracotomy is chosen, the skin incision should be centered over the lesion in a proximal to distal direction. The intercostal space should be incised at the cranial aspect of the rib in effort to avoid the intercostal neurovascular structures that reside immediately caudal to each rib. If a rib resection technique is used, the incision should be started 20 cm dorsal to the costochondral junction centered over the middle of the longitudinal aspect of the rib. The incision can be elongated dorsally to the desired working length. Care must be taken not to extend the incision ventral to the costochondral junction to prevent inadvertent transection of the cranial epigastric vessels. The incision is extended to the periosteum, which is sharply incised. The periosteum is elevated by using a periosteal elevator. At the most proximal extent of the incision, a Gigli wire is passed subperiosteally around the rib. After transecting the proximal aspect, the rib is resected by dislocating it distally at the costochondral junction insertion. Alternatively, an oscillating bone saw, osteotome and mallet, or large rongeurs can be used to remove part of a rib. The axial rib periosteum is incised along with the parietal pleura to reach the thoracic cavity. Handheld or mechanical retractors can be used to increase the observable area of the affected hemithorax. Partial lung lobectomy can be effective in removing solitary abscesses and other types of confined masses. Unfortunately, most neoplastic diseases do not present with readily resectable masses. The affected lung should be elevated to define the interface between normal and abnormal tissue. Stapling instruments* can be used to place overlapping staple lines at the resection site to effectively seal the remaining lung tissue. This can also be hand-sutured with overlapping mattress sutures to prevent air loss. Depending on location, larger-diameter airways may require suture closure independent of pulmonary parenchymal closure.

Before closure, an intercostal block should be performed. Five ml of a long-acting local anesthetic (Bupivacaine hydrochloride 0.5%) is administered at the caudal aspect of the dorsal remnant of the resected rib as well as two ribs cranial and caudal. The injection is made with a 19-gauge needle and flexible tubing. Proper needle placement is facilitated by placing a hand in the thorax and identifying the caudal aspect of the ribs.

---

*TA 90, US Surgical, Tyco Health Care; Norwalk, CT.

Some animals exhibit substantial postoperative pain if the pleural cavity is left open after surgery, which allows air to rush in and out of the pleural cavity. Therefore, if possible, the incision should be partially closed with drainage and lavage enhanced by using drains. However, in all cases with an intact pleural cavity where an abscess is marsupialized, the incision should be left open. The thoracic wall is closed by apposing the pleura and intercostal muscles with the periosteum using number-2 absorbable sutures, such as polyglactin 910, in a simple continuous pattern. Suction through a teat cannula in the pleural space is used to reinflate the collapsed lung. If general anesthesia was used, positive pressure ventilation during closure will express most of the air from the pleural space and facilitate this procedure. The subcutaneous tissue and skin can be routinely closed. The placement of a drain and Heimlich valve in the dorsal aspect of the thorax is optional but in the authors' experience increases the animal's comfort by decreasing the postoperative pneumothorax.

In cattle with large, caudally oriented pulmonary abscesses in which partial lung lobe resection is considered impossible, marsupializing the abscess capsule to the skin may be possible. A similar intercostal or rib resection approach can be employed. Most lung abscesses adjacent to the thoracic wall are adhered to it allowing safe marsupialization. If not, the fibrous wall of the abscess should be initially secured to the thoracic wall and skin with sutures. The sutures should effectively seal the abscess from the pleural cavity while leaving access for a drainage incision. The abscess capsule should then be incised to produce an exit portal for the accumulated purulent exudate and debris or foreign material. The abscess cavity can then be lavaged if necessary and the surgical wound left to heal by second intention.

Lung biopsy is rarely desired; however, percutaneous techniques can be frustrating as appropriate diagnostic tissue samples may be difficult to obtain. Surgical biopsy can be successfully performed under direct observation by using a thoracoscopy or thoracotomy. Thoracoscopy is less invasive and requires little knowledge of the lesion site. On the other hand, a thoracotomy for a lung biopsy is far more invasive and requires an accurate anatomical diagnosis to locate abnormal tissues.

Thoracoscopy is performed with the animal standing after the affected hemithorax is prepared for aseptic surgery. Local infiltration of anesthetic is done over the junction between the middle and dorsal third of the tenth intercostal space. A 1-cm skin incision is made slightly caudal to the intended intercostal space entry. The laparoscopic trocar (10 mm diameter) is inserted into the intercostal space, and a pneumothorax is created after opening the port. At that time, the animal's response is observed closely in the unlikely event the mediastinum is incomplete. The laparoscope (10 mm diameter) is then inserted and the thoracic cavity examined. A second port can usually be made for instrument handling. The entry site is determined by thoracoscopic guidance by using an 18-gauge spinal needle to verify the optimal port location. After the instrument port is created, a blunt probe is used to evaluate the pleural cavity. Instead of a laparoscope, an endoscope can be used. If a flexible endoscope is used, a 6-cc syringe barrel is used to manufacture a thoracoscopic port. The tip of the syringe barrel is cut and beveled to serve as a port. The sterilized syringe case is then inserted into the intercostal space and used as an entry site for the flexible endoscope. This also gives some rigidity that helps direct the endoscope toward the cranial or caudal aspect of the thoracic cavity. Because of farm animals' tendency to create fibrous adhesions, observation of the chest area may be limited in cases with extensive adhesions, and ultrasonographic examination would be preferable.

DIAPHRAGMATIC HERNIA

This disease is another indication, although rare, for surgical treatment of the pleural cavity in cattle. This can result from trauma, dystocia, or traumatic reticuloperitonitis. Buffalo appear to be over-represented in affected bovine populations. The clinical signs associated with diaphragmatic hernia include decreased production, weight loss, dysphagia, colic, bloat, and respiratory difficulties. Physical examination may indicate muffled thoracic auscultation with borborygmi sounds audible from the thorax. Palpation per rectum may indicate a forward position of abdominal viscera and an empty feel to the caudal abdomen in general.

Radiography and ultrasonography can help confirm the presence of abdominal viscera in the thoracic cavity. Treatment is surgical or salvage. Affected cattle should be fasted 2 to 3 days before surgical repair. Various approaches have been described to reach the diaphragm for repair, including ventral midline, paramedian, paracostal celiotomies starting just caudal to the xiphoid, and caudal rib resection thoracotomy. Thoracoscopy, as described above, can be used to determine the optimal site for rib resection to repair a diaphragmatic hernia. One should consider one of the ventral approaches for hernias in the ventral third of the diaphragm, and thoracoscopy and thoracotomy for hernias in the dorsal 2/3 of the diaphragm. A standing rumenotomy to empty the rumen and reticulum has been recommended before using recumbent approaches to the diaphragm. Direct suture repair is suggested when possible. Large (#2 or 3), monofilament, absorbable or nonabsorbable sutures in simple continuous or continuous mattress patterns are recommended. Mesh can be used to repair diaphrag-

matic defects but should not be placed into a contaminated wound environment.

DISORDERS OF THE PERICARDIUM

Thoracotomy is indicated for drainage and debridement of the pericardium, foreign body removal, and rare surgical manipulation of the heart, major vessels, and lungs. Thoracotomy can be done with affected cattle standing or by using general anesthesia in sternal or inclined recumbency. In the authors' experience, general anesthesia in lateral recumbency in cattle with pericarditis is associated with a high mortality rate. A reticular foreign body may enter the thorax from either the left or right side (see Figure 9-7); therefore an accurate diagnosis is essential for surgical success.

The most typical approach to the pericardium is to enter the thorax at the left fifth or sixth ribs or intercostal spaces or at the sixth or seventh ribs by the approach described in the section pertaining to diseases of the lungs and pleural cavity. Upon entering the chest, the pericardium is often adhered to the regional pleura with advancing disease. Therefore incising into the pleural cavity must be carefully performed. Presurgical ultrasound examination may provide the necessary forewarning of this possibility. Before draining the pericardium, the surgeon should look for a fibrous tract that enters the pericardium caudally. Septic pericarditis is most commonly the result of foreign body penetration from the reticulum. If preoperative radiographs indicate a foreign body present in the chest, early identification of this tract is critical for successful removal of the foreign body and a successful procedure. Pericardial drainage will be unsuccessful if the foreign body is left in the thorax. The key is identifying the fibrous tract encircling the foreign body early to prevent its cranial or caudal displacement. The fibrous tract is clamped with a large Oschner clamp to immobilize the foreign body as soon as the tract is identified. The surgeon then incises the fibrous tract with large scissors until the center is identified. The foreign body is then grasped and removed. The pericardium is sutured to the skin at the incision edge. This can be accomplished with large (#2 or 3), monofilament, absorbable or nonabsorbable sutures in an interrupted or continuous patterns. The pericardium is often quite fibrotic and capable of holding suture tension; however, sepsis can render it friable and frustrating to suture. The pericardium is then incised and drained manually. Depending on the duration of septic pericarditis, there can be thick caseous purulent exudates that must be manually removed from the pericardium (Figure 9-18). After drainage, lavage with warm isotonic fluid is used as needed. Because of the postoperative pain and delayed healing, it is best to reinflate the lungs and use a drain to manage the pleural space as described in the previous section. The pericardial cavity

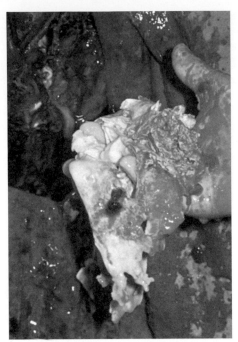

Figure 9-18 Thick caseous purulent exudates being removed from around the pericardium.

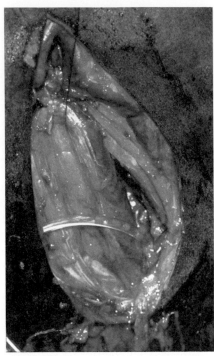

Figure 9-19   The incision is being partially closed and drains are placed in the pleural space and pericardium for postoperative lavage and drainage.

may be left open to drain or be partially closed and managed with drains if this allows appropriate lavage and adequate drainage (Figure 9-19). Extensive chronic pericarditis will often require marsupialization of the pericardium for postoperative drainage. Drains can be placed in the pericardial sac for targeted lavage.

Postoperatively, continued access and good hygiene practice with repetitive lavage is necessary if the resulting wound is left open. Chest bandages to cover the wound or local bandages secured with loops of suture can work well. If the foreign body returned into the reticulum during the manipulation, a rumenotomy to remove the foreign body may be necessary at the same restraint or anesthetic episode. It may be preferable to delay a rumenotomy and place a magnet in the reticulum until the initial surgical morbidity of the thoracotomy has resolved.

CARDIOVASCULAR DISORDERS
Diseases of the cardiovascular system amenable to surgical treatment are not common in cattle.

Long-term catheterization or problematic jugular injections can result in thrombosis and septic thrombophlebitis of the cervical jugular veins of cattle. Clinical signs associated with these disorders include warm, firm, "corded" distention of an affected jugular vein, venous distention of the affected side of the head, fever, and possible cardiac abnormalities. Local and systemic

antibiotic and antiinflammatory therapy is indicated but may not resolve advanced aggressive thrombophlebitis. Ultrasonography can be very beneficial in defining the extent of a lesion. Surgical treatment should be considered if a septic process fistulates through the skin or the thrombotic process advances toward the thoracic inlet. The surgical goal is resection of the abnormal infected section of the jugular vein. This preferably is performed with the patient under general anesthesia. The affected region of the jugular vein should be aseptically prepared. An incision should be made in the skin through the entire length of the targeted aspect of the jugular vein. The vein can be bluntly elevated and isolated from surrounding tissues. The interface between thrombotic and normal vein should be identified. Vascular forceps or circumferential ligatures can be applied across the normal aspects of the vein at the cranial and caudal ends to isolate the diseased aspect of the jugular vein. The vein should then be transected with only normal venous tissue left. The remaining ends of the jugular vein can be oversewn or left with ligatures in place. The incision should be left open to heal by second intention. Close attention to wound hygiene is important until normal granulation tissue covers the wound. Quite satisfactory and cosmetic results can be achieved if the vascular disorder is confined to the cervical jugular vein.

Patent ductus arteriosus (PDA) is a rare congenital malformation in calves. This disease results from the ductus arteriosus (which allows blood to flow from the pulmonary artery to the descending aorta in a fetus, bypassing the nonfunctional lungs) failing to close. In most cases, because the ductus arteriosus remains patent after birth, differential blood pressure forces blood from the aorta to reenter the pulmonary circulation through the pulmonary artery. This results in left ventricular hypertrophy, and possibly failure, as the heart attempts to increase cardiac output to systemic circulation. If the pulmonary pressure is elevated, the differential blood pressure forces poorly oxygenated blood into systemic circulation through the aorta. Calves are presented for decreased stamina, growth, and exercise intolerance. The diagnosis is suspected by ausculting a holosystolic murmur and confirmed by angiography or echocardiography outlining the PDA. Prostaglandin inhibitor has been used successfully in humans to resolve PDA. No data are available for cattle. We have only treated one calf surgically in which a PDA was ligated with umbilical tape through a fifth rib left thoracotomy. Ligation assisted by thoracoscopy and intraarterial occlusion devices is now available and should be considered first if the ductus arteriosus fails to close after administering flunixin.

RECOMMENDED READINGS

Anderson DE, St. Jean G: Surgery of the respiratory system, *Vet Clinics of North America, Food Animal Practice* 13: 593-645, 1997.

Blood DC, Radostits OM, Henderson JA: Diseases of the cardiovascular system. In *Veterinary medicine*, ed 6, London, 1985, Bailliere Tindall.

Blood DC, Radostits OM, Henderson JA: Diseases of the respiratory system. In *Veterinary medicine*, ed 6, London, 1985, Bailliere Tindall.

Ducharme NG, Fubini SL, Rebhun WC, Beck KA: Thoracotomy in adult dairy cattle: 14 cases (1979-1991), *J Am Vet Med Assoc* 200: 86-90, 1992.

Gasthuys F, Verschooten F, Parmentier D, De Moor A, Steenhaut M: Laryngotomy as a treatment for chronic laryngeal obstruction in cattle: a review of 130 cases, *Vet Rec* 130: 220-223, 1992.

Krishnamurphy D, Deshpande KS, Nigan JM, et al: Repair of diaphragmatic hernia in bovine: transthoracic approach, *Ind J Vet Surg* 1: 7-11, 1980.

Krishnamurphy D, Nigan JM, Peshin PK et al: Thoracopericardectomy and pericardiectomy in cattle, *J Am Vet Med Assoc* 175: 714-718, 1979.

Malone ED, Farnsworth K, Lennox T, Tomlinson J, Sage AM: Thoracoscopic assisted diaphragmatic repair using a rib resection, *Vet Surg* 30: 175-178, 2001.

Panter KE, James LF, Gardner DR: Lupines, poison-hemlock, and *Nicotiana* spp: toxicity and teratogenicity in livestock, *J Nat Toxins* 8: 117-134, 1999.

Panter KE, Weinzweig J, Gardner DR, Stegelmeir BI, James LF: Comparison of cleft palate induction by Nicotina Glauca in goats and sheep, *Teratology* 61: 203-210, 2000.

Ramakrishna O, Krishnamurphy D, Nigan JM: Constrictive pericarditis in cows, *J Vet Surg* 4: 36-39, 1983.

Rings DM: Surgical treatment of pleuritis and pericarditis, *Vet Clinics of North America, Food Animal Practice* 11: 177-182, 1995.

Smith JA: Ruminant respiratory system. In Smith BP, *Large animal internal medicine*, St Louis, 1990, Mosby.

Ward JL, Rebhun WC: Chronic sinusitis in dairy cattle: 12 cases (1978-1989), *J Am Vet Med Assoc* 201: 326-328, 1992.

CHAPTER 10

SURGERY OF THE BOVINE DIGESTIVE SYSTEM

10.1—Surgical Diseases of the Oral Cavity

Norm G. Ducharme

Many surgical diseases can interfere with an animal's ability to prehend and transfer food material to the esophagus. The cause of dysphagia can be a congenital abnormality or diseases acquired through pain and/or mechanical obstruction. Of course, pain itself can prevent an animal from eating or drinking (e.g., severe oral inflammations, mandibular fracture, glossitis, foreign body penetration, temporohyoid arthropathy, etc.). Mechanical causes of dysphagia include a foreign body, anatomical defects such as cleft palate, or peripharyngeal masses such as neoplasia and abscess. Although this chapter focuses on surgical diseases, when evaluating an animal with dysphagia, one should consider a variety of centrally mediated neuromuscular disorders such as listeriosis and rabies. Peripheral neurological diseases such as neuropathy of the lingual and hypoglossal nerves should also be considered. Probably the most common cause of muscular disorders is white muscle disease. The following sections propose a diagnostic and therapeutic approach to surgical diseases of the oral cavity.

Anatomical Considerations

The lips of cattle play an important role in prehension of food and, of course, suckling, but their shape varies significantly. They are relatively immobile and insensitive, which presumably contributes to the indiscriminate eating habits of cattle. The relatively immobile lips and rostral position of the commissure limits the extent the mouth can open and therefore interferes with a thorough oral exam. On the other hand, small ruminant lips are much more mobile and serve to prehend much better than cattle.

The mouth of cattle is long and narrow with the hard palate being narrowest rostral to the cheek teeth. The wide gap between the incisors and cheek teeth (diastema provides a hand grip for restraining the head and opening the mouth. Paired dental pads replace the upper incisors seen in most other species. Unlike that of small ruminants, the tongue is most important for prehension in cattle: the tongue grasps forage and drags it into the mouth where the ventral incisors' pressure against the dental pads cuts it. The tongue's importance in prehension explains why tongue amputation after laceration causes greater morbidity in cattle than in horses or small ruminants. Small ruminant lips have replaced the tongue's function as a prehension organ.

The dental formula of farm animals is summarized in Tables 10.1-1 through 10.1-4, but breeds may differ significantly. The canine tooth is also called the fourth or corner incisor. A significant anatomical characteristic is the shallow depth of the alveolar socket and associated tooth root in cattle. This leads to dental attrition in older cattle more readily than in horses but also facilitates tooth excision in advance of dental disease.

The large quantity of salivary glands in ruminants (Figure 10.1-1) and swine (Figure 10.1-2) contribute to large amounts of saliva being produced, estimated to be as much as 100 liters per day in adult cattle. The left and right parotid glands are located ventral to the ear, extend along the caudal border of the mandible, and drain into the mouth by a single large duct (i.e., the parotid or Stenson's duct). The parotid duct continues rostrally along the ventral border of the mandible following the rostral aspect of the masseter muscle and finally opening in the caudal aspect of the mouth at the level of the

TABLE 10.1-1

Summary of Teeth and Their Eruption Patterns in Cattle

TOOTH	DECIDUOUS			PERMANENT		
	NUMBER IN UPPER ARCADE	NUMBER IN LOWER	ERUPTION PATTERN	NUMBER IN UPPER ARCADE	NUMBER IN LOWER ARCADE	ERUPTION PATTERN
Incisor	0	3	First 2 weeks	0	3	I1 = 1.5-2 years I2 = 2-2.5 years I3 = 2.5-3 years
Canine	0	1	First 2 weeks	0	1	3.5-4 years
Premolar	3	3	First 2 weeks	3	3	P2 = 2-2.5 years P3 = 1.5-2 years P4 = 2.5-3 years
Molar	0	0	NA*	3	3	M1 = 5-6 months M2 = 1-1.5 years M3 = 2-2.5 years

Modified from Oehme, Prior, and Dyce et al: *Large animal surgery,* Baltimore, 1974, Williams and Wilkins.
These are given as general guidelines; breeds may differ significantly.
*NA = not applicable.

TABLE 10.1-2

Summary of Teeth and Their Eruption Patterns in Sheep

TOOTH	DECIDUOUS			PERMANENT		
	NUMBER IN UPPER ARCADE	NUMBER IN LOWER	ERUPTION PATTERN	NUMBER IN UPPER ARCADE	NUMBER IN LOWER ARCADE	ERUPTION PATTERN
Incisor	0	3	Birth	0	3	I1 = 15 months I2 = 21 months I3 = 27 months
Canine	0	1	First 3 weeks	0	1	3 years
Premolar	3	3	First 12 weeks	3	3	17-20 months
Molar	0	0		3	3	M1 = 5-6 months M2 = 8-10 months M3 = 18-24 months

Modified from Dyce KM, Sack WO, Wensing CJG: *Veterinary anatomy,* Philadelphia, 1996, WB Saunders.
These are given as general guidelines; breeds may differ significantly.
*NA = not applicable.

TABLE 10.1-3

Summary of Teeth and Their Eruption Patterns in Goats

TOOTH	DECIDUOUS			PERMANENT		
	NUMBER IN UPPER ARCADE	NUMBER IN LOWER	ERUPTION PATTERN	NUMBER IN UPPER ARCADE	NUMBER IN LOWER ARCADE	ERUPTION PATTERN
Incisor	0	3	First 1 week	0	3	I1 = 1-1.5 years I2 = 1.5-2 years I3 = 2.5-3 years
Canine	0	1	First 3 weeks	0	1	3-4 years
Premolar	3	3	First 4 weeks	3	3	1.5-2 years
Molar	0	0		3	3	M1 = 3-4 months M2 = 8-10 months M3 = 18-24 months

Modified from Dyce KM, Sack WO, Wensing CJG: *Veterinary anatomy,* Philadelphia, 1996, WB Saunders.
These are given as general guidelines; breeds may differ significantly.
*NA = not applicable.

TABLE 10.1-4

Summary of Teeth and Their Eruption Patterns in Swine

TOOTH	DECIDUOUS			PERMANENT		
	NUMBER IN UPPER ARCADE	NUMBER IN LOWER	ERUPTION PATTERN	NUMBER IN UPPER ARCADE	NUMBER IN LOWER ARCADE	ERUPTION PATTERN
Incisor	3	3	I1 = First 3 week I2 = 8-14 weeks I3 = birth	3	3	I1 = 12-17 months I2 = 17-18 months I3 = 8-12 months
Canine	1	1	Birth	1	1	8-12 months
Premolar	3	3	P1 = 7-10 weeks P2 = 1-5 weeks P4 = 1-7 weeks	4	4	P1 = 3.5-6.5 months P2 = 12-16 months
Molar	0	0		3	3	M1 = 4-6 months M2 = 7-13 months M3 = 17-22 months

These are given as general guidelines; breeds may differ significantly.
Modified from Nickel, Schumacher, and Seiferle: *The viscera of domestic animals*, New York, 1979, Springer Verlag.
*NA = not applicable.

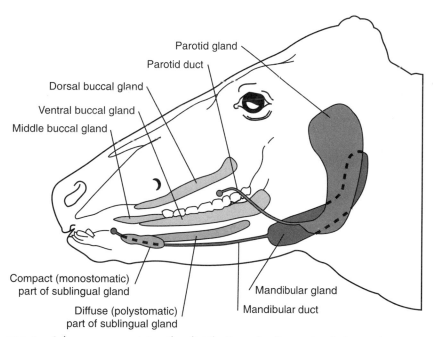

Figure 10.1-1   Schema summarizing the distribution of salivary glands in ruminants.

(Redrawn from Dyce KM, Sack WO, Wensing CJG: The digestive system. In *Veterinary anatomy*, Philadelphia, 1996, WB Saunders.)

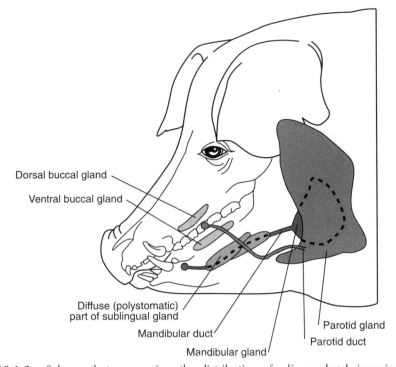

Dorsal buccal gland

Ventral buccal gland

Diffuse (polystomatic)
part of sublingual gland

Mandibular duct

Mandibular gland

Parotid gland

Parotid duct

Figure 10.1-2   Schema that summarizes the distribution of salivary glands in swine.

(Redrawn from Dyce KM, Sack WO, Wensing CJG: The digestive system. In *Veterinary anatomy*, Philadelphia, 1996, WB Saunders.)

second to last cheek tooth. The left and right mandibular glands are more axial than the parotid glands but also more ventral they are and centered on the angle of the jaw (mandible). Each gland drains into the mouth by its own single duct. These mandibular ducts extend rostrally submucosally and open on their respective sublingual caruncle on either side of the frenulum of the tongue. The left and right sublingual salivary glands contain two parts: a monostomatic and a polystomatic. The polystomatic glands lie on either side of the tongue on the floor of the mouth and drain to many stomas beside the frenulum. The left and right monostomatic glands are located rostral to their respective ipsilateral polystomatic gland and drain into the mouth through a single duct alongside—or joining—the mandibular duct. Many other small salivary glands exist in various locations of the oral cavity.

Diagnosis and Treatment

DENTAL

Because of the importance placed on maintaining producing animals' body condition and on maximizing growth potential in animals intended for human consumption, a dental examination is an important veterinary service. This is especially of concern when animals

are grazing on short grass. Dental disease occurs because of abnormal wear associated with various forms of malocclusion, grazing short grass on sandy soil, dental injuries and decay, or dental loosening in an older animal, presumably because of periodontal or endodontal disease. Clinical signs include salivation, pain during mastication, and dropping food. Use of a headlight or flashlight is important to perform a good oral examination. When examining an animal with a tooth abscess, the mouth has a malodorous odor, and the involved tooth can be recognized by its discoloration and associated discharge. Radiographic examination can also indicate the site of the lesion.

With the animal under heavy sedation or general anesthesia, a mouth speculum is used to keep the mouth open while a forceps is used to grasp the tooth. With repeated lateral to medial movement, the tooth is progressively loosened and finally removed. Digital inspection of the alveolar socket is necessary to confirm that no tooth fragments persist. For a few weeks postoperatively, daily mouth lavage, systemic antibiotics and feeding a soft diet may be beneficial.

LACERATIONS

Oral lacerations in cattle are associated with the same indiscriminate eating habit which results in traumatic reticulopericarditis. Lacerations are more common in calves because of their oral prehension and suckling habits on objects in their environment such as barbed wire, needles, and thorns. The lacerations may involve the lips, buccal membranes, and the tongue. Animals usually present with excess salivation, which may be mixed with blood, decreased appetite, and various degrees of dysphagia, depending on the severity of the laceration. The animal's tongue often protudes past its lips.

The diagnosis is based on physical examination. First, the head is grasped with one hand on the maxilla at the level of the interdental space. The rostral aspect of the mouth can then be inspected and palpated using the other hand. Most lacerations heal without surgical intervention by using daily mouth lavage and systemic antibiotics and by feeding a soft diet.

Severe tongue lacerations sometimes require a partial glossectomy. Because of the tongue's crucial role in prehension of food, as much of the tongue as possible should be preserved. In preparation for surgery The animal is anesthetized and placed in lateral recumbency. A tourniquet (made of rolled gauze) is applied proximal to the intended transection site. The tongue is transected so that the dorsal and ventral aspects protrude beyond the center (Figure 10.1-3A). The ventral and dorsal aspects are sutured together with an interrupted horizontal mattress pattern with a no.-1 or no.-2 absorbable sutures (Figure 10.1-3B and C). The animal should receive systemic antibiotics postoperatively and should be fed a soft diet (not pasture) for best results.

Soft palate lacerations present with nasal regurgitation of water and feed material and tracheal aspiration of this material. For further details on diagnosing and treating cleft palate lacerations, please see the cleft palate chapter (Section 9.2.1.1.3).

Buccal fistulae result from lacerations or other traumatic incidents and result in loss of saliva and feed material as well as cosmetic defects. While the animal is ruminating, the cud may be dropped during mastication. The diagnosis is obvious; one needs to inspect the lesion to determine the optimal time of repair. Surgery should be done on fresh lacerations or after any inflammation and infection in the local musculature has been resolved. The fistula edges are debrided while the animal is under sedation following infiltration of a local anesthetic or under general anesthesia. The defect is closed in three layers. The muscles (usually buccinator) are reapposed with absorbable suture material (no. 1 or 2) in a simple interrupted pattern. The oral mucosa is closed with a simple continuous pattern using no. 00 absorbable sutures. Finally, the skin is reapposed with a simple interrupted suture (no. 1). Postoperatively, systemic antibiotics are indicated along with a soft gruel or liquid diet, preferably for 10 to 14 days.

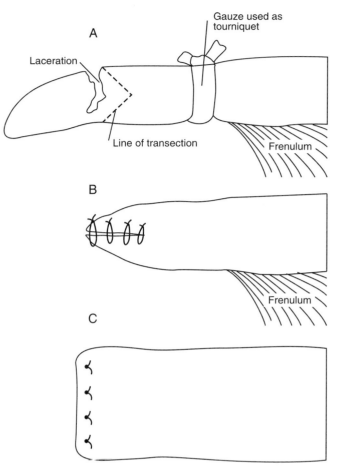

Figure 10.1-3   The tongue is transected so its dorsal and ventral aspects protrude beyond its center. *A,* Lateral view of the tongue, showing laceration and intended transection line. *B,* Lateral view of tongue, which shows position of horizontal mattress suture. *C,* Dorsal view, which shows position of horizontal mattress suture.

Oropharyngeal trauma and subsequent retropharyngeal cellulitis and dysphagia can occur after improper administration of medication with a balling gun. Animals are presented because they become anorectic and have an associated decrease in milk production (when relevant). On examination, they have varying degrees of cervical swelling and associated signs of infections—elevated temperature, leukocytosis, and hyperfibrinogenesis. The cervical swelling may interfere with respiration (see disorders of the nasopharynx, Section 9.2.1.1.3); the animal will extend its head and neck while trying to straighten their upper airway (Figure 10.1-4). A foul-smelling odor indicative of necrotic tissue may originate from the mouth. Endoscopic, or open-mouthed, examination of the nasopharynx and oropharynx will reveal the laceration and/or abscess (Figure 10.1-5). The

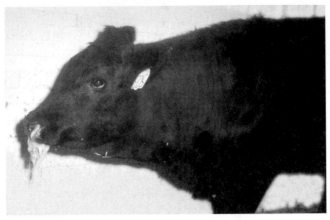

Figure 10.1-4   Adult Holstein-Friesian cow with perilaryngeal abscess caused by pharyngeal trauma. Note the extended head and swollen shaved perilaryngeal area.

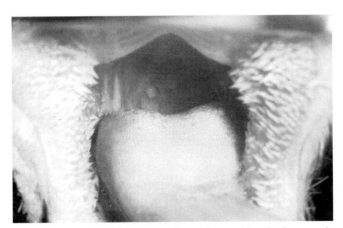

Figure 10.1-5   Oral examination of a calf, which reveals abscessation of oropharynx.

cervical area is swollen, and crepitus can sometimes be palpated if the area is not too severely distended. Ultrasonographic evaluation will reveal pockets of fluids in the subcutaneous tissue of the proximal cervical area. Radiographic evaluation will reveal air and fluids in the cervical area (Figure 10.1-6). These animals may aspirate feed and saliva and develop signs of lower airway disease. Therefore the lower airway should be evaluated for signs of mediastinitis (Figure 10.1-7) and aspiration pneumonia.

The treatment principle is to limit the extension of the cellulitis with appropriate parenteral antimicrobials and surgical drainage. If cellulitis is not controlled, it will proceed alongside the trachea and may result in septic mediastinitis (see Figure 10.1-7). Therefore if there is significant accumulation of fluid and feed material in the cervical area, the accumulated fluid is surgically drained under general anesthesia. See disorders of the nasophar-

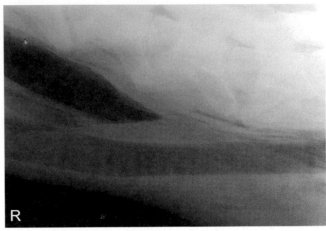

Figure 10.1-6   Right lateral mid cervical radiographs in a mature cow that is suffering from nasopharyngeal perforation associated with balling gun injury. Note fluid line, a large gas pocket, and linear gas pattern as air dissects between cervical fascias.

(Courtesy Dr. Anthony P. Pease, Cornell University.)

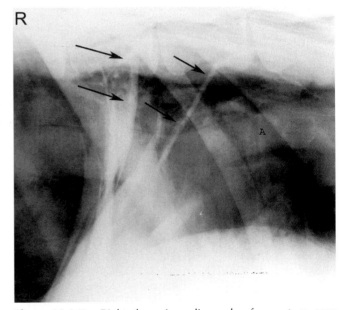

Figure 10.1-7   Right thoracic radiograph of a mature cow with pneumomediastinum, and pneumoretroperitoneum. Thoracic cavity on left; abdominal cavity on right; *A*=aorta; arrows identify each crura of the diaphragm.

(Courtesy Dr. Anthony P. Pease, Cornell University.)

ynx (Section 9.2.1.1.3) for a description of this procedure.

SELF-SUCKLING

Self-suckling is most commonly treated by using a nasal ring with a burr (Figure 10.1-8) or nasal flap and

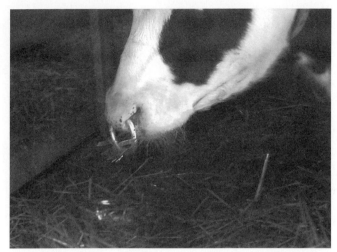

Figure 10.1-8 *A,* Weaning ring used to prevent self-suckling.

(Courtesy of Dr. Lorin Warnick, Cornell University.)

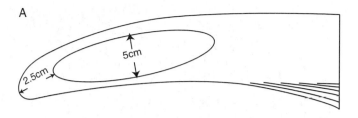

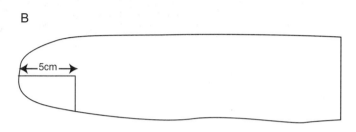

Figure 10.1-9 *A,* Ventral glossectomy; note elliptical excision of a section of the tongue. *B,* Lateral glossectomy: note unilateral excision of the first two inches of the tongue.

individual housing. If these more conservative treatments are not successful, a partial glossectomy can be considered.

Partial Glossectomy

Two surgical techniques have been created to perform a partial glossectomy to prevent self-suckling in animals. The techniques are performed with sedation and local infiltration of lidocaine or general anesthesia. Both techniques alter the tongue's contour to prevent the animal from forming a U-shaped tongue for suckling. For the ventral glossectomy technique, an elliptical incision is made that is approximately 5 cm at its widest part and starts rostral to the frenulum attachment on the tongue and extends rostrally 2.5 cm caudal to the tip of the tongue (Figure 10.1-9A). Each side of the ellipse is incised at an angle toward the midline to facilitate closing the defect, as shown in Figure 10.1-3B. The lateral glossectomy technique removes half of the tip of the tongue (Figure 10.1-9B). Again, the incision is extended at an angle to facilitate closing the tongue similar to what is shown in Figure 10.1-3B, except in a different plane.

SALIVARY GLANDS

Diseases of the salivary glands can be divided into two categories: congenital and acquired. Congenital abnormalities of the salivary glands are associated with agenesis or atresia of the parotid duct, resulting in a fluid-filled swelling proximal to the obstruction site.

Acquired diseases are usually secondary to lacerations or other trauma to the parotid gland that ruptures the salivary gland/or duct. Sometimes a rumen cud obstructs the parotid duct and results in back pressure in the duct, which leads to rupture. The ruptured duct may accumulate saliva in the subcutaneous tissue (salivary cyst or mucocele [mucous cyst or retention cyst of the salivary gland]) or form a fistula if it was ruptured by a laceration. Secondary ascending infections of the glands may also result from any ruptured salivary gland or duct.

Diagnosis of these various diseases is made by physical examination and salivary diagnostic imaging, such as ultrasound exam or sialogram. Palpating a soft fluctuant swelling within the confines of a parotid duct (Figure 10.1-10) strongly suggests an obstructed duct with a secondary distension of the duct. An example of a normal sialogram is shown in Figure 10.1-11.

Generally, salivary gland duct obstruction is unilateral. Therefore treatment mainly focuses on correcting a cosmetic defect, because the effect on digestive activity from unilateral loss of saliva is inconsequential. First, the duct's opening in the mouth should be examined to ensure that it is not obstructed. One can cannulate the duct to estimate the length of the obstructing membrane. A sialography study can also be performed at the same time if ultrasound examination combined with physical examination is not conclusive. Although aspiration of the duct may confirm the diagnosis if saliva is present, it may also result in contamination and secondary infection. Therefore, this procedure is not done routinely.

Many surgical options are available for treating an obstructed duct or salivary gland fistula. Congenital salivary duct obstruction can be left untreated and simply

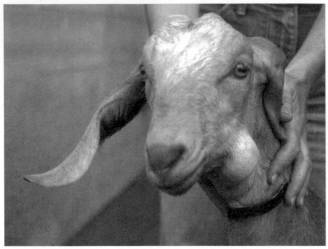

Figure 10.1-10   A soft fluctuant swelling can be palpated within the confines of a salivary duct in this young goat.

(Courtesy of Dr. Mary Smith, Cornell University.)

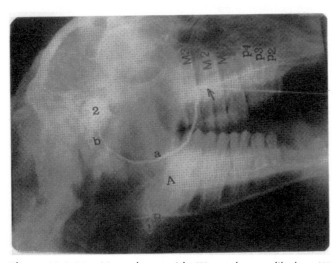

Figure 10.1-11   Normal parotid (2) and mandibular (1) sialography in a ewe. (a) main parotid duct their smaller branches (b), and the parotid duct opening (arrow), main mandibular duct (*A*), and their smaller branches (*B*), premolar 2 (P2), premolar 3 (P3), premolar 4 (P4), molar 1(M1), molar 2 (M2), and molar 3 (M3).

(Reproduced with permission from Deghani et al, *Res Vet Sci* 68: 3-7, 2000).)

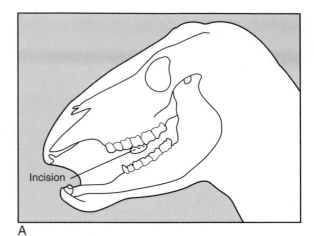

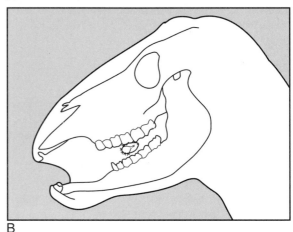

Figure 10.1-12   *A,* A longitudinal incision is made in the oral cavity at the level of the distended duct. *B,* The mucosa edge of the duct is sutured to the buccal mucosa in a simple interrupted pattern.

be monitored. The salivary function loss in a unilateral case is insignificant and results mainly in a cosmetic defect.

The duct proximal to the obstruction can be marsupialized to the oral cavity. This is technically difficult because the duct's unobstructed section is always more caudal than the anatomical opening. The marsupializa-

tion is done as follows. A longitudinal incision is made in the oral cavity at the level of the distended duct (Figure 10.1-12A). The incision is extended to the axial wall of the parotid duct in the same plane. Saliva will leak out into the incision. The incision is enlarged so the stoma created is 1 to 1.5 cm. The oral mucosa is sutured to the parotid duct mucosa with a simple interrupted pattern of absorbable monofilament suture material of appropriate size (2-0 or 3-0) (Figure 10.1-12B). A size-5 to size-8 French polyethylene catheter should be passed through the newly formed stoma and sutured to the buccal mucosa to prevent unwanted closure. The catheter is removed 7 to 10 days later.

The gland may be injected with a caustic agent to destroy all secreting cells until the fistula resolves and heals. Use of 10 to 15 ml of Lugol's iodine or up to 35 ml of 10% buffered formalin (check with local regulatory veterinarian) injected through a catheter placed into the duct for this procedure has been reported. The duct must be held closed for a few minutes to achieve diffusion of the caustic agent throughout the gland. Posttreatment glandular and periglandular swelling may require an antiinflammatory agent such as acetylsalicylic acid or flunixin meglumine.

Excising the parotid gland is the last surgical option. This procedure is done under general anesthesia with meticulous care in the dissection because of the proximity of the salivary gland to important neurovascular bundles.

The surgeon should weigh each procedure's advantages and disadvantages. Although creating a new stoma is the preferred physiological approach, the morbidity is higher because the created stoma may close or stricture, and the condition recurs. Destroying the gland by injecting caustic material causes temporary discomfort and requires analgesia but usually resolves the problem; the resulting loss of gland function appears to be inconsequential. Gland excision is the most complicated approach and requires careful dissection.

Acquired salivary diseases such as fistula and lacerations offer many surgical options: simple duct ligation, destruction of the gland, resection of the gland, or primary repair of the defect. Under appropriate anesthesia (sedation plus local infiltration or general anesthesia), the duct is surgically isolated and ligated with a nonabsorbable suture material. Failure of the ligature as a result of pressure buildup and ascending gland infection is a complication associated with this procedure. Resection of the gland is even more complicated in these cases because of the associated fibrosis and inflammation caused by the laceration. Gland destruction is the simplest form of treatment. As previously described, this treatment is associated with some discomfort, but no long-term complications have been reported.

Primary repair of the lacerated duct is physiologically the best approach but is associated with a greater risk of morbidity from causes such as failed repair and ascending infection. Under appropriate anesthesia, the lacerated duct is isolated. A size-5 to size-8 French polyethylene catheter is passed through the defect into the mouth. A portion of the catheter is passed retrograde proximal to the laceration, thus bridging the defect. The laceration in the duct is sutured over the stent with absorbable monofilament suture (3-0 or 4-0) in a simple continuous pattern. The end of the stent that exits into the oral cavity is sutured to the buccal mucosa.

FRACTURES

Mandibular fractures and, very rarely, maxilla and incisive bone fractures are seen occasionally in ruminants. These traumatic injuries lead to difficulty or inability to eat, dripping of saliva, and prolapsed tongue. The

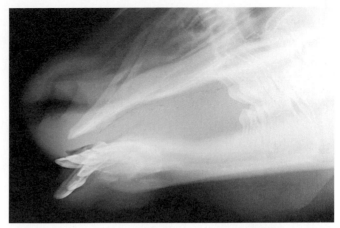

Figure 10.1-13 Calf with a fracture of the rostral mandible, involving three incisors.

diagnosis is made by clinical examination, although radiographic examination will confirm the diagnosis and the extent of the fracture. One should attempt to evaluate tooth integrity in any oral fracture. For a fracture that involves an alveolus with an intact tooth, medically speaking, the tooth should be stabilized in place rather than being removed. However financial factors may dictate removal rather than stabilizing the tooth with an acrylic cap. If the tooth is stabilized, the periodontal ligament will heal at the same time as the alveolar fracture; the tooth will be preserved in many cases. A tooth root abscess remains a possibility, and this should be assessed at the time of reevaluation. However, a tooth with a fractured root should be removed.

In calves, common fractures involve the rostral aspect of one mandible (Figure 10.1-13) or along the mandibular symphysis. If the fracture is minimally displaced, it often heals without treatment. Some calves fracture the rostral aspect of both mandibles in the interdental space, thus resulting in significant displacement that requires treatment (Figure 10.1-14A). In adult ruminants or in any cases in which significant displacement is present, reduction and immobilization is indicated. In all cases, stabilization reduces pain and allows eating to be resumed more quickly.

The treatment goal is to reduce the fracture into normal or near normal anatomical alignment and to stabilize the fracture. One should remember that eating or ruminating applies disruptive forces against the fracture, and the tension side is on the oral surface of the mandible, maxilla, and incisive bone. Implants should be placed on the tension side.

SURGICAL OPTIONS FOR FRACTURES

Surgical options to reduce and immobilize a fracture of the mandible, maxilla or incisive bone are acrylic, wires,

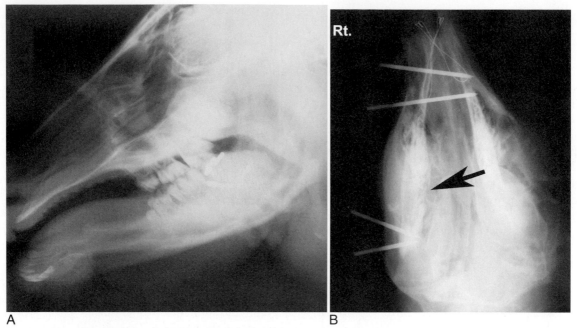

Figure 10.1-14   *A,* Lateral radiograph of 1-year-old Ayrshire heifer with bilateral rostral mandibular fracture and caudal right mandibular fracture (visible on dorsoventral view). *B,* Dorsoventral radiograph that shows repair of a caudal right mandibular fracture (black arrow) with a type I fixator. Converging IM pins are placed on either side of the fracture and are stabilized by a connecting rod made of a 2.5-cm scavenger hose filled with acrylic. The rostral bilateral mandibular fracture is repaired with two figure-8 orthopedic wires.

U-bar, Kirchner apparatus, and internal plates. The techniques are described in the following discussions. In general, using the simplest treatment method is far better. For most (if not all) fractures of the rostral mandible, a wire applied in a figure-eight fashion around incisors on either side of the fracture is sufficient. A wire cannot be appropriately tightened around the incisor and canine teeth of some animals because the teeth are too short, so an acrylic bridge or cap is added. This applies to the majority of ruminant orofacial fractures.

Figure-Eight Wiring

This technique consists of placing an orthopedic wire (1-1.2 mm) around the base of one or more teeth on either side of the fracture in a figure-eight pattern (Figures 10.1-14B and 10.1-15A-B). A 14-gauge needle can be placed to help pass the wire between two teeth (Figure 10.1-15A). Alternatively, a drill can make a canal through which the wire is passed. The knot is twisted and secured on the rostral aspect of the mandible. If the fracture extends caudal to the four incisors (canine teeth) or extends into the interdental space, the wire is secured to the first cheek tooth or a canal is drilled into the bone (incisive or mandibular) in the interdental space (Figure 10.1-16) between the incisors rostral and caudal to the fracture.

Acrylic

This is normally used to provide additional stability to a fixation, generally a figure-eight wire. Although dental acrylics are available, for economic reasons the acrylic* used to secure blocks on cattle hooves is adequate. Because of the exothermic properties of this nondental acrylic, a layer of petroleum gel is applied to the buccal mucosa to protect the soft tissue before the acrylic is applied.

Screw Fixation

Screws can be used to stabilize any rostral mandibular fracture. Aside from the risk of penetrating the root of the incisors or canine teeth, the costs and need for specialized equipment are strong deterrents for using this technique. Nevertheless, screw fixation is an effective means of stabilizing a fracture (see Section 11.5.1 for details on internal fixation). The author has used screw fixation of mandibular fractures in large bulls.

Screws should be applied in a lag fashion at approximately 90 degrees to the fracture plane. Using a drill guide to protect the soft tissue, the surgeon over drills the proximal fragment through stab incisions with an

*Technovit, Jorgensen Laboratories; Loveland, CO

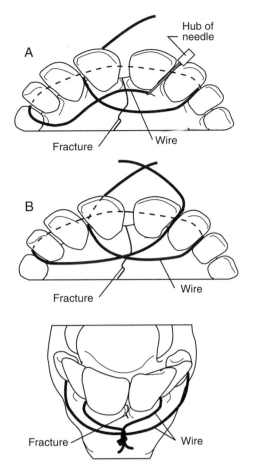

Figure 10.1-15 *A,* An orthopedic wire is guided between the teeth bases with a 14-gauge needle. *B,* The wire is placed in a figure-eight pattern around the base of one or more teeth on either side of the fracture.

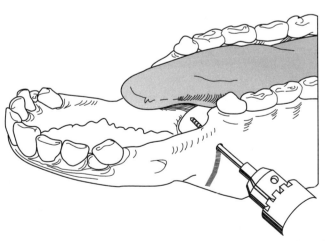

Figure 10.1-16 A 3.2-mm drill bit is used in the interdental space to make a canal through which the orthopedic wire is passed.

appropriate sized drill bit (4.5 mm or 5.5 mm, respectively, for cortical screws of these diameters). An insert is placed, and the distal far fragment is drilled with a 3.5- or 4-mm drill bit, respectively, for the previously mentioned screw diameters. If 6.5-mm partially threaded cancellous screws are used, a 3.5- or 4-mm drill bit is used through the proximal and distal fragment. The drill hole length is measured, and a screw that length minus the fracture gap is measured. After a tap the same size as the screw diameter is used, the appropriate length screw is inserted and tightened. In young animals, a washer under the screw head may be needed. Screws may be used in combination with figure-eight wires using tension band principles.

U-bar

This technique is rarely used because of its difficulty in application. A smooth, round ¼ inch (6.35 mm) rod is bent into the shape of a "U." Holes are drilled into this rod to allow passage of orthopedic wires. The U-bar is inserted on the outside of the mandible or maxilla (Figure 10.1-17). Orthopedic wires are passed around the base of various incisors and cheek teeth and secured to perforations in the U-bar. This is readily done around

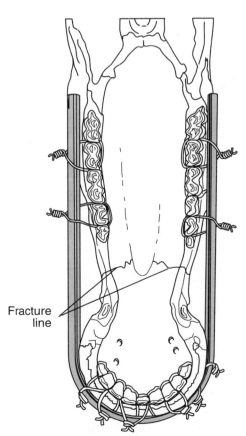

Figure 10.1-17 Drawing that shows placement of "U" bar used to treat caudal mandibular fractures.

the incisors, but is particularly difficult when securing the wire to the cheek teeth. Because ruminants have a small commissure, one needs to pass a 14-gauge needle through the cheek and guide it between the teeth of interest. The wire is placed through perforations in the U-bar after it has been secured between the cheek teeth. A small buccostomy that *avoids* the commissures of the lips is sometimes needed, but it increases the technique's morbidity rate.

Kirschner-Ehmer

The primary indication for this technique is a fracture of the mandible caudal to the symphysis. Type I or II immobilization can be used. With general anesthesia, the animal is placed in dorsal recumbency unless additional fixation is required through the oral cavity; in the latter case, lateral recumbency is selected to keep the fractured side uppermost. The goal is to place two intramedullary (IM) pins (9.53 or 6.35 mm) on each side of the fracture through stab incisions placed on the lateral and ventral aspect of the mandible. After the stab incisions, the soft tissue is retracted with a curved hemostat or drill guide to protect the soft tissue overlying the mandible. Using a smaller drill bit than the IM pins, the surgeon drills a hole into the lateral and ventral aspect of the fractured mandible (type I fixator) on the rostral end of the fracture. The drill hole must be placed in the ventral third of the mandible to avoid tooth roots. Radiographic guidance is helpful in preventing later complications. An IM pin, preferably a positive profile pin, is then placed. A second IM pin is placed at a converging angle. The procedure is repeated on the caudal mandibular fragment. The pins are stabilized by a connecting rod made from a 2.5-cm scavenger hose filled with acrylic (see Figure 10.1-14B). The connecting rods are wrapped with bandage material* to fill the defect between the connecting rod and mandible. This prevents the object from inadvertently violating this space and causing disruption of the repair. Alternatively, a commercially made connecting rod can be used, but this is usually not economically justifiable. In all cases, the pins must be cut close to the connecting rod and a rubber hose or other protective material is used to cover their sharp ends.

If bilateral fractures of the mandible exist, the pins are passed through both mandibles (type II fixator), and connecting bars are placed on both sides.

A pinless external fixator[†] was recently introduced. The system consists of pinless clamps in different sizes and geometries. The clamps are applied to the bone cortex (without penetrating the medullary cavity) and fixed in place by tightening a nut. The universal clamps connect to a connector bar, thus creating an external fixator. The advantages of the technique are that it avoids penetrating the medullary cavity and damaging the tooth root as well as its ease of application and minimal surgical time. The pinless system's disadvantage in comparison to the previously described techniques is its increased cost.

Plating

This surgical option is rarely used in ruminants because of the cost of implants and satisfactory outcomes achieved with other methods. If elected, plates are applied as follows. Under general anesthesia, a linear skin incision is made along the ventrolateral aspect of the mandible. The incision is extended to the mandible. A single narrow dynamic compression plate is placed on the ventral aspect of the mandible. In this position, the plate is actually applied on the compression site of the fracture, but given the position of the cheek teeth, no alternative is available. Plates can also be used on the lateral aspect of the vertical ramus of the mandible. The plates are applied by using an appropriate drill guide so that they compress the fracture site (see Section 11.5.1) Screws should be carefully placed to ensure they do not enter any cheek tooth's root, particularly in young animals.

In all cases, postoperative antibiotics (7 to 10 days) and a short course of analgesics are recommended. Once to twice daily, the mouth is lavaged with mild antiseptic to remove accumulated debris around the implants and/or in the fracture site. If IM pins are used, the incision site around the pins is cleaned with an antiseptic solution, and a dressing is applied to minimize the risk of osteomyelitis. A soft diet is recommended for 10 to 14 days.

Most mandibular fractures heal rapidly enough to allow implant removal at 1 to 2 months after surgery, although radiographic confirmation of healing can take up to 4 months. Except for screws and plates, implants are always removed. Plates and screws can be left in place if the fracture has healed and no evidence of foreign body (implant) reaction or infection is present. Implants are removed under general anesthesia.

COMPLICATIONS

Although most fractures heal uneventfully, complications include early implant loosening, osteomyelitis, sequestration, and tooth root abscess. Implant loosening is rarely a problem because oromaxillary fractures stabilize relatively quickly. Depending on the clinical condition of the fracture when loosening occurs, implants are either removed or replaced.

Osteomyelitis, sequestration, and tooth root abscess are treated with surgical debridement and curettage under general anesthesia. Systemic antibiotics are needed

---

*Powerflex, Andover Coated Products; Salisbury, MA
[†]Pinless External Fixator, Synthes; Paoli, PA

for osteomyelitis cases. Tooth root abscesses are treated by excision as described earlier in this chapter.

Osteomyelitis

Other than osteomyelitis secondary to fracture, trauma can result in soft tissue damage, periosteal devitalization, and secondary infection. Treatment involves surgical debridement and antibiotics described in complications of internal fixation (Section 11.5-4).

A sporadic cause of mandibular or maxillary osteomyelitis is actinomycosis infection (lumpy jaw) in cattle and sheep. Pathologically, this results from an opportunistic infection by *Actinomyces bovis* after trauma. Animals present with a painful bony swelling that progresses if untreated and eventually shows an eroded ulcerated area devoid of skin and progressively increasing facial deformation (Figure 10.1-18). After biopsy of the mass, the diagnosis is made by gram stain evaluation where sulfur granules are observed. The sulfur granules of actinomycosis are large and oval or horseshoe-shaped. There are also a number of gram-positive, filamentous or short rodlike hyphae beneath clubs. The radiographic appearance of this lesion is typical: an enlarging osseous mass with a honeycomb appearance (Figure 10.1-19). These masses have reportedly resolved solely through medical treatment consisting of penicillin G (22,000 IU/kg sid) and isoniazid (10-20 mg/kg sid), both for 30 days. In addition, sodium iodine is admin-

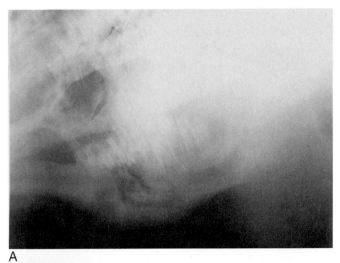

A

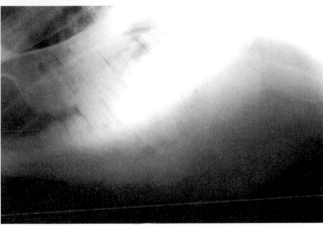

B

Figure 10.1-19 *A* and *B,* Typical radiographic appearance of *Actinomyces* osteomyelitis in 2 cows. Note the honeycomb appearance of the enlarging osseous mass.

(Courtesy of Dr. Nathan Dykes, Cornell University.)

istered (30 g/450 kg, IV) every 2 to 3 days until signs of toxicity (i.e., iodism—dry skin, head, neck, and shoulder) are noted.

In extensive cases of mandibular actinomycosis, surgery can be used as adjunct therapy. Under general anesthesia, the protruding pyogenic granuloma can be removed and sections of infected bone curetted. Antibiotic therapy must be continued because surgery alone is not curative. As an alternative to parenteral administration of antibiotics, local implantation of polymethylmethacrylate (PMMA) beads containing penicillin G (see Section 11.5.2.9) (after debridement) has been used with success in a limited number of cases.

MISCELLANEOUS
Cleft Palate

Cleft palate (Figure 10.1-20) is described in Section 9.2.1.1.4.

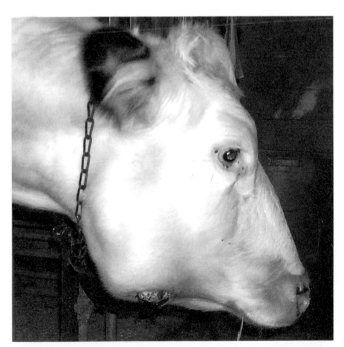

Figure 10.1-18 Mandibular osteomyelitis caused by actinomycosis infection (lumpy jaw) in a Holstein-Friesian cow. Note ulcerative lesion on the mandible.

(Courtesy of Dr. Mary Smith, Cornell University.)

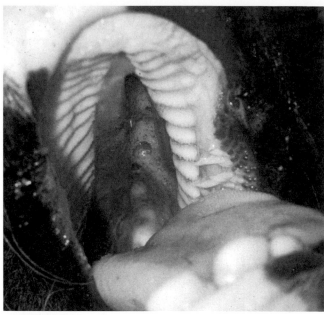

Figure 10.1-20   Cleft palate in a young calf that involves the hard palate.

(Courtesy of Dr. Mary Smith, Cornell University.)

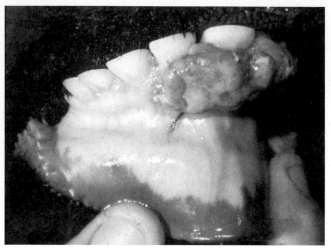

Figure 10.1-21   Oral mass (hamartoma) in a young calf.

Neoplasia

Chapter 3 discusses neoplasia. Tumors of dental origin (odontoma and ameloblastoma or adamantinoma) have been reported in cattle and sheep. In addition, hamartomas are sometimes seen (Figure 10.1-21). The term *hamartoma* refers to a mass composed of normal cellular elements that originates from the tissue where it is found. Unlike normal tissue, hamartomas are poorly organized and are believed to be developmental abnormalities rather than true neoplasms. They have been seen on the maxilla but are more common on the rostral aspect of the lower jaw. Their position interferes with mastication. These are usually seen in young animals (<3 years of age). Osteosarcoma and lymphosarcoma should be considered if a hard swelling on the mandible or maxilla is detected on physical examination. It can be differentiated from *Actinomycosis* because of the latter's characteristic radiographic pattern and typical presence of skin ulceration and pyogenic granulomas. In all of the aforementioned cases, the diagnosis is confirmed by histopathological evaluation of a biopsy.

The key to successful management is early surgical resection. Early treatment has a better chance of success (lesion-dependent) because the lesion can be entirely removed without significant mandibular loss. If treatment is delayed too long, the tumor will invade the mandibular symphysis and require a rostral mandibulectomy, a treatment with significant morbidity.

To perform mass removal the animal is anesthetized and placed in lateral recumbency with the mass uppermost. Depending on the type of tumor, the mass is transected at its junction on the mandible/maxilla with a surgical blade, oscillating saw, Gigli wire, or osteotome. A partial hemimandibulectomy may be required for "en bloc" mandibular resection in certain tumors. All abnormal bone/tissue is removed or curreted. The gingiva is sutured with absorbable sutures in a simple interrupted pattern wherever possible, and the rest of the defect is left to heal by second intention. Postoperatively, antibiotics (7 to 10 days) and a short course of analgesics are recommended. The mouth is lavaged with water or mild antiseptic once or twice daily.

An unusual but characteristic swelling seen in young (1 to 2 years) cattle is a neurofibroma (see Chapter 3). Typically, it consists of a mucocutaneous lesion(s) in young cattle around the head and neck (Figure 10.1-22A). They present as nonpainful masses that enlarge progressively in size. The mass results in a cosmetic defect and gets traumatized because of its location and size. It has been suggested that this is a heritable defect caused by a mutation at the bovine neurofibromatosis type 1 locus.

Ultrasound examination reveals a multilobular appearance to the mass, and when cut in cross-section, reveals the typical appearance as shown in Figure 10.1-22B. Needle aspiration fails to yield purulent material. The diagnosis can be confirmed by biopsy and is usually treated by surgical excision. The author has treated such lesions by excision, as biological progression in untreated patients can cause clinical problems, especially in periorbital lesions.

The animal is anesthetized and placed in lateral recumbency. A fusiform incision is made around the base

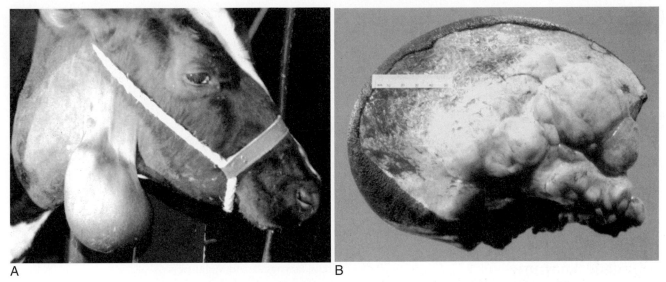

Figure 10.1-22   *A,* Large unilateral swelling in the cervical area seen in a cow. The swelling is firm but is not painful. *B,* Appearance of neurofibroma on cross-section.

(Courtesy of Dr. Donald Smith, Cornell University.)

of the mass. The neck of the mass is identified and isolated via blunt dissection and ligation of transected vessels. Following transaction closure is routine, except in lesions involving the eyelid where careful reconstruction is required. Recurrences have not been encountered in our limited experience but are biologically possible.

Oropharyngeal Membrane

Similar to choanal atresia, a persistent membrane can obstruct the oropharynx, thus preventing any milk, saliva or other liquid from reaching the esophagus. This rare congenital anomaly prevents an animal from ingesting any nutrients. Newborns present with this history and a progressive loss of condition. Treatment has not been reported in large animals, but presumably would consist of membrane resection as described in humans.

RECOMMENDED READINGS

Amstuz HE. Dental problems, *Modern Vet Pract* 60: 639-640, 1979.

Bent JP 3rd, Klippert FN, Smith RJ: Management of congenital buccopharyngeal membrane. *Cleft Palate Craniofac J* 34: 538-541, 1997.

Davidson HP, Rebhun WC, Habel RE: Pharyngeal trauma in cattle, *Cornell Vet* 71: 15-25, 1981.

Dehghani SN, Tadjalli M, Masoumzadeh MH: Sialography of sheep parotid and mandibular salivary glands, *Res Vet Sci* 68: 3-7, 2000.

Dyce KM, Sack WO, Wensing CJG: The head and ventral neck of ruminants. In Dyce KM, Sack WO, Wensing CJG, editors: *Veterinary anatomy,* Philadelphia, 1996, WB Saunders.

Henninger RW, Beard WL, Schneider RK, Bramlage LR, Burkhardt HA: Fractures of the rostral portion of the mandible and maxilla in horses: 89 cases (1979-1997), *J Am Vet Med Assoc* 214: 1648-1652, 1999.

Hofmeyr CFB: The digestive system. In Oehme FW, Prier JE, editors: *Large animal surgery,* Baltimore, 1974, Williams and Wilkins.

Horney FD, Wallace CE: Surgery of the bovine digestive tract. In Jennings PB: *The practice of large animal surgery,* Philadelphia, 1984, WB Saunders.

Kubo M, Osada M, Konno S: A histological and ultrastructural comparison of the sulfur granule of the actinomycosis and actinobacillosis, *Natl Inst Anim Health Q (Tokyo)* 20: 53-59, 1980.

Lischer CJ, Fluri E, Kaser-Holtz B, et al: Pinless external fixation of mandibular fracture in cattle, *Vet Surg* 16: 14-19, 1997.

Parks AH, Baskett SA: Salivary gland disease. In Robinson NE: *Current therapy in equine medicine,* Philadelphia, 1997, WB Saunders.

Plumlee KH, Haynes JS, Kersting KW, Thompson JR: Osteosarcoma in a cow, *J Am Vet Med Assoc* 202: 95-96, 1993.

Rebhun WC: Infectious diseases of the gastrointestinal tract. In Rebhun WC: *Diseases of dairy cattle,* Baltimore, 1995, Williams and Wilkins.

Sartin EA, Doran SE, Riddell MG, Herrera GA, Tennyson GS, D'Andrea G, Whitley RD, Collins FS: Characterization of naturally occurring cutaneous neurofibromatosis in Holstein cattle: a disorder resembling neurofibromatosis type 1 in humans, *Am J Pathol* 145: 1168-1174, 1994.

Schmotzer WB, Hultgren BD, Huber MJ, et al: Chemical involution of the equine parotid salivary gland, *Vet Surg* 20: 128-132, 1991.

Smoak IW, Hudson LC: Persistent oropharyngeal membrane in a Hereford calf, *Vet Pathol* 33: 80-82, 1996.

Singh JIT, Singh AP, Patil DB: The digestive system. In Tyagi RPS and Singh JIT: *Ruminant surgery,* Shandara, 1993, CBS.

St-Jean G, Basaraba RJ, Kennedy GA, Anderson DE: Maxillary lymphosarcoma in a cow, *Can Vet J* 35: 56-57, 1994.

Wiggs RB, Lobprise HB: Acute and chronic alveolitis/osteomyelitis ("lumpy jaw") in small exotic ruminants, *J Vet Dent* 11: 106-109, 1994.

Wilson RB: Gingival vascular hamartoma in three calves, *J Vet Diagn Invest* 2: 338-339, 1990.

10.2—Esophageal Surgery

Susan L. Fubini and Anthony P. Pease

Only a few diseases have been documented that cause esophageal disorders in the bovine, the most common being foreign body obstruction. Other differential diagnoses include esophageal diverticula, esophageal stricture, esophageal ulceration, esophageal perforation, hypoplasia of the esophageal musculature, megaesophagus, and esophageal obstruction by an extraesophageal mass. One study estimated that esophageal disorders in the bovine account for 0.8% of the clinical cases.

Esophageal Anatomy

The bovine esophagus measures 90 to 105 cm from the pharynx to the cardia. Because the rumen is closely related to the diaphragm, no appreciable intraabdominal portion of the esophagus exists. In sheep, the esophagus measures about 45 cm long.

In the cranial third of the bovine neck, the esophagus travels dorsal to the trachea. From the third to sixth cervical vertebrae, it moves left of the trachea. By the thoracic inlet, the esophagus has traveled to the dorsolateral surface of the trachea. It courses in the mediastinum, passing dorsal to the base of the heart and tracheal bifurcation. The esophagus crosses the aortic arch and continues caudally through the esophageal hiatus at the level of the eighth or ninth intercostal space.

Structures that accompany the cervical esophagus include the carotid sheath, recurrent laryngeal nerve, tracheal lymphatic trunk, and deep cervical lymph nodes. In the caudal mediastinum, the esophagus is adjacent to the dorsal and ventral trunks of the vagus nerve. Dorsally, it is in proximity to the large caudal mediastinal lymph nodes. These nodes can become enlarged and exert pressure on the vagal trunks.

The esophagus comprises four layers that include the outer adventitial layer (tunica adventitia), muscular layers (tunica muscularis), submucosa (tela submucosa), and mucosal layer (tunica mucosa). In the thoracic esophagus the adventitial layer is replaced by a serosal covering (tunica serosa), which is formed by the mediastinal pleura. In ruminants, except at the cranial and caudal ends, the tunica muscularis comprises outer and inner spiral layers of striated muscle fibers that run throughout the length of the esophagus. At the cranial and caudal ends, the inner muscle layer consists of circular fibers, whereas the outer layer consists of longitudinal fibers. The outer layer of elliptical fibers at the pharyngeal end of the esophagus is incomplete ventrally, where it attaches to the cricoid cartilage. At this site, the overlapping pharyngeal and esophageal musculature forms a pharyngoesophageal sphincter.

The tela submucosa consists of loose connective tissue, which allows longitudinal folds to form in the tunica mucosa when the esophagus is contracted. A thick layer of stratified squamous epithelium lines the esophagus. Blood is supplied from the cranial thyroid, common carotid, bronchoesophageal, and reticular arteries. Branches of the cranial and middle thyroid veins, the caudal part of the external jugular vein and the cranial vena cava provide venous drainage. Esophageal veins drain into the azygos veins, reticular vein, and left ruminal vein. Esophageal branches of the vagus nerve innervate the cranial half of the esophagus. The caudal half is innervated by esophageal branches off the recurrent laryngeal and vagal nerves.

Because the esophagus courses medial to the left jugular groove, a visible and palpable bulge is evident in the left jugular groove when a bolus is swallowed or an orogastric tube is passed.

Clinical Signs of Esophageal Disease

Obstructive esophageal disease, or choke, is typically manifested in cattle by bloat and salivation. The salivation can be exacerbated by foreign material. Gaseous distention of the rumen results from the inability of the cow to eructate and release gas. The animal's head and neck are extended. Coughing is common, and the tongue often protrudes. Retching is sometimes seen. The animal is often dehydrated and may be anxious or very agitated. Cattle lose tremendous quantities of saliva, which contains a large amount of bicarbonate; therefore cattle often develop metabolic acidosis with an esophageal obstruction.

Diagnosis of Esophageal Disease

Physical examination findings are used to diagnose esophageal disease along with endoscopy, radiography, and ultrasound examination.

The cow's vital signs hydration status should be assessed along with hydration status. Pharyngeal trauma and rabies must be considered and kept in mind as differential diagnoses. The laryngeal area and neck should be palpated for swelling, cellulitis, or subcutaneous emphysema. An oral examination should be performed to evaluate the pharynx and rule out cleft palate, dental disease, foreign body, or neoplasia.

The lower airway should be auscultated carefully to determine if there is any sign of aspiration pneumonia. Passage of a stomach tube through a Frick speculum would be the next step to help localize an intraluminal obstruction (detailed in Chapter 1). The tube should be passed gently to avoid damage to the potentially compromised mucosa.

ESOPHAGOSCOPY

Esophagoscopy is indicated to help localize an obstruction, identify obstructing material, and assess damage to the esophagus, especially when the problem has been resolved. A 2- or 3-m flexible fiberoptic endoscope permits evaluation of the entire esophagus in most animals. The cow should be restrained, ideally in a chute and head gate, to protect the examiner and equipment. If possible, the endoscope is passed through to the cardia and the esophagus insufflated with air and examined as the endoscope is being withdrawn. The normal esophagus has longitudinal mucosal folds. The mucosal folds and swallowing artifacts should not be construed as abnormal. Because of saliva accumulation and the tendency for the esophagus to collapse periodically, it is easy to miss or overinterpret a lesion. Therefore any lesion found should be reexamined by repeatedly passing over the area to eliminate any artifacts.

BOVINE ESOPHAGEAL RADIOLOGY

Survey and contrast radiographs are recommended to characterize lesions in the bovine esophagus (Figure 10.2-1). Fluoroscopy can be used to evaluate the swallow

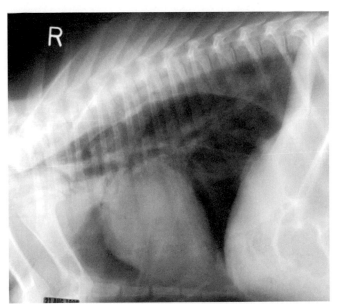

Figure 10.2-1   Right lateral thoracic radiographs of a calf with mega-esophagus. Note that the esophagus is markedly dilated with gas and fluid. A tracheal stripe sign is present.

(Courtesy of Dr. Peter Scrivani, Cornell University.)

reflex in farm animals, but the difficulty in restraining patients can be technically challenging. Esophagraphy is considered the method of choice for evaluating bovine esophageal disorders.

Survey radiographs should be obtained to determinate an adequate technique and help classify the disorder before contrast material is administered. Lateral survey radiographs of the neck can be obtained by using a regular screen and film holder. Stocks are recommended to eliminate the need for a handler to hold the patient. Exposure factors of 20 to 40 mAs and 70 to 77 kVp at 90-cm focal distance have been described for radiographs of the cervical esophagus. For the thoracic portion of the esophagus, an exposure factor of 90 mAs and 90 to 96 kVp can be used with a 1:20 grid. Ventrodorsal and dorsoventral radiographs of patients that weigh more than 60 kg are usually not diagnostic because of the large amount of musculature and difficulties obtaining radiographs, as positioning would probably require general anesthesia. Left and right lateral radiographs of the thoracic cavity have been recommended in place of a ventrodorsal or dorsoventral radiograph. To image the thoracic portion of the esophagus, high-speed film-screen combinations and larger X-ray units are required to achieve adequate exposure. The published exposure factor for thoracic radiographs in a bovine is 21-42 mAs and 78-118 kVp with a 1:7 grid.

Contrast administration in the esophagus (esophagraphy) is relatively easy in the bovine. Barium suspension (60% w/vol) is administered via an oroesophageal or nasal esophageal tube placed in the cranial third of the esophagus or cranial to the obstruction. Barium suspension is preferred because of the ease of administration in comparison to paste and lack of inflammatory response if some barium is aspirated. it Iodinated contrast medium can cause a severe inflammatory process if aspirated. Barium paste (70% w/vol) is preferred if mucosal ulceration is suspected because the paste coats and better delineates the mucosal surface. Barium has been documented to cause a granulomatous response if it dissects into the soft tissues; therefore iodinated contrast medium can be considered if esophageal perforation is suspected.

No standard dose for esophagraphy in the bovine exists. However, 300 ml to 3 liters of a barium suspension can be administered, and the contrast can be given at full strength or diluted 1:1 with water, thus making a 30% w/vol suspension. The amount administered should be altered based on the suspected disorder. For example, an esophageal obstruction does not require the same volume as a flaccid megaesophagus does. Radiographs should be obtained as soon after contrast administration as possible.

Surgical Considerations

Unfortunately, esophageal surgery in any species is fraught with complications. Most of the esophagus does not have a serosal covering, which is important in forming a fibrin seal. Furthermore, the esophageal lumen is not "clean"; constant movement occurs during swallowing, and its location causes tension on any suture line. The proximity of the recurrent laryngeal nerve to the esophagus can have deleterious effects on manipulations. Some procedures, such as a standing cervical esophagotomy, can be performed by using sedation and local anesthesia. For more extensive manipulations, general anesthesia is preferable.

Most esophageal disorders can be managed conservatively; thus few reports of surgical intervention in the ruminant esophagus exist. A lateral or ventrolateral approach is typically described for performing a cervical esophagotomy; a left-sided rib resection is usually performed on the thoracic esophagus. General anesthesia and positive pressure ventilation are essential for a thoracotomy.

A longitudinal incision is used to incise the esophagus. Once the muscular coat is incised, the esophagus separates into two layers: the elastic inner layer, which is composed of mucosa and submucosa, and the outer muscular layers and adventitia. The inner layer provides the greatest tensile strength during esophageal closure. Preservation of blood supply, aseptic technique, apposition of tissues without tension, and appropriate preoperative and postoperative management are essential for a successful outcome.

ESOPHAGEAL CLOSURE

Primary esophageal closure involves a 2-layer technique. The mucosa and submucosa are closed together in either a simple continuous or simple interrupted pattern. A nonabsorbable (e.g., polypropylene or nylon) or long-lasting absorbable (e.g., polyglactin 910, polydioxanone, or polyglyconate) suture material is used (Figure 10.2-2). It is recommended the knots be tied within the esophageal lumen to prevent contamination of the wound by ingesta migrating along suture tracts. The muscular layer can be closed by using either an absorbable or nonabsorbable noncapillary suture with a simple interrupted or mattress pattern (see Figure 10.2-2). A suction drain* may be placed to allow evacuation of contaminated exudate. The lack of serosal covering may contribute to complications after surgery, including leakage and dehiscence.

In 1988 Dallman suggested that the holding layer of the canine esophagus might be the submucosa. If this is

*J-Vac Drain, Johnson & Johnson; New Brunswick, NJ

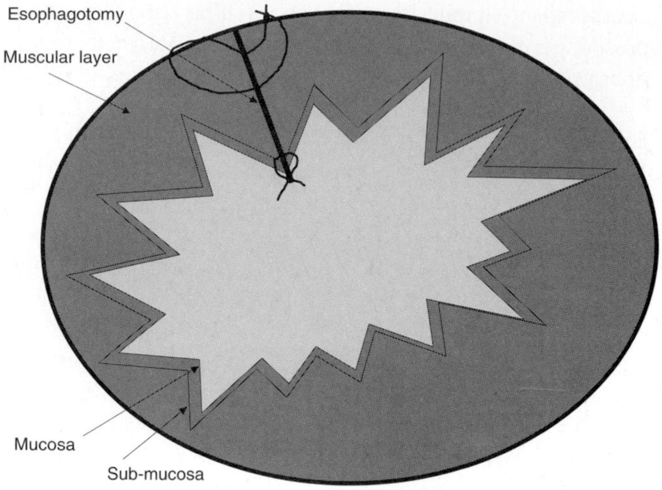

Figure 10.2-2   Schematic representation of surgical closure of the esophagus.

true, suturing the submucosa and muscle in one or two layers while avoiding penetration of the mucosa could reduce the incidence of complications in esophageal surgery.

FOREIGN BODY OBSTRUCTION

Foreign body obstruction, or "choke," a common esophageal disorder in cattle, results from incomplete mastication and rapid ingestion. Cattle produce large quantities of saliva, which makes a smooth-skinned potato or apple difficult to masticate, so it can slip into the pharynx and esophagus. Other common sources of obstruction include cabbage, beets, turnips, and ears of corn. Infrequently, sharp foreign bodies such as glass or irregular metallic objects can be swallowed and lodged in the esophagus.

The clinical signs of "choke" mentioned earlier include ruminal tympany, excessive salivation, coughing, tongue protrusion, and extension of the head and neck. The animal may be dehydrated and anxious.

Obstructions in the cervical esophagus can usually be palpated externally. After rabies has been ruled out, a thorough oral examination should be performed to evaluate the pharynx and check for any foreign bodies. Passage of a nasogastric tube helps determine swallowing ability and localize the obstruction site. If the esophagus is filled with fluid proximal to the obstruction, visualization can be difficult.

Plain radiographs can show esophageal distention with gas or deviation of the esophagus (see Figure 10.2-1). Feed material impactions (Figure 10.2-3A or radioopaque foreign bodies may show up on plain survey films. Contrast studies help delineate nonmetallic foreign bodies (Figure 10.2-3B). Gas accumulation in the soft

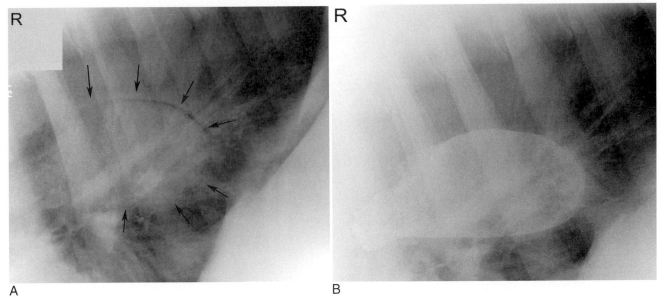

Figure 10.2-3   Five-year-old shorthorn cow with esophageal obstruction. *A,* Right lateral thoracic radiograph showing soft tissue density in the esophagus. Note air density (black arrows) outlining the junction of the obstruction and the esophageal wall. *B,* After barium administration, which emphasizes the size and shape of the esophageal obstruction.

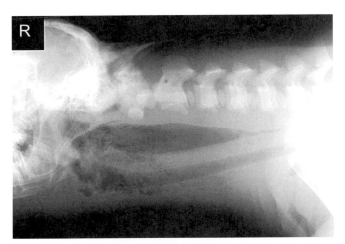

Figure 10.2-4   Right cervical radiograph of a calf with a cranial cervical esophageal rupture. Note accumulation of gas in the subcutaneous tissues.

(Courtesy of Dr. Ned Dykes, Cornell University.)

tissues adjacent to the esophagus (Figure 10.2-4) may indicate an esophageal perforation or rupture. If choke is present, a soft tissue opacity may be seen within the esophagus contrasted by gas (see Figure 10.2-3A). If choke is present for more than 48 hours, gas within the esophageal wall may be detected as a result of necrosis of the mucosa. If the obstruction is present in the cervical portion of the esophagus, the trachea and larynx may

be ventrally displaced. Contrast radiography can be used; however, the obstruction is usually palpated and diagnosed during passage of an orogastric or nasogastric tube. Esophagraphy is more useful for evaluating the mucosal wall for strictures or perforation after the obstruction has been cleared. If esophagraphy is performed, the cranial portion of the obstruction will be delineated, and contrast medium may be detected in the trachea because of aspiration.

Extraesophageal masses diagnosed in the bovine include hematoma, cervical abscess, and extraesophageal tumors. Primary esophageal tumors have not been reported, and congenital abnormalities of the esophagus are extremely rare. We have seen one calf with chronic bloat associated with a tracheoesophageal fistula (Figure 10.2-5). Extraesophageal lesions usually displace the larynx, trachea, and esophagus ventrally. On survey radiographs, gas is occasionally detected in the cervical esophagus. If contrast medium was administered, ventral deviation of the esophagus with mild dilation and difficulty swallowing the barium suspension can be observed.

The initial treatment of choke is aimed at resolving the ruminal tympany by using a needle attached to a suction apparatus. Alternatively, a small trocar or cannula can be used to decompress the rumen. The animal should be held off feed and water to lessen the risk of aspiration pneumonia until the obstruction is removed.

Spontaneous resolution of an esophageal obstruction may occur with or without sedation. If the object is in

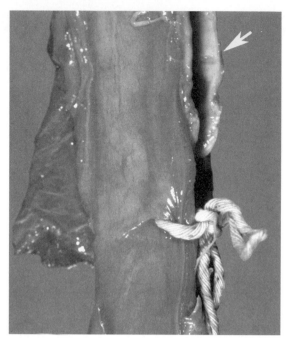

Figure 10.2-5 Tissues from a calf with chronic bloat associated with a tracheoesophageal fistula. Arrow shows lumen of the trachea while rope is seen exiting through the esophageal mucosa.

the proximal or midcervical portion of the esophagus, it may be gently moved into the proximal esophagus and eventually the oral cavity. The cow should be restrained in a stanchion or chute while the operator gently places his or her fingers into the jugular furrow just distal to the obstruction. Steady uniform pressure should be applied, especially when the esophageal musculature is relaxed, to slowly move the foreign body toward the pharynx. Once the foreign body reaches the proximal esophagus, it may be possible to grasp the foreign object with the help of a mouth speculum and by pulling the tongue out of the oral cavity. Mild sedation (xylazine at .01-.02 mg/kg/IV) can be helpful as well.

A wire snare has been used with success in some instances to encircle and retrieve foreign objects in a more distal obstruction. This procedure does risk damaging the esophageal mucosa.

The thoracic esophagus widens slightly, making it possible to use a smooth stomach tube to advance some distal thoracic obstructions into the rumen where foreign materials can be retrieved via rumenotomy. Ideally, the site should be observed first via esophagoscopy to determine whether such manipulations would be detrimental (e.g., if the obstruction has sharp edges).

Repeated warm water lavage may help break up feedstuff in a feed impaction. The animal should be sedated with the head lowered to prevent aspiration pneumonia during the warm water lavage. Alternatively, a large-diameter, malleable endotracheal tube may be passed through the nose into the esophagus, where the cuff is inflated, and a smaller nasogastric tube is passed through the lumen of the endotracheal tube to perform the lavage. This technique allows lavage fluids to drain through the endotracheal tube, minimizing the risk of aspiration. Although it may take several hours and repeated attempts to dissolve an impaction, gentle manipulation is essential to minimize further damage to the esophagus.

If the feed impaction cannot be resolved in the standing animal or the patient cannot be adequately restrained, other techniques are used. The endotracheal tube technique can be performed with the cow under general anesthesia. Esophagoscopy with the cow standing can be used. If all manipulative attempts fail, surgery, such as an esophagotomy, should be considered because prolonged obstruction can cause permanent mucosal damage. After the obstruction is removed, the esophagus should be evaluated to assess mucosal damage.

CERVICAL ESOPHAGOTOMY

The cow is restrained in stocks or chute to perform a standing procedure or positioned in right lateral recumbency if using sedation or, ideally, general anesthesia. The stomach tube is placed to the level of the obstruction prior to anesthesia. The neck is prepared for aseptic surgery.

After approaching the esophagus, pediatric Balfour retractors are applied to obtain exposure of the esophagus. The affected area is isolated from the surgical field using moist sponges. The esophagus is incised, and the foreign body is removed. The incision should be made in healthy esophageal tissue if possible. If the esophageal wall has a normal appearance, primary closure is recommended as described previously. Food and water are withheld for 48 hours after surgery, and maintenance intravenous fluid therapy is instituted. If considerable dead space exists, a closed suction drain is advisable for the first 48 to 72 hours. If the esophageal wall is compromised, it should be allowed to heal by second intention with daily wound care. If the animal loses too much feed material and water through the esophageal defect and cannot maintain body condition, a rumen fistula can be placed (see Section 10.3.1). The animal can then be fed via rumen fistula until the esophageal defect is small enough to allow oral alimentation.

TRANSTHORACIC ESOPHAGOTOMY

Isolated reports of successful transthoracic esophagotomy procedures in ruminants have been made. General anesthesia and positive pressure ventilation are essential. The animal is placed in right lateral recumbency. A 35 to

40 cm skin incision is made over the seventh or eighth rib. Usually, it is necessary to perform a partial rib resection (see Section 9.3.1) by dissecting under the rib 4 cm proximal to the costochondral junction. Blunt dissection is done along the pleural surface of the rib; thus a Gigli wire can be passed and worked in a proximal direction. While the site is lavaged with warm saline, the Gigli wire transects the rib. The distal portion of the rib is easily removed at the costochondral junction. All soft tissues are packed off with moist, sterile bath towels. A Penrose drain or umbilical tape loops can be placed around the esophagus and used for manipulation. The esophageal incision and closure are as previously described. A chest drain is placed before closing the thoracic cavity. The parietal pleura are closed, followed by muscle, subcutaneous tissues, and skin.

ESOPHAGEAL PERFORATION OR LACERATION

Esophageal perforation or rupture is caused most often by overzealous use of an instrument to dislodge an obstruction. The foreign body itself can also cause pressure necrosis of the esophageal wall. Other causes include pharyngeal trauma, extension of a soft tissue infection, and cervical trauma.

Affected animals usually develop impressive subcutaneous emphysema. They are inappetent and depressed. Swelling develops at the site of the rupture and can progress to a sizable infection of the surrounding area. Migration of infection down fascial planes to the mediastinum and thoracic cavity can be catastrophic (see Figure 10.1-7). The diagnosis can be confirmed with esophagoscopy, ultrasound, or a contrast radiographic study. On survey radiographs, irregular gas opacities may be detected in the soft tissues of the neck, surrounding the esophagus and trachea, and/or within the mediastinum. If esophagraphy is performed, iodinated contrast medium should be used to delineate the perforation but may be cost-prohibitive. For large patients barium suspension can be used (diluted 1 : 1 with water) as long as the potential complication of granuloma formation is explained to the client. If the esophagus is perforated, contrast medium is detected in the soft tissues outside the esophagus.

Tissues healthy enough to be closed after esophageal perforation are rare, but primary closure can be attempted with a lesion less than 12 hours old. Closed suction drainage should be used to avoid serum and blood accumulation at the surgical site. Therapeutic antibiotics, nonsteroidal antiinflammatory drugs, and tetanus prophylaxis are administered. If primary closure is not possible, ventral drainage is provided, and the wound is allowed to heal by contraction and epithelialization. Adequate ventral drainage is mandatory to prevent septicemia and cellulitis extending along fascial

planes and causing lower airway disease—possibly generalized septicemia. The patient can be fed via a rumen fistula. Healing these tissues can be a long, drawn-out process and is rarely warranted.

STRICTURE

Stricture or stenosis of the esophagus can occur after extramural or intramural lesions, extramural compression, or extension of an infectious process. Stenosis secondary to a developmental abnormality such as a persistent right aortic arch is rare but has been reported. Other extramural causes of compression include lesions in the cranial abdomen, such as an abscess or adhesion that results in a narrowing of the esophageal hiatus. Rarely, esophageal granulomas can occur secondary to *Actinobacillus* or *Arcanobacterium pyogenes* infection or neoplasia. Healing after esophageal rupture and surgery can all result in stricture.

Full-thickness mucosal or submucosal defects heal predominantly by contraction and fibrosis. The resulting annular lesions are categorized as the following three types, depending on the location, duration, and fibrosis: 1) mural lesions involve only the adventitia and muscularis; 2) esophageal rings or webs involve only the mucosa or submucosa; and 3) annular stenosis involves all layers of the esophageal wall. The survey radiographs are usually normal, unless the condition is chronic and a focal dilation (has formed cranial to the stricture). An esophageal stricture appears as a focal narrowing of the lumen that persists on sequential radiographs. Strictures should not be confused with peristalsis; therefore multiple radiographs should be taken to confirm the diagnosis. A double contrast esophagram can be performed by placing a cuffed orogastric tube (such as an endotracheal tube) proximal to the stricture and administering barium suspension, followed by a similar volume of room air. A radiograph is obtained while the esophagus is distended.

Nonsurgical Management

Clinical and experimental studies in horses indicate that stricture formation may occur as soon as 15 days after circumferential mucosal loss. The lumen diameter is not expected to change for 30 days, but between 30 and 60 days, the lumen diameter increases, with the greatest change occurring between 30 and 45 days. Therefore acute equine strictures are managed with antibiotic therapy, nonsteroidal antiinflammatory drugs, and frequent feedings with small quantities of a pelleted mash. By extrapolation, we recommend similar guidelines for ruminants.

Bougienage and pneumatic or hydrostatic dilators have been successful in humans with chronic esophageal strictures. These techniques have been used very little to date in domestic or farm animals. It would be possible to feed a ruminant via a rumen fistula while managing an esophageal stricture.

Surgical Management

Surgery can be considered if the stricture diameter does not change by 60 days and clinical signs are progressive. To some extent, the nature of the esophageal stricture dictates the method of surgical correction. Described surgical methods include esophagomyotomy; partial esophageal resection; complete resection and anastomosis, esophagoplasty, esophageal replacement, muscle or synthetic patch grafting, and fenestration of the cicatrix through an esophageal fistula.

ESOPHAGOMYOTOMY

Esophagomyotomy is indicated for an esophageal stricture that involves only the muscularis and adventitia. A nasogastric tube is positioned before surgery. The esophagus is approached and gently freed from surrounding tissues, and the strictured area is identified. One or more longitudinal incisions are made in the esophageal musculature without incising the mucosa. The nasogastric tube should be able to easily cross the surgical site inside the mucosa. The musculature can be separated from the mucosa around the entire circumference of the esophagus if necessary. The myotomy may or may not be sutured. The remainder of the surgical incision is closed and drained in a routine manner.

PARTIAL ESOPHAGEAL RESECTION

Partial esophageal resection combines a longitudinal esophagomyotomy with a mucosal resection. The procedure is ideal for strictures confined to the submucosa and mucosa but may also be used for full-thickness strictures. A longitudinal esophagomyotomy is performed, and the diseased submucosa and mucosa are identified and resected. If the lesion is confined to the submucosa and mucosa, only the muscular layer and adventitia are closed. The mucosa is closed only if achievable without excessive tension. It is advantageous to suture the muscularis because the mucosa can then regenerate along the inside of the muscular tube.

COMPLETE ESOPHAGEAL RESECTION

Esophageal resection and anastomosis have been recommended if the stricture involves all layers, and the muscularis is damaged extensively and useless as a scaffold for mucosal regeneration. Minimizing tension on the anastomosis is essential for a favorable result.

A routine approach is made to the esophagus. Healthy tissue cranial and caudal to the lesion is transected. A two-layer anastomosis is performed by closing the submucosa and mucosa in a simple continuous or interrupted pattern and the muscular layer in a simple interrupted pattern. Gentle tissue handling and careful use of retractors are essential to avoid damage to the carotid sheath, vagosympathetic trunk, and recurrent laryngeal nerve.

After surgery, extraoral alimentation can be through a rumen fistula in an adult cow, an esophagotomy tube distal to the surgery site in a young ruminant, or by daily passage of a nasogastric tube.

FENESTRATION THROUGH A CICATRIX

A final option for surgical repair of an esophageal stricture involves an esophagostomy, followed by fenestration of the mucosal and submucosal cicatrix. The esophagostomy heals as a traction diverticulum, thereby increasing the lumen size. The animal can again be fed via a rumen fistula or via a tube placed in the esophagostomy site.

Esophageal Diverticulum

OCCURRENCE AND DIAGNOSIS

Esophageal diverticula is the second most common esophageal disorder in the bovine. There are two types of esophageal diverticula, and both are usually acquired conditions. *Traction (true) diverticula* results from contraction of periesophageal fibrous scar tissue, often secondary to a wound or previous surgery. Traction diverticula are usually asymptomatic. *Pulsion (false) diverticula* results from protrusion of mucosa and submucosa through a defect in the esophageal musculature. These diverticula may result from external trauma, fluctuation in esophageal intraluminal pressure, and overstretch damage to esophageal muscle fibers by impacted foodstuffs. Affected animals are often dysphagic but able to drink. They may regurgitate after eating. Coughing, salivation, and ruminal distention are typical. The diverticulum may enlarge over time and become evident as a large swelling in the neck, which results in dysphagia or choke. Esophagoscopy helps define the relative size of the opening of the diverticulum. This disorder can usually only be seen during esophagraphy as a focal accumulation of contrast material. Occasionally, an esophageal stricture can be detected just caudal to the focal dilation. If a diverticulum is present within the thoracic portion of the esophagus, the most common clinical sign is regurgitation. In one study, 86% of cases with thoracic diverticula had radiographic evidence of pneumonia.

TREATMENT

Repair of a pulsion diverticulum involves mucosal inversion with reconstruction of the muscular layer or diverticulectomy. The former is preferred because the mucosa is left intact, which minimizes the risk of postoperative leakage, infection, or fistula formation.

ESOPHAGEAL FISTULA

Esophageal fistulae may result from healing esophagotomy incisions or after esophageal perforation. They are diagnosed with contrast radiographs. Clinical signs include cervical swelling, fever, and dysphagia. The lesions may be difficult to demonstrate with esophagoscopy, and passage of a nasogastric tube is usually possible. Most fistulas heal once ventral drainage is established. If healing does not occur, resection of the sinus tract and closure of the stoma may be necessary.

ESOPHAGEAL ULCERATION

Ulcerations in the esophagus are typically lesions associated with viral-diarrhea complex. Esophagraphy may assist with early detection and diagnosis before results obtained from serology. Barium paste (70% w/vol) is generally used and is placed on the tongue of the calf. Ulcerations will appear as a filling defect along the longitudinal lines of the mucosa.

Mucosal damage can also follow resolution of an esophageal obstruction. These are treated with time and a diet avoiding longstem rough hay. As mentioned earlier, extrapolation from equine studies indicates possible increase in the diameter of a traumatized esophagus for as long as 60 days.

MEGAESOPHAGUS

Sporadic reports of segmental and generalized megaesophagus in cattle have been documented. Affected animals are dysphagic, salivate, and cough. Aspiration pneumonia is common. The esophagus is dilated on imaging studies, and the longitudinal folds of mucosa are not evident. This disorder is usually described in weanling calves that have an atonic esophagus that accumulates solid food that may occlude the esophagus and cause bloat However, one case has been described in an adult heifer. Regardless of age, survey radiographs reveal air or an air-fluid interface within an atonic esophagus (see Figure 10.2-1). Esophagraphy shows a large accumulation of contrast material in the esophagus. In the adult case report, a large amount of eosinophils were present in the esophageal wall, and a hypothesis of roundworm larval migration that impaired esophageal function was suspected.

Treatment is supportive. Animals should be frequently fed small amounts of easily digestible feeds. White muscle disease should be ruled out. Long-stemmed hay should be avoided. Antibiotics are indicated for pneumonia. The prognosis is unfavorable.

RECOMMENDED READINGS

Aanes WA: The diagnosis and surgical repair of diverticulum of the esophagus, *Proc Am Assoc Equine Pract* 21: 211, 1975.

Alexander JE: Esophageal stricture in a heifer, *J Am Vet Med Assoc* 145: 699-700, 1964.

Bargai U, Nathan AT, et al: Acquired megaesophagus in a heifer, *Vet Radiol* 32: 259-260, 1991.

Bargai U, Pharr JW, et al: The esophagus. In Morgan JP, editor: *Bovine radiology*, Ames, Iowa, 1989, Iowa State University Press.

Butler JA, Colles CM, Dyson SJ, et al: The alimentary and urinary system. In Butler JA, Colles CM, Dyson SJ, Kold SE, Poulos PW, editors: *Clinical radiology of the horse*, ed 2, Oxford, Blackwell Science Limited, Oxford, 1993, pp. 529-562.

Craig DR, Todhunter RJ: Surgical repair of an esophageal stricture in a horse, *Vet Surg* 16: 251, 1987.

Dallman MJ: Functional suture-holding layers of the esophagus in the dog, *J Am Vet Med Assoc* 192: 638, 1988.

Derksen FJ, Stick JA: Resection and anastomosis of esophageal stricture in a foal, *Equine Pract* 5: 17, 1983.

Fox FH: The esophagus, stomach, intestines, and peritoneum. In Amstutz HE, editor: *Bovine medicine and surgery*, ed 2, Santa Barbara, 1980, American Veterinary Publications.

Fubini SL, Starrak GS, Freeman DE: Esophagus. In Auer JA, Stick JA, editors: *Equine surgery*, ed 2, Philadelphia, 1999, WB Saunders.

Greet TRC: Observations on the potential role of oesophageal radiography in the horse, *Equine Vet J* 14: 73, 1982.

Hackett RP, Dyer RM, Hoffer RE: Surgical correction of esophageal diverticulum in a horse, *J Am Vet Med Assoc* 173: 998, 1978.

Kasari TR: Dilatation of the lower cervical esophagus in a cow, *Can Vet J* 25: 177-179, 1984.

McGavin MD, Anderson NV: Projectile expectoration associated with an esophageal diverticulum in a cow, *J Am Vet Assoc* 166: 247-248, 1975.

Meagher DM, Mayhew IG: The surgical treatment of upper esophageal obstruction in the bovine, *Can Vet J* 19: 128-132, 1978.

Morgan JP: Esophageal obstruction and dilation in a cow, *J Am Vet Med Assoc* 147: 411-412, 1965.

Roberts SJ, Kennedy PC, Delahanty DD: A persistent right aortic arch in a Guernsey Bull, *Cornell Vet* 43: 57, 1953.

Ruben JMS: Surgical removal of a foreign body from the bovine esophagus, *Vet Rec* 100: 220, 1977.

Singh AP, Nigam JM: Radiography of bovine esophageal disorders, *Mod Vet Pract* 61: 867-869, 1980.

Stick JA, Derksen FJ, Scott GA: Equine cervical esophagotomy: complications associated with duration and location of feeding tubes, *Am J Vet Res* 42: 727, 1981.

Stick JA: Surgery of the equine esophagus, *Vet Clin North Am Large Anim Pract* 4: 33, 1982.

Stone SJ: Oesophagotomy in the bovine, *Irish Vet News* 9: 20-21, 1987.

Thrall DE, Brown MD: Esophageal stenosis and diverticulum in a calf, *J Am Vet Med Assoc* 159: 1040-1042, 1971.

Todhunter RJ, Stick JA, Slocombe RF: Comparison of three feeding techniques after esophageal mucosal resection and anastomosis in the horse, *Cornell Vet* 76: 16, 1986.

Todhunter RJ, Stick JA, Trotter GW, et al: Medical management of esophageal stricture in seven horses, *J Am Vet Med Assoc* 185: 784, 1984.

Verschooten F, Oyaert W, et al: Radiographic diagnosis of lung disease in cattle, *J Am Vet Radiol Soc* 15: 49-59, 1974.

Verschooten F, Oyaert W: Radiological diagnosis of esophageal disorders in the bovine, *J Am Vet Radiol Soc* 18: 85-89, 1977.

Vestweber JG, Leipold HW, Knighton RG: Idiopathic megaesophagus in a calf: clinical and pathological features, *J Am Vet Med Assoc* 187: 1369-1370, 1985.

Watson E, Selcer B: Use of radiographic contrast media in horses, *Comp Cont Educ Pract Vet* 18: 167, 1996.

10.3—Surgery of The Ruminant Forestomach Compartments

Norm G. Ducharme and Susan L. Fubini

Anatomy and Physiology

The three nonglandular forestomach compartments in the cow are the rumen, reticulum, and omasum. The abomasum is the true "stomach" and has a glandular mucous membrane. The rumen occupies most of the abdomen's left side; its long axis extends from ribs seven to eight to the pelvis. The reticulum lies against the diaphragm left of midline opposite the sixth to eighth ribs, and the omasum is right of midline at the ventral aspect of ribs 7 to 11. The abomasum lies mostly right of midline and extends from the xiphoid area to the ninth or tenth intercostal space in the nonpregnant cow. The cardia opens dorsal to the fundus of the reticulum. The reticular groove is located on the right wall of the reticulum and joins the reticuloomasal orifice. The omasal groove is on the left wall of the omasum and joins the omasoabomasal orifice.

In the newborn calf, the abomasum is twice as large as the rumen. The rumen becomes about nine times as large as the abomasum over the first year of life as a result of the mechanical stimulus of roughage in the diet and the chemical charges associated with fermentation.

The vagus nerve, which is made up of 90% sensory fibers, is the primary innervation of the forestomach compartments and abomasum. The dorsal vagal trunk innervates the rumen, caudal aspect of the reticulum, omasum, and visceral surface of the abomasum. The ventral vagal trunk supplies the reticulum, parietal side of the reticuloomasal junction, omasum, and abomasum.

The forestomach compartments, especially the rumen, are sites of microbial fermentation. The rumen or reticulum movement allows mixing of ingesta as well as regurgitation, eructation, and passage of ingesta into the omasum. The omasum acts as a pump that aspirates ingesta and transfers it to the abomasum. The abomasum behaves similarly to the stomach of a nonruminant. Digestive enzymes in the abomasum are responsible for the next phase of digestion.

Etiology and Pathogenesis

Disorders of the rumen and forestomach compartments in adult cattle can result from a variety of causes,
including those that are dietary, inflammatory, and/or mechanical. A diet inadequate in roughage, coarse feed, and grain overload are examples of dietary causes of forestomach disease. Cattle's indiscriminate eating habits make them susceptible to inadvertent ingestion of foreign bodies with subsequent penetration of a forestomach compartment. Foreign body ingestion results in localized reticuloperitonitis, which is called *traumatic reticuloperitonitis* (TRP). Wires account for approximately 70% of ingested foreign bodies. Nails and steel objects make up the other 30%. Regardless, most foreign bodies are ferromagnetic, which argues for therapeutic or prophylactic administration of magnets. The use of magnets placed in feeders or administered prophylactically to cattle explains why the prevalence of TRP has noticeably decreased in the last two decades.

Acute TRP results in stasis of the forestomach compartments. If the foreign body continues to migrate, many disease entities can result, including perforation of a gastrointestinal viscus, pericarditis, and myocarditis. A more chronic possible sequela to TRP is the formation of adhesions that physically interfere with the vagal nerve, thus resulting in permanent forestomach dysfunction. Another sequela to TRP is cranial abdominal or thoracic abscess formation. In addition to clinical signs associated with chronic infection, the cranial abdominal abscess results in mechanical obstruction of the reticuloomasal passage and forestomach dysfunction until it is treated. Depending on its size and location, a thoracic abscess may impair ventilation or result in cardiac signs if compression of the pericardium occurs. Other causes of forestomach dysfunction are seen when trichobezoars or ingested foreign bodies, such as plastic bags or placenta, cause a mechanical obstruction by lodging in the reticuloomasal orifice. In addition, neoplasia, predominately lymphosarcoma, can affect vagal innervation by infiltration or, more commonly, involvement of the pyloric area, thus mechanically obstructing the abomasum. Finally, it must be remembered that the vagus nerve can be damaged or inflamed in areas other than the abdomen (including the pharynx, larynx, esophagus, and thoracic cavity), so a disease process near the vagal nerve in any of these locations can result in ruminal dysfunction and is termed *vagal indigestion*. Therefore many forestomach disorders that are termed *vagal indigestion* are not caused by actual damage to the vagal nerves but may be mechanical, inflammatory, or functional disorders that result in an outflow obstruction. Regardless, clinical presentation of vagal indigestion encompasses most common forestomach disorders.

Vagal Indigestion

Historically, vagal indigestion has been classified two ways by different authors. Hoflund's classification is as follows:

Type 1—functional stenosis between reticulum and omasum with atony of the rumen and reticulum

Type 2—functional stenosis between reticulum and omasum with normal or hypermotile rumen and reticulum

Type 3—permanent functional stenosis of the pylorus with atony or retained activity of the reticulum

Type 4—incomplete pyloric stenosis.

Ferrante and Whitlock's classification is as follows:

Type 1—failure of eructation or free-gas bloat

Type 2—omasal transport failure

Type 3—abomasal impaction

Type 4—Partial obstruction of the stomach.

Hoflund's classification was introduced after experimentally sectioning various segments of the vagal nerve. In our experience with Ferrante and Whitlock classifications, the clinical differentiation between types 3 and 4 is unclear. We have modified the Ferrante and Whitlock classification based on our clinical experience to align it better with treatment strategies.

CORNELL CLASSIFICATION OF VAGAL INDIGESTION IN CATTLE

Type I involves failure of eructation, which results in gaseous distension of the rumen. This may result from mechanical obstruction of the esophagus and cardia. Type I indigestion may also result from physiological disturbance of the eructation mechanism associated with diet or immaturity. Treatment entails placing a rumen fistula (see Section 10.3) to remove the obstruction and/or ruminal gas until normal physiological function returns.

Type II involves failure of omasal transport that results in distension of the reticulum and rumen with gas and well-mixed feed and fluid. The causes are multiple and range from mechanical intraluminal obstruction of the reticuloomasal orifice, mechanical extraluminal obstruction of the reticuloomasal groove by a mass (abscess) and adhesions, and neurogenic denervation of the ruminoreticulum innervation (i.e., vagal nerve). Efforts should be directed toward identifying and removing the cause. A left paralumbar fossa exploratory and rumenotomy are typically required.

Type III involves failure of normal abomasal outflow, which results in dilation of the forestomach compartments with fluid and ingesta; the abomasum is filled with fluid or firm ingesta. This may be caused by neurologic or neuromuscular deficits of the abomasum caused by damage to its innervation (vagal nerve, long pyloric nerve); mechanical obstruction of the pylorus or proximal duodenum; coarse feed or adhesions (secondary to TRP) that result in abomasal impaction; or severe abomasal volvulus that caused neuromuscular damage to the

wall of the abomasum. Treatment entails right paralumbar fossa or paracostal celiotomy to correct the primary problem if possible.

CLINICAL FINDINGS

General clinical signs include decline in milk production and appetite. Rumen motility is decreased or absent, and ruminal distention may occur. Feces become scant. With chronic cases, feed intake and fecal output decrease. Milk production is low, and a rough hair-coat develops. Chronic left flank distension and weight loss may become apparent. Other clinical signs are related to the initial causes of forestomach dysfunction. Cattle affected with acute traumatic reticuloperitonitis often have fever with mild elevations in heart and respiratory rates. The decline in milk production and appetite is sudden. A sharp cranial abdominal pain may be noted when xiphoid pressure is applied or the withers are pinched. By 3 to 4 days, the abdominal pain and pyrexia may subside to some extent as the inflammatory reaction lessens and the cow localizes the process.

From a surgical perspective, forestomach disorders manifest in three main ways. In the three types of vagal indigestion (Cornell classification as described above), clinical signs of outflow obstruction from the rumen and/or forestomach compartments occur. These can be detected clinically by external examination of the contour of the abdomen, rectal examination, and identification and characterization of the source of the distended abdomen: which organ is distended and is the source of distension fluid or gas. Type I animals develop distension high and low in the left paralumbar fossa, and if untreated eventually develop respiratory dyspnea caused by compression of the diaphragm. Simultaneous auscultation with percussion and rectal examination identify the rumen as being gas-distended. Cattle with type II and III vagal indigestion develop abdominal distention high and low in the left paralumbar fossa and low in the right as the rumen distends (Figure 10.3-1). Rectal examination identifies the rumen as being distended by liquid ingesta and gas. In addition, enlargement of the ventral sac of the rumen extending to the right side of the abdomen is identified. Distension of the abomasum differentiates type II from III and can be assessed by ultrasonography. Cattle may have bradycardia (HR <60 beats/min.) with both these types of disorders, presumably because of increased vagal tone and anorexia.

Once the diagnosis of a forestomach disorder is made, signs of the primary cause of the disease should be sought. For type I disorders, signs of esophageal obstruction, such as head extension and salivation, may be present. In type II, carbohydrate overload could lead to fluid distension of the rumen and reticulum, low ruminal pH, and metabolic acidosis. Lesions of the reticulum

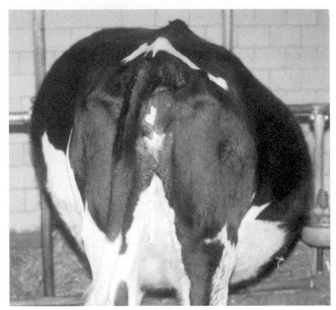

Figure 10.3-1 Cow with distension high and low in the left paralumbar fossa and low in the right as the rumen distends as seen in Type II and III vagal indigestion forestomach disorder.

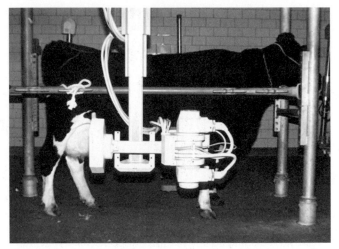

Figure 10.3-2 A dairy cow in place for a standing radiographic study of the cranial abdomen.

that involve the vagus nerve are typically located on the right or medial wall of the reticulum and include traumatic reticuloperitonitis (presence of radiodense foreign body in the cranial abdomen), adhesions in the cranial abdomen (ultrasonographic or surgical findings), reticular and liver abscesses (ultrasound or radiographic examination, elevated serum total protein), and neoplasia—such as lymphosarcoma—located around the reticuloomasal junction.

Type III vagal indigestion can be associated with a primary abomasal impaction, a foreign body obstruction, pyloric lymphosarcoma, or a functional duodenal obstruction. It can be related to previous surgery for abomasal volvulus that caused a stretch or ischemia of the vagal nerves. In many instances, a specific diagnosis can only be made after a left paralumbar fossa exploratory celiotomy and rumenotomy is performed.

CLINICAL PATHOLOGY

In cattle with acute traumatic reticuloperitonitis, a neutrophilia (neutrophils >4000/ul) with a left shift is typically seen. Plasma fibrinogen levels are often elevated (>1000 mg/dL, normal 300-600 mg/dL). With chronic disease, elevations in total protein (TP) and serum globulins are expected. One author reported that TP elevation was so important that an elevation above 10 g/dl in cattle with abdominal disease was highly suggestive of TRP. Acid base and electrolyte abnormalities will vary depending on the location of the obstruction, (Type 1-III), duration of disease, and nature of treatment

given. Therefore cows with acute, untreated type I vagal indigestion generally have no electrolyte disturbance. Severe cases or those suffering from ventilation failure associated with severe abdominal distension require immediate attention. Cattle with type II initially have no electrolyte disturbance initially. Over a few days, hypokalemia occurs because of decreased feed intake and extracellular fluid shifts. Apparently, ruminal function can no longer maintain the normal plasma/rumen chloride gradient; therefore rumen chloride ions increase. This leads to a hypochloremic, hypokalemic metabolic alkalosis. This metabolic disturbance will be exaggerated if the cow is given saline laxatives. Type III indigestion has chloride ions sequestered (to various degrees) in the abomasum so hypochloremic, hypokalemic metabolic alkalosis is typical.

Abdominal fluid analysis may help determine if there is an inflammatory process in the abdomen. The technique is described in the physical examination chapter (Chapter 1). Elevations in white blood cells (>6,000 cells/ul) and total protein (>3.0 g/dL) indicate an inflammatory response. It is important to remember that cattle are efficient in localizing an infectious abdominal process, so the amount of abdominal fluid can vary in different regions of the abdomen. Therefore, ultrasound examination is useful to increase the value of abdominocentesis in cattle.

Radiography can help identify perforating foreign bodies in the reticular area. With the animal standing, a horizontal beam is centered on the reticulodiaphragmatic region in the cranioventral abdomen/caudoventral thorax (Figure 10.3-2). Radiographs obtained allow the identification of radiopaque foreign bodies and gas/fluid interfaces typical of an intraabdominal abscess (Figure 10.3-3, A and B). However, false negatives and false pos-

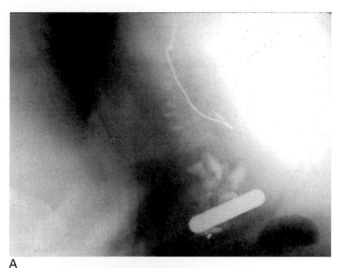

A

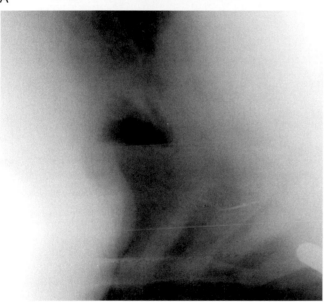

B

Figure 10.3-3 *A,* Radiographs of the cranial abdomen of a cow with traumatic reticuloperitonitis allows identification of radiopaque foreign bodies and gas fluid interfaces typical of an intraabdominal abscess. *B,* Radiographs of the cranial abdomen of a cow with traumatic reticuloperitonitis and thoracic abscess. Note that the foreign body is in the thoracic cavity and there is gas fluid interface typical of a thoracic abscess.

(Courtesy of Dr. Stephanie Nykamp.)

itives are possible. Diagnosis of a foreign body penetration can only be made with certainty if the foreign body can be seen beyond the confines of the reticulum. In one study, if a foreign body was detected as superimposed within the reticular wall and not on the floor of the reticulum, the probability of perforation was almost 100%. Another report of radiographs of the reticulum in a large number of cattle showed that the most reliable features

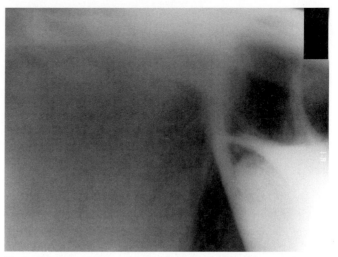

Figure 10.3-4 Radiographs of the cranial abdomen of a cow with suspected traumatic reticuloperitonitis. Even though no foreign body is seen, the image quality obtained when a cow is in dorsal recumbency prohibits any certainty that no penetrating foreign body nor abscess is in the area.

of a perforating foreign body were those that were positioned atypically and had abnormal gas shadows and depressions in the cranioventral margin of the reticulum. Obtaining standing lateral, horizontal-beam radiographs on an adult cow requires specialized equipment (machines capable of 125 kVp and 40 mAs (see Section 2.1). Another less convenient option is to place the cow in dorsal recumbency with the beam centered over the same area. Penetrating foreign bodies do not move with the ingesta; thus they become surrounded by gas in the reticulum. A foreign body seen in the ventral aspect of the reticulum while the animal is in dorsal recumbency (Figure 10.3-4) confirms the penetrating foreign body diagnosis. A portable unit can yield diagnostic radiographic films of the reticulum with the animal in dorsal recumbency, but not with the animal standing. (Equipment would need capabilities of 75 kVp and 30 mAs; more details in Section 2.1.)

Ultrasound examination of the normal reticulum has been described (Braun, 1994). In another report the same author described diagnosis of a cranial abdominal abscess in five cattle examined with a 3.5 MHz linear transducer. An example of this is given in Figure 10.3-5. Abscesses such as these can be drained either with percutaneous drain placement or via rumenotomy into the rumen as described later. The abscesses can be followed after surgery, with ultrasound, to determine the success of the drainage procedure.

MEDICAL TREATMENTS

Type I medical treatment is directed at gas decompression of the rumen. Orogastric intubation is performed

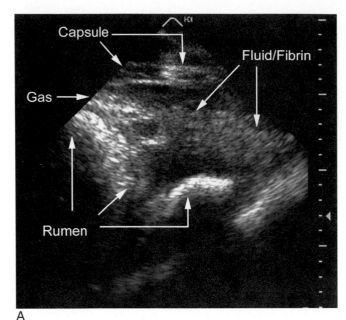

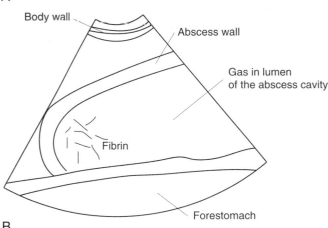

Figure 10.3-5   *A,* Transverse sonogram made on the ventral midline of the cranial abdomen obtained from an adult Holstein cow with a 4-2 MHz convex linear probe. Between a forestomach compartment and the body wall, a peritoneal abscess cavity contains fibrin, fluid, and gas. Surrounding this cavity is a well-circumscribed capsule. *B,* Schematic line diagram of sonogram in *A.*

first to ensure a patent digestive tract oral to the reticulum-rumen. If an obstruction is found in the esophagus, attempts should be made to push the obstruction into the rumen by using a stomach tube and water. Care must be taken to prevent inadvertent aspiration of lavage fluid and secretion into the trachea (i.e., the head is kept low, and a conservative amount of fluid is used only if necessary). Dietary changes are instituted if no obstruction or other abnormality is found during examination.

In Types II and III, a search is made for the cause. In traumatic reticuloperitonitis cases, medical treatment is directed at preventing perforation of the reticulum and treating the septic reticulitis and peritonitis. Oral admin-

istration of a good-quality magnet fixes ferromagnetic foreign bodies. A magnet administered orally falls into the cranial sac of the rumen, but normal ruminal contractions usually bring the magnet to the reticulum. Foreign bodies still partially in the lumen of the reticulum that have injured the reticular wall are attracted to and fixed to the magnet, thus preventing their migration from continuing and most times returning the foreign body into the lumen of the reticulum. Ancillary therapy includes stall confinement, fluid therapy, and broad-spectrum antibiotics. In approximately half the cases, the perforating foreign body does not remain in the wall of the reticulum but returns to the lumen, which makes medical treatment of traumatic reticuloperitonitis successful.

Use of a magnetic metal retriever to remove ferromagnetic foreign bodies has been advocated by some. This instrument consists of a large magnet attached to a wire cable that passes through a plastic tube. It is passed orally through the esophagus into the reticulum where the magnet attracts ferromagnetic foreign bodies. Concern about esophageal and pharyngeal trauma has limited this instrument's popularity.

In cases of abomasal impaction (Type III), mineral oil and other laxatives can be administered in an attempt to relieve the impaction. Water restriction can occur in a cold climate from freezing, so one should ensure a good water supply. Other causes of Types II and III forestomach disorders usually require surgical intervention.

Surgical Treatment

Three surgical approaches are used to treat cattle with vagal indigestion. For type I vagal indigestion (failure of eructation and free gas bloat), placing a rumen trocar or cannula is indicated. The reader is referred to the chapter on ruminal distension in calves (see Section 14.1). Left flank celiotomy and rumenotomy is used as a diagnostic procedure for type II and III vagal indigestion in cases of traumatic reticuloperitonitis in which an animal fails to respond to conservative therapy or if a perireticular abscess is suspected. A right flank, right paramedian (in lateral recumbency) or right paracostal celiotomy is used in type III vagal indigestion as a diagnostic procedure, to treat abomasal impaction, or to manage pyloric obstruction and dysfunction. These procedures are described in Sections 10.4.3 and 10.4.4.

LEFT FLANK CELIOTOMY
The left flank is prepared for aseptic surgery. Anesthesia is achieved by infiltration with a local anesthetic in a line block, inverted L block, or paravertebral block.

A 20- to 25-cm dorsoventral skin incision is made 4 cm caudal and parallel to the last rib and 6 to 8 cm ventral to the transverse process of the lumbar vertebrae.

It is important to locate the incision as close to the ribs as possible to allow a more complete examination of the cranial abdomen. The few centimeters gained over a mid-paralumbar incision may be critical when the surgeon's arm is placed through the incision and rumenotomy to palpate the reticulum and reticuloomasal canal, especially in a large cow. However, one must be careful not to place the incision any closer to the ribs than described previously, because rumenotomy is a clean-contaminated procedure and postoperative incisional infection with osteomyelitis are possible. The subcutaneous tissues, external and internal oblique muscles, transversus muscle, and peritoneum are incised in the same plane. When possible, a sterile, impervious sleeve should be used for palpating the abdominal cavity. The caudal abdominal cavity is explored first including the urinary bladder, uterus, left kidney, dorsal and ventral sacs of the rumen, and intestinal mass. To reach the cranial abdomen the arm is passed ventral to the superficial layer of the greater omentum and directed cranially to locate the pylorus and pyloric part, body, and fundus of the abomasum, the omasum, and the reticulum. All parts of the reticulum must be palpated to verify whether adhesions and/or abscesses are present. The right side of the reticulum and left lobe of the liver (Figures 10.3-6 and 10.3-7), where abscesses are most often found, must be especially evaluated. The diaphragm, apex, and parietal surface of the spleen are also palpated.

Any adhesions found in the cranial abdomen must be assessed with gentle palpation to avoid disruption and minimize the risk of spreading inflammation. Adhesions in the cranial abdomen are more typical of traumatic reticulitis as the cause of peritonitis. Adhesions along the ventral body wall are more likely to be caused by perforating abomasal ulcers. If extensive cranial abdominal adhesions or ruminal distention prevent adequate palpation, a rumenotomy should be performed. Two procedures have been used to secure the rumen to the skin: the rumen board, or Weingarth apparatus, and suturing the rumen to the skin. The rumenotomy site is in the dorsal sac of the rumen using both techniques.

RUMENOTOMY WITH THE RUMEN BOARD OR WEINGARTH APPARATUS

Because use of the rumen board and Weingarth apparatus is similar, only use of the rumen board will be described.

The wall of the dorsal sac of the rumen is grasped with two large noncrushing rumen forceps. These forceps are hooked on the dorsal and ventral aspect of the rumen board. This allows exteriorization of a portion of the rumen wall (Figure 10.3-8). The rumen wall is incised dorsally. The rumen hooks are implanted in the cut edges of the rumen and attached securely to screws and nuts placed at regular intervals along the rumen board. The

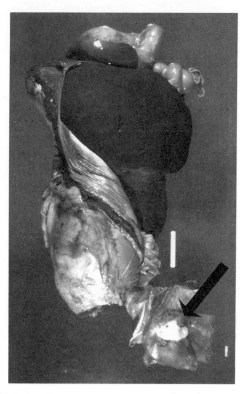

Figure 10.3-6   *Post mortem* specimen that shows an abscess adjacent to the left lobe of the liver with a draining tract at the skin (arrow).

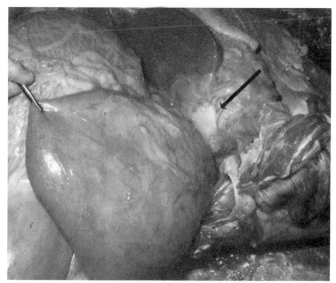

Figure 10.3-7   *Post mortem* specimen viewed from the right side. The reticulum is reflected caudally. Note the abscess (arrow) adjacent to the ventral part of the left lobe of the liver.

incision is continued ventrally, and the hooks are placed at regular intervals to secure the rumen wall to the rumen board down to the level of the ventral forceps (Figure 10.3-9). This procedure can be done quickly without assistance. Care must be taken during

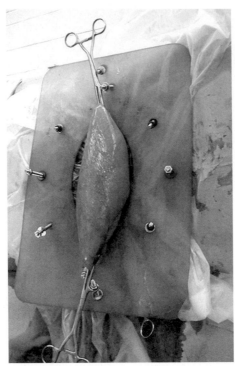

Figure 10.3-8   Rumen forceps are hooked on the dorsal and ventral aspect of the rumen board. This allows exteriorization of a portion of the rumen wall.

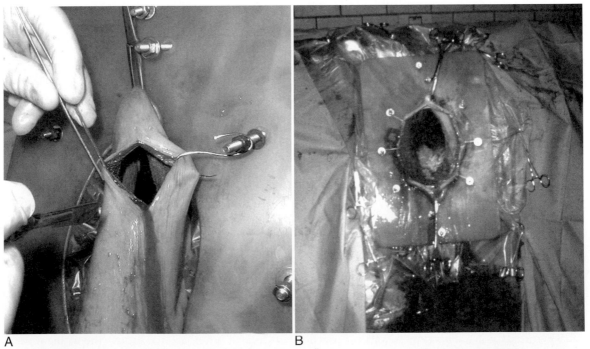

A   B

Figure 10.3-9   *A,* After incising the rumen wall, *B,* rumen hooks are implanted in the cut edges of the rumen and attached securely to screws and nuts placed at regular intervals along the rumen board.

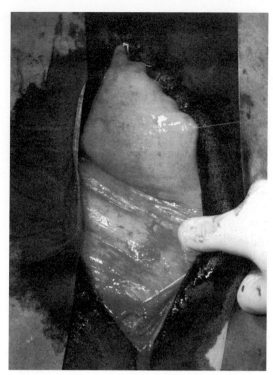

Figure 10.3-10   The rumen is sutured to the skin with a Cushing-type pattern to form a seal between the rumen and the skin.

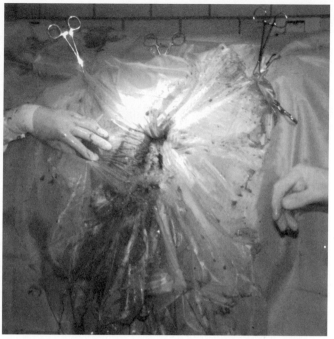

Figure 10.3-11   A rumenotomy has been performed and a plastic wound protector applied. Solid contents of the rumen are removed manually.

intraruminal palpation not to contaminate the inner surface of the board, which is in direct contact with the abdominal cavity. Placing a wound ring* before exploring the lumen of the rumen helps decrease contamination.

RUMENOTOMY AFTER SUTURING THE RUMEN WALL TO THE SKIN

The goal of rumenotomy is to obtain a good seal between the skin and rumen, so that even if ruminal contents escape the incision, no abdominal contamination will occur. As one makes the seal, it is important to exteriorize a generous part of the rumen so the rumenotomy incision can be closed without disrupting the rumen-to-skin seal. Otherwise, the seal will have to be undone to close the rumen, which increases the possibility of abdominal contamination. The dorsal sac of the rumen is grasped by an assistant and exteriorized with forceps or moist sponges. Starting at the dorsal aspect, the rumen is sutured (usually with a nonabsorbable #1 suture) to the skin with a simple continuous pattern and to the rumen with a Cushing-type pattern (Figure 10.3-10). A cutting needle should be used so that the skin is penetrated. Care should be taken not to penetrate the ruminal mucosa, although the authors have not recognized complications when penetration has occurred.

*Steri-Drape TM, wound edge protector; 3M Health Care, St Paul, MN, 55144-1000

Once the rumen has been sutured to the skin, the site is checked to verify a good "seal" between rumen and skin. An incision is made in the rumen, starting 3 cm ventral to the dorsal commissure and extending ventrally to 3 cm dorsal to the ventral commissure, with care taken not to inadvertently incise the sutures that form the rumen and skin seal. A rumen shroud or wound ring* is placed in the incision to protect the incised ruminal wall and to prevent ingesta from accumulating at the junction of the rumen and skin (Figure 10.3-11).

TRANSRUMINAL EXPLORATION

After the rumen has been stabilized and incised, enough contents should be emptied to permit a thorough exploration (see Figure 10.3-11). If the contents of the rumen are mostly fluid it is possible to drain them by creating a siphon with a large bore stomach (Kingman) tube (Figure 10.3-12). The position, size, and consistency of the reticulum, omasum, and abomasum can be defined by transruminal palpation. The ruminoreticular fold, esophageal orifice, and omasal orifice should be palpated for lesions.

The reticulum is meticulously explored for foreign bodies. If all parts of the reticulum cannot be palpated, more ruminal ingesta can be removed to reduce the cranial displacement of the reticulum caused by ruminal distention. A guarded prognosis should be given when a perforating foreign body is found if the thoracic cavity has

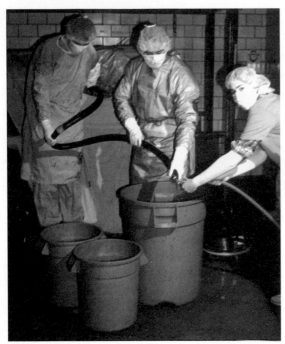

Figure 10.3-12   A rumenotomy has been performed. A Kingman tube is used to drain fluid from the rumen.

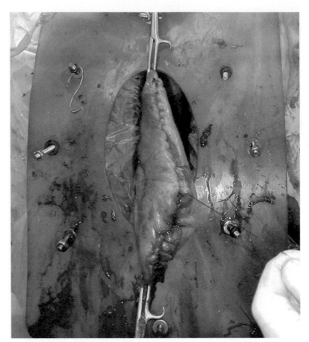

Figure 10.3-13   The rumen is closed with a two-layered (at least one converting) inverting pattern.

been penetrated. Exploration of the reticulum should be continued in case there is more than one foreign body present; all foreign bodies should be removed regardless of whether they are penetrating. Normally the reticulum can be inverted into the rumen by manually grasping its cranioventral aspect. If a penetrating foreign body is not found, the surgeon should try to invert the reticulum. This helps determine the presence, location, and extent of adhesions. The surgeon's finger must probe all the honeycomb cells of the reticulum at the site of adhesions in search of foreign bodies. The surgeon can also sweep the reticular wall with a magnet in an attempt to find ferromagnetic foreign bodies. Another possible enhancement of diagnostic capabilities is to carry an ultrasound probe (5 MHz sector scanner) into the lumen of the rumen in a rectal sleeve. In all but the largest cows, the left hand can usually reach through the reticuloomasal orifice into the omasal canal to evaluate the consistency of omasal contents. In some cases, the abomasal lumen can be entered by directing one's hand ventrally from the omasal orifice. The leaves of the abomasum normally feel very smooth and slippery upon palpation. Adhesions that limit reticulum mobility would be typical of traumatic reticulo-peritonitis. The ventral sac of the rumen adhered to the body wall is more typical of localized peritonitis after a perforated ruminal or abomasal ulcer.

Occasionally, an abscess will be found tightly adhered to the reticular wall. These feel like a ball. A spherical mass with uniform consistency can be imaged with ultrasound. Lack of experience may cause confusion in differentiating an abscess from the omasum. An abscess can

be distinguished from the omasum by identifying the reticuloomasal groove, and using several fingers to delineate the omasum. The presence of purulent material in the abscess can be confirmed by inserting a 14-gauge needle, connected by an extension set to a syringe, through the reticular wall into the mass adhered to the reticular wall to aspirate the abscess. Once the abscess has been positively identified, it can be lanced into the reticulum, where the abscess is tightly adhered to the reticular wall. A scalpel blade is secured by umbilical tape to the surgeon's hand before it is introduced through the rumen into the reticulum (Figure 10.3-14). After the abscess is lanced, the abscess cavity is searched for a foreign body.

If the abscess is not tightly adhered to the reticulum wall, the rumenotomy site and abdomen are closed and a ventral (midline or paramedian) exploratory celiotomy performed to either resect or drain the abscess. A 28 French trocar catheter* is inserted into the abscess for drainage lateral to the ventral incision. The catheter must be carefully inserted so that it does not penetrate the mammary vein, which is often collapsed when a cow is in dorsal recumbency. The catheter must be passed through the adhesions or omentum to prevent abdominal contamination if leakage occurs around the catheter. This latter procedure could also be done percutaneously

*Pleur-Evac thoracic catheter; Genzyme Biosurgery, Genzyme Corporation, Fall River, MA 02720

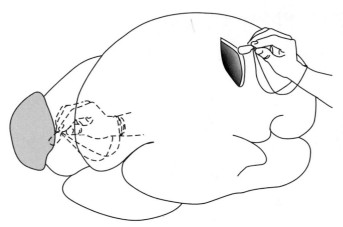

Figure 10.3-14   A schematic diagram that shows a scalpel blade secured to a surgeon's hand as the surgeon prepares to drain a cranial abdominal abscess adhered to the reticulum.

using ultrasonographic guidance with the cow standing. After the drain's intended entry point is identified, local anesthetic is placed at that site. A short (1-cm) incision through the skin and external sheath of the rectus abdominis is made with a blade. The drain is placed into the opening and guided into the abscess. Holding the drain by its shaft near the skin not at the end is important so that it does not enter the abdomen any deeper than desired once it has passed the resistance of the internal sheath or abscess wall. The only difference between the surgical and ultrasound-guided approach is that ultrasound cannot ensure the catheter is passing through adhesions, so any purulent contamination around the drain may result in localized peritonitis. However, economical and medical reasons may justify a nonsurgical approach for placing a drain. The trocar is then removed from the catheter, and the catheter is clamped. The catheter is secured to the skin (Figure 10.3-15). The ventral incision is closed (if performed), and the animal is allowed to stand; after which the catheter is unclamped and the abscess drained. The catheter is flushed daily until drainage is minimal (approximately 10 to 14 days), at which time the catheter is removed.

CLOSURE

After gross contamination has been removed, the rumen wall is closed with No. 2 absorbable sutures with a two-layer closure; at least one layer of which should be an inverting pattern (see Figure 10.3-13). The surgery site is thoroughly lavaged, and all soiled instruments are discarded. If the rumen was sutured to the skin, the suture is cut, and one quadrant at a time is freed. A moist sponge is used to wipe off ingesta trapped between the rumen and skin. The surgeon dons fresh sterile gloves.

The abdominal musculature is usually closed in two or three layers by using a simple continuous pattern of

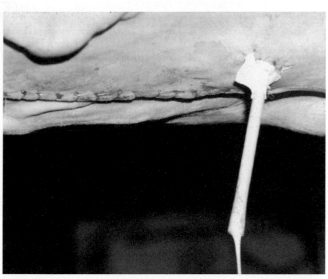

Figure 10.3-15   Drainage of a liver abscess through a 28 French Foley catheter placed adjacent to a right paramedian celiotomy.

absorbable sutures in the muscle layers. The skin layer is closed with a continuous Ford interlocking pattern. It is wise to close the ventral aspect of the skin incision with two to three simple interrupted sutures. The possibility of incisional infection is obvious, and drainage can be easily obtained by removing these ventral two-to-three sutures if necessary.

POSTOPERATIVE MANAGEMENT

Antibiotics are administered systemically to treat the septic reticuloperitonitis. Oral or intravenous fluids may be needed to correct dehydration and metabolic alkalosis, if present. Rumen transfaunate can be given to reestablish normal flora and stimulate ruminal motility.

Postoperative complications include swelling and discharge at the incision site. Because of the nature of the surgery, contamination of the incision site occurs easily. If recognized, these infections respond well to ventral drainage.

PROGNOSIS

The prognosis depends on the location of the reticular perforation. If the foreign body has penetrated the diaphragm, a poor prognosis should be given; septic pericarditis, myocarditis, and thoracic abscesses are possible sequelae. If perforation involves the right wall of the reticulum, a guarded prognosis is given; adhesions that involve the ventral branch of the vagus nerve may result in vagal syndrome type II or III. A favorable prognosis is given when the perforation does not affect the thoracic cavity and right side of the reticulum. Single abdominal abscesses (reticulum, liver) also carry a favorable prognosis if they can be drained or resected (see Figure 10.3-15). Unfortunately, liver abscesses have a

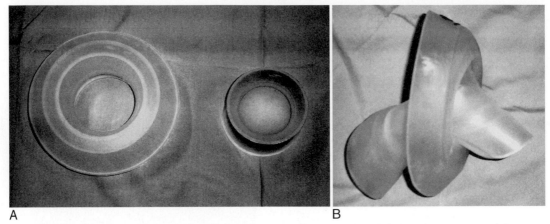

Figure 10.3-16   *A,* Commercial rumen fistula (right) and plug (left). *B,* The top part of the inner flange of the fistula is passed through the lumen of the cannula, toward the outside flange, to form a cone to facilitate insertion through the surgically created stoma.

fairly high (30%) recurrence rate. Extensive adhesions in the cranial abdomen are not necessarily associated with a poor prognosis in the authors' experience. If the adhesions do not involve the vagus nerve, ruminal motility does not appear to be greatly impaired by the presence of adhesions. This may be because the rumen wall is protected from restricting adhesions by the superficial layer of the greater omentum.

PLACEMENT OF A COMMERCIAL RUMEN FISTULA IN ADULT CATTLE

The left paralumbar fossa is clipped and prepared for aseptic surgery. Perioperative antibiotics are administered. A 15-cm skin incision is made in the midparalumbar fossa, starting 6 cm ventral to the transverse processes. This incision length is appropriate for a 10 cm fistula.* It is critical that the length be precise to ensure a snug fit with the fistula. The incision is extended sharply through the skin and external abdominal oblique muscle. The internal abdominal oblique and transverse abdominis muscles are opened in the direction of their muscle fibers. The peritoneum is tented and incised with scissors.

The peritoneum and abdominal musculature are sutured together for the first layer of closure with a synthetic absorbable suture. This effectively creates a muscular ring about 12 cm in length that will snug down around a 10-cm fistula, thus preventing leakage of ruminal contents. For the second layer, a portion of the dorsal sac of the rumen is exteriorized and anchored to the subcutaneous tissues or dermis by using an absorbable suture material. If secured to the dermis a cutting needle is essential. A good seal should be obtained before proceeding to open the rumen. This will

*Bar Diamond, Inc., Parma, ID, 83660-0060 (www.bardiamond.com)

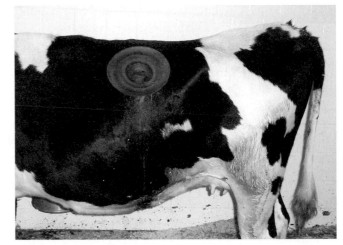

Figure 10.3-17   Cow with surgically placed rumen fistula.

prevent abdominal contamination with rumen contents. For the third layer, the rumen is incised and the mucosa sutured to the skin in an interrupted pattern with a nonabsorbable suture material on a cutting needle. This provides the stoma to insert the commercial fistula.

Placing the fistula can be very difficult because the site has been prepared to ensure a tight fit. The fistula can be warmed in very hot water to improve pliability (Figure 10.3-16A). The inner flange of the fistula is inverted into the outer flange (Figure 10.3-16B) to serve as an entry into the stoma. After being placed through the surgically created opening, the inner flange is rotated into its correct position (Figure 10.3-17).

After surgery the site should be cleaned daily, and the cow should be kept on antibiotics for 5 to 7 days. Some pressure necrosis is inevitable between the cannula and the rumen-to-skin seal, but over time this will improve; the site will enlarge slightly to accommodate the fistula.

Lactic Acidosis

The consumption of a large amount of rapidly fermentable concentrate feed or a sudden diet change to such food can result in severe indigestion. This syndrome has been termed *lactic acid indigestion, grain overload, rumen overload,* and *acute carbohydrate engorgement.*

This is a condition most commonly seen in feedlots but can occur in other instances such as inadequately mixed rations or cattle getting loose in the feed room. Within 6 hours of ingestion, the easily fermentable concentrate is broken down to lactic acid isomers of both the D and L forms. The L isomer is used rapidly, whereas the D isomer persists and results in D-lactic acidosis. *Streptococcus bovis* is the primary organism responsible for this conversion. The pH of the rumen contents decreases to 4.5 to 5.0, at which time microbes other than *Streptococcus bovis* have been destroyed. Rumen stasis occurs. *Streptococcus bovis* continues to exist at this low pH and produces more lactic acid. Rapid accumulation of lactic acid in the rumen osmotically draws water into the rumen, thus accentuating the cow's dehydration. In addition, the acidic fermentation produces excessive amounts of volatile fatty acids (VFA), which are absorbed and contribute to a metabolic acidosis. Eventually, the rumen mucosa is damaged, allowing transudation of protein into the rumen. Affected cattle are inappetent, dehydrated, and tachycardic, with a sudden decline in milk production. The rumen is distended and fluid filled. Eventually, diarrhea develops, and untreated animals become weak and recumbent.

A sample of rumen fluid in the acute stages will show a pH of 4.5 to 5.0 (normal is 6.5 to 7.0). This may be less evident with time as the rumen contents are buffered by the high bicarbonate content of swallowed saliva. A severe metabolic acidosis with neutropenia is typical.

The prognosis and treatment plan will depend on the duration of the insult. In the acute stage, a rumenotomy may be indicated to empty as much foodstuffs as possible. Recommendations for surgery include an animal with a rumen pH of 5.0 or less, a heart rate greater than 100 beats per minute, dehydration greater than 8%, and marked rumen distention, which indicates a severe grain overload. The rumen is emptied and lavaged with water several times to remove as much lactic acid as possible. Additional therapy includes laxatives, fresh hay in the rumen, repeated rumen transfaunates if available, parenteral calcium, nonsteroidal antiinflammatory drugs, and intravenous fluid therapy. Intravenous fluids should be balanced electrolyte solutions such as lactated Ringer's solution, and supplemental sodium bicarbonate is added if acidemia is suspected or confirmed by acid-base/electrolyte values. Prognosis for these cattle is guarded.

Other treatments may be attempted for animals that show less severe signs and higher rumen pH values; or if such a significant number of animals are affected, rumenotomies for all is precluded. These include rumen warm water lavage with a Kingman tube, antacid solutions such as 2 to 4 quarts of milk of magnesia, fluid therapy, and calcium solutions. Other empirical treatments include: antihistamines, penicillin solutions administered via a stomach tube in an effort to reduce the number of *Streptococcus bovis* organisms in the rumen, and roughage-only diets until the animals recover. Vitamin B supplementation is indicated because of thiaminase production by microorganisms and broad spectrum antibiotics may be given to prevent untoward sequelae.

Surgery may not benefit cattle in which signs have been present for more than 24 hours because the amount of rumen mucosal injury has been determined. Cattle affected with lactic acidosis that survive the acute phase and whose rumen pH returns to normal are still at risk for sequelae to the chemical rumenitis that has occurred. Over the next several days, bacterial opportunists such as *Fusobacterium necrophorum* may invade the areas of chemical damage and cause a bacterial rumenitis. This can progress to a bacterial and/or mycotic rumenitis that can enter the portal circulation and cause embolic infection of the liver, lungs, brain, or other viscera.

RECOMMENDED READINGS

Dubensky RA, White ME: The sensitivity, specificity and predictive value of total plasma protein in the diagnosis of traumatic reticuloperitonitis, *Can J Comp Med* 47: 241-244, 1983.

Ducharme NG: Surgical considerations in the treatment of traumatic reticuloperitonitis, *Compend Contin Educ Pract Vet* 5: S213-S224, 1983.

Ducharme NG: Surgery of the bovine forestomach compartments, *Vet Clin North Am (Food Anim Pract)* 6: 371-397, 1990.

Ducharme NG, Dill SG and Rendano V: Reticulography of the cow in dorsal recumbency: an aid in the diagnosis and treatment of traumatic reticuloperitonitis, *J Am Vet Med Assoc* 182: 585-588, 1983.

Ferrante PL, Whitlock RH: Chronic vagal indigestion in cattle, *Comp Cont Ed* 3: S231-S237, 1981.

Fubini SL, Ducharme NG, Erb HN, Smith DF, Rebhun WC: Failure of omasal transport attributable to perireticular abscess formation in cattle: 29 cases (1980-1986), *J Am Vet Med Assoc* 194: 811-814, 1989.

Fubini SL, Ducharme NG, Murphy JP, Smith DF: Vagus indigestion syndrome resulting from liver abscess in dairy cows, *J Am Vet Med Assoc* 186: 1297-1300, 1985.

Fubini SL, Smith DF: Failure of omasal transport due to traumatic reticuloperitonitis and intraabdominal abscess: *Compend Contin Educ Pract Vet* 4: S492-S494, 1982.

Fubini SL, Yeager AE, Mohammed HO, Smith DF: Accuracy of radiography of the reticulum for predicting surgical findings in adult dairy cattle with traumatic reticuloperitonitis: 123 cases (1981-1987), *J Am Vet Assoc* 197: 1060-1064, 1990.

Habel RE: A study of the innervation of the ruminant stomach, *Cornell Vet* 46: 555-633, 1956.

Neal PA, Edwards GB: "Vagus Indigestion" in cattle, *Vet Rec* 82: 396-402, 1968.

Rebhun WC: Vagus indigestion in cattle, *J Am Vet Med Assoc* 176: 506-510, 1980.

Rebhun WC: Lactic acidosis. In Rebhun WC: *Diseases of dairy cattle.* Philadelphia. 1995, Williams & Wilkins.

Rebhun WC: Abdominal diseases. In Rebhun WC: *Diseases of dairy cattle,* Philadelphia, 1995, Williams & Wilkins.

von Dirksen G, Stober M: Contribution to the functional disorders of the bovine stomach caused by the lesions of the nervus vagus-Hoflund's syndrome summary, *DTW Dtsch Tierarztl Wochenschr* 69: 213-217, 1962.

Ward JL, Ducharme NG: Traumatic reticulo peritonitis in cattle: a clinical update, *J Am Vet Med Assoc* 6: 874-877, 1994.

10.4—Surgery of the Abomasum

Ava M. Trent

Normal function of the abomasum is critical for the health and productive success of beef and dairy cattle. Altered abomasal function is one of the most common indications for abdominal surgery in adult dairy cows and, to a lesser extent, in calves, bulls, and beef cattle. Many of the abomasal disorders in cattle can be managed effectively in a field setting with a solid understanding of abomasal physiology and abdominal anatomy.

Abomasal Physiology and Abdominal Anatomy

DEVELOPMENTAL ANATOMY

The abomasum is the most distal of the four stomach compartments in all cattle. However, the size, position, intake path of ingesta, and digestive function change dramatically from birth to early adulthood, creating different diagnostic and therapeutic challenges for the veterinarian. In the neonatal calf, the abomasum is the primary functioning stomach compartment. At birth, it is the largest of the four compartments, with a volume twice that of the combined ruminoreticulum. It fills the right cranioventral abdomen, extending caudally on and to the right of midline to a point well beyond the 13th rib. In the young calf, stimulation of pharyngeal receptors by milk components and suckling diverts all milk through the reticular groove into the abomasum, bypassing the poorly developed rumen. As the calf begins to consume solid feed, the ruminoreticular compartments assume a more active role in digestion and begin to increase in size. At 8 weeks of age, the volume of the abomasum is equal to that of the ruminoreticulum, and by 12 weeks of age the ruminoreticulum is twice the size of the abomasum. By the time a cow is 1.5 years of age, all compartments have reached their mature total capacity of 95 to 230 L with relative volumes of 80% (rumen), 8% (abomasum), 7% (omasum), and 5% (reticulum).

ABOMASAL FUNCTION

The abomasum, in coordination with the activities of the proximal and distal intestinal tract, plays a critical role in digestion. Alterations in secretions or motility can result in significant disruption of digestion and major disturbances in systemic fluid and electrolyte balance. Conversely, changes in systemic or gastrointestinal homeostasis that result from natural events or therapeutic intervention for other disease processes can produce direct or secondary disturbances in abomasal motility. Fortunately, many of the local and systemic effects on abomasal function and abomasal dysfunction's effect on local and systemic processes can be predicted through an understanding of abomasal function.

The abomasum is the only stomach compartment with glandular mucosa that can secrete digestive juices, including hydrochloric acid, pepsin, and rennin. Alkaline chyme stimulates abomasal emptying, and acidic chyme inhibits emptying via release of local peptides and hormones. The uniquely long distance between the pylorus and where the duodenum allows of highly alkaline bile and pancreatic fluids entrance in ruminants helps maintain the low duodenal pH necessary for ruminant digestion.

In the adult ruminant, the abomasum functions in a manner similar to the simple stomach of monogastric animals. The luminal pH is maintained at a 3.0 level in healthy cattle by the physical features mentioned above and by coordination of secretions with abomasal motility. The normally low pH of the abomasum does not support viable pathogenic microorganisms, although abomasal lesions can be colonized by a variety of opportunistic organisms. Secretion of digestive fluids is relatively continuous, but volume and acidity are affected by several local and systemic neurohumoral factors, including gastrin (increases fundic secretion of HCl and pepsin) and somatostatin (decreases gastrin secretion). The volume and acidity of secretions are also reduced when the abomasal or duodenal pH is decreased, flow of ingesta into the abomasum is prevented, or stimulation by the vagal nerve occurs. Distention of the abomasal body, injection of histamine, infusion of buffered fatty acids into the abomasal lumen, and stimulation by parasympathomimetic agents, such as atropine, increase the volume and acidity of secretions.

Abomasal motility and clearance in the adult are also regulated by local and systemic factors. Contractions (aborad and orad) must be coordinated with opening and closing of the pyloroduodenal junction and aborad and orad contraction patterns in the cranial duodenum to ensure appropriate timing for mixture and digestion of contents as well as to clear ingesta into the distal intestinal tract. The strength of peristaltic contractions is normally greatest in the pyloric antrum, with variable contractions in the body and minimal activity in the fundic region. Whereas flow of ingesta from the ruminoreticulum into the abomasum is relatively constant, abomasal emptying appears to occur 18 to 20 times a day and corresponds to strong antroduodenal contractions. Motility is increased in anticipation of, during, and for several hours after a meal. Motility can be depressed by many factors, including high-roughage meals, duodenal distention, introducing volatile fatty acids in the rumen, ruminal absorption of histamine, low rumen pH, and extreme or chronic abomasal distention. Gastric outflow reflects a balance between propulsive abomasal contraction and a braking action at the gastroduodenal juncture, often called the *duodenal brake.* The composition of chyme (specifically acidification), the volume of material entering the duodenum, and local and systemic neurohumoral mediators such as gastrin and somatostatin appear to inhibit abomasal outflow through this mechanism. Narcotic and alpha-2 adrenergic agents such as xylazine hydrochloride may also inhibit abomasal outflow by affecting the duodenal brake. Vagal nerve function plays a role in normal abomasal motility, although it has been difficult to determine the specific nerves and pathways involved because local intrinsic control mechanisms can compensate and reestablish abomasal motility even after complete cervical vagotomy. Nonetheless, vagal nerve injury is commonly implicated as a cause of abomasal dysfunction.

A variety of systemic factors have also been associated with decreased abomasal motility including endotoxemia, alkalemia, systemic histamine release, epinephrine release, prostaglandin I_2, hyperinsulinemia, tumor necrosis factor, decreased cholinergic tone, decreased nitroxergic activity, and pain. Normal abomasal motility requires adequate serum levels of several key electrolytes. Decreases in serum calcium and potassium specifically are potential causes of depressed gastric and intestinal motility in many species. Although experimental depression of abomasal motility in cattle through hypocalcemia appears to require lower serum calcium levels than typically encountered in clinical cases, the potential role of hypocalcemia in combination with other depressant factors remains a concern. Ketosis is also associated with decreased abomasal motility, although whether ketosis is a cause, effect, or incidental event of hypomotility is unclear.

The relatively continuous nature and composition of abomasal secretions results in fairly characteristic changes in systemic fluid and electrolyte balances in adult ruminants with impaired abomasal outflow. Accumulation of hydrogen and chloride in the abomasal lumen leads to a hypochloremic metabolic alkalosis. Hyponatremia is common, even in the face of dehydration. Hypokalemia can result from reduced food intake as well as from a cellular exchange for hydrogen in the face of alkalosis. Paradoxical aciduria may occur in hypovolemic cattle with concurrent hypochloremic alkalosis, hypokalemia and hyponatremia. The severity of the dehydration and electrolyte disturbances depends upon the duration and degree of outflow disturbance and the presence or absence of vascular compromise. In cases of severe vascular compromise with tissue necrosis, as may be seen with prolonged abomasal volvulus, a metabolic acidosis may develop and result in a blood pH return toward more normal values. Concurrent conditions may also superimpose metabolic disturbances. Specifically, severe ketosis or diarrhea may result in a metabolic acidosis despite changes directly resulting from a displacement.

Surgical Conditions of the Abomasum

A variety of digestive and inflammatory conditions affect abomasal function. Two major categories of abomasal abnormalities that either indicate the need for surgery or must be managed when encountered during abdominal surgery are conditions primarily recognized because of altered abomasal outflow and conditions associated with loss of abomasal wall integrity. These categories are not mutually exclusive.

ALTERED ABOMASAL OUTFLOW

Most abomasal disorders ultimately are recognized because of a disturbance in normal abomasal outflow with resulting alterations in digestion, systemic fluid and electrolyte balances, and fecal production. Abomasal outflow can be altered by a wide range of mechanical and functional factors or, in many cases, a combination of both. The disorders can be grouped into two categories: those associated with repositioning of the abdomen in the abdominal cavity (i.e., displacements) and those that occur without a significant change in abomasal position.

Abomasal Displacement Syndromes

The abomasum has the capacity for major changes in volume and location. The abomasum is mobile because it is suspended in the distal turn of a U supported by the lesser omentum (Figure 10.4-1). Three syndromes that involve movement of the abomasum are commonly recognized: left abomasal displacement (LDA), right abomasal dilation/displacement (RDA), and volvulus of the abomasum on the right side (RVA). The conditions called RDA and RVA may be two stages in a progression

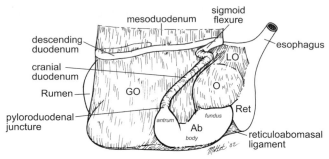

Figure 10.4-1 Schematic diagram representing the normal anatomical position of the abomasum in relation to adjacent viscera. GO, greater omentum; LO, represents lesser omentum.

rather than separate syndromes, with RDA developing first and developing in some but not all cases into a RVA. A fourth displacement syndrome of cranial displacement of the abomasum between the liver and diaphragm has also been described as an incidental finding but is seldom recognized and will not be discussed further in this text.

The abomasum can displace without volvulus to the left or right of its normal position by swinging, folding, or stretching of the lesser omentum and attached structures. The result is a partial outflow obstruction as the narrow duodenum is compressed by stretching and, in the case of an LDA, by compression under the rumen. If the movement of the abomasum involves a rotation of structures around an axis through the lesser omentum, the resulting volvulus can produce complete outflow obstruction as well as compressing vessels and nerves as they pass along the neck of the omasum.

All of the abomasal displacement syndromes occur more commonly in high-production dairy cows but also appear sporadically in calves, dairy bulls, and beef cattle. Abomasal displacement to the left is by far the most common of the recognized displacement syndromes. Left displacements are significantly more common than either right displacement or volvulus and represent 85% to 96% of all displacement conditions. In a study of over 100,000 cattle admitted to 17 veterinary teaching hospitals in North America, LDAs were 7.4 times more common than right abomasal volvulus. This ratio is somewhat lower than that reported in field studies, which presumably reflects a higher referral rate for abomasal volvulus than for left displacement.

Abomasal displacement conditions have some common features in pathogenesis, effect, and treatment. Although the bulk of the research has focused on factors that predispose to left abomasal displacement, the etiopathogenesis of right abomasal dilation and abomasal volvulus are thought to be similar. The potential for abomasal displacement exists whenever conditions support gas accumulation in the abomasum. Any of the local or systemic factors described under Abomasal Development and Function that alter abomasal motility can predispose to displacement.

Left Abomasal Displacement (LDA)—General Considerations

Definition and Incidence Left displacement of the abomasum (LDA, refers to the abomasum relocating to the left side of midline between the rumen and left body wall. It was first reported in 1950 and is currently one of the most common surgical problems encountered in modern production dairies, with an incidence of 0.35% to 4.4% in large population studies—and as high as 15% in some herds. The number of reported LDAs appears to have increased in production dairy cattle over the last two decades, indicating an increase in incidence, in recognition, or both.

Left displacements occur sporadically in beef cows and in beef and dairy bulls. In data from over 100,000 admissions to 17 veterinary teaching hospitals in North America, dairy cattle were found to have an adjusted odds ratio of 95.2 of developing an LDA in comparison to beef cattle, and female cattle in general have a 29.1 adjusted odds ratio in comparison to males.

Predisposing Factors The majority of LDAs in adult dairy cows occur in the first month of lactation, with 57% reported in the first 2 weeks *postpartum,* 80% within the first month, and 85% to 91% within the first 6 weeks *postpartum.* The risk of development increases with age and is highest in dairy cows between 4 and 7 years of age. Predisposition in Guernsey, Holstein-Friesian, and Ayrshire breeds has been suggested, although some variation exists between studies. A genetically linked predisposition has been suggested in Holstein cattle but has been disputed. A phenotypic predisposition in cattle with large abdominal cavities has also been suggested. A seasonal predisposition for developing LDAs has been identified in North American cattle, with the highest incidence in spring (March through June) and the lowest in fall (September through October).

The high incidence of left displacement during the early stages of lactation in mature dairy cows presumably reflects the simultaneous occurrence of a number of factors that set the stage for abomasal dilation and displacement to the left. Common periparturient events, such as rapid changes in diet (decreased fiber and increased concentrates), decreased exercise, hypocalcemia, ketosis, fatty liver, and conditions potentially associated with endotoxemia such as mastitis, retained placenta, stillbirth, and metritis are among the factors that potentially lead to decreased gastrointestinal motility and gas build-up in the abomasum. Although these factors are commonly implicated as predisposing factors, studies have not consistently confirmed most of these nondietary factors to be risk factors for left displacement, and some may prove to be concurrent but not causally related events. Rapid changes in abdominal topography in the periparturient period may also favor left displacement. In the late stage of pregnancy, the distended uterus can elevate the rumen off the ventral body wall and push the abomasum into a more cranial and transverse position. As the uterine volume suddenly decreases with parturition and the rumen is allowed to fill, the abomasum may become trapped on the left. Delivery of twins and large maternal body size have been implicated as risk factors in some studies and may act by further increasing the room for abomasal displacement to the left.

Whether it is causally related or incidental, the veterinarian must recognize that concurrent diseases are very commonly present and must be identified and addressed for successful case management of cows with an LDA. A large multi-institute study identified concurrent diseases in 53.6% of cattle with LDAs; ketosis and uterine disease were most commonly identified. Thirteen percent of cows with concurrent disease had more than one disorder. Other studies report as much as 64% of cases have concurrent disease, with one study reporting 44.1% of cases had multiple concurrent diseases. In addition to ketosis, metritis and retained placenta, other concurrent conditions commonly reported are mastitis, hypocalcemia, fatty liver, lameness, and abomasal ulcers.

Predisposing factors are not well established in cattle other than in adult female dairy cows. Abomasal ulcers, foreign bodies, and geosediments have been reported as factors in the pathogenesis of LDAs in calves, mature bulls, and beef cows.

Diagnosis Adult dairy cows with an LDA typically are noticed when their milk production and/or feed consumption is less than expected or they have a sudden drop in milk production and/or feed consumption later in their lactation. Classically, cows with LDAs selectively go off concentrates first, although this may vary with individual animals. Other commonly recognized signs include depression and loose or pasty, scant feces that may be darker in color than normal. The nature of feces is an important indicator of possible concurrent diseases. Although often called *diarrhea,* fecal volume generally decreases in cows with only an LDA. When fecal volume and fluidity increases, concurrent intestinal diseases such as Johnes or bovine viral diarrhea should be considered, with the prognosis and plan adjusted accordingly. Dark feces (melena) may occur as a result of abomasal hemorrhage from ulcers, with a similar need for an altered prognosis and plan.

The veterinarian most commonly diagnoses LDA by using simultaneous auscultation and percussion to detect a tympanic ping on the left side of the cow. The ping is usually centered over the last few ribs on a line from the elbow to the tuber coxae. With extreme distention, the abomasal ping can be detected in the left flank as far caudally as the tuber coxae and as far cranially as the ninth rib. Occasionally, the ping will be located more ventral or cranial than expected. This may occur transiently because of repositioning of structures as gas enters or leaves the abomasum. However, if the abnormal ping location is consistent, the possibility of abomasal adhesions caused by concurrent abomasal ulcers should be considered. In some cases, the ping will disappear completely for a period of time only to recur at a later time. This is commonly called a *floating DA,* which suggests the abomasum moves back and forth from displaced to normal position. It is more likely the ping comes and goes as gas builds then passes temporarily out of the abomasum, which remains left of the rumen.

The ping caused by an LDA must be differentiated from other sources of left-sided pings, including ruminal tympany, pneumoperitoneum, and rumen void. By combining information about the ping's location and results from abdominal palpation per rectum, veterinarians can make most diagnoses in adult cattle with a high degree of reliability. It is uncommon for a left displaced abomasum to distend to a size that can be directly palpated per rectum; however, the rumen is usually palpably displaced to the right of the body wall. This often causes a sharp depression of the flank behind the last left rib visible on external examination. This depression commonly is called a *slab-side.* Ruminal tympany causes a ping that is typically more dorsally and caudally placed along the dorsal left paralumbar fossa than an LDA ping. A distended rumen should be palpable per rectum against the left body wall, and the left paralumbar fossa will appear full—not sunken—on external examination. The ping associated with pneumoperitoneum is also more dorsally located and may be less resonant than an LDA or ruminal ping, although ping intensity is not a highly reliable method of differentiation. Pneumoperitoneum may produce a ping on either or both sides of the cow, with right-sided pings more common than left. The characteristic "tight" feeling of the collapsed descending colon on one's arm and the readily movable descending colon without the normal abdominal resistance during palpation per rectum should also suggest pneumoperitoneum. It is possible for both LDA and pneumoperitoneal pings to be present, in which case concurrent left displacement and perforating abomasal ulcers should be suspected. On occasion, a dull ping in the typical location of an LDA can be detected in association with a very small rumen. Sometimes called a *rumen void ping*, this ping is generally not very resonant. Palpation by rectum should confirm the small rumen size (collapsed dorsal sac of the rumen).

On occasion, the veterinarian may also detect a tympanic ping on the right side of the abdomen in cows with a characteristic left-sided LDA ping. In most cases, this represents a transient accumulation of gas in the cecum, ascending colon, or duodenum. This gas may accumulate in these sites from generalized ileus or may represent boluses of gas that have escaped from the displaced abomasum during movement or transportation. In either case, frequent changes in location and size of these right-sided pings help differentiate them from signs of an intestinal obstruction. If the right-sided ping is constant in location and steady or increasing in area, palpation per rectum to check for the presence of a distended viscus is indicated. The characteristic loss of definition of abdominal structures during palpation per rectum would support a diagnosis of pneumoperitoneum.

If a question about the diagnosis of LDA still remains, several additional diagnostic steps can be taken. A nasogastric tube can be passed into the rumen. While an assistant blows on the external end of the tube, the left flank immediately caudal to the last rib can be ausculted. The bubbling sound in the rumen will be soft and distant if the abomasum is displacing the rumen toward midline but loud and close if the rumen is adjacent to the body wall. Decompression of gas from the rumen may allow more diagnostic evaluation per rectum. Fluid can be collected by stomach tube to evaluate for elevated rumen chloride (normal is less than 30 mEq/L) consistent with abomasal outflow obstruction and ruminal reflux if laboratory resources are available. Alternatively, centesis can be used to collect a small amount of fluid from the viscus adjacent to the left flank to evaluate the pH. A 6- to 8-cm or longer 10- to 14-gauge needle is passed through the body wall into the center of the area defined by a ping. The odor of the gas escaping through the needle may suggest rumen or abomasum, but digestive disturbances can alter contents of either structure enough to make use of this evaluation alone unreliable. A purulent odor suggests peritonitis with pneumoperitoneum or abscess formation. A 20-cm length of polypropylene tubing with an attached syringe is quickly passed through the needle, and a small amount of fluid is aspirated for evaluation by using standard pH paper. A pH less than 3.5 indicates a displaced abomasum, whereas a pH greater than 5.5 suggests a ping originating from the rumen. This test is known as *the Liptac test*. Although helpful, it should be used only if differentiation cannot be made with standard methods. This is because some local peritoneal contamination will occur, which increases risk of infection if

exploratory surgery follows. The procedure should be avoided on the right side of the abdomen, where the small intestine can be penetrated and cause peritonitis. The growing availability of ultrasound yields an additional practical diagnostic tool.

In addition to identifying an LDA, the veterinarian must also assess the cow for concurrent conditions and metabolic status. In the absence of immediate laboratory access, the degree of electrolyte disturbance can be roughly correlated to the level of dehydration. Adult cattle with 4% to 5% dehydration can be expected to have mild metabolic hypochloremic alkalosis with normal to slightly low potassium and/or sodium. These changes generally resolve after restoration of normal abomasal position if cattle have access to water. Cattle with more severe dehydration can be expected to have more significant disturbances, and a laboratory evaluation would be beneficial. In a field setting, cows with 8% to 10% dehydration can be expected to be hypokalemic as well as hyponatremic and hypochloremic. A paradoxical aciduria, detectable with a pH strip, may be present. Hypocalcemia is a common causative or concurrent condition that should be evaluated and addressed. Early signs of hypocalcemia include slow pupillary light response and cool or cold ear tips in comparison to ear base. Muscle fasciculations and weakness suggest advanced hypocalcemia. Assessment for metritis, mastitis, udder edema and abomasal ulcers are important components of the decision process for case management. The presence of abomasal ulcers is suggested by anemia and a positive fecal occult blood test (bleeding ulcer), cranial right abdominal pain on pressure, pneumoperitoneum, fever of undetermined origin, an elevated peritoneal fluid white blood cell count (>3000 cells/μl) with neutrophilia and degenerative neutrophils and possibly bacteria, or an abnormally located left sided ping (see the section, Abomasal Ulcers, in this chapter).

Treatment Effective management of a cow with an LDA requires a number of decisions, the first being whether to treat the individual cow at all. This decision should be based on the cost of treatment, anticipated economic losses from the LDA and concurrent conditions, prognosis for return to production, expected future income from production, immediate slaughter value, and—perhaps of greatest impact—the owner's interest in treating the specific animal in question. Use of decision analysis can help weigh the variable economic factors, although the owner may ultimately make his or her decision based on factors that do not fit directly into an objective formula.

Recent studies have provided useful information for predicting treatment costs, prognosis, and expected economic gains and losses in general terms. Without travel, examination or concurrent disease treatment expenses, the cost of a minimally invasive closed procedure for treatment was estimated to be half that of a conventional open procedure. The prognosis for return to function varies slightly with the treatment approach chosen (see discussions of each technique) and the nature of concurrent conditions. The prognosis for return to function ranges from 77% to 91% after closed surgical procedures and 80% to 100% after conventional surgical procedures. A large study of cattle presented to 17 North American teaching hospitals for treatment of an LDA showed an overall hospital fatality rate of 5.6%, indicating that short-term survival is high. In one randomized treatment study, 6 of 37 (15.2%) cows treated by a closed technique and 12 of 35 (34.3%) cows treated by conventional surgery were lost from the herd through death or culling within 120 days of the procedure. The prognosis for cows with concurrent perforating ulcers is even lower. Only 8 of 21 (38%) cows survived to discharge, and only 14% remained in the herd one year after surgery in one study.

Most losses from the herd after treatment have been attributed to concurrent disease processes rather than from events directly related to the LDA or treatment method. A drop in milk production can be expected in lactating cows diagnosed with an LDA, with recovery to expected production levels within 120 days of surgical (conventional or closed) treatment. The milk loss (after an adjustment for decreased feed cost) was estimated in one case-control study to be 10% more for closed procedure than for conventional surgery. Losses from delayed conception, loss of genetic potential, and other consequences of the LDA and concurrent diseases are more difficult to factor into a formula, but may be important considerations in the decision to treat or not treat an individual cow. Finally, the amount of potential income from slaughter should be considered. The cost of treating LDAs by toggle-pin was 65% of omentopexy cost in a case-control study that considered the cost of treatment, milk loss, and livestock loss (replacement cost and slaughter value based on percent of treated animals lost to the herd within 120 days).

A variety of methods have been used to correct and stabilize abomasal displacements. Selection of a specific approach should take into account the likelihood the process will do the following: 1) effectively return the abomasum to its normal position; 2) stabilize the abomasum in a functional position; 3) allow management of concurrent pathology in the abdomen; 4) minimize additional risk to the patient; 5) be possible with the available restraint options; and 6) be economically reasonable for the owner. Although each technique has unique features, approaches can be grouped into three main categories: medical management, minimally invasive closed procedures, and conventional open surgical procedures.

Left Abomasal Displacement (LDA): Medical Management

The common goal of medical approaches is to restore abomasum motility sufficiently to allow it to expel gas and spontaneously return to its normal position. Although some aspects of medical therapy are valuable adjuncts to surgical treatment, the likelihood of effectively resolving an LDA with medical therapy alone is very low (less than 5%). Pharmaceutical approaches include oral or systemic calcium, parasympathomimetic agents, various oral intestinal stimulants, fluid therapy to correct dehydration and electrolyte imbalances, and agents to treat ketosis (dextrose, insulin, propylene glycol corticosteroids). Although correcting fluid imbalances and treating ketosis and hypocalcemia in affected animals are valuable adjuncts to surgically managing an LDA, there is little evidence to suggest that pharmaceutical treatments alone have any permanent effect on correcting a displacement. Acid-base disturbances can be exacerbated if magnesium-based intestinal stimulant use is continued in an uncorrected displacement. Withholding feed for 48 hours, feeding high fiber diets, forced exercise, and truck rides have been suggested treatments generally acknowledged to have little long-term effect. A transient reduction or loss of the characteristic LDA ping after transportation is a phenomenon well recognized by food animal practitioners at referral centers. The rapid return of the ping (generally within 6 to 8 hours) suggests that transportation helps expel gas from the abomasum but does not restore normal abomasal position or function.

The typical fluid disturbances in adult cattle with LDAs are dehydration with hypochloremic metabolic alkalosis and often hypokalemia and hyponatremia. Adult cattle with an LDA and clinically mild (<6%) dehydration without other metabolic disturbances do not necessarily require systemic fluid therapy if surgical correction of the displacement is planned within a few hours, although systemic fluid therapy may speed recovery. These cows can generally self-correct their fluid imbalances through oral intake after surgery if adequate water is available. Provision of two water sources is recommended for 48 to 72 hours after surgery: plain water as well as water supplemented with electrolytes (including potassium) and dextrose. Most cattle will select the electrolyte solution as needed; however, plain water should always be available to avoid accidentally exacerbating dehydration in those few cattle that will not drink electrolyte solution. Supplementing water or water plus electrolyte solution by stomach tube after correcting the displacement is also an option if access to water sources for spontaneous intake is unreliable. Preoperative or postoperative intravenous fluid therapy is encouraged for moderately dehydrated adult cattle and strongly recommended, if not mandatory, for severely dehydrated animals. Administration of 20 to 40 L of isotonic saline with 20 to 40 mEq/L of KCl given IV over 4 to 6 hours is ideal but is generally only practical when the cow is brought to a clinic or referral site. Hypertonic saline (1 to 2 L) is a more practical initial approach in a field setting, assuming that surgical correction of the displacement is planned within several hours and that oral supplementation can be provided after surgery. Because of its rapid rate of administration, potassium should not be added to hypertonic saline .

The method chosen for correction of concurrent hypocalcemia and ketosis should also reflect the severity of disturbance and condition of the cow. Adult cattle with clinical signs of hypocalcemia, including muscle fasciculations and weakness, will benefit from intravenous calcium borogluconate or calcium dextrose solution, particularly if a standing surgical approach is planned. Subcutaneous calcium borogluconate or oral formulations are appropriate for stable, mildly dehydrated cattle in the perioperative period. Intravenous dextrose (1-2 L of 50% dextrose or a calcium/dextrose solution) is the preferred initial treatment for cattle with moderate to severe ketosis. Return to full feed consumption after surgery is an important goal for control of ketosis as well as for recovery of milk production. Oral propylene glycol (300 ml PO sid or bid for 4 to 5 days) can increase ruminal alkalosis and decrease appetite. Therefore it is only recommended in postoperative cattle with mild ketosis that are eating and have good ruminal motility. More aggressive therapy such as corticosteroids (10 to 20 mg dexamethasone once), protomine zinc insulin (200 U SQ every 48 hours while receiving intravenous 5% dextrose), or continuous IV 5% dextrose infusion may be indicated for cows with nonresponsive ketosis after surgery. A recent controlled study suggests that administration of 500 mg of recombinant bovine somatotropin after surgical correction of LDA may improve recovery from ketosis after surgery.

Left Abomasal Displacement (LDA): Minimally Invasive Closed Procedures Minimally invasive closed procedures include rolling, blind tack, toggle pin, and laparoscopy-assisted toggle pin. All rely on the concept that gas trapped in the displaced abomasum causes the abomasum to shift to the highest available space in the abdomen when a cow is on its back. This position approximates the abomasum's normal position on or slightly to the right of ventral midline. Repositioning requires that the abomasum be free to move, which will not occur if the abomasum is adhered in an abnormal position or lacks sufficient gas to float it back to its normal position during the procedure. These procedures share many similar advantages and disadvantages.

The short time needed for the nonlaparoscopic procedure (<15 minutes in most cases) in comparison to the time for conventional open surgical procedures reduces the risk of dorsal recumbency and allows its use in most cows without withholding feed and water. Dorsal recumbency may also increase drainage of the uterus in cases with concurrent metritis. Invasion of the peritoneal cavity is minimal in comparison to conventional surgery, thus decreasing the risk of surgical complications related to peritonitis and incisional healing. However, reports of infections ascending along the toggle or suture that have resulted in localized but catastrophic peritonitis have been made. The minimal equipment required and short surgical time results in lower cost for the initial nonlaparoscopic procedure than for conventional surgical approaches. As a consequence, nonlaparoscopic closed procedures may be more economical than open procedures in cattle with limited long-term value in the herd or with medical problems that temporarily preclude more involved surgical procedures.

Except for the laparoscopy-assisted toggle pin, the primary disadvantage shared by these approaches is the veterinarian's inability to confirm return of the abomasum to a functional position at the time of the procedure. These approaches cannot be used for prophylactic stabilization of the abomasum in the absence of gas, because the abomasum would not be adjacent to the body wall and available for fixation. In addition, a complication of this approach is unintentional penetration of gastrointestinal viscus (rumen, cecum, small intestine, omasum, and others), which can lead to devastating consequences. Rolling has the additional disadvantages of a high recurrence rate and lack of stabilization. Because of the difficulty of differentiating between RDA and RVA without surgical exploration, these approaches should not be considered for treating right-sided abomasal pings. Because these closed techniques have a high statistical success rate in a herd, an occasional failure can be accepted as financially justifiable. The risk to individual animals prohibits using minimally invasive techniques other than laparoscopy-assisted procedures in very valuable cattle, except possibly rolling for temporary relief of displacement. Evaluating and treating concurrent abdominal pathology is not possible with these approaches. Arterial oxygen in a nonanesthetized cow without supplemental oxygen support drops from a baseline standing mean of 85.9 ± 2.06 mm Hg to a dorsal recumbency mean of 64.7 ± 2.92 mm Hg to 40 to 0 mm Hg within 15 minutes and 61.5 ± 2.29 mm Hg at 30 minutes. Even a limited period of dorsal recumbency carries significant risk in animals with preexisting pneumonia or ruminal distention, and an alternative standing approach should be considered in these cases. Sufficient personnel to safely cast and position the cow must be available, although judicious use of tranquilizers and experience reduces the number of people needed.

Rolling Rolling does not involve a direct method of restoring or stabilizing the abomasum in its normal position but instead relies on the gas in the displaced abomasum to float it to its normal location. Because of the limited security of this procedure, it is only recommended for short-term relief of symptoms in cows that do not warrant or cannot tolerate another procedure at the time. The rolling approach is contraindicated in cows with marked respiratory compromise (although the short duration makes it safer than conventional open surgery that uses recumbent approaches) when a ping is not currently present, or in cattle with concurrent abdominal disease. A more secure stabilization method is justified for animals with long-term value in the herd.

Preparation Several preparatory steps can improve the success and safety of the procedure in adult cows. Preoperative administration of calcium (IV) to cows with signs of hypocalcemia will help improve abomasal motility and can decrease the risk of musculoskeletal injury during recovery. A single preoperative dose of prophylactic antibiotics may be indicated if needle decompression is planned. Preoperatively clipping the right cranioventral abdomen from xyphoid to umbilicus between midline and the right mammary vein also reduces the amount of contamination if needle decompression is planned. Placing ropes on the front and back legs on the side that will be down initially (typically right) helps control the casting process and allows quick control of all feet as the cow is placed in dorsal recumbency. A rapid-acting sedative such as xylazine HCl (0.05-0.1 mg/kg IV) administered immediately before casting facilitates the process of dropping and stabilizing the cow on its back. Xylazine HCl use should be avoided during the last trimester of pregnancy because of its potential stimulatory effect on uterine myometrium. It is not recommended with abdominal distention because of its tendency to promote ruminal distention.

The cow should be cast in right lateral recumbency and rolled in a clockwise direction onto her back. If ropes were not preplaced on the front and back legs, they can be placed at this time. Alternatively, the process can be done without ropes by placing a person on either side of the withers to stabilize the cow on her back.

Procedure Once the cow is in dorsal recumbency, the veterinarian should confirm the abomasal location by simultaneous auscultation and percussion of the cranioventral abdomen. The cow should be maintained on its back until the ping is no longer detectable, thus indicating that most or all of the gas has been cleared from the abomasum. Rocking the cow gently in a 60° to 70° arc while it is in dorsal recumbency may help evacuate gas and return the abomasum to its normal position. The veterinarian can speed gas clearance by placing a large-gauge (14- or 16-gauge), 6- to 12-cm needle through the ventral body wall into the center of the area of the ping until gas flow has ceased. The needle should be rapidly removed as soon as gas flow ceases to minimize tissue trauma and peritoneal contamination. Suction, if available, accelerates the process and may allow more complete decompression. Local infusion of an antibiotic through the needle during removal is not recommended, although it is anecdotally described. If decompression is planned, a single prophylactic dose of antibiotic before the procedure would be a more effective method of controlling infection.

After decompression, the cow should be carefully and slowly rolled onto her left side and into sternal recumbency. Once in a sternal position, the cow should be allowed to stand when ready. Pushing a cow to stand while it is hypoxic and disoriented may increase the risk of incoordination and injury. Examination per rectum after recovery is not a routine procedure but is an advisable precaution for cows in the last trimester of pregnancy to identify early uterine torsion. Examination per rectum is mandatory in any adult cow that demonstrates signs of abdominal pain after recovery to rule out uterine torsion or intestinal volvulus.

Prognosis and Complications Long-term studies of rolling alone as a treatment indicate that, despite apparent initial improvement in a high percentage of cows, 70% to 75% of cows redevelop an LDA, often within several days. Therefore rolling is recommended only as a temporary means of relief for adult cattle that do not warrant a more aggressive approach.

Blind Tack/Toggle Pin The blind tack suture procedure was described by Hull in 1972. Sterner and Grymer first described the toggle pin technique in 1982. Like the rolling procedure, the blind tack and toggle pin techniques rely upon the gas in a displaced abomasum to carry it to a normal position when the cow is placed in dorsal recumbency. However, these approaches add a step to stabilize the abomasum once it has returned to its normal position. Although this increases the long-term success of these procedures over rolling alone, complications are more severe if complete repositioning does not occur. The primary advantages of the toggle pin technique over a blind tack are the ability to confirm penetration of the abomasum before fixation and remove most of the gas from the abomasum.

The toggle pin technique shares many of the limitations described for the blind tack, including being contraindicated for cows with marked respiratory compromise (although the short duration makes it safer than open recumbent approaches), a ping not currently present, and having concurrent abdominal disease. Identifying additional large gas-filled structures (rumen, cecum) before surgery would be another contraindication because these structures may also "rise" to the highest position in the ventral abdomen and be mistakenly identified and "pexied" as the abomasum once the cow is on its back. Neither technique can be used to stabilize the abomasum prophylactically in an animal without an existing displacement.

Preparation Preoperative considerations are similar to those described for rolling, but a few additional steps are recommended. Clipping the right cranioventral abdomen from umbilicus to xyphoid before casting, although not absolutely necessary, decreases the risk of infection, facilitates identification of the appropriate location, and minimizes the time the cow must spend in dorsal recumbency. Identifying the milk well and milk vein locations on the right with a marker before casting the cow may be helpful.

The cow should be cast and positioned in dorsal recumbency (see Rolling). Tying the front and hind limbs in an extended position increases the safety of the procedure. Hay bales can be used to support the shoulders if a ditch or gutter is not available. Use of local anesthesia is possible; however, the benefit of analgesia must be weighed against the increased time and risk of premature abomasal decompression.

Procedures It is important to work quickly once the abomasum returns to a functional position before the gas is cleared from the abomasum. As soon as the cow is restrained in dorsal recumbency, the position of the abomasum must be confirmed by locating a ping in the right cranioventral abdomen, and the area should be quickly scrubbed. *If a distinct ping cannot be identified in the appropriate location, the procedure should be aborted without placing any sutures or pins.* By following this simple guideline, accidental tacking of structures other than the abomasum can be avoided in most cases.

For a blind tack, a large, 9- to 20-cm, curved, handheld needle (originally an upholstery needle) should be placed in the center of a long (30-cm) strand of no. 2 to no. 4 nonabsorbable suture material. The needle is pushed through the body wall into the abomasal lumen and back out through the body wall at a site in the center of the ping area between the midline and milk vein and several centimeters caudal to the xyphoid. The doubled suture is tied and auscultation and percussion repeated to identify the remaining area of ping. If the area is large enough, a second suture is placed 4 to 6 cm cranial or caudal to the first within the area that still pings. Once the suture or sutures have been placed and tied, the cow is rolled slowly onto her left side and then into sternal recumbency. The cow is allowed to stand when ready.

Placement of toggle pins begins by pushing a 4-mm (12 French) cannula and trocar (Figure 10.4-2) into the abomasum through the body wall in the area of ping. Placement of the first pin at the most cranial aspect of the ping has been suggested to facilitate penetration of the abomasum. The trocar is removed and penetration of the abomasum is confirmed by the abomasal gas odor passing through the cannula. If the veterinarian is in doubt, polyethylene tubing passed through the cannula

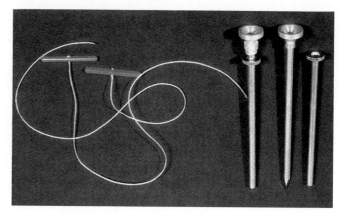

Figure 10.4-2 Picture of toggle pin and attached suture material, and, from right to left, cannula, trocar, and assembled cannula and trocar.

can be used to aspirate a small amount of fluid from the penetrated lumen for evaluation with a wide-range pH paper. A fluid pH of 2 to 3 would confirm penetration of the abomasum. In practice, the time necessary to collect fluid must be weighed against the risk of losing contact with the abomasum as gas escapes. If confirmation by fluid pH is performed, gas escaping from the cannula should be minimized until the bar is placed. Once the position has been confirmed, a 3-cm long 10-French (3.3 mm diameter) polypropylene toggle pin with a centrally attached 30-cm polyamide suture should be pushed through the cannula with the trocar into the abomasal lumen. The cannula is then removed, the bar is pulled firmly against the abomasal wall (Figure 10.4-3), and a hemostat is placed on the suture near its exit from the skin. If gas is still present, a second pin should be placed 5 to 10 cm caudal (or cranial if that is where the ping remains) to the first. Once the second pin is pushed through the cannula, the cannula should be left in place until all gas has escaped from the abomasum. The cannula is then removed; the second pin is pulled firmly against the abomasal wall; and the two sutures are tied together, leaving room for 1 to 2 fingers under the suture. Tighter placement increases the risk of the bars necrosing through the abomasal wall. If the ping disappears before the second pin is placed, the sutures attached to the first pin can be sutured to the skin. Once the pins have been placed, the cow can be rolled slowly onto its left side and on into sternal recumbency.

Postoperative Care Concurrent diseases should be treated accordingly. If antibiotic prophylaxis was administered before surgery, no need to continue after surgery exists unless indicated for treatment of concurrent diseases. The cow should be closely monitored during the first week after surgery for signs of restored abomasal function (appetite, milk production). In some cases of left abomasal displacement, the abomasum only partially

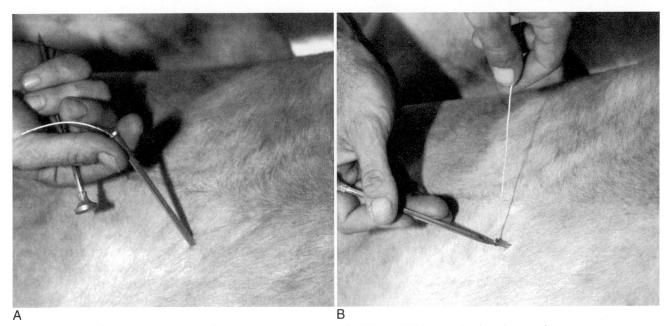

Figure 10.4-3 Use of toggle pin in a cow with LDA. *A,* With cow in dorsal recumbency, the trocar is placed at the intended pexy site. The toggle is placed. *B,* The trocar is removed and the sutures grasped.

repositions when the cow is placed in dorsal recumbency, thus leaving its long axis perpendicular to the cow's midline. This may still produce a ping in the right paramedian area. If the abomasum is tacked in this position, function will be mildly to moderately impaired. Incomplete repositioning also increases the risk of accidentally catching the greater omentum with the suture or toggle pin, thereby fixing the abomasum in an abnormal position. If significant progress is not evident, the sutures or toggle pins should be released by cutting the sutures as close to the skin as possible within 48 hours after surgery and allowing the suture ends or pins to slide into the abomasal lumen. An open procedure should be considered at this point if the cow is to remain in the herd.

One of the more serious and avoidable complications of the blind tack and toggle pin techniques is abomasal fistulation along the suture tract (Figure 10.4-4). This complication can be avoided by releasing the sutures at the skin surface after a stable adhesion has formed but before the track for a fistula develops. A stable fibrous adhesion should be present by 10-14 days after suture placement. Sutures should be cut as close to the skin as possible 2-3 weeks after placement. The portions remaining in the abdomen will either slide back into the abomasum and be passed through the intestinal tract or be incorporated into the fibrous adhesion. Delaying release of the sutures or pins for more than 3 weeks after surgery increases the risk of fistulation (see Figure 10.4-4).

Prognosis and Complications An initial success rate of 77% to 93% has been reported for blind tacks. The reported initial success rates for cows treated with toggle pins vary from 80% to 88%. The reports generally refer to short-term survival and do not usually take into account the percentage of cows (4%-7%) for which a planned blind procedure could not be performed in the absence of a ping. Toggle pin stabilization of LDAs compared favorably with right paramedian abomasopexy in postoperative feed intake, milk production, and survival in the herd in one randomized study. More cows treated by toggle pin stabilization remained in the herd 120 days after treatment (31/37) than those treated by standing right pyloroomentopexy (23/35).

The blind tacks and toggle pin procedures have high success rates that are comparable to those for open techniques, but potential complications can be more severe (sometimes castrotrophic). Reported complications include redisplacement (caused by failure to catch the abomasum or suture pull out), abomasal rupture at the suture site (Figure 10.4-5), local or diffuse peritonitis (caused by leakage along the suture line, laceration of a viscus during needle or pin placement, or suture pull out), cellulitis, pexy of structures other than the abomasum (Figure 10.4-6), partial or complete abomasal obstruction (caused by pexy of the abomasum without full return to a normal position, placement of pexy sutures too close to the pylorus, or pexy of omentum that results in a forced displacement), fistulation, and thrombophlebitis of the subcutaneous vein. Despite the purported severity of complications associated with minimally invasive procedures, controlled studies indicate failures tend to be most commonly

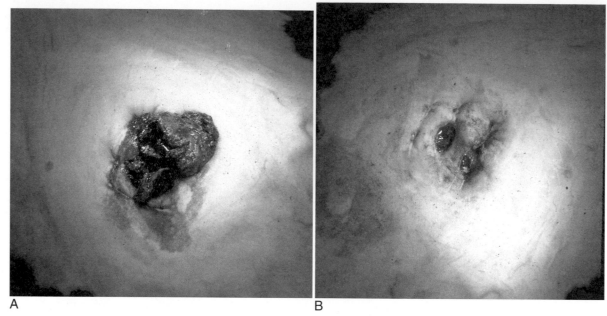

Figure 10.4-4   Cow in dorsal recumbency after blind tack. *A,* Failure to remove the sutures has resulted in an abomasal fistula along the suture tract with herniation of some of the folds of the abomasum. These folds have become ulcerated and necrotic. *B,* After resection of the prolapsed abomasal mucosa two fistulous tracts are apparent at the site of the previous blind stitch.

(Courtesy of Dr. Norm G. Ducharme; Cornell University.)

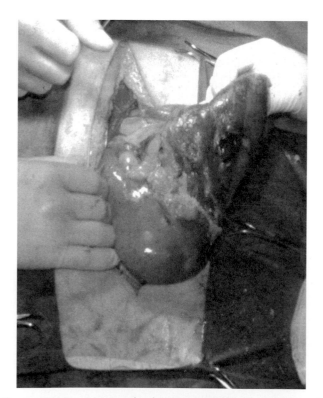

Figure 10.4-5   Lacerated abomasum after a blind tack procedure (as seen through a ventral right paramedian incision).

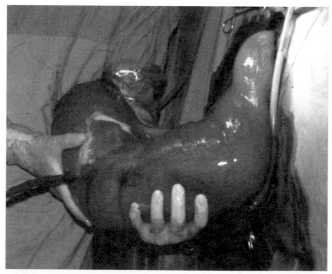

Figure 10.4-6   Inadvertent perforation of the cecum during toggle pin placement was apparent when viewed during a right paralumbar fossa exploratory celiotomy.

(Courtesy of Dr. Susan L. Fubini; Cornell University.)

due to factors unrelated to the surgical technique. In the original report of the blind tack procedure, 5 of the 40 treated animals were considered failures. Four of the failures were related to concurrent diseases, and the fifth was a complication of casting the animal for recumbency.

In one study of 96 cows scheduled for treatment by toggle pin, six cows died within 1 to 11 days of treatment, and six procedures failed. Seven of the 12 deaths/failures were directly related to the surgical procedure. Four procedures were cancelled in the absence of a detectable ping in dorsal recumbency, and three bar sutures were pulled out, thus resulting in one animal with fatal peritonitis and two redisplacements corrected in subsequent procedures. Of the five remaining deaths/failures, three were unrelated to the procedure, and two were lost to follow-up. In a second study, 13 of 31 cows treated with toggle pins died or were culled by 60 days of lactation after treatment. Of the 13 losses, only one case, an obstruction of the pylorus by misplacement of the caudal pin was attributable to the procedure itself. All others were lost because of concurrent or subsequent diseases or poor production.

Laparoscopy-Assisted Toggle Pin In addition to a laparoscope, additional equipment* as shown in Figure 10.4-7, is needed to place a modified stronger safety toggle pin (see Chapter 4.6). This procedure's main advantage is ensuring that the abomasum is the viscus being pexied and that any inadequate toggle positioning can be immediately identified and corrected.

Procedure With the animal in an appropriate restraining device, the dorsal third of the left paralumbar fossa and the 11th intercostal space are clipped and prepared for aseptic surgery; two entry points are needed in the dorsal third of the left flank. The laparoscope is inserted into the paralumbar fossa, and the trocar is inserted through the eleventh intercostal space. After administering local anesthesia at the intended laparoscope entry point, an 8- to 10-mm strap incision is made in the paralumbar fossa. A blunt insufflation needle is inserted into the abdomen, and insufflation is performed. The laparoscopic blunt trocar is inserted into the abdomen, and an 8 or 10 mm laparoscope is placed in the abdomen. The abomasum is identified and differentiated from the rumen by its smooth contour and position more lateral than the rumen (Figure 10.4-8). Under laparoscopic guidance, the trocar and its stylet are inserted into the most dorsal aspect of the abomasum (greater curvature) to a depth sufficient enough that the trocar remains within the lumen of the abomasum when the stylet is removed (see Figure 10.4-8). After the stylet is removed without allowing much gas to evacuate, the modified toggle is inserted into the abomasum. All gas is then allowed to evacuate from the abomasum. The laparoscope and trocar are removed without deinsufflating the abdomen, and one skin suture is placed to close each site.

*Dr. Fritz GmbH, 975 TU Tuttlingen, Germany (*http://www.dr-fritz.de*) and Spectrum Surgical Instruments, Stow, OH 44224 (www.spectrumsurgical.com)

The cow is then sedated with xylazine hydrochloride and placed in dorsal recumbency. A 30 cm by 15 cm section of the ventral paramedian abdomen is prepared for aseptic surgery, and local anesthesia is placed at the intended surgical site. The laparoscope is introduced into the cranial aspect of the abdomen approximately 7 cm

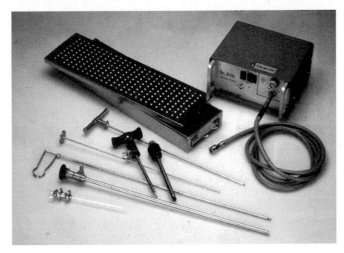

Figure 10.4-7 Equipment used for laparoscopic abomasopexy. Note: a long (35 cm) trocar is needed to place the modified toggle pin.

(Courtesy of Dr. Heinz Janowits, Holland)

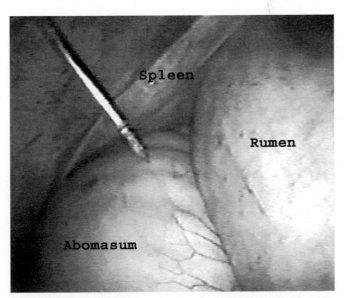

Figure 10.4-8 Laparoscopic view of the left paralumbar fossa of a cow with an LDA. The laparoscope is placed more caudal in the abdomen than the trocar. Trocar is about to be inserted into the abomasum to place the modified toggle pin.

(Courtesy of Dr. RM. Fritz; Tuttlingen, Germany)

caudal to the xiphoid and 7 cm lateral to the midline (insufflation is not needed if only minimal deinsufflation occurred during the first procedure). Under laparoscopic control, an instrument portal is placed 10 cm caudal, and the toggle sutures are grasped with laparoscopic forceps, exteriorized, and clamped. All laparoscopic instruments are removed; the portal closed with a single skin suture; and the cow placed in right lateral recumbency. Each suture is threaded through a sponge and tied together loosely (Figure 10.4-9). Alternatively, the toggle sutures may be tied with the animal in dorsal recumbency. The animal is allowed to stand. The toggle sutures are cut flush with the skin 3 to 4 weeks after surgery. A one step laparoscopic procedure is described in Section 4.6.

In the United States these procedures are not yet used routinely mostly due to the cost of the instrumentation. There are no published reports that we are aware of that use laproscopic aided pin placement on a large number of cows. If there are extensive adhesions or ulcers present in addition to the abomasal displacement they would be difficult to mange with laparoscopy alone. Furthermore there is a learning curve with the laparoscopic equipment. It may be that as more familiarity is gained with the laparoscopic procedures and the costs of the equipment drops the usage of the techniques will become more widespread.

Left Abomasal Displacement (LDA): Conventional Open Surgical Procedures The conventional open surgical procedures group includes all procedures that involve a surgical approach to the abdomen. They share diagnos-

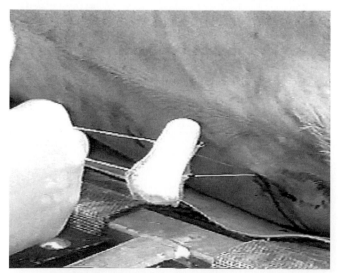

Figure 10.4-9 Each end of the toggle sutures is placed through a sponge before being tied for completion of laparoscopic assisted abomasopexy.

(Courtesy of Dr. R.M. Fritz; Tuttlingen, Germany)

tic and therapeutic advantages over closed procedures (except for laparoscopy-assisted) by allowing direct visualization and/or manual examination of the abomasum and other structures in the abdomen, but they share the disadvantages of cost and risks associated with abdominal surgery. These procedures differ from each other by the cow's position during surgery, location of the approach incision, quality of access to the abomasum and other structures in the abdomen, and structure(s) used to stabilize the abomasal position. The commonly used open procedures that meet the goals of treatment for LDAs include right paralumbar fossa omentopexy, right paralumbar fossa pyloropexy, right paramedian abomasopexy, and left paralumbar fossa abomasopexy. Other techniques described in the literature—including rumenopexy, pyloromyotomy, left paralumbar fossa omentopexy and right paralumbar fossa abomasopexy—have significant disadvantages over the four described procedures and have largely fallen out of use in favor of the other more reliable techniques.

The open procedures share a similar risk of peritoneal and/or incisional infection. In otherwise healthy cattle where good technique is used, all open procedures would be considered clean, and prophylactic antibiotics would not be warranted. However, a high percentage of cows with an LDA either have a concurrent infectious process (mastitis, metritis) or a concurrent condition that may decrease the host response to surgical contaminants (ketosis, hypocalcemia, dehydration). Limitations in restraint and the surgeon's ability to control the surgery site in a field setting also increase the risk of surgical contamination. If any of these risk factors exist, a single broad-spectrum preoperative prophylactic dose of antibiotics given IM (1 hour) or IV (15 minutes) before surgery would be indicated. Preoperative calcium supplementation is particularly important if a recumbent approach is planned or if the cow is at risk of going down during a standing approach. Fluid therapy should be initiated before surgery in moderately and severely dehydrated cattle.

Right Paralumbar Fossa (Flank) Omentopexy or Pyloropexy The standing right paralumbar fossa approach for either omentopexy and/or *pyloropexy* is probably the most versatile approach for repositioning and stabilization of the many types of abomasal displacement and provide the best access to most other intraabdominal structures. As a standing procedure, this approach is somewhat safer than recumbent procedures in cows with respiratory disease, with increased abdominal pressure caused by late-term pregnancy or ruminal distention, or with musculoskeletal problems that might make rising after surgery difficult. It is also preferred in bulls because the traditional stocks provide sufficient restraint and therefore are very practical. Minimal restraint is required for this approach, and the small number of people needed for restraint and positioning make this approach very popular. The right paralumbar fossa approach allows access to more abdominal structures for diagnostic and therapeutic procedures than any other approach in adult dairy cattle and should be considered when evaluation of other structures is needed. The status of the *postpartum* uterus can be evaluated, and, to a limited degree, purulent material can be drained by uterine elevation and massage. The combination of access and relatively low stress on the cow make this a common choice for prophylactic stabilization of the abomasum in cows at high risk for displacement.

Although the majority of the abomasum can be palpated in its normal position from this approach, only the most distal pyloric region can be seen. Access to the abomasum is even more limited while the abomasum is displaced to the left. Therefore this approach is not indicated when direct access to the abomasal fundus or body is needed. Correction of left displacement from this approach requires the abomasum to be movable with space for the abomasum to slide ventrally under the rumen. Therefore this is not a viable approach if focal adhesions caused by ulcer perforation are holding the abomasum in the left displaced position or if peritonitis from any source has resulted in accumulation of fibrin or fibrous tissue in the cranioventral abdomen. This approach is also not appropriate if the cow is too weak or lame to remain standing for the time needed for surgery.

Preparation The cow should be restrained in a head gait with an immobile wall or gait on its left side and with surgical access to the flank and paralumbar fossa on its right side. The right flank should be clipped and prepared for aseptic surgery. A right paravertebral or inverted-"L" block is recommended for analgesia. A line block can also be used but may increase incisional swelling, difficulty of incisional closure, and the risk of incisional complications. If the cow is in danger of lying down during surgery due to weakness or hypocalcemia, leg ropes can be placed on the left front and hind limbs before surgery. This will allow a nonsterile assistant to help reposition the cow without disturbing the sterile field. The cow's head should be tied with the head turned slightly up and to the right to increase the likelihood that any cow that goes down will be on its left side and minimize contamination of the surgical field. Sedation increases the risk of recumbency and is not recommended unless the cow is intractable and a recumbent approach is not possible.

Procedure A 15- to 20-cm vertical (or up to 20-degree craniodorsal to caudoventral) incision should be made through the body wall in the right paralumbar fossa. The incision starts a hand's breadth from the transverse processes of the lumbar vetebra in the middle of the right paralumbar fossa and extends ventrally (with the ventral end of the incision placed 3 to 4 cm caudal to the caudal curve of the last rib). In large cows or bulls, the incision can be made 3 to 4 cm caudal to and parallel to the last rib. Unless specifically required for certain manipulations, the incision should not extend ventral to the caudal curve of the last ribs. This minimizes the likelihood of the small intestine exiting through the incision.

When the abomasum is in its normal position, the descending duodenum will be one of the first structures encountered deep to the peritoneum crossing the dorsal aspect of the incision in a standing right paralumbar fossa approach. With a left displacement, the descending duodenum will be pulled ventrally and appear at the ventral aspect of the incision. Care should be taken to avoid accidental injury to the duodenum during the approach. Once the peritoneum has been incised, the location of the abomasum in a left displaced position should be confirmed by first reaching caudally with the left arm around the omental sling to the caudal dorsal sac of the rumen on the left side of the abdomen. The dorsal sac of the rumen is followed as far cranially as possible to palpate the dorsal aspect of the abomasum between the cranial aspect of the rumen and the left body wall. Before one attempts to replace the abomasum, the cranioventral abdomen between the greater omentum and ventral midline should be palpated to confirm freedom from adhesions. Adhesions can indicate the presence of abomasal ulcers, traumatic reticuloperitonitis, or other sources of peritoneal contamination. Regardless of their source, they can prevent relocation of the abomasum, and an alternative approach should be considered. The area of the umbilicus should be palpated specifically to check for an umbilical vein remnant running from the umbilicus to the visceral surface of the liver. If present, this fibrous, cordlike remnant can interfere with correction of the displacement and should be transected sharply. Once the path for replacement is clear, the process of relocation can begin. Either before or after the abomasum is repositioned a quick but systematic exploration of the rest of the abdomen should be performed to identify other lesions.

Decompression of the gas in the abomasum to facilitate repositioning and minimize tension and omental tearing is strongly recommended before attempting to move the abomasum. A large gauge (14- to 10-gauge) needle securely attached to a 40-cm or longer piece of sterile tubing should be placed in a guarded position in the left hand and carried caudally around the omental sling and to the left, over the dorsal rumen sac, to the dorsal bulge of the abomasum. The needle tip should be repositioned from its guarded position so it can be pushed at a fairly shallow angle into the lumen at the dorsal-most aspect of the abomasum. The free end of the tubing should be external to the cow and directed away from the sterile field in case fluid is evacuated as well as gas. The left hand should keep the needle in the abomasum and apply mild ventral pressure until just before the abomasum falls out of reach. The tubing should be occluded to prevent reflux of contents into the peritoneal cavity by folding the tube with the right hand, and the tubing and needle should be drawn in one smooth motion out of the abdomen and placed away from the sterile fields. Inserting the needle at an angle offsets the holes in the serosal and mucosal surfaces and minimizes leakage when the needle is withdrawn. Although the bacterial count in the abomasum is normally low, the low pH of the fluid can initiate peritoneal inflammation and increase the risk of peritoneal infection, even with a low number of organisms.

Two common techniques are used to move an abomasum from the left side via a right paralumbar fossa approach. In some cases the surgeon can reach around the omental sling and rumen with the left arm, place the left hand on the dorsal aspect of the abomasum, and physically push the viscus ventrally under the rumen. In the author's experience this is only possible for surgeons with fairly long arms in small cows with minimal rumen fill. In most cases it is more feasible to pull the abomasum under the rumen by grasping and placing traction on the omentum. To perform this technique, the surgeon should push the left hand with the palm facing down between the omentum and ventral body wall under the rumen and as far as possible toward the left elbow. This will generally place the hand ventral to the pyloroduodenal juncture or the thick greater omentum adjacent to the pylorus. The hand is turned over with the palm up and the hand open. The open hand will be filled with either the thick greater omentum or the pylorus. The pylorus may be identified by its relative firmness associated with the thick *torus pyloricus* muscle. These are the most stable structures that can be reached from this approach and can tolerate the most tension. Once a handful of thick greater omentum or pylorus is grasped, steady traction is applied to the right, with care taken to keep the fingers together to minimize the concentration of pressure and decrease the risk of tearing fragile omentum. By turning the palm ventrally again and flexing the wrist while pulling, the dorsal surface of the wrist elevates the rumen, which may help ease the path for the abomasum. If the surgeon can feel the tissue tearing in his or her hand at any point, traction should be stopped, the tissue released, and an attempt made to grasp more solid tissue, or preferably the pylorus, by repeating the reaching process again. If the omentum

continues to tear and the abomasum is not replaced after several attempts, the possibility of abomasal adhesions should be considered, and the procedure should be aborted in favor of an alternative approach. Persistent traction on an adhered abomasum carries a high risk of disrupting a fibrinous or fibrous seal over a perforating ulcer and causing extensive peritoneal contamination. Minor tears in the omentum carry minimal risk, but full-thickness tears adjacent to the greater curvature of the abomasum can damage the vessels and nerves in the greater omentum that supply the abomasum, thus leading to significant hemorrhage and possible neurovascular injury as well as limiting or eliminating the use of the omentum for a pexy.

Once the abomasum has moved to the right side of the rumen, it is important to ensure the normal position has been fully restored and no additional pathology is present. The ventral tension on the descending duodenum should be decreased, and it should move more dorsally in the incision. The surgeon should be able to identify the pylorus and confirm the absence of twists by placing caudodorsal tension on the greater omentum and working hand over hand from its attachment on the ventral aspect of the descending duodenum in a cranioventral direction until the pylorus is visible (usually) or palpable (always) at the cranioventral aspect of the incision. The omentum can be torn if mishandled, especially in overconditioned or underconditioned cattle. Damage usually occurs when pressure is concentrated in a small area, such as at the fingertip. Keeping all fingers together to distribute pressure on the omentum as evenly as possible and using a moistened, spread-gauze sponge in each hand, if necessary, can help minimize the risk of tearing. Once the pylorus has been identified, the caudodorsal tension on the greater omentum should be maintained with the right hand while the left hand is passed cranioventrally along the greater curvature or parietal surface of the abomasum to the reticulum. This allows the surgeon to palpate the abomasum for thickenings or adhesions suggestive of ulcers and to confirm the reticulum is free of adhesions. The omasum should be palpated dorsal to the lesser curvature of the abomasum and against the visceral surface of the liver. If the omasum is positioned medial to the abomasum, it should be lifted into its normal position by reaching cranially, medial and ventral to the abomasum and pushing up on the omasum with the palm of the left hand.

Once repositioned the surgeon has two choices: stabilize the abomasum with an omentopexy or a pyloropexy:

Omentopexy The keys to a stable omentopexy are the following: 1) choosing a site as close as possible to the pyloroduodenal juncture without interfering with duodenal function; 2) distributing the pexy over as wide an area as possible; 3) incorporating peritoneum in the pexy;

and 4) using a suture that lasts long enough for a firm fibrous adhesion to form that does not promote infection. A variety of suture techniques have been used to pexy the greater omentum to the body wall. Most are effective if placed in an appropriate location, although they vary in ease of placement and impact on incisional closure. The one described in this text meets all of the requirements described above and is easily placed.

A 6- to 8-cm vertical section of thick greater omentum located no more than 3-4 cm caudal to the pyloroduodenal juncture is identified. An appendage of the omentum, commonly called the "sow's ear," has been cited as a landmark for the pexy, but this feature is highly variable in development and proximity to the pylorus and is not recommended as the primary target for pexy location. If the paralumbar fossa incision was placed appropriately, this site on the omentum, when positioned at the ventral aspect of the incision, will allow the pylorus to fall with only slight tension into a functional position cranioventral to the incision and just inside the ninth to tenth intercostal space. If the incision is too dorsal for this to occur, it should be extended ventrally. If it is too caudal, the surgeon will have to make a choice between choosing a more caudal site on the omentum and allowing more room for the abomasum to swing, or pulling the desired site more caudally and increasing the tension on the omentum. Placement of the pexy in the omentum either too far caudal or dorsal to the pylorus and fatty omentum are considered the primary reason for dilation and redisplacement and should be avoided.

The omentum is stabilized by incorporating a 1.5-cm fold of omentum in the closure of the peritoneum and tranversus abdominal muscle (Figure 10.4-10). Nonabsorbable sutures are desired for lasting adhesions. The most commonly used suture is number-3 polyamide* placed on a half-circle taper needle because of its low cost. Principles of surgery would indicate that a monofilament nonabsorbable material such as nylon would be preferable. Number-2 chromic catgut has also been used because of its initial inflammatory effect, which is thought to promote the formation of adhesions. Absorbable suture material should have the advantage of not staying around too long should the surgical site become contaminated; however, chromic gut is rapidly absorbed and produces less stable adhesions than non-absorbable materials. Other than polydiaxonone, common absorbable materials do not maintain their integrity long enough to stimulate optimum adhesions and are not recommended. Braided and coated nonabsorbable materials do form strong adhesions but increase the risk of infection and are not recommended if other

*Supramid, S. Jackson Inc., Alexandria, WA 22303

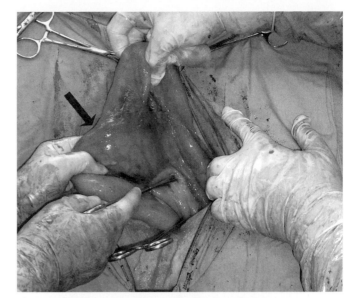

Figure 10.4-10   Standing right flank celiotomy in a cow. Cranial is to the right. The fold of the omentum normally used for the omentopexy is held in the surgeon's hand (arrow). The intended pylopexy site is held by Lahey thyroid forceps.

(Courtesy of Dr. Brett Woodie; Cornell University.)

risk factors such as peritonitis, inflammation, or remote infection are present.

The selected site on the greater omentum can be grasped with two Lahey thyroid clamps or penetrating towel clamps placed in a vertical plane 15 cm apart. This facilitates incorporation of the fold of omentum in the closure of the peritoneum and transverse abdominal muscle. However, care must be taken to avoid using the clamps for traction as they can easily tear through the omentum and prevent a stable pexy. The closure starts at the ventral aspect of the incision and moves dorsally. If it is difficult to include omentum in the most dorsal part of the incision it can be excluded. Gas can be evacuated from the peritoneal cavity by having a helper compress the abdominal wall in the left paralumbar fossa as the first layer of closure is tied to minimize the amount of postoperative pneumoperitoneum. Alternatively, if available, gas suction applied through a blunt teat cannula placed through the dorsal aspect of the incision after the first layer is closed will resolve the pneumoperitoneum. Postoperative pneumoperitoneum adds confusion during postoperative evaluation for pings and can also delay return to full feed. The remainder of the incision can be closed in 2 or 3 layers with an absorbable material for the muscle layers and a nonabsorbable material for the skin.

Prognosis and Complications   The prognosis for successful treatment of left abomasal displacement with omentopexy is good with reports of 86% to 90% of treated cattle returning to the herd. A higher success rate of 93.8% for omentopexy was reported in a study that

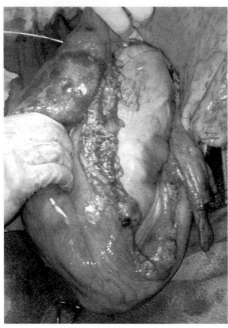

Figure 10.4-11   Torn omentum near the pylorus. This is one of the reasons an omentopexy fails.

(Courtesy of Dr. Norm G. Ducharme; Cornell University.)

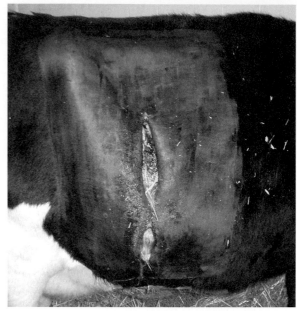

Figure 10.4-12   Cow with incisional infection postpyloropexy. To establish drainage of the retroperitoneal abscess, the middle and ventral part of the incision has been opened. The extent of the infection and depth of the drainage needed will vary and should be determined with ultrasound and rectal examinations.

(Courtesy of Dr. Susan L. Fubini; Cornell University.)

combined 411 LDAs and 43 right-sided displacements. As for other open and minimally invasive techniques, early treatment failures are more commonly a result of concurrent diseases rather than the displacement or method used for treatment. Cows treated for LDA by omentopexy compared favorably to those treated by abomasopexy at 1-, 3-, and 6-month follow-ups with respect to milk production, reproductive performance, surgical complications, and length of time retained in the herd, although there was a trend (p ≤ 0.1) for better milk production at the 1-month follow-up in cows treated by abomasopexy.

The most commonly reported complications are recurrence of dilation and displacement to the left or right, incisional infection (Figure 10.4-12), and peritonitis. A redisplacement rate of 3.6% to 4.2% was cited in one study of LDAs, whereas a rate of 5% was cited in a larger study that included 411 LDAs and 43 right-sided displacements. A group of 25 (78%) out of 32 cattle operated on a second time for recurrence of abomasal displacement initially were treated by omentopexy, and 18 out of the 25 cattle were originally treated for LDA. The recorded reasons for omentopexy failure included omental tearing (Figure 10.4-11) or stretching. The risk of omental breakdown leading to redisplacement is thought to be increased by faulty technique (most commonly related to placing the pexy too far caudal or dorsal in the omentum relative to the pylorus), and in cows with damaged, very thin, or extremely fat omentum. Subjectively, redisplacement may be more common

when performed in cows in their last trimester of pregnancy because of the altered visceral positions of late pregnancy and changes in position during and immediately after parturition.

If a left-sided ping that is not consistent with pneumoperitoneum develops after surgery, it is likely the pexy has failed and an LDA has recurred. Dilation and displacement to the right around a persistent but stretched omentopexy are also possible, as are right-sided displacement or volvulus with complete loss of the pexy. However, one study of repeat surgeries found that 78% of redisplacements, regardless of the method of fixation, occurred on the same side as the original displacement. Dilation on the right in the face of an existing pexy may occur with ileus from persistent hypocalcemia and, if the cow is otherwise stable and can be closely monitored, IV calcium may resolve the problem. However, reexploration is indicated in other cases of left or right-sided pings if the cow is to remain in the herd. A right paramedian approach for abomasopexy is the current preferred method for stabilization in the case of redisplacement after a failed omentopexy. In those cases, it is not necessary to release any remaining omentopexy from the right flank approach to be able to perform an abomasopexy. Occasionally an incisional infection will develop into a large abscess and produce a right-sided ping that must be differentiated from an RDA or RVA (Chapter 10.8).

Pyloropexy A right paralumbar fossa pyloropexy may be performed alone or used in conjunction with an omentopexy to stabilize the abomasum. The pyloropexy is a more secure, direct fixation method; however, one should be aware that the risk of penetration of the lumen may be slightly greater than with a right paramedian abomasopexy because the mucosa in the pyloric area is more adherent to the submucosal area. Several methods can be used to perform a pyloropexy. Methods differ by the location of suture placement in the abomasum or pylorus and in the incision or body wall. A common form of pyloropexy involves placement of 1 or 2 sutures through all muscle layers and the peritoneum cranioventral to the incision and in a cruciate pattern through the thick torus pyloricus muscle. Sutures are tied subcutaneously. The omentum caudal to the pylorus can then be included in the incisional closure as described for right flank omentopexy. When a pyloropexy is performed without omentopexy, sutures placed in the pyloric antrum may be directly incorporated in the incisional closure. The pylorus is identified as described above. The site of the pyloropexy should be at least 5 cm proximal to the pylorus to prevent secondary stenosis. After slipping the mucosa away from the seromuscular layer, a penetrating towel clamp or Lahey thyroid forceps are placed 5 cm proximal to the pylorus in the seromuscular layer of the pyloric antrum (see Figure 10.4-10). A second clamp is placed 10 cm proximal to that one. With these two clamps, the portion of pylorus to be used in the pexy is placed in the ventral aspect of the incision. A suture is placed to reappose the tranversus abdominal muscle and peritoneum. The next bite of this continuous suture line incorporates the portion of the abomasum identified by the clamps. Before each bite is placed into the abomasum, the mucosa is "slipped" away from the seromuscular layer to prevent inadvertent penetration of the lumen and its potentially disastrous consequence.

Prognosis and Complications Reports that describe the technique and outcome of right flank pyloropexy, with or without omentopexy, are limited, although the procedure is fairly common in certain areas of North America. In one randomized study that compared a modified pyloropexy with toggle-pin fixation for treatment of LDAs, 23 of 35 (65.7%) cows in the pyloropexy group remained in the herd 120 days after surgery, in comparison to 29 of 37 (78.3%) treated by toggle pin. Anecdotal reports suggest that using a pyloropexy decreases the risk of redisplacement in comparison to omentopexy alone; however, controlled comparisons are lacking. Potential complications include peritonitis (localized or diffuse), redisplacement, and physical or functional interference with motility at the pyloroduodenal juncture.

Right Paramedian Abomasopexy The right paramedian approach provides the most direct access to the greatest surface area of the abomasum, and an aboma-sopexy theoretically allows a more secure stabilization of the abomasum than an omentopexy or a pyloropexy. In addition, the fundus is the more important part of the abomasum to secure; this area distends first and leads to the displacement. The tendency of the abomasum to return to normal position once the cow is in dorsal recumbency reduces the need for abomasal manipulation and decreases the risk of iatrogenic omental or serosal trauma. The proximity of the abomasum to the incision makes this approach possible for the smallest surgeon and largest cow. It is the approach most likely to allow safe correction of a left displacement with concurrent adhesions. The right paramedian abomasopexy is usually the preferred procedure to stabilize a failed omentopexy or pyloropexy. Although available personnel and facilities will occasionally make dorsal recumbency difficult to safely achieve or maintain, experience and judicious use of tranquilizers make this approach viable in most settings. The paramedian incision scar is not apparent in the standing cow, and owners who have cosmetic concerns may prefer this approach. Finally, an added benefit of this technique (for the cow but not necessarily the adjacent surgeon) is spontaneous drainage of purulent fluid from the uterus in cows with metritis.

The need for dorsal recumbency does add to the requirements for restraint and may not be appropriate if help is unavailable or if facilities or equipment for restraint in this position are limited. Dorsal recumbency also places an added strain on the cow's cardiopulmonary system (see Closed Procedures) and would be contraindicated in cows that will not safely tolerate this position, including those with pneumonia, hypotension, a distended rumen, a heavily gravid uterus, or major musculoskeletal problems that may be exacerbated during casting or recovery. Injury during recovery is a possibility that can be minimized by picking a site with good footing, allowing the cow to take its time to stand after returning to sternal recumbency, and judicious use of hobbles in cows with signs of hypocalcemia or preexisting musculoskeletal disorders. This approach also provides very limited access to other structures in the abdomen and is not indicated if a more complete exploration is needed. The presence of periparturient edema that extends cranial to the umbilicus will interfere with delineation of tissue layers and make closure more difficult; therefore the right paramedian approach should be avoided when ventral edema is extensive unless other options present more significant disadvantages. In some freestall housing conditions, the amount of fecal contamination may make an adequate clip and preparation extremely difficult to achieve. The procedure does require the surgeon to kneel and may be physically challenging for individuals with knee or back problems.

Preparation The procedure can be performed without withholding food or water in cows that have been anorexic. However, a fasting period (24 to 36 hours) may be considered if the cow's rumen is distended or a complicated procedure is anticipated (i.e., suspected ulcers, previous attempt at fixation, etc.). Withholding food will exacerbate any existing ketosis and supplementation with IV dextrose may be necessary. Prophylactic antibiotics should be considered before surgery. If possible, clipping the cranioventral abdomen before casting the cow will decrease the time in dorsal recumbency and decrease respiratory stress. The right paramedian area should be examined for scars that might indicate previous surgery. Large vessels in this area can make hemorrhage a problem.

The cow must be positioned and restrained in dorsal recumbency. In a field setting, this can be done by casting the cow and rolling it with its left side against a wall, fence-line or other stable structure, or by rolling the cow into a ditch or gutter padded with bedding that is deep enough to limit lateral movement. Hay bales can be used to limit rolling at the withers but used alone are usually not adequate. With either option, the front and hind limbs should also be tied in an extended position. A sedative such as xylazine HCl (0.05-0.1 mg/kg IV), acepromazine (0.025-0.075 mg/kg IV) or butorphanol tartrate (0.0025-0.005 mg/kg IV or IM) can be administered to help cast the cow and minimize struggling. Xylazine is the most commonly used sedative. Sedation is not mandatory unless the individual cow in question is fractious or the facilities available for restraint are limited. The benefits of improved restraint must be weighed against the undesirable tendency of xylazine to produce ruminal atony and stimulate uterine contractions. Xylazine is not recommended for use in the last trimester of pregnancy in cattle because of its uterine stimulatory effects. However, it is extremely useful in cattle that are difficult to handle. Analgesia can be achieved with an "L" block or line block. The "L" block is preferred because it minimizes swelling at the actual site of the incision. The "L" should extend from ventral midline 1 to 2 cm caudal to the xiphoid process, laterally to the right 5 to 8 cm and then continued caudally parallel to ventral midline and medial to the milk well and milk vein.

Procedure A 15- to 20-cm incision should be made parallel and 3 to 4 cm to the right of midline, extending caudally from a point 4 to 5 cm caudal to the xiphoid. The incision must be long enough to allow insertion of the surgeon's arm to the proximal humerus but not so long that it causes unnecessary hemorrhage or additional time in closure. In this location, the incision will be continued through six distinct layers: the skin, subcutaneous fascia (including the caudal deep pectoral muscles in the cranial $\frac{1}{3}$ of the incision), thick external fascia of the rectus sheath, rectus abdominus muscle (which can usually be separated rather than incised), thinner internal fascia of the rectus sheath, and peritoneum. A relatively large branch of the superficial epigastric vein often crosses the caudal half of this incision in the subcutaneous layer and should be ligated before transection if possible.

A quick but thorough exploration of the abdomen is strongly recommended before proceeding with abomasal repositioning and stabilization. This step can identify additional problems as well as adhesions or other situations that might interfere with abomasal repositioning. Adhesions should only be disturbed as necessary to restore the abomasum to its normal position.

Once exploration is complete, the surgeon can concentrate on identifying the abomasal regions and related structures. If the abomasum has returned to its normal position, the parietal serosal surface of the abomasum or its attached greater omentum will be the first structures observed deep to the peritoneum. The greater omentum attaches along the greater curvature of the abomasum and continues to the left of midline to completely cover the ventral sac of the rumen. The serosal surface of the abomasum can be followed caudally and dorsally along the right body wall as it narrows approaching the pylorus. The pylorus can be identified by the attachment of omentum on both sides and the palpable firmness of the torus pyloricus muscle. The pylorus is a common site for focal lymphosarcoma and should be carefully evaluated for enlargement or irregularities. Fat necrosis can also occur in the omentum surrounding the pylorus and interfere with abomasal outflow. In either case, masses in this region should be biopsied. If either lymphosarcoma or fat necrosis is present, the prognosis is poor, although it is theoretically possible to provide temporary relief by bypassing the pylorus with an abomasoduodenostomy (descending duodenum) via a subsequent right flank or right paracostal approach. After evaluation of the pylorus, the greater curvature of the abomasum should be followed cranially along the insertion of the greater omentum and reticuloabomasal ligament directly to the distinctively honeycombed reticulum positioned against the diaphragm. When following the greater curvature of the abomasum to the reticulum the parietal serosal surface of the abomasum should be visually and manually examined for scarring or thickening that might suggest previous or impending penetrating ulcers, focal bleeding ulcers, or lymphosarcoma. The location of the omasum dorsal to the body of the abomasum against the right body wall and the visceral surface of the liver should also be confirmed by palpation.

To find the abomasum, if it is not immediately obvious at the incision, the surgeon palpates cranially and then left and right along the diaphragm and body wall, while he or she checks for the smooth serosal surface of the abomasum and adhesions to the body wall that might be interfering with relocation of the abomasum. If the abomasum is still not identified, one returns to the reticulum and follows any connected structure to the left or right. Alternatively, an arm can be swept to the left and right and used to sweep any mobile structure to the midline. Finally, the location of the greater omentum is confirmed by beginning on the left side of the rumen and following it cranially and to the right to the next serosal surface. The greater omentum may be fragile and care should be taken not to tear it. Complete repositioning must be confirmed before suture placement by identifying the pylorus, the insertion of the greater omentum on the greater curvature of the abomasum, and identifying the ligament between the abomasum and reticulum.

Adhesions associated with an LDA are commonly a result of abomasal ulcers. Many focal adhesions can be broken down with careful manual pressure. Manipulation of adhesions is painful and analgesia will not be provided by standard local nerve blocks (see Section 10.9.1). Topical lidocaine applied with a lidocaine-soaked gauze sponge may decrease pain in some cases, but application to the specific areas needed is often difficult, and manual lysis is often performed without additional analgesia. If manual lysis is possible, the ulcer site should be pulled to the incision and oversewn. If manual lysis is not considered possible without risking abomasal penetration and the site is close enough to place a curved intestinal clamp across the ulcer site, the adhesion can be separated with Mayo scissors as close to the body wall as possible. The ulcer and clamp can then be drawn to the celiotomy incision to allow oversew of the ulcer. If the site is not accessible for safe lysis and oversew, one should consider leaving the site undisturbed and consider culling the cow. Indeed, transection of a fibrous abomasal adhesion is associated with significant morbidity. If the farmer chooses to pursue surgery to "free" the abomasum, it is done carefully. The goal is to dissect the weaker adhesions so only a fibrous core remains to hold the abomasum in place. Then the fibrous core is transected at the body wall; this procedure is done blindly with a large scissor with a long handle that is kept as close to the body wall as possible. As soon as the abomasum is released it is brought to the incision and any perforation is oversewn.

Adhesions localized around the cranial abdomen in the area of the reticulum may be associated with traumatic reticuloperitonitis (TRP). It may be possible to allow reposition of the abomasum without transecting the adhesions. If possible, the adhesions and reticulum should be palpated to identify any inciting foreign body. If the foreign body has partially penetrated the reticulum, it may be possible to extract it through the adhesions, although successful isolation through extensive adhesions is rarely possible. A small incision in the reticular wall can be used, if necessary, to facilitate foreign body removal.

Once the abomasum has been identified and all landmarks confirmed, the site for pexy should be identified. The optimum site for pexy is a 10- to 12-cm section on the serosal surface, 2 to 4 cm to the right of the insertion of the greater omentum and extending caudally from a site 5 to 8 cm caudal to the reticuloabomasal ligament. To locate the desired site, caudal tension is placed on the abomasum near its juncture with the greater omentum until the connection to the reticulum, often identified by the thin reticuloabomasal ligament, can be visualized or palpated. The site can be marked by placing towel clamps through the seromuscular layer of the abomasum at the cranial and caudal ends of the planned suture line.

Partial or total decompression of gas from the abomasum can facilitate manipulation, palpation, and suture placement if the abomasum is taughtly distended. A 14- to 16-gauge needle securely attached to a section of sterile tubing should be inserted at a shallow angle at the most dorsal site on the serosal surface of the abomasum, with the free end of the tubing held away from all sterile surfaces. Application of suction can speed the rate of decompression but is generally not necessary for an LDA.

The standard suture pattern for an abomasopexy is a simple continuous pattern initiated at the caudal aspect of the incision through the internal layer of the rectus sheath and peritoneum. Inclusion of the peritoneum is specifically indicated in this approach to enhance the stability of the adhesion at the incision (see Section 10.9.1). As the pattern is continued cranially the seromuscular layer of the abomasum should be incorporated in at least six subsequent bites with the peritoneum and internal fascia. Care should be taken to avoid penetrating the mucosa by pinching the abomasal wall with each bite and feeling the mucosa slip out of the fingers before suture placement in the abomasum. Towel clamps preplaced in the seromuscular layer to mark the site of the pexy can also help separate the seromuscular layer. While the caudal clamp must be removed after the first bite in the abomasum, the cranial clamp can be used to help elevate and depress the abomasum to facilitate suture placement. A no. 1- to no. 3-gauge nonabsorbable nonreactive suture material is recommended for the first layer of closure to establish the most permanent adhesion; monofilament such as nylon or polypropylene is preferable. Polyamide is frequently used even if it contains multiple strands because of its low cost. Polydiaxonone is also acceptable but economically less practical. As for omentopexy, more rapidly absorbed materials do not persist long enough to consistently cause a stable longterm adhesion and are not recommended. Braided and coated nonabsorbable materials will cause very stable adhesions in the healthy cow but carry an increased risk of infection or fistulation and are not recommended in the presence of peritoneal inflammation or remote infection. Particular care should be taken to avoid penetration of the lumen if a multifilament suture is used.

The remainder of the incision should be closed in 3 to 5 layers. Closure of the rectus abdominus muscle adds little strength to the incision but does close dead space and may facilitate closure of the next layer. A #1- to 2-gauge absorbable suture such as chromic gut in a continuous pattern is recommended for this layer. The external fascial layer is considered to be the most critical strength-holding layer in this incision, and particular attention should be paid to its closure. As a layer that is primarily dense connective tissue, slow return of maximum tensile strength can be expected. For this reason, a nonreactive nonabsorbable suture material may be most appropriate for this layer. However, high-tensile strength absorbable materials such as polyglycolic acid or polyglactin 910 are also commonly used. Choice of a suture pattern should reflect the quality of the tissue, tension on the incision, stability of the cow, and technical skill of the surgeon. An interrupted pattern is specifically recommended when the tissue is not holding sutures well and surgeon experience is not high. A continuous pattern is indicated when time is critical. Horizontal mattress patterns may be indicated when wound tension is high to help avoid suture pull out between the fibers of the external fascia. Otherwise, the choice may be personal preference. A separate subcutaneous layer, including any cutaneous muscle involved in the cranial aspect of the incision, should be added if the gap between fascia and skin is wide. Chromic gut (#0 or #1) is adequate for this layer. A nonabsorbable material is typically used for skin, with suture removal indicated 10 to 14 days after surgery.

A modification of the right paramedian abomasopexy uses 3 horizontal mattress sutures through the abomasal wall and the peritoneum and transverse abdominus muscle. These 3 sutures are placed lateral to the incision, and the incision is closed without inclusion of the abomasum. The modification was proposed to decrease the risk of fistulation because the abomasopexy is not part of the incision. This technique is more complicated and therefore not used routinely. At present, there is no objective information is available about whether this modified procedure is more or less successful than the more commonly used procedure described earlier.

Prognosis and Complications Reported initial success rates for cows treated by right paramedian abomasopexy range from 83.5% to 95%. Right paramedian abomsopexy is often considered the most stable fixation method for treating LDAs, although controlled comparisons with other treatment options are limited. Repeat surgeries for correction of abomasal redisplacement were more common after omentopexies than abomasopexies

in one study. Another study that compared 48 cows treated by abomasopexy and 52 treated by omentopexy in a randomized trial of LDAs found similar results for incisional complications, reproductive performance, and loss from the herd in follow-up at 1, 3, 6, and 12 months after surgery. Milk production was also similar, although a trend for better milk production at 1 month after surgery was noted for the right paramedian abomasopexy group.

Recognized complications after right paramedian abomasopexy include incisional hemorrhage, dehiscence, herniation or fistulation, redisplacement, and, rarely, intestinal or uterine volvulus associated with shifting of viscera during recovery from dorsal recumbency. Incisional hemorrhage is a common risk that results from the high vascularity of the ventral abdomen of lactating cattle. While in dorsal recumbency, vessels are under less pressure, and ligatures that appear adequate during closure may not maintain hemostasis as pressure increases in the standing cow. Although incisional hemorrhage can be significant, it can be controlled by a pressure wrap or stent and is rarely life-threatening. Acute dehiscence generally reflects technical failure (torn sutures, torn external rectus fascia, poor suture placement), whereas delayed dehiscence is more commonly associated with incisional infection (potentially caused by contamination from the abomasal lumen, ulcer related inflammation, or surgical contamination). Herniation involves loss of integrity of one or more incisional layers deep to the skin and occurs days to weeks after surgery as a consequence of dehiscence. *Fistulation* refers to the development of a patent track between the abomasal lumen and skin surface, and typically takes weeks to develop. Fistulation is most commonly attributed to placement of sutures, particularly multifilament nonabsorbable sutures, completely into the abomasal lumen. Leakage of abomasal fluid along the suture lines begins the development of a tract that progresses gradually toward the skin surface. Left untreated, the fistula enlarges, and the mucosal leaves of the abomasum herniate through the fistula (Figure 10.4-13). These abomasal leaves become ulcerated, and chronic blood loss can result in anemia. Body wall hernias without fistulae or signs of intestinal compromise can be left without treatment if economics warrants a more conservative approach. However, dehiscence and fistulation must be treated surgically if the cow is to be kept in the herd. Because of the loss of fluid, electrolytes, and blood, one should evaluate the blood gas and electrolyte status and perform a packed cell volume and total serum or plasma protein determination before surgical repair of an abomasal fistula. The surgical approach for treating incisional herniation, dehiscence, and fistulation is similar and is described later under Mechanical Obstructions (hernia-

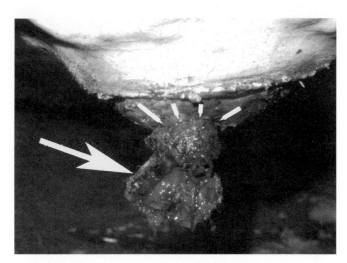

Figure 10.4-13 Cow with postabomasopexy fistula with herniation of abomasal leaves. Note edge of fistula (small arrows) and the herniated swollen abomasal leaves (large arrow) contaminated with bedding material.

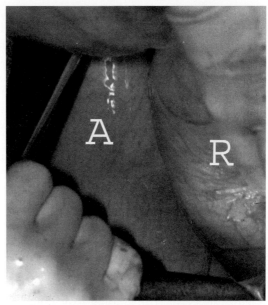

Figure 10.4-14 Standing left flank celiotomy to correct an LDA. Note the smooth contour of the abomasum (*A*, adjacent to the body wall, in comparison to the more axial rumen (*R*).

(Courtesy of Dr. Norm G. Ducharme; Cornell University.)

tion, dehiscence) and under ulcers and fistulation. In addition to local insision-related complications, one should remember the rare complications associated with placing a cow in dorsal recumbency—uterine torsion and small intestinal volvulus. The uncommon complication of uterine torsion is most likely to occur when the uterine mass is greatest and is therefore a greater risk in the last trimester of pregnancy. Intestinal volvulus is also a rare complication and appears to be a spontaneous event that would be difficult to predict or prevent, but cows with ileus and distended small intestine may be more at risk.

Redisplacement after right paramedian abomasopexy is uncommon and generally reflects improper technique, including use of absorbable suture material with premature absorption, suturing of the greater omentum rather than the seromuscular layer, incomplete penetration of the seromuscular layer, or placement of too few sutures leading to suture pull out. A repeat surgery that uses the same right paramedian approach is typically the preferred approach to correct a redisplacement after abomasopexy because it allows good access to release any remaining sutures and apparently provides greater stabilization.

Left Paralumbar Fossa (Flank) Abomasopexy The left flank abomasopexy provides the surgeon with some access to the greater curvature and parietal surface of the abomasum when it is in a left displaced position (Figure 10.4-14). The procedure provides the safety of a standing approach and in cows with adhesions secondary to ulcers and LDA may provide limited access to the greater curvature of the abomasum to permit adhesiolysis. This approach has been cited as the safest method of stabilization for left displacements in cows in the last trimester of pregnancy, although accurate repositioning can be

challenging and requires experience. It allows correction during performance of a left paralumbar fossa exploratory celiotomy if the clinician misidentified an LDA as a ruminal bloat. This is more likely to occur in cases of chronic LDA in yearling heifers. Although the need is uncommon, this approach is the only one that allows treatment of an LDA and traumatic reticuloperitonitis in one surgical episode. It is also a practical method of managing the even less common concurrent LDA and dystocia that require cesarean surgery. It is possible to evaluate a *postpartum* uterus and, to a limited extent, to facilitate drainage of purulent fluid by manual elevation and massage using the standing left flank approach.

The left flank approach provides poor access to intestinal structures distal to the abomasum and is not indicated if evaluation and possible manipulation of other structures is necessary. Adequate access to the abomasum for suture placement depends on a fairly dorsal displacement of the abomasum on the left; therefore this approach should not be considered if the ping is absent, relatively low (below midabdomen) or cranial (cranial to the tenth rib) on the left side at the time of surgery. *This approach is not indicated for right displacements of any kind.* Placement of the pexy sutures in the right paramedian area from the left flank approach requires a fairly long reach. While access can be improved by extending the flank incision further ventrally, an alternative fixation method may be preferable for surgeons with very short arms or in very large cows with deep abdominal cavities. A distended rumen will also increase the difficulty of suture placement and may be reason to consider another approach. Unlike other stabilization procedures, this approach requires a capable assistant to help with suture placement and stabilization to ensure both efficiency and asepsis. An untrained herdsman or other assistant can be prepared to perform these tasks, although the assistance of a trained technician is preferable.

Preparation Preparation is similar to that for a standing right flank omentopexy, with appropriate substitutions for the left-side approach. Prophylactic antibiotics should be considered if risk factors for infection are present. In addition, steps to prepare the assistant to aid in the procedure and to ensure correct and safe placement of the pexy sutures should be taken. If the assistant is knowledgeable about the relevant anatomy, minimal preparation is necessary. Otherwise, several steps should be taken to prepare the assistant, including explaining their role and placing a mark at the target sites for suture placement and a mark to indicate hazards including the right milk well and milk vein.

Procedure A 15- to 20-cm vertical incision should be made in the left flank 2 to 4 cm caudal to the last rib. The ventral aspect of the standard incision should be at the level of the caudoventral curve of the costochondral arch but can be extended more ventrally if the ping is relatively low, the cow large, or the surgeon's arms short.

The parietal surface of the greater curvature of the abomasum should be visible at the cranioventral aspect of the incision. The abomasal serosal surface faces the left body wall. The greater omentum attaches along the dorsal and caudal border of the visible abomasum (see Figure 14.1-1) and continues medially between the abomasum and the medially displaced rumen.

A straight needle should be threaded on each end of a 1- to 2-m length of #2 monofilament nonabsorbable suture. Suture with swaged on curved needles at both ends may also be used. One needle should be used to take 5 to 8 bites in a continuous pattern through the seromuscular layers of the parietal surface of the abomasum 2 to 3 cm away from but parallel to the attachment of the greater omentum and as far cranially on the abomasum as possible (Figure 10.4-15). The bites should be placed at the center of the suture segment, and two long ends of suture are left. The needle attached to the most cranial aspect of the suture line in the abomasum should be guarded in the right hand and carried ventrally along the left body wall to a site 3 to 4 cm to the right of the midline and 4 to 5 cm caudal to the sternum. The assistant can use the end of a syringe case pressed up against a premarked site to help the surgeon identify the appropriate site for needle placement. Once the surgeon reaches the desired site, they should push the needle

quickly through the ventral body wall, where the assistant should grasp the needle with a hemostat, pull it completely through the ventral body wall, clamp it with a hemostat, and maintain moderate ventral tension.

After successful placement of the cranial suture, the procedure should be repeated with the needle on the caudal end of the suture, taking care to avoid crossing sutures or perforating omentum or other viscera that can be present on the ventral body wall. Once both suture ends have been passed through the ventral body wall and stabilized with hemostats by the assistant, the surgeon can decompress the gas from the abomasum with a 10- to 14-gauge needle with attached tubing. The surgeon should then manually push the abomasum to the ventral body wall as the assistant maintains tension on the sutures. The assistant, if skilled in tying surgical knots, should place the first throw on the knot while the surgeon confirms that the abomasum is pulled firmly to the ventral body wall without any entrapped tissue. The assistant can then complete the knot. If the assistant is not skilled in tying surgical knots, he or she should make a simple throw on a knot and clamp the throw with a hemostat. The surgeon can complete the knot after closing the incision.

Closure of the incision is routine. If prophylactic antibiotics were administered before surgery, no postoperative antibiotics are indicated. To avoid fistulation, exposed suture must be cut and allowed to retract into the abdomen once a stable adhesion has been allowed to form but before the process of fistulation has begun—optimally between 14 and 21 days after surgery.

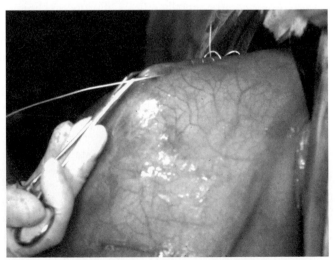

Figure 10.4-15   Standing left flank celiotomy to correct an LDA. A continuous pattern is placed through the seromuscular layers of the parietal surface of the abomasum 2 to 3 cm from the attachment of the greater omentum.

(Courtesy of Dr. Susan L. Fubini; Cornell University.)

Prognosis and Complications Less information is available on the success rate of the left flank abomasopexy than for other techniques. The most commonly recognized complications of this technique are accidental damage to the milk vein, entrapment of omentum or small intestine between the abomasum and the ventral body wall, and improper positioning of the abomasum leading to partial outflow obstruction. Structures, particularly omentum, can be easily caught by the needle as the surgeon passes it blindly from the incision to the ventral body wall, or trapped between the abomasum and ventral body wall between the two sutures as the abomasum is pulled down. Structures may also be trapped between abomasum and ventral body wall if the abomasum is allowed to slip back away from the ventral body wall before it is tied. Redisplacement can occur if the sutures break, are placed in the omentum rather than the seromuscular layer, or pull through the abomasal wall. The risk of suture breakage increases when a clamp is used to stabilize the suture ventral to the abdomen in an area that will be involved in the knot. An inadequate number of bites in the abomasal wall or failure to pull the abomasum snugly to the ventral body wall increases the risk of suture pullout. Suture pullout can also result in localized or generalized peritonitis. Abomasal fistulation is of particular risk if multifilament nonabsorbable sutures are used to penetrate the mucosa. Proper technique and release of sutures 2 to 3 weeks after surgery can minimize the risk of these complications. In the author's experience, this technique has one of the steepest learning curves.

Abomasal Displacements to the Right (RDA and RVA): General Considerations

Definition and Incidence When the abomasum dilates on the right side of the cow, it has the potential to float dorsally with a relatively flat (Figure 10.4-16) or folded

(Figure 10.4-17) lesser omentum (RDA), or to twist on the lesser omentum that supports it, creating an abomasal volvulus (RVA; Figure 10.4-18). Historical descriptions of the RVA referred to it as an abomasal *torsion*. However, the omental attachments prevent the abomasum from twisting around its own luminal axis as would be required for a torsion, and the term **volvulus** more accurately describes the condition.

The direction and amount of twist necessary to be considered a volvulus have been much discussed and are a source of much confusion. It is most accurate to describe the process as a volvulus of the abomasum and

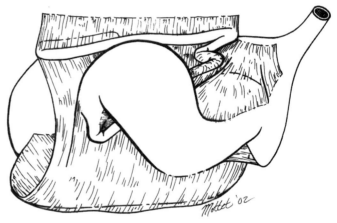

Figure 10.4-17   As gas accumulates in the abomasum, the abomasal body may float dorsally along the right body wall.

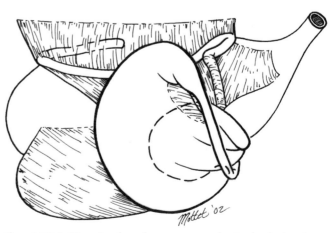

Figure 10.4-18   As the abomasum and attached structures rotate in a counterclockwise direction around an axis through the center of the lesser omentum, the cranial duodenum becomes trapped by the distended abomasal body, either between the abomasal fundus and omasum or more cranially between the omasum and reticulum.

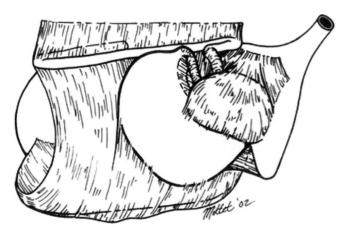

Figure 10.4-16   As gas accumulates in the abomasum, the pyloric antrum may begin to move dorsally.

attached structures around an axis through the center of the lesser omentum on which they are suspended. A volvulus can only occur around the center axis in the lesser omentum in a clockwise or counterclockwise direction relative to the fixed points along the dorsal border of the lesser omentum. The vast majority of cases of abomasal volvulus occur in a counterclockwise direction. In most cases, the duodenum becomes trapped ventrally between the cranial aspect of the abomasum and the omasum, and aside from some medial and ventral displacement, the omasum is relatively uninvolved (see Figure 10.4-18). In some cases the cranial duodenum is actually entrapped ventrally between the omasum and reticulum. In these cases the omasum is clearly displaced medial to the abomasum, and the reticulum is pulled caudally, craniomedial to the abomasal body (see Figure 10.4-18). In either case, the weight of fluid in the abomasal body and fundus is sufficient to prevent the duodenum from sliding free caudal to the abomasum.

The amount of twist necessary to be a volvulus is also a common topic for debate. Technically, any degree of rotation around the lesser omentum could be called a volvulus. The real question is not the number of degrees of rotation but whether the positional change will produce complete luminal obstruction and irreversible neurovascular damage if left uncorrected. Once the change in position has progressed to the point at which the abomasum cannot fall back into its normal position even after excessive gas has been relieved, it may be presumed to be at risk of permanent damage. From the surgeon's perspective, this allows a functional definition based on the ability or inability of the surgeon to correct the displacement after gas decompression by placing direct caudodorsal traction on the greater omentum from a point ventral to the descending duodenum. If the displacement cannot be corrected by traction (barring adhesions or entrapment), then the rotation has been sufficient to entrap the duodenum, complete outflow obstruction has occurred, neurovascular compromise is probable, and, if left uncorrected, progressive rotation and death are essentially ensured.

An accurate comparison of the incidence of RDA to RVA is hampered by the overlap of clinical parameters in affected animals, making *ante mortem* differention of the two conditions, without surgical exploration, impossible. The variations in definition and application of diagnostic criteria used during surgery also make the differentiation difficult. In a review of case records at a single institution using a uniform set of surgical/*post mortem* criteria, 280 cases of RVA and 123 cases of RDA were identified and suggested a ratio of approximately 2 to 1. The tendency to refer more compromised cases and the potential for an RDA to progress to an RVA during the time between on-farm diagnosis and arrival at a referral

institution may result in a higher ratio of RVA to RDA in this study that used referral centers than would be expected in practice.

Displacements to the right (including both RDAs and RVAs) are far less common in dairy cows than those to the left. In a comparison with RVAs only, left displacements were found to be 7 times more common in a large North American multiinstitute study. Like LDAs, right-sided disorders (RDAs and RVAs) are more commonly identified in dairy cows than in dairy bulls, beef cattle, or calves of any breed. Abomasal volvulus specifically was found to be more common in dairy than in beef cattle (adjusted odds ratio of 36.4) and more common in female than male cattle (adjusted odds ratio of 3.3).

Predisposing Factors Although less information on predisposing factors for RDAs and RVAs is available, the etiopathogenesis is considered similar to an LDA. Factors that alter abomasal motility and lead to gas accumulation also presumably predispose to displacement to the right. Reports of RVA, like those of LDA, show that cases are more likely in the first two weeks after parturition (28.3% of cases), although cases are generally more evenly distributed across the rest of the lactation period. Both abomasal volvulus and LDA develop most commonly between 4 and 7 years of age, although volvulus is relatively more common than LDA in cattle less than 1 year of age. The normal position of the abomasum on or slightly to the right of midline (as well as the normal weight and position of the rumen) presumably makes displacement to the right the easier path outside of the periparturient period. Concurrent diseases (such as ketosis, uterine diseases, mastitis and pneumonia) are also found commonly in cattle with abomasal volvulus. Perforating ulcers with adhesions are less common in cows with right abomasal displacements than in those with LDAs. Two of 21 cases of concurrent abomasal displacement and perforating ulcers involved right-sided displacements. In contrast to LDAs, abomasal volvulus occurs most commonly in January.

Diagnosis Cows with either an RDA or RVA typically present to the herdsman with signs very similar to those described for LDAs (i.e., partial or complete anorexia, decreased milk production, and decreased fecal output with altered consistency [fluid or pasty]). However, in the case of an RVA, the progression of signs may be very rapid and a subset of affected cows will first present to the herdsman with signs of severe depression, anorexia, and dehydration.

The presence of a tympanic area (ping) centered over the tenth to 13th ribs and on a line from elbow to tuber coxae is the primary diagnostic sign of an RDA or RVA. This ping must be differentiated from other sources of right-sided pings that include cecal dilation/torsion, gas accumulation in the duodenum, spiral colon, ascending colon or small intestine, or right flank abscess. An abomasal ping can generally be differentiated from pings associated with other structures by combining information about ping location, size and pitch. The cecum, colon, and small intestine are limited in their mobility by their mesenteric attachments to the dorsal body wall while the abomasum and ascending duodenum are limited by more cranial attachments at the duodenal sigmoid flexure and the reticular connection to the diaphragm. Cecal, colonic, and small intestinal pings will be centered on a point in the paralumbar fossa, more caudal than that for the abomasum or duodenum. The cecum is the only structure that has the potential to dilate to a size comparable to the abomasum and is the primary differential for single-pitched pings greater than 10 cm in diameter. In addition to differentiation by locating the ping, the cecum is usually palpable by examination per rectum while the abomasum rarely distends far enough caudally to be palpable, and if it does, it is attainable by fingertips only. Small intestinal pings are typically a collection of small-diameter pings of varying pitch. Spiral colon pings also tend to involve multiple areas that vary in pitch. The cranial and descending sections of the duodenum can accumulate gas and may ping at or dorsal to the location for an abomasal ping, although the maximum diameter of a ping the duodenum can produce is about 10 cm.

Preoperative differentiation with any degree of reliability between RDA and RVA is difficult in an individual animal. Although severe electrolyte disturbances are more typical of abomasal volvulus, the size of the ping and degree of most fluid imbalances overlap, with both conditions associated with dehydration and a hypochloremic, hypokalemic, hyponatremic metabolic alkalosis. Prolonged RDAs can produce severe fluid and electrolyte disturbances, while early RVAs may have relatively mild disturbances. Some disturbances tend to follow a progression that reflects the severity of disease, but overlap is possible. In a study that included RDAs and RVAs, the following parameters on average reflected the progression of disease: decreasing body temperature, increasing heart rate, hyponatremia, and anion gap. In severe cases of volvulus, tissue ischemia and necrosis can produce a metabolic acidosis that superimposes on the metabolic alkalosis common to abomasal outflow obstructions. As a result, the blood pH, chloride, and potassium values may return toward normal in the most severe cases of volvulus, even in the face of a very high anion gap. Definitive diagnosis can only be made by exploratory or *post mortem*. The difficulty of differentiating between RDA and RVA preoperatively, the potential risk that an RDA will progress to an RVA given time, and the difference in prognosis should a volvulus develop are all reasons to support surgical exploration within

several hours after identifying any right-sided abomasal ping.

General Treatment Considerations Treatment options must take into account the possibility of either an RDA or RVA, and the risk of rapid and potentially uncorrectable deterioration if treatment is delayed when a volvulus is present. If treatment is to be pursued, surgical intervention for definitive diagnosis and position correction is essential. Two different approaches allow correction and stabilization of an RDA or RVA in adult cattle. The standing right-flank omentopexy or pyloropexy is the most universally effective approach for adult cows with right-sided pings consistent with RDA or RVA and provide optimal access for abomasal evaluation, decompression, and position correction with minimal stress on the cow. Some information suggests that adult cows with RDA or RVA treated by right-paramedian abomasopexy may have better in-hospital survival than those treated by right flank omentopexy. The right paramedian abomasopexy can also be used if a cow cannot stand for the right flank approach. One should avoid right paramedian abomasopexy in very sick animals with ruminal distension because of the risk of regurgitation and the added stress of compromising ventilation with the animal in dorsal recumbency.

Some evidence suggests that, regardless of approach, redisplacement is more common after surgical correction of displacements to the right than after surgical correction of LDAs. Redisplacement is more likely to occur on the same side as the original displacement. Medical management of fluid and electrolyte disturbances in conjunction with surgery is a critical part of management.

Regardless of the approach selected, thorough preoperative evaluation is necessary to identify concurrent conditions that might affect the approach selection or interfere with the success of surgery. Specific evaluation for conditions that may have predisposed to altered abomasal motility—such as hypocalcemia, endotoxemia, and ketosis—is indicated. Correction of hypocalcemia, ketosis, and other fluid imbalances is initiated before surgery, if possible. Fluid therapy is similar to that described for LDAs earlier, although disturbances may be greater and more aggressive therapy is frequently needed. Preoperative prophylactic antibiotics are indicated due to the risk of ischemic injury.

Abomasal Displacements to the Right (RDA and RVA): Specific Procedures

Right Flank Omentopexy/pyloropexy The preparation and approach for a right flank omentopexy is as described above for LDA. In addition to the standard surgical equipment and a 10- to 14-gauge needle with attached tubing needed for an LDA, a 3- to 6-cm diameter sterile stomach tube should be available in case fluid decompression of the abomasum is necessary.

Procedure A standing right flank approach is performed, as previously described for the LDA. The distended abomasum will be the first structure encountered after the peritoneum is incised, and care must be taken to avoid accidental incision during the approach.

The first step in correcting the displacement is to determine if the abomasum is simply dilated and/or displaced, or if a volvulus has occurred. First locate the greater omentum ventral to the descending duodenum and place caudal tension on the omentum by walking hand over hand along the omentum in a cranial direction. If the abomasum is dilated and displaced dorsally without volvulus it will usually be possible to follow the omentum directly to a site of attachment on the greater curvature of the pylorus or abomasum. Occasionally the displaced abomasum will be too distended to allow the surgeon to follow the greater omentum all of the way from the descending duodenum to its attachment to the pylorus without decompression. However, inability to follow the omentum to the abomasum or pylorus after decompression indicates the presence of a volvulus. Additional findings that suggest the presence of a volvulus include large amounts of fluid in the abomasum, medial displacement of the omasum, and caudal displacement of the reticulun medial to the abomasum. In a counterclockwise volvulus, the omentum will be pulled from the ventral descending duodenum into a taut narrow band as it passes cranioventrally (medial to the abomasum), and then ventral to the twist between the abomasoomasal (see Figure 10.4-18) or omasoreticular juncture, cranial to the distended abomasal body. In the case of a clockwise volvulus, the omentum will be pulled cranially, then lateral dorsal to the twist between the abomasum and omasum. The direction of the volvulus can be determined in many cases by placing the left hand palm down on top of the omentum with fingers in two folds of the omentum and following the omentum forward. If it is a counterclockwise volvulus, the hand will be forced to turn clockwise, with thumb down. The reverse will occur with a clockwise volvulus. The direction the hand is forced to turn is the direction that the abomasum must be pushed to correct the volvulus.

Reducing the size of the abomasum is occasionally necessary to differentiate between an RDA and RVA and almost always to allow safe repositioning. In most cases of RDA and RVA, the abomasum is primarily distended with gas and can be decompressed with a needle and attached tubing as described for LDA. However, it is important to remove the fluid from an abomasum that is primarily distended before all the gas is removed. If gas is removed first, the abomasum tends to fall ventrally, making access for fluid removal difficult and greatly increasing the potential for peritoneal contamination. Fluid should be removed by first placing a 4- to 7-cm diameter circular purse string suture in the exposed serosal surface of the abomasum at a location as far dorsal to the ventral aspect of the paralumbar fossa incision as possible. A high–tensile strength, low–tissue drag suture material, such as polyglactin 910 or polydiaxonone, is indicated. After the purse string suture first throw is placed, a stab incision is made in the center of the purse string pattern. A 3- to 6-cm diameter sterile stomach tube is quickly inserted through the stab incision into the abomasum while the purse string suture is tightened to minimize leakage. The surgeon or assistant should place his or her left arm ventral to the abomasum to help maintain elevation of the site during drainage. Fluid should be siphoned from the abomasum until flow ceases or the site of tube insertion begins to fall ventral to the incision. When this occurs, the tube should be kinked to reduce backflow and removed from the abomasum while the purse string is tightened. Gross debris should be removed from the area of the purse string if possible, the purse string tied, and the site of the purse string oversewn with an absorbable suture material. If gas distension still prevents repositioning, gas decompression should be performed with needle and tubing.

Once an RDA or RVA has been decompressed, the surgeon should attempt to expose the pylorus by placing caudodorsal tension on the greater omentum. If the pylorus cannot be exteriorized at the incision by this process, an RVA is confirmed and manual correction will be necessary. The process of correcting a dilatation is the same as a volvulus, except that it is much easier. The goal is to push the abomasal body manually in the correct direction to free the cranial duodenum and pylorus. The direction the dilated abomasal body should be moved is indicated by the direction the surgeon's hand turns during the omentum examination, the same as a volvulus. If in doubt, the surgeon should assume the counterclockwise volvulus occurred, the most common direction. To correct a counterclockwise volvulus, the surgeon should place the left arm medial to the abomasal body as far cranially as possible and dorsal to the path of the greater omentum (Figure 10.4-19A). Keeping all fingers together with the palm facing laterally against the dilated abomasal body, the palm and heel of the left hand should be used to rock the dorsal aspect of the abomasal body in a large loop, first laterally, then ventrally and caudally (Figures 10.4-19B and C). A long, sweeping motion is usually most effective. Several tries may be necessary. This method works well for the more common volvulus in which the pylorus and duodenum pass between abomasum and omasum but may not be effective when the duodenum is entrapped cranial to the omasum. If no progress has been made after 3 to 4 tries, a change to the second approach is indicated. In this approach, the left hand is placed medial and ventral to the abomasum and ventral to the omasum, which will have been drawn medially by the volvulus. In a volvulus,

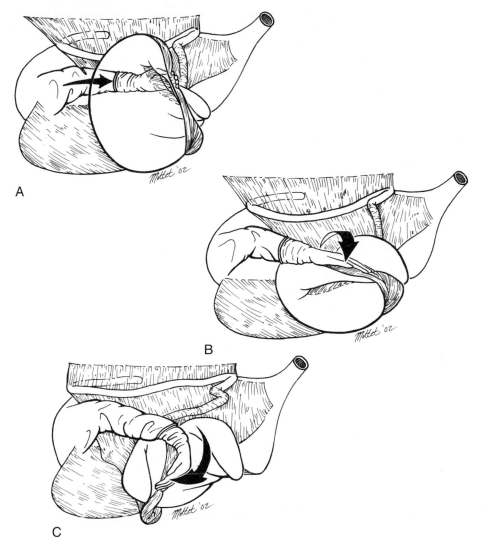

Figure 10.4-19   Correction of a counterclockwise abomasal volvulus by abomasal manipulation from a right paralumbar fossa approach. A counterclockwise abomasal volvulus can be corrected by placing the left forearm medial to the distended abomasal body (*A*) and rocking the distended body laterally, ventrally (*B*), and finally caudally (*C*) to free the duodenum from its site of entrapment ventral to the abomasoomasal juncture. Once freed, the greater omentum can be traced from the descending duodenum to the pylorus.

the omasum tends to accumulate more fluid than usual, but its thick walls still make it distinguishable by palpation. With the left hand and arm placed medial to the abomasum and ventral to the omasum, the omasum should be lifted dorsally and cranially toward the diaphragm (Figure 10.4-20). This typically frees the duodenum and allows exposure of the pylorus when tension is placed on the greater omentum. After repositioning the omasum, the abomasal body can be rocked cranially, then ventrally and caudally, to return it to normal position (see Figure 10.4-19).

Clockwise volvulus is relatively uncommon, and descriptions of correction procedures are limited; however, the principles of correction are similar to those used to correct a counterclockwise volvulus. After fluid and/or gas decompression have been completed, the surgeon should attempt to expose the pylorus by placing caudodorsal tension on the greater omentum. If unsuccessful, the surgeon should place their left or right arm between the dorsal aspect of the abomasal body and right body wall. The palm should face the abomasum while cupping the cranial aspect of the abomasal body. With the palm and forearm, the dorsal aspect of the body should be rocked medially then ventrally and laterally.

After the duodenum has been freed and the pylorus exteriorized by traction on the greater omentum, the remaining landmarks should be checked as described above for LDA. The pylorus, greater omentum, parietal

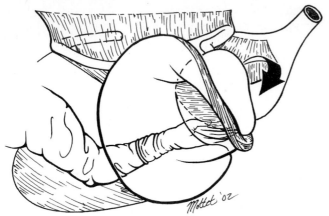

Figure 10.4-20   Correction of counterclockwise abomasal volvulus by omasal manipulation from a right paralumbar fossa approach. As a second method for correcting a counterclockwise abomasal volvulus, the surgeon can place his or her left forearm ventral to the omasum in its position medial to the abomasum and then lift the omasum dorsally and then laterally. This method is particularly valuable for correcting a volvulus where the cranial duodenum is entrapped between the omasum and reticulum but can also be a valuable tool for managing the more common form of volvulus (Figure 10.4-18). This method may be combined with abomasal manipulation as described in Figure 10.4-19.

abomasal surface, reticulum, and omasum should each be identified and evaluated for correct location and freedom from lesions. The greater omentum should be carefully inspected for any tears that may have occurred as a result of the volvulus or from efforts to reposition the abomasum (see Figure 10.4-11). Incomplete tears through one of the two serosal surfaces can and should be left without closure. Full-thickness tears should be closed with an absorbable material to protect the vasculature to the greater curvature and prevent entrapment of small intestine in the rent. Once all landmarks have been identified and evaluated, an omentopexy/pyloropexy can be performed as described above for an LDA. In some cases the omentum has been so severely traumatized that an omentopexy is not advised; therefore pyloropexy is performed. Alternatively, performance of a right paramedian abomasopexy 24 hours later may be the best method of stabilization for cows with long-term value. Incisional closure is as described above for LDA.

Right Paramedian Abomasopexy   The preparation and approach is as described earlier for an LDA. When a cow or bull is positioned in dorsal recumbency, the unsupported ventral body wall caudal to the rib cage collapses dorsally, and viscera are more difficult to distinguish and manipulate. In addition, the relationship of structures is less familiar to most veterinarians from this approach. Nonetheless, identification of key landmarks is critical

for successful diagnosis and correction of abomasal displacement disorders to the right. Decompression is usually mandatory to allow accurate evaluation and repositioning.

If the abomasum is displaced without a volvulus, it will often return to its normal position once the cow is placed in dorsal recumbency. In this case, the surgeon will encounter a gas-distended viscus immediately deep to the peritoneum. After gas is removed from the viscus, it will be possible to identify the reticulum cranially at the diaphragm and trace from the reticulum caudally along the greater curvature of the abomasum (marked by the attachment of the greater omentum) to the pylorus as described for LDA. The firmer omasum should be palpable but not visible dorsal to the abomasum and against the right body wall. A brief but thorough exploration of the accessible parts of the abdomen should be completed before performing an abomasopexy.

If a volvulus is present, following a direct and continuous path from reticulum along the greater curvature to the pylorus will be impossible. With a counterclockwise volvulus, the surgeon will first encounter either the serosal surface of the abomasum or the greater omentum covering the abomasum deep to the peritoneum. The reticulum will often be pulled caudally, medial to the abomasum. The distended body of the abomasum will fill the right side of the abdomen. The descending duodenum will cross the ventral aspect of the right abdomen but be buried between the abomasum and omasum or between the omasum and rumen ventral to the caudally pulled reticulum.

In most cases gas decompression alone provides enough room and flexibility to manually correct the volvulus. The goal is to shift the fluid from the abomasum to the pylorus: this can be done in multiple ways. The surgeon places the right hand palm up, fingers together, underneath the abomasum and attempts to rock the abomasum forward and toward the incision; this should move some fluid through the duodenum and lessen the weight of the abomasum. Significant effort is needed here. An alternative option is to grasp the duodenum with the left hand and move it laterally and dorsally so it is lower than the fluid level in the abomasum. A third method involves applying pressure on the omasum toward the dorsum of the cow (slightly caudally); this will transfer pressure to the abomasum so it either rocks forward or its fluid content moves ventrally toward the duodenum. A combination of these techniques is needed and it may be necessary to extend the incision so that both arms can be used. The right arm pushes the omasum caudally and the left arm rocks the abomasum out of the incision. If correction is not obtained, one can drain the abomasum similarly to what is described in the standing approach. The key difference is the duodenum is the only available structure (the abomasum is against the dorsal body wall). The duodenum is easily elevated to the incision, and a purse string is placed as previously described. A stomach tube is then passed into the duodenum through the pylorus and on into the abomasum, so the fluid can be evacuated.

After correction of the volvulus, all of the landmarks described for the right paramedian approach to LDAs previously described should be evaluated to ensure correct repositioning. Tears in the greater omentum are possible and should be managed as described above in the right-flank approach. Debris from fluid decompression should be carefully removed before placing the abomasopexy layer, as described for LDAs. Additionally, a water-soluble antibiotic can be used to lavage the incisional layers. Closure of the remaining incisional layers is as described for LDAs.

Abomasal Displacements to the Right (RDA and RVA): General Postoperative Care Regardless of the approach used, the cow should be carefully monitored after surgery. Return to normal water and feed consumption after treatment of an RVA is expected to be slower than with RDAs and LDAs. Continuous fluid therapy is often necessary to fully restore normal hydration and electrolyte balances. If preexisting infection or contamination was found or excessive contamination occurred during surgery, a therapeutic course of antibiotic therapy should be initiated after surgery until at least 3 days after the last clinical sign (3 days after surgery if signs do not occur). Analgesics may improve comfort and speed return to feed.

General Prognosis and Complications The prognosis for survival and return to productive function with right-sided complications is largely determined by the degree of tissue damage, which is in turn a reflection of the amount and duration of the volvulus. Complications related to tissue damage include those associated with direct tissue damage (abomasal perforation, peritonitis, septicemia, omental tearing) and persistent abomasal neuromuscular dysfunction (decreased or altered abomasal motility, intermittent bloat, dehydration, electrolyte disturbances, poor nutrient absorption, abomasal impaction). Complications related to the surgical procedure itself (redisplacement, malpositioning) are less significant in comparison to those associated with tissue damage but are still important considerations for the surgeon.

Adult cattle with a surgical diagnosis of RDA would be expected to have minimal vascular compromise and a favorable prognosis for short-term survival and return to successful production similar to that for cattle with LDAs. In one of the few studies that used a consistent surgical definition to differentiate between RDA and RVA, 99% of the 218 cows diagnosed with RDA were discharged from the hospital. Of those discharged, the majority (199; 92%) returned to their expected levels in attitude, feed consumption, fecal production, and milk production at the time of discharge. Information on long-term productivity in the herd was not collected in this study and is difficult to reliably isolate RDAs specifically from other studies. Long-term productivity similar to LDAs, if not better is expected because the concurrent diseases responsible for the majority of LDA losses from the cattle herd are less common in RDAs.

More information on short-term survival and long-term productivity is available for cows with RVA, although the variation in definitions used between and sometimes within, studies suggests the need for caution, particularly when interpreting data from multiple institutions, over extended periods of time, or both. One study reported a 99% short-term survival until discharge for cows with RDA, and 218 of 240 cows (91%) with a surgical diagnosis of RVA survived until discharge, making the in-hospital fatality rate 9%. Of the 218 that were discharged, only 147 (71%) were considered to have returned to their expected levels in attitude, feed consumption, fecal production, and milk production at the time of discharge. In another study of 100 surgically corrected RVAs that used a similar classification system, 18% died or were euthanatized before discharge; 14% were discharged but had not met expectations for feed intake, defecation, or milk production; and 68% had returned to expected levels before discharge. A multi-institutional study of veterinary teaching hospital admissions showed an even higher in hospital fatality rate of 23.5%, with an additional 15.7% of cattle discharged after surgery failing to become productive in the herd. Reported in-house fatality rates from several smaller studies of cows with abomasal volvulus ranged from 24% to 31%. Phone follow-up 1 to 6 months after surgical treatment of 80 cattle with right abomasal volvulus classified 59 (73.8%) as productive, 10 (12.5%) as salvaged for slaughter, and 11 (13.7%) as dead or euthanized by the time of follow-up.

The difference in survival rates is significant and must be considered before the decision to proceed with treatment is pursued. Despite the difficulty of preoperatively differentiating between RDA and RVA in an individual animal, several clinical and biochemical parameters can be used with caution as prognostic indicators. At least one study has shown the following biochemical parameters as predictive of nonsurvival due to death, euthanasia, or slaughter as a result of poor production: preoperative tachycardia (>100/min), dehydration (>6%), hypochloremia (<79 mEq/L), hyponatremia, hypokalemia, decreasing base excess, base excess plus serum lactate concentration, base excess plus hypochloremia, increasing anion gap, serum ALP greater than 100 IU/L, and superimposed metabolic acidosis with a high anion gap. Tissue ischemia and necrosis in cows with a prolonged or extremely tight volvulus can develop a concurrent metabolic acidosis. As a result, the blood pH returns toward normal, the anion gap increases and the base excess may fall into a negative range. These findings as a group are indicators of an extremely poor prognosis in adult cattle. Surgical findings that may be associated with a poor prognosis include a large volume of fluid in the abomasum that requires fluid decompression and serosal inflammation or necrosis.

Conversely, when cattle with RVA were divided into productive (expected appetite, weight, and milk production) and nonproductive (slaughtered for low production, died, or were euthanized) groups at follow-up 1 to 6 months after surgery, several factors were found to have significant positive predictive value for productivity. These factors included normal hydration status, serum creatinine ≤1.5 mg/dl, serum ALP activity ≤100 IU/L, serum Cl ≥95 mEq/L, and heart rate ≤80 beats/minute.

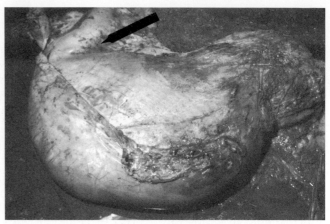

Figure 10.4-21   Abomasal impaction diagnosed on gross *post mortem* examination. Arrow points to the pyloric part of the abomasum.

(Courtesy of Dr. John King; Cornell University.)

Abomasal Outflow Obstructions

Abomasal outflow can be disrupted in a number of ways that do not involve displacement. These conditions are typically categorized as either mechanical or functional disturbances, based on the etiology. Classically, obstructions that result from an identifiable physical obstruction to aborad flow are classified as mechanical, while all others are believed to result from chemical or neurologic interference with normal motility and are considered functional. In practice, many cases of abomasal outflow obstruction involve both mechanical and functional mechanisms at some stage in their course. Effective management decisions require that all mechanisms be addressed.

Mixed Mechanical and Functional Obstructions: Abomasal Impaction   The term *impaction* is typically reserved to describe distention of a viscus beyond its normal volume with contents that have less fluid content than normal. This definition is consistent with the syndrome of abomasal impaction (Figure 10.4-21) as it is seen in cattle. However, the condition called *abomasal impaction* in sheep involves abomasal distention with contents varying in consistency from fluid to dry. It is likely that the term is used to describe two different conditions in the two species.

The abomasum can theoretically become impacted as a result of a variety of mechanical and neurologic etiologies. Potential mechanical causes include abnormal or dry luminal contents (hair, placenta, sand, gravel, and poor-quality roughage in the face of restricted water intake) that lodge in the pyloric region, mural lesions (lymphosarcoma, fibrosis) that prevent normal contraction and dilation of the pyloric antrum or cranial duodenum, and extraluminal lesions (adhesions, masses) that

distort or compress the abomasal outflow tract. Multiple cases of abomasal impaction have been identified during severe winter weather in range cattle with poor-quality roughage and limited access to water and in groups of cattle with high concentrations of indigestible materials, such as sand and gravel, in their diet. Sand and gravel impaction may be of particular risk in cattle maintained in dry lots with bunker silos and with limited access to fiber. Pregnant cattle near the end of gestation appear to be more commonly affected. Alternatively, lesions that might interfere with the normal function of the abomasum or coordination of orad and aborad flow at the pyloroduodenal juncture have been implicated in many cases without a clear initiating mechanical cause. These include vagal nerve irritation in the thoracic or abdominal cavity, focal mural lesions at key foci, peritoneal inflammation with secondary ileus, and direct nerve or neuromuscular damage after abomasal volvulus. Individual cases of impaction have been specifically linked with traumatic reticuloperitonitis, perforating abomasal ulcers, and abomasal volvulus. The wide range of proposed and confirmed etiologies suggests that multiple factors may result in a similar clinical result.

Clinical signs of abomasal impaction develop gradually and include right or bilateral ventral abdominal distention, progressive anorexia, decreased fecal production, and loss of condition. In some cases ruminal hypomotility with or without distention will also be present. The pulse rate may be normal or slow throughout much of the course, although an elevated rate has been reported in the terminal stage of the condition and is considered a poor prognostic sign. Dehydration may be mild to severe. Electrolyte disturbances vary from none to severe hypochloremic metabolic alkalosis with normal or decreased sodium and potassium. Metabolic

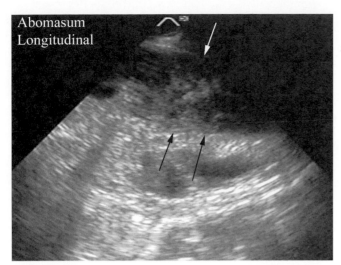

Figure 10.4-22 Longitudinal sonogram of the abomasum in an adult Holstein cow with a 3-2 MHz phased array sector probe. The wall of the abomasum is very thick (3.5 cm) and hypoechoic with loss of the normal layering. Necropsy confirmed the presence of lymphosarcoma within the abomasum.

(Courtesy of Dr. Amy Yeager; Cornell University.)

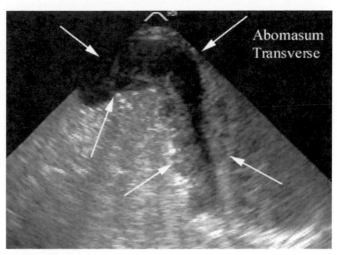

Figure 10.4-23 Transverse sonogram of the abomasum near the level of the pylorus in an adult Holstein cow with a 3-2 MHz phased array sector probe. Note the very thick hypoechoic wall with loss of discernable layers (arrows). Necropsy confirmed the presence of lymphosarcoma within the abomasum.

(Courtesy of Dr. Amy Yeager, Cornell University.)

acidosis can develop in chronic cases from starvation or tissue necrosis. Elevated anion gap and elevated ruminal chloride may also be present.

Abomasal impaction should be considered as a differential in cases with the clinical signs described and an appropriate history. However, diagnosis is often difficult to make in adult cattle without exploratory surgery. A firm distended viscus can often be detected by ballottement in the right paracostal region, although it may be difficult to differentiate with physical exam alone the impacted abomasum from a fetus in cattle in their last trimester of pregnancy. Ultrasound can be used to confirm the presence of the impacted viscus or a thickened abomasal wall, as seen in abomasal lymphosarcoma (Figures 10.4-22 and 10.4-23). In extreme cases, it may be possible to palpate the impacted abomasum in the right cranioventral abdomen, but in most cases the abomasum is not detectable by rectal palpation.

Cows with abomasal impaction have a guarded to poor prognosis. The prognosis worsens with the chronicity of the impaction and increasing age of the cow. The prognosis is poor to grave in cases for which the cause can be identified but not eliminated (lymphosarcoma, pyloric strictures) and in many cases for which a cause is never identified. Even in cases initiated by intraluminal materials that can be removed, severe prolonged distention can lead to abomasal perforation or permanent neuromuscular damage. However, some cases in the early stages of distention can be treated successfully by relieving distention and eliminating the cause.

Several options for managing abomasal impaction exist. Slaughter and euthanasia should be considered initially in all cases because of the relatively poor overall prognosis. If the owner considers the animal to be economically worth treatment, two basic approaches to management exist: medical management and surgical decompression.

Medical Management Medical management of early cases of abomasal impaction associated with intraluminal causes has been reported to be effective in a few cases and may be the only option available to manage multiple cases in herd outbreaks. However, a significant risk exists that reliance on medical management alone will delay surgical exploration to confirm the diagnosis and may delay more definitive treatment beyond the point of salvage. Prolonged administration of lubricants and stimulants in animals with untreatable etiologies such as lymphosarcoma is neither effective nor humane. No evidence suggests that lubricants administered per os or by stomach tube reach the abomasum in sufficient quantities to improve outflow. Motility stimulants alone have been reported to be unsuccessful and carry the risk of inducing a rupture if outflow is physically obstructed. The limited evidence of success is unsurprising in that materials administered orally in mature ruminants are unlikely to be transferred into the abomasum before deactivation in the rumen. Administration of intravenous fluids is an important tool in managing dehydration and electrolyte disturbances but will not in itself restore function and must be continued as long as the impaction persists. Metoclopramide (0.3 mg/kg subcutaneously 4 to 6 times daily) may improve ingesta movement through the pylorus.

Medical therapy may be a useful adjunct to surgical therapy in some cases. In addition to providing access for more specific diagnosis and possible therapy, surgical exploration provides the opportunity to establish a direct route of administration for parenteral agents into the abomasum. This can be done at the time of a rumenotomy by manually directing the distal end of a nasogastric tube through the reticuloomasal orifice and stabilizing the nasal end for continued infusion of lubricants (procedure description below). Better success has been anecdotally reported when lubricants (mineral oil, magnesium hydroxide, magnesium sulfate, dioctyl sodium sulfasuccinate) were introduced directly into the abomasum (or omasum) in small doses over an extended period of time. Use of neostigmine, cascara sagrada, carbamylcholine chloride, and a variety of systemic stimulants have been of some value in conjunction with the direct infusion of lubricants, but administration should be delayed at least 24 hours until the lubricants have had time to soften the intraluminal contents.

Surgical Management Although most reports suggest a poor outcome with surgical management, it has been the more successful approach in the author's hands. The following three surgical approaches exist: 1) rumenotomy to access content of the fundus of the abomasum and remove luminal obstruction such as foreign bodies (plastic materials, etc.) or deliver lubricants into the abomasum; 2) right paracostal or paramedian approach to allow access to extraluminal and intraluminal cause of impaction as well as examination of most of the abomasum and to allow emptying of the abomasum through abomasotomy; 3) in very selected cases a right flank celiotomy may be useful because it allows access to the pylorus and cranial duodenum. The benefits of electing surgical treatment include the following: First, it is the best available way to differentiate between potentially treatable and untreatable causes of impaction, granting that a cause may not be determined for a significant number of cases. Secondly, it may allow direct management of the cause in a few cases. Thirdly, it can allow more direct—and potentially more effective—administration of adjunctive medical therapy. Finally, it provides the quickest means of relieving pressure on the distended abomasal wall, a critical consideration if abomasal function is to be preserved.

Surgical intervention is not without risks. Affected animals are often in poor systemic condition. This is particularly true for direct approaches to the abomasum that require recumbency since many affected cattle have a distended rumen as well as abomasum and omasum. Even when apparently successful surgery is completed, unidentified or poorly addressable causes may persist in interfering with abomasal function. Finally, the abomasal wall may be too badly damaged to recover even if the initial source of obstruction can be removed.

The risk of recumbent abomasotomy can be reduced by first performing a rumenotomy to decompress the rumen before considering an abomasotomy. This adds two surgeries to the potential cost but enhances the prognosis and should be an option understood by the owner in their decision for therapy vs. slaughter. If the decision is made to treat a suspected case, the following two-step process of rumenotomy and abomasotomy is recommended.

Surgical Management: Left Flank Exploratory/ Rumenotomy (Step 1) The cow should be prepared for a standing left flank exploratory and potential rumenotomy as described in Section 10.3.

An initial and thorough exploration to confirm abomasal impaction and to identify any potential extraluminal cause of impaction is critical. Reexploration after completion of a rumenotomy carries an unacceptably high risk of causing peritonitis; therefore every effort to palpate all accessible structures of interest should be taken at the beginning of the surgery. Initial palpation of the caudal abdomen should include close evaluation of lymph nodes and the uterus for enlargement or irregularities suggestive of lymphosarcoma or lymphadenitis. The size, position, and consistency of the abomasum should be evaluated by reaching around the caudal aspect of the rumen and palpating the visceral surface of the abomasum. The pyloric region should be palpated for irregularities that might suggest lymphosarcoma (Figure 10.4-24), ulceration, or post-ulcer scarring. Firm masses in the omentum adjacent to the pylorus might suggest fat necrosis (Figure 10.4-25). The cranial abdomen is examined for masses or signs of inflammation that might indicate traumatic reticuloperitonitis, liver abscesses, abomasal ulceration, or neoplasia.

Once exploration has been completed to the best of the surgeon's ability, he or she should proceed to a rumenotomy (see Section 10.3). Once the rumen is stabilized, transruminal palpation should be performed to verify exploratory findings and to examine poorly accessible areas. Next, intraluminal structures should be examined. The position, size, and consistency of the abomasum can be easily defined by transruminal palpation. The rumenoreticular fold, esophageal orifice and omasal orifice should be palpated for lesions and to assess the strength of contractions against the hand. Abnormalities at multiple sites might help localize a neurologic lesion. In all but the largest cows, it is usually possible to reach with the left hand through the reticuloomasal orifice into the omasal canal to evaluate the consistency of omasal contents. In some cases of abomasal and omasal impaction, the omasal canal will be packed with dense,

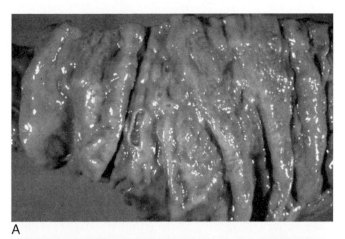

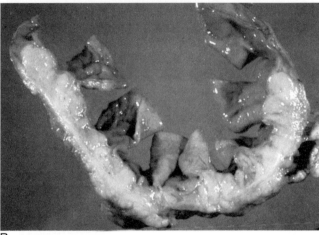

Figure 10.4-24 Abomasal lymphosarcoma. *A,* Note the thickened mucosal leaves of the abomasum. *B,* Note the thickened abomasal wall on cross section.

(Courtesy of Dr. John King; Cornell University.)

dry material that must be manually scraped back into the reticulum to allow palpation of the canal.

A nasogastric tube passed by an assistant into the reticulum can be manually redirected by the surgeon through the omasal orifice and, if the canal is clear or can be cleared, all the way into abomasum. Once the tube tip is at its desired location in the abomasum, the assistant should mark the tube's point of entry into the nostril. The external tip of the tube can be stabilized by suturing the tube or attached tape to the nares or taping the tube to a halter after completion of the celiotomy. Repeated abomasal infusion of lubricants or motility stimulants can be administered via the tube after surgery.

At this stage, a decision should be made whether to follow the rumenotomy by an abomasotomy. An abomasotomy would be indicated to relieve abomasal pressure if distention is severe and may have therapeutic value if a probable cause is not identified during exploration, thus leaving the possibility of an intraluminal obstruction. If

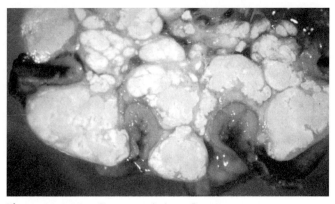

Figure 10.4-25 Fat necrosis in a Guernsey cow.

(Courtesy of Dr. John King; Cornell University.)

an abomasotomy is planned, ruminal content should be reduced to a small volume to minimize the risk of aspiration and respiratory stress during abomasotomy. Regardless of subsequent plans, decreasing the volume of a distended rumen will improve the animal's comfort level and may enhance the quality of contractions and improve appetite. Closure of the rumenotomy and flank incisions is described in Section 10.3.

Surgical Management: Abomasotomy (Step 2) Ideally abomasotomy should be performed within 12 to 24 hours of a rumenotomy to take advantage of the empty rumen. Surgical antibiotic prophylaxis should be repeated before surgery. The safest approach is a low right paracostal or right paramedian celiotomy with the cow positioned in left lateral recumbency. A paracostal approach is preferred if access to the pylorus and cranial duodenum is also needed, as this incision can be extended into the right paralumbar fossa. Transection of two nerves (ventral thoracic and lumbar nerves) is of no clinical consequence, but transection of a third nerve can result in abdominal wall denervation, which can cause bulging of the abdominal wall after surgery. Therefore efforts should be made not to transect more than two ventral thoracic nerves. The abomasum can only be partially exteriorized; therefore removal of ingesta requires repeated movements of hand or instruments in and out of the lumen. Careful isolation of the abomasotomy site with sterile impervious drape is needed because the risk of abdominal contamination is high. Alternatively, a large sterile plastic bag (which is by nature impervious) can be used as a wound protector. The middle of the bag is first fenestrated and placed over the intended incision site. The edge of the bag is sutured to the wall of the abomasum before the abomasotomy to prevent abdominal contamination. A large (no. 1) suture material is placed into the seromusucular wall of the abomasum (avoiding the lumen) in a simple continuous pattern encircling the intended abomasotomy site and incorporating the plastic bag. Once the abomasum has been exposed and isolated, a 12- to 15-cm incision can be made in the exposed serosal surface of the abomasum while at least 2 cm is left between the abomasal incision and drape or plastic bag at each end of the incision.

Once hemorrhage from large submucosal vessels has been controlled, ingesta should be removed from the abomasum and omasal canal to allow assessment of mucosal surfaces and ingesta composition. The composition of ingesta at the pyloric antrum should be closely examined for possible intraluminal obstructions, and the lumen of the pyloroduodenal juncture should be palpated for patency, masses, or scarring. In many cases of impaction from poor-quality feed, a compacted ball of feed will be present at the pyloric antrum, and the duodenum will be empty. Whether motility disturbances caused the compaction or the compacted ball initiated the obstruction is difficult to tell. Ruptures, ischemic necrosis, and ulceration are fatal complications of abomasal impaction. The lesser curvature of the abomasum is a common site for these complications to occur and should be examined closely.

After the lumen has been thoroughly evaluated, the exposed serosa should be lavaged with sterile isotonic fluid, and the abomasal incision should be closed using a double inverting pattern. Care should be taken to fully invert the mucosa between serosal surfaces during abomasal wall closure. The serosa should be lavaged again before removing the isolating drapes or the plastic bag serving as wound protector.

While the right paracostal approach provides access to the pyloric portion of the abomasum, it does not allow complete exploration of the proximal abomasum or omasum in large cows and may not allow safe exteriorization of the pylorus if the abomasum is extremely distended. If either of these conditions exist, a right paramedian approach is recommended. With the cow in left lateral recumbency, a 25-30 cm cranial right paramedian incision is made. The serosal surface of the abomasum is sutured to the skin circumferentially around the incision using the same process described for rumenotomy (chapter 10.3). Once the suture line is complete and a good seal is confirmed, the abomasum is incised and mucosal hemorrhage controlled. A wound protector is recommended to minimize contamination and serosal trauma. Content may be removed and the abomasal lumen can be explored at this point. Particular attention should be paid to the proximal lesser curvature of the abomasum which is a common site for ischemic necrosis and perforation in chronic impaction cases. Following exploration, the wound protector should be removed, the abomasal surface lavaged, and the abomasal incision closed in a double inverting pattern with an absorbable suture material such as polygalactin 910 or polydiaxonone. The sutures between the skin and abomasum can

be removed and any debris removed before the abomasum is allowed to return to the abdomen.

Postoperative care should include analgesics and supportive care. Antibiotics initiated prophylactically before surgery should be continued at therapeutic levels for at least 3 days beyond clinical signs of infection if significant contamination occurred or if signs of preexisting infection were identified during surgery. If the abomasal wall has been permanently damaged or the original cause of the impaction persists, the abomasum will gradually refill. The process may take weeks to become apparent, and the owner should be made aware that an initial improvement in signs might not indicate full recovery.

Alternative Surgical Management: Right Flank Exploratory Surgery is typically performed with both diagnostic and therapeutic goals. The standing right flank approach provides adequate access for diagnosis and identification of lesions in the pyloroduodenal region. Successful treatment of two cases that resulted from gravel ingestion has been reported with this approach. In one case, with an accumulation of gravel in the pyloric antrum, manually breaking down the mass and massaging the material back into the abomasal body was possible. In a second case with gravel in the descending duodenum, the material was removed by enterotomy. However, this approach does not provide adequate access for abomasotomy, and, if material in the abomasum cannot be disrupted manually, a second surgery will be necessary. If the rumen is distended, an intermediate step of a left flank rumenotomy may be indicated to improve safety for the abomasotomy.

Mixed Mechanical and Functional Obstructions: Adhesions Adhesions secondary to perforating abomasal ulcers or periabomasal inflammatory foci can create partial or complete abomasal outflow obstruction by preventing the normal wall motility necessary for contractions or by distorting the normal position of the outflow tract. Iatrogenic adhesions caused by improper placement of an omentopexy, abomasopexy, or pyloropexy can also impair outflow by the same mechanisms. Adhesions to the abomasum or adjacent structures can also produce pain by placing tension on parietal or visceral surfaces, or interfere with abomasal innervation, thus creating some degree of functional motility impairment.

The treatment goals for inflammatory and iatrogenic adhesions are to restore the normal functional position of the abomasum and maintain or restore the integrity of the abomasal wall. This usually requires lysis (separation) of the adhesions. Early fibrinous adhesions (<10-14 days) are relatively fragile and can generally be lysed by blunt dissection. In the case of poorly placed left flank abomasopexy, blind tack, or toggle pin surgeries, external release of the sutures within the first week of placement is often sufficient to allow the abomasum to return to a more functional position. Other methods of surgical stabilization require reexploration, generally through the original incision, for release.

After 10 to 14 days, spontaneous and artificial adhesions will generally have sufficient fibrous tissue to make lysis by blunt dissection difficult and, in some cases, impossible. The integrity of the abomasal wall must be carefully protected because it is often difficult to see or feel a separation between the adhesion and wall. Excessive tension is as likely to tear through the abomasal wall as it is to lyse the adhesion. Techniques for management of mature adhesions are described in management of LDA with adhesions (see Section 10.4.1). If control of the site cannot be achieved, a decision to abort the procedure and recover the cow for another approach or for slaughter should be considered. The right paramedian or right paracostal approaches tend to provide the best access for adhesions involving the abomasum. Defects in the abomasal wall should be oversewn and any full-thickness defects in the omentum should be closed.

If adhesions were producing an outflow obstruction by changing the position of the outflow tract without otherwise compromising the lumen, release of the adhesions and restoration of the abomasum to its normal position will generally be sufficient to restore function. Adhesions commonly recur at the site of adhesion lysis, but, in the case of the bovine abomasum, no adjacent small diameter bowel loops could be occluded by new adhesions. If the abomasum has been replaced in a normal position, new adhesions should stabilize the abomasum in the desired location. Performance of an abomasopexy or omentopexy may not be essential because of the presence of freshly broken adhesions in the area, but we feel it should still be performed in most cases. Inflammation is, by definition, present at the site of adhesion lysis, and multifilament nonabsorbable sutures should be avoided (see discussion of omentopexy and abomasopexy for LDAs (in Section 10.4.1).

If the adhesions were producing an outflow obstruction by constricting the lumen in the narrow parts of the outflow path, it may be appropriate to decrease or prevent development of postlysis adhesions. In general terms, this will involve efforts to minimize tissue trauma by gentle tissue dissection and precise hemostasis, use of tissue lubricants (carboxymethylcellulose, 1% solution, molecular weight from 250 to 1000 kd) to avoid serosal and peritoneal abrasion, minimizing the amount of foreign material (i.e., sutures) and blood left at the wound site, and leaving peritoneal defects (with the exception of full-thickness omental tears) unsutured. Addition of surface-coating agents that protect surfaces and/or promote plasminogen activation should be considered.

Mechanical Obstructions

Intraluminal Obstructions Purely mechanical intraluminal obstructions are relatively uncommon causes of abomasal obstruction in the adult cow. The reticuloomasal orifice in adult cattle normally prevents passage of material that has not been reduced to the small size necessary for digestion and also serves as a filter for many metal objects that might lodge in the pylorus or duodenum. Bailing twine, placenta, and trichobezoars do occasionally lodge in the pyloric region and cause an obstruction in adult ruminants. Compacted solid ingesta is often present in the pyloric antrum of cattle with abomasal impactions, although the compacted material is probably secondary to an initial neuromuscular dysfunction rather than the primary cause of the obstruction (see Abomasal Impaction). Other causes of intraluminal obstruction are uncommon and sporadic in nature.

Intraluminal obstruction of the abomasum in adult cattle can be expected to result in the same fluid and electrolyte disturbances described above for left abomasal displacement (i.e., hypochloremic metabolic alkalosis with possible hyponatremia and hypokalemia). In the rare case in which the intraluminal material penetrates the wall or causes pressure necrosis, signs of peritoneal inflammation and possibly infection may be present.

Treatment involves surgical removal of the obstructing object, correction of fluid and electrolyte imbalances, and management of any associated inflammation or infection. Surgical access to the primary site of obstruction (i.e., the pylorus) is limited in adult cattle to a right paracostal or right paramedian approach with the cow positioned in left lateral recumbency These approaches are described in detail in Abomasal Impaction. If the pylorus has been obstructed because of fibrosis or perforation, an abomasoduodenostomy can be performed between the serosal parietal surface of the abomasum and the descending duodenum as described in the following discussion.

Mural Lesions Mural lesions can obstruct outflow by several mechanisms, including narrowing or distortion of the lumen, interference with normal contractions, and damage to intrinsic nerves and signaling mechanisms. Lesions must generally be in the narrow distal end of the abomasum to produce a mechanical obstruction. Mural lesions include tumors, abscesses, and fibrosis. Intestinal tumors are relatively uncommon in cattle in comparison to man or dogs, but several have been reported in the abomasum. The most common is lymphosarcoma (see Figure 10.4 24). Adenocarcinoma can occur in the abomasum but is more typically found in the small and large intestine. Fibrosis and intramural abscesses most commonly result from ulcers. Intraluminal obstructions that create pressure necrosis and loss of the mucosal barrier can also lead to fibrosis of the wall.

Cows with mural tumors of the abomasum have a very poor prognosis and treatment is not generally recommended. Small mural lesions in the proximal pyloric antrum or abomasal body may be resectable, although bypass is often the only method of restoring aborad flow. A side-to-side anastomosis can be performed between the parietal surface of the abomasum and the descending duodenum or proximal jujenum via a standing right flank (adults only), or recumbent right paracostal or right flank approach. In the authors' experience this has been successful in a very limited number of cases when the anastomosis is between the pyloric part of the abomasum and the descending duodenum and is best done in standing animals by using stapling instruments. On the contrary, anastomosis between the pyloric part of the abomasum and the jejunum has not been successful. If the proximal jejunum is used, the omental sling must be transected at the intended level of the anastamosis and the edge of the transected omentum sutured together to close the omental bursa. Access is more limited in adult cattle than in calves, and, if possible, cows should be held off feed for up to 48 hours before surgery to improve access.

Extraluminal Masses Any extraluminal mass adjacent to the pyloric antrum or proximal duodenum that compresses the lumen can lead to a partial or complete outflow obstruction. Omental fat necrosis (see Figure 10.4-25) and abscesses are the most commonly recognized extraluminal masses that produce abomasal outflow obstruction. Drainage or marsupialization of abscesses may improve motility by decreasing the diameter of the abscess and decreasing pressure on the abomasal outflow tract. Care must be taken to maintain a relatively normal anatomical relation for the abomasum and duodenum if abscess marsupialization is planned. If fat necrosis has become extreme enough to impair pyloric outflow, bypass of the pylorus to the descending duodenum might relieve the obstruction.

Functional Obstructions Functional obstructions can develop from any stimulus that interferes with the normal coordination of contractions in the abomasum and outflow tract. Diagnosis is generally based on eliminating all mechanical sources of obstruction and identifying signs consistent with possible physiologic disturbances. Regardless of the source and extent of the functional motility disturbance, involvement of the abomasum is likely to produce the characteristic fluid and electrolyte changes associated with abomasal outflow obstruction (i.e., dehydration with a hypochloremic metabolic alkalosis with or without hyponatremia and hypokalemia). Identification of these changes alone does not usually help differentiate between mechanical and functional outflow obstructions. Although surgery is often involved during diagnostic evaluation to rule out mechanical disturbances and may be of some benefit in temporarily relieving abomasal distention, it does not commonly play a role as a primary treatment method of most functional obstructions.

Functional Obstructions-Ileus Abomasal motility is regulated by a range of local and systemic mediators, as discussed in the introductory section Physiology and Function. Although the role of many causative factors is still under debate, evaluation and treatment of potential contributing factors should be a routine part of case care. Hypocalcemia, hypokalemia, alkalosis, and ketosis are all possible primary causes of depressed abomasal motility, and correction of these disturbances can restore motility in some cases. Nutritional factors commonly are implicated as a cause of altered abomasal motility that leads to displacement in adult cattle and calves (see Left Abomasal Displacement). Adjustment of diet to eliminate or reduce risk factors may resolve some cases. Gastrointestinal motility can be depressed by painful or inflammatory stimuli located elsewhere in the peritoneal cavity or body. Conditions associated with endotoxemia are an example and include such widespread problems as liver abscesses, endometritis, coliform mastitis, and septicemia. Treatment should focus on correcting potential initiating causes, including relief of pain and control of inflammatory stimuli.

LOSS OF ABOMASAL MUCOSA INTEGRITY

Loss of the abomasal mucosa barrier leading to potential leakage of abomasal content can occur as a result of persistent luminal pressure from stationary intraluminal objects (trichobezoars, foreign bodies, etc.), abomasal ulcers, mural lesions that interfere with mucosal blood flow or expand through the wall (lymphosarcoma, abscesses, etc.), and extraluminal lesions that invade the lumen (surgical incisions, suture material, foreign bodies). Diagnostic and therapeutic approaches for intraluminal and expansile mural lesions were discussed earlier under Outflow Obstructions. Abomasal ulcers and fistulation are reviewed in the following discussion.

Abomasal Ulcers

Definition Abomasal ulcers are lesions that penetrate the basement membrane of the abomasal mucosa. Erosion of the mucosa presumably precedes the development of an ulcer. Once the basement membrane has been invaded, the clinical presentation is based on the depth of penetration and the structures involved. Four different types of abomasal ulceration have been described: Type 1) nonpenetrating ulcers; Type 2) ulcers with profuse intraluminal hemorrhage; Type 3) perforations with localized peritonitis (Figure 10.4-26); and Type 4) perforations with diffuse peritonitis. The Type 1 category of ulcers has been used to describe both erosions and true ulcers that have penetrated the basement membrane but have not fully broken through the abomasal wall (nonpenetrating ulcers). Perforation on the visceral surface of the abomasum can lead to the syndrome

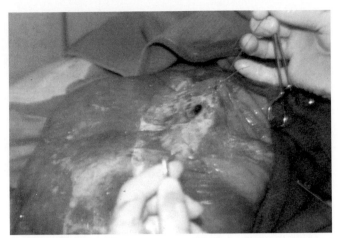

Figure 10.4-26 Abomasal perforation with localized contamination.

known as *omental bursitis* (see Section 10.8.1), considered in this text as a subset of Type 3 ulcers. An individual cow may have multiple ulcers that fall into more than one category.

Incidence and Predisposing Factors Abomasal ulcers have been recognized in cattle of all ages and breeds but are more common in cattle in intensive management settings. Specific groups recognized to be at risk for ulcers in general include high production dairy cows, feedlot cattle, veal calves, and beef calves. Abomasal ulceration in calves is of sufficient concern in Europe to receive attention in the recommendations of the Council of the European Community's minimum standards for protection of calves. Some reports indicate that the incidence of clinically significant abomasal ulcers is increasing.

Diffuse nonperforating erosions/ulcers are commonly recognized in some groups of cattle, including veal calves, 2- to 8-week-old calves, weanling calves, and fattening cattle, primarily at the time of slaughter. Stress from a variety of sources including changes in housing or feed, straw ingestion, exposure to infectious agents, and high milk production have been implicated as predisposing factors. The overall prevalence of Type I ulcers in veal calves in one study that compared the effects of different types of housing was 86.8%. However, because most cases of Type I ulcers are believed to be subclinical, the incidence in groups of cattle that are not routinely seen at slaughter or necropsy is difficult to estimate.

Type 2 (bleeding) ulcers may be multiple or single, but the category is generally reserved for ulcers that cause severe intraluminal blood loss. Cows with bleeding ulcers represented 26 (0.41%) of 6385 cattle admitted to one referral center over a 14-year period. Bleeding abomasal ulcers can be divided into two groups based on etiology: those associated with lymphosarcoma and those that are not. Cows with lymphosarcoma-associated bleeding ulcers are generally over 5 years of age and are diagnosed

throughout the lactation period. Cows with ulcers unassociated with lymphosarcoma generally are less than 4 years of age, present in the first few weeks after parturition, and typically have one or more concurrent postparturient diseases (LDA, metritis, mastitis, and ketosis).

The occurrence of perforating ulcers in adult cattle appears to be more sporadic and associated with episodes of metabolic stress, including recent parturition, peak milk production, and one or more concurrent diseases (abomasal displacement, metritis, mastitis, and ketosis). Diets high in concentrate and corn silage have also been implicated. In a review of cases over a 14-year period in one referral hospital, 43 cases of perforating ulcers were admitted and represented 0.63% of cases admitted during this period. One early study reported that 85% of perforating ulcers resulted in localized peritonitis in the omental bursa, although a more recent study showed an equal or greater percentage of perforating ulcers resulting in diffuse peritonitis.

Diagnosis The clinical signs produced by abomasal ulcers depend largely on the category of ulcer and range from vague signs of digestive disturbance to signs consistent with peritonitis or anemia.

Type I Ulcers Type I ulcers often lack any detectable clinical signs. However, the presence of Type I erosions/ulcers may be suspected in cattle known to be at risk and that show signs of poor appetite, decreased weight gain, and decreased ruminal motility. Concurrent disease is common. Affected animals may be positive for fecal occult blood, but a negative test does not rule out the diagnosis. Erosions do not penetrate the mucosal basement membrane and can heal without contraction or scarring. They produce little detectable change when viewed from the serosal surface of the abomasum and can only be diagnosed with certainty at necropsy or during abomasotomy. However, when erosions progress to ulcers, they produce a local inflammatory response with peripheral thickening and occasional serositis that can be detected by palpation of the abomasal wall during abdominal exploration. The contraction and scarring that occurs as a part of healing is also detectable by palpation during exploratory surgery. Nonperforating ulcers are also commonly associated with concurrent diseases, but up to 50% of affected animals may have clinical signs associated with ulceration, including abdominal pain, melena, or pale mucous membranes.

Type II Ulcers The hallmark signs of bleeding abomasal ulcers are melena caused by blood digested in the abomasum and a positive fecal occult blood test. This test is very sensitive and fresh feces should be collected for examination before performing abdominal palpation per rectum to avoid false positive results. Other sources of gastrointestinal hemorrhage must be considered as differentials.

Cows with bleeding ulcers unrelated to lymphosarcoma are initially identified by the herdsman based on an acute drop in milk production and the appearance of dark loose feces. Pale mucous membranes are common. Cows with non–tumor-associated ulcers are usually anemic (PCV < 25%) and are likely to have severe anemia (PCV < 15%) with signs of regeneration (nucleated red blood cells and/or increased reticulocyte counts). Signs of abdominal pain may also be present. Ulceration over large submucosal arteries or veins can produce acute severe blood loss that leads to death before external signs are detectable in either adults or calves.

The initial signs in cows with lymphosarcoma are more variable and depend on the effect of the tumor on abomasal function, the amount of bleeding, and the involvement of other viscera. Cows with tumors isolated to the abomasum are typically recognized based on signs associated with altered abomasal motility (abomasal displacement, anorexia, or hemorrhage, depression, dark loose stool, pale mucous membranes, and tachycardia). Only 50% of cows with lymphosarcoma-associated abomasal ulcers were found to be anemic in one study, and only 25% had severe anemia (PCV < 15%). Other signs of lymphosarcoma—including lymphadenopathy, lymphocytosis, and abnormal lymphocytes in peritoneal fluid—may also be present in some cases.

Types III and IV Ulcers The outlook for cattle that present with perforating ulcers depends upon the perforation depth, ulcer location, the animal's age, and the presence and nature of concurrent diseases. Ulcers that penetrate slowly in areas covered by omentum are more likely to produce localized peritonitis or omental bursitis (Type III Ulcers) with less noticeable clinical signs. Cases of perforation associated with LDA also fall in this category, even though they may occur on the uncovered serosal surfaces of the abomasum. It has been hypothesized that the distended abomasum enhances the contact between the perforation site and the body wall, thus allowing better localization of the contamination. Ulcers that occur rapidly in areas that are not covered by omentum are more likely to produce generalized peritonitis (Type IV Ulcers) with severe acute clinical signs (Figure 10.4-27).

In Adult Cattle, type III ulcers may lack any clinical signs specific to the perforation, with identification occurring during investigation of concurrent diseases. Signs, when present, include intermittent anorexia, ruminal stasis and/or distention, abdominal distention, abdominal pain, melena, and anorexia. Perforation on the visceral surface of the abomasum can lead to the syndrome known as *omental bursitis,* with partial confinement of contaminants between the two layers of the greater omentum. In these cases clinical signs tend to progress gradually and include anorexia, decreased milk

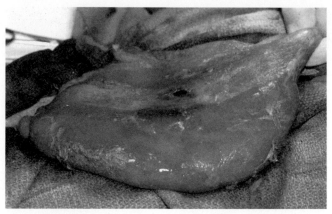

Figure 10.4-27   Abomasal perforation with diffuse peritonitis (Type IV). Note extensive contamination on the abomasal wall.

production, bilateral ventral abdominal distention, decreased rumen contractions, loose or scant feces, and loss of body condition.

Physical examination with manual pressure on the ventral abdomen may localize abdominal pain to the right cranioventral body wall. This can help distinguish the localized peritonitis caused by Type III Ulcers from that caused by traumatic reticuloperitonitis, which is more commonly associated with left cranioventral pain. Localization is not always possible, and overlap in location does occur; therefore results should be considered as supportive rather than diagnostic.

Laboratory results are also seldom diagnostic but may provide supportive information. Feces will be positive for occult blood in some but not all cases. Nonspecific systemic signs of inflammation (pyrexia, neutrophilia, hyperfibrinogenemia, may be present in the acute stages of perforation and intermittently afterward. Peritoneocentesis can indicate peritonitis, but the adult cow's ability to localize peritoneal contaminants results in many false negatives in the face of established infection. Elevated peritoneal white blood cell counts and normal to increased peritoneal protein in the face of a systemic hypoproteinemia suggest peritonitis. Cows with Type III localized perforating ulcers in one study were observed to have a mild hypochloremic, hypokalemic metabolic alkalosis. However, 83% of the cows in this group also had LDAs, and the metabolic and electrolyte changes may reflect the abomasal displacement rather than the ulcer. In cows with a diagnosis of LDA or RDA/RVA, the presence of pneumoperitoneum, signs of abdominal pain (arched back, pain on abdominal pressure), and pyrexia that is not explained by other concurrent disease suggests the presence of perforating ulcers. Ultrasonography can be used to help identify or confirm cranial right abdominal peritonitis. Ultrasonography can also help identify fibrin accumulation along the cranioventral abdomen and in some cases can help determine if the accumulation is concentrated on the right or left side of midline.

Cows with Type IV abomasal ulcers present with acute signs of depression, anorexia, agalactia, and systemic shock. Tachycardia, tachypnea, pyrexia, and abdominal pain are common clinical signs. Other gastrointestinal disturbances, including left abomasal displacement and ruminal tympany, are less common than in cows with type III ulcers but still present in about half the cases. A normal- or low-serum total protein in the face of hemoconcentration that results from loss of protein into the peritoneal cavity is often present in cows with diffuse peritonitis. Leukocytosis, neutrophilia, and left shift are also common in affected cattle. Elevated white cell counts and protein concentrations in peritoneal fluid can be expected in some—but not all—cases. Cows with Type IV ulcers may show a metabolic acidosis with hypokalemia and hypocalcemia.

Cows that survive an acute episode of either Type III or Type IV abomasal ulcers may develop chronic recurrent signs associated with adhesions or chronic abscessation.

Management Treatment of individual animals with Type I or multiple Type II ulcers should focus on medical management tools directed at reduction of metabolic stress, resolution of concurrent diseases, and supportive care for systemic disturbances. Management changes to reduce stress should be considered for the herd in general. Treatment is not recommended for cows with Type II ulcers associated with lymphosarcoma because of the poor prognosis for lymphosarcoma in general. Medical management tools are also important as the sole means of management or as an adjunct to surgical therapy for isolated Type II, III, or IV ulcers.

Surgical therapy is rarely the first choice for managing ulcers of any type, even when an isolated ulcer is suspected. By the time of diagnosis, cattle with isolated bleeding ulcers are often in poor condition and may not tolerate the recumbent approach necessary for access to the abomasum. The extensive omentum and propensity for fibrin deposition in adults provide a reasonably effective initial seal for ulcers that perforate gradually. Surgical intervention can disrupt tentatively localized infection, which leads to more diffuse distribution and increases the risk of septicemia and systemic shock. In most cases the cow's own defense mechanisms are better capable of safely localizing and sealing a perforating abomasal ulcer than is the surgeon. However, surgery is commonly involved in treating concurrent abomasal displacements and diagnostic evaluation of cases with nonspecific signs of forestomach motility disturbances. The goals when surgical therapy is used are to control hemorrhage, eliminate further peritoneal contamination, eliminate any outflow obstruction produced by ulcers or

their sequellae, and ensure a functional abomasal position. The primary surgical procedures performed are submucosal vessel ligation, ulcer resection, or ulcer inversion and oversew.

Surgical access to the abomasum for therapy is limited. The standing left flank approach will allow separation of adhesions from some Type III ulcers with concurrent LDA and restoration of normal abomasal position but does not provide adequate access for any other procedure, with or without abomasal displacement. The preferred approaches in adult cattle are low right paracostal or right paramedian incisions with the animal positioned in left lateral or dorsal (right paramedian only) recumbency. Surgical antibiotic prophylaxis is indicated when planning surgery in which ulcers may be encountered.

Type II Ulcers Surgical intervention is not generally recommended as the primary approach for treatment of bleeding ulcers. However, when bleeding ulcers are encountered during surgery (thickened and discolored area, Figure 10.4-28) for treatment of abomasal displacement or diagnostic exploratory, in some cases identifying the site of hemorrhage and decreasing or eliminating bleeding may be possible. This requires identifying the site or sites of hemorrhage and ligating or compressing the involved submucosal vessels. The quantity of hemorrhage seems to decrease once the abomasum is returned to its normal position.

After the abomasum is exposed, the site of hemorrhage should be identified by palpating focal abomasal wall thickening. Whenever possible, the involved area should be exteriorized, packed off from the adjacent

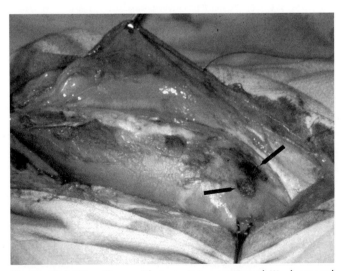

Figure 10.4-28 Cow with type II (arrows) and III abomasal ulcer with localized peritonitis.

(Courtesy of Dr. Norm G. Ducharme; Cornell University.)

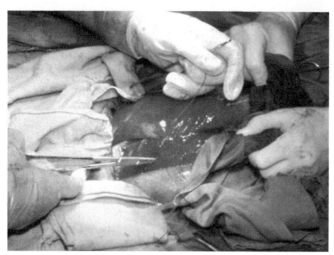

Figure 10.4-29 Abomasal ulcer being oversewn with a double inverting pattern.

tissues, and isolated with intestinal forceps before full-thickness excision of the ulcerated area (Figure 10.4-29). Stay sutures (#1 monofilament) should be placed at either end of the exposed site to support the intestinal forceps and maintain control of the site, should it be necessary to release the forceps to identify and ligate submucosal vessels. The abomasal serosa should be lavaged to remove debris if the lavage fluid can be directed out of the peritoneal cavity. The abomasal defect should be closed with a single or double inverting and penetrating suture pattern.

If the ulcer is located in the lesser curvature or near the omasal orifice, gaining direct access to the serosal surface over the lesion may be possible. In a few of these cases, it may be possible to oversew the lesion and compress the involved vessels without entering the abomasal lumen. Large-gauge (#1 or #2) synthetic absorbable suture material should be used to place large overlapping horizontal mattress pattern sutures across the course of the involved vessels. Alternatively, exposing the luminal surface of the lesion on the lesser curvature may be possible by suturing the parietal surface of the abomasum to the skin as described above for treatment of abomasal impactions. This technique will allow ligation of bleeding ulcers and will potentially allow the site to be oversewn, although it carries an increased risk of peritoneal contamination and peritonitis.

Types III and IV Ulcers The majority of Type III ulcers that are identified *ante mortem* are found during exploratory surgery for left abomasal displacement. Type IV ulcers that perforate rapidly on the parietal surface are often impossible for the peritoneal cavity to contain and lead to rapid deterioration and death. However, no reports suggest that surgical intervention can improve the outcome. Acute perforation of a partial-thickness or fibrin-sealed ulcer during exploratory surgery is an exception to the rule. If the ulcer can be quickly isolated and oversewn, a combination of debridement, extensive abdominal lavage, antibiotic, and supportive care can be successful.

Adult Cattle and Feedlot Steers After exposure of the abomasum, the site of ulceration should be identified. The perforation is generally located at the site of the most well-established adhesions. Once the site has been identified, it should be isolated from as many surrounding adhesions as possible and elevated toward the incision. Before beginning adhesion lysis, the abomasal wall in the vicinity of the perforation should be clamped with atraumatic intestinal forceps or, if this is not possible, isolated manually and the surrounding tissues packed off to help control accidental leakage. Thin fibrinous adhesions may be gently separated manually, whereas thicker fibrous adhesions may require sharp incision. If the ulcer is in a location that cannot be safely isolated, the adhesions should be left in place and the cow recovered. At this time, a decision to treat medically, perform a second surgery through another approach, or elect slaughter/euthanasia will be needed.

Once the site has been isolated, the area of ulceration should be resected and oversewn with a double inverting pattern with an absorbable suture material such as polyglycolic acid, polyglactin 910, or polydiaxanone. Chromic gut has been used for this purpose but is not recommended because of the potential for premature absorption in the presence of abomasal acid and the enzyme activity of bacteria and white blood cells. Some authors have described successful management of perforated ulcers by inverting the ulcer site without resecting the ulcer, and oversewing the site with a double inverting pattern. Care should be taken to avoid spreading debris or contaminated fluid beyond the local site of contamination. The incision should be closed routinely, taking care to lavage each layer of the incision thoroughly before closure. Antibiotic therapy should be continued to treat the peritonitis as indicated based on the level and stage of infection.

If ulceration has produced a localized abscess adjacent to the ventral body wall or within the omental bursa, it may be possible to marsupialize the abscess and treat it by drainage and lavage. Once drainage has stopped, it may be necessary to surgically close the artificial tract.

Prognosis

Type II Ulcers The prognosis for cows with bleeding ulcers associated with lymphosarcoma is grave. The prognosis for cows with non–tumor-associated bleeding ulcers is guarded to poor. Nine of 12 cows survived in one study, while 0 of 4 survived in another study. The

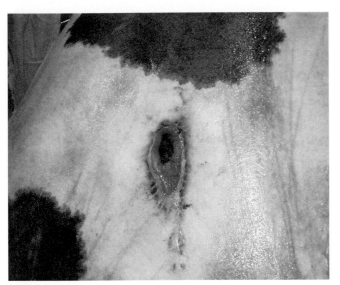

Figure 10.4-30 Ventral abdomen of a cow with an abomasal fistula after a right paramedian abomasopexy.

(Courtesy of Dr. Brett Woodie; Cornell University.)

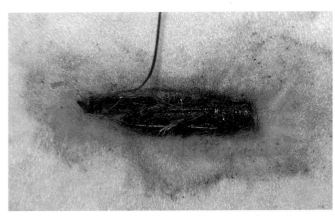

Figure 10.4-31 Ventral abdomen of a cow with an abomasal fistula after a toggle pin application. The sutures of the toggle were tied through a needle case and left in place inadvertently. Note the needle case is still in the fistula.

(Courtesy of Dr. Brett Woodie; Cornell University.)

author of the latter study reports better results in cases presented after the study period.

Type III Ulcers The prognosis for adult cattle with localized peritonitis is guarded to fair with surgical intervention if the ulcer can be isolated and oversewn without disseminating contaminants throughout the abdomen, and if the inflammatory response does not permanently impair normal function. Ten of 17 cows (59%) approached surgically in one study were successfully discharged. The other seven cows were euthanized because of abomasal rupture during manipulation (n = 3) and extensive adhesions that interfered with digestive function (n = 4). Seven of 12 cases (58%) with localized peritonitis and concurrent abomasal displacement treated surgically were discharged in a second study. Little information is available on prognosis for cows treated conservatively.

Type IV Ulcers The prognosis for adult cattle with diffuse peritonitis is very poor. Two of 22 (9%) affected cattle survived to discharge in one study. One of 9 (11%) cases with concurrent abomasal displacement treated surgically survived to discharge in a second study.

Abomasal Fistulae

Definition and Predisposing Factors Abomasal fistulae are tracts that communicate from the lumen of the abomasum to the skin surface or occasionally to the lumen of another viscus (reticulum, rumen, and omasum), organ (liver), or body cavity (thorax). Fistulae between the abomasum and skin are most commonly recognized as a technique-related complication of right paramedian abomasopexy (Figure 10.4-30) or of blind tack (see Figure

10.4-4B) or toggle pin (Figure 10.4-31) fixation of abomasal displacement. The primary predisposing factor that leads to fistulation after abomasopexy is most likely penetration of abomasal mucosa, particularly with multifilament nonabsorbable materials. Failure to release the tack suture 2 to 4 weeks after surgery is considered the major reason for fistulation after a blind tack or toggle pin procedure (see Figure 10.4-4B). Most cases of fistulation after right paramedian abomasopexy occur within several months; cases can occur as early as 2 weeks and occasionally as late as 8 months after surgery. Fistulation typically takes longer to develop (10 to 12 months) after a blind tack. Abomasal fistulation in association with ventral body wall hernias—particularly umbilical hernias in calves—have also been reported. Other fistulae have been attributed to abomasal ulcers or penetrating foreign bodies migrating from the reticulum to the abomasum or out of the abomasal lumen.

Diagnosis Internal fistulae have a wide variety of clinical signs based on the fistula path, including signs consistent with local or diffuse peritonitis and motility disturbances. A specific diagnosis is seldom made before exploratory. On the other hand, external fistulae are quite easy to diagnose based on the drainage of abomasal fluid and/or blood from the center of an area of cellulitis, usually located in the right paramedian area of the abdomen. Necrotic abomasal mucosa may also protrude through the fistula. Other clinical signs vary with the duration and amount of abomasal fluid lost and amount of blood lost from eroded submucosal vessels. Fluid and blood loss can be severe with extreme electrolyte disturbances (hypochloremia, hypokalemia, hyponatremia, metabolic alkalosis, dehydration) and hemorrhage (anemia, hypovolemia, and tachycardia).

Treatment The continued loss of abomasal fluid through a fistulous tract will eventually lead to life-threatening fluid and electrolyte disturbances. Hemorrhage from exposed submucosal vessels can rapidly lead to severe anemia and hypovolemic shock. Treatment goals are to adequately stabilize the cow for surgery, which is done with the cow in dorsal recumbency. The fistulous tract is isolated and resected, with care taken to minimize contamination of adjacent structures and restore luminal integrity of the abomasum.

Preparation The amount of preparation that can be completed before surgery will depend on the severity of ongoing hemorrhage. Ideally, surgery is delayed for 24 to 48 hours to allow correction of fluid imbalances (including a blood transfusion if there is severe anemia and to reduce rumen fill. This is possible when ongoing hemorrhage is minimal or when the surgeon can control hemorrhage in the standing cow. If hemorrhage cannot be controlled, it may be necessary to proceed more quickly to surgery and administer fluids and blood before and during surgery. Perioperative antibiotics are indicated because of the potential for contamination of adjacent tissues during surgery.

The cow should be restrained in dorsal recumbency under general anesthesia or cast and restrained with ropes. General anesthesia has the distinct advantages of better airway control, better immobilization, and reliable analgesia but has the obvious disadvantage of cost. Manual restraint should be combined with an inverted "L" block with 2% lidocaine for analgesia. Light sedation with xylazine hydrochloride can be used in manually restrained animals to help control movement but is not recommended in animals in poor systemic condition.

As much of the cranioventral abdomen as possible should be clipped while the cow is standing to minimize time in recumbency. It will usually be necessary to complete clipping around the tract once the cow is in dorsal recumbency. Any exposed necrotic tissue should be removed and the tract oversewn, if possible (Figure 10.4-32). If the tract cannot be oversewn, the exposed contaminated tissue should be isolated as much as possible from the adjacent surgical field by covering it with an adhesive drape or towel.

Procedure An elliptical or fusiform incision should be made around the tract through skin and body wall. The dissection continues into the peritoneal cavity (Figure 10.4-33). Limited mobility exists in the tissues in this location, and the incision should be as close to the tract as possible without entering the tract lumen. Elevating the tissues during the entry into the abdomen is helpful to avoid inadvertent perforation of underlying structures. Once in the peritoneal cavity, it may be necessary to separate adhered omentum and, occasionally, other structures from the tract. This is usually possible with

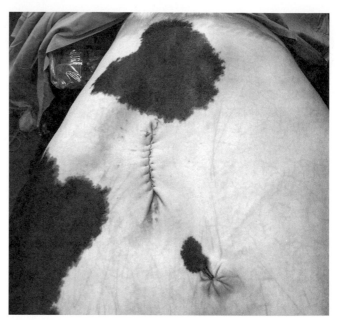

Figure 10.4-32   Same cow as in Figure 10.4-26 after oversewing the fistula before surgical excision.

(Courtesy of Dr. Brett Woodie; Cornell University.)

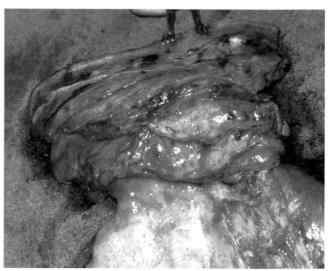

Figure 10.4-33   En bloc resection of an abomasal fistula and body wall.

(Courtesy of Dr. Norm G. Ducharme; Cornell University.)

blunt dissection alone, but firmly adhered structures may require sharp resection with subsequent defect repair. Once the tract and attached abomasum have been freed (see Figure 10.4-33), the tract and abomasum should be elevated to the incision. Stray sutures should be placed in the abomasal wall 2 to 4 cm from either end of the tract to help maintain control of the abomasum. Noncrushing intestinal forceps can then often be placed across the abomasum at the base of the tract. Laparotomy sponges or sterile bath towels should be used to pack off adjacent tissues before resecting the tract and attached abomasal wall. The abomasal wall is then sharply incised and the tract removed. The resulting defect in the abomasum should be closed in a double inverting pattern with an absorbable suture material such as polygalactin 910 or polyglycolic acid. Chromic gut has been used but the absorption rate is less reliable because of the action of hydrochloric acid in the lumen of the abomasum.

Closure of the body wall can be difficult with the limited mobility of tissues, size of the defect, and loss of defined tissue layers around the fistula. The areas should be copiously lavaged, and surgeons should change gloves and instruments for closure. New, sterile drapes should be applied. Use of 18-gauge, stainless steel wire in a through-and-through vertical or horizontal mattress pattern provides the most secure closure under these circumstances (Figure 10.4-34). The steel mattress sutures can be used as the sole means of closure or in conjunction with primary closure. Quills (rubber, buttons) can be used to help distribute tension from the steel sutures on the skin surface (see Figure 10.4-34). In cases with defined tissue layers and reasonable tension, standard primary closure patterns have been used with good success. However, the through-and-through pattern has been recommended in cases with significant wound contamination to facilitate drainage.

Postoperative antibiotics are recommended to treat cellulitis associated with fistula development, and analgesics are advised to relieve discomfort and speed return to feed. Supportive therapy, including fluids and calcium, may be indicated for a period of time after surgery as well. Nonsteroidal antiinflammatory agents are recommended for 2 to 3 days after surgery to ease discomfort and encourage eating but should not be continued indefinitely because of their potentially ulcerogenic effect on abomasal mucosa. If through and through steel stuctures were used, they are loosened periodically as the body wall granulates closed. The incision must be cleaned daily.

Prognosis and Complications In a report on nine adult cows with abomasal fistula secondary to right paramedian abomasopexy (6), blind tack (2), and unknown cause (1), one cow was euthanatized at surgery because of extensive peritonitis and pyloric involvement; one cow was euthanatized 8 days after surgery because of peritonitis secondary to abomasal rupture; and seven were discharged. Three subsequently died or were culled for apparently unrelated reasons 8 to 12 months after discharge, and the rest were productive members of the milking herd.

RECOMMENDED READINGS

Ames S: Repositioning the displaced abomasum in the cow, *J Am Vet Med Assoc* 153: 1470-1471, 1968.

Baker JS: Abomasal impaction and related obstructions of the forestomachs in cattle, *J Am Vet Med Assoc* 175: 1250-1253, 1979.

Baker JS: Diagnosis and surgery of right displacement of the abomasum in the bovine, *Proc 14th World Congress Diseases Cattle* 1: 30-35, 1986.

Bartlett PC, Kopcha M, Cowe PH, Ames NK, Ruegg PL, Erskine RJ: Economic comparison of the pyloro-omentopexy vs the roll-and-toggle procedure for treatment of left displacement of the abomasum in dairy cattle, *J Am Vet Med Assoc* 206: 1156-1162, 1995.

Begg H: Diseases of the stomach of the adult ruminant, *Vet Rec* 62: 797-808, 1950.

Blikslager AT, Anderson KL, Bristol DG, Fubini SL, Anderson DE: Repeat laparotomy for gastrointestinal disorders in cattle: 57 cases (1968-1992), *J Am Vet Med Assoc* 207: 939-943, 1995.

Cable CS, Rebhun WC, Fubini SL, Erb H, Ducharme NG: Concurrent abomasal displacement and perforating ulceration in cattle: 21 cases (1985-1996), *J Am Vet Med Assoc* 212: 1442-1445, 1998.

Cebra CK, Cebra ML, Garry FB: Gravel obstruction in the abomasum or duodenum of two cows, *J Am Vet Med Assoc* 209: 1294-1296, 1996.

Constable PD, Miller GY, Hoffsis GF, Hull BL, Rings DM: Risk factors for abomasal volvulus and left abomasal displacement in cattle, *Am J Vet Res* 53: 1184-1192, 1992.

Constable PD, St. Jean G, Hull DM, et al: Preoperative prognostic indicators in cattle with abomasal volvulus, *J Am Vet Med Assoc* 198: 2077-2065, 1991.

Erb HN, Martin SW: Age, breed, and seasonal patterns in the occurrence of ten dairy cow diseases: a case control study, *Can J Comp Med* 42: 1-9, 1978.

Fubini SL, Ducharme NG, Erb HN, Sheils RL: A comparison in 101 cows of right paralumbar fossa omentopexy and right paramedian abomasopexy for treatment of left displacement of the abomasum, *Can Vet J* 33: 318-324, 1992.

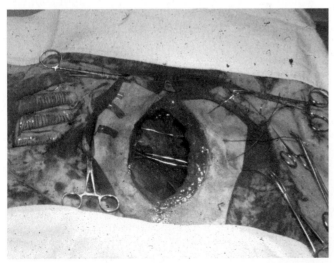

Figure 10.4-34 Following en bloc resection of an abomasal fistula and body wall resection, the body wall is closed by preplacing stainless steel sutures in a vertical mattress pattern and using plastic tubing to distribute the tension on the skin underneath the steel sutures.

(Courtesy of Dr. Norm G. Ducharme; Cornell University.)

Fubini SL, Gröhn YT, Smith DF: Right displacement of the aboma-sum and abomasal volvulus in dairy cows: 458 cases (1980-1987), *J Am Vet Med Assoc* 198: 466-464, 1991.

Garry F, Hull BL, Rings DM, Hoffsis G: Comparison of naturally occurring proximal duodenal obstruction and abomasal volvulus in dairy cattle, *Vet Surg* 17: 226-233, 1988.

Garry FB, Hull BL, Rings DM, et al: Prognostic value of anion gap calculation in cattle with abomasal volvulus: 58 cases (1980-1985), *J Am Vet Med Assoc* 192: 1107-1112, 1988.

Geishauser TH, Diederichs M, Failing K: Vorkommen von Labma-genverlagerung bei Rindern in Hessen, *Dtsch Tierarztl Wschr* 103: 142-144, 1996.

Gertsen KE: Surgical correction of the displaced abomasum, *Vet Med Small Anim Clin* 62: 679-682, 1967.

Getty R: *Sisson and Grossman's the anatomy of the domestic animals;* vol 1, ed 5, Philadelphia, 1975, WB Saunders.

Grymer J: Displaced abomasum: a disease often associated with con-current diseases, *Comp Cont Ed* 11: S290-S295, 1980.

Grymer J, Johnson R: Two cases of bovine omental bursitis, *J Am Vet Med Assoc* 181(7): 714-715, 1982.

Grymer J, Sterner KE: Percutaneous fixation of left displaced aboma-sum, using a bar suture, *J Am Vet Med Assoc* 180: 1458-1461, 1982.

Guard C: Metabolic diseases: a herd approach. In Rebhun WC, editor: *Diseases of dairy cattle.* Philadelphia, 1995, Williams and Wilkins.

Hoffsis GF, MacGuirk SM: Diseases of the abomasum and intestinal tract. In JL Howard, editor: *Veterinary therapy 2: food animal prac-tice.* Philadelphia, 1988, WB Saunders.

Hull BC: Closed suturing technique for correction of left abomasal dis-placement, *Iowa State Univ Vet* 34: 142-144, 1972.

Janowitz H: Laparoscopic reposition and fixation of the left displaced abomasum in cattle, *Tierarztl Prax Ausg G Grosstiere Nutztiere* 26: 308-313, 1998.

Jensen R, Pierson RE, Braddy PM, et al: Fatal abomasal ulcers in year-ling feedlot cattle, *J Am Vet Med Assoc* 169: 524-526, 1975.

Kelton DF, Garcia J, Guard CL, et al: Bar suture (toggle pin) vs open surgical abomasopexy for treatment of left displaced abomasum in dairy cattle, *J Am Vet Med Assoc* 193: 557-559, 1988.

Klein L, Fisher N: Cardiopulmonary effects of restraint in dorsal recumbency on awake cattle, *J Am Vet Res* 49: 1606-1608, 1988.

Mitchell KJ: Dietary abomasal impaction in a herd of dairy replace-ment heifers, *J Am Vet Med Assoc* 198: 1408-1409, 1991.

Müller KE: Some aspects of pathogenesis and therapy of abomasal dis-placements in cattle, *Cattle Practice* 6: 41-44, 1998.

Palmer JE, Whitlock RH: Bleeding abomasal ulcers in adult dairy cattle, *J Am Vet Med Assoc* 183: 448-451, 1983.

Palmer JE, Whitlock RH: Perforated abomasal ulcers in adult dairy cows, *J Am Vet Med Assoc* 184: 171-174, 1984.

Parker JE, Fubini SL: Abomasal fistulas in dairy cows, *Cornell Vet* 77: 303-309, 1987.

Rebhun WC, Fubini SL, Peek SF, Ducharme NG: Presurgical diagno-sis of abomasal displacement and perforation, *Bov Pract* 30: 75-78, 1996.

Saint Jean GD, Hull BL, Hoffsis GF, Rings MD: Comparison of the different surgical techniques for correction of abomasal problems, *Comp Cont Ed Food Animal* 9: F377-F383, 1987.

Sali G, Sali A, Sali M: Zwanzigjährige Erfahrungen mit Labmagenver-lagerungen beim Rind, *Tierärztl Umschau* 6: 438-440, 1987.

Simpson DF, Erb HN, Smith DF: Base excess as a prognostic and diag-nostic indicator in cows with abomasal volvulus or right displace-ment of the abomasum, *Am J Vet Res* 46: 796-797, 1985.

Smith DF. Right-side torsion of the abomasum in dairy cows: classifi-cation of severity and evaluation of outcome, *J Am Vet Med Assoc* 173: 108-111, 1978.

Smith DF: Treatment of left displacement of the abomasum, part I, *Comp Cont Ed* 3: S415-S423, 1981.

Smith DF, Munson L, Erb HN: Abomasal ulcer disease in adult dairy cattle, *Cornell Vet* 73: 213-224, 1983.

Sterner KE, Grymer J: Closed suturing techniques using a bar-suture for correction of left displaced abomasum: a review of 100 cases, *Bov Pract* 17: 80-84, 1982.

Trent AM: Surgery of the bovine abomasum, *Vet Clinics North America* 6: 399-448, 1990.

Van der Velden MA: Functional stenosis of the sigmoid curve of the duodenum in cattle, *Vet Rec* 112: 452-453, 1983.

Wallace CE: Left abomasal displacement: a retrospective study of 315 cases, *Bov Pract* 9: 50-58, 1974.

Whitlock RH: Bovine stomach diseases. In NV Anderson, editor: *Veterinary gastroenterology,* Philadelphia, 1980, Lea & Febiger.

10.5—Small Intestine Surgery in Cattle

Susan L. Fubini and Ava M. Trent

Anatomy

The small intestine of the cow measures from 27 to 49 meters. The cranial part of the duodenum runs dorsally from the pylorus towards the liver, where it takes an S-shaped turn and is adhered tightly to the visceral surface at the hepatic duodenal ligament. It continues dorso-caudally across the abdomen as the descending duode-num and is suspended by the mesoduodenum. The fused superficial and deep walls of the greater omentum attach to its ventral surface. This portion of the duodenum is usually seen upon entry into the abdomen when a right paralumbar fossa celiotomy is performed in an adult dairy cow. At the level of the fifth and sixth lumbar ver-tebrae the duodenum turns around the caudal edge of the greater omentum at the caudal duodenal flexure and continues as the ascending duodenum in a cranial direc-tion. This portion of the duodenum terminates as it passes to the right side of the mesenteric root and con-tinues as the jejunum. The duodenocolic fold attaches the duodenojejunal flexure to the descending colon.

The jejunum is 26 to 48 meters long and is tightly coiled at the edge of the sheetlike mesentery that sus-pends it. The mesentery of the most proximal jejunum is short, which makes it impossible to exteriorize this portion of the bowel from the abdomen. The mesentery lengthens at the more distal segments of jejunum and at the ileum. The distal jejunum and proximal ileum are suspended by a narrow, mobile portion of the mesentery, which has been termed the *distal flange*. The majority of the small intestine is contained within the supraomental recess on the right side of the abdomen. The distal flange may extend caudad outside the recess.

The ileum consists of proximal coiled and distal straight segments that form the terminal portion of small intestine. The ileocecal fold runs from the jejunum and ileum junction to the cecum. For purposes of relevant surgical anatomy, the combined jejunum and ileum has been called the *jejunoileum*. The ileum enters the cecum obliquely at its ventral surface at the ileocecocolic junction. In the adult cow, this junction is obscured by fat.

The cranial mesenteric artery and vein and its branches provide the blood supply to the jejunum and ileum. Proximal branches of this major vessel include the pancreatic branches, caudal pancreaticoduodenal artery, middle colic artery, and ileocolic artery. In the cow, a large collateral branch leaves the cranial mesenteric artery, crosses the right side of the spiral colon, and rejoins the cranial mesenteric artery distally. This vessel is not present in small ruminants. The continuation of the cranial mesenteric artery supplies jejunal arteries that form a series of anastomosing arches. Branches from this vessel supply the proximal part of the ileum and anastomose with the mesenteric ileal branch of the ileocolic artery. In the cow the mesenteric lymph nodes are located between the jejunum and the last centrifugal coil of the spiral colon. In small ruminants they are located between the first centripetal and last centrifugal coils of the spiral colon.

Small Intestinal Accidents

Obstructive lesions of the small intestine are not common but are still seen on a regular basis. In many instances, it is difficult to tell a true obstruction from a functional disorder such as indigestion or enteritis, thus making discussion of a differential diagnosis useful.

The cause of small intestinal accidents is not always apparent. Intussusception has been associated with viral enteritis, alteration of diet, and a nidus such as a small polyp or nodule that causes aberrant intestinal motility. Torsion of the mesenteric root has been reported rarely after casting and rolling a cow for surgery.

Severe abdominal pain is apparent when a strangulating intestinal obstruction is present. This results from tension on the mesentery and bowel distention proximal to the lesion. If the strangulated tissue becomes nonviable, the pain may become less intense for a period of time if left untreated. A localized peritonitis develops; fluid and protein are lost into the abdominal cavity; and eventually the animal deteriorates rapidly as more generalized sepsis ensues. Endotoxemia, shock, and a metabolic acidosis are present when the animal becomes terminal.

The most common location of small intestinal obstruction in the adult cow is the distal jejunum and ileum, which results in ileus and sequestration of fluids

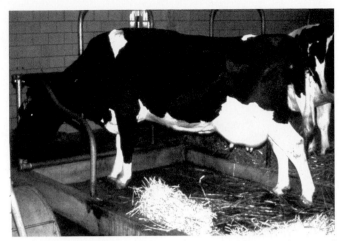

Figure 10.5-1   Abdominal pain manifested by stretching and treading in a cow with a small intestine obstruction.

in the upper gastrointestinal tract. The obstruction in combination with decreased water intake results in dehydration. Because transit of abomasal fluid rich in hydrochloric acid is impeded, hypochloremic metabolic alkalosis is typical. Hypokalemia results from the lack of dietary intake of potassium-rich foods and extracellular fluid shifts.

Calves have lesions in the small intestine as well but also throughout the gastrointestinal tract. Depending on a calf's age, the electrolyte derangements may be less pronounced than an adult's.

CLINICAL SIGNS

A characteristic sign of cattle with obstructive small intestinal diseases is abdominal pain manifested by treading and stretching out (Figure 10.5-1). They may kick at the ventral abdomen and become recumbent if pain is severe (Figure 10.5-2). Affected animals are depressed and anorexic, with decreased rumen contractions and a precipitous drop in milk production. Fever is atypical unless generalized peritonitis occurs, although the heart rate is usually elevated. The respiratory rate is usually normal unless the abdominal distention is severe.

As the disease progresses, fluid accumulates in the bowel proximal to the obstruction and cattle develop abdominal distention, usually low and bilateral. Succussion of the abdomen yields a fluid wave. Small areas of tympanitic resonance may result from gas accumulation in bowel proximal to the obstruction. Manure becomes scant or absent. In some cases melena is passed, presumably from sloughing of devitalized intestine mixed with mucus and fecal material (Figure 10.5-3). Abdominal fluid analysis may be helpful in determining if an inflammatory process is present. Fluid can be obtained from an avascular portion of the abdomen (avoid ventral

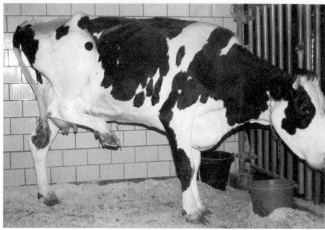

Figure 10.5-2 Abdominal pain characterized by kicking at the abdomen in a cow with an intussusception.

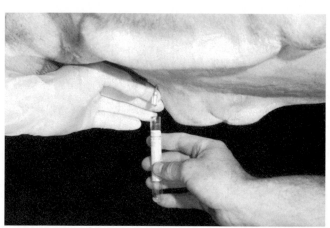

Figure 10.5-4 Abdominal fluid collected using an 18-gauge 3.81-cm needle.

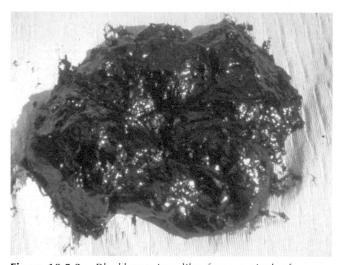

Figure 10.5-3 Blackberry jam–like feces typical of a cow with a small intestine strangulating obstruction.

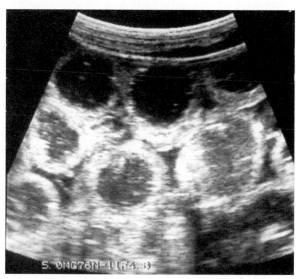

Figure 10.5-5 A transabdominal ultrasound image of a calf with a 5 MHz probe. Note the multiple loops of thickened small intestines filled with a mixture of fluid and gas. This image represents small intestines orad to a small intestinal obstruction.

abdominal vessels), either close to the midline or in front of the udder (Figure 10.5-4). Elevations in total protein (>2.5 g/dL) and cell count (>10,000 cell/μl) are indicative of inflammation.

Ultrasound and rectal examination can be very helpful in identifying distended viscera and, in some cases, the actual cause of the obstruction (Figure 10.5-5). For example, it may be possible to image or palpate the coiled loops of involved intestine with intussusceptions, and fibrin surrounding the lesion may be detectable at later stages of the disease.

Ultrasound is especially useful in small calves when a rectal examination is not possible. Calves with small intestinal obstruction behave similarly to cattle, although

the signs of colic and abdominal distention may be more subtle. Enteritis is common in calves and can be very difficult to distinguish from other obstructive diseases. Signs of abdominal pain, scant or absent manure, progression of signs, and ultrasound findings of bowel distention are reasons to consider surgical exploration.

Intussusception

Intussusception is the invagination of a portion of intestine (intussusceptum) into the lumen of adjacent bowel (the intussuscipiens). This action drags the mesentery and associated blood vessels of the intussusceptum into the neighboring bowel creating an intestinal obstruction. Eventually, the affected bowel becomes nonviable because of its compromised blood supply, and peritonitis results. Untreated cattle usually die 5 to 8 days after the onset of clinical signs.

A paper published by Constable and associates in 1997 discusses 336 cases of intussusception from seventeen veterinary medical teaching hospitals between March 1, 1964, and December 31, 1990. No sex or seasonal predilection for developing intussusception was found, although an increased prevalence in Brown Swiss cattle relative to Holsteins was found. A decreased risk existed for Hereford cattle. The most common locations of intussusception were the small intestine (84%): colocolic (11%), and ileocolic (2%). Calves 1 to 2 months of age were at greater risk for developing intussusception, and animals with intussusceptions distal to the ileum were more likely to be calves. It has been suggested that more fat in the mesentery and a prominent ileocecal ligament may stabilize the bowel and prevent intestinal invagination in adult cattle. The length and mobility of the jejunal mesenteric attachments, especially the distal third, may be why the majority of cattle have jejunojejunal or jejunoileal intussusceptions.

Cattle with intussusception usually show the low grade abdominal pain mentioned previously. This is manifested by treading, stretching out, and kicking at the abdomen. Fecal material that contains mucous or melena is scant and may eventually be absent all together. A pronounced fluid wave upon succussion of the right side of the abdomen and low bilateral abdominal distention is typical, except for cattle with proximal intussusception. Cattle show no interest in feed, stop cleaning their noses, and eventually become dehydrated and metabolically deranged. Rectal and ultrasound examination may reveal distended proximal small intestine, and the intussusception may be discerned in some instances. The lesion is almost never reducible. Single intussusceptions are most common, although a double intussusception has been described. A few reports of cattle surviving after sloughing an intussusception exist, but this is rare. Tumors, polyps, or some other intramural or intraluminal mass may induce abnormal peristalsis, thus facilitating induction of an intussusception. Overeating on lush pasture has been suggested as another cause for abnormal motility and development of intussusception.

Affected cattle should be stabilized with appropriate fluid therapy, nonsteroidal antiinflammatory drugs, and calcium solutions preoperatively. Broad-spectrum perioperative antimicrobials are indicated. An epidural should be given before a standing procedure if the cow is straining. Epidural anesthesia is discussed in the anesthesia chapter, but a low dose should be used so that the cow does not suffer from any hind limb weakness, especially if standing surgery is to be done.

A right paralumbar fossa celiotomy provides the best exposure to the intestinal tract distal to the pylorus. It is possible to perform an exploratory celiotomy and resection and anastomosis in a standing cow, but a more complete, thorough procedure can be done with a recumbent or anesthetized animal. Unfortunately, this requires more people and specialized facilities. Some clinicians advocate starting with a standing celiotomy. If the lesion is too extensive or complicated or exposure is inadequate, the incision can be temporarily closed, and the cow anesthetized or sedated in left lateral recumbency before continuing the procedure. In lateral recumbency, the incision will extend further ventrally so the right lower flank needs to be prepared. It is always a quandary as to whether to attempt an exploration standing. A standing approach may be more appropriate when the nature of the problem is known. If a complete exploratory is necessary, it is more easily accomplished in the anesthetized (preferably) or sedated, recumbent animal. Calves should be explored in lateral recumbency under sedation and a local anesthetic or general anesthesia (Figure 10.5-6).

The abdominal incision should be located halfway between the tuber coxae and the last rib. In a standing cow, it is recommended that the incision not be carried too far ventrally because of the risk of viscera prolapsing out of the abdomen. If the cow is recumbent or anesthetized, a more ventral incision can be made so the majority of the intestinal mass can be exteriorized and inspected.

The surgeon should explore the abdomen *in situ* while palpating for any obvious bowel distention, tight bands, adhesions or mass lesions. The color and quantity of peritoneal fluid should be noted. To access the caudal abdomen, the omental sling is pulled forward,

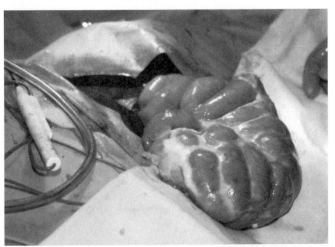

Figure 10.5-6 A severe fibrinous peritonitis in a calf explored from a right paralumbar fossa celiotomy.

and the apex of the cecum, usually in the pelvic inlet, is identified and exteriorized. The cecum is rotated 90 degrees outside of the abdomen bringing the ileum into view. The ileum can be followed to the distal flange of the intestine, which can be rocked out of the abdomen. In a standing cow, the rest of the small intestine is palpated in the abdomen and any abnormal finding brought to the incision. In the recumbent cow, the majority of the small intestine and cecum can be delivered and evaluated. Bowel proximal to the obstruction is usually distended, and bowel distal to the lesion is empty. An intussusception will usually present as tightly coiled loops (Figure 10.5-7). The lesion is typically nonreducible, and attempts to manipulate the bowel are contraindicated because it may be friable and rupture is a risk. The vasculature should be ligated close to the affected bowel to avoid impinging on the blood supply of adjacent bowel. In edematous mesentery, it can be difficult to visualize the individual mesenteric vessels. Much of the dissection can be done bluntly with a gauze sponge gently separating the fat to see the vasculature. Before the resection, a Penrose drain is placed proximal and distal to the diseased bowel to minimize spillage of intestinal contents. The area should be isolated from the rest of the abdomen with moist, sterile towels or laparotomy pads.

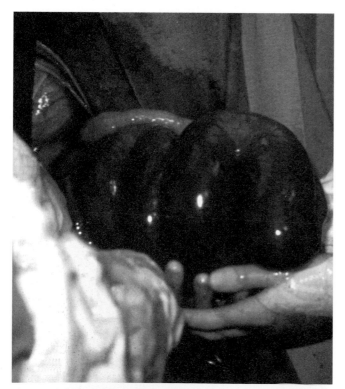

Figure 10.5-7   This is a jejunal intussusception in an adult cow exteriorized through a right paralumbar fossa celiotomy. Note the coiled loops typical of an intussusception.

(From Rebhun WC: *Diseases of dairy cattle*, Philadelphia, 1995, Williams & Wilkins.)

A one- or two-layer end-to-end anastomosis is usually performed, although some surgeons prefer a side-to-side anastomosis. A suggestion to rotate the ends of the bowel has been made in the literature to offset the mesenteric regions when performing an end-to-end anastomosis. This is because cattle have a large serosal-free area at the mesenteric attachment to the small intestine and the rotation provides at least one serosal-covered surface for the entire anastomotic circumference, thus allowing subsequent fibrin deposition and healing. A 2-0 absorbable suture on a taper needle is an appropriate choice for an anastomosis in adults. Young calves have friable small intestine, and a 3-0 suture should be used.

After the anastomosis, the mesenteric defect is closed, the site rinsed copiously with sterile fluids, and the bowel replaced into the abdomen. Surgeons should change gloves and instruments. Replacing the distended intestine back into the abdomen can be difficult, especially in the recumbent cow. It is helpful to decompress the rumen with gas suction and to gently replace handfuls of small intestine starting proximal and working distally. Closure of the abdomen is routine.

Passing large amounts of liquid manure within 24 hours after surgery is a good sign because it signifies a patent intestinal tract. Manure should return to normal over the next 3 to 4 days. Reports of small numbers of cattle doing well after surgery have been made, but Constable's report with a larger number of cattle may be more realistic. He found a postoperative survival rate of 43%, and an overall survival rate of 35%. Reasons for such a poor outcome most likely include the cattle being sick for a long time before admission, peritonitis present at the time of surgery, postoperative ileus, and/or too much devitalized bowel to remove.

Intestinal Volvulus

SEGMENTAL SMALL INTESTINAL VOLVULUS

Volvulus results from twisting of a segment of intestine upon itself, thereby creating an obstruction and strangulation of the blood supply. Some refer to these conditions as a *volvulus of the intestine* and *torsion of the mesentery*. The cause of the twist is not known but may be secondary to ileus. Because of the long mesentery of the distal jejunum and ileum—the so-called *distal flange*—these sections of intestine are more mobile and prone to volvulus. All ages can be affected. Abdominal pain is apparent with signs similar to—but generally more severe than—those of cattle with intussusception. Abdominal distention develops as the proximal intestine fills with gas and fluid. Feces are passed initially, then become scant, and finally absent or mucoid. Rectal and ultrasound examinations usually show distended small intestine often wedged in the pelvic inlet. Cows become tachycardic and dehydrated. Initially a hypochloremic metabolic alkalosis is typical, but as the disease progresses, bowel may become nonviable, and a metabolic acidosis results.

TREATMENT

Cattle should be hydrated and prepared for surgery. Perioperative antibiotics and nonsteroidal antiinflammatory drugs are indicated. A right paralumbar fossa celiotomy is performed as described previously. Affected animals are painful enough that they may be reluctant to stand, thus making left lateral recumbency desirable. However, the final decision for standing vs. down surgery will depend on the surgeon's preference, available facilities, and the temperament of the animal. Upon the surgeon's entry into the abdomen, the nature of the abdominal fluid is noted, and an *in situ* palpation is performed by feeling for any tight bands or mass lesions. The proximal bowel usually is greatly distended with fluid and gas. The twisted bowel feels turgid and, if it is distal small bowel, is typically knotted up in the pelvic inlet. With the animal in lateral recumbency, exteriorizing the majority of the small intestine, correcting any displacement, and checking its orientation is possible (Figure 10.5-8). In the

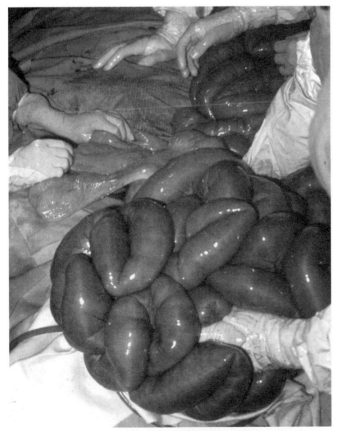

Figure 10.5-8 Volvulus of the distal jejunum and ileum in a cow explored under general anesthesia from the right paralumbar fossa. The cecum is empty; the distal small intestine is compromised; and the proximal small intestine is dilated proximal to the obstruction.

standing animal, the bowel is gently untwisted as it is delivered to the incision. A line of demarcation between noninvolved and involved bowel confirms the diagnosis. The surgeon should be able to tent the mesentery and sweep it up to the root of the mesentery, and it should feel straight. Usually the bowel color and contractility will improve within five minutes of correcting a twist.

There are very few reported methods to determine intestinal viability in cattle, and often these techniques are not practical. It is important not to condemn the bowel without first considering whether the fluid sequestered within the thin-walled, dilated intestine is dark and blood-tinged. This fluid can make the intestine look very dark and congested. The surgeon should push the fluid away from the wall of the intestine and evaluate the color. Because of the convoluted loops of small intestine, it is not practical to perform an enterotomy and "milk" out intestinal contents so that the small intestine is less distended. The bowel is too friable, and its coiled nature makes moving fluid and ingesta difficult. It can be extremely difficult to replace the distended intestine. The rumen should be decompressed and the bowel kept moist. It is replaced in handfuls from proximal to distal with a gentle rocking motion.

The prognosis depends on the duration of the obstruction and the viability of the bowel. A resection and anastomosis can be performed if indicated, but it lengthens the surgery time and makes the procedure more complicated. Furthermore, the amount of bowel involved may preclude a resection. It is easy to contaminate the site as the proximal intestine is usually greatly distended with fluid and gas. If not already given, it is appropriate to administer nonsteroidal antiinflammatory drugs to interrupt the arachidonic cascade and hopefully minimize absorption of endotoxin.

Torsion of the Mesenteric Root

This is a dramatic illness because so much of the bowel is involved in the twist. Only part of the duodenum and dorsal colon are spared. Affected animals experience profound pain. They may actually throw themselves on the ground, get up, and go down again. Bilateral abdominal distention becomes apparent, and cows are tachycardic and tachypneic. Tight bands can be palpated per rectum. Distended viscera can be palpated rectally or imaged by ultrasound.

TREATMENT

Prompt surgical intervention is essential. Perioperative fluids, antibiotics, and analgesics are indicated. This is a major insult, and affected adult cattle rapidly deteriorate and die. A liberal right paralumbar fossa celiotomy is made. Any gas in viscera is decompressed, and by following the mesenteric root, the twist is identified and corrected. Some surgeons do this procedure standing.

The author's preference is lateral recumbency. Untwisting such a massive intestinal mass can predispose the intestine to absorb large amounts of endotoxin, and death may ensue. The rapid progression of signs makes the prognosis for adult cattle grave. A few calves have been saved in our hospital when astute owners recognized the early signs of abdominal discomfort.

MISCELLANEOUS CAUSES OF SMALL INTESTINAL OBSTRUCTION

Incarceration, Entrapment

Sporadic reports of the small intestine becoming entrapped in adhesions, embryonic remnants, or mesenteric rents have been made. Some specific examples include the following:

1. Persistent vitelloumbilical band that runs from the ileum to the umbilicus.
2. Persistent round ligament of the liver that runs from the liver to the umbilicus (Figure 10.5-9).
3. Urachal remnant traveling from the urinary bladder to the umbilicus.
4. Paraovarian bands run from the ovary or broad ligament to the omentum (Figure 10.5-10).
5. Remnants of the ductus deferens in steers.

The small intestine can either become wrapped around one of these bands or entrapped within a loop. The bowel becomes obstructed, and the band can compromise the blood supply at the site of the incarceration.

Clinical signs are similar to those of cows with intussusception. It may be possible to palpate a taut band per rectum. As with other small intestinal obstructions, a

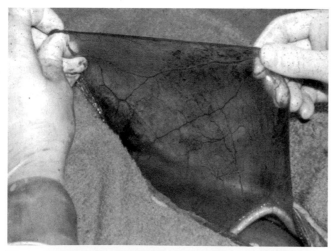

Figure 10.5-9   This was an incidental finding of a persistent round ligament on a right paramedian approach. Small intestine has been reported to twist around such bands.

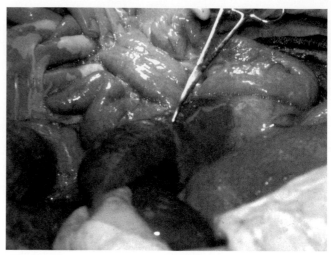

Figure 10.5-10   A right paralumbar fossa celiotomy being performed in a cow with a small intestinal obstruction. The hemostat is pointing out a paraovarian band that was blindly broken down at surgery. No resection was necessary.

right paralumbar fossa celiotomy is performed. The abdomen is explored. The band is palpated and, if possible, exteriorized. If it cannot be visualized, the band may have to be transected blindly. The bowel that was entrapped should be examined to determine if an area of ischemia was created that might necessitate a resection and anastomosis. If it was a narrow band, inverting the affected segment is another surgical option. Fortunately, this is rarely necessary.

The small bowel can become entrapped in a mesenteric rent, either spontaneously or secondary to intestinal surgery in which the mesentery was not closed properly. In some cases, the internal hernia has been corrected by enlarging the defect, replacing the bowel in normal position, and then closing the defect. It has been reported that three cows had proximal jejunum become obstructed in a mesenteric rent, thought to have developed following parturition. The lesions were inaccessible from a standing right paralumbar fossa celiotomy. None of the cows was saved.

Duodenal Outflow Obstruction

Sporadic cases of duodenal outflow obstruction caused by inflammation of the duodenum that results from ulcers, penetrating foreign bodies, intraluminal or extraluminal masses, or adhesions in the vicinity of the sigmoid flexure have been reported. In 1980, Van der Velden from Utrecht described a syndrome of functional duodenal outflow obstruction, which he hypothesized resulted from a disturbance in normal retrograde motility patterns that originate at the sigmoid flexure. Van der Velden subsequently reported eighteen cases in 1983.

Reports of spontaneous obstructions and those with identified lesions have a number of similarities. Cases have been reported predominately in female dairy breeds from 1 to 8 years of age. Common clinical signs in both groups include anorexia, decreased milk and fecal production, tachycardia, variable degrees of depression, and decreased ruminal contractions. Other signs present in some cattle include abdominal distention, colic, scant feces, and ruminal distention. In contrast to the occasional right ventral abdominal distention found with right-sided abomasal volvulus, cows with duodenal outflow obstructions tend to have bilateral ventral abdominal distention. Tympanic pings on the right side are also common findings in a position consistent with or dorsal to right abomasal displacement/volvulus.

Cattle with identified duodenal lesions all had marked fluid and electrolyte disturbances, including dehydration, hyponatremia (127.8 +/− 6.2 mEq/L), hypokalemia (3.2 +/− 0.7 mEq/L), hypochloremia (51.2 +/− 14.8 mEq/L), hyperphosphatemia (9.9 +/− 1.6 mg/dL), hyperglycemia (618.2 +/− 243.3 mg/dL), hyperproteinemia (9.1 +/− 0.5 g/dL), metabolic alkalosis (42.4 +/− 11.2 mEq/L HCO3; 16.0 +/− 10.8 mEq/L base excess), and elevated anion gap (36.6 +/− 7.9 mEq/L). Electrolyte disturbances were comparable to—or more severe than—values reported for cows with abomasal volvulus; however, the anion gap was attributed to accumulation of a different set of anions in the two conditions. Protein and phosphate increases were considered to account for most of the anion gap in cows with duodenal obstruction, as opposed to increases in sulfates and organic acid anions resulting from tissue necrosis and anaerobic metabolism in abomasal volvulus. Van der Velden's report included less complete information on fluid and electrolyte disturbances, but the available information is consistent with that reported by Garry with additional information on base excess (10-32 mmol/L), serum chloride (45-90 mmol/L), and elevated rumen chloride concentrations (up to 75 mmol/liter).

A definitive diagnosis requires exploration from the right side, preferably a standing right flank exploratory. The characteristic sign of this condition is distention of the cranial portion of the duodenum with a flaccid descending duodenum. The abomasum may also be dilated and dorsally displaced. The initial cases of spontaneous duodenal obstruction were actually diagnosed as right abomasal displacement and treated by omentopexy without success. Careful palpation of the area of the sigmoid flexure may reveal a specific lesion that can account for the outflow obstruction. However, the normal ligamentous thickening in this area supports the fragile pancreatic and biliary ducts that should not be misinterpreted as an adhesion.

Treatment/Prognosis/Complications Treatment involves removal of any identified obstructing lesions (adhesions, masses) or, if the lesion cannot be removed or identified, a duodenal bypass around the site of obstruction needs to be done. The cranial part of the duodenum is anastamosed to the descending duodenum usually in a side-side manner. Supportive fluid and/or antibiotic therapy are usually indicated based on the cause of obstruction and the status of the patient.

Although this syndrome appears to be uncommon and bears many similarities to an RDA, definitive treatment for a functional or mechanical duodenal obstruction should be considered if, on initial exploration for an RDA, abomasal dilation/displacement without volvulus and proximal duodenal distention to but not beyond the sigmoid flexure is identified. Reexploration with definitive treatment is also a legitimate consideration if a cow with the above signs has been treated by omentopexy, and fluid and electrolyte disturbances have progressed during the first 2 days after surgery.

Jejunal Hemorrhage Syndrome

In the past five years, reports of a disease in dairy cows called *jejunal hemorrhage* or *acute death syndrome* have increased. Descriptions of this disease vary from acute death with no premonitory signs to animals that show visible signs of colic shortly before death. At necropsy, the major finding consistent within these animals has been severe hemorrhage of the jejunum. Most often, this is seen as an intraluminal blood clot, but some cases have been reported with subserosal hemorrhage (Figure 10.5-11). The only reliable finding seems to be the presence of *Clostridium perfringens* type A at the site of the jejunal lesion. It has been proposed that *C. perfringens* type A is the causative organism of this disease; however, this is quite controversial. If the animal lives long enough for observation, clinical signs include vocalization, diaphoresis, bruxism, enophthalmia, tachycardia, pale mucous membranes, and small bowel distention. Eventually, shock, recumbency, and death ensue. Occasionally, an animal is seen early enough with a localized lesion and has had a resection and anastomosis performed. In most instances, medical therapy with a blood transfusion, fluid therapy, and antimicrobials are essential.

This can present as a herd problem. One study surveyed dairy practitioners in Iowa, Minnesota, and Wisconsin and found that risk factors included advanced age and early lactation. The syndrome was reported more frequently in herds that milked more than 100 cows and fed total mixed ration. This was only one study, and it could involve biases such as large herds being more likely to perform necropsy examinations. More information regarding this disease should become available in the future.

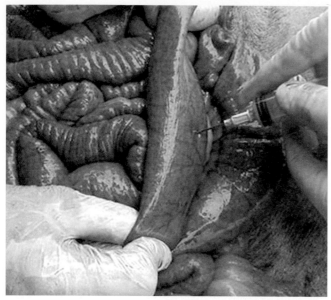

Figure 10.5-11   This is a *post mortem* specimen showing loops of jejunum affected with the spontaneous hemorrhage syndrome. An aspirate is being obtained for bacterial culture.

(Courtesy of Dr. Gillian Perkins; Cornell University.)

FAT NECROSIS

It is rare—but possible—for fat necrosis or lipomatosis to encroach on the intestinal lumen, especially in older overconditioned animals. Affected cattle have a very insidious onset of disease with decreased amounts of loose manure, abdominal distention, and mild colic. It may be possible to palpate hard intraabdominal masses rectally or image them with ultrasound. In valuable animals, an exploratory celiotomy or ultrasound-guided biopsy may be indicated. The prognosis is grave, although resecting or bypassing the affected bowel may be possible in some instances.

NEOPLASIA

Another cause of extraluminal intestinal obstruction is neoplasia. The most common tumors found in cattle include adenocarcinoma and lymphosarcoma. In rare instances, it may be able to resect or bypass a localized neoplasm. Lymphosarcoma has a predilection for the pylorus (see abomasal section, Chapter 10.4), but can occur at other locations. Signs are vague as with fat necrosis. The prognosis is grave. Surgical resection in most cases is impractical.

SPONTANEOUS RUPTURE OF THE SMALL INTESTINE

Dr. John King (Professor Emeritus of Pathology at Cornell University) has observed spontaneous rupture of

jejunal segments at postmortem, which he postulated might be secondary to entrapment between the uterus and body wall during parturition.

RECOMMENDED READINGS

Anderson DE, Constable PD, St Jean G, Hull BL: Small-intestinal volvulus in cattle: 35 cases (1967-1992), *J Am Vet Med Assoc* 203: 1178-1183, 1993.

Baxter GM, Darien BJ, Wallace CE: Persistent urachal remnant causing intestinal strangulation in a cow, *J Am Vet Med Assoc* 191: 555-558, 1987.

Constable PD, St. Jean G, Hull BL, Rings DM, Morin DE, Nelson DR: Intussusception in cattle: 336 Cases (1964-1993), *J Am Vet Med Assoc* 210: 531-536, 1997.

Dennison AC, Van Metre DC, Callan RJ, Dinsmore P, Mason GL, Ellis RP: Hemorrhagic bowel syndrome in dairy cattle: 22 cases (1997-2000), *J Am Vet Med Assoc* 5: 686-689, 2002.

Ducharme NG, Smith DF, Koch DB: Small intestinal obstruction caused by a persistent round ligament of the liver in a cow, *J Am Vet Med Assoc* 180: 1234-1236, 1982.

Fubini SL, Smith DF, Tithof PK, et al: Volvulus of the distal part of the jejunoileum in four cows, *Vet Surg* 15: 150-152, 1986.

Garry F. Hull BL, Rings DM, et al: Comparison of naturally occurring proximal duodenal obstruction and abomasal volvulus in dairy cattle, *Vet Surg* 17: 226-233, 1988.

Godden S, Frank R, Ames T: Survey of Minnesota dairy veterinarians on the occurrence of and potential risk factors for jejunal hemorrhage syndrome in adult dairy cows, *Bov Pract* 35: 97-103, 2001.

Kirkpatrick MA, Timms LL, Kersting KW, Kinyon JM: Case report: jejunal hemorrhage syndrome of dairy cattle, *Bov Pract* 35: 104-116, 2001.

Koch DB, Robertson JT, Donawick WJ: Small intestinal obstruction due to persistent vitelloumbilical band in a cow, *J Am Vet Med Assoc* 173: 197-200, 1978.

Levine SA, Smith DF, Wilsman NJ, Kolb DS: Arterial and venous supply to the bovine jejunum and proximal part of the ileum, *Am J Vet Res* 48: 1295-1299, 1987.

Levine S et al: Comparative healing of mesenteric and antimesenteric incisions in the bovine jejunum, *Am J Vet Res* 49(8): 1339-1343, 1988.

Pearson H: Intussusception in cattle, *Vet Rec* 89: 426-437, 1971.

Pearson H: The treatment of surgical disorders of the bovine abdomen, *Vet Rec* 92: 245-254, 1973.

Pearson H, Pincent PJN: Intestinal obstruction in cattle, *Vet Rec* 101: 162-166, 1977.

Richardson DW: Paraovarian-omental bands as a cause of small intestinal obstruction in cows, *J Am Vet Med Assoc* 185: 517-519, 1984.

Robertson JT: Differential diagnosis and surgical management of intestinal obstruction in cattle, *Vet Clin North Am {Large Anim Pract}* 1: 377-394, 1979.

Serteyn D, Mottart E: Resection of an ileocecal intussusception in a cow, *Agri-Practice* 30-31, 1987.

Smith DF: Intussusception in adult cattle, *Comp Cont Ed Pract Vet* II: S49-S53, 1980.

Smith DF: Bovine intestinal surgery, part 1, *Mod Vet Pract* 65: 705-710, 1984.

Smith DF: Bovine intestinal surgery, part 5: intussusception, *Mod Vet Pract* 66: 405-409, 1985.

Smith DF: Bovine intestinal surgery, part 6: intussusception (continued), *Mod Vet Pract* 66: 443-446, 1985.

Van der Velden MA: Functional stenosis of the sigmoid curve of the duodenum in cattle, *Vet Rec* 112: 452-453, 1983.

10.6—Surgery of the Cecum

Adrian Steiner

Anatomy

The cecum is a large, mobile tube with the apex directed caudally. Cranially, the cecum is continuous with the proximal loop of the ascending colon (PLAC), and no valve exists between these two segments of the large intestine (Figure 10.6-1). The ileocecocolic (ICC) junction represents the division between the cecum and colon. The main part of the cecum is situated within the supraomental recess. The free cecal apex is directed toward the pelvic cavity. The cecum is attached dorsally to the PLAC by the short cecocolic fold and ventrally to the ileum by the ileocecal fold (Figure 10.6-1). The PLAC extends cranially from the cecum to the level of the 11th rib and then doubles back to the level of the caudal flexure of the duodenum. There, it turns from the right to the left of the mesentery and is continuous with the spiral colon. The ileocolic artery with its three colic branches is responsible for the blood supply of the ICC area. The cecal artery, which arises from the first colic branch, supplies the ileum by the ileal branches and the cecum by the cecal branches. The cecal artery crosses the ileum near the ICC junction and progresses along the ileocecal fold parallel to the cecum. At the free end of the ileocecal fold, the cecal artery has anastomoses with the first ileal artery. The arteries are accompanied by their corresponding veins and nerves.

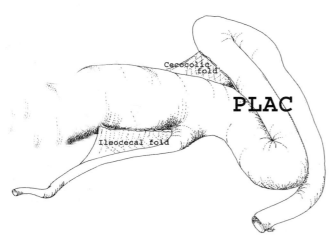

Figure 10.6-1 Diagrammatic representation of the normal anatomy of the ileum, cecum, and proximal loop of the ascending colon (PLAC). The ileocecal and cecocolic fold are labeled.

Physiology

In cattle, the cecum and colon are the main sites for microbial digestion besides the reticulorumen. In the cecum and the colon of the cow, 11.6% to 17% of the total dietary cellulose, 2% to 11 % of the total starch, and 20% of the soluble carbohydrates are digested. Cecocolic fermentation accounts for 8.6% to 16.8% of total volatile fatty acid (VFA) production in sheep. The efficiency of the large intestine for VFA production is similar to that of the rumen. Principal end-products of microbial carbohydrate fermentation in the hindgut are acetate, propionate and butyrate, which are found up to 99% in the dissociated form because the pH of large intestinal contents is usually considerably higher than pKa values of the individual VFA. VFA are absorbed through the cecal epithelium. Absorption takes place by passive diffusion of the undissociated ions through the cell membrane, whereas the anions are absorbed at a considerably slower rate by diffusion through hydrophilic pores. The absorption of VFA from the cecum of sheep is about twice as high at pH 6.2 (equilibrium-shift towards undissociated ions) as at pH 7.7 (equilibrium-shift towards anions). The cow is able to partially compensate for the removal of the cecum, including the ICC junction. In a study of five steers, digestibility of dry matter and cellulose returned to preoperative values within 16 weeks after cecal amputation. Consistency of feces, however, did not return to preoperative firmness, thus illustrating the importance of this segment of the gut for water resorption.

Cecal Dilatation/Dislocation

ETIOPATHOGENESIS

Hypocalcemia or/and an inhibitory effect of elevated VFA concentrations in the cecum on cecal motility has been reported. Diets excessively rich in rumen-resistant starch have therefore been implicated in the development of spontaneous cecal dilatation and dislocation (CDD), as a consequence of increased carbohydrate fermentation in the large intestine. In a controlled study on VFA concentrations in the large intestine of cows, dissociated and undissociated VFA were elevated in the contents of cecum, PLAC, and rectum of cows with CDD in comparison to healthy control cows. However, whether this elevation of VFA was the cause or the consequence of reduced motility and stasis of digesta remained unclear. In a subsequent study, contractility of *ex vivo* intestinal wall specimens from the cecum and spiral colon of healthy cows was found not to be affected by preincubation with butyric and valerianic acid.

Myoelectric activity patterns similar to that observed orad to an intestinal obstruction were recorded from the cecum and PLAC of cows with delayed recovery or recurrence after surgical correction of spontaneous CDD. Hence, it was hypothesized that some motility disturbance of the spiral colon rather than the cecum itself might be implicated in the development of spontaneous CDD. Physiologic myoelectric motility patterns of the spiral colon were described in detail. After an abrupt increase of starch-rich concentrates in diet from hay to a ration of 50% hay and 50% starch-rich concentrates within 60 hours, pH values decreased, and VFA concentrations increased significantly in the colon of healthy experimental dairy cows. Significant changes in patterns of myoelectric activity of the spiral colon, however, were restricted to phases III and IV of the bovine migrating myoelectric complex and to propagation velocity. The classical hypothesis that an abrupt increase of the concentration of VFA might be responsible for atony of the cecum, and spontaneous occurrence of CDD was not supported by the aforementioned recent findings. Etiology and pathogenesis of spontaneous CDD are still unknown.

EPIDEMIOLOGICAL FACTORS

In a recent epidemiological study realized in Switzerland, similar prevalences of CDD and abomasal displacement (DA) were found. Breed predilection for occurrence of CDD does not exist, but there is an increased risk for development of CDD during the production phase until the end of lactation and in cows without supplementation of stock salt and/or minerals.

CLASSIFICATION OF CECAL DILATATION/DISLOCATION

Cecal *dilatation* is distention of the cecum without twist. The cecal apex is directed caudad and positioned in front of or within the pelvic cavity. Rotation along its long axis is called cecal *torsion* (Figure 10.6-2), and rotation in the area of the ICC junction or the PLAC—when viewed from the right side of the cow—is termed *clockwise or counterclockwise twist or volvulus*. The author prefers the

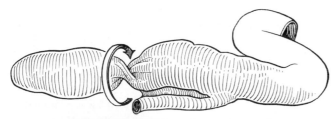

Figure 10.6-2   Schematic representation of cecal torsion.

(Reprinted with permission from Fubini SL: Surgery of the bovine large intestine. In Bristol DG, editor: *Surgery of the bovine digestive tract, Vet Clin North America, Food Animal Practice*, Philadelphia, 1990, WB Saunders.)

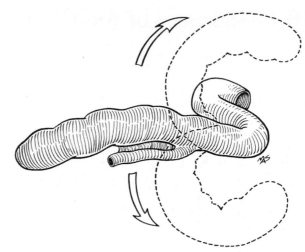

Figure 10.6-3   Schematic representation of cecal dislocation or volvulus. *Dorsal retroflexion* (retroflexio at dorsam) and *ventral retroflexion* (retroflexio ad ventram) of the cecum may occur.

(Reprinted with permission from Fubini SL: Surgery of the bovine large intestine. In Bristol DG, editor: *Surgery of the bovine digestive tract, Vet Clin North America, Food Animal Practice*, Philadelphia, 1990, WB Saunders.)

terms *dorsal retroflexion* (retroflexio at dorsam) and *ventral retroflexion* (retroflexio ad ventram) to better define the previously used terms *clockwise* and *counterclockwise twist/volvulus*, respectively (Figure 10.6-3). The degree of rotation in cases of retroflexion may vary from 90 degrees to more than 360 degrees. The term *dislocation* can refer to any twist, torsion, volvulus, or retroflexion.

SYMPTOMS AND DIAGNOSIS

Symptoms of simple cecal *dilatation* are not specific. They include a drop in milk yield, reduced appetite and amount of feces, and occasionally discrete signs of colic. Ruminal motility and small intestinal peristalsis may be reduced. The right paralumbar fossa is distended (Figure 10.6-4); percussion (ping) and succussion auscultation in the right flank are positive, extending from the tuber coxae to the last rib. The distended cecum is identified through rectal examination. The apex of the cecum reaches the pelvic cavity and can be palpated as a tense dome-shaped hollow organ with a smooth surface. It can be difficult to tell a distended cecum from an enlarged right displaced abomasum. The cecum usually has thinner walls than the abomasum, and is oblong in shape. A distended right-sided abomasum, is a rounded structure located more cranially in the abdomen. Hematological and serum biochemical parameters are usually within normal range. These signs become more severe in case of *retroflexion* or *torsion*. In case of *retroflexion*, animals are anorectic and have more obvious signs of

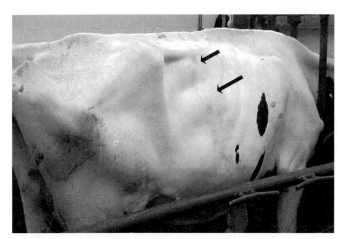

Figure 10.6-4 Mature white Holstein-Friesian cow with cecal dislocation. The distended cecum has resulted in two outlines of distended viscera (arrows) in the right paralumbar fossa.

(Courtesy of Dr. GA Perkins, Cornell University.)

colic. Reduction of milk yield is more pronounced; heart rate is elevated; and atony of the rumen is common. Feces are absent or very sparse and of dry consistency covered with mucus. The area of the ping and the positive succussion auscultation is larger, extending further craniad than in a case of simple dilatation. Upon rectal examination, the body—but not the apex—of the cecum can be palpated in the right upper quadrant as a tense tubular hollow organ with a diameter of about 15 to 20 cm. Biochemical analysis of blood may rarely reveal a hypochloremic, hypokalemic metabolic alkalosis caused by stasis or even reflux of intestinal contents.

Torsion of the cecum occurs less often than retroflexion, but symptoms are similar. Cecal torsion can be diagnosed through rectal examination. The cecal apex is directed caudad, and the tense ICC ligament, which may have pain elicited upon palpation, is identified as a tense structure that spirals around the cecum.

THERAPY AND PROGNOSIS

Medical therapy is indicated if the general condition of the animal is normal or only slightly disturbed, defecation is still present, and rectal examination does not reveal any torsion or retroflexion. If the prerequisites for medical therapy are not fulfilled or medical treatment is revealed as unsuccessful within 24 hours after initiation, typhlotomy is indicated. Cecal amputation is indicated only in cases of CDD recurrence or devitalization of the cecal wall.

Medical treatment consists of intravenous fluid administration supplemented with potassium chloride as needed, purgatives, and NSAIDs as needed. Bethanechol

may be administered subcutaneously at 0.07 mg/kg bwt, TID for 2 days. Alternatively, some authors have reported beneficial effect from oral administration of one pound of instant coffee. Supplementary medication may include correction of calcium deficiency and treatment of ketosis. Feed is completely withheld for at least 24 hours, and small amounts of hay is then gradually offered, provided defecation is present and CDD has resolved. In a retrospective study, only 13 of 111 cows (12%) with spontaneous CDD fulfilled the criteria for medical treatment. One of those required surgical treatment 2 days after initiation of medical treatment because of deterioration of the general condition. If recovery does not become evident within 24 hours after initiation of medical treatment, surgical intervention is recommended.

Typhlotomy

Surgery is performed through a right flank approach, preferably in the standing animal under local anesthesia. The abdomen is opened through a 25-cm incision that starts dorsally about 8 cm below the lateral processes of the lumbar vertebrae and 8 cm cranial to the tuber coxae, extending slightly oblique in a cranioventral direction parallel to the internal oblique abdominal muscle. The abdomen is then thoroughly explored, and the cecum, PLAC, and spiral colon positions identified (Figure 10.6-5). Decompression of any large gas-filled viscus

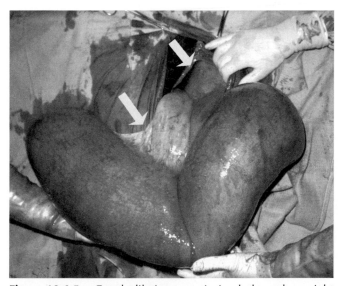

Figure 10.6-5 Cecal dilation exteriorized through a right paralumbar fossa celiotomy. In addition to the distended cecum one can see the cecocolic fold (bottom arrow) and proximal loop of the ascending colon (top arrow).

(Courtesy of Dr. SL Fubini; Cornell University.)

may make more room for manipulations and decrease the possibility of intestinal rupture. If the cecum is simply dilated, the apex is found in or in front of the pelvic cavity, directed caudally. In case of (dorsal or ventral) retroflexion of 180 degrees, the apex of the cecum is directed craniad, and in case of torsion, the apex is directed caudad. Manipulation of the ICC ligament is painful and reveals spiraling around the cecum along its longitudinal axis.

Dislocations are carefully corrected intraabdominally. The cecum and as much of the PLAC as possible are exteriorized (Figure 10.6-6) by gently pushing with the palm(s) of one or both hands from the inside toward the outside of the abdomen to reduce the risk of rupture and/or perforation of the distended bowel. If the bowel is compromised or severely distended, it may be appropriate to perform a typhlotomy before any attempt is made to untwist the dislocation. The apex of the cecum is isolated from the rest of the abdomen, and a typhlotomy is performed at the most ventral location (Figure 10.6-7). Digesta are first passively drained from the extraabdominal part of the cecum and then gently milked from the intraabdominal part of the cecum and the PLAC to the incision site. The exteriorized cecum is rinsed with copious amounts of prewarmed 0.9% saline solution and the incision site closed with a simple inverting continuous or an inverting seromuscular suture pattern (i.e., Cushing or Lembert) with size USP 3-0 or 2-0 monofilament absorbable suture material. The exteriorized sections are again copiously rinsed and placed

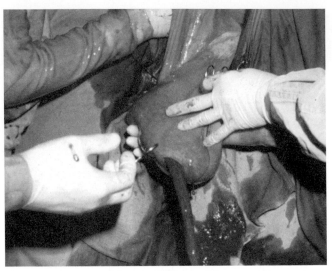

Figure 10.6-7   Typhlotomy performed from a right paralumbar fossa celiotomy

(Courtesy of Dr. SL Fubini, Cornell University.)

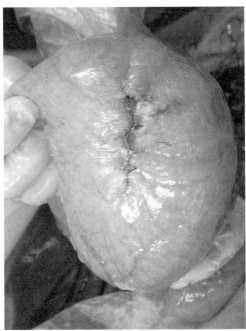

Figure 10.6-8   Intraoperative view of the cecal apex after the incision has been closed with two continuous inverting seromuscular suture patterns.

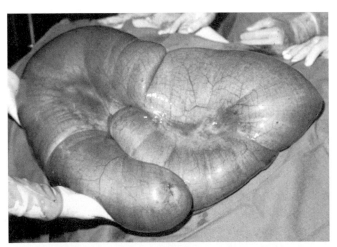

Figure 10.6-6   Cow under general anesthesia in left lateral recumbency. Intraoperative view of the dilated cecum and proximal ascending colon (PLAC) in a case of spontaneous cecal dilatation/dislocation exteriorized through a right paralumbar fossa celiotomy

(Courtesy of Dr. SL Fubini; Cornell University.)

back into their physiologic position within the supraomental recess. The cecum is evaluated again 10 minutes later; and if it has refilled, a second typhlotomy is done to relieve the cecum and PLAC of digesta that may have accumulated within these segments by propulsion from the ileum or reflux from the spiral colon. The typhlotomy site is finally oversewn twice (one layer should be in an inverting pattern) (Figure 10.6-8). At this point,

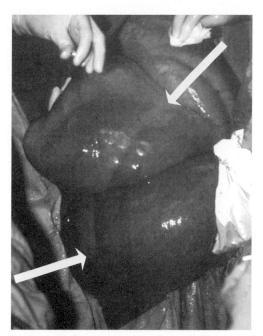

Figure 10.6-9 Right paralumbar fossa celiotomy showing the spiral loops of the ascending colon (top arrow) located abaxially and dorsal to the cecum (bottom arrow). This indicates that correct anatomical positioning has not yet been achieved.

(Courtesy of Dr. SL Fubini; Cornell University.)

the orientation of the distal flange of small intestine and the spiral loop of the ascending colon should be checked for correct anatomical positioning. The spiral loop of the ascending colon should be axial to the cecum and PLAC (Figure 10.6-9). Closure of the abdominal wall is performed in a routine manner.

Postoperatively, bethanechol (0.07 mg/kg bwt, sc, tid, for 2 days) may be administered to help restore intestinal motility. Antimicrobials (e.g., sodium penicillin, 30,000 IU/kg bwt, IV) are administered perioperatively. If contamination is severe, prolonged administration of a broad-spectrum antimicrobial for 3 to 5 days may be indicated. If necessary, intravenous or oral rehydration to correct electrolyte imbalances, calcium deficiency and to treat ketosis should be performed. Operated cows are put on a restricted diet for 24 to 48 hours. The restricted diet is followed by a medium coarse forage ration of increasing quantity to finally reach the normal ration within 5 to 7 days. Manure is usually very loose initially and becomes more formed over time. Recovery (i.e., restoration of appetite and gastrointestinal motility) may be expected within 2 to 5 days after the surgical intervention.

Possible complications after typhlotomy include septic peritonitis as a result of severe intraoperative contamination or suture line leakage and persistent motility disorder of the large intestine leading to short-term recurrence of CDD. In the latter case, cows should be reoperated on, and cecal amputation, leaving the ileocecal junction intact, should be performed. Overall, long-term recurrence rates after typhlotomy have been reported to range from 10% to 22.5%. Although recurrence is theoretically impossible after cecal amputation, this procedure is not recommended during the initial surgical intervention because the long-term success rate is not significantly different from that after typhlotomy alone. In a retrospective study with 80 cows treated surgically for CDD within a period of 19 months, short-term (release from the clinical) survival rate was 91%. With a mean of 11 months after surgery, 67.5% of cows were still productive members of their herds. Anecdotal reports describe dilation of the cecal stump after amputation anywhere from 3 months to a year after typhlectomy distal to the ileocecal junction. In these cows, recurrence was treated by resection of the remaining cecal stump.

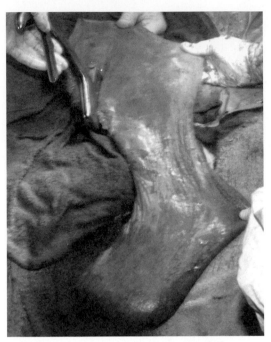

Figure 10.6-10   Resection of the apex of the cecum for recurrence of CDD. The cow is under general anesthesia, in left lateral recumbency. Autosuture equipment (the TA-90) is being used to place a double row of staples across the lumen of the cecum. A second application of the stapling instrument would be necessary before transection of the cecum

(Courtesy of Dr. SL Fubini; Cornell University.)

Cecal Intussusceptions

Because cecal intussusception is primarily a disease of calves, it is described in detail in Section 14.2.2.

Amputation of the Cecum

In case of recurrence of CDD or devitalization of the cecal wall, cecal amputation immediately distal to the ICC junction is recommended. This procedure may be performed in the standing animal after local analgesia of the right flank. The cecum is evacuated as described before, and the ICC ligament is anesthetized by infiltration of 30 ml of a 2% lidocaine solution, injected near the ICC junction to block the cecal nerve. The cecal branches of the cecal artery and vein are ligated close to the attachment of the ICC ligament to the cecum to preserve blood supply to the ileum. Ligature of the blood vessels may be accomplished either by direct visualization after blunt dissection of the overlying fat or by blind mass

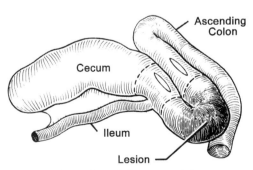

Figure 10.6-11   Resection of the apex of the cecum and the devitalized bowel located at the first turn of the PLAC. A side-to-side anastomosis is done to reestablish intestinal continuity.

(Reprinted with permission from Fubini SL: Surgery of the bovine large intestine. In Bristol DG, ed: *Surgery of the bovine digestive tract, Vet Clin North America, Food Animal Practice,* Philadelphia, 1990, WB Saunders.)

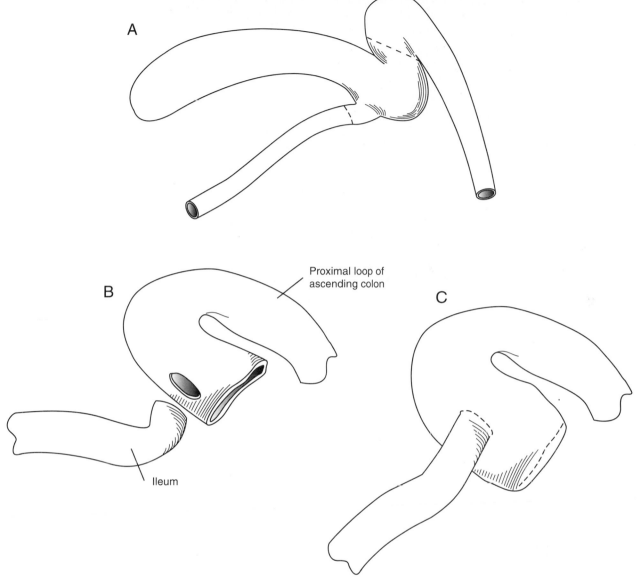

A

Proximal loop of
ascending colon

B

C

Ileum

Figure 10.6-12 *A,* Dotted lines indicate the lines of transection in preparation for a complete typhlectomy. The vasculature between the cecum and ileum should be ligated during the preparation process. B, Commencing an end-to-side anastomosis between the ileum and ascending colon. C, Anastomosis completed.

ligatures of the ligament. The ICC ligament is transected. Two intestinal clamps—one from the mesenteric and one from the antimesenteric side—are placed a few centimeters aboral to the intended site of amputation, just proximal to the ICC junction. The cecum is transected, and the cecal stump closed with two continuous inverting seromuscular suture patterns (i.e., Cushing or Lembert) with size USP 2-0 or 3-0 resorbable (calves) suture material. Alternatively, the stump may be closed by using a stapling instrument* and two linear 90-mm

*Auto Suture, TA-90, United States Surgical Corporation; Norwalk, CT 06850

cartridges of 3.5-mm staples. The staple lines overlap in the center of the stump (Figure 10.6-10).

If retroflexion has been present for a prolonged period of time and/or the degree of rotation exceeds 270°, vascular compromise and concurrent hemorrhagic strangulating obstruction of the PLAC may occur. This condition requires partial resection of the PLAC, followed by side-to-side anastomosis. The ICC junction is left intact (Figure 10.6-11). This procedure is technically difficult and is preferably performed under general anesthesia with the cow positioned in left lateral recumbency to minimize contamination and facilitate manipulation of the intestinal segments being operated. Aftercare is according to that described for typhlotomy.

A complete typhlectomy with ileocolic anastomosis has been reported as a surgical treatment for severe cecal dislocation with devitalization of the entire cecum (Maala, 1983). This is a difficult, long procedure in most instances and should be done under general anesthesia. The entire cecum is resected and an end-to-side or side-to-side anastomosis performed as shown in Figure 10.6-12.

RECOMMENDED READINGS

Abegg R, Eicher R, Lis J, et al: Concentration of volatile fatty acids in digesta samples obtained from healthy cows and cows with cecal dilatation and dislocation, *Am J Vet Res* 60: 1540-1545, 1999.

Allemann M, Eicher R, Mevissen M, et al: Effect of sodium butyric acid, sodium valerianic acid, and osmolarity on contractility of specimens of intestinal wall obtained from the cecum and spiral colon of healthy cows, *Am J Vet Res* 61: 678-683, 2000.

Braun U, Eicher R, Hausammann K: Clinical findings in cattle with dilatation and torsion of the caecum, *Vet Rec* 125: 265-267, 1989.

Braun U, Hermann M, Pabst B: Haematological and biochemical findings in cattle with dilatation and torsion of the caecum, *Vet Rec* 125: 396-398, 1989.

Braun U, Marmier O: Ultrasonographic examination of the small intestine of cows, *Vet Rec* 136: 239-44, 1995.

Braun U, Steiner A, Bearth G: Therapy and clinical progress of cattle with dilatation and torsion of the caecum, *Vet Rec* 125: 430-433, 1989.

Breves G, Diener M, Ehrlein H, et al: Physiologie des Magen-Darm-Kanals. In von Engelhardt W, Breves B, editors: *Physiologie der Haustiere*, Stuttgart, 2000, Enke im Hyppokrates Verlag GmbH.

Bristol D, Fubini S: Surgery of the neonatal bovine digestive tract, *Vet Clin North Am (Food Anim Pract)* 6: 473-493, 1990.

Constable P, St. Jean G, Hull B, et al: Intussusception in cattle: 336 cases (1964-1993), *J Am Vet Med Assoc* 210: 531-36, 1997.

Doll K, Klee W, Dirksen G: Blinddarminvagination beim Kalb, *Tierärztl Prax* 26: 247-253, 1998.

Eicher R, Audigé L, Braun U, et al: Epidemiologie und Risiko-Faktoren von Labmagenverlagerungen und Blinddarmdilatation bei der Milchkuh. Internationaler Workshop Ätiologie, Pathogenese, Diagnostik, Prognose, Therapie und Prophylaxe der Dislocatio abomasi, 1998.

Fubini SL: Surgery of the bovine large intestine, *Vet Clin North Am (Food Anim Pract)* 6: 461-471, 1990.

Fubini SL, Erb HN, Rebhun WC, et al: Cecal dilatation and volvulus in dairy cows: 84 cases (1977-1983), *J Am Vet Med Assoc* 189: 96-99, 1986.

Goodall ED, Kay RNB: Digestion and absorption in the large intestine of the sheep, *J Physiol* 176: 12-23, 1965.

Julian R, Hawke T: Cecal colic intussusception in a calf, *Can Vet J* 4: 54-55, 1963.

Klein WR, van der Velden MA, Ensink JM: Single intraoperative administration of antibiotic to cows with caecal torsion: wound infection and postoperative performance: a retrospective and prospective study, *Vet Quart* 16: S111-S113, 1994.

Maala CP, Sack WO: The arterial supply to the ileum, cecum and proximal loop of the ascending colon in the ox, *Zbl Vet Med C* 10: 130-146, 1981.

Maala CP, Sack WO: Nerves to the cecum, ileum, and proximal loop of the ascending colon in cattle, *Am J Vet Res* 43: 1566-1571, 1982.

Maala CP, Sack WO: The venous supply of the cecum, ileum, and the proximal loop of the ascending colon in the ox. *Zbl Vet Med C* 12: 154-166, 1983.

Maala CP, Smith DF, Hintz HF, et al: Removal of the cecum, including the ileocecocolic junction, and its effects on digestibility in cattle, *Am J Vet Res* 44: 2237-2243, 1983.

Matthé A, Lebzien P, Flachowski G: Zur Bedeutung von Bypass-Stärke für die Glucoseversorgung von hochleistenden Milchkühen, *Übers Tierernährg* 28: 1-64, 2000.

Meylan M, Eicher R, Blum J, et al: Effects of an abrupt increase of starch-rich concentrates in the diet of dairy cows on volatile fatty acid concentrations in rumen and intestine: significant association with myoelectric activity of the spiral colon, *Am J Vet Res* 63: 857-867, 2002.

Meylan M, Eicher R, Röthlisberger J, et al: Myoelectric activity of the spiral colon in dairy cows, *Am J Vet Res* 63: 78-93, 2002.

Nickel R, Schummer A: Mittel- und Enddarm. In Nickel R, Schummer A, and Seiferle E (eds.): *Lehrbuch der Anatomie der Haustiere.* Berlin und Hamburg, 1975, Paul Parey, pp. 169-177.

Pankowski RL, Fubini SL, Stehman S: Cecal volvulus in a dairy cow: partial resection of the proximal portion of the ascending colon, *J Am Vet Med Assoc* 191: 435-436, 1987.

Pearson H: Intussusception in cattle, *Vet Rec* 89: 426-437, 1971.

Ridges A, Singleton A: Some quantitative aspects of digestion in goats, *J Physiol* 161: 1-9, 1962.

St. Jean G: Decision making in bovine abdominal surgery, *Vet Clin North Am (Food Anim Pract)* 6: 335-358, 1990.

Siciliano-Jones J, Murphy M: Production of volatile fatty acids in the rumen and cecum-colon of steers as affected by forage: concentrate and forage physical form, *J Dairy Sci* 72: 485-492, 1989.

Steiner A, Braun U, Lischer C: Blinddarmdilatation/ -torsion bei der Kuh:80 Fälle (1988-1990), *Wien Tierärztl Mschr* 79: 41-46, 1992.

Steiner A, Braun U, Waldvogel A: Comparison of staple and suture techniques for partial typhlectomy in the cow: a prospective clinical study of 40 cases, *J Vet Med Assoc* 39: 26-37, 1992.

Steiner A, Oertle C, Flückiger M, et al: Was diagnostizierten sie? Welche Massnahmen schlagen sie vor? *Schweiz Arch Tierheilk* 131: 577-578, 1989.

Steiner A, Roussel A, Martig J: Effect of bethanechol, neostigmine, metoclopramide, and propranolol on myoelectric activity of ileo-ceco-colic area in cows, *Am J Vet Res* 56: 1081-1086, 1995

Stocker S, Steiner A, Geiser S, et al: Myoelectric activity of the cecum and proximal loop of the ascending colon in cows after spontaneous cecal dilatation/dislocation, *Am J Vet Res* 58: 961-968, 1997.

Svendsen P: Inhibition of intestinal motility by volatile fatty acids, *Nordisk Veterinaer medicin* 24: 123-131, 1972.

Svendsen P: Inhibition of cecal motility in sheep by volatile fatty acids, *Nord Vet Med* 24: S393-S396, 1972.

Svendsen P, Kristensen B: Cecal dilatation in cattle: an experimental study of the etiology, *Nord Vet Med* 22: 578-583, 1970.

Weller R, Gray F: The passage of starch through the stomach of sheep, *J Exp Biol* 31: 40-48, 1954.

10.7—Surgery of the Colon

Adrian Steiner

Anatomy

In cattle, the colon consists of the ascending, transverse, and descending parts. The ascending colon is divided into three sections: proximal loop, spiral colon, and distal loop (Figures 10.6-1 and 10.7-1). The proximal loop of the ascending colon (PLAC) communicates orally with the cecum on the lateral side of the mesenteric root and aborally with the spiral colon on the medial side. The spiral colon in cattle consists of two centripetal coils, the central flexure, and two centrifugal coils (see Figure 10.7-1). The distal loop of the ascending colon represents the communication between the spiral and transverse colon. The short transverse colon is situated cranial to the cranial mesenteric artery and passes from right to left. The descending colon courses in a caudal direction and is continuous with the longer peritoneal and shorter retroperitoneal part of the rectum. The colon terminates

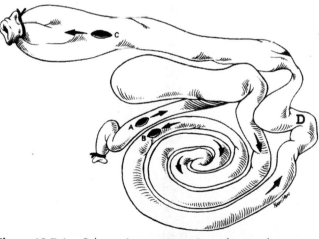

Figure 10.7-1 Schematic representation of normal anatomy of three parts of the ascending colon (proximal, spiral, and distal [D]), transverse colon, descending colon, and rectum. Arrows show the flow of ingesta. The cecum has been elevated dorsally to allow a better view of the spiral colon. If extensive adhesions exist in the outermost loop of the spiral colon, the ileum (A) or the spiral colon (B) can be anastomosed to the descending colon (C).

(Reprinted with modifications by permission from Smith DF, Donawick WJ: Obstruction of the ascending colon in cattle: 1, clinical presentation and surgical management, *Vet Surg* 8:93-97, 1979.)

at the level of the anus, which is surrounded by internal and external anal sphincter muscles, which are responsible for opening and closing the anus. The fat-filled mesentery in adult cattle is theorized to maintain the relationship of the large intestine's various segments, thus minimizing the occurrence of intussusception (IS) in this region. The calves' mesenteric fat is usually minimal, which may allow increased mobility of the slings of the colon. This explains why intussusception of the cecum and colon is nearly exclusively seen in calves, not in adult cattle.

Physiology

Three major functions of the colon are the following: 1) together with the cecum, the main site of microbial digestion besides the reticulorumen; 2) an important site of water absorption; and 3) aboral transportation of digesta to the rectum. The rectal ampulla is able to store considerable amounts of intestinal contents before defecation. Motility of the spiral colon in healthy dairy cows was recently described in detail. Myoelectric activity of the spiral colon was closely associated with motility of the ileum and proximal colon, and it showed the typical phases and organization of migrating myoelectric complexes (MMC). The MMC in the bovine spiral colon was termed *bcMMC* and had a mean duration of 188.6 ± 30.8 minutes.

Intussusception of the Spiral Colon

Intussusception of the spiral colon is rare but has been seen more commonly in calves than adult cattle. It may be that the fat in the mesentery of the adult intestinal tract prevents invagination of the bowel (see Section 14.2.3).

Obstruction of the Spiral Colon

ETIOPATHOGENESIS
Obstruction of the spiral colon is either a consequence of dysmotility, sequelae of cecal dilatation/dislocation, or caused by lesions extrinsic to the bowel. Extraluminal constriction may be caused by fat necrosis; lymphosarcoma; hematoma from an expressed corpus luteum; or adhesions that resulted from perimetritis, traumatic reticuloperitonitis, perforating abomasal ulcer, intraperitoneal injection of irritating drugs, or previous intraabdominal surgery.

CLINICAL SIGNS AND DIAGNOSIS
Clinical signs occur gradually over several days or weeks and include reduced milk yield, appetite, and fecal

output. Adhesions may be palpated at rectal examination and visualized by ultrasonographic examination through the right paralumbar fossa.

SURGICAL MANAGEMENT

Surgical correction is performed in the standing animal by a right flank laparotomy. Because adhesions usually involve more than just one part of a spiral colon loop, resection and anastomosis is rarely a useful surgical option. The involved bowel is left *in situ,* and the obstruction is bypassed with a side-to-side anastomosis between the bowel proximal and distal to the obstruction. This can be between loops of spiral colon or between the ileum and outermost centrifugal loop of the spiral colon. If the latter is involved in the adhesion, a side-to-side anastomosis between the ileum and descending colon may be performed (see Figure 10.7-1). For side-to-side anastomosis, a side-to-side stainless steel stapling instrument (the GIA or ILA)* may be used after the two bowels to be anastomosed have been adapted with stay sutures, or the bowel can be sutured by hand.

PROGNOSIS

Prognosis depends on the cause of the extraluminal obstruction. In one report, three of four cows with adhesions of the spiral colon that underwent this surgical procedure survived. Depending on the extent of the loss of absorptive function of the spiral colon, fecal consistency may not return to normal at all or not until after significant delay. In an experimental bypass procedure (side-to-side anastomosis of the ileum with the outermost centrifugal loop of the spiral colon) in four calves, fecal dry matter had not reached preoperative values by 4 weeks after surgery.

Rectal Prolapse

OCCURRENCE AND CLASSIFICATION

Any breed, sex, or age can be affected; however, rectal prolapse occurs most commonly in feedlot cattle from 6 months to 2 years of age. In a type I prolapse, only the rectal mucosa projects through the anus. A type II prolapse is a complete prolapse of all layers of the rectum. In a type III prolapse, a variable amount of descending colon intussuscepts into the rectum in addition to a type II lesion. In a type IV prolapse, variable lengths of the peritoneal rectum and/or descending colon form an intussusception through the anus. Types I and II are much more common than types III and IV.

*Autosuture, US Surgical Corp., Norwalk, CT 06850

PATHOGENESIS AND PREDISPOSING FACTORS

Rectal prolapse generally results from an increase of the pressure gradient between the abdominal/pelvic cavity and the anus. In normal conditions, the sphincter effectively creates a barrier for the normal pressure gradient. Conditions that cause inadequate tone of the sphincter and/or a high pressure gradient can result in eversion of mucosa. Exposure of the mucosa to the environment further irritates the mucosa and may initiate a vicious cycle of straining until a complete prolapse of the rectum occurs. Short exposure causes damage to the superficial layer, which quickly resolves when the prolapsed tissue is replaced. Prolonged exposure results in progressively deeper involvement. Unreduced prolapses become edematous, hemorrhagic, and finally necrotic. Predisposing factors that contribute to rectal prolapse include increased abdominal pressure or fill, excessive coughing, colitis, cystitis, diarrhea, and tenesmus from dystocia.

CLINICAL SIGNS AND DIAGNOSIS

The usual presentation of a prolapse is a mucosal mass protruding beyond the anus with a variable amount of edema, inflammation, and necrosis (Figure 10.7-2). On manual palpation, types I to III are continuous with the mucocutaneous junction of the anus, whereas type IV represents a protrusion with a palpable trench inside the rectum.

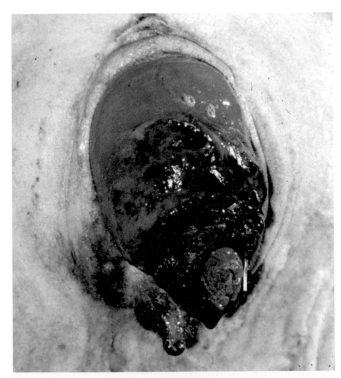

Figure 10.7-2   Type II rectal prolapse in a ewe.

(Courtesy of Dr. RP Hackett; Cornell University.)

MANAGEMENT

Generally, management of rectal prolapse includes elimination of predisposing factors, soothing of the irritated mucosa, elimination of straining, and resolving the prolapse. The condition of the prolapsed tissue plays the most important role in choosing the treatment method. The color of the membranes, degree of edema/hemorrhage, and presence and depth of erosions are the parameters used to decide whether the tissue is salvageable. In general, the rectum recovers from injury well, and attempts should be made to salvage the prolapsed tissue unless deep necrosis or trauma to the tissue exists. Caudal epidural anesthesia is performed first. This temporarily eliminates straining, allows evaluation of the tissue, facilitates repositioning, and allows surgical intervention, if necessary. The prolapsed tissue is cleaned with a mild antiseptic. The tissue is evaluated for necrosis, trauma, or tears. The treatment options include replacement and purse-string suture, submucosal resection, or amputation. For management of a type IV prolapse, celiotomy, resection of the affected tissue, and end-to-end anastomosis would be indicated.

REPLACEMENT AND PURSE-STRING SUTURE

This technique is indicated for treatment of salvageable rectal prolapses. After caudal epidural anesthesia is performed and the mucosa is cleaned, the edema is reduced by temporary topical application of a hyperosmotic solution, such as a sugar solution. Lidocaine jelly is applied, and the tissue is manipulated back into its normal position. A purse-string suture is applied to the perirectal tissue with 0.2 to 0.5 cm umbilical tape. The rectal opening is tightened to two-to-three fingers' width to prevent recurrence of the prolapse while allowing passage of fecal material. The umbilical tape is tied in a bow that is placed laterally and readily allows adjustment of the suture. Usually, the purse-string suture is removed within one week after placement to reduce fecal contamination and the severity of suture tract infection. If straining recurs, the caudal epidural may need to be repeated.

SUBMUCOSAL RESECTION

Submucosal resection is the preferred technique if the prolapsed mucosa is necrotic, ulcerated, or traumatized, but the underlying tissue is healthy. This technique includes removal of the affected mucosa and salvage of the healthy underlying tissue. After placing caudal epidural anesthesia and cleaning the mucosa, the edema is reduced by temporary topical application of a hyperosmotic solution, and a final preoperative evaluation is performed (Figure 10.7-3). A piece of flexible tubing of appropriate diameter is inserted into the lumen of the prolapse and cross-pin fixation performed to control movement of the prolapse during surgery. For this

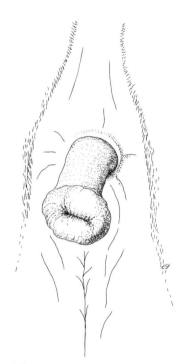

Figure 10.7-3 Schematic representation of a rectal prolapse type II before submucosal resection.

purpose, two 15-cm, 18-gauge needles are inserted at a 90° angle to each other, close to the anal opening across the prolapse and tubing, exiting at the opposite site (Figure 10.7-4). Two circumferential incisions are made through the mucosa on either side of the tissue to be removed. A longitudinal incision at the same depth is then made to connect the circumferential incisions. The collar of affected tissue is removed in the healthy submucosal plane by using blunt dissection (Figure 10.7-5). Hemorrhage may be controlled by ligature of individual vessels. The mucosa is aligned with four simple interrupted sutures that are placed equidistant around the circumference of the prolapse (Figure 10.7-6). The four quadrants are apposed separately with one simple continuous suture pattern for each quadrant (Figure 10.7-7). Size #2-0 to 3-0 monofilament absorbable material with a taper point swaged-on-needle is used. The specific type of suture pattern and tubing that acts as a place holder prevents the occurrence of a purse-string effect at the suture site that might decrease the lumen and provoke postoperative stricture formation. Several advantages of this technique in comparison to amputation have been described and include the following: not exposing the serosal lining minimizes the possibility of peritonitis or perirectal abscess formation; not transecting the main blood supply minimizes the danger of

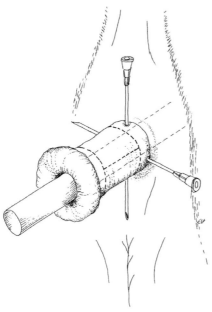

Figure 10.7-4   A piece of flexible tubing is inserted into the lumen of the prolapse, and cross-pin fixation is performed with two 18-gauge needles. The dashed lines represent the intended sites of mucosal incision.

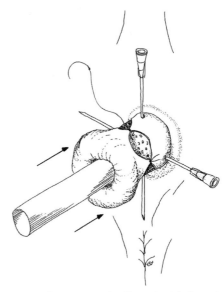

Figure 10.7-6   The mucosa is aligned with four simple interrupted sutures placed equidistant around the circumference of the prolapse.

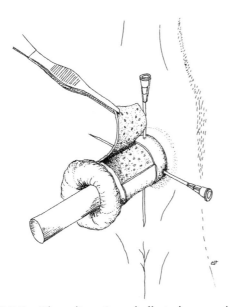

Figure 10.7-5   Blunt dissection of affected mucosal tissue in the healthy submucosal plane.

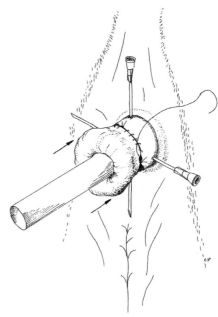

Figure 10.7-7   Final alignment of the mucosa with continuous sutures.

postoperative hemorrhage; less postoperative straining occurs; the lumen is only minimally constricted; healthy tissue is not sacrificed; and healing is faster.

STAIRSTEP AMPUTATION

When the prolapsed tissue is severely damaged, amputation may be the only alternative. Although several tech-

niques of amputation have been described and accepted, the authors prefer the stairstep technique because the tendency for stricture formation is kept minimal. Preparations—including epidural anesthesia, insertion of tubing, and needle fixation—are identical to those described for submucosal resection. A circumferential incision is made just cranial to the necrotic area. All tissues except the inner mucosa and parts of the inner submucosa are incised (Figure 10.7-8). With blunt dissection, a plane is created towards the caudal aspect of the prolapse within the inner submucosa between the inner and outer segment (Figure 10.7-9). The outer segment is pulled forward, and the inner segment amputated 2 to 3 cm more distal than the outer segment (Figure 10.7-10). This allows salvage of extra mucosa and facilitates adaptation of the mucosal layers over the bulging fat tissue. Suture pattern and material for adaptation of the mucosal layers are identical as described for submucosal resection (Figure 10.7-11).

AFTERCARE AND COMPLICATIONS

After amputation and mucosal resection, the cross-pins are removed and a routine purse-string suture is applied and removed within one week. Lidocaine jelly may be applied topically for the first few days after surgery. Potential postoperative complications include stricture formation, perirectal abscess formation, dehiscence, peritonitis, or evisceration of intestines after dehiscence.

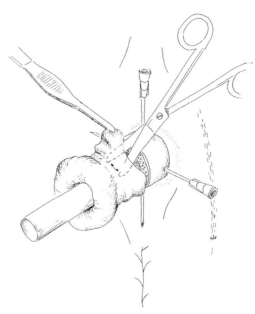

Figure 10.7-9   A plane is created towards the caudal aspect of the prolapse.

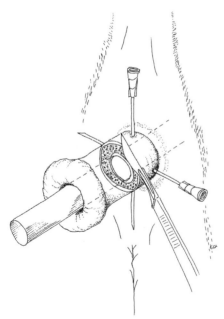

Figure 10.7-8   Schematic representation of the first step of stair-step amputation to correct rectal prolapse type II. A circumferential incision is made just cranial to the necrotic area. All tissues except the inner mucosa and parts of the inner submucosa are incised.

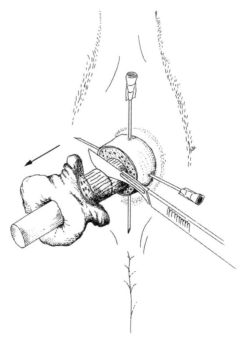

Figure 10.7-10   The inner segment is amputated.

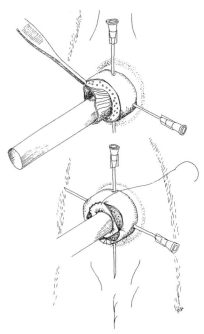

Figure 10.7-11 Adaptation of the mucosal layers as described for submucosal resection.

RECOMMENDED READINGS

Hess H, Leipold G, Schlegel F: Zur Genese des angeborenen Darmverschlusses des Kalbes, *Monatsheft Veterinärmed* 37: 89-92, 1982.

Johnson H: Submucous resection, surgical resection prolapse of the rectum, *J Am Vet Med Assoc* 102: 113-115, 1943.

Maala CP, Smith DF, Hintz HF, et al: Removal of the cecum, including the ileocecocolic junction, and its effects on digestibility in cattle, *Am J Vet Res* 44: 2237-2243, 1983.

Meylan M, Eicher R, Röthlisberger J, et al: Myoelectric activity of the spiral colon in dairy cows, *Am J Vet Res* 63: 78-93, 2002.

Nickel R, Schummer A: Mittel- und Enddarm. In Nickel R, Schummer A, Seiferle E, editors: *Lehrbuch der Anatomie der Haustiere*, Berlin und Hamburg, 1975, Paul Parey.

Smith DF, Donawick WJ: Obstruction of the ascending colon in cattle, I: clinical presentation and surgical management, *Vet Surg* 8: 93-97, 1979.

Smith DF, Donawick WJ: Obstruction of the ascending colon in cattle, II: an experimental model of partial bypass of the large intestine, *Vet Surg* 8: 98-104, 1979.

Strand E, Welker B, Modransky P: Spiral colon intussusception in a three-year-old bull, *J Amer Vet Med Assoc* 202: 971-972, 1993.

Turner T, Fessler J: Rectal prolapse in the horse, *J Am Vet Med Assoc* 177: 1028-1032, 1980.

Von Willer S, Müller W, Schlegel F: Untersuchungen über die genetisch bedingte Variabilität der angeborenen partiellen Kolonaplasie beim Rind, *Monatsheft Veterinärmed* 39: 473-476, 1984.

Williams D, Tyler D, Papp E: Abdominal fat necrosis as a herd problem in Georgia cattle, *J Am Vet Med Assoc* 154: 1017-1021, 1969.

Welker B, Modransky P: Rectal prolapse in food animals, part I: cause and conservative management, *Compend Cont Educ Pract Vet* 13: 1869-1884, 1991.

Welker B, Modransky P: Rectal prolapse in food animals, part II: surgical options, *Compend Cont Educ Pract Vet* 14: 554-558, 1992.

10.8—Intraabdominal and Retroperitoneal Abscesses

Susan L. Fubini

Cattle can have intraabdominal abscesses associated with the reticulum, liver, omentum, or uterus, and retroperitoneal abscesses secondary to intraabdominal medication, surgical intervention, or pyelonephritis.

Perireticular Abscesses

In most instances, abscess formation adjacent to the reticulum is secondary to hardware disease. Cows with cranial abdominal abscesses often show signs typical of vagal indigestion, including abdominal distention high on the left and low on the right, bradycardia, irregular rumen motility, hypophagia, and hypogalactia.

The chronic antigenic stimulation results in high total protein, gamma globulin, and fibrinogen concentrations. The white blood cell count may be elevated, and total protein in the abdominal fluid is high in some cases. Venous blood gas and plasma electrolyte concentrations are usually within normal limits because the interruption in motility is at the reticuloomasal junction (e.g., proximal to the abomasum). A mild hypochloremic metabolic alkalosis present in some cows is most likely a result of ileus or previous treatment with antacids.

If available, radiography of the cranial abdomen may show a radiopaque foreign body and a gas/fluid interface characteristic of an abdominal abscess (see Figure 10.3-3). In some instances, ultrasound of the right cranial abdomen can depict a suspicious mass (Figure 10.8-1). Sections 10.3 and 10.8.2 discuss treatment of reticular or liver abscess.

Omental Bursa Abscess

ANATOMY

The greater omentum consists of superficial and deep layers that are connected caudally. The superficial wall arises from the greater curvature of the abomasum, cranial part of the duodenum, and ventral border of the descending duodenum (see Figure 10.4-1). From the right side, it descends along the abdominal wall, crosses ventrally to the left side, and ascends between the ventral sac of the rumen and left abdominal wall to the left longitudinal groove of the rumen. The deep wall of the greater omentum attaches to the right longitudinal

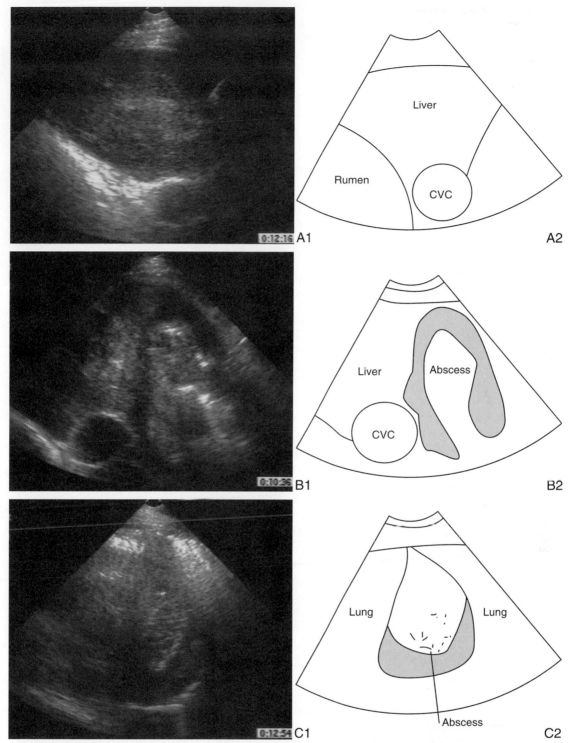

Figure 10.8-1 Transverse sonograms of the right dorsal abdomen and adjacent thorax obtained from a 1-year-old Holstein bull with dyspnea and an abscess of the liver, diaphragm, and right lung. A 3-2 MHz phased array sector probe was used. The left side of the sonogram is ventral. *A1,* At the right eleventh intercostal space, there is normal liver, caudal vena cava (CVC), and rumen. *A2,* Schematic representation of *A1. B-1,* At the right tenth intercostal space, the abscess is contiguous with the liver. During respiration, the abscess did not slide against the liver, suggesting adherence to or origin from the liver. *B2,* Schematic representation of *B1. C1,* At the ninth intercostal space, the abscess is contiguous with the lung. The abscess did not slide independently of the lung, thus suggesting adherence to or origin from the lung. *C2,* Schematic representation of *C1.*

(Courtesy of Dr. Amy Yeager; Cornell University.)

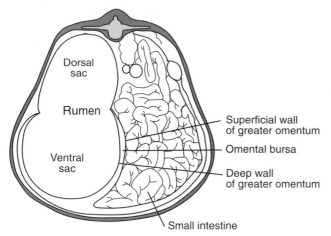

Figure 10.8-2 A line diagram that shows how the forestomach compartments and abomasum relate to the omentum and the omental bursa.

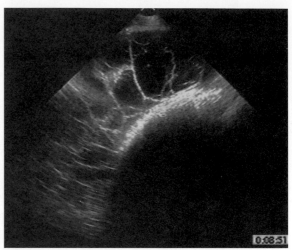

Figure 10.8-3 Transverse sonogram of the left caudal abdomen obtained from a 2-year-old Ayrshire cow with omental bursitis secondary to previous rumenotomy. A 5-3 MHz phased array sector probe was used. The left side of the sonogram is ventral. The image of the left side of the abdomen has an extensive collection of fluid and fibrin (8 cm thick) located between the body wall and rumen. This fluid and fibrin collection extended from the dorsal left abdomen across the ventral abdomen to the right side of the abdomen.

(Courtesy of Dr. Amy Yeager; Cornell University.)

groove of the rumen. The omentum passes ventrally in contact with the visceral surface of the ventral sac of the rumen and then goes dorsally around the ventral aspect of the intestines and ascends on the right side of the abdomen to unite with the superficial layer on the ventral surface of the descending duodenum. The walls of the greater omentum enclose the caudal recess of the omental bursa, which contains the ventral sac of the rumen and is a potential space in a live animal (Figure 10.8-2). The omental bursa communicates with the peritoneal cavity via the epiploic foramen. Dorsal to the sling formed by the deep wall of the greater omentum is the extensive supraomental recess that is open caudally and contains most of the intestinal tract. Portions of the intestinal tract, such as the apex of the cecum and distal flange of the small intestine, protrude from the recess and lie in the region of the pelvic inlet.

Etiopathogenesis

The exact cause of omental bursitis is not known; however, most reports speculate that an ulcer perforating the medial wall of the abomasum along the lesser curvature could result in ingesta spillage into the omental bursa. A perforation of the ventral wall of the rumen or reticulum by a foreign body could also result in omental bursitis. The foreign body seeds the omental bursa and can result in infection. Necrotic rumenitis, secondary to a bacterial or mycotic infection, could cause necrosis of the rumen wall and allow seepage of ruminal fluid into the omental bursa. The spread of an umbilical infection to the greater omentum, extension of another abdominal abscess into the omental bursa, or omental bursitis

secondary to *postpartum* perimetritis are less likely causes.

Regardless of the etiology and treatment options attempted, this disease has vague presenting signs and is difficult to treat, which makes the prognosis guarded.

Clinical Syndrome

Omental bursitis is an uncommon clinical condition in cattle. It is also difficult to make a definitive preoperative diagnosis. Affected animals usually have vague signs of a chronic illness, including decreased appetite, scant manure, and depressed milk production. They may be febrile. In most instances, abdominal distention and a viscus are detectable on the right side of the abdomen. The right-sided viscus may be palpable per rectum and may "ping" when simultaneous auscultation and percussion are performed. Ultrasound may reveal an accumulation of fluid and exudate that can extend all the way from mid paralumbar fossa on the right to a similar position on the left (Figures 10.8-3 and 10.8-4). If it is a valuable cow, a right-sided exploratory celiotomy is indicated. Exploration will reveal a large viscus covered by the superficial layer of omentum. An aspirate will show a transudate or, in some cases, purulent exudate (Figure 10.8-5). If the omental bursitis was caused by abomasal

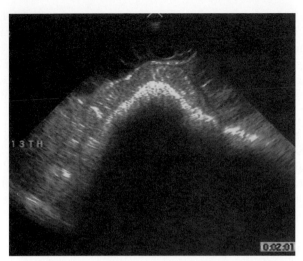

Figure 10.8-4 Transverse sonogram of the right caudal abdomen obtained from a 2-year-old Ayrshire cow with omental bursitis secondary to previous rumenotomy. A 3-2 MHz phased array sector probe was used. The left side of the sonogram is ventral. In the right abdomen, fluid and fibrin are located between the body wall and intestines. Unlike peritonitis, the fluid contained within the omental bursa did not mingle between segments of intestine.

(Courtesy of Dr. Amy Yeager; Cornell University.)

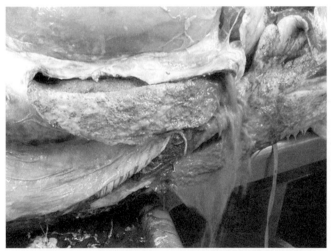

Figure 10.8-5 A postmortem specimen of a case of omental bursitis in a cow. The cow is in left lateral recumbency, and the superficial layer of the omentum has been opened showing the large amount of purulent exudate.

perforation as a result of a moderate or large ulcer, feed material may also be present in the omental bursa.

Surgical Treatment

Surgery is not very rewarding, but it is possible in some instances to marsupialize the omental bursa to the right and/or left lower abdomen. Drainage at the most ventral aspect of the abdomen should be avoided for fear of herniation of viscera through the wall of the omental bursa into the abdominal incision. Furthermore, an incision at the most ventral part of the abdomen can become occluded by the pressure of intraabdominal contents, which prevents adequate drainage. The omental bursa can compartmentalize the infection so the purulent exudate is localized to one part of the bursa. Surgical drainage should be done at the site that exhibits the most distension, as determined by ultrasound or rectal examination before surgery or by intraabdominal exploration during surgery. After aseptic preparation of the ventral abdomen, local anesthesia is infiltrated at the intended drainage site. The aim is to create a seal between the omental bursa and body wall at the drainage site. A 10-cm incision is made over the swelling on the lower abdomen. The incision is extended through muscle layers and peritoneum by using a combination of blunt and sharp dissection. The omental bursa is identified and aspirated to confirm the presence of purulent material. The superficial sheet of omentum is secured circumferentially to the subcutaneous tissues or dermis of the skin incision, which effectively isolates the site from the rest of the abdomen. The bursa is opened, and the incised edges are sutured to the skin with a simple interrupted pattern. This creates a defect in the body wall that is usually well tolerated. The omentum can be friable and difficult to handle, thus making this procedure difficult. If the capsule around the omentum is thickened, the surgery is more straightforward because stronger tissue holds the sutures better. Furthermore, a thick capsule allows lavage of the abscess cavity during and after surgery without causing worry about seeding the abdomen or tearing the omentum away from the body wall. In general, postoperative lavage of the omental bursa should be avoided because its wall is so thin it may rupture. Instead, the clinician should keep the incision open with daily gentle manual debridement of the surgical site. The abscess will contract over time. Perioperative antibiotics are appropriate.

OTHER ABDOMINAL ABSCESSES

Abscesses associated with the omentum or uterus may be excised through a celiotomy at the appropriate site. In some instances, it may be necessary to remove a portion of the uterus or omentum at the same time (see Section 12.3). When the location of an abscess prevents removal or drainage (either into a forestomach compartment or through the body wall), treatment with single aspiration and lavage with a dilute antiseptic solution and chronic systemic antibiotic therapy may be successful. This is accomplished by placing a large 14 to 28 French catheter* through the omentum or adhesions into the abscess cavity. Suction is applied to the catheter and as much material as possible is drained from the abscess. Following this, the drain is removed and the site where it was placed oversewn if necessary.

SINGLE LARGE LIVER ABSCESS

It has been reported that a single, large liver abscess can cause very similar signs to those described for perireticular abscess formation (see Figure 10.8-1). The major difference found at surgery in cattle affected with liver abscess was the absence of adhesions to the forestomach compartments, making drainage into the forestomach compartment impossible (see Figure 10.3-6). These liver abscesses are usually diagnosed on rumenotomy when a mass adjacent to the omasum is felt through the rumen wall. Palpation of the reticular wall shows no adhesions to the mass. These cows must be closed and approached in a different manner. The abscesses are on the right side of the abdomen, usually associated with the left lobe of the liver. Access to them can be gained by a cranial right paramedian approach with the cow in dorsal recumbency, a right paracostal approach with the cow in the left lateral recumbency, or a ventral midline approach with the cow in dorsal recumbency. A celiotomy is made, and the abscess is identified. A small 3-cm incision is made adjacent to the original incision; a large (20 to 24 French) chest trocar* is placed through the body wall and fed through any omental adhesions available into the abscess cavity. The catheter is aspirated to ensure infected material exists within the cavity before it is sutured into place. The cattle are allowed to stand up, and the abscess is drained. It may be helpful to gently lavage the abscess cavity over the next few days to drain out any infected material. An approximate 30% recurrence rate has been reported in cattle infected with these single, large liver abscesses. Because of the recurrence problem, a number of modifications have been tried, including lavaging the abscess during surgery and placing more than one drain. Anecdotally, results with these other treatment scenarios have not proven to be much more rewarding. Therefore we still place one large-bore catheter to provide drainage and warn the client recurrence is a possibility. We have tried placing a percutaneous catheter directly into the abscess of one cow with ultrasound guidance. Peritonitis ensued because the catheter was not passed through adhesions, which allowed purulent exudate to leak into the abdomen at the site of the drain placement.

If the abscess recurs, a partial resection of the left lobe of the liver and its associated abscess can be attempted under general anesthesia through a right paramedian or right paracostal approach. This should be reserved for very valuable cows that suffer a recurrence because of the difficulty associated with the procedure and the possibility of severe intraoperative hemorrhage.

RETROPERITONEAL ABSCESSES

Cattle can get infected material accumulated in the retroperitoneal space secondary to pyelonephritis (Chapter 12), previous surgery, or intraperitoneal treatments.

Affected cattle present with nonspecific clinical signs that may include fever, inappetence, distention at the site of the infection, a drop in milk production, elevated total protein levels, and a leukocytosis. Transabdominal ultrasound and rectal examination are useful in determining the nature and size of the retroperitoneal fluid accumulation. Accumulations of fluid and exudate in the retroperitoneal space can be quite large. The large fluid pocket should be aspirated to confirm that exudate is present. The abscessed cavity wall can be very thick, thus necessitating aspiration with a 14-g, 14-cm (5 1/2″) intravenous catheter. Once the pocket is identified and infection confirmed, aggressive ventral drainage is required. This means identifying the infected area, approaching it with sharp dissection, and continuing to use a combination of sharp and blunt dissection until adequate drainage is achieved. In some instances, it is necessary to follow the infected tracts along fascial planes until the full extent of the contamination is identified. An outlet for drainage at the most ventral part of the pocket is required to prevent pooling of exudate and lavage fluids. The defect must heal from the inside out and should be lavaged carefully (a risk of creating peritonitis by rupturing the wall surrounding the fluid accumulation exists) on a daily basis. If the abdominal cavity is not involved, nonsterile fluids can be used for lavage. If there is a risk deeper tissues are involved, sterile fluids should be used. With appropriate wound care, the outcome is favorable.

INCISIONAL INFECTION

One often can detect a fluid pocket around surgical incisions in the first postoperative week; these are usually seromas that should be monitored for 10 to 14 days. The incisional fluid pocket should be aspirated only if the animal is one or more weeks postsurgery and is showing signs consistent with infection, such as inappetence, fever, a drop in milk production, or a large retroperitoneal pocket detected on rectal or ultrasound examination.

---

*Pleur-Evac Thoracic Catheter, Genzyme Biosurgery, Genzyme Corporation; Fall River, MA 02720

If an incisional infection is apparent, waiting until it localizes and matures into a discrete pocket before draining it is ideal. This is best determined by ultrasound. It may be possible to simply remove the most ventral skin sutures and establish drainage, especially for flank incisions. This usually requires some blunt dissection with a sterile, long hemostat and sterile gloves.

As mentioned in the retroperitoneal abscess section, some of the infected pockets can be huge requiring some bold, blunt dissection to achieve adequate drainage. However, ultrasound is the best guide for this critical task to avoid lacerating large vessels or other vital structures or entering a body cavity inadvertently.

As with any infection, adequate ventral drainage is the treatment mainstay. At the clinicians' discretion, parenteral antibiotics may be indicated, especially with involvement of deeper tissues. Lavage of the infected cavity is appropriate as discussed in the retroperitoneal section in Section 10.8.2.

More invasive surgery may be necessary (Section 10.4-4) for complicated incisional infections, such as an abomasal fistula after right paramedian abomasopexy (see Section 10.4.1).

RECOMMENDED READINGS

Baxter GM: Omental bursitis in a cow, *Modern Veterinary Practice* 67: 729-731, 1986.

Ducharme NG: Surgery of bovine forestomach compartments. In *The Vet Clinics of North America Surgery of the Bovine Digestive Tract*, Philadelphia, 1990, WB Saunders.

Ducharme NG: Surgical considerations in the treatment of traumatic reticuloperitonitis, *Compend Contin Educ Pract Vet* 4: S213-S219, 1983.

Ferrante PL, Whitlock RH: Chronic (vagus) indigestion, *Compend Contin Educ Pract Vet* 38: S231-S237, 1981.

Fubini SL, Ducharme NG, Murphy JP, et al: Vagus indigestion syndrome resulting from a liver abscess in dairy cows, *J Am Vet Med Assoc* 186: 1297-1300, 1985.

Grymer J, Johnson R: Two cases of bovine omental bursitis, *J Am Vet Med Assoc* 181: 714-715, 1982.

Hekmati P, Zakarian B: Bursitis omentalis in cattle: three case reports, *Vet Rec* 89: 138-139, 1971.

Neal PA, Edwards GB: "Vagus" indigestion in cattle, *Vet Rec* 82: 396-402, 1968.

Nickel R, Schummer A, Seiferl E, et al: The viscera of domestic animals, *The Nickels Viscera book*, ed 2, New York, 1979, Springer Verlag.

Ogilvie TH, Butler DG, Gartley CJ, et al: Magnesium oxide induced metabolic alkalosis in cattle, *Can J Comp Med* 17: 108-110, 1983.

Parker JB, Gaughan EM: Partial resection for treatment of a single liver abscess in dairy heifer, *Vet Surg* 17: 87, 1988.

Rebhun WC, Fubini SL, Lesser FR, et al: Clinical results of 12 cattle affected with vagal indigestion, *Proceedings. 14th World Congr Dis Cattle* 2: 1146-1151, 1986.

Rebhun WC: Vagus indigestion in cattle, *J Am Vet Med Assoc* 176: 506-510, 1980.

Whitlock RH: Bovine stomach diseases. In Anderson NV, editor: *Veterinary gastroenterology*, Philadelphia, 1980, Lea & Febiger.

10.9—Surgery and the Peritoneum

Ava M. Trent

Disorders of the peritoneum are only occasionally recognized as a primary reason for surgery of the abdomen in cattle. However, veterinarians depend on the healing properties and host defense mechanisms of the peritoneum for success in every abdominal surgery performed. Despite the apparently simple nature of the peritoneum, mishandling during surgery can result in a negative treatment outcome regardless of the nature of the surgery.

Basic Structure and Function

ANATOMY
Gross Anatomy

The peritoneum is a continuous tissue layer that lines the internal surface of the body wall and diaphragm (parietal layer) and has continuous coverage of the surface of all abdominal viscera (visceral layer) in the abdominal cavity. The visceral peritoneum wraps around the neurovascular pedicles and surfaces of viscera and omentum that extend into the abdominal cavity. Structures broadly attached to the body wall, such as the right kidney, are only partially covered by peritoneum and are called *retroperitoneal*. Caudally, the peritoneal reflection extends slightly into the pelvic cavity and leaves the caudal portion of the rectum uncovered. Similar folds in the peritoneum admit the esophagus (esophageal hiatus) and aorta (aortal hiatus) through the diaphragm. The peritoneum extends through the inguinal rings to cover the testicles and spermatic cords in males. The visceral and parietal surfaces normally lie in close apposition within the abdominal cavity and glide easily along each other to allow viscera to reposition in the abdomen with peristaltic contractions and changes in visceral volume. The space enclosed by the visceral and parietal peritoneum is called *the peritoneal cavity*. This space is normally filled with a small volume of fluid transudate that contains a limited number of mature cells and protein.

Histology

The peritoneum is a serosal membrane that consists of a single layer of mesothelial cells and is supported by a basement membrane. The mesothelial cells are normally squamous in shape and have cilia that trap cellular products to help maintain the necessary gliding surfaces. The layer is attached to the body wall and viscera by a glycosaminoglycan matrix that contains collagen fibers, vessels, nerves, macrophages, and fat cells. The parietal submesothelial layer varies in thickness and cell concentrations among species and has a moderate thickness in the cow. The visceral submesothelial layer is thin, and the visceral peritoneum (serosa) closely adheres to the underlying viscera. The parietal peritoneum can be grossly separated from the underlying muscle and fascia. Except for the peritoneum that covers omentum, the visceral peritoneum cannot be manually separated intact from the underlying viscera.

Histological studies in laboratory animals show that junctures between peritoneal cells are tight, and passive diffusion limits bidirectional passage to relatively small molecules, including water, glucose, and electrolytes. Distinct openings (stomata) up to $12\,\mu m$ in diameter are present in the parietal peritoneum that covers the diaphragm. These stomata are adequately sized to allow passage of large molecules and cells, primarily to remove cells, bacteria, particles, and molecules less than $10\,\mu m$ in diameter. Similar openings occur in the visceral peritoneum that covers both sides of the omentum over focal aggregates of lymphoid tissue called milk spots. Lymphoid and myeloid originating cells move into the peritoneal cavity through these openings, and cells and particulate matter move out of the peritoneal cavity through these openings.

Blood and Lymphatic Supply

The peritoneal cells receive oxygen and other nutrients by passive diffusion along a concentration gradient from vessels in the submesothelium. A low molecular weight transudate from these submesothelial vessels is the source of the small amount of fluid found in the healthy peritoneal cavity. The omental milk spots appear to be the primary source of phagocytes in the peritoneal cavity. The volume of fluid and often the protein concentration increases as an apparently normal physiologic process in late pregnancy. The volume, protein, and cellular content of this fluid increase dramatically in the presence of inflammatory stimuli.

Lymphatic vessels accompany the arteries and veins in the submesothelium, with specialized accumulations in sites corresponding to peritoneal stomata. Lymphatic vessels carry fluid through substernal and thoracic lymph nodes into the thoracic duct and general circulation. Lymphatic fluid can also drain via the wall of the omental bursa to the specialized lymphatic vessels in the diaphragm.

Innervation

Parietal peritoneum is supplied by fibers from spinal nerves able to detect sharp and deep pain stimuli. Standard nerve blocks used for incisional analgesia (paravertebral, line, "L") do not provide analgesia for the parietal peritoneum during a standing flank incision. The surgeon should expect a painful and accurately localized response to the incision through the peritoneal layer and be prepared to work quickly through this layer to minimize discomfort. Inflammatory processes that originate in or extend to the parietal peritoneum also stimulate a localizable painful sensation at the contact site.

The visceral peritoneum is innervated by the same afferent (sensory) nerves that supply the underlying viscera. These nerves are primarily type C pain fibers that pass along visceral sympathetic nerves into the spinal cord. The viscera and visceral peritoneum can detect stimuli that trigger the deep burning pain sensation characteristic of type C fibers, including stretch, chemical irritation, and anoxia but cannot detect sharp pain or touch. The most severe visceral pain results from rapid distention of the smaller diameter bowel or tension on the mesentery, both of which produce rapid stretching of visceral peritoneum. Distention of larger diameter viscera such as the rumen and abomasum is less likely to create the rapid peritoneal stretch that producees pain. Unlike spinal nerve fibers, stimulation of visceral afferent pain fibers does not result in accurate localization of the pain source. Consequently, the animal's behavior (posture, kicking, etc.) is unlikely to accurately reflect the pathology location, unless an inflammatory stimulus has extended to the parietal peritoneum. This occurs commonly in cases of traumatic reticuloperitonitis and abomasal ulceration and allows localization of pain to the cranioventral abdomen by manual pressure on the ventral body wall. Lack of sharp pain sensation allows the surgeon to manipulate and incise viscera without any analgesia beyond the local block for the approach.

PHYSIOLOGY AND FUNCTION

Several peritoneal functions are critical to the health of all abdominal structures, including production of peritoneal fluid, maintenance of a gliding surface, removal of waste products, and repair of tissue defects. These functions are usually adversely affected by surgical invasion of the peritoneal cavity. A surgeon's ability to minimize the adverse effects of surgery and disease and to maximize desirable effects is critical for surgical success.

Peritoneal Fluid Production

Peritoneal fluid is produced by transudation from submesothelial vessels across the peritoneal membrane. The amount of fluid is normally small (less than $50\,ml$ in man) and contains neutrophils, mononuclear cells, eosinophils, macrophages, lymphocytes, desquamated mesothelial cells, and an average of $3.0\,gm/ml$ of protein. The volume often increases during late pregnancy. A significant increase in volume without notably abnormal changes in cellularity or protein concentration can occur in animals with heart failure and ascites or in early uroperitoneum.

Electrolytes and other small molecules enter the peritoneal cavity by diffusion along a concentration gradient and remain in equilibrium with the extracellular fluid of the body. As a result, the concentration of electrolytes in peritoneal fluid is normally similar to that in serum.

Gliding Surface

The peritoneum maintains a gliding surface for peritoneal surfaces in the abdomen through several mechanisms. Peritoneal cells secrete a mixture of phospholipids with lubricating and surfactant properties. These lipids and glycoproteins form a 2- to 15-μm-thick glycocalyx that is trapped against the mesothelial surface and provides very efficient boundary lubrication. The small amount of free fluid in the peritoneal cavity plays a limited role in supporting this gliding surface. In addition, peritoneal cells in most species produce a baseline level of tissue plasminogen activator (tPA), a substance that converts plasminogen to a potent fibrinolytic agent called plasmin. The baseline level of peritoneal tPA production does vary by species, and the cow appears to have one of the lowest levels. Bovine peritoneum also produces relatively large amounts of fibrinolytic inhibitors. As a result, the cow peritoneum may be predisposed to allow formation of fibrinous adhesions, which is a potential advantage for controlling the relatively common problems of forestomach perforation from traumatic reticuloperitonitis and abomasal ulcers. This process will be discussed further in Peritoneal Repair and Peritoneal Adhesions.

Host Defenses

The peritoneum and peritoneal cavity are protected from contaminants and tissue damage by three main mechanisms: phagocytosis as part of the inflammatory response, physical removal through openings in the peritoneal membranes, and functional localization by omentum and fibrin.

Inflammatory Response and Phagocytosis The inflammatory response in the peritoneal cavity is similar to that in other tissues, although most of the responding cells and mediators must be brought into the cavity across the peritoneal membrane. Initial degranulation of mast cells with release of vasoactive agents results in submesothelial vessel dilation and a large volume of fluid influx into the peritoneal cavity. The initial fluid contains inflammatory mediators, including complement, opsonins, immunoglobulins, chemotaxins, and protein precursors of fibrin and proteases. A cascade of cytokines is also initiated with the inflammatory process. These cytokines,

which are produced by mesothelial and other cells, help regulate the inflammatory response, phagocytosis, and wound healing. Mesothelial cells express adhesion molecules that promote adherence of both inflammatory cells and bacteria to the surface.

Thrombin conversion of soluble fibrinogen in the inflammatory fluid to insoluble fibrin begins within minutes of fluid entry into the peritoneal cavity. Neutrophils enter the peritoneal cavity in large numbers within 2 hours of contamination and peak at 24 hours. This is followed by a gradual decline. The first wave of neutrophils is followed by macrophages that peak by the second day after contamination. In a study of peritoneal fluid changes after a clean abdominal surgical procedure in adult cattle, the average neutrophil and mononuclear cell counts rose from 1312 and 770 cells/μl averages, respectively, before surgery to 10,619 and 1216 cells/μl averages at 6 days after surgery. Mesothelial cells are able to ingest bacteria but do not efficiently kill the ingested pathogens. The ability of phagocytes to efficiently locate, engulf, and kill pathogens depends on the presence of complement and opsonins in the peritoneal cavity. Phagocytes are most efficient when both the phagocytes and bacteria are surface-bound. The effectiveness of phagocytosis can be impaired by the presence of adjuvants. Adjuvants are agents that promote pathogen survival by a variety of mechanisms—including impeding host responses and improving the local environment for pathogen survival. Large volumes of fluid, including those associated with the initial inflammatory response, serve an adjuvant role by decreasing the ability of phagocytes to find and engulf suspended pathogens. Pathogens trapped in fibrin are less accessible to phagocytes and systemic or locally administered antibiotics and antiseptics. The antimicrobial agents capable of penetrating the fibrin are not always active in the local environment. Fibrin prevents physical transport of entrapped pathogens to exit portals in the peritoneal membrane for physical removal.

Physical Removal Waste and breakdown products can be physically removed from the peritoneal cavity by either diffusing across the peritoneal membrane or traversing stomata in the diaphragmatic and omental peritoneum. Diffusion is limited to water, electrolytes, and smaller molecules such as urea nitrogen. Larger molecules and cells can only leave the peritoneal cavity intact by way of the stomata. In laboratory species and man, a normal circulation of peritoneal fluid carries material in a general route from dorsal, caudoventrally and then cranially along the ventral abdomen to the diaphragm. Once through the diaphragmatic stomata, waste is picked up by lymphatic vessels in the diaphragm and carried dorsally via substernal and thoracic lymph nodes into the thoracic duct. Bacterial contaminants not filtered by lymph nodes along the route can appear in the systemic circulation within 12 minutes of introduction into the peritoneal cavity. Clearance through the diaphragmatic stomata can be impaired by accumulations of fibrin or fibrosis in the cranioventral abdomen.

Peritoneal circulation also carries waste products past the omentum where they can pass through areas of discontinuity into underlying capillaries and lymphatic vessels. The extensive surface area of the omentum potentially increases its role in waste clearance in cattle.

Functional Isolation of Waste by Omentum and Fibrin

Complete physical removal of peritoneal contaminants is not always possible. A third form of host defense functionally isolates pathogens and contaminants from peritoneal tissues by localization in either fibrin or omentum.

The rapid accumulations of fibrin in the peritoneal cavity are capable of trapping local contaminants in their matrix. The efficiency of trapping varies with the specific bacteria, degree of fibrin organization, and presence of other factors in serum. Once there, pathogens are partially isolated from peritoneal tissues as well as other host defenses. Over time, the fibrin can be organized into a fibrous capsule or abscess cavity. The healthy peritoneum of most species possesses an intrinsic control mechanism to help remove fibrin deposits before they can be organized into fibrous tissue and persistent adhesions or abscesses (see Peritoneal Repair and Peritoneal Adhesions). The cow's ability to produce extensive volumes of fibrin and its relative lack of peritoneal fibrinolytic activity suggest a greater role for fibrin trapping in this species.

The omentum commonly migrates to sites of waste production or accumulation, either incidentally as part of its normal movement pattern or actively through as yet undefined mechanisms. It is often the first tissue to adhere to or surround the initial site of contamination. An angiogenic factor identified in the lipid fraction of omentum is believed to play a role in the omentum's ability to adhere to sites of tissue damage and serve as a source of rapid neovascularization. As a result, omental attachments become stable very rapidly. In addition to enhancing omental contact for waste removal and functional isolation, these attributes have been applied in the therapeutic use of omentum to seal and provide initial vascular supply for damaged tissue inside and outside of the abdominal cavity.

Peritoneal Repair

Peritoneal damage occurs whenever natural disease or invasive diagnostic or surgical procedures traumatize the parietal or visceral peritoneum. If the trauma is sufficient, mesothelial cells will be lost or physically removed. Successful recovery requires restoration of a functional peritoneal surface. The surgeon makes a number of diagnostic and therapeutic choices that can either facilitate or impede peritoneal healing.

The first step in appropriate peritoneal management is to recognize the peritoneum does not heal like other tissues. Rather than following the skin's contraction and epithelialization processes of healing, peritoneal defects heal diffusely across the defect area. Sharply excised experimental defects, irrespective of size, are diffusely filled by fibrin, cellular debris, and neutrophils within 12 hours of resection. By 24 to 36 hours, the number of cells on the wound surface has increased, and macrophages have become the predominant cell type. Macrophages supported by fibrin cover the wound surface by the second day after injury. In the absence of other adhesion stimuli, this initial inflammatory exudate will begin to resolve and the first immature mesothelial cells will appear within 48 to 72 hours. Islands of mesothelial cells proliferate into connecting sheets. A functionally mature mesothelial surface with a smooth juncture with adjacent mesothelium is evident within 4 to 6 days after resection. By 7 to 10 days after resection both surface cells and submesothelial tissues are histologically and functionally mature. Whether these immature cells are seeded from submesothelial tissues or cells in the peritoneal fluid has been a topic of debate. Injuries such as abrasion, drying, and ischemia, which do not directly remove mesothelial tissue, result in mesothelial cell death and defoliation. The process of healing following defoliation is similar, although often less successful.

Peritoneal healing requires the coordination of fibrin and phagocyte deposition, mesothelial cell colonization and proliferation, and fibrin removal (lysis). Removal of the fibrin after it has served the functions of initial wound seal and matrix for cell deposition and migration is a critical step for wound healing without adhesion formation. Plasmin is the primary agent responsible for fibrin lysis in the peritoneal cavity and is activated primarily by tissue plasminogen activator. The mesothelium is considered responsible for 95% of peritoneal tPA activity in man. Macrophages also produce tPA. A urokinase-type plasminogen activator (uPA), prevalent in urine but also found in other tissues, and nonspecific proteolytic enzymes may also play minor roles in fibrin removal in peritoneal wounds. Agents that either inhibit fibrin formation or fibrin lysis help balance the process of fibrinolysis. Antithrombin III and protein C impede fibrin formation. Several fibrinolytic inhibitors (FI) are produced by mesothelial cells as well as by other tissues in the body. Plasminogen activator inhibitor 1 (PAI-1) is considered the most important fibrinolytic inhibitor in the peritoneal cavity in man and laboratory animals.

Under optimal circumstances with mild and transient peritoneal trauma, the peritoneal environment supports temporary involvement of fibrin in wound repair. Mesothelial cell production of tPA decreases or ceases entirely immediately after wounding and remains low until new mesothelial cells enter the wound site. Fibrinolytic inhibitor levels do not usually decrease during this early stage and in some cases may actually increase. This allows fibrin to enter and temporarily seal the wound so that it serves as a scaffold for new cell deposition. The local tPA levels begin to increase 3 to 4 days after wounding and will increase above baseline by 7 to 10 days after injury when the wound is covered with new and metabolically active mesothelial cells. The increasing tPA levels support lysis of the now unnecessary fibrin.

Factors that interfere with initial deposition of fibrin can prevent wound closure, whereas factors that interfere with—or overwhelm—the process of fibrinolysis promote the development of fibrous adhesions (see Peritoneal Adhesions). However, failures in peritoneal healing under clinical conditions typically reflect a persistent inflammatory stimulus (visceral leakage or fistulation) rather than an imbalance in intrinsic tPA and FI activity. Surgical procedures can also interfere with peritoneal healing by this mechanism. Incomplete visceral closure with leakage or accidental incorporation of omentum in a body wall incision can prevent complete peritoneal healing. Attempts to control undesirable adhesions by artificially enhancing fibrinolysis can also interfere with necessary incisional healing (see Peritoneal Adhesions).

Species variation is recognized in mesothelial production of tPA. Bovine mesothelium does not produce tPA either before or within 10 days of wounding but does produce fibrinolytic inhibitors before and after injury. Although this is consistent with the observation of large quantities of fibrin in the peritoneal cavities of cattle with inflammatory lesions, it does not explain the equally valid observation that many peritoneal lesions heal successfully without persistent fibrin or fibrous tissue.

PHYSICAL EXAMINATION

The primary clinical signs of peritoneal disease detectable by physical examination are signs of abdominal pain, altered visceral position or motility, abnormal gas accumulation, and fibrin accumulation.

Pain occurs as a result of stretching of the visceral peritoneum or inflammation of parietal or visceral peritoneum. Common signs of both visceral and peritoneal pain include elevated pulse and respiratory rate, ileus, and anorexia. Visceral pain may also cause agitation, occasional kicking at the abdomen, or frequent changes in position. Discomfort may be more evident during palpation per rectum. These signs are usually more marked in calves than in adult cattle and can include violent rolling and kicking. Inflammation of parietal peritoneum typically causes a decrease in movements that would stretch the parietal inflamed region. Adult cattle with inflammation of the ventral parietal peritoneum may be reluctant to lie down and will resist arching their backs when pinched on their dorsal spinous processes caudal to the withers, occasionally producing an audible or auscultable grunt. The site of parietal inflammation can be localized in some cattle by pushing a fist or blunt object of similar width firmly into the abdomen in an organized pattern along the body wall. Pain is indicated by the cow's effort—often subtle—to shift away from pressure in affected areas. The process of applying focal abdominal pressure is helpful in differentiating between inflammatory foci concentrated in the caudal, central, or cranial abdomen or between the right and left sides.

The presence of adhesions may be suggested by several additional findings. Nonreducible or partially reducible umbilical, inguinal, or traumatic body wall hernias generally indicate the presence of adhesions. Immobile structures or sheets of adhesions may be detectable on palpation per rectum. A roughened surface on viscera or the body wall from fibrin deposits may also be palpable. Detection of pneumoperitoneum by auscultation or palpation per rectum without a history of recent abdominal surgery would indicate loss of normal barriers and/or peritoneal infection. Abscesses adjacent to the body wall can produce a tympanic sound on simultaneous auscultation and percussion similar to that produced by an obstructed abomasum or intestinal segment. An example of this situation is the uncommon development of a large right-sided abscess following omentopexy or pyloropexy, as described in Section 4.5.1

PERITONEAL IMAGING

Transabdominal ultrasonography can be used to evaluate the structural integrity of the body wall, identify fluid or fibrin adjacent to the body wall, and evaluate motility in viscera adjacent to the body wall in calves and adult cattle. Transrectal ultrasonography can provide similar information on the pelvic and caudal abdominal cavity in adults. Transabdominal ultrasonography is particularly useful in characterizing the contents of intraabdominal umbilical remnants and the nature of adhered structures in calves with umbilical infections. Ultrasound also allows differentiation between umbilical infection and herniation, edema, hemorrhage, or free fluid accumulation (including urine) in calves with swelling of the abdominal wall. Ultrasonography can also be used to help guide fluid collection from the peritoneal cavity or from abscess cavities adjacent to the body wall (Figure 10.9-1). Ultrasound is used effectively to follow the

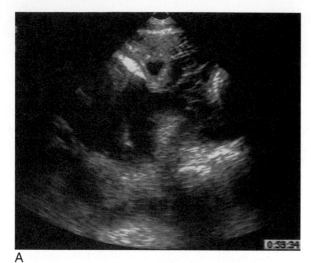

A

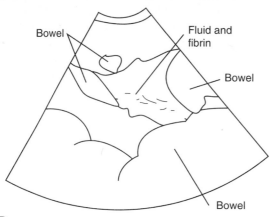

B

Figure 10.9-1 *A,* Sonogram of the ventral abdomen obtained from an adult Holstein cow with a 3-2 MHz phased array sector probe. The image illustrates fluid and fibrin within the peritoneal cavity. This cow was diagnosed with diffuse peritonitis secondary to a perforated reticulum. *B,* Schematic representation that illustrates the structure seen in *A.*

(Courtesy of Dr. Amy Yeager; Cornell University.)

resolution of abscesses after transcutaneous or transreticular drainage in adult cattle.

Radiography can provide valuable information about the structural and functional integrity of the peritoneum in the neonate and adult. Radiographs can help characterize structures in body wall defects and may identify accumulations of peritoneal fluid, abscesses, or abnormally positioned structures in the neonatal calf. The increase in body size and the extensive development of the forestomach compartments and greater omentum limit the value of radiography in adult cattle. It has been used most extensively for evaluation of the cranioventral abdomen, in which accumulations of fibrin or multiple small gas pockets and persistent dorsal displacement of

the reticulum indicate peritonitis. More details are provided in Section 2.1 and 10.3.

PERITONEAL FLUID
Fluid Collection

The unique development of the ruminant stomach, expansive omentum, and the species' propensity for fibrin deposition place some constraints on collection of peritoneal fluid in cattle. Ideally, abdominocentesis is done under ultrasonographic control at or near the disease process. Otherwise, there are four abdominal sites that can be used. These include: 3 to 6 cm to the right and left of the caudal midline, 3 to 6 cm cranial to the mammary gland in the female or 3 to 6 cm caudal to the preputial opening in the male. Two cranial sites 3 to 6 cm to the right and left of the cranial midline at the most dependent site of the abdomen, usually 5 to 6 cm caudal to the xiphoid process, can be alternative sites. In general, one of the two recommended caudal sites in the standing adult is preferred. Using all four sites has been suggested to provide better localization of the lesion.

Samples can be collected with an 18-gauge, 1.5-inch needle in most adult cattle. Longer needles are occasionally indicated for highly conditioned beef cows and adult bulls. In young calves, a 20-gauge, 1-inch needle is more appropriate. A teat cannula may be used instead of a needle if preferred. All penetration should be performed in the center of a clipped and aseptically prepared area.

Fluid is normally limited in volume and a small (3 ml) EDTA tube and sterile 3-cc syringe should be immediately available to collect fluid by gravity. Attempts to aspirate fluid are typically not successful, presumably because the negative pressure created is sufficient to plug the needle or cannula with the omentum. Excessive amounts of EDTA will cause cell lysis, a false depression of the PCV and total protein, and altered serum electrolyte values.

Fluid Evaluation

The fluid should be evaluated grossly for clarity, color, opacity and odor. A centrifuged anticoagulated sample (EDTA or heparin) can be used to determine packed cell value and plasma protein concentration. An anticoagulated sample should also be stained and evaluated microscopically for cell characteristics and the presence of intracellular or extracellular bacteria or parasites. If initial evaluation indicates that bacteria are present, a gram stain should be performed to differentiate between gram-negative and gram-positive organisms for selection of initial antibiotic therapy. Sterile samples should be submitted for aerobic and anaerobic cultures if possible.

Cytology

Normal peritoneal fluid is clear to slightly turbid and clear to light yellow in color, with a potential slight pink tinge normal in late gestation. The specific gravity should be less than 1.016, and the pH should be between 6 and 8. A pH of less than 4 would suggest accidental abomasocentesis. The total protein is typically less than 3 gm/dl. Fibrinogen in normal bovine peritoneal fluid may be sufficient to clot on exposure to air.

The cell count in peritoneal fluid is normally less than 10,000 white blood cells/μl. Mature neutrophils and monocytes are the predominant cells and are fairly equal in number. Up to 60% mature neutrophils with a total cell count of <10,000 cells/μl would be considered within normal parameters. Greater than 60% neutrophils, particularly with an elevated total cell count, would be abnormal and suggests contamination, infection, or trauma. The presence of degenerating neutrophils is abnormal and suggests infectious or toxic changes. Eosinophils are commonly detected in peritoneal fluid of cattle in some geographical areas. Other than the potential implication of parasite migration or other antigenic stimulation, eosinophils are not considered indicative of peritoneal pathology. Lymphocytes, macrophages, and desquamated mesothelial cells may also be present in normal fluid. Platelets are not normal components of peritoneal fluid, and their presence suggests the sample has been contaminated with blood.

Special Chemistry Evaluation

The concentration of common serum enzymes in normal peritoneal fluid is determined by their molecular weight, with smaller molecules such as urea nitrogen in equilibrium with serum. The relative elevation of electrolytes and enzymes that are concentrated in urine in the peritoneal fluid are useful aids in diagnosing urinary tract rupture (see Section 12.3.2).

Disorders of the Peritoneum

PERITONEAL INFECTION

Peritonitis, or peritoneal inflammation, is a common finding in both adult cattle and calves. Inflammation without infection can occur from mechanical trauma during surgery or from chemical irritation caused by urine leakage or poorly balanced or caustic lavage solutions. Peritonitis from infectious agents is more common.

Categories of Infectious Peritonitis

Primary peritonitis refers to peritoneal infection without an evident intraabdominal source of infection. Primary peritonitis is relatively rare in cattle in comparison to secondary peritonitis. The fibrinous peritonitis associated with sporadic bovine encephalomyelitis (*Chlamydia psittaci*) and septicemia caused by *Haemophilus spp.* are examples. Contamination by passive diffusion or forced flow of organisms from the uterus through patent oviducts in the postparturient period has also been recognized as a source of peritonitis in cattle.

Secondary Peritonitis Secondary peritonitis is the most common source of peritonitis in cattle. Secondary peritonitis includes cases of bacterial peritonitis secondary to intraabdominal lesions. In cattle, sources of bacterial peritonitis include lesions that disrupt normal barriers between a visceral lumen and the peritoneal cavity (foreign body perforations, ulcers, ischemia) and extension of preexisting infection through the peritoneal membrane (umbilical remnant infection, liver or renal abscesses, retroperitoneal infections, body wall infections).

Tertiary Peritonitis Tertiary peritonitis is defined as a recurrent peritoneal infection after an appropriately managed episode of primary or secondary peritonitis. A single organism or a limited number of synergistic organisms are typically involved. This category clearly exists in cattle, although differentiation between cases of recurrent peritonitis after appropriate management of secondary peritonitis versus unresolved cases of secondary peritonitis would be difficult.

Pathophysiology Regardless of the source of contamination, peritoneal infection occurs when the number and virulence of contaminating organisms exceeds the ability of available host defenses to control or eliminate the organisms before they are able to multiply and invade tissue to cause tissue damage. The number of organisms necessary to cause peritonitis appears to depend on a variety of factors, including the nature of the organism, method of introduction, local environment, and available defenses.

The number of organisms necessary to cause infection can be decreased by the presence of adjuvants—agents that either decrease the availability or efficacy of host defenses or increase the survivability of invading pathogens. A number of specific adjuvants have been identified in the peritoneal cavity, including increased fluid levels, blood, hemoglobin, and foreign bodies. Inadequate hemostasis, incomplete removal of lavage fluid, inadequate debridement, traumatic surgical technique, and use of excessive or reactive suture material or surgical mesh by the surgeon all act as adjuvants in the peritoneal cavity and increase the risk of infection. Some organisms act synergistically in the peritoneum, and their concurrent presence increases the survival of both. The frequency of polymicrobial infections with *E. coli, Arcanobacter pyogenes,* and *Fusobacterium necrophorum* suggests that a synergistic relationship may exist.

Once contaminants have entered the peritoneal cavity, they can move through one of several stages based on the nature of contamination, available host defenses, and the nature and timing of therapeutic intervention. The first contamination stage (Stage 1, "golden period") represents a delay of 4 to 6 hours between the introduction of bacteria into a tissue and establishment of infection. All surgical abdominal procedures initiate this stage unless infection has already developed from a previous source of contamination.

Stage 1 is characterized by a rapid inflammatory response with fluid influx that contains complement, opsonins, chemotaxins, fibrinogen, and thrombin. Physical removal is the primary host defense mechanism against bacteria and inert contaminants during this period, with the greatest rates of removal during the first 3 hours after contamination. Neutrophil influx and phagocytosis become significant within hours of initial contamination and remain high throughout this stage. Soluble fibrinogen is rapidly converted to insoluble fibrin, thus allowing fibrin entrapment of contaminants. The presence of adjuvants can interfere with one or more of the available waste removal methods and decrease the ability of the host to eliminate contaminants before infection can develop.

Mortality is very low during the contamination phase of peritonitis. Clean surgeries (elective, no invasion of a lumen) in generally healthy animals without breaks in technique would normally introduce so few organisms that host defenses alone are sufficient to control the contaminants. Addition of therapeutic assistance in the form of antimicrobial therapy and removal of adjuvants can help host defenses eliminate more extensive contaminant loads. However, if bacteria are not physically removed or effectively neutralized by the combination of host defenses and therapeutic intervention, infection will develop and enter stage 2.

Stage 2 (acute generalized peritonitis) occurs between 3 to 4 hours and 4 to 5 days after initial contamination. The peritoneal circulation has distributed at least some contaminants away from the original site of inoculation in route to the diaphragmatic stomata. Active infection may be present throughout the peritoneal cavity if the number of contaminating organisms is high. When contamination occurs outside of the supraomental bursa in adult cattle, the extensive omentum may help decrease the concentration of organisms carried into the bursa by physically separation. This is consistent with the clinical observation that contamination originating in the bovine cranioventral or craniolateral abdomen (traumatic reticuloperitonitis, liver abscesses, some abomasal ulcers) tends to spare the viscera within the supraomental bursa, whereas sources that originate in the caudal region or within the supraomental bursa are more commonly associated with generalized peritonitis.

Physical removal of contaminants is still the predominant host defense mechanism in early Stage 2, but the volume of material removed decreases later as fibrin deposits limit fluid flow. Functional trapping by omentum and fragile, easily disrupted fibrin strands and clots begin to play a role. Phagocytosis is active, with neutrophils peaking 24 hours after infection and decreasing slowly afterward. Macrophages begin to play a significant role the second day after contamination. The process of selective reduction begins during this stage, but the flora from polymicrobial contamination remains. Mortality is high during this stage and accounts for the majority of deaths attributed to peritonitis. The primary cause of death in Stage 2 is bacteremia that results from the rapid transfer of specific pathogens from the peritoneal cavity into the general circulation. Gram-negative aerobes/facultative anaerobes such as *E. coli* are by far the most common agents identified in the circulation in man and the laboratory species for which this information is available. Adjuvants in the peritoneal cavity typically increase the mortality rate. The presence of anaerobes in the peritoneal cavity at this stage appears to be necessary for abscess formation in stages 3 and 4 and also improves the environment for survival of synergistic organisms. Experimental inoculation of contaminants in a fibrin clot decreases acute mortality in laboratory animals, although it also increases the incidence of abscess formation in later stages. The cow's ability to rapidly deposit large volumes of fibrin in response to contaminants may contribute to its apparent success in surviving the early stages of peritonitis.

Once this stage has been entered, three possible outcomes are the following: 1) host defenses may still overcome pathogens, thus leading to complete resolution of infection (typically in animals with good host defenses, relatively small numbers of contaminating organisms, and few adjuvants) but often leaving residual changes in the peritoneal cavity such as adhesions; 2) pathogens may clearly overwhelm host defenses, thus leading to fulminant peritonitis and death (typically from bacteremia); or 3) pathogens and host defenses may achieve a standoff, thus leading to the third stage of peritonitis.

Stage 3 (acute localizing peritonitis) is a transitional period for cases that have survived stage 2 but were incapable of completely eliminating organisms from the peritoneal cavity. This stage occurs between 4 and 10 days after contamination in laboratory animals and man, although the propensity for fibrin formation may shift the schedule forward or shorten its duration in cattle. Selective reduction is complete, and the number of initial contaminants has been typically reduced to one or two organisms capable of long-term survival in the peritoneal environment. Single organisms or a combination of two to three synergistic organisms are most common.

The predominant method of waste control is functional removal by fibrin and omental entrapment. Regional differences may occur in the distribution of fibrin based on the concentration of organisms distributed in stage 2 as well as the location of necrotic tissue or persistent inflammatory stimuli, such as foreign materials. Physical removal of contaminants continues at a reduced level, which is limited by obstruction of stomata and interference with contaminant mobility by fibrin accumulations. However, fibrin also impedes access of phagocytic cells to entrapped organisms.

Mortality is lower in this stage than in stage 2 and is more sporadic. Cows that survive stage 3 will either move on to stage 4 or effectively resolve the infection with persistent adhesions and/or sterile abscesses. If pathogenic organisms are effectively eliminated, the potential for return to full health will depend on the location and nature of persistent adhesions (see Peritoneal Adhesions).

Cases that survive stage 3 by localizing persistent pathogens into organized abscesses enter stage 4 (chronic abscessing peritonitis). This stage begins anytime at or after the 8th day following contamination. The propensity of the bovine abdomen for fibrin deposition may increase the likelihood of encountering this stage in cattle. Selective reduction is complete, and a relatively small number of organisms, typically anaerobes (obligate or facultative), capable of abscess formation can be found. In some cases, organisms will be eliminated, thus leaving a sterile abscess. Mortality is low in this stage, but the persistent infection can create a continued strain on the animal's system evidenced by poor weight gain, suboptimal food consumption, and decreased milk production. Intermittent escape of bacteria from abscesses can occur and cause episodes of pyrexia, neutrophilia and depression. Depending on location, abscesses and adhesions may suddenly produce complete obstruction or serve as a focus for intestinal volvulus, resulting in more acute and severe clinical signs. In humans, death in this stage is commonly attributed to multiple organ failure. Although not commonly acknowledged in cattle, bacterial endocarditis and pyelonephritis have been recognized in association with peritonitis at *post mortem* evaluation.

Clinical Signs and Diagnosis

The clinical presentation of cattle with peritonitis depends largely on the source and magnitude of contamination and the stage of infection.

Clinical signs during stage 1 are primarily associated with the initiating lesion rather than the peritoneal insult.

Identification of the specific onset of this stage in naturally occurring cases is usually impossible unless the animal was being monitored for progression of a suspected visceral lesion by serial peritoneocentesis. Sudden relief of severe abdominal pain consistent with visceral distention/obstruction followed by gradual signs of depression and shock may mark the time of visceral rupture and peritoneal contamination. Cases initiated by surgical intervention have a more reliable identification of the initial time of contamination, although recognition of excessive contamination is not always immediate. By the end of this stage, peritoneocentesis would typically demonstrate neutrophilia and hyperfibrinogenemia.

Cows in stage 2 usually demonstrate both systemic and abdominal signs. Systemic signs include depression, anorexia, dehydration, elevation or depression of temperature and pulse rate, and signs of systemic shock. Feces are usually decreased in volume and may vary from loose to pasty in consistency. Rumen motility is often depressed, and rumen distention may be present. Pain from peritoneal inflammation may be detectable. Surgical exploration would often reveal large volumes of fluid with loose disorganized accumulations of fragile fibrin clots and erythematous surfaces.

Systemic neutrophilia with or without a left shift or neutropenia is common. However, hematological changes are variable, and normal neutrophil counts do not rule out peritonitis. Plasma fibrinogen is typically elevated. Serum chemistry changes parallel the cow's lactation cycle and intestinal ileus. These changes include hypocalcemia, hypochloremia, and hypokalemia. Serum urea nitrogen and creatinine are commonly increased because of dehydration and prerenal azotemia. Serum protein may be increased or decreased in this stage, depending on the rapidity with which protein is lost into the peritoneal cavity balanced by inflammatory increases in serum fibrinogen and globulins. A marked increase in peritoneal total white blood cell and neutrophil counts is typical during this stage; however, care should be taken not to overinterpret an increased count as a definite sign of infection. In a study of peritoneal fluid after clean surgical exploratory celiotomy and omentopexy in adult cattle, total nucleated white blood cell and neutrophil counts rose as high as 17,800 and 11,125 cells/μl, respectively, at 1 day after surgery and as high as 65,000 and 46,800 cells/μl 2 days after surgery.

Clinical signs in stages 3 and 4 are similar and vary in severity based on the location of infection and its duration. Depression, anorexia, dehydration, changes in fecal consistency, depressed ruminal motility, depressed milk production, and weight loss may be intermittently present. Temperature, pulse rate, and respiratory rate vary from above to below normal limits. If the process involves the parietal peritoneum, localized pain may be detectable on physical examination. If the normal motility patterns of viscera are disturbed, the resulting tension on bowel can produce signs of visceral pain.

Intermittent seeding of organisms into the circulation may produce fluctuating fever or signs of septic shock consistent with stage 2.

Hyperfibrinogenemia is the most consistent hematological finding. Systemic cytology and serum chemistries will often be within normal limits, although changes seen in earlier stages may be present. The results of peritoneocentesis may vary greatly by location. Cytology for fluid collected from areas of active inflammation will be consistent with an active or sterile abscess (degenerative neutrophils, occasional bacteria), whereas cytology of adjacent sites may be normal or may reflect mild inflammation.

Grossly, accumulations of fibrin are becoming more localized and more organized in stage 3, but some may still be disrupted manually. By stage 4, adhesions and abscess walls are primarily fibrous and distinctly localized. Intermittent disturbance of adhesions or abscesses may reinitiate an inflammatory reaction with some less organized fibrin interspersed among the fibrous adhesions.

Common Organisms in Cattle

An accurate description of pathogens involved in peritonitis in cattle is hampered by lack of consistent culture procedures in clinical cases of peritonitis, particularly for anaerobes. Without regard for the source of contamination and methods of culture, the most common agents identified in peritonitis of adult cattle are *Arcanobacterium pyogenes* (previously identified as *Corynebacterium/Actinomyces pyogenes*), *Fusobacterium necrophorum, E. coli* and—less commonly—*Staphylococcus* spp. and *Streptococcus* spp. Less information is available about the organisms associated with specific sources of contamination; therefore prediction of probable contaminants for prophylaxis and initial therapy is often based on knowledge of normal local flora.

The flora of the gastrointestinal tract varies greatly based on distance aborad. The ruminoreticulum contains a large number of potentially pathogenic obligate and facultative anaerobes necessary for the digestion process—and relatively few viable pathogenic aerobes. Cases of peritonitis resulting from traumatic reticuloperitonitis are typically attributed to *Arcanobacterium pyogenes, Fusobacterium necrophorum,* and *E. coli.* The acidic environment of the healthy abomasum maintains an essentially sterile environment, although lesions such as ulcers can be colonized by a variety of organisms. Moving from proximal to distal in the intestinal tract, the flora shifts from low numbers of gram-positive aerobes

to increasing numbers of gram-negative aerobes (Enterobacteriaceae) in the ileum, and very large numbers of gram-negative aerobes and anaerobes in the cecum and colon. Similar flora are present in the urogenital viscera, with the additional consideration of *Moraxella* spp., *Proteus* spp., *Pasteurella multocida,* and *Bacteroides* spp. in the uterus and *Corynebacterium renale, Pseudomonas aeruginosa* in the urinary tract. Organisms associated with persistent infection of the umbilical remnants of calves include *Arcanobacterium pyogenes, E. coli,* and, less commonly, *Proteus* spp. and *Enterococcus* spp. Several nematodes migrate through the peritoneal cavity, including *Setaria* spp. These nematodes typically cause a mild and transient fibrinous peritonitis and may be associated with an increase in peritoneal eosinophils.

TREATMENT

The four goals of peritonitis treatment are 1) eliminate sources of contamination; 2) eliminate infectious agents; 3) minimize detrimental effects of the host defense process; and 4) provide systemic support. The relative importance of each and appropriate therapeutic steps vary with the three stages of infection.

Contamination—Stage 1

Therapy in stage 1 is directed at preventing the development of infection from recently introduced organisms. Prophylactic antibiotics—if not on board already—can be of some benefit but should be given intravenously to achieve high serum and tissue levels as soon as possible. If a source of contamination first develops intraoperatively, rapid steps to minimize the amount and distribution of contamination are indicated. Gross contamination should be localized whenever possible by exteriorizing the site of leakage or packing it off with laparotomy sponges; physically removing all accessible contaminants; and avoiding palpation unless absolutely necessary so that contaminants are not physically transported from the site of leakage to other sites in the abdomen. If the site can be adequately exteriorized to allow external drainage, localized lavage with a sterile isotonic fluid can help remove contaminants. However, generalized lavage is more likely to distribute high concentrations of organisms to potentially clean areas and is only recommended if the site cannot be exteriorized or dissemination has already occurred. Effective removal of lavage fluid is very difficult in the adult cow, and any remaining fluid will interfere with host defenses after closure. There is no proven benefit in adding antibiotics to the lavage fluid if appropriate systemic antibiotics have been administered.

Acute Diffuse Peritonitis—Stage 2
(e.g., traumatic reticuloperitonitis)

Intervention during this stage should focus on preventing death from potential gram-negative bacteremia and eliminating continuing sources of contamination and adjuvants. Systemic antibiotics (Appendix 1) should have good efficacy against the gram-negative aerobes that are most likely to enter and survive in the general circulation and, if consistent with the source of contamination, against anaerobes. Intraperitoneal organisms have not yet been fully localized by fibrin or omentum and are accessible to systemic antibiotics. Nonsteroidal antiinflammatory drugs should be considered to help manage possible endotoxemia. The use of peritoneal lavage appears to be of limited or no value during this stage and carries the risk of adding adjuvant fluid to the cavity. Surgical exploration is not indicated at this stage unless it is necessary to identify and eliminate a persistent source of contamination.

Acute Adhesive Peritonitis—Stage 3
(e.g., LDA with perforating ulcer)

This stage presents a number of challenges to the surgeon. Systemic antibiotics protect against sporadic shedding of organisms into the systemic circulation, although the developing fibrin accumulations will interfere with access to entrapped bacteria for either systemically or locally administered drugs (Appendix 1). Cattle that have survived to this point will have established some seal over sites of contamination to minimize or eliminate further contamination. However, the seal is tentative and may be disrupted by surgical exploration, peritoneal lavage, or normal activities of the cow, potentially sending the peritonitis back into stage 2 with an increased risk of septicemia and related risks. Unless the cow's condition takes a sudden turn for the worse, surgical intervention is not usually recommended.

Chronic Abscessing Peritonitis—Stage 4

At this point a distinct abscess (or abscesses) has formed, and the goal is to either remove or marsupialize the infection before multiple organ failure occurs. Cranial abdominal abscesses (in the liver or caused by traumatic reticuloperitonitis) that are directly or indirectly (by way of a solid sheet of adhesions) connected to the ventral body wall may be drained transcutaneously using a large-gauge (28-32 French) drain. Ultrasound can be used to guide drain placement in the standing animal, or the drain may be placed during ventral midline celiotomy. Perireticular abscesses that are firmly attached to the reticulum, are located at or above the ventral floor of the reticulum, and are caused by traumatic reticuloperitonitis may be effectively drained into the reticulum by an incision through the reticular wall from the luminal side using a rumenotomy approach. Intestinal resection and/or bypass may be necessary if viscera are obstructed. Antibiotic access to organisms is poor in this stage, and antibiotic use may even be contraindicated if it obscures clinical signs or results in a delay of definitive surgical treatment. Nonetheless, abscesses not amenable to either resection or marsupialization have been managed in other species by long-term therapy (4 to 6 weeks) with antibiotics that have good penetration into and efficacy in the environment of an abscess (Appendix 1). This option is seldom possible in cows for economic and antibiotic regulation reasons. Clinically, it would appear that organisms may be eliminated from some abscesses by the host and, if the abscess wall itself does not interfere with other critical structures, no further action is required.

PROGNOSIS

The prognosis for cases of peritonitis that reach stage 2 or 3 is fairly low, whereas for stage 4 it is approximately 30%. Mortality is highest in the early, acute diffuse stage of peritonitis, primarily because of gram-negative septicemia.

Noninfectious Diseases of the Peritoneum

NONSEPTIC PERITONITIS

Chemical peritonitis can be initiated by any body fluid or exogenous fluid that contains toxic elements or has a pH significantly different from relatively neutral peritoneal fluid. Many therapeutic agents that can be administered safely by intravenous or other parenteral routes will induce some degree of inflammatory reaction in the peritoneal cavity, including nonaqueous and many acidic or basic aqueous antibiotics, concentrated fluids such as hypertonic calcium and dextrose, and antiseptic solutions such as povidone iodine solution. Lavage fluids that are either more basic or acidic than peritoneal fluid can also induce chemical peritonitis. Introduction of normally separate body fluids, such as bile, can initiate a marked inflammatory reaction. Chemical peritonitis as a result of urine contamination is the most common form of mild chemical peritonitis in cattle.

UROPERITONEUM

The uroperitoneum is discussed in Section 12.3.2.

Peritoneal Adhesions

Peritoneal adhesions are physical connections between normally separate peritoneal surfaces caused by bridging fibrinous or fibrous tissue. Peritoneal adhesions form as an extension of the healing process in response to damaged tissue that cannot be rapidly replaced or restored to normal function.

SIGNIFICANCE

Peritoneal adhesions can have both beneficial and detrimental effects, although the detrimental sequelae are more commonly acknowledged. Intestinal obstruction is the most commonly recognized detrimental effect. Neonates are considered to be at particularly high risk of obstruction. Other undesirable effects of peritoneal adhesions include abdominal pain caused by traction on mobile viscera, infertility from extraluminal compression of the oviducts, and urinary dysfunction caused by extraluminal compression of ureters or traction on the bladder.

It is important to remember the process of adhesion formation is an extension of the normal healing process. Although the location and extent of adhesions can interfere with visceral function, they also can provide a seal for breaks in continuity of viscera and the body wall, thus serving a potential life-saving function. Adhesions, particularly to omentum, provide a route of neovascularization to areas of ischemia. Adhesions around a site of contamination can help seal the site and limit dissemination of material throughout the abdominal cavity. The surgeon can also intentionally create adhesions to stabilize large-diameter viscera in functional positions (i.e., abomasopexy).

The incidence of peritoneal adhesions in cattle is unknown, but the ability of adhesions to help localize contamination from foreign body perforation of the reticulum and abomasal ulcers in cattle is well recognized. The extensive omentum in cattle helps separate these common sites of contamination in the cranioventral abdomen from the small and large intestines within the supraomental bursa. This anatomical variation probably accounts for the relatively rare event of intestinal obstruction from adhesions in cattle. Intestinal obstruction is a greater risk with lesions that originate within the supraomental bursa or pelvic region, although these are less common sites of contamination. Infertility associated with adhesions in the region of the ovary and oviducts has been recognized in cows. Dysuria or pollakiuria have been recognized as a result of bladder or urachal adhesions, most commonly in calves.

The cow may be uniquely designed to benefit from the positive effects of peritoneal adhesions. The relatively low fibrinolytic activity of bovine mesothelium would promote adhesion development, while the extensive omentum helps separate the most common sites of contamination from viscera more sensitive to their detrimental effects. As surgeons, we use adhesions intentionally to stabilize the abomasum with a variety of abomasopexy and omentopexy techniques. These procedures form stable adhesions by suturing the target structure to the body wall. Preexisting adhesions provide a protective wall that allows us to marsupialize cranial abdominal abscesses into the reticulum or through the ventral body wall. Rapid formation of localized adhesions also serves a protective function during transabdominal bladder catheterization for urinary tract obstruction in steers. The extensive omentum can also be used to help revascularize ischemic tissues that cannot be removed, while limiting leakage and preventing formation of more detrimental adhesions at the same time.

PATHOPHYSIOLOGY

Fibrin deposition is part of the initial response to peritoneal injury or contamination. When the stimulus is localized and transient, fibrin deposits are typically limited to the wound surface and are resolved as new mesothelial cells fill the wound (see Peritoneal Repair). When more extensive areas of tissue damage occur, fibrin deposition is more extensive. If two damaged peritoneal surfaces covered by fibrin matrix come into contact during the early healing period, the matrices can connect, thus forming a fibrinous adhesion. If this fibrin scaffold persists, fibroblast invasion will begin within 3 to 4 days. Collagen deposition by fibroblasts and subsequent infiltration of capillaries create the more solid and potentially detrimental fibrous adhesion, usually within 7 to 14 days after injury. Once a fibrous adhesion is formed, it is considered relatively stable aside from maturation of the collagen and remodeling along principle lines of force. Lysis may be possible through collagenase activity, although the process would be very slow (many months to years).

CONTROL AND TREATMENT
Promotion
Promotion of adhesions may be necessary to help stabilize a mobile viscus, provide a source of neovascularization for damaged tissue, or help seal potential leaks from areas of contamination. Abomasal displacements are the most common reason to promote adhesions in cattle. The surgeon can increase the likelihood of establishing a stable, long-lasting, localized adhesion between the body wall and either the abomasum or omentum by using a nonabsorbable suture material and incorporating parietal peritoneum in the incision line.

The extensive omentum can be used effectively to create potentially beneficial adhesions in a variety of situations in the cow. By suturing omentum over sites of questionable viability, the surgeon can provide a source of vascularization, help prevent leakage through ischemic visceral walls or poorly sealed anastomotic sites, and block adhesion to other viscera. Care should be taken to avoid interposing sections of omentum between incision edges because this can interfere with incisional healing, thus leading to partial or complete dehiscence.

Prevention

Adhesion prevention may be approached at a number of levels, including the following: 1) decreasing trauma to peritoneal surfaces; 2) decreasing the inflammatory response; 3) decreasing conversion of soluble fibrinogen to fibrin; 4) decreasing contact between traumatized surfaces; 5) controlling the nature of traumatized surface contact; 6) enhancing natural fibrinolytic activity; 7) decreasing fibrinolytic inhibitor activity; 8) decreasing fibroblast invasion and collagen deposition; and 9) enhancing collagenase activity. Specific preventative measures may act at one or more levels and generally fall into the following six categories: 1) surgical techniques; 2) antiinflammatory agents; 3) anticoagulants; 4) fibrinolytic agents; 5) coating solutions; and 6) solid barriers. Some measures are practical and appropriate for adhesion control under all surgical conditions. Others are limited by cost or feasibility to situations of increased risk in animals of significant value to the owner.

Routine Preventative Measures A number of practical measures are available to decrease the risk of undesirable adhesions and should be applied routinely. These include limiting serosal trauma, avoiding stimuli that promote inflammation, and controlling contact between traumatized surfaces. Gentle tissue handling and prevention of tissue drying, abrasion, or ischemia are all important steps that decrease peritoneal trauma. Leaving parietal peritoneum unsutured will decrease serosal ischemia and the risk of adhesion without decreasing wound strength or the rate of healing. Minimizing the amount of fluid, blood, ischemic tissue, and foreign material left in the abdomen will also decrease the stimulus for adhesions. When it is necessary to leave surgical foreign material such as sutures in the abdomen, absorbable materials are less likely than nonabsorbable materials to lead to fibrous adhesions. Nonsteroidal antiinflammatory agents decrease a number of factors that promote adhesion formation (including vascular permeability, plasmin inhibitor, platelet aggregation, and coagulation) and reduce adhesion formation in some animal models. Steps to prevent infection are indicated as part of inflammation control and include prophylactic antibiotics, good aseptic technique, minimizing the presence of adjuvants, and avoiding elective abdominal surgery until remote infections can be eliminated.

The extensive omentum and the compartmental nature of the adult bovine abdomen are perhaps the greatest potential tools in protecting against detrimental adhesions. Efforts to limit serosal trauma and contamination to areas outside of the supraomental bursa are indicated whenever possible. Particular care should be taken to avoid inadvertently tracking contaminants from sites of poorly localized infection into the caudal abdomen or supraomental bursa. If lesions exist that cannot be resolved without fully removing ischemic tissue, an omental patch should be considered. If the omentum can be easily mobilized to the site of ischemia, suturing the omentum to the site may seal potential sites of leakage and provide a source of neovascularization. Although omental adhesions are not without potential complications, they are less likely to cause physical or functional problems than adhesions to other serosal surfaces are.

Increased Adhesion Risk and Value Although the routine precautions described earlier are sufficient in most conditions, some situations merit further preventative measures because the risk of deleterious adhesions is high and the value of extra prophylactic measures are economically warranted for that animal in the owner's opinion. Adult cattle with potentially increased risk include those with lesions in the supraomental bursa or pelvic canal, particularly those in both genders involving the small intestine or spiral colon, or the uterus or pelvic canal in females with high reproductive potential. Calves younger than 3 months of age may have increased risk regardless of the location of the lesion because of their limited omental development and minimal compartmentalization. The relative value of the animal is determined by the owner's assessment of its potential future value. The decision of which options to use should be based on cost and relative benefit in consultation with the owner.

Coating solutions used as a dip or wash for surgical gloves and sponges—or as a local lavage—have been used with some frequency in human surgery and less frequently in equine abdominal surgery. Coating agents decrease serosal trauma primarily by reducing the friction between gloves, sponges, and tissues through mechanical lubrication. The most commonly used coating agent in veterinary practice is 1% sodium carboxymethylcellulose (SCMC), a high molecular weight substitute polysaccharide. It is relatively inexpensive in its powder form but must be converted to a sterile solution for application. Coating agents have been of some benefit in decreasing adhesions in man and horse but can make viscera slippery and difficult to handle. Their use may be indicated when surgical manipulation of viscera in a controlled environment such as the supraomental bursa is necessary. A precipitate has been found in the blood of horses and cows in which SCMC was administered as a peritoneal infusion at a dose of 0.96 to 11.7 ml/kg. A direct correlation between the concentration of precipitate and the concentration of solution administered was found. No specific pathologic effect was identified. Solid barrier agents (see Potential Tools) may also be beneficial in preventing adhesions in selected cases but, with the exception of omentum, have not yet been tested in cattle.

Potential Tools A variety of techniques have been explored in human surgery or experimentally in laboratory species and may prove either detrimental or beneficial for future use in cattle. Other coating solutions tested in laboratory animals and man with variable success include chondroitin sulfate, 32% dextran 70, poloxamer solutions, hyaluronic acid, hyaluronic acid with phosphate-buffered saline, and polyvinylpyrrolidone. In addition to natural barrier agents such as omentum, a number of natural and synthetic solid barrier agents such as fat, amnion, Gelfilm® and Gelfoam®*, Surgicel®[†], polytetrafuoroethylene mesh[‡], oxidized regenerated cellulose[§], and a chemically derived sodium hyaluronate and carboxymethylcellulose bioresorbable membrane (Seprafilm®; Genzyme) have had limited use in cattle.

Recombinant forms of tissue plasminogen activators have reached second (Alteplase, Activase®; Genentech) and third (Reteplase, Retevase®; Boehringer Mannheim) generations and have shown particular promise in adhesion prevention in human and laboratory animal studies. These agents have significant advantages over earlier fibrinolytic agents such as urokinase and streptokinase. They are absorbed specifically into fibrin clots and show little or no effects on hemostasis if absorbed into the general circulation. They are not antigenic and do not induce an inflammatory response. Although not currently tested for use in bovine abdominal surgery, these may emerge as potentially useful agents in the future, despite the differences in baseline plasminogen activator activity in cattle. Emerging areas of adhesion prevention include prevention of collagen deposition, inhibition of angiogenesis, use of gene therapy, and use of anti-transforming growth factor-β and antitumor necrosis factor-α.

Treatment

Treatment of peritoneal adhesions typically involves separating detrimental adhesions and may involve additional procedures to restore the function of affected viscera. Perhaps the most difficult aspect of treating existing adhesions is preventing recurrence. Separation, or *lysis,* of adhesions can be performed bluntly, by sharp incision, or by other methods of incision—including electrocautery and laser. The risk of adhesion recurrence is high regardless of the method of lysis, and preventative meas-

ures described previously should be considered if the recurrence of adhesions is a concern. This is more likely to be the case for adhesions in the supraomental bursa or pelvic canal. Lysis of adhesions to the abomasum may be of less concern if the abomasum is secured in a functional position, in which case new adhesions may be beneficial.

Blunt dissection, usually manual, is commonly used to lyse fibrinous and early fibrous adhesions in cattle, particularly when adhesions cannot be exteriorized or well exposed. Particular care must be taken to protect connected viscera. As the adhesion matures, it will be intimately integrated into the wall of connected viscera. A distinct line of separation between fibrous tissue and visceral wall may not be apparent, and the fibrous adhesion often has greater tensile strength than the visceral wall. Uncontrolled tension on a mature adhesion is more likely to pull a hole in the visceral wall than to break the adhesion. To safely break a maturing fibrous adhesion, the surgeon should firmly hold the site of adhesion attachment to a viscus and use his or her thumb and first fingers of both hands to break the adhesion as close to its center and as far from attached viscera as possible. It is often necessary to manually split the adhesion longitudinally into bands with smaller cross-sectional areas that are easier to break. Sharp incision will be necessary for mature fibrous adhesions not amenable to manual disruption and may be advisable for less mature thick adhesions that can be safely exposed. Although laparoscopic laser lysis has shown lower recurrence rates in comparison to other methods in many studies of man and laboratory species, it is seldom a practical option in food animals. Electrocautery carries similar practical limitations.

RECOMMENDED READINGS

Ahrenholz DH, Simmons RL: Differential binding of *Escherichia coli* and *Staphylococcus aureus* by polymerizing fibrin, *Surg Forum* 31: 74-75, 1980.

Ahrenholz DH, Simmons RL: Fibrin in peritonitis, I: beneficial and adverse effects of fibrin in experimental *E. coli* peritonitis, *Surgery* 88: 41-47, 1980.

Anderson DE, Cornwell D, St.-Jean G, Desrochers A, Anderson LS: Comparison of peritoneal fluid analysis before and after exploratory celiotomy and omentopexy in cattle, *Am J Vet Res* 55(12): 1633-1637, 1994.

Braun U, Iselin U, Lischer C, Fluri E: Ultrasonographic findings in five cows before and after treatment of reticular abscesses, *Vet Rec* 142: 184-189, 1998.

Brown GL, Stone HH: Intraperitoneal infections. In Polk HC Jr., ed: *Clinical surgery international, 4: infection and the surgical patient,* New York, 1982, Churchill Livingstone.

Burkhard MJ, Baxter G, Thrall MA: Blood precipitate associated with intraabdominal carboxymethylcellulose administration, *Vet Clin Path* 25: 114-117, 1996.

---

*Upjohn, Kalamazoo, MI
[†]Johnson & Johnson, New Brunswick, NJ
[‡]PTFE, Gore-Tex®; Gore & Associates, Flagstaff, AZ
[§]ORC, Interceed®; Johnson & Johnson.

Di Paolo N, Sacchi G: Anatomy and physiology of the peritoneal membrane. In Scarpioni LL, Ballocchi S, editors: Evolution and trends in peritoneal dialysis, *Contrib Nephrol Basel Karger* 84: 10-26, 1990.

Ducharme NG, Dill SG, Rendano VT: Reticulography of the cow in dorsal recumbency: an aid in the diagnosis and treatment of traumatic reticuloperitonitis, *J Am Vet Med Assoc* 182: 585-588, 1983.

Dunn DL, Barke RA, Ahrenholz DH, Humphrey EW, Simmons RL: The adjuvant effect of peritoneal fluid in experimental peritonitis: mechanisms and clinical implications, *Ann Surg* 199: 37-43, 1984.

Ebeid M, Rings DM: Generalized peritonitis in cattle: 31 cases (1993-1997), *Bov Practitioner* 33: 144-148, 1999.

Entriken TL, editor: *Veterinary pharmaceuticals and biologicals,* ed 12, Lenexa, Kan., 2001, Veterinary Healthcare Communications.

Farthmann EH, Schöffel U: Epidemiology and pathophysiology of intraabdominal infections (IAI), *Infection* 26: 329-334, 1998.

Goldsmith HS, Griffith AL, Catsimpoolas N: Increased vascular perfusion after administration of an omental lipid fraction, *Surg Gynecol Obstet* 162: 579-584, 1986.

Hellebrekers BWJ, Trimbos-Kemper TCM, Trimbos JBMZ, Emeis JJ, Kooistra T: Use of fibrinolytic agents in the prevention of postoperative adhesion formation, *Fert Steril* 74: 203-212, 2000.

Hirsh DC, Zee YC: *Veterinary microbiology,* Malden, Mass., 1999, Blackwell Science.

Holmdahl L, Ivarsson M-L: The role of cytokines, coagulation, and fibrinolysis in peritoneal tissue repair, *Eur J Surg* 165: 1012-1019, 1999.

Hosgood G: The omentum, the forgotten organ: physiology and potential surgical applications in dogs and cats, *Comp Cont Ed* 12: 45-50, 1990.

Kopcha M, Schultze AE: Peritoneal fluid, part II: abdominocentesis in cattle and interpretation of nonneoplastic samples, *Comp Cont Ed* 13(4): 703-709, 1991.

Liakakos T, Thomakos N, Fine PM, Dervenis C, Young RL: Peritoneal adhesions: etiology, pathophysiology, and clinical significance, *Digestive Surgery* 18: 260-273, 2001.

Moll HD, Schumacher J, Wright JC, Spano JS: Evaluation of sodium carboxymethylcellulose for prevention of experimentally induced abdominal adhesions in ponies, *Am J Vet Res* 52: 88-91, 1991.

Petrities-Murphy MB: Mammary carcinoma with peritoneal metastasis in a cow, *Vet Pathobiol* 29: 552-553, 1992.

Platell C, Papadimitriou JM, Hall JC: The influence of lavage on peritonitis, *J Am Coll Surg* 191: 672-680, 2000.

Plumb DC: *Veterinary drug handbook,* ed 4, Ames, Iowa, 2002, Iowa State Press.

Radostits OM, Blood DC, Gay CC: *Veterinary medicine,* ed 8, Philadelphia, 1994, Baillière Tindall.

Simmons RL, Ahrenholz DH. Pathobiology of peritonitis: a review, *J Antimicrobial Chemotherapy* 7 (Suppl A): 29-36, 1981.

Skau T, Nyström P-O, Öhman L, Stendahl O: The kinetics of peritoneal clearance of *Escherichia coli* and *Bacterioides fragilis* and participating defense mechanisms, *Arch Surg* 121: 1033-1039, 1986.

Steinberg B, Goldblatt H: Studies on peritonitis, II: passage of bacteria from the peritoneal cavity into lymph and blood, *Arch Intern Med* 32: 449-493, 1927.

Such J, Runyon BA: Spontaneous bacterial peritonitis, *Clin Infec Dis* 27: 669-676, 1998.

Timoney JF, Gillespie JH, Scott FW, Barlough JE: *Hagan and Bruner's microbiology and infectious diseases of domestic animals,* ed 8, Ithaca, 1988, Comstock Publishing Associates.

Trent AM, Bailey JV: Bovine peritoneum: fibrinolytic activity and adhesion formation, *Am J Vet Res* 47: 653-655, 1986.

Trent AM, Smith DF: Surgical management of umbilical masses with associated umbilical cord remnant infections in calves, *J Am Vet Med Assoc* 185: 1531-1534, 1984.

Vaala WE, House JK: Neonatal infection. In Smith BP, editor: *Large animal internal medicine,* St Louis, 2001, Mosby.

Van Metre DC, Divers TJ: Urolithiasis. In Smith BP, editor: *Large animal internal medicine,* St Louis, 2001, Mosby.

Watkins FH, Drake DB, Holmdahl MD, Cox MJ, Fay MF, Edlich RF: Peritoneal healing with adhesion formation: current comment, *J Long-Term Effects Med Implants* 7: 139-154, 1997.

Watson D: *The Henston large animal and equine veterinary Vade Mecum,* ed 11, Peterborough, England, 1999, Veterinary Business Development, Ltd.

Weibel MA, Majno G: Peritoneal adhesions and their relation to abdominal surgery: a postmortem study, *Am J Surg* 126: 345-354, 1973.

Wilkins BM, Spitz L: Incidence of postoperative adhesion obstruction following neonatal laparotomy, *Br J Surg* 73: 762-784, 1988.

Wilson AD, Hirsch VM, Osborne AD: Abdominocentesis in cattle: technique and criteria for diagnosis of peritonitis, *Can Vet J* 26: 74-80, 1985.

Wilson DG, MacWilliams PS: An evaluation of the clinical pathologic findings in experimentally induced urinary bladder rupture in preruminant calves, *Can J Vet Res* 62: 140-143, 1998.

Wittman DH: Operative and nonoperative therapy of intraabdominal infections, *Infection* 26: 335-341, 1998.

Wolfe DF, Carson RL, Hudson RS, et al: Mesothelioma in cattle: eight cases (1970-1988), *J Am Vet Med Assoc* 1999: 486-491, 1991.

CHAPTER 11

SURGERY OF THE BOVINE MUSCULOSKELETAL SYSTEM

11.1—Musculoskeletal Examination in Cattle

David E. Anderson and
André Desrochers

Musculoskeletal examination of cattle lacks uniformity, and many techniques for lameness examination have been described. Veterinarians most often subjectively evaluate the animal to determine which limb or region is affected and then rely on physical examination to determine the diagnosis. This system is useful in identifying lameness sites in most cases because the temperament and lack of training of cattle prevents a thorough lameness exam and necessitates consideration of other information, such as most commonly affected sites, diseases more common to a given age group, and historical data. In horses, flexion and extension tests, selective perineural anesthesia, and intraarticular anesthesia are used to isolate a focal area of pain. These techniques can be adapted to use in cattle, but they have not become commonplace because cattle are infrequently halter trained, often do not tolerate limb handling followed by controlled walking and trotting, and commonly are housed on surfaces that have a higher risk of falling (e.g., wet concrete). Further, cattle are less commonly presented to the veterinarian for examination of subtle diseases that cause mild lameness (e.g., osteochondrosis, bowed tendons, stress fracture). Thorough history, observation of stance and stride, and physical examination is critical to the diagnosis of lameness in cattle. The clinician should remember that 80% to 90% of lameness

in cattle originates distal to the fetlock. For this particular reason, unless there is an obvious lesion on the limb, such as a swollen joint or fracture, examination of the claws should always be performed.

History

Historical data for the affected individual and of the farm are important to refining differential diagnosis of lameness. The veterinarian should obtain a detailed knowledge of production levels, nutrition programs, vaccination regimens, origin of the animal and length of residence at the facility, any changes in management, and occurrence of other diseases on the farm. Questions more specific to the affected animals should be posed to determine the duration of lameness, when the first clinical signs were observed, what the initial signs were, how the animal's condition has progressed, what medications have been administered—at what dose, by what route, and for how long—and what response was noted after giving medications.

Lameness Examination

OBSERVATION

Significant information can be gained by taking a few minutes to look at the animal quietly in its stall or in its normal environment. Lameness most easily can be assessed when the cow is observed in motion. Certain types of walking surfaces may exacerbate some lameness (e.g., grass vs. dirt vs. gravel vs. concrete). A cow with a sole lesion may experience more pain to walk on concrete or gravel rather than grass because concussion is more pronounced.

283

POSTURE

Many lamenesses are obvious by observing the cow's stance. Attention should be paid to the posture of the cow—including the back, shoulders, pelvis, and major limb joints. Back posture was a primary factor in a lameness scoring system proposed by Sprecher et al. (Table 11.1-1). With the animal standing, observe the general stance first and more specifically of each limb and digit. Compare one region to the opposite side and determine whether obvious swelling, wounds, shifting of weight, and foot posture such as toe touching or displacement of weight-bearing onto the medial or lateral claw are present. A cow with heel lesions (Figure 11.1-1) will have a tendency to relieve its pain by standing on the toes. A cow with laminitis will tend to place the feet such that weight is shifted to the heels. Cows with sole lesions of the medial digits of the front limbs tend to place their feet such that weight is shifted to the lateral digit. Cows in which bilateral sole lesions are present may cross their forelimbs (Figure 11.1-5).

If only one of the digits is affected and the disease is not severe, the animal will bear weight on the sound digit of the same foot. Examination of the foot reveals excess wear of the wall and sole of the healthy digit. In longstanding diseases with severe lameness, the heels are taller and the wall longer on the affected digit in comparison to that of the healthy claw. A dropped fetlock (e.g., hyperextension of the fetlock joint) may be noticed on the sound limb because of excessive load on the flexor tendons and suspensory ligament (Figure 11.1-2). In young animals, angular limb deformities secondary to uneven weight-bearing occur rapidly with chronic lameness. When chronic lameness occurs in a hind limb, the contralateral tarsus typically will develop varus deformity (the limb is bowed outward so the convex surface occurs in the lateral aspect of the limb; see Figure 15.3-3). When chronic lameness occurs in a forelimb, the carpus typically develops a valgus deformity (the limb is bowed inward so the lateral aspect of the limb has a concave appearance, Figure 11.1-3).

TABLE 11.1-1
Lameness-Scoring Systems Described for Cattle

ANDERSON DESCRIPTION	GREENOUGH	SPRECHER ET AL, 1997	WELLS DESCRIPTION
0—Normal gait	1—Normal: gait	1—Normal: Stands and walks normally, flat back topline	0—Gait abnormality not visible at a walk: not reluctant to walk
1—Mild: walks easily, readily; bears full weight on foot and limb but has an observable gait alteration; stands on all four limbs; line of back bone normal	2—Slightly abnormal: stiff uneven gait	2—Mildly lame: Stands with flat back topline; arches back during ambulation; slightly abnormal gait	1—Mild variation from normal gait at walk; includes intermittent mild gait asymmetry of mild bilateral or quadrilateral restriction in free movement
2—Moderate: reluctant to walk and bear weight but does use the limb to ambulate; short weight-bearing phase of stride; rests the affected limb when standing; increased periods of recumbency, may see arching of back bone	3—Slight lameness: Moderate and consistent lameness	3—Moderately lame: Stands and walks with arched back topline; shortened phase of stride	2—Moderate and consistent gait asymmetry or symmetric gait abnormality but able to walk
3—Severe: reluctant to stand; refuses to walk without stimulus, non–weight-bearing on affected limb; "hoops" over limb rather than bear weight; does not use limb when standing and lies down most of the time; backbone arched with caudoventral tip to pelvis	4—Obvious lameness: Still weight-bearing	4—Lame: Arched back topline when standing and walking; obvious diminished weight-bearing in one or more limb(s)	3—Marked gait asymmetry or severe symmetric abnormality
4—Catastrophe: recumbent; unable to rise; humane euthanasia often indicated	5—Severe lameness: non–weight-bearing	5—Severely lame: constantly arched back; difficulty moving	4—Recumbent

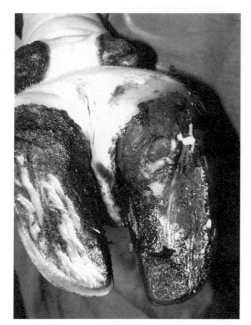

Figure 11.1-1   Cow with sole ulcer in medial claw.

(Courtesy Norm G. Ducharme; Cornell University.)

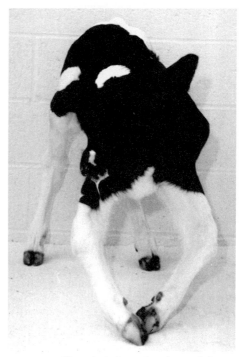

Figure 11.1-3   Calf with bilateral valgus deformity of the carpi.

(Courtesy Norm G. Ducharme; Cornell University.)

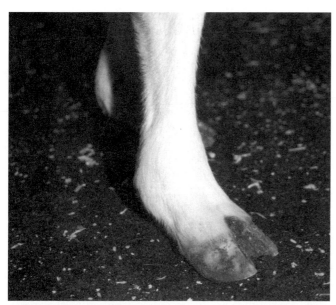

Figure 11.1-2   Dropped fetlock as a result of excessive weight-bearing.

(Courtesy Michael Wildenstein; Cornell University.)

Cows with laminitis often stand with the back arched and the feet placed under the body (Figure 11.1 4A and B). They are reluctant to walk. Draining tracts above a swollen coronary band associated with a severe lameness is typical of septic arthritis of the distal or proximal interphalangeal joint (see Figure 11.4-12). Cattle affected with heel erosion or inderdigital dermatitis will tend to keep their heels just on the border of the gutter in a tie stall barn to relieve the pain. They shift weight constantly because of the discomfort. On certain occasions, the animal will relieve the pain on the affected claw by bearing weight on the sound claw only. If both front medial claws are affected, they may cross their legs (Figure 11.1-5).

Differential diagnoses for non–weight-bearing lameness should always include the following: sole abscess, fracture, joint luxation, weight-bearing ligament or tendon injury, nerve injury (e.g., radial nerve, femoral nerve, sciatic nerve), septic arthritis, and septic tenosynovitis. An abnormal deviation of the limb is usually related to a fracture, collateral ligament rupture or joint luxation. The stance and position of the limb is abnormal with nerve damage, tendon rupture, or a severe ligament injury. Cattle affected with a radial nerve paralysis will have a dropped elbow, but this must be differentiated from a humerus fracture, radius/ulna fracture, or septic arthritis of the elbow joint. A rupture of the muscular or tendinous portion of the gastrocnemius muscles is shown by hyperflexion of the hock and a dropped

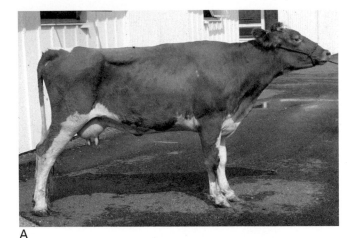

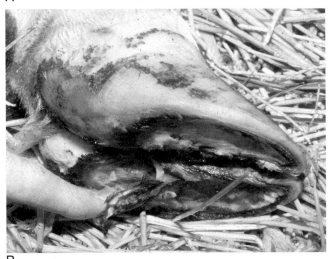

Figure 11.1-4 *A*, Guernsey with laminitis in the hind limbs. Laminitis results in underrun heels with the characteristic stance on the toes. *B*, Underrun heels of same cow.

(Courtesy Thomas J. Divers; Cornell University.)

calcaneus (e.g., hock is horizontal rather than vertical during weight-bearing; see Figure 11.4-29), but this must be differentiated from a fractured calcaneus or sciatic nerve paralysis (Figure 11.4-31). Careful attention should be paid to muscle atrophy because this may be caused by nerve injury or disuse atrophy. Neurogenic muscle atrophy occurs rapidly and is severe. Muscle atrophy caused by disuse occurs over a longer period of time. Chronic lameness of the front limb will usually bring atrophy of the triceps, biceps, and scapular muscles. The consequence of this atrophy is a more apparent shoulder with joint instability and the animal may be falsely diagnosed with shoulder joint diseases. Similarly, atrophy of the muscles of the rear limb causes pronounced greater trochanter of the femur that may be misdiagnosed as a coxofemoral joint luxation.

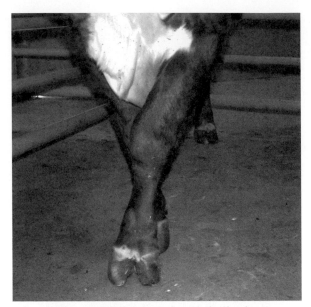

Figure 11.1-5 Bull with bilateral medial sole abscesses; note crossing of limbs to avoid medial weight-bearing.

(Courtesy Thomas J. Divers; Cornell University.)

EXAMINATION IN MOTION

In certain cases, lameness is subtle, and other procedures are necessary to localize the lesion. The characteristics of the lameness can more easily be assessed with the animal walking. The observer should attempt to describe the severity of the lameness and assess the individual components of the gait including the arc of flight, position of the digit when it touches or leaves the ground, and the relative time spent in each phase of the stride. An example is a sole ulcer of the left front medial digit (see Figure 11.1-1). This disease may cause a shortened weight-bearing phase of stride and a prolonged non–weight-bearing phase of stride in the affected limb because the cow is reluctant to place the foot down and quick to relieve pressure by picking the foot up off the ground. This animal may place the foot with the limb carried further under the body in an attempt to transfer weight to the lateral digit and may place the foot closer to the body, rather than extending the limb in an attempt to spare the pressure on the heel.

When diseases of the proximal limb, such as the hip, stifle, or shoulder, are suspected, the individual structures should be palpated as the animal walks. Bone-on-bone crepitation may be felt if a luxation or fracture is present. Soft tissue crepitation may be felt if tendon or ligament injury is present. Gas crepitation may be felt if emphysema of the tissues is present (e.g., sucking wound, clostridial myositis). It is sometimes difficult to pinpoint the location of the crepitation because it can be felt some distance from the lesion. Marked bone-on-bone crepitation that originates from the stifle often feels similar to the coxofemoral joint; they can be difficult to distinguish. Identification of swelling over the greater trochanter and rectal palpation of the hemipelvis and region of the coxofemoral joint during ambulation may help localize the lesion to the coxofemoral joint. Alternatively, auscultation of the suspected regions with a stethoscope during walking or manipulation of the limb may help localize the point of maximum intensity of the crepitus.

Conformation is involved in certain types of lameness. Cattle that have a post-legged conformation (e.g., hyperextended joints during weight-bearing, usually tarsus and stifle) are more subject to degenerative changes in the joints. The animal does not have the same capacity of shock absorption because hyperextension causes weight-bearing on cartilage that is not designed for weight-bearing and insufficient flexion of those joints exacerbates the cartilage insult. Sickle-hocked (e.g., hyperflexion of the hock during weight-bearing) cows endure excessive stress in flexor tendons that may result in a drop in the fetlock and rapid wearing of the heels.

GRADING OF LAMENESS

Assessment of the severity of the lameness is helpful to classify lameness and monitor responses to treatment. For this reason, lameness-scoring systems have been created. Equine lameness-scoring systems have been well standardized. However, these systems are difficult to extrapolate for use in cattle because of the need to control the gait (e.g., walk, trot) and perform various tests (e.g., circling, flexion tests). These tests may be performed in show cattle, but no standardization has been established for cattle. Various scoring systems have been described for use in lameness examination of cattle, and these scoring systems are based more on locomotion rather than responses to specific tests. Greenough and Wells, Sprecher et al, and Anderson (see Table 11.1-1) have described lameness-scoring systems that use grades of 1-to-5 or 0-to-4, but none has been universally accepted in practice. Multiple variations of lameness scoring have been published. Whatever the system used, veterinarians should be consistent and coherent to evaluate with precision. All associates in the same practice should agree on a grading system to facilitate communication within the practice and with the clients.

LIMB EXAMINATION

At this point, the clinician should have an idea of which leg is affected and an estimation of the affected region of the limb. Now, the affected limb must be examined carefully. Unless an obvious lesion is apparent, the authors start by a palpation of the limb. The clinician should watch for pain reaction and determine whether swelling, deformation, crepitation, warmth, and wounds are present. A hoof tester may be used to evaluate pain of the claw. The hoof tester should be applied where the common lesions of the sole surface are usually situated, including the apical region of the sole, the white line zone, and the prebulbar region. The hoof tester may be used to impact the dorsal and abaxial hoof wall to evaluate for a pain response that suggests laminitis, submural infection, and fracture of the distal phalanx. These manipulations can be performed with the animal standing and by picking up the affected limb for a short time. Alternatively, these procedures may be done with the animal free-standing and rope restraints used on the limb, restrained in a head gate or chute (see Figure 4.4-29), restrained in a standing hoof-trimming chute, restrained in lateral recumbency on the ground after a casting rope is used, or restrained in lateral recumbency on a tilt table. Sedatives and tranquilizers should be avoided whenever observations of pain responses are desired. After localization of the lesion, local anesthesia or sedation may be required to complete the examination.

Examination of long bones is performed by applying firm pressure in regions of minimal soft tissue presence (e.g., medial aspect of tibia and radius, greater trochanter of femur, greater tubercle of humerus, etc). If the animal has an adverse response—as evidenced by withdrawal, avoidance, attempts to kick the evaluator, or muscular flinching—the opposite leg should be palpated for comparison. Most fractures are obvious, but incomplete nondisplaced fractures can be suspected if deep palpation of the limb elicits a pained reaction. Each joint should be palpated separately, and complete flexion, extension, abduction, and adduction of the limb should be done. Isolation of the shoulder and elbow or of the stifle and tarsus is difficult when flexion or extension movements are performed because muscle tendon units unite these joints.

Special techniques are employed when injuries to the coxofemoral joint or cruciate ligaments are suspected.

Examination of the coxofemoral joint requires manipulation of the rear limb. These tests can be performed with the animal standing, but they are easier to perform with the animal in lateral recumbency with the affected limb uppermost. The relative position of the greater trochanter to that of the tuber coxae and the tuber ischii should be determined before than animal is laid down. The normal position of the greater trochanter is ventral to both of these bony prominences and imaginary lines drawn between them will create a "triangle" (Figure 11.1-6). Failure to palpate the greater trochanter may suggest a ventral luxation of the coxofemoral joint. Positioning of the greater trochanter in-line with the tuber coxae and tuber ischii suggests dorsal luxation of the

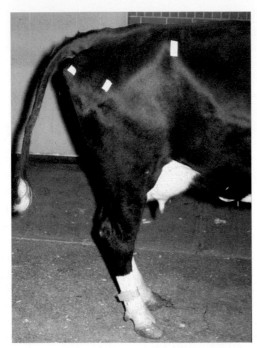

Figure 11.1-6   Lateral view of a cow with white tape on the greater trochanter, tuber coxae, and tuber ischia. Note the relative position of the greater trochanter is ventral to the tuber coxae and tuber ischia.

(Courtesy Norm G. Ducharme; Cornell University.)

coxofemoral joint. After the animal is laid down with the affected leg uppermost, the foot or the metatarsus III/IV is grasped and the entire limb rotated while performing repeated abduction and adduction motions. Fracture of the physis of the head of the femur (i.e. capital physeal fracture) should elicit crepitation of the hip that can be felt and occasionally heard. Coxofemoral joint luxation should elicit more crepitation, excessive movement of the greater trochanter, and ease of abduction if the luxation is ventral.

Cranial cruciate ligament (CCL) rupture is more difficult to diagnose. Typically, the stifle is swollen and painful to palpation. A "drawer" test can be performed with the animal standing and is easier to perform when the injured limb is weight-bearing. The examiner should stand immediately behind the affected leg and place both hands on the tibial crest by encircling the limb. Then, the examiner's knee is placed on the back of the calcaneus (see Figure 11.4-20). A drawer test is positive if displacement or crepitation can be felt after firm caudal traction on the tibial crest followed by a sudden release. The anatomy and function of the rear limb of cattle is such that the tibia is already displaced cranial to the femur when the CCL is ruptured. Thus caudal movement of the tibia is a sign of "positive drawer." The examiner must be careful when performing this test to avoid being

kicked. An alternative technique is for the examiner to stand cranial and lateral to the affected limb and place both hands on the tibial crest. Then, a firm, rapid thrust is applied to the proximal tibia, and the limb is observed for displacement and felt for crepitus. Although this test is safer to perform, we have found this technique to be less sensitive for detecting injury to the CCL.

USE OF SELECTIVE ANESTHESIA

Selective perineural anesthesia with lidocaine HCl 2% solution is common practice in equines for lameness diagnosis but is uncommon in cattle. Nonetheless, selective perineural anesthesia can be used to isolate regions of lameness. The clinician must be familiar with the anatomy of the nerves of cattle because these are quite different from those of the horse. The authors often employ regional anesthesia by placing intravenous lidocaine distal to a tourniquet (intravenous regional anesthesia, IVRA). The tourniquet is left in place for 10 to 20 minutes, released, and the lameness reevaluated. IVRA induces anesthesia for a significantly shorter period of time in comparison to that of selective perineural anesthesia. Therefore lameness evaluation must be expedited. This technique is useful when the clinician wants to rule out the digits as a source of pain that has failed to be localized by previously mentioned diagnostic tests. With selective perineural anesthesia, each digit can be anesthetized individually, and this procedure aids in more specific isolation of lameness. Occasionally, intraarticular anesthesia is desired to isolate subtle lameness to a specific joint. We have found this to be most useful for diseases that affect the coxofemoral joint, scapulohumeral joint, femoropatellar and femorotibial joints, and the elbow. In complex joints, the examiner should pay special attention to the frequency of joint communication, depending upon which joint is injected (Table 11.1-2).

EXAMINATION OF THE FOOT

Adequate restraint is critical to performing a thorough examination of the claw. Fortunately, claw-trimming chutes have become commonplace and facilitate the ease, safety, and efficiency of examination (see Figure 4.4-29). If a chute is not available, different techniques have been described for restraining the animal. Certain animals require sedation either for restraint or to complete the examination. Xylazine HCl is commonly used because of its rapid onset of action, short duration, and the availability of reversal drugs. It is preferable to withhold feed from these animals for 12 to 24 hours before sedation to avoid bloating and reduce the risk of regurgitation while in lateral or dorsal recumbency. However, we routinely place cattle in lateral recumbency for short periods of time (e.g., <30 to 45 minutes) without restricting feed. Close monitoring of the patient is required to

TABLE 11.1-2

Joint Communications in Cattle

JOINT	COMMUNICATION	FREQUENCY (%)
Fetlock	Medial to lateral digit	99%
Stifle	Femoropatellar to medial femorotibial	100%
	Lateral femorotibial to medial femorotibial and femoropatellar	65%
	All three together	57%
Carpus	Antebrachiocarpal—no communications	96%
	Middle carpal to carpometacarpal joint	86%
	Middle carpal joint to antebrachiocarpal and carpometacarpal joints	14%
	Carpometacarpal joint to middle carpal joint	86%
	Carpometacarpal joint to middle carpal and antebrachiocarpal joints	22%
Tarsus	Tibiotarsal to proximal intertarsal	100%
	Proximal intertarsal to distal intertarsal	0%
	Distal intertarsal to tarsometatarsal	21%
	Tarsometatarsal joint to distal intertarsal joint	43%

Adapted from Desrochers A: Characterization of the anatomic communications of the carpus, fetlock, stifle, and tarsus in cattle using intraarticular latex and positive contrast arthrography. Master's Thesis. Kansas State University, Manhattan, Kan, 1995.
Frequency of communication is based on communication when the first joint listed is injected. The phrase *all three together* indicates that communication did not depend upon which joint was injected.

prevent respiratory compromise or regurgitation. Immediately after application of restraint, the foot is thoroughly cleansed. Thorough examination is difficult to perform when mud, manure, and debris contaminate the foot. The total time the animal is maintained in lateral recumbency should be minimized to reduce the likelihood of development of muscle or nerve injury. Heavily muscled and obese cattle are at increased risk of developing myopathy or neuropathy after prolonged periods of lateral recumbency. Excessively thin animals are at increased risk of developing nerve injury. These conditions are caused by direct compression injury and by indirect injury resulting from compression of vessels that causes hypoxia to the tissues.

A hoof tester is applied to the different areas of the claw. Firm pressure should be applied, but the examiner must be cautious to apply similar degrees of pressure to each point and—most importantly—on each claw. Without consistency of application, response to hoof pressure tests can misinterpreted. When hoof testers are applied with consistent pressure, they can be reliable.

Corrective trimming may be performed first, followed by detailed inspection of the lesions. Each blackened area (e.g., cavity filled with manure, dirt, debris or necrotic tissue) should be explored. This is particularly important along the white line or the apical region of the sole. A pinpoint lesion is often similar to the "tip of an iceberg," and further trimming may reveal large defects or an abscess. The interdigital space is inspected for redness, abnormal proliferation, or necrotic tissue. The heel bulbs are closely inspected for the presence of erosions, separation, digital dermatitis, or other lesions. Any draining tract should be inspected with a malleable probe or a teat cannula.

Selected Diagnostic Tests

Ancillary diagnostic tests for lameness evaluation in cattle include radiography, arthrocentesis, ultrasonography, CT scan, scintigraphy, histopathology, microbial culture, and thermography. Each test has specific indications to be performed, but we most commonly perform radiography, ultrasonography, microbial cultures, and arthrocentesis. If a joint or tendon sheath is suspected to be involved, sterile saline may be injected into the joint, after aseptic preparation of the skin. The lesion is observed for drainage as evidence that a communication with the wound exists. This must be done aseptically to prevent iatrogenic infection of the joint or tendon sheath. In many areas, nuclear scintigraphy is banned in all food-producing species. This has greatly limited use of scintigraphic bone scans as diagnostic tools to discover bone inflammation or bacterial infection.

RECOMMENDED READINGS

Amstutz HE: Assessment of the musculoskeletal system, *Vet Clin N Am Food Anim Pract* 8: 383-396, 1992.

Clarkson MJ, Downham DY, Faul WB, Hughes JW, Manson FJ, Merrit JB, Murray RD, Russell WB, Sutherst JE, Ward WR: Incidence and prevalence of lameness in dairy cattle, *Vet Rec* 138: 563-567, 1996.

Desrochers A: Characterization of the anatomic communications of the carpus, fetlock, stifle, and tarsus in cattle using intraarticular latex and positive contrast arthrography. Master's Thesis. Kansas State University, Manhattan, Kan, 1995.

Farrow CS: Digital infections in cattle: their radiographic spectrum, *Vet Clin N Am Food Anim Pract* 15: 411-423, 1999.

Farrow CS: The radiographic investigation of bovine lameness associated with infection, *Vet Clin N Am Food Anim Pract* 15: 425-441, 1999.

Goggin JM, Hoskinson JJ, Carpenter JW et al: Scintigraphic assessment of distal extremity perfusion in 17 patients, *Vet Radiol & Ultrasound* 38: 211-220, 1997.

Greenough PR: Lameness in cattle, *Basic concepts of bovine lameness*, ed 3, Philadelphia, 1997, WB Saunders.

Kofler J: Application of ultrasonic examination in the diagnosis of bovine locomotory system disorders, *Schweizer Archiv fur Tierheilkunde* 137: 369-380, 1995.

Ley SJ, Waterman AE, Livingston A: Measurement of mechanical thresholds, plasma cortisol, and catecholamines in control and lame cattle: a preliminary study, *Res Vet Sci* 61: 172-173, 1996.

Manson FJ, Leaver JD: The influence of concentrate amount on locomotion and clinical lameness in dairy cattle, *Animal Production* 47: 185-190, 1998.

Philipot JM, Pluvinage P, Luquet F: Clinical characterization of a syndrome by ecopathology methods: an example of dairy cow lameness, *Vet Res* 25: 239-243, 1994.

Raven ET: **Parage.** In *Soins des onglons des bovins, parage fonctionnel,* Ontario, Canada, 1992, Collège de Technologie Agricole et Alimentaire d'Alfred.

Scott GB: Changes in limb loading with lameness for a number of Friesian cattle, *Vr Vet J* 145: 28-38, 1989.

Singh SS, Ward WR, Lautenbach K, et al: Behavior of lame and normal dairy cows in cubicles and in a straw yard, *Vet Rec* 133: 204-208, 1993.

Sprecher DJ, Hostetler DE, Kaneene JB: A lameness scoring system that uses posture and gait to predict dairy cattle reproductive performance, *Theriogenology* 47: 1178-1187, 1997.

Tryon KA, Clark CR: Ultrasonographic examination of the distal limb of cattle, *Vet Clin N Am Food Anim Pract* 15: 275-300, 1999.

Weaver AD. Lameness in cattle: investigational and diagnostic checklists, *Vr Vet J* 141: 27-33, 1985.

Wells SJ, Trent AM, Marsh WE, Robinson RA: Prevalence and severity of lameness in lactating dairy cows in a sample of Minnesota and Wisconsin herds, *J Am Vet Med Assoc* 202: 78-82, 1993.

Whay HR, Waterman AE, Webster AJF: Associations between locomotion, claw lesions and nociceptive threshold in dairy heifers during the peri-partum period, *Vet J* 154: 155-161, 1997.

11.2—Internal Fixation

Steven S. Trostle

In the past, simple forms of orthopedic treatment have been used to treat long bone fractures in farm animals. In the last decade, three major factors have advanced ruminant orthopedics. As veterinarians, we have developed a better understanding of bone physiology and biomechanics related to fracture repair. Implants and equipment available to treat animals have increased in size and dimension; therefore mechanical support can be provided to large animals by internal fixation devices in appropriate situations. As the economic value and potential of selected ruminants have increased via advances in assisted reproductive technology, clients have demanded that conditions once thought irreparable be treated.

Selection of Cases for Internal Fixation

Guidelines have not been defined to help determine when internal fixation should be selected to repair orthopedic conditions in ruminants. Internal fixation's major advantages are that it provides rigid stabilization of the fracture and immediate, functional use of the limb. This point cannot be overemphasized; ruminant orthopedic patients are generally weight-bearing and ambulatory early, if not immediately, in the postoperative period. The disadvantages of internal fixation are the associated costs of general anesthesia, the implants, and equipment required to apply internal fixation devices. Aside from economic issues, internal fixation requires a basic understanding of orthopedic fixation principles and first-hand knowledge of the implants and equipment, which generally requires advanced training or extensive experience to be proficient.

Internal fixation should be considered for ruminant long bone fractures proximal to the carpus and tarsus, because these bones are more difficult to stabilize with other forms of fixation. Highly comminuted fractures distal to the carpus and tarsus may also benefit from the rigid stability offered by internal fixation.

SPECIAL CONSIDERATIONS FOR CALVES

Ruminant neonatal bones have a low bone density and thin bony cortices; and their ability to support and sustain implants such as intramedullary pins and screws is a primary concern (Fessler and Adams, 1996). The bone/implant interface is very weak (Figure 11.2-1A-C). Recent studies have evaluated various screws' holding power in neonatal bones (Kirpenstein et al, 1992; Kirpenstein et al, 1993). No difference between the holding power of 4.5-mm cortical, 5.5-mm cortical, and 6.5-mm fully threaded cancellous screws in neonatal femurs was found, but a direct correlation between the screws' holding power and bone cortical thickness was found. The 6.5-mm fully threaded cancellous screws had greater holding power than either 5.5-mm or 4.5-mm cortical screws in neonatal metacarpal and metatarsal bones, particularly the metaphysis. No difference between the holding power of 4.5-mm and 5.5-mm cortical screws in the diaphysis or metaphysis was found. In a recent study, the force required for screw pullout seemed to be more directly related to bone mineral density than cortical bone thickness (Shettko et al, 2001). Washers and bolts have been used with screws for calf internal fixation to overcome pullout problems and prevent bony failure at the screw-to-bone-to-implant interfaces in neonatal bone (Ferguson, 1985). Regardless of whether bone mineral density, cortical bone thickness, or both are responsible for a screw's holding power, it remains a concern in calf internal fixation.

Many fractures that occur in young farm animals involve the physis (growth plate). It has been proposed that younger animals are predisposed to physeal-type fractures because the physis cartilaginous makeup is weaker than bone and the surrounding support struc-

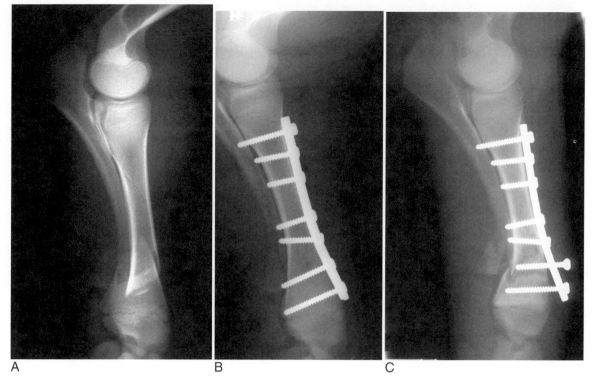

A   B   C

Figure 11.2-1 *A,* Lateral radiograph of 3-day-old calf with a Salter-Harris type II fracture of the distal radius. *B,* Lateral radiograph of same fracture treated with a dorsally placed bone plate and screws. *C,* Lateral radiograph of previously described repair 14 days postoperatively. The distal two screws are backing out, and there was loss of contact between the distal radius and bone plate.

(Courtesy of Dr. Ryland B. Edwards III, University of Wisconsin.)

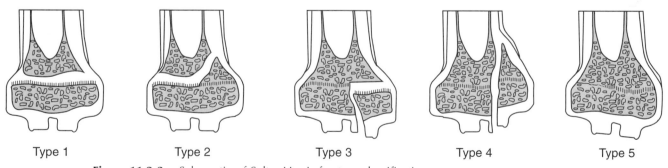

Type 1   Type 2   Type 3   Type 4   Type 5

Figure 11.2-2 Schematic of Salter Harris fracture classification system.

tures. The Salter-Harris classification (Figure 11.2-2) is used to describe fractures that involve the physis and adjacent metaphysis. In clinical practice, Salter-Harris type I and II fracture in farm animals makes up a large majority (>95%) of physeal fractures. Type I fractures, which are not as common, involve complete separation of the epiphysis from the metaphysis through the physis. A typical type I physeal fracture is the *slipped capital femoral physis,* which occurs through the femur prox-

imal growth plate (Figure 11.2-3A). Other, even less common Salter-Harris type I fractures occur in the tuber calcaneus and olecranon. These latter two fractures occur through traction growth plates (i.e., where muscles or tendons insert or originate). In Salter-Harris Type II fractures (the most common farm animal physeal fracture), the epiphysis separates from the metaphysis through the physis with a small corner of the metaphysis fractured as well. These most commonly occur in the

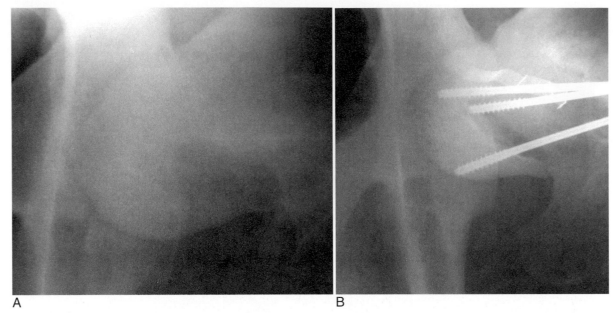

Figure 11.2-3   *A,* Ventrodorsal radiograph of a slipped capital femoral physeal fracture in a 14-month-old bull. *B,* Previously described fracture repaired with 7-mm cannulated screws.

(Courtesy of Dr. Ryland B. Edwards III; University of Wisconsin.)

distal metatarsus and metacarpus, distal femur and radius, or proximal tibia (Figure 11.2-4A).

Salter-Harris type I and II physis fractures in farm animals generally have a favorable prognosis, but concern about how healing may impact long bone growth and an angular limb deformity developing always remains. Salter-Harris type III (through the physis and metaphysis) and Salter-Harris type IV (through the physis, epiphysis and metaphysis) fractures are very rare in ruminants because they involve a joint surface, and have a more guarded prognosis. Type V physeal fracture, the least common, is seen as a crushing injury to the physis.

Clinicians dealing with younger animals must be careful not to forget the rest of the body while concentrating on the fracture. It is important to assess the immunological status of newborn calves and be assured passive transfer has occurred before attempting any form of surgical intervention. Lack of a competent immune status will predispose the calf to postoperative infection. Other common calf diseases, such as pneumonia, omphalophlebitis, or septic polyarthritis, should also be evaluated before giving owners a prognosis.

SPECIAL CONSIDERATIONS FOR ADULTS

The primary concern for internal fixation in adult cattle is implants, unlike calves, in which the bone may be a limiting factor for successful internal fixation. Much progress has been made in implant design and material properties, but most are still adaptations from human surgery. Because early ambulation in adult ruminants is generally necessary, implants bending or failing during the postoperative period is not uncommon. The clinician who attempts internal fixation in adults must have substantial knowledge and pay attention to details. Because a lot of force is required to cause an adult long bone fracture, disruption of soft tissue and skin integrity is a concern. Open fractures are more difficult to treat successfully. Bone grafting should be strongly considered in all adult cattle fractures.

Evaluation of a Fracture for Internal Fixation Repair

RADIOGRAPHY

Preoperative radiographs provide the definitive diagnosis of fractures in most farm animals. In selected cases, other imaging modalities—such as nuclear medicine, computed tomography, and magnetic resonance imaging—increased diagnostic accuracy over radiography. Radiographs should be of high quality and carefully evaluated for fissure fractures. Multiple views of the affected area should be taken to provide a complete study and minimize the risk of missing a lesion(s).

Intraoperative radiography should also be considered when one is using any form of fixation—but particularly internal fixation. Intraoperative radiography can assess the positioning and placement of implants as well as the reduction of the fracture. Intraoperative radiographs

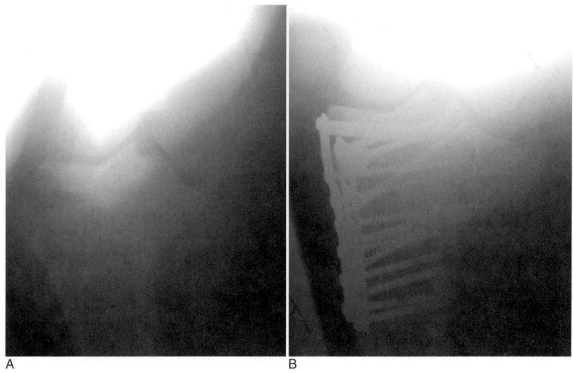

Figure 11.2-4 *A,* Craniocaudal radiograph of a 16-month-old, 490-kg bull with a Salter-Harris type II fracture of the proximal tibia. *B,* Previously described fracture repaired with two T-plates placed medially across the physis.

(Courtesy of Dr. Ryland Edwards III; University of Wisconsin.)

should be completed in more than one view whenever possible to ensure that the repair is appropriate.

GENERAL

All ruminants should be held off feed for at least 24 hours and ideally 48 hours to minimize regurgitation and decrease the likelihood of aspiration pneumonia. If this cannot be completed, ruminal decompression should be attempted before general anesthesia by oral passage of a Kingman tube. Internal fixation is a time-consuming process, and complications associated with ruminal distension during anesthesia should be minimized. The surgical team should consider alternative plans in case the primary surgical plan cannot be completed. All equipment and supplies potentially needed in surgery should be readily available at the start of the operation.

EVALUATION OF THE PATIENT

The veterinarian must give as complete and accurate an assessment of the fracture and potential outcome of the repair to the client as possible. Both veterinarian and client must consider a "risk-benefit" ratio. The size, weight, age and disposition of the animal should always

be considered. In general, a successful outcome for internal fixation repair is inversely related to age, weight and size. The fracture must be evaluated to give an accurate prognosis. The more highly comminuted fractures generally have a less favorable prognosis. However, not all simple fractures are candidates for internal fixation; and not all comminuted fractures are hopeless because of farm animals' ability to rapidly produce significant periosteal bone and their more passive demeanor protecting the repair. Generally, transverse fractures are more amenable to repair than comminuted fractures. Although most fractures in adult cattle can be treated successfully, they are always more difficult to repair than identical fractures in calves.

The condition of the surrounding soft tissues should be considered in evaluation of a fracture. The surrounding soft tissues are responsible for extramural blood supply to the fracture site. Open or closed fractures with severely traumatized soft tissues often become infected, which significantly complicates the repair. Infection as a complication is discussed later in this chapter. However, it is paramount to remember that infection and instability are intolerable together. If contamination of the fracture site occurs and persistent infection develops, instability and failure of the repair are highly probable. This is the primary reason open fractures have a much less favorable prognosis than closed fractures. Broad spectrum, preoperative antibiotics are always recommended before fracture repair with internal fixation. Antimicrobials' duration and withdrawal time needed to achieve proper care must be carefully considered during the selection process because of human public health concerns. The duration and frequency of antimicrobial coverage is controversial among surgeons but should be directly correlated to the type of fracture (open vs. closed) and extent of soft tissue damage.

ANESTHESIA
Chapter 6 discusses anesthesia.

POSITIONING
Positioning is a more relevant issue for adult cattle because they are prone to radial nerve paralysis and torn adductor musculotendinous structures. The down forelimb should always be extended as much forward as possible with adequate padding. Likewise, the hind limbs should be properly supported and padded as myopathy in the hind limbs may predispose the animal to slip and tear the adductor musculature. When possible, place the animal in right lateral recumbency, which allows needle decompression of the rumen if necessary. During positioning, cautiously pull on the tail; it is relatively easy to create coccygeal fractures by using manual traction. Finally, marked tension is required to reduce certain long bone fractures. A rope should be placed around the front and rear quarters to prevent the animal from changing position while traction is applied. Be careful to properly pad the areas where traction or countertraction will be applied.

SURGICAL APPROACH
The optimal surgical approach should minimize soft tissue trauma while allowing direct visualization of the fractured bone and site. In general, the greater the trauma is to soft tissues and surrounding area, the longer the surgical approach necessary to gain adequate exposure. After the fracture is exposed, debride the clotted blood and devitalized tissue. A culture of the deep surrounding soft tissues is recommended for open fractures to define potential pathogens and select appropriate antimicrobials. The fracture site should be continuously lavaged during the surgical procedure with a solution containing an antibiotic such as cephalosporin to reduce contamination. Aseptic techniques should be maintained throughout the surgical procedure. The surgery team should plan and use a time-efficient procedure to decrease the risk of anesthetic and surgical complications.

FRACTURE REDUCTION
The goal of a successful internal fixation is accurate, rigid anatomic reduction. Anatomic reduction allows the bone to share the load transfer and restore function to the leg. Nonanatomical and/or inaccurate reduction predisposes the implant to migration and/or failure. Reduction should be performed by gradually fatiguing the inverse myotactic reflex. Reduction may be achieved by tenting the bone ends out of the incision and toggling them against one another until they align anatomically. However, mechanical devices such as a large animal fracture distractor,* a calf jack, or other pulley system may be needed to provide consistent tension and resultant muscle fatigue in cases in which reduction cannot be performed manually (Ames, 1995). Reduction can be maintained by using bone reduction forceps, placing a lag screw across the fracture gap, or using cerclage wire. The efficacy of neuromuscular blocking agents used is not always predictable, and they do require positive pressure ventilation to overcome respiratory depression.

General Principles of Internal Fixation

BONE PLATES
Several basic principles regarding use of bone plates in fracture fixation are important (Trostle and Markel, 1996). These include bone properties, plate material and geometry, screw-bone interface, number of screws, screw material and tension, plate-bone interface, placement of the plate relative to loading, and compression between fragments. A bone plate's bending stiffness is related to the third power of the plate's thickness. Therefore changing the plate thickness does more to change plate rigidity. The mechanical properties of bone also affect the behavior of the plate-bone system. For example, less stiff bone will increase the load-sharing contribution of the plate. Loads can be transmitted between the plate and bone through bone screws and friction-type forces between the plate surface and bone.

In large animal orthopedics, a bone plate is a device that shares the load by passing some of the load from the plate to bone fragments. Subjected to bending loads, a plated bone can take on a bending open (compressive surface) or bending closed (tensile surface) configuration (Figure 11.2-5). The plate's placement relative to the loading direction determines the load proportion supported by the plate. The plate/bone composite is far stiffer in the bending closed position than in the bending open position. This makes it important to anatomically reconstruct the bone cortex opposite the bone plate placement.

Plating provides the most rigid form of internal fixation used in ruminant orthopedics. Application of bone

---

*Synthes, PO Box 1766; Paoli, PA 19301-1262

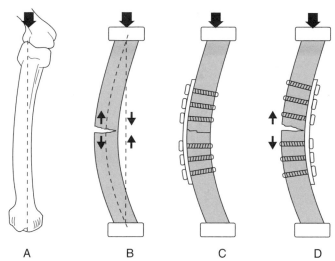

A B C D

Figure 11.2-5 Illustration of the principle of placing a bone plate on the tension surface of a bone, so the bone receives compressive forces. For example, the long bone *(A)* can be compared to a bent column *(B)*. A plate applied to the convex or tension side of the bone when it is loaded counteracts the tension forces and provides rigid internal fixation in the bending closed position. If the plate is applied on the concave surface *(D)*, it does not give as rigid fixation, and the plate is subjected to excessive bending forces that predispose it to failure.

(Modified with permission from Brinker WO, Piermattei DL, Flo GL, editors: *Handbook of small animal orthopedics and fracture treatment,* ed 1, Philadelphia, 1983, WB Saunders.)

plates should be performed on the tension surface whenever possible because of the biomechanical advantages previously noted. In younger, lighter-weight animals, one plate may be used to achieve stabilization. Oftentimes, two plates are used in larger animals in an effort to obtain adequate stabilization of the fracture. The surgeon should contour the plate(s) to ensure that the entire surface of the plate is in contact with the bone (bone-plate interface). Every effort should be made to optimize the bone-plate interface because this provides a more rigid and stable fracture repair and enhances the likelihood of a positive outcome. Plate(s) should span from the proximal to distal metaphysis to enhance the bone-plate interface and minimize stress concentrated at the bone ends. When two plates are used, they should be placed at 90 degrees to one another and end in a staggered fashion to prevent stress concentration at the bone end and facilitate easier screw placement.

The standard plates used for repair fractures of the long bones are the 4.5-mm narrow and 4.5-mm broad dynamic compression plates; however, other specialty plates are available (Table 11.2-1). The oval shape of the holes in dynamic compression plates allows them to be used to compress fracture fragments. Narrow plates have holes aligned in a straight line, whereas the holes in broad plates are staggered. Narrow plates have a smaller width (12 mm vs. 16 mm) and thickness (3.6 mm vs. 4.5 mm) in comparison to broad plates. Recent reports cite success-

TABLE 11.2-1

Standard and Special Plates Used in Farm Animal Surgery

Name	3.5-mm broad DCP	4.5-mm narrow DCP	4.5-mm broad DCP	Broad LCDCP	ABP	DCS plate	DHS plate	One-third tubular plate
Plate type	Standard	Standard	Standard	Special	Special	Special	Special	Special
Plate cross-section								
Width (mm)	12	12	16	17	16	16	19	0
Thickness (mm)	3.6	3.6	4.5	6.0	5.6	5.4	5.8	1
Length (mm)	85 (7 holes) to 265 (22 holes)	39 (2 holes) to 263 (16 holes)	103 (6 holes) to 359 (22 holes)	106 (6 holes) to 322 (18 holes)	100 (6 holes) to 260 (16 holes)	92 (5 holes) to 204 (12 holes)	46 (2 holes) to 270 (16 holes)	25 (2 holes) to 145 (12 holes)
Plate angle	Straight	Straight	Straight	Straight	95 degrees	95 degrees	135 degrees (140, 145, 150 degrees)	Straight
Screw size (mm)	3.5	4.5, 5.5 (6.5)	4.5, 5.5 (6.5)	4.5, 5.5 (6.5)	4.5, 5.5 (6.5)	4.5, 5.5 (6.5)	4.5, 5.5 (6.5)	3.5
Hole arrangement	Straight	Straight	Offset	Offset/DCU	Offset	Offset	Offset	Straight
Angled portion	—	—	—	—	U-shaped cross-section	Barrel 25 and 38 mm long	Barrel 38 mm long	—
Special screw through barrel	—	—	—	—	—	Yes	Yes	—
Hole distance (mm)	12	16	16	18	16	16	16	12
Center holes (mm)	16	25	25	18	—	—	—	16
Material	Stainless steel	Stainless steel	Stainless steel	Titanium	Stainless steel	Stainless steel	Stainless steel	Stainless steel

DCP, dynamic compression plate; LCDCP, limited contact dynamic compression plate; ABP, angled blade plate; DCS, dynamic condylar screw; DHS, dynamic hip screw; DCU, dynamic compression unit.
From Auer JA: Principles of fracture treatment. In Auer JA, Stick JA, editors: *Equine surgery,* ed 2, Philadelphia, 1999, WB Saunders.

ful use of dynamic condylar screw (DCS) and dynamic hip screw (DHS) plates in long bone fracture repair (Auer et al, 1993) (Figure 11.2-6). The DCS and DHS plates are identical in width to the 4.5-mm broad plates but thicker at 5.6 mm and 5.8 mm, respectively. Other plates—such as the angled, Cobra head, T-, and semitubular plates—have been used in special circumstances.

The use of bone plate luting has been recommended to augment fracture repair in large animal surgery (Nunamaker et al, 1991). Bone plate luting involves placing bone cement (polymethylmethacrylate) between the plate and bone as well as the screw head and plate. To lute a bone plate, one must loosen all the screws in the plate and lift the plate off the bone. The bone cement is then placed between the plate and bone, and the screws are immediately retightened. Bone cement should be kept out of the fracture site as it may delay or prevent healing. After the screws are retightened, the bone cement redistributes into the unoccupied space in the plate screw holes. The two proposed mechanisms behind plate luting are the following: 1) plate luting enhances the bone-plate interface; and 2) decreases shear stress at the screw head in the plate. Bone plate luting does not compensate for poor contouring of plates. The additional use of antimicrobials (with consideration for public health standards) in the bone cement may provide sustained local antimicrobial activity.

Comminuted fractures should be converted to two-part fractures by attaching the fragments to the parent bone with lag screws. Screws (3.5 mm) are recommended for this procedure because the head can be sufficiently countersunk to prevent interference with bone plate application. Ideally, if one plate is used, it should be placed on the tension surface of the bone and loaded in compression. Plates placed on a tension surface should be prestressed before they are applied to ensure transcortical compression and stability. Plates are prestressed by slightly overbending the plate to leave a gap between the fracture line and plate at the level of the fracture line. When screws are applied, prestressing brings the bone to the plate, creating compression up to the far cortex and along the entire fracture line. If a second plate is used, it may be loaded in compression or neutralization. Screws should be placed in every hole of a bone plate to maximize the bone-implant interface. Lag screw principles may be used within the bone plate and should be performed with large comminuted fragments.

SCREWS

Two basic types of screws (cancellous and cortical) are used in ruminant orthopedic surgery (Table 11.2-2). The parts of a screw include head, shaft, core, thread, pitch, shaft length, thread length, and total screw length,

TABLE 11.2-2

Screw, Drill Bit, Tap Chart

SCREW NAME	3.5-MM CORTEX	4.5-MM CORTEX	4.5-MM SHAFT	4.5-MM CANNULATED		5.5-MM CORTEX	5.5-MM SHAFT	6.5-MM CANCELLOUS			7.0/7.3-MM CANNULATED
Screw ø	3.5	4.5	4.5	4.5		5.5	5.5	6.5			7.0/7.3
Gliding hole ø	3.5	4.5	4.5	4.5	None	5.5	5.5	(4.5)			None
Thread hole ø	2.5	3.2	3.2	3.2		4.0	4.0	3.2			Self-tapping
Screw tap ø	3.5	4.5	4.5	4.5		5.5	5.5	6.5			Self-drilling
Screw shape											
Cannulation/guide pin	—	—	—	175 mm/1.6 mm		—	—	—			2 mm/2.8 mm
Type thread	Cortical	Cortical	Cortical	Cancellous		Cortical	Cortical	Cancellous			Cancellous
Pitch	1.25	1.75	1.75	1.75		2.0	2.0	1.75			2.75
Screw head ø	6.0	8.0	8.0	6.5		8.0	8.0	8.0			8.0/8.2
Thread length	Entire length	Entire length	Variable	16.0	Entire length	Entire length	Variable	16.0 32.0	Entire length		16.0/32.0
Shaft ø	—	—	4.5	3.1	—	—	5.5	4.5 4.5	—		4.5/4.8
Core ø	2.4	3.1	3.1	2.7		4.0	4.0	3.0			4.5
Self-tapping	Planned	Yes	Yes	Yes		Planned	Planned	—			Yes

From Auer JA: Principles of fracture treatment. In Auer JA, Stick JA, editors: *Equine surgery*, ed 2, Philadelphia, 1999, WB Saunders.
Manufacturer: Synthes, 1690 Russell, Paoli, PA 19301-1262.

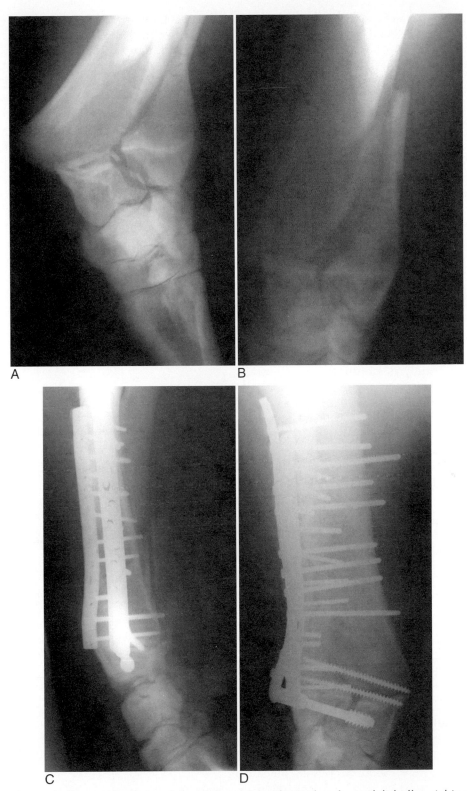

Figure 11.2-6 *A*, Lateral and *B*, craniocaudal radiographs of an adult bull weighing 900 kg with a comminuted distal radius fracture. *C*, Lateral and *(D)* craniocaudal radiographs of the previous fracture repaired with a dynamic condylar screw and plate system.

(Courtesy of Dr. Ryland B. Edwards III; University of Wisconsin.)

which vary among the different screw sizes. Cortical screws are completely threaded and have a relatively thin thread width. Cancellous screws are available in various thread lengths and have a wider thread diameter and pitch than cortical screws.

Screws are also commonly classified by their diameter. In general, 4.5-mm and 5.5-mm cortical and 6.5-mm cancellous screws are used in ruminant orthopedics. The 5.5-mm cortical screws have demonstrated superior strength characteristics in comparison to the 4.5-mm cortical and 6.5-mm cancellous screws. The 6.5-mm cancellous screws are available in three different thread lengths (16-mm, 32-mm, and fully threaded). The 3.5-mm cortical screw also has been used to achieve interfragmentary compression, since the head is small enough that it may be completely countersunk in the adult bovine cortex and covered by a bone plate.

A 7-mm cannulated screw system has been advocated to repair slipped capital femoral physeal fractures in adult bulls (Wilson et al, 1990). A study biomechanically compared 7-mm cannulated screws to 5.5-mm cortical and 6.5-mm cancellous screws in a femoral head fracture model. Results of this study demonstrated that 7-mm cannulated screws had greater holding power than 6.5-mm cancellous screws but their holding power was similar to 5.5-mm cortical screws. The study also noted that the cannulated screw systems (4.5-, 7-, and 7.3-mm) offer added flexibility when screw placement is critical. This is because smaller-diameter guide wires (1.5- to 2.8-mm) are used to place the cannulated screws, and these small guide wires can be replaced easily if they are not in the optimal position.

Screws should be placed so the near (cis) and far (trans) cortices are engaged to achieve optimal stability. Interfragmentary compression may be achieved by using screws within and outside the bone plate. Ideally, three screws each should be placed proximal and distal to the fracture fragments to achieve security. The use of power assistance in tapping and placing the screws does not alter the pullout strength when proper technique is utilized (Gillis et al, 1992). Power assistance can greatly reduce surgical and anesthetic times with their subsequent risk of complications.

INTRAMEDULLARY PINS AND INTERLOCKING NAILS

Intramedullary devices have several advantages in fracture treatment, including restoration of bony alignment and early recovery of weight-bearing in young, light-weight animals. These devices are intended to stabilize a fracture by acting as an internal splint, thus forming a composite structure of bone and rod in which both contribute to fracture stability. This load-sharing property is fundamental to the rods' design and should be recognized when they are used for fracture treatment (Figure 11.2-7).

Several material and structural properties of intramedullary rods alter their axial, bending, and torsional rigidities. These include cross-sectional geometry, rod length, the presence of a longitudinal slot, and the elastic modulus of the material. The cross-sectional geometry of the rod significantly affects all rigidities. In general, the overall rigidity of intramedullary rods increases with rod diameter, because the "moment of inertia" is approximately proportional to the fourth power of the rod's radius. The contact distance between an implant and bone at the proximal and distal segments of bone is the unsupported length of intramedullary fixation. This distance shortens as the fracture heals. The unsupported length of the rods is important in the initial stages of fracture healing. The interfragmentary motion is proportional to the square of the unsupported length in bending; therefore a small increase in unsupported bent length can lead to a larger increase in interfragmentary motion.

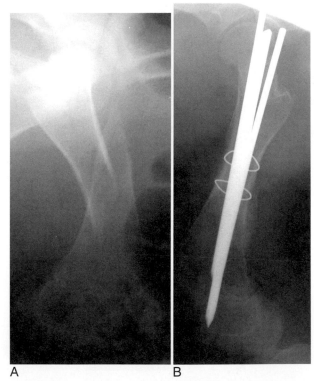

Figure 11.2-7 *A,* Lateral radiograph of a 2-day-old calf with a middiaphyseal femoral fracture. *B,* Previously described fracture repaired by using intramedullary pins (stack pinning) and cerclage wire.

(Courtesy of Dr. Ryland B. Edwards III; University of Wisconsin.)

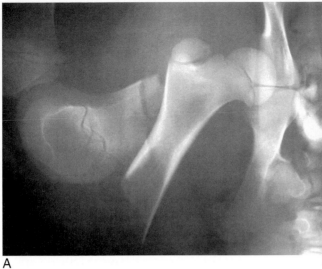

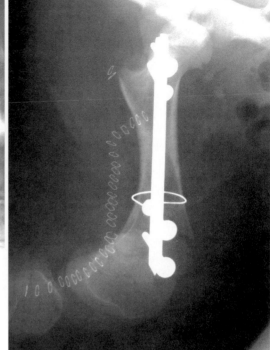

Figure 11.2-8 *A*, Lateral radiograph of a 1-day-old calf with a diaphyseal femoral fracture. *B*, Previously described fracture repaired using an interlocking nail.

(Courtesy of Dr. Ryland B. Edwards III; University of Wisconsin.)

With torsional loading, the unsupported length is determined by the points at which sufficient mechanical interlocking occurs between bone and implant to support torsional loads. The concept of unsupported length is not applicable to simple rod designs without proximal or distal locking mechanisms, since there may be little resistance to torsion. Clinically, placing multiple pins (stack pinning) is recommended to increase intramedullary contact and enhance torsional and bending stability when one uses simple rod designs.

The most commonly used intramedullary pins are Steinmann pins, which range in size from 3.2 mm up to 6.35 mm. Intramedullary pins are available with trocar, chisel, or trocar-threaded tips. Threaded pins are recommended to repair neonatal bone, which is less dense and more prone to migration. Intramedullary pins can be applied by using a hand-driven or power-assisted device. Single or multiple stack pins may be used and placed in normograde or retrograde fashion, depending on the nature of the fracture. Stack pins increase frictional forces between the pins and the cortical surface, thus decreasing rotational instability. Intramedullary pins should be secured in the subchondral epiphysis, and care should be taken not to introduce or maintain intramedullary pins through the articular surface because of ensuing risk of degenerative joint disease.

In general, intramedullary pins should be used for diaphyseal fractures of relatively straight bones. Intramedullary pins are contraindicated for the repair of long oblique, spiral, or comminuted fractures without the use of devices that augment the primary repair and prevent overriding or rotation of the fracture fragments. Commonly used devices include cerclage wire and screws. Intramedullary pins have also been "tied in" with external skeletal fixators to provide additional stability (St-Jean et al, 1992b).

Interlocking nails have been used in human surgery to repair fractures of the humerus, tibia, and femur (Figure 11.2-8). Similar to intramedullary pins, interlocking nails provide stiffness in bending. The use of both proximal and distal locking with screws can prevent axial displacement of the bone along the rod and provide enhanced torsional rigidity. For interlocking nails, the distance between the proximal and distal locking points typically determines the unsupported length. Interlocking nail systems for large animal surgery are commercially available.* Interlocking nails have a single trocar point, are 13 mm in diameter, and vary in length. The interlocking nails have 5.7-mm diameter screw holes placed 16.5 mm apart over their entire length. An open surgi-

*Innovative Animal Products, 6256 34th Avenue NW; Rochester, MN

cal technique is recommended with interlocking nails because of their large diameter. A 6.35-mm diameter intramedullary pin placed in normograde fashion from the proximal location into the medullary cavity and seated distally in the subchondral bone of the distal epiphysis creates a pathway for interlocking nail insertion. The intramedullary pin is then removed. The interlocking nail replaces the intramedullary pin in the same pathway, which decreases the likelihood of the bone fracturing during interlocking nail placement. A slightly smaller-diameter (11 or 12 mm) reaming device is an alternative. The interlocking nail is inserted as described above with a large hand chuck. The aiming device is then attached to the proximally exposed portion of the interlocking nail. The aiming device ensures that drilling and tapping the bone is achieved within the screw holes of the interlocking nail. Longer-shanked drills and taps may need to be used to accomplish this task. Generally two screws each are placed in the distal and proximal primary fracture fragments. Interlocking nails have been used to repair humeral and femoral fractures in calves. The quality of the surrounding bone in neonates may determine the strength of repairs that use interlocking nails. Distal placement of intramedullary devices should be checked by intraoperative radiography or stifle arthrotomy. Intramedullary pins should be cut proximally at the level of the skin to allow for pin removal and prevent impingement of the sciatic nerve. Intramedullary pin removal can be difficult to perform in rapidly growing animals that have achieved clinical union but poses no problem to the animal if they remain *in situ*. Removal should be considered if the intramedullary pins have migrated or are associated with an infective process. Interlocking nail length should be selected so soft tissues and skin can cover the proximal end. Interlocking nails cannot be removed without a second surgical procedure.

Fractures of the Femur

CLINICAL PRESENTATION

Fractures of the femur are the second most common fracture that occurs in cattle—particularly in neonatal calves. Femur fractures result in extensive swelling, hematoma formation, and crepitus of the proximal hind limb (Trostle and Markel, 1996b). Cattle are lame on the injured leg, and the degree of lameness depends on the age and weight of the animal as well as displacement of the fracture fragments. Cattle often toe-touch with the affected leg and may appear to have a shortened leg if the pull from the quadriceps muscles causes marked overriding of fracture fragments. A differential list of other considerations for cattle with proximal hind limb lameness should include coxofemoral luxation, cranial cruciate rupture, and septic arthritis of the coxofemoral or stifle joints.

The definitive diagnosis of a femoral fracture is made by radiography (see Figures 11.2-7 and 11.2-8). At least two standard radiographic views should be performed to assess the fracture. This is most easily accomplished if the animal is tranquilized and placed in lateral recumbency to obtain both mediolateral and craniocaudal views. The most commonly reported femur fractures are an oblique-to-spiral fracture of the mid-to-distal diaphysis or a short transverse-to-oblique fracture of the distal metaphysis, although proximal diaphyseal fractures have been reported (Ferguson, 1994). Comminution is usually present, and high-quality radiographs should be obtained to accurately evaluate the degree of comminution. Spiral and oblique fractures are generally thought to be caused by torsional and bending forces acting upon the bone. Reasons for the high prevalence of distal metaphyseal/physeal region fractures are not completely understood but may be related to the high torsional forces placed on the distal femur.

SURGICAL APPROACH

To facilitate the surgical approach, cattle should be positioned in lateral recumbency, with the affected limb upward. A lateral approach is employed, and a liberal superficial dissection should be performed because the large muscle masses of the proximal hind limb limit femur exposure. A linear incision is made starting slightly caudal to the greater trochanter and extending to the lateral epicondyle of the femur. The plane of dissection parallels the cranial border of the biceps femoris through the tensor fascia lata muscle. Exposure to the diaphysis is gained by incising through the vastus lateralis muscle parallel to its muscle fibers.

METHODS OF INTERNAL FIXATION REPAIR

Dynamic compression, Cobra head, angled blade, and condylar bone plates and screws have had limited success in repairing femoral fractures. The tension surface of the femur is generally considered to be the lateral to craniolateral aspect of the bone from the middiaphysis proximally. Torsion is the predominant distal force on the femur. For maximum stabilization, applying bone plates to the femur at these sites is recommended. In calves, generally one laterally placed plate may be used. In older animals, two plates placed at ninety degrees to one another on the lateral and cranial surfaces are recommended.

Retrograde, intramedullary stack pinning has been used to repair neonatal bovine femoral fractures with success (St-Jean et al, 1992a). In a recent report, 83% of the fractures treated in this manner were considered to have healed satisfactorily. However, complications such as pin migration occurred in 50% of the cases, and osteomyelitis developed in one case. The authors suggested the use of partially threaded pins to aid in preventing pin migration. All calves in this study had considerable callus formation present, thus suggesting instability. Although intramedullary pins are noted for their strength and stiffness in bending, fracture fragments tend to rotate or displace axially along single intramedullary pins. Stack pinning, external fixators, and cerclage wires have been used to help stabilize the torsional and compressive instability of single intramedullary pin fixation repair; but the results have been variable (Figure 11.2-9).

Intramedullary pins may be placed in either a normograde or retrograde fashion. A closed surgical technique can be used to place intramedullary pins in normograde fashion in minimally displaced fractures, but ensuring proper placement in the distal fragment requires care. Both normograde and retrograde placement of intramedullary pins can be performed with open surgical techniques.

Interlocking nails have been proposed as a possible alternative repair method for diaphyseal fractures of the femur (Trostle et al, 1994). Interlocking, intramedullary nails provide rigid fixation in bending similar to intramedullary pins. The addition of screws helps lock fracture fragments and provides enhanced compressive and torsional stability. The bone-plating problems associated with bone quality, as seen in neonatal calves, may persist. The author has had several successful clinical outcomes after using interlocking nails as a fixation technique for neonatal femoral fractures.

Fractures of the Femoral Head

CLINICAL PRESENTATION

Fractures of the femoral head or slipped capital physeal (Salter-Harris type I) fractures occur in two primary populations. One is young calves after forced fetal extraction associated with hip lock and shear forces placed across the coxofemoral region. The second population is young (1 to 2 years old) bulls in group housing. Blunt trauma in a lateromedial direction to the coxofemoral region results in shear force across the physis and ultimately failure. Cattle with slipped capital femoral physis have

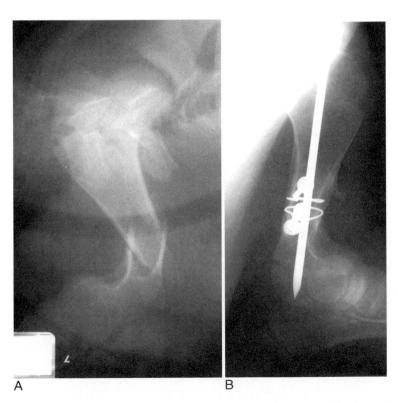

A   B

Figure 11.2-9   *A,* Lateral radiograph demonstrating a middiaphyseal fracture of the humerus in a 2-day-old calf. *B,* Previously described fracture 30 days after being repaired with a single intramedullary pin, lag screws and cerclage wire.

(Courtesy of Dr. Ryland B. Edwards III; University of Wisconsin.)

lameness but generally bear weight on the affected leg. In chronic cases, marked muscle atrophy may appear, but visually it is difficult to distinguish between it and other abnormalities. Palpation of the right coxofemoral joint while the left is being placed through a full range of motion typically elicits crepitus. If an assistant is not available, one can often detect a noticeable clicking and crepitus by placing one hand over the coxofemoral joint while pulling the animal's tail towards the affected side with the other hand. Ventrodorsal or lateral positioned radiographs with the affected leg up, flexed, and abducted (frog-legged) provide a definitive radiographic diagnosis (see Figure 11.2-3, A).

SURGICAL APPROACH

The animal is placed in lateral recumbency with the affected leg uppermost. A dorsolateral approach just cranial to the greater trochanter is used to expose the coxofemoral joint. The incision is extended distally to the distal aspect of the femur. A plane of dissection is created through the fascia lata and cranial border of the biceps femoris. A partial tenotomy of the origin of the vastus lateralis and sometimes middle gluteal and gluteus accessorius is required to provide exposure of the joint capsule (Figure 11.2-10).

METHODS OF INTERNAL REPAIR

The leg is internally rotated to facilitate reduction of the fracture. The fracture can then either be stabilized with 5- to 6.32-mm Steinman pins or 7- or 7.3-mm cannulated screws (Wilson et al, 1994; Hull, 1996) (see Figure 11.2-3, B). The implants are inserted retrograde from the insertion of the accessory gluteal through the femoral neck and into the fragment. Care should be taken not to invade or leave implants in the joint. Radiographic guidance (including fluoroscopy) at surgery is extremely helpful when one is placing implants. Devascularization of the femoral head may occur as a result of fracture or surgical dissection. This is because the blood supply to the femoral head flows through the round ligament of the head of the femur, joint capsule, and femoral neck. The latter two are disrupted by a fracture. During a surgical procedure, every effort should be made to preserve the blood supply to prevent femoral head necrosis from occurring. This is followed by revascularization, bone resorption, flattening of the femoral head, and osteoarthritis (Figure 11.2-11).

In case of irreversible damage to the articular cartilage of the acetabulum and/or femoral head, femoral head excision should be considered (Squire et al, 1991). In this case an osteotomy of the greater trochanter is performed. Before the osteotomy, the greater trochanter is drilled and tapped, and two or three 6.5 mm cancellous screws are inserted into the intended proximal fragment before the osteotomy. A Gigli wire is used to perform the osteotomy. The femoral neck is transected with an oscillating saw or Gigli wire. The greater trochanter is put back in place with a 1.2-mm wire in a tension band fashion (see Figure 11.4-35). Closure is done by reapposition of the various anatomical planes.

Fractures of the Humerus

CLINICAL PRESENTATION

Fractures of the humerus are relatively uncommon, but they do occur, most often secondarily to trauma (Rakestraw, 1996). Cattle with fractures of the humerus typically have a "dropped elbow" appearance and drag the effected limb in the flexed position. Other differentials for cattle with a dropped elbow appearance include olecranon fracture, triceps myopathy, and radial nerve paralysis. Palpation of the limb demonstrates extensive soft tissue swelling around the fracture site with associated crepitation when the limb is passively adducted and abducted. Concurrent damage to the radial nerve is often present because the radial nerve runs adjacent to the musculospiral groove off the humerus. The integrity of the radial nerve is critical for a positive outcome. It is difficult to clinically assess the function of the radial nerve with electrodiagnostics such as electromyography and nerve conduction velocity. Transient functional interruption is common because of the inflammation surrounding the nerve (neuropraxia). Clinical signs generally provide strong support for the diagnosis of a humeral fracture, and the diagnosis is confirmed by radiography. Radiographs of the humerus are difficult to obtain in healthy standing animals and can be even more difficult to obtain with extensive soft tissue swelling and pain. Short-acting anesthesia may be required to obtain quality images.

The most common types of fractures of the humerus include diaphyseal fractures that typically have a spiral-to-long oblique configuration. Fractures of the humerus are seldom open because of the extensive soft tissue surrounding the bone. Fractures can also occur through the distal physis and usually are a Salter-Harris type II configuration. Fractures of the deltoid tuberosity and greater tubercle can occur but are extremely rare in ruminants.

SURGICAL APPROACHES

The two described surgical approaches to the humerus include a lateral and cranial approach. The radial nerve is the most important vital structure that must be identified and preserved when either surgical approach is performed. The lateral approach provides exposure to the irregular lateral surface of the humerus and is not a desirable surface for plating the humerus. However, this approach is useful for assisting in placement of

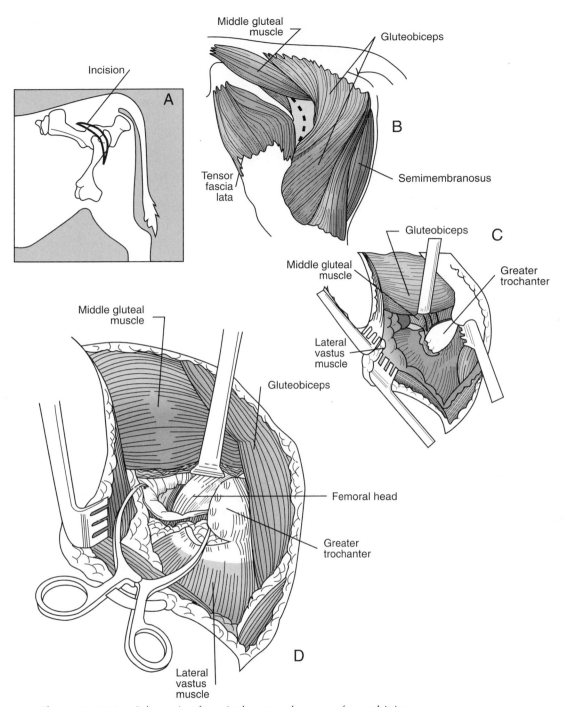

Figure 11.2-10   Schematic of surgical approach to coxofemoral joint.

intramedullary pins or interlocking nails. The cranial approach provides access to the straighter and more regular surface of the humerus.

For the cranial approach, the animal is placed in lateral position with the affected leg uppermost (Figure 11.2-12). The skin and subcutaneous tissue is incised from the cranial aspect of the greater tubercle of the humerus dis-tally over the cranial aspect of the extensor carpi radialis muscle. The plane of dissection is established by proxi-mally splitting the brachiocephalicus muscle cranial to the deltoid tuberosity. At the distal half of the incision, the caudal border of the brachiocephalicus is separated from its attachment to the brachial fascia. The cephalic vein is identified, double-ligated, and transected. The

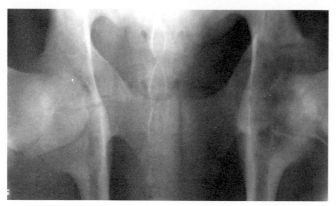

Figure 11.2-11   Femoral head necrosis as viewed on a ventrodorsal radiograph.

(Courtesy of Dr. Ryland B. Edwards III; University of Wisconsin.)

insertions of the brachiocephalicus muscle on the crest of the humerus distal to the deltoid tuberosity are transected. The underlying deltoid muscle is elevated from the deltoid tuberosity, thus exposing the brachialis muscle along the lateral aspect of the humerus in the musculospiral grove. The belly of the biceps muscle is elevated from the humerus. To gain further access to the distal part of the humerus, a portion of the origin of the extensor carpi radialis muscle is elevated from its attachment to the lateral humeral condyle. The radial nerve is identified along the caudal border of the brachialis muscle and distally between the brachialis and extensor carpi radialis muscle. Retraction of the brachialis muscle caudally and the biceps brachii muscle medially provides sufficient exposure to the cranial cortex. Retraction of

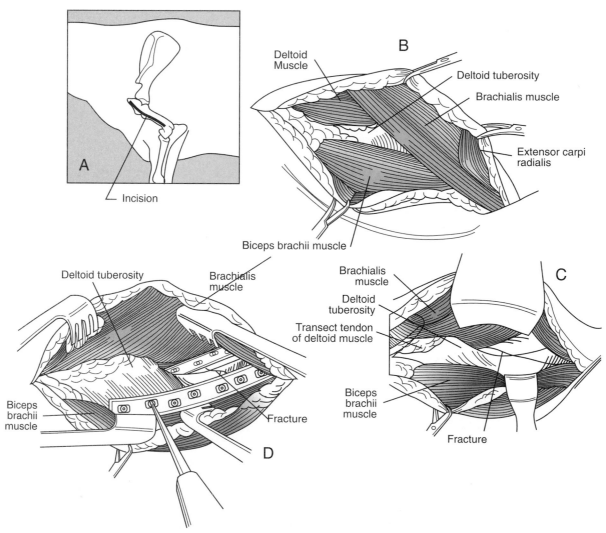

Figure 11.2-12   Schematic of surgical approach to humerus.

the brachialis muscle cranially allows exposure to the lateral aspect of the humerus.

In the lateral approach, the animal is positioned in lateral recumbency with the affected leg uppermost. The skin and subcutaneous tissues are incised from the greater tubercle to the lateral epicondyle of the humerus. The incision lies cranial to the cranial border of the triceps brachii muscle. To gain exposure to the proximal humerus, a plane of dissection is created under the caudal border of the brachiocephalicus muscle. The brachiocephalicus muscle is reflected cranially to reveal the cranial border of the brachialis muscle. The cranial border of the brachialis muscle is retracted caudally and the brachiocephalicus muscle cranially to expose the proximal third of the humerus. The close approximation of the brachialis muscle to the musculospiral groove of the humerus makes exposure of the middle third of the humerus difficult. To expose the distal third of the humerus, the brachialis muscle must be retracted cranially, the triceps brachii muscle caudally, and the extensor carpi radialis muscle caudoventrally. The radial nerve runs craniodistally in close approximation to the musculospiral groove of the humerus and deep to the triceps brachii and extensor carpi radialis muscles.

METHODS OF INTERNAL FIXATION REPAIR

Intramedullary pins or interlocking nails may be used to treat diaphyseal fractures of the humerus. Intramedullary pins can be placed in either normograde fashion starting proximally from the greater tubercle passing distally to the medial side of the humeral condyle. Care should be taken to avoid driving pins into the olecranon fossa of the humerus. A single intramedullary pin can be used, or multiple stack pins can be used to increase rotational stability and decrease the likelihood of longitudinal collapse of the fragments. Cerclage wire or interfragmentary compression with lag screws is also commonly performed when utilizing intramedullary pins (see Figure 11.2-8B). Interlocking nails can also be used to repair diaphyseal and distal fractures of the humerus. Interlocking nails insertion and placement landmarks are similar to those of intramedullary pins.

Bone plate fixation and screws can be used to treat humeral fractures. In younger calves, single-plate application to the cranial aspect of the humerus usually provides enough support for healing. In animals above 200 kg, double-plating techniques that use both the cranial and lateral surfaces should be attempted. If possible, 4.5-mm broad DCP plates should be used because of their strength. Contouring the plate on the lateral side is extremely difficult because of the deltoid tuberosity, and for that reason, use of a lateral plate as the sole means of repair is not recommended.

Fractures of the Radius/Ulna

CLINICAL PRESENTATION

Fractures of the radius are not very common in cattle. Fractures of a cow's radius usually occur because a leg in a fixed position is struck, typically either in a lateral-to-medial or cranial-to-caudal direction. Fractures of the radius commonly occur in the mid diaphysis or distally through the growth plate as a Salter-Harris type II fracture (see Figure 11.2-1). In adults, fractures of the radius are commonly highly comminuted. Because of the large amount of soft tissue covering the radius, most radial fractures are typically closed. Cattle with fractures of the radius have an appreciable lameness with associated soft tissue swelling of the antebrachium. They tend to rest with the leg pointed and are minimally weight-bearing. On occasion, marked angulation is visible at the fracture site; it is best viewed with a cranial-to-caudal leg position. Radiographs provide the definitive diagnosis. Olecranon fractures are extremely rare (Hague et al, 1997) and present as severe forelimb lameness and an inability to bear weight. The elbow is dropped because of the lack of functional triceps activity. Palpation of the olecranon reveals pain and swelling. The diagnosis is confirmed by radiography (Figure 11.2-13).

SURGICAL APPROACH TO RADIUS

The animal is positioned in lateral recumbency with the affected leg uppermost. A curvilinear incision through the skin and subcutaneous tissue is started at the lateral epicondyle of the humerus and extended distally to the lateral tuberosity of the radius where the collateral ligament of the carpal joints originates (Figure 11.2-14). The apex of the curvilinear incision is directed cranially to help gain exposure to the dorsal aspect of the radius. The skin is reflected, and the plane of dissection is established between the common digital extensor muscle and extensor carpi radialis muscle. Care must be exercised not to damage the radial nerve as it courses the most proximal aspect of the radius. The cranial and lateral surfaces of the radius are readily exposed by this surgical approach. The abductor digiti I longus closely adheres to the lateral aspect of the distal radius and may need to be bluntly reflected.

METHODS OF INTERNAL REPAIR

The radius does not lend itself to intramedullary fixation. Bone plating is the only form of internal fixation that should be considered when one is fixing a fracture of the radius. The tension surface of the radius is located along the cranial cortex. In calves less than 200 kg, a single 4.5-mm broad DCP can easily be contoured to the cranial

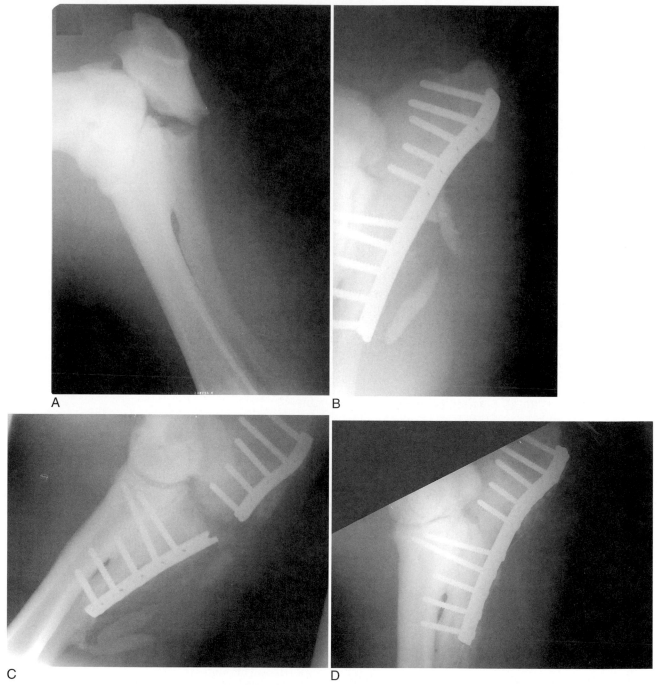

A   B

C   D

Figure 11.2-13   *A,* Lateral radiograph of the olecranon of a 3-year-old 500-kg Hereford cow with an acute olecranon fracture. *B,* After repair with a narrow DCP plate. *C,* Implant failed and *D,* was repaired by removing the broken plate and replacing it with 2 DCP plates using the same screw holes. In addition, bone grafting was performed.

(Courtesy of Dr. Ned Dykes; Cornell University.)

aspect of the radius. In heavier and older calves, double plating should be considered. Plates can be placed craniolaterally and craniomedially or cranially and laterally. True placement of a lateral plate is difficult because of natural cranial-to-caudal bowing of the radius. If plates are applied to the radius, external coaptation proximal to the carpus should be avoided because this changes the tension surface of the radius from the cranial-to-caudal cortex and significantly weakens the mechanical advantage of the repair.

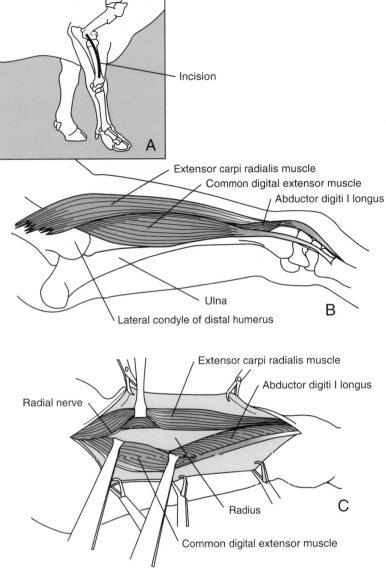

Figure 11.2-14 Schematic of lateral approach to radius.

In Salter-Harris type II fractures of the distal radial physis, dynamic condylar screw (DCS) plates and screws should be considered in adult cattle (see Figure 11.2-6). In young calves, lag screw fixation with 5.5-mm cortical screws or 6.5-mm cancellous screws and application of a cast up to the elbow level has also been successful.

SURGICAL APPROACH TO OLECRANON

The animal is positioned in lateral recumbency with the affected leg uppermost. A curvilinear incision through the skin and subcutaneous tissue is started at the cranial most proximal aspect of the olecranon curving caudally to the caudal aspect of the olecranon just below the joint of the elbow and extending distally on the caudal

midline. The incision is extended so a plane of dissection is developed between the flexor carpi ulnaris and ulnaris lateralis. A section of the attachment of the triceps tendon on the olecranon is elevated with a no. 15 blade to allow implant placement.

METHODS OF INTERNAL REPAIR

The methods of internal fixation are based on tension band principles with either orthopedic wires or narrow DCP plate. After appropriate reduction and debridement of the fracture site, the fracture is reduced. The ulna in cattle is a very thin bone, so one has to be careful with inserting an intramedullary nail. Likewise, because the ulna is very thin, one must chisel the caudal aspect of the ulna to create a flat surface to receive a bone plate. In addition, because of the size of the ulna, screws applied through the plate must also engage the caudal cortex of the radius for adequate holding power (see Figure 11.2-13B and D). In larger animals two plates, one on top of the other, may be needed (see Figure 11.2-13C and D). The addition of bone cement on either side of the thin ulna helps stabilize the plate in position and prevents the plate from displacing in an axial-abaxial plane.

Fractures of the Tibia

CLINICAL PRESENTATION

Tibia fractures occur in all age groups, and affected cattle have marked soft tissue swelling around the tibia. A significant lateral deviation of the limb at the fracture site is often found on visual examination of the affected leg. Survey radiographs of the entire tibia are most informative. Care should be taken to ensure radiographs of the entire tibia, especially the proximal tibia, are obtained so fractures or fissure lines are not missed. Fractures of the tibia are often highly comminuted and at risk of opening along the medial surface because of the lack of soft tissue covering. Fractures occur typically in the middiaphysis (Figure 11.2-15); however, Salter-Harris type II fractures of the proximal and distal physis do exist (see Figure 11.2-4).

SURGICAL APPROACHES

Both the lateral and medial surgical approach may need to be used to gain exposure to fractures of the tibia. For the lateral approach, the animal is positioned in lateral recumbency with the affected leg uppermost (Figure 11.2-16). A curvilinear incision through the skin and subcutaneous tissues is made from the proximolateral aspect of the tibia to the lateral malleolus of the distal tibia. A plane of dissection is created by displacing the long digital extensor muscle cranially and the fibularis longus and lateral digital extensor muscles caudally. Care should be taken to avoid the peroneal nerve. The superficial peroneal nerve lies in the proximal aspect between the long and lateral superficial digital extensor tendons. The deep peroneal nerve is located between the long digital extensor muscle and the cranial tibial muscle.

For the medial approach, the animal is positioned in lateral recumbency with the affected leg down (Figure 11.2-17). A curvilinear incision through the skin and subcutaneous tissues is made from the proximomedial aspect of the tibia to the medial malleolus of the distal tibia. The apex of the curvilinear incision is directed caudally. The saphenous vein, artery, and nerve are located in the proximal aspect of the incision in the superficial fascia between the popliteus muscle and the deep digital flexor muscle. The saphenous complex is reflected cau-

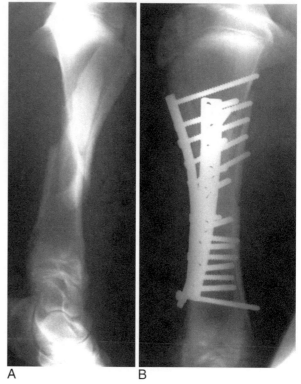

Figure 11.2-15   *A,* Lateral radiograph of an 8-month-old bull that weighed 440 kg with a comminuted diaphyseal fracture of the tibia. *B,* Previously described fracture repaired using craniomedially and craniolaterally placed bone plates and screws.

(Courtesy of Dr. Ryland B. Edwards III; University of Wisconsin.)

dally with the superficial fascia. An incision is made through the deeper layer of the fascia from the medial malleolus proximally to the tendinous attachment of the gracilis muscle to the tibial crest. The cranial tibialis muscle can be reflected laterally to expose the medial aspect of the tibia.

METHODS OF INTERNAL REPAIR

Fractures of the tibia can be difficult to repair because of the bone's unique geometry and the loading forces applied to it being located between two high range-of-motion joints: the tarsus and stifle. For diaphyseal fractures, double plating is recommended (see Figure 11.2-15B). Plates should be placed on the craniomedial and craniolateral surfaces and extend from the proximal to the distal metaphysis. Interlocking nails may be used to treat diaphyseal fractures by retrograde placement of the nail, proximally from the fracture site to the tibial plateau, or normograde placement from the tibial plateaus. Salter-Harris type II fractures of the tibia are difficult to repair because of the lack of bony purchase in the epiphysis. Proximal Salter-Harris type II fractures

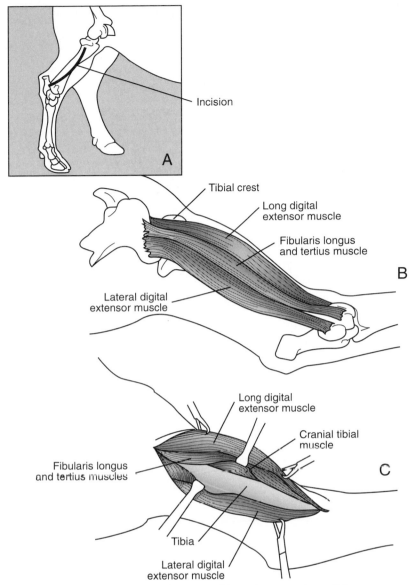

Incision

A

Tibial crest

Long digital
extensor muscle

Fibularis longus
and tertius muscle

Lateral digital
extensor muscle

B

Long digital
extensor muscle

Cranial tibial
muscle

Fibularis longus
and tertius muscles

C

Tibia

Lateral digital
extensor muscle

Figure 11.2-16   Schematic of lateral approach to tibia.

have been repaired using medial placed T-plates or multiple DCP plates in a tension band principle (see Figure 11.2-4B).

Fractures of the Metacarpus and Metatarsus

CLINICAL PRESENTATION

Fractures of the large metacarpal and metatarsal bones are the most common type of fractures in cattle. Most of the fractures that occur in neonatal calves are associated with the placement of devices on the distal extremities to facilitate fetal extraction. The incidence of metacarpal fractures is slightly higher in the metacarpus than the metatarsus. Most fractures of the metatarsus that are associated with forced fetal extraction occur in the distal metaphysis and are treated by either external coaptation or external skeletal fixation. Fractures of the metacarpus and metatarsus in nonneonates usually occur as a Salter-Harris type I or II fracture of the physis or a middiaphyseal fracture. Fractures of the mid diaphysis of adults can be highly comminuted and are at risk of opening because of the general lack of soft tissue covering (Figure 11.2-18A). Affected animals are not weight-bearing, and the definitive diagnosis is obtained by radiography of the affected limb. External fixation can be used to successfully treat many fractures of the

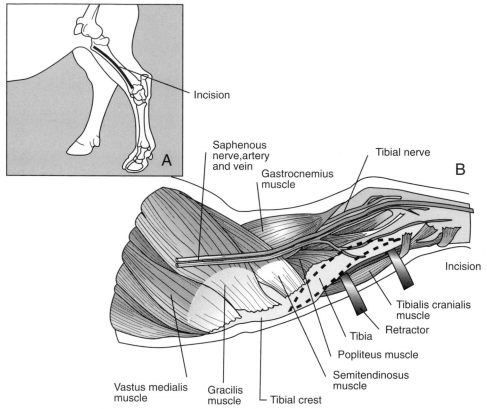

Figure 11.2-17   Schematic of medial approach to tibia.

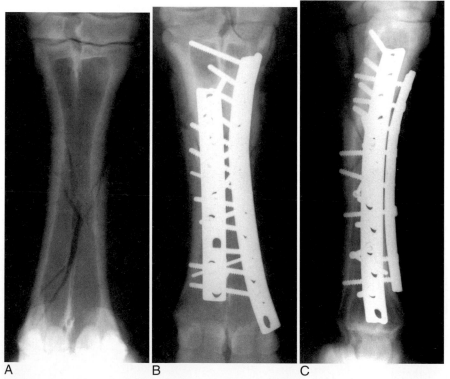

Figure 11.2-18   *A,* Dorsoplantar radiograph of a 550-kg bull with a comminuted metatarsal fracture. Previously described fracture repaired by using dorsally *(B)* and laterally *(C)* placed bone plates and screws.

(Courtesy of Dr. Ryland B. Edwards III; University of Wisconsin.)

metacarpus and metatarsus in cattle. However, internal fixation with bone plates should be considered for larger-sized adult animals with comminuted fractures.

SURGICAL APPROACH

The animal is positioned in lateral recumbency with the affected leg uppermost. Either a dorsomedial or dorsolateral approach is used. A curvilinear incision through the skin and subcutaneous tissues is made from the carpometacarpal joint to the metacarpo/metatarsophalangeal joint. The apex of the curvilinear incision should be directed dorsally, and the plane of dissection is between the lateral digital extensor tendon and the common or long digital extensor tendon. Alternatively, a linear incision can be used that is made directly over one of the extensor tendons. The extensor tendon can then be split longitudinally. This technique allows increased soft tissue coverage of the plates. The tendons are elevated away from the metacarpus/tarsus with blunt dissection to provide direct exposure to the bone.

METHODS OF INTERNAL REPAIR

In adults, double plating is advised, with one plate being placed dorsally (Figure 11.2-18B and C). The true tension surface of the metacarpus and metatarsus is not known, and considerable debate exists as to whether a second plate should be placed laterally or medially. The author's opinion is that the plate should be placed on the side where the bony cortex is least likely to be anatomically constructed, thereby promoting plate placement in the bending closed position and decreasing the likelihood of implant fatigue or failure. A single bone plate placed on either the medial, dorsal, or lateral bone surface may be the best treatment for older calves. Internal fixation with bone plates may be supplemented by external coaptation.

Intramedullary devices cannot be readily used as a means of repairing fractures of the metatarsus or metacarpus. Normograde or retrograde placement of intramedullary devices cannot occur without significant damage to either the proximal carpus or tarsus, or distal (metacarpo/metatarsophalangeal) joint surface.

Other Fractures

PELVIC FRACTURES

In general, fractures of the pelvis occur in adults and most commonly involve the wing of the ileum, sometimes called *knock down hip* (Cox, 1978). Often dairy cattle in confined housing have these fractures associated with direct trauma from another animal or striking an immovable object. When the animal is viewed from behind, one can notice the asymmetry of the tuber coxae (Figure 11.2-19). On palpation, the fractured tuber coxae can be palpated ventral to its normal position. Pal-

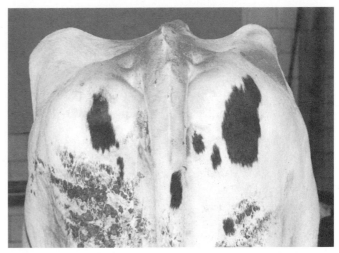

Figure 11.2-19   Caudal view of a cow with a right fracture of the ileal wing (tuber coxa).

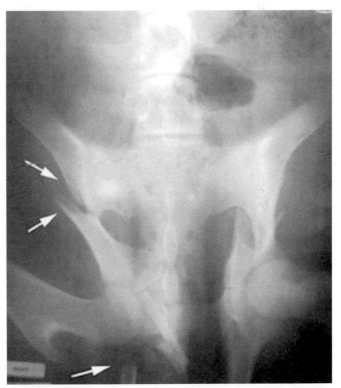

Figure 11.2-20   Ventrodorsal radiograph of the pelvis of a 7-month-old heifer hit by a car. There are ilial and ischial body fractures (arrows).

pation also reveals edema, hematoma, and pain. Conservative treatment consists of stall rest for approximately 60 days. In some cases, the fragment becomes infected or develops into a sequestrum, in which case surgical debridement is recommended. Very rare fractures of the pubis and ischium have been reported as a result of being hit by a moving vehicle (Figure 11.2-20). Owners should be advised not to breed females that have suffered these fractures unless prior rectal exam determines that callus formation has not reduced the diameter of the pelvic cavity, a potential cause of calving problems. Alternatively, embryo transfer or a planned cesarean section should be considered. Pubic symphysiotomy is another technique used to handle difficult dystocia in young heifers.

SCAPULA FRACTURES

Fractures of the scapula are rare and are frequently associated with major trauma such vehicular collisions. Clinical signs vary by the location. Conservative management often successfully treats fractures of the body of the scapula. Fractures of the scapular neck and glenoid are typically associated with a readily appreciable lameness because of the articular component. Treatment of these fractures is difficult and involves internal fixation methods (Adams) that reconstruct the scapulohumeral joint (see Internal Fixation section in this chapter) The location makes these fractures' prognosis poor. Fractures that involve the scapular neck or glenoid require that injuries to the subscapular nerve also be considered.

Sacral Fracture

Norm G. Ducharme

Sacral injuries and fractures are traumatic and are associated with mounting injury during estrus or excessive traction on the tail. The fracture may result in clinical signs including an abnormal contour of the dorsal sacrococcygeal area (Figure 11.2-21). In addition, depending on the location of the injury, various neurological deficits may be seen. Fracture to the most cranial aspect of

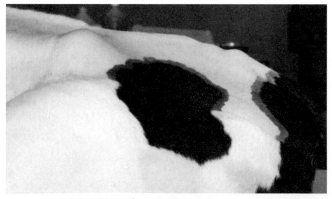

Figure 11.2-21   Loss of normal smooth contour of the dorsal sacrococcygeal area of a heifer with a sacral fracture.

sacrum may result in damage to the sciatic, and obturator nerves; therefore clinical signs may also be seen in the pelvic limbs. Damage to the obturator nerves results in adductor muscle deficit. Finally, deficit to the sciatic nerve results in knuckling at the fetlock. Pelvic and pudendal nerve injuries may result in disorders in micturition and defecation. In addition, flaccidity of the anus and vulva can be seen. Caudal neurological damage to the coccygeal nerve can lead to deviation of the tail if unilateral damage is present. If bilateral damage to the innervation is present, a decrease or lack of tail tone is seen with soiling of the tail by fecal material.

Treatment options include the following: conservative management (which allows time for fibrous or bony union of the fracture and restoration of nerve function), antiinflammatory agents, avoidance of tail manipulation, and placing the animal in a box stall with excellent footing is recommended. If an adductor muscle deficit is present, the hind limb should be tied (hobbling—use commercial hobbles or a rope tied just above the fetlock while giving about 2 feet of movement between each leg). If return of tail function does not occur, tail soiling will cause unsanitary conditions in the milk parlor, thus requiring tail amputation.

A tail amputation is performed as follows. In the average adult cow 5 or 6 cc of lidocaine hydrochloride is placed between two coccygeal vertebrae proximal to the intended amputation site. A tourniquet is applied and the amputation area prepared for aseptic surgery. The intent is to transect between two coccygeal vertebrae and close the skin over the defect. The skin is incised 2 to 3 cm more caudal than the intervertebral space to be incised. The intervertebral space is identified, and the blade inserted under the skin flap until the space is reached and transected. The coccygeal vein and artery are identified at the ventral aspect of the remaining vertebra and ligated. The tourniquet is temporarily released to identify additional significant vessels. The skin is reapposed over the coccygeal vertebra with simple interrupted sutures.

Surgical repair of sacral fractures can also be done by using internal fixation (see Internal Fixation section in this Chapter). The fracture is stabilized by using either internal fixation (narrow DCS plate) on the vertebral body adjacent to the fracture or by placing a spinous process plate* on the spinous process adjacent to the fracture. The procedure is performed under general anesthesia, and the animal is placed in sternal or lateral recumbency. The caudal sacral area is prepared for aseptic surgery. An incision with a dorsal midline approach is made until the dorsal spinous process is identified. The

*Lubra plate, Lubra Co; Fort Collins, CO

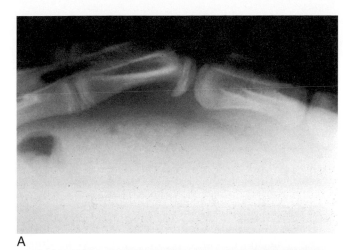

A

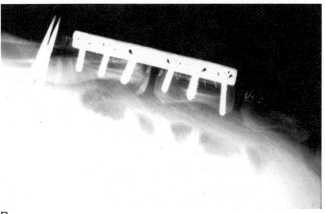

B

Figure 11.2-22 *A,* Lateral radiograph of physeal fracture of last sacral fragment of heifer. *B,* Intraoperative view after surgical repair with narrow plate placed in the vertebral body of last sacral vertebra and first caudal vertebra.

(From McDuffee et al: Repair of sacral fracture in two dairy cattle, *J Am Vet Med Assoc* 202: 1126-1128, 1993 [Reproduced with permission].)

incision is extended along either side of the dorsal process if spinous process plates are to be used. If fixation will be made on the vertebral body, an incision of the sacrotuberous ligament on the appropriate side is needed to allow adequate exposure (Figure 11.2-22A and B).

CARPUS AND TARSUS FRACTURES

Fractures of the carpus and tarsus small bones are very rare (Welker, 1989). These fractures are extremely difficult to treat because of degenerative joint disease development. To salvage an animal, external forms of fixation should be considered. If continued production for the animal is a goal, anatomic reconstruction with bone screws for internal fixation of the bone(s) that comprise the joint surface(s) provides the best chance for a positive outcome.

MANDIBLE AND MAXILLA FRACTURES

Fractures of the mandible and maxilla are secondary to trauma and occur in younger farm animals more often than in adults. In general, fractures of the mandible are more common than those of the maxilla. The most common form of mandibular fracture occurs rostral to the interdental space.

Clinical signs associated with mandible and maxilla fractures are highly variable. Clinical signs can be as minimal as localized swelling to obvious bony malalignment, often associated with oral wounds, ptyalism, and failure or difficulty with prehension and mastication. Radiography provides the definitive diagnosis, and oblique films of the dental arcades as well as intraoral images should be considered to obtain a complete study. The head blood supply is very good, and mandible and maxilla fractures generally heal well if the fracture can be immobilized for a period of time. Minimally displaced fractures that do not impede the animal's ability to masticate, swallow, or breath can be treated conservatively. Rostral fractures of the mandible can be treated by circumdental wiring, cross pinning, tension band wiring, external skeletal fixators, or intraoral splints (Colahan and Pascoe, 1983; Lischer et al, 1997). Fractures of the mandibular symphysis can be treated by circumdental wiring or lag screw fixation. Fracture of the horizontal ramus of the mandible or maxilla can be treated by using some form of external skeletal fixation or placement of a laterally placed bone plate (Wilson et al, 1990) (see section 10.1).

SEQUESTRUM

Osseous sequestration does occur in cattle and is associated with localized trauma that results in cortical bone ischemia and bacterial invasion secondary to the loss of periosteal and soft tissue integrity. Clinically, cattle with sequestration vary from nonhealing wounds or fistulous tracts (cloaca) to large defects with exposed bone (Valentino et al, 2000). Most sequestrums occur in cattle between 6 months and 2 years of age and are localized to the distal extremities, commonly the metacarpal or metatarsal bones.

Cattle with sequestration at the distal extremities are usually lame. The diagnosis is confirmed by radiographic examination (Figure 11.2-23). Treatment of osseous sequestrum includes surgical debridement of the sequestrum, involucrum, and cloaca (sequestrectomy). Significant debridement is often required to gain adequate exposure of the sequestrum because bovine periosteum has a reactive nature. Radiographic guidance during surgery is helpful in completely identifying the devitalized bone. After surgical debridement, a primary closure can be performed. Alternatively, the wound can

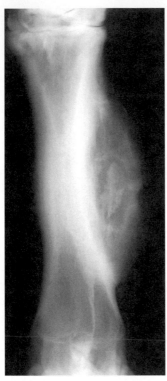

Figure 11.2-23 Dorsopalmar radiograph of an osseous sequestration in a 16-month-old bull. Note where the involucrum and cloaca are located.

(Courtesy of Dr. Ryland B. Edwards III; University of Wisconsin.)

be allowed to heal by second intention with the wound protected by a bandage or cast. Some large cortical defects may compromise the bone's strength and require a cast application.

Complications of Internal Fixation

The postoperative care of ruminants with internal fixation of fractures includes stall confinement until clinical union is achieved. This time period may be as short as 30 to 60 days in immature animals but may require up to 6 to 9 months in adults, particularly if the repair is unstable. The only currently available methods for evaluating fracture healing other than clinical assessment are radiography and computed tomography (Trostle and Markel, 1996).

The two most common reasons for repair failure after fixation are infection (osteomyelitis, septic arthritis) and implant migration or breakage. The clinical signs of these two postoperative complications are similar and include localized pain and soft tissue swelling, exudate from the incision or a tract in the granulation tissue, and exacerbation of the previous lameness. Radiography aids in the assessment of implant migration and infection. Obvious implant migration is readily detected on follow-up radiographs; however, comparisons with the initial, postoperative radiographs may be needed to detect subtle changes. Osteolytic changes of the bone near the fracture margins or near the implants are indicative of osteomyelitis.

INFECTION

Osteomyelitis and septic arthritis are serious and potentially devastating complications of internal fixation. The best method of managing infection is to prevent its occurrence. Broad-spectrum, therapeutically dosed, antimicrobials should be administered in the perioperative period. The length of postoperative antimicrobial administration is controversial and depends upon many factors. These factors include the following: whether the fracture was open or closed, the degree of surrounding soft tissue trauma before and during surgery, surgical time, soft tissue coverage of the implant, and response to initial antimicrobial therapy.

The three goals in the treatment of osteomyelitis are the following: 1) establishment of drainage through debridement of the infected bone and tissue; 2) culture and selection of appropriate antimicrobial agent(s); and 3) removal of the implant after union has occurred. Management of osteomyelitis is particularly frustrating and often unrewarding. Most cases involve a profound, long-term financial and time commitment from the owner and veterinarian. Despite valiant efforts, the prognosis for successful treatment and resolution of osteomyelitis is poor.

IMPLANT FAILURE OR MIGRATION

Implants fail similarly to bone, either by a single catastrophic event or by cyclic fatigue (see Figure 11.2-13C). Catastrophic failure usually occurs in the immediate recovery period and is initiated at the weakest point of fixation or at a point of stress concentration. Cyclic fatigue usually results in screw loosening or failure from shear forces at the screw-plate interface and may eventually continue the complete length of the repair. This emphasizes the need to choose the appropriate size and implant at the time of treatment (see Figure 11.2-13D).

The most common form of implant migration in femur fracture repairs is associated with pins used for either intramedullary repair or external skeletal fixation in neonatal calves. Because of the relative softness of the bone, intramedullary pins can migrate either proximally or distally within the intramedullary cavity. Migration into a joint may predispose the calf to degenerative joint disease or septic arthritis. External skeletal fixator pins may also loosen and migrate in the soft tissues. Pin migration through the skin predisposes the fixation to osteomyelitis, since the pin tract serves as a direct communication from the outside to the medullary cavity.

Prognosis

The reported success rate for fracture repair in cattle varies widely. It is difficult to compare results between studies because the end point of success or satisfaction is not clearly defined. Each individual animal should be evaluated on its own merits. Open fractures (regardless of type, location, and bone) always have a less favorable prognosis because of the problems associated with infection and implants used with internal repair. The prognosis primarily depends on the size and age of the animal. Because a lot of energy is required to fracture an adult cattle bone and the fractures are typically highly comminuted, the prognosis is less favorable because fixation devices often cannot overcome the mechanical forces of larger-sized animals. Older calves carry a fair to good prognosis because their size and weight relative to the implant is more favorable. In younger calves the prognosis is good to excellent, but problems associated with a neonatal bone's ability to support fixation devices remain a primary concern.

RECOMMENDED READINGS

Adams SB: Fractures of the scapula. In Nixon AJ, editor: *Equine Fracture Repair*. Philadelphia 1996, WB Saunders, pp 254-258.

Ames NK: Use of a fracture distractor in two cattle, *J Am Vet Med Assoc* 207: 478, 1995.

Auer JA et al: Internal fixation of long bone fractures in farm animals, *Vet Comp Ortho Traumatology* 6: 36-35, 1993.

Colahan PT, Pascoe JR: Stabilization of equine and bovine mandibular and maxillary fractures, using an acrylic splint, *J Am Vet Med Assoc* 182: 1117-1119. 1983.

Cox VC: Pelvic fracture in a cow, *J Am Vet Med Assoc* 172: 1316-1317, 1978.

Cox VS, Breazile JE, Hoover TR: Surgical and anatomic study of calving paralysis, *Am J Vet Res* 36: 427-430, 1975.

Crawford WH, Fretz PB: Long bone fractures in large animals, *Vet Surg* 14: 295, 1985.

Ferguson JG: Management and repair of bovine fractures, *Comp Contin Educ Pract Vet* 4: S128, 1982.

Ferguson JG: Special considerations in bovine orthopedics and lameness, *Vet Clin North Am [Food Anim Pract]* 1: 131, 1985.

Ferguson JG: Femoral fractures in the newborn calf: biomechanics and etiological considerations for practitioners, *Can Vet J* 35: 626-630, 1994.

Fessler JF, Adams SB: Decision making in ruminant orthopedics, *Vet Clin North Am [Food Anim Pract]* 12: 169-180, 1996.

Gillis JP et al: Holding power of cortical screws after power tapping and self-tapping, *Vet Surg* 21: 362, 1992.

Hague BA et al: Tension band plating of an olecranon fracture in a bull, *J Am Vet Med Assoc* 211: 757-758, 1997.

Hull BL: Advances in ruminant orthopedics: fractures and luxations of the pelvis and proximal femur, *Vet Clin North Am [Food Anim Pract]* 12: 47-57, 1996.

Kirpenstein J et al: Holding power of orthopedic screws in femora of young calves, *Vet Comp Orthop Traumatol* 6: 16-20, 1993.

Kirpenstein J et al: Holding power of orthopedic screws in metacarpal and metatarsal of young calves, *Vet Comp Orthop Traumatol* 5: 100-103, 1992.

Lischer CJ et al: Pinless external fixation of mandible fractures in cattle, *Vet Surg* 26: 14-19, 1997.

McDuffee LA, Ducharme NG, Ward JL: Repair of sacral fracture in two dairy cattle, *J Am Vet Med Assoc* 202: 1126-1128, 1993.

Nunamaker DM et al: Mechanical and biological affects of plate luting, *J Orthop Trauma* 5: 138, 1991.

Rakestraw PC: Advances in ruminant orthopedics: fractures of the humerus, *Vet Clin North Am [Food Anim Pract]* 12: 153-168, 1996.

Reif U et al: Long-term results of bovine mandibular fractures involving the molar teeth, *Vet Surg* 29: 335-340, 2000.

Schneider RK et al: Multidirectional *in vivo* strain analysis of the equine radius and tibia during dynamic loading with and without a cast, *Am J Vet Res* 43: 1541, 1982.

St-Jean G et al: Intramedullary pinning of femoral diaphyseal fractures in neonatal calves: 12 cases (1980-1990), *J Am Vet Med Assoc* 200: 1372, 1992a.

St-Jean G et al: Repair of a proximal femoral fracture in a calf using intramedullary pinning, cerclage wire, and external fixation, *J Am Vet Med Assoc* 200: 1701, 1992b.

Shettko DL et al: Effects of age, location, screw size, and bone mineral density on screw pullout force in neonatal bovine femurs, *Vet Surg* (in press).

Squire KRE, Fessler JF, Toombs JP, Van Sickle DC, Blevins WE: Femoral head osteotomy in horses and cattle, *Vet Surg* 20: 453-458, 1991.

Trostle SS, Wilson DG, Dueland RT et al: In vitro biomechanical comparison of solid and tubular interlocking nails in neonatal bovine femora, *Vet Surg* 24: 235-243, 1995.

Trostle SS, Markel MD: Advances in ruminant orthopedics: fractures of the femur, *Vet Clin North Am [Food Anim Pract]* 12: 19-46 and 169-180, 1996.

Trostle SS et al: Management of a radius fracture in an adult bull, *J Am Vet Med Assoc* 206: 1917-1919, 1995.

Tulleners EP: Management of bovine orthopedic problems: part I, fractures, *Compend Contin Educ Pract Vet* 8: S69, 1986.

Tulleners EP: Metacarpal and metatarsal fractures in dairy cattle: 33 cases (1979-1985), *J Am Vet Med Assoc* 189: 463-468, 1986.

Tulleners EP: Advances in ruminant orthopedics: metacarpal and metatarsal fractures in cattle, *Vet Clin North Am [Food Anim Pract]* 12: 199-210, 1996.

Valentino LW et al: Osseous sequestration in cattle: 110 cases (1987-1997), *J Am Vet Med Assoc* 217: 376-383, 2000.

Welker FH: Tarsal fractures in a heifer and a bull, *J Am Vet Med Assoc* 195: 240-241, 1989.

Wilson DG et al: Fixation of femoral physeal fractures with 7.0mm cannulated screws in five bulls, *Vet Surg* 20: 240, 1990.

Wilson DG, Ulm MJ: Holding power of orthopaedic screws in bovine femoral heads: a comparison of 7.0-mm cannulated screws to 5.5-mm cortical and 6.5-mm cancellous screws, *Vet Comp Orthop Traumatol* 6: 160, 1993.

Wilson DG et al: A surgical approach to the ramus of the mandible in cattle and horses: case reports of a bull and a horse, *Vet Surg* 19: 191-195, 1990.

11.3—External Fixation

Guy St. Jean and David E. Anderson

General Principles

Temporary stabilization of limb fractures may be performed before moving the animal or attempting to get the animal to stand. As a general rule, fractures below the level of the midradius or midtibia may temporarily stabilized with splint or casts. In our experience, field stabilization of fractures proximal to this level should not be attempted. These efforts often result in the creation of a "fulcrum effect" at the fracture site and result in increased soft tissue trauma, damage to neurovascular structures, or compounding of the fracture. Cattle with these fractures should be carefully loaded into the trailer and allowed time to lie down before beginning transport. For these proximal injuries, cattle will usually protect the limb adequately for transport and any additional trauma that occurs is less severe than that which may occur as a result of the "fulcrum effect."

External coaptation for temporary stabilization may be done by using splints or a cast. Two boards of a large PVC pipe cut in half, placed 90 degrees to each other (e.g., caudal and lateral aspect of the limb), create a stable external coaptation. A padded bandage is placed on the limb, the splints positioned and elastic tape applied firmly. Circular clamps (e.g., hose clamps) may be used to achieve firm placement of the splints on the limb. All external coaptation devices should extend to the ground. For injuries distal to the carpus or hock, the splints should be placed to the level of the proximal radius or tibia, respectively. For injuries proximal to the carpus or hock and distal to the midradius or midtibia, the lateral splint should extend to the level of the proximal scapula or pelvis, respectively.

The location of the fracture, presence of soft tissue and neurovascular trauma, closed or open fracture environment, behavioral nature of the animal, and experience of the veterinarian are important factors for considering the type of treatment to choose. For fractures that involve the appendicular skeleton, the following questions must be answered:

1. Is treatment required?
2. Can the fracture be acceptably reduced or closed, or is internal reduction required?
3. Can the fracture be adequately immobilized by using external coaptation alone, or is internal fixation—with or without external coaptation—required?
4. What is the cost-benefit analysis?

In farm animals, external coaptation as a practical, relatively easy approach should be considered as an option for many fractures (except humeral and femoral fractures). Casts and splints—separately or in combination—have been used successfully in all types and sizes of ruminants. Closed treatment is the preferred method for many types of fractures. The more distal the injury, the more external fixation becomes the optimal method for success. The materials for fabricating casts and splints are readily available, and ruminants usually become accustomed to fixation within a few days, so reasonable locomotion is possible.

Transfixation pinning with some type of external fixation has been used successfully in ruminants. The technique involves limited surgical invasiveness with reduced cost, improved stability over external coaptation alone, and prospects for early ambulation while preserving joint mobility. It is simple and useful, even in field situations. Over the years, external fixators have improved and all manner of external supports have been used successfully, including cast material, metal rods, steel plates, and acrylics. Either external coaptation alone—or combined with transfixation pins—provides the veterinarian techniques to manage virtually all fractures distal to the elbow and stifle in most ruminant patients.

CASTING

Ideally, the cast should be extended at least a joint above and a joint below the fracture site to reduce distracting forces. This ideal aside, some relatively stable physeal and distal metaphyseal fractures of the metacarpus and metatarsus can be immobilized with a short limb cast that incorporates the digit and extends to just below the carpus. Unstable physeal, distal metaphyseal, and all diaphyseal and proximal metaphyseal fractures require the use of a full-limb cast extending to the proximal radius or tibia.

Placement of the cast is facilitated by use of rope restraint. Sedation or general anesthesia is used as needed. An assistant should help maintain alignment of the limb during application while checking the position of the limb in craniocaudal and lateromedial planes. Tension on the limb during casting may be achieved by placing wires through holes drilled in the hoof wall and applying traction. The holes should be placed such that the hoof is positioned in a normal to slightly flexed position.

The thick skin and heavy hair coat of ruminants help prevent serious cast sores. The hair is brushed clean of any debris or dirt. The dewclaws and top of the cast are padded with a wide strip of orthopedic felt, but only stockinette or foam resin padding is placed on the remainder of the limb. Thick padding, placed along the entire limb, will quickly become compressed, thus leaving room for the limb to move within the cast so displacement of the fracture occurs. Full-limb casts are used for fractures that occur at or proximal to the mid-metacarpus or metatarsus but distal to the midradius or midtibia. Full limb casts are placed similarly to half limb casts, but the bony prominences of the accessory carpal bone, styloid process of the ulna, calcaneus, and medial and lateral malleolus of the tibia must be padded.

Fresh 3-, 4-, or 6-inch quick-setting polyurethane resin-impregnated knitted fiberglass fabric cast material is extremely strong and easy to apply. It is lightweight, porous, waterproof, and quick-setting on warm water. Gloves must be worn to protect the operator's hands. The cast material is completely immersed in very warm water for approximately 20 seconds, and excess water is allowed to drip off. The casting tape is applied in even overlapping spirals, including the foot; however, one must be certain to avoid creases, binding, or finger impressions, particularly in the first layers. Additional rolls are added in an even manner as needed to increase cast thickness and—consequently—strength.

The thickness of the cast is usually based on clinical judgment. Casts 4 to 6 layers thick may be adequate for ruminants less than 150 kg body weight, but adults may require casts 8 to 12 layers thick. Casts used on the hind limbs must be made thicker because of stress concentration by the angulation of the hock. Incorporation of metal rods within the cast (two rods placed 90 degrees to each other) can increase the strength of the cast but is only needed in the largest of patients. The distal aspect of the cast (weight-bearing surface) should be protected from excessive wear and moisture with a layer of acrylic. Elastic bandage tape is placed circumferentially around the top of the cast and applied to the limb to prevent dirt, straw, and debris from getting between the cast and the limb. The animal should be restricted to a box stall or pen with good footing, preferably a dirt floor. The animal's general well-being and appetite should be evaluated daily. Ideally, the animal should ambulate comfortably at a walk, and the cast should be checked daily to be certain no heat, excessive looseness, exudate, or cast fractures are present. Any significant changes in the animal's level of comfort with the affected limb may be grounds for cast removal and reevaluation.

Ruminants younger than 1 month old should have a cast change and reevaluation every 3 weeks because of their growth. Uncomplicated healing usually occurs in 3 to 6 weeks. Ruminants 1 to 6 months of age should be reevaluated at approximately 4-week intervals. Uncomplicated fracture healing in animals 6 to 12 months old usually occurs in approximately 6 weeks with one cast needed. Yearlings and adults usually can tolerate a properly fitting cast between 6 to 8 weeks with radiographic evidence of fracture healing after 12 to 16 weeks (one cast change). Fracture healing after casting is usually characterized radiographically by extensive circumferential periosteal new bone growth.

After cast removal, flexor tendon laxity must be expected. Usually during this transition time the limb is supported with a short-limb bandage constructed of several pounds of rolled cotton, 6-inch-wide rolled gauze, and elastic adhesive bandage material. The bandage usually can be removed after 2 weeks. Confinement should be continued for 4 to 8 weeks after cast removal, depending on the animal's comfort, palpable limb stability, and radiographic evidence of fracture healing.

Metacarpal and metatarsal fractures are among the most common fractures in ruminants. Fortunately extensive orthopedic experience and great skill are not necessary in dealing with these fractures. They are amenable to external coaptations using a fiberglass cast. The prognosis for long-term, pain-free survival is excellent for closed fractures and fair for open fractures managed in this manner. Surviving animals generally are not lame, do not have significant limb deformity or shortening, and generally become productive. Even considering the narrow profit margin involved in treating cattle with serious injuries, this method of fracture management usually is economically profitable.

Open fractures can sometime be resolved with casting, but the prognosis for a successful outcome diminishes substantially in comparison to a closed fracture and the expense of fracture management is significantly higher. Owners must be strongly advised of the difficulties and expense of treating open fractures.

For the treatment of an open fracture with casting, the hair adjacent to the wound should be clipped and the affected area prepared for sterile surgery. All devitalized tissue must be excised sharply, and, when necessary, the bone is exposed and curetted. The wound can be lavaged by using several liters of balanced polyionic solution. The wound is wrapped with a sterile gauze bandage, and the cast is then applied. Broad-spectrum antimicrobial therapy should be instituted before surgery and continued for at least 10 to 14 days. Adjustments in antimicrobial therapy can be made based on results of culture sensitivity of fluid and tissue obtained at surgery.

THOMAS SPLINT CAST COMBINATION

Tibial fractures account for approximately 12% and radial fractures account for approximately 7% of long bone fractures diagnosed in ruminants. These fractures may result in significant economic loss to an individual producer if inadequate fixation methods are employed that result in failure of bony union or creation of an open fracture.

The Thomas splint (Figure 11.3-1) and cast combination is an economical method for obtaining fracture stability that does not require specialized equipment. Construction of a Thomas splint can be challenging at the time an animal is presented with a fracture. We prefer to have multiple sizes of Thomas Splints premade with adjustable sidebar length. These are not perfectly fitted to the individual animal but are adequate for fracture stability and are time-efficient. To custom make a Thomas splint, one must measure the circumference of the groin or axillary region with an orogastric tube. The medial ring should be firmly positioned against the groin or axilla. The lateral and dorsal ring should extend dorsal to the greater trochanter of the femur or the greater tubercle of the humerus and spine of the scapula.

The ring should not impinge on the tuber coxae or tuber ischii. White tape can be used to conform the ring and mark where the cranial and caudal bars of the splint will exit the ring. The ring is removed from the animal. Construction of the splint is started with a 12-foot length of tubular steel. The size of tubular steel is correlated with the size of the animal. For ruminants less than 140 kg, we recommend one-quarter-inch (6.35 mm) outer diameter steel. For animals between 140 kg and 500 kg, use half-inch outer diameter steel, and for ruminants above 500 kg use 1-inch steel (2.5 cm).

A vise or round surface is used to bend the steel rod (larger rods may be heated to facilitate bending). The rod must be bent, starting in the center of the rod, 540 to 630 degrees to complete the ring and project the sidebars distally along the limb. Forelimb splints have straight sidebars. For hindlimb splints, the caudal bar is bent to accommodate the hock. The distal aspect of the splint may be completed by bending the bars beneath the digits and overlapping them in a "U" configuration.

If the splint is too long, the animal will have difficulty ambulating, and this may lead to angular deformities in the contralateral limb. The bars are then welded together for stability. Alternately, a solid foot-plate may be constructed from tubular steel of a small enough diameter to telescope inside the major sidebars. Holes may be drilled through the two bars at 2.5-cm intervals to make an adjustable splint. The ring of the splint is padded with roll cotton and tape. If the padding is too thick, however, the splint may become loose with time.

Xylazine hydrochloride (0.05 mg/kg, IV) is administered, and the animal is positioned in lateral recumbency with casting ropes. For tibial fractures, the limb is cast from the distal metatarsus to the proximal tibia. The cast material should be carefully applied as far proximally on the tibia as possible. Then, the splint is placed on the limb; one must be sure to apply the splint fully into the axilla or groin. Holes are drilled into the hoof walls and bailing wires are used to attach the digits to the base of the splint. Two to three wires per digit should be placed to prevent loosening caused by wire breakage. The wires on the base are encased in methylmethacrylate to protect them. Then, the cast is placed into the splint to maximize stability and prevent proximal and distal motion within the splint.

After application of the Thomas splint and cast combination, the animal should be confined to a small pen for 6 to 10 weeks before removal (Figures 11.3-2 and 11.3-3). The animal must be examined by the owner several times each day during the first 2 to 3 days. The

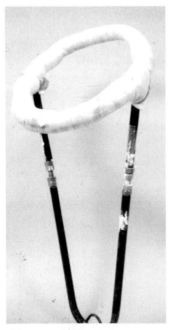

Figure 11.3-1   Thomas splint.

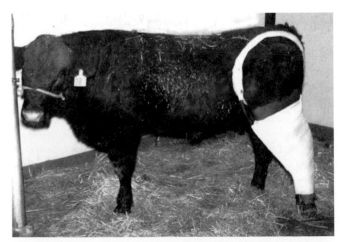

Figure 11.3-2   Application of the Thomas splint and cast combination for a fracture of the tibia in a bull.

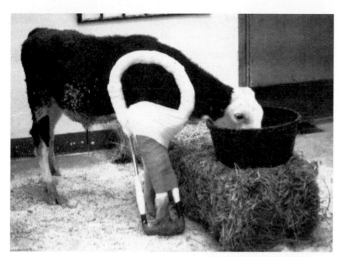

Figure 11.3-3 Application of the Thomas splint and cast combination for a fracture of the radius in a calf.

splinted limb must remain uppermost when the animal is lying down. Otherwise, the animal could become cast with the limb trapped beneath it and bloat. The animals usually learn to manage the splint well by day 2 or 3. The cast should be examined frequently for the first week. If the cast becomes loose after swelling associated with the fracture trauma is reduced, it should be replaced. A loose cast may allow enough motion to create an open fracture or delayed union.

Tibial and radial fractures in animals under 1 year of age or less than 500 kg can be given a good prognosis with the Thomas splint cast combination. The owner should be prepared for up to 8 weeks of confinement for affected animals with the splint applied, and an additional 2 weeks of confinement during the accommodation period after the splint has been removed. Short- and long-term complications have been reported with the use of the Thomas splint cast combination. These include prolonged recumbency, tympany of the rumen, skin abrasions, pressure sores, osteoporosis, muscular atrophy, joint stiffness, and delayed union of the fracture.

EXTERNAL SKELETAL FIXATION (ESF)

External skeletal fixation (ESF) refers to the stabilization of a debilitating musculoskeletal injury (typically fractures but also joint luxation or tendon rupture) by using transfixation pins (or transcortical pins) and any external frame connecting the pins and spanning the region of instability.

Fracture stability therefore is obtained by transferring the biomechanical forces endured by the bone around the fracture environment and through the external device.

The goal of the ESF is to provide a sustainable, comfortable means to return the patient to weight-bearing (or function) as soon as possible after surgery, to maintain normal joint mobility, if possible, and to provide an optimal environment for osteosynthesis and wound healing.

Cast immobilization of fractures in ruminants is chosen, whenever appropriate, because of economic considerations. However, when cast immobilization is not appropriate or does not provide optimal management of fractures, other modalities must be considered. Soft tissue injuries and open fractures may not be managed optimally by use of casts, or splint-cast combinations. ESF may be chosen based on fracture configuration, soft tissue injuries, or open fractures. Usually, ESF is used in purebred animals, show animals, or other ruminant of high perceived economic value. ESF is being increasingly used in cattle, sheep, and goats.

BIOMECHANICS OF EXTERNAL SKELETAL FIXATION

External fixator design is the most important factor that affects fracture stability. External skeletal fixator stability is increased by increasing the number of pins placed in each fracture fragment, angling the pins in each fragment, increasing the size of the pins used, increasing the number of connecting bars, increasing the size of the connecting bars used, using bilateral or multiplanar fixator designs instead of unilateral designs, and minimizing the distance between the connecting bar and the bone.

Diverging pins increase the torsional stability of the fixator in comparison to parallel pins. Pin diameter must be carefully chosen not to exceed a safe pinhole size in relation to the diameter of the affected bone. In most cases, the authors used quarter-inch (6.35 mm) pins in ruminants. Positive profile threaded pins have superior axial extraction forces in comparison to smooth pins.

Regardless of the frame configuration, the distance between the connecting bars and the bone should be minimized. Doubling the bone-to-connecting bar distance reduces the resistance to compressive loads of approximately 25%. The pin clamp of the external fixator is a potential "weak link" in the fixator if improperly applied and may result in pin-bone junction motion, pin loosening, and loss of fracture stability. Concerns over potential clamp failure, owner monitoring of fixator clamps, clamp fatigue with repeated use, and economic constraints in veterinary surgery have prompted the use of acrylic polymers and casting to replace the sidebar-clamp assembly.

Transfixation pinning and casting (TPC) has been used for many years in veterinary surgery, particularly in cattle. The advantages of TPC include minimal bone-to-external frame distance, pin placement restricted only by fracture configuration and anatomic considerations (not by the design of the fixator), biomechanical forces shared with the cast and application to patients (age, weight, height) not limited by availability of standard equipment. Also, fiberglass casts are not as brittle as acrylic polymers and therefore may be less likely to suffer catastrophic failure. Disadvantages of TPC include poor access to soft wounds, greater difficulty in removal, potential for cast-induced soft-tissue injuries, and cost proportional to amount of cast material needed (no reusable parts).

CLINICAL APPLICATION OF EXTERNAL SKELETAL FIXATOR

ESF has many advantages for the treatment of fractures. ESF provides early return to function of the affected limb, management of soft tissue wounds on the limb, preservation of local blood flow to the fracture site, preservation of bone-stimulatory proteins that exude into the fracture site at the time of initial injury, diversity in design for comminuted fractures, ease of implant removal after clinical union of the fracture, and relatively few complications resulting from the implants. ESF has been applied to most of the long bones of the domestic species. Transarticular application of external fixators has been used in the presence of severe soft tissue trauma or severe comminution of the proximal or distal ends of the affected bone and for arthrodesis of joints. Transarticular use of external fixators must be done with consideration for the potential of inducing damage to the involved joint because of immobilization.

Disadvantages of ESF are suboptimal fracture reduction and poor anatomic alignment, absence of interfragmentary compression, less rigid stabilization of the affected bone in comparison to bone plates, increased postoperative management in comparison to bone plates or casting, pain associated with micromotion at the pin-bone interface, and potential failure of the implants before clinical union of the fracture.

We routinely use antibiotics for 7 days after surgery during application of an external fixator for a closed fracture. Antibiotic selection for use in cattle must be made with consideration for extra-label use and potential antibiotic residues. The authors usually repair fractures of the metacarpus/metatarsus, radius, ulna, and tibia with the patient in dorsal recumbency and the limb suspended from an overhead frame. Fractures of the humerus and femur are approached with the animal in lateral recumbency. Excessive soft-tissue swelling and inflammation is typical of fractures in large animals. After the animal is clipped and aseptically prepared for surgery, the authors place marker needles (18-gauge, 3.8-cm for most fractures; 18-gauge, 8.9-cm for the tibia in adults) at the sites proposed for placement of the transcortical pins. Radiograph images are obtained and the pin sites are chosen based on the relationship of the marker

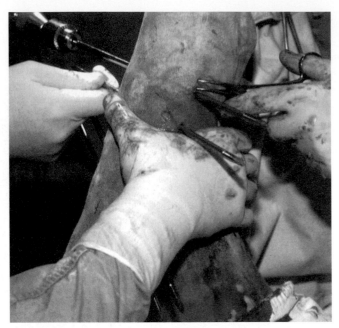

Figure 11.3-4   Two transcortical pins have been implanted in a calf with a tibial fracture. The patient is in dorsal recumbency with the limb suspended.

needles with the fracture, fissure lines, adjacent joints, and intact cortical bone.

A 1-cm incision is made through the skin at the chosen pin site. A hole is then drilled through the bone and another incision is made for the exit site of the pin (for bilateral transcortical pins). We use a pneumatic orthopedic drill with variable speeds up to 700 rpm. Pins are implanted with the drill at low speed. However, standard electric or battery-powered drills may be used after appropriate sterilization. During drilling, the drill bit should be continuously flushed with a sterile isotonic solution to help decrease thermal injury to the bone. Finally the pin is implanted (Figures 11.3-4 and 11.3-5). A tissue protector, or pin guide, is beneficial to prevent excessive soft-tissue trauma during drilling and implantation.

ESF was designed so transfixation pins, sidebars, and clamps could be used to stabilize fractures unsuited for external coaptation alone or for internal fixation. The main limitation of sidebars and clamps is the ability of the assembly to resist failure during loading. We have used commercially available fixator frames in animals that weigh less that 150 kg. We do not recommend the use of traditional sidebar-clamp assemblies for cattle weighing more than 150 kg because of the higher risk the pin-clamp sidebar unit will fail.

Welding the transfixation pins to the sidebar has been proposed as a means to decrease postoperative management and strengthen the attachment of the pin to the sidebar for use in cattle. Welding may result in thermal

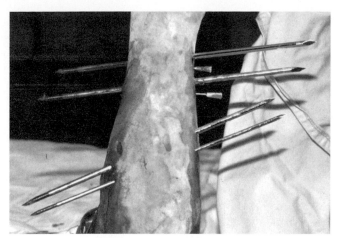

Figure 11.3-5 Four transcortical pins have been implanted in a calf with a tibial fracture.

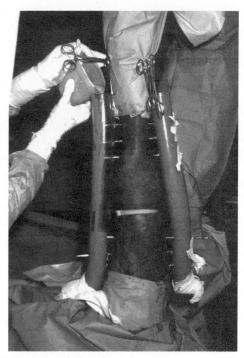

Figure 11.3-6 Methylmethacrylate side-bar used in a Type 2 external fixator in a cow with an open radial fracture. The patient is in dorsal recumbency.

injury to the bone because of heat conduction in the transfixation pins and may also result in electric shock to the patient. Also, the sidebars are not reusable, and poorly applied welds may break, thus leading to failure of the assembly.

The use of methylmethacrylate as an inexpensive, conformable sidebar has biomechanical advantages in comparison to the standard steel sidebars and clamps (Figure 11.3-6). Use of acrylic sidebars has advantages similar to those of traditional ESF. However, acrylic sidebars cannot be adjusted after the resin has hardened and must be replaced if an error in configuration of the frame occurs. Acrylics harden with an exothermic reaction. Therefore potential thermal injury to the skin and bone must be considered. Transfixation pins should be rinsed with fluids during the exothermic period to help dissipate heat. An adequate supply of acrylic should be readily available at the time of surgery, and the acrylic must be poured into the tubing mold while it is relatively liquid. Pouring the acrylic in multiple layers or while it is firming up causes air pockets or cracks in the sidebar and may result in catastrophic failure. Though acrylics have good biomechanical stiffness, they are brittle. Therefore acrylic sidebars must be inspected daily to ensure that failure of the fixator does not occur. The acrylic sidebars may be removed in sections by using obstetrical wire to cut the acrylic surrounding the pins.

TRANSFIXATION PINNING AND CASTING (TPC)
Transfixation pinning and casting allows minimal postoperative case management with a high degree of success. This advantage is particularly suited to food animals. We exclusively use fiberglass casting tape for TPC. Pin position and fixator configuration cannot be adjusted after the cast has been applied when using TPC. Also, open wounds or open fractures are difficult to

manage with TPC. Complications during TPC, such as creation of an open fracture or development of cast sores, are difficult to assess, and some delay may result before these problems are addressed. We recommend using resin-impregnated foam* on the limb before casting. This foam padding conforms to the limb, provides excellent protection, and its porous structure allows the limb to remain dry under the cast. We have observed a decrease in the severity of pin tract complications when foam padding was used.

Management of Specific Fractures

RADIUS/ULNA
Cattle have a complete ulna that articulates with the antebrachiocarpal joint. Fracture of the radius therefore is nearly always complicated by fracture of the ulna. The radius is well suited to ESF by using TPC when the fracture is closed. When fracture configuration allows placement of multiple pins proximal and distal to the fracture and the patient weighs less than 150 kg, we place the cast spanning the antebrachium only. This allows free movement of all joints in the forelimb. In patients that weigh more than 150 kg, we use a full-limb cast to provide additional support. When the fracture is open, we use ESF with metal or acrylic sidebars to provide access to

---

*3M Custom Support Foam, 3M Animal Care Products; St. Paul, MN

the wound for daily fracture management. Clinical union is expected within 4 to 6 weeks in calves and within 8 to 10 weeks in adults after stabilization. Open fractures may require 12 weeks or more for clinical bone union.

TIBIA

In the experience of the author, fracture of the tibia is the most common fracture treated by ESF/TPC in ruminants (Figure 11.3-7). TPC of tibial fractures is highly successful in cattle. Transfixation pins are difficult to place correctly in the tibia because of the extensive soft tissue coverage of the cranial, lateral, and caudal aspects of the bone. The principle neurovascular structures of the pelvic limb are located on the caudomedial aspect of the tibia. Therefore lateral-to-medial transfixation pins may be placed with minimal risk of neurovascular trauma. Ideally, transfixation pins should be implanted, from lateral to medial, between the fibularis longus and lateral digital extensor and long digital extensor muscles proximally and the lateral digital extensor and long digital extensor muscles distally. However, the fascial planes between muscles surrounding the tibia are difficult to palpate, and extensive swelling associated with inflammation and fracture hematoma make palpation difficult. Therefore we place transfixation pins based on the fracture configuration, often placing pins through muscles. Although significant complications were observed in foals when pins interfered with muscle movement, we have not observed a clinically significant problem in ruminants. When using TPC, we advocate

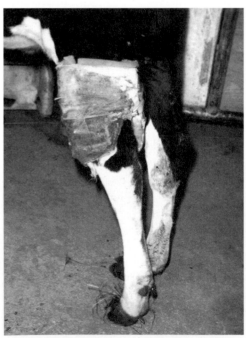

Figure 11.3-7 Transfixation pinning and casting used for immobilization of a tibial fracture in a calf.

placing pins proximal and distal to the fracture to maximize stability. In calves with diaphyseal fracture of the tibia, three pins are placed proximal and distal to the fracture. Cast material is applied to span the length of the tibia, and a segment is cut out of the distal caudal cast to allow free movement of the calcaneal tendons. Normal ambulation is afforded by this technique. Distal fractures may be stabilized by placing pins in the metatarsus and applying a transarticular cast. In adult cattle, we place pins similarly, but a full limb cast should be applied to increase the stability of the assembly.

MANAGEMENT OF OPEN FRACTURES

We consider all fractures with a penetrating skin wound associated with the fracture to be infected because of the severity of contamination with dirt and manure typical of farm animals. After induction of anesthesia, we clean and superficially debride the wound, prepare the limb for aseptic surgery, and copiously lavage the wound. We then obtain aerobic and anaerobic cultures of the bone and medullary cavity. This procedure decreases contamination with transient, surface bacteria and yields a more reliable indication of true pathogen(s). Empiric antibiotic therapy is initiated at the time of surgery and continued until bacterial culture and sensitivity results are obtained. Based on our clinical experience and bacterial susceptibility results, we routinely initiate antibiotic therapy with procaine penicillin G.

After initial debridement and cleaning, we perform copious lavage one to two times daily, depending on the degree of contamination and the severity of the infection. After daily lavage (and debridement as indicated) the wound, limb, and ESF are wrapped with clean bandage materials. Sterile gauze padding is applied to the wound. We often use topical antiseptic ointments to cover the external wound. We feel the potential benefit of topical antiseptics in preventing superinfection of the wound outweighs any inhibitory effects on wound healing. Daily lavage is continued until granulation issue has covered the wound. The wound is then cleaned every 48 to hours until the defect has been "filled in" by granulation tissue and no longer requires cleaning.

Chronic infection (osteomyelitis) of the fracture can be more difficult to resolve. Often these infections are associated with osseous sequestra and resolve after removal of the sequestered bone. Infected fractures that progress to septic nonunion should be treated aggressively. Aerobic and anaerobic cultures and microbial susceptibility tests are repeated, and the fracture site is extensively debrided. The debridement is continued until healthy bone is exposed. A fresh, autologous cancellous bone graft is then harvested and implanted into the fracture site. We have harvested autologous cancellous bone from the ileum of calves and adult cattle without complications. We use a 4.5- to 6.0-mm drill bit to enter the medullary cavity of the bone. A bone curette is used to collect the cancellous bone. This bone graft is packed into the fracture and the skin is closed over the site, if possible.

When the infection is too excessive for routine debridement and cancellous bone grafting or when the wound does not have a healthy granulation bed to provide blood supply to the graft, we perform extensive debridement and implant hand made antibiotic impregnated beads. We prepare methylmethacrylate bone cement and then mix in powdered penicillin, sodium ceftiofur, cefazolin or ampicillin before implanting the cement. Septic nonunion may be successfully treated by rigid immobilization and the surgical techniques described above. However, the economic limitations of an individual animal may be encountered before clinical union of the fracture has occurred.

RECOMMENDED READINGS

Adams SB, Fessler JF: Treatment of radial-ulnar and tibial fractures in cattle, using a modified Thomas splint-cast combination, *J Am Vet Med Assoc* 183: 430-433, 1983.

Anderson De, St. Jean G, Vestweber JG, et al: Use of a Thomas splint-cast combination for stabilization for tibial fractures in cattle: 21 cases (1973-1993), *Agri-Practice* 15: 16-23, 1994.

Anderson DE, St. Jean G, Desorchers A: Repair of open, comminuted fractures of the radius and ulna in a calf with transarticular Type II external skeletal fixator, *Agri-Practice* 15: 24-28, 1994.

Anderson DE, St. Jean G: Repair of fractures of the radius and ulna in a ewe using positive profile transfixation pins and casting, *Can Vet J* 34: 686-688, 1993.

Baxter GM, Wallace CE: Modified transfixation pinning of compound radius and ulna fracture in a heifer, *J Am Vet Med Assoc* 198: 665-688, 1991.

Kaneps AJ, Schmotzer WB, Huber MJ, et al: Fracture repair with transfixation pins and fiberglass cast in llamas and small ruminants, *J Am Vet Med Assoc* 195: 1257-1267, 1989.

McClure SR, Watkins JP, Bronson DG, et al: In vitro comparison of the standard short limb cast and three configurations of short limb transfixation cast in equine forelimbs, *Am J Vet Res* 55: 1331-1334, 1994.

St. Jean G, St. Pierre H, Lamothe P, et al: Fractures epiphysaires et des os longs chez les ruminants, *Med Vet Quebec* 15: 63-77, 1985.

St. Jean G, DeBowes RM: Transfixation pinning and casting of radial-ulnar fractures in calves: a review of three cases, *Can Vet J* 33: 257-262, 1992.

St. Jean G, Clem MF, DeBowes RM: Transfixation pinning and casting of tibial fractures in calves: five cases (1985-1989), *J Am Vet Med Assoc* 198: 139-143, 1991.

Tulleners EP: Management of bovine orthopedic problems, part 1: fractures, *Compend Contin Educ Pract Vet* 8: S69-S79, 1986.

Willer RL, Egger EL, Histand MB: Comparison of stainless versus acrylic for the connecting bar of external skeletal fixators, *J Am Animal Hosp Assoc* 27: 541-548, 1991.

Wilson DG, Vanderby R: An evaluation of six synthetic casting materials: strength of cylinders in bending, *Vet Surg* 24: 55-59, 1995.

Wilson DG, Vanderby R: An evaluation of fiberglass application techniques, *Vet Surg* 24: 118-121, 1995.

11.4—Treatment of Pathological Diseases
Foot and Digits

Guy St. Jean and André Desrochers

Digital disease in cattle is common. The hind lateral digit is most commonly involved. Lameness that originates from the digits is a multifactorial disease. Parity, stage of lactation, abnormal hoof growth, exclusion of dry hay from the diet, age and weight of the animal, and rear claw angle are all risk factors that can contribute to lameness.

The most common lesions in lameness that originates from the digits are sole ulcer, sole abscess, and interdigital necrobacillosis or interdigital phlegmon. These lesions can often be treated with local debridement, topical antiseptic on the wound, and, if necessary, a wooden block applied with polymethylmethacrylate* on the healthy digit of the affected limb to alleviate pain. However, a sole ulcer and abscess can result in deep sepsis of the digits if neglected. This sepsis can spread to the distal sesamoid bone and its synovial bursa and to the distal and proximal interphalangeal joints. A thorough examination of the digits and radiographic evaluation helps the clinician choose the appropriate treatment and surgical approach. Age, sex, weight, type of production, and environment of the cattle also should be considered in the choice of therapy.

Vertical Crack

This condition is secondary to excessive drying of the superficial layers of the hoof wall and subsequent trauma. The crack starts from the weight-bearing surface of the hoof and extends proximally. If the coronary band is traumatized, the opposite situation is observed; a vertical crack starts from the coronary band and extends distally. The animal will be lame if the sensitive laminae or other deep structures of the hoof are affected.

The first part of treatment is thorough debridement of the crack. This can be done with a curved hoof knife or motorized burr. Debridement should be carefully done, so that the intact sensitive lamina is not too traumatized. A 1-cm bar or triangle may be used to make grooves at the end of the crack to redistribute the force and prevent the crack from extending further. Wiring of the crack also prevents further extension and decreases the pain engendered by movement of the wall on the sensitive laminae. If the dermis is not infected, polymethylmethacrylate can

---

*Technovit, Jorgensen Laboratories; Loveland, CO

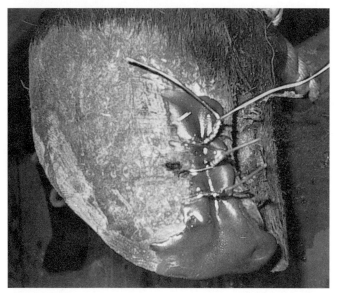

Figure 11.4-1 Vertical crack in the dorsal wall filled up with polymethylmethacrylate and tighten with wires.

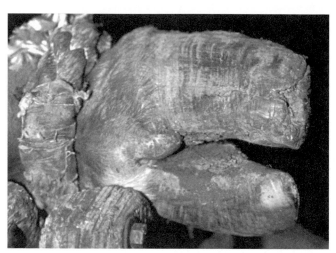

Figure 11.4-2 Interdigital hyperplasia lesion with a vertical crack on the lateral digit.

be applied to fill the defect (Figure 11.4-1). If the sensitive laminae are exposed or infection is present, polymethylmethacrylate application should be delayed until the infection is controlled and the exposed laminae are covered with keratinized tissue (i.e., dry surface). In severe cases, a wooden block should be applied on the healthy digit, and the animal should be rested in a stall. The prognosis is good to excellent if the sensitive laminae are not infected. Hoof ointment may be applied to the hoofs to prevent further desiccation.

Amputation of the Accessory Digit (Dewclaw)

Amputation of the accessory digit of the hind limb has been described to prevent self-inflicted teat laceration. The technique is simple and easily performed on calves 4 to 8 weeks old. The animal is sedated and kept in lateral recumbency. The area around the accessory digit is prepared aseptically, and a local block is performed around the dewclaw. The dewclaw is pushed proximally to avoid resection of the plantar annular ligament and plantar common digital artery. Sharp dissection with a scalpel is used to remove the dewclaw. Hemostasis is performed, and a bandage with antiseptic ointment is placed on the wound. If the surgery is performed on older cattle, a tourniquet around the distal metatarsus may be used to control hemorrhage.

Interdigital Hyperplasia (Corn)

Interdigital hyperplasia is a proliferative reaction of the interdigital skin. The incidence of lameness caused by

interdigital hyperplasia is between 1% and 4.8%. Excessive outward spreading of the digits secondary to an underdeveloped ligamentous structure overstretches the interdigital skin and causes hyperplasia. Males are affected more often than females. The animal affected by this disease is moderately to severely lame. A foul odor may be present during physical examination because of erosive lesions and secondary infection. The proliferative mass is hairless, ulcerated secondary to pressure trauma, and painless to palpation (Figure 11.4-2). The lesions can be found on one or all four limbs. Treatments with either *en bloc* resection of the growth, cryosurgery, and electrocautery have been successful. The procedures should be performed after administration of intravenous regional anesthesia. If *en bloc* resection is chosen, an Allis tissue forceps is used to grasp the interdigital corn. A wedge-shaped excision is made on each side of the mass. All hyperplastic tissues should be removed to minimize the risk of recurrence. The interdigital fat should also be removed to avoid its interposition between the incised skin edges. Hemorrhage is controlled, and a bandage is applied. The toes are wired together by drilling two holes through the hoof wall at the point of the toes. The bandage is left in place for 5 days, and the animal is kept in a small, clean stall.

Fracture of the Distal Phalanx

Fracture of the distal phalanx is secondary to trauma or fluorine intoxication. Pathologic fracture secondary to osteitis of the distal phalanx has also been reported. Cattle show a sudden onset of severe lameness and a typical stance: bearing weight on the healthy digit of the affected leg. The lateral hind digit or medial front digit

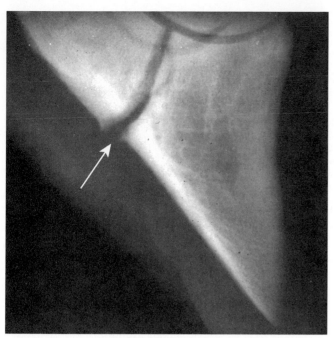

Figure 11.4-3 Interdigital radiograph of a digit. There is a displaced articular fracture of the distal phalanx (arrow) extending from the solar surface to the coffin joint.

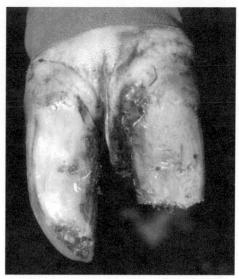

Figure 11.4-4 Severe pedal osteitis of the lateral digit treated with partial amputation.

often is affected. In the authors' experience, the front digits are affected more commonly. Examination is important to rule out sole abscess, white line abscessation, or digital interphalangeal (DIP) joint abnormalities that cause similar clinical signs.

Radiographic images of the affected digit are important to diagnose this condition. Radiographs usually show a fracture that extends vertically from the middle aspect of the distal interphalangeal joint to the solar surface with a fracture gap superior at the solar aspect of the distal phalanx (Figure 11.4-3). The palmar or plantar fragment may rotate because of the pull of the deep digital flexor (DDF) tendon. Treatment consists of immobilizing the affected digit by putting a wooden block on the healthy digit of the affected limb. The affected digit is wired in slight flexion to the wooden block to prevent separation of the palmar or plantar fragment from the parent bone caused by tension from the DDF tendon on the flexor process of the distal phalanx. The wooden block should be left in place for 6 to 8 weeks, with the animal confined to a small well-bedded stall. After 6 weeks, the block is removed, and the animal is reassessed. Determination of improvement should be based upon clinical signs, not on radiographic evaluation. The fracture gap can take 4 to 5 months to heal and sometimes 8 months. The prognosis for return to normal function is good if the cattle are treated promptly. If bony proliferation and signs of degenerative joint disease are visible on radiographs or a septic process caused the

fracture, facilitated ankylosis of the distal interphalangeal joint or digit amputation should be considered.

Pedal Osteitis

Pedal osteitis is defined as a septic process of the distal phalanx. The infection originates from solar trauma (such as a puncture wound or severe abrasion at the toe) or extension of an existing infection around the distal phalanx. The incidence could be high in feedlot cattle on a concrete floor. Cattle recently placed in a feedlot will fight around a feed bunk, and their hind digits will slip on the concrete floor, thus causing severe abrasion at the toe region and secondary infection.

A preoperative radiograph is helpful to evaluate the extent of the infection. The sole and infected corium is debrided first (Figure 11.4-4). The infected part of the distal phalanx is curetted. Lavage is performed, and the wound is bandaged. A wooden block is applied on the healthy digit of the affected limb. Bandaging and lavage should be continued until the infection is controlled and granulation tissue covers the distal phalanx. Amputation could be performed for economic reasons or if the infection is extensive.

Septic Arthritis of the Distal Interphalangeal Joint

Cattle affected with DIP joint sepsis have a history of chronic lameness and often have been previously treated. The clinical signs vary with the function of the structure involved in the process and the chronicity of the disease.

Sepsis of the DIP joint is caused mainly by extension of sole disease, such as pododermatitis circumscripta or traumatica and white line disease (Figure 11.4-5). A penetrating foreign body in the interdigital space or interdigital phlegmon is also often implicated in sepsis of the DIP joint. The distal sesamoid bone and its bursa, the tendinous portion of the deep digital flexor (DDF) muscle, the tendon sheath of the DDF muscle, and the superficial digital flexor (SDF) muscles are in close relationship; uncontrolled solar infection may affect these structures.

Cattle with DIP joint sepsis usually are very lame. The coronary band is swollen and red, and the adjacent horn is of poor quality. A fistula tract may be present on the dorsal palmar or plantar aspect of the abaxial collateral ligament of the middle and distal phalanx. Another fistula tract may be seen dorsoproximally to the coronary band and axial to the tendinous portion of the common or long digital extensor muscle. Examination of the hooves and interdigital spaces may show the origin of the septic arthritis. A swollen heel suggests infection of the distal sesamoid bone and its bursa and the digital cushion pad, and a fistula tract may be present at the heel skin junction. Cattle with deep sepsis of the digit show signs of pain when the heel is palpated or the digit is extended. Severe necrotic process may extend into the tendinous portion of the DDF tendon so it ruptures and causes the affected digit to tilt upward.

Radiographic evaluation of the DIP joint is helpful in determining the extent and duration of the process. Septic arthritis is apparent on radiographs 10 days after onset of the infection. Widening of the joint space from increased intrasynovial pressure, soft tissue swelling, and the presence of gas may be the only abnormalities seen on radiography of acute septic arthritis. Radiographic views of a DIP joint with chronic septic arthritis first show a decreased joint space because of cartilaginous degeneration followed by an increased joint space because of subchondral bone lysis. Distal and proximal periosteal proliferation is present (Figure 11.4-6). The distal sesamoid bone may show lysis of its articular surface or may be destroyed completely. The proximal interphalangeal (PIP) joint also might be involved in the process. If a fistula tract is present, communication with the DIP joint is confirmed by inserting a sterile probe into the tract or with positive arthrography.

Acute septic arthritis of the DIP joint is rare but possible. Arthrocentesis is indicated, and synovial fluid may be submitted for cytologic examination and bacterial culture. Treatment consists of systemic and local antibi-

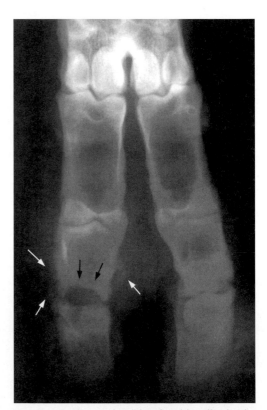

Figure 11.4-6   Radiograph of the distal hindlimb, dorsoplantar view. There is subchondral bone lysis, widening of the distal interphalangeal joint (black arrows), and new bone formation (white arrows). This is compatible with a chronic septic arthritis of the distal interphalangeal joint.

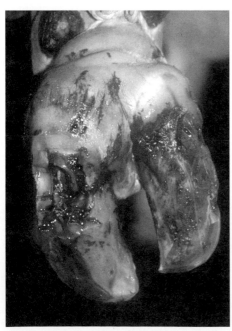

Figure 11.4-5   The lateral digit has a chronic sole ulcer. The heel and the coronary band are swollen, which is compatible with a septic arthritis of the distal interphalangeal joint.

otics and thorough joint lavage. A 14-G 5-cm needle is inserted dorsoproximal to the coronary band, axial or abaxial to the tendinous portion of the extensor muscle, and at a 60-degree angle to the coronary band. The joint is distended with 10 ml of 0.9% NaCl solution. A second needle is then inserted plantar or palmar to the abaxial collateral ligament of the DIP joint, above the coronary band, at a 45-degree angle. Lavage of the joint is performed until the synovial fluid is clear and without fibrin clots.

Five hundred ml of 0.9% NaCl solution under pressure usually is enough to lavage the joint. Arthrotomy should be considered if fibrin is abundant and lavage difficult.

After completion of joint lavage, 100 mg of ceftiofur is injected intraarticularly. Joint lavage is performed a minimum of 3 days subsequently or longer if needed. Joint lavage is discontinued based on clinical improvement, clarity of the synovial fluid, or negative bacterial culture. In the authors' experience, *Arcanobacterium pyogenes*, *Escherichia coli* and *Staphylococcus* spp. are the most common bacteria isolated from an infected DIP joint. Systemic antibiotics should be administered for 1 to 2 weeks after disappearance of clinical signs.

Chronic presentation of septic arthritis of the DIP joint is a more common situation (Figure 11.4-7). Surgery is the treatment of choice to provide debridement and drainage of the DIP joint. The two surgical options are digit amputation and facilitated ankylosis of the joint.

DIGIT AMPUTATION

Digit amputation has been used successfully to treat pedal osteitis, luxation, or fracture of the distal phalanx, deep sepsis of the digit, and septic arthritis of the DIP or PIP joint. The advantages are that it is a rapid and inexpensive procedure, all the infected tissues are resected, and cattle usually return rapidly to their previous level of production. The disadvantages are that expected production life is reduced, heavy animals do poorly, and cosmetic result is poor. The production life of cattle that have a digit amputated depends on which digit was removed, weight of the animal, and type of housing. Cattle that weigh more than 680 kg and have a digit amputated will have a short production life. The site of amputation should be chosen based on the extent of the infection. Digit amputation through the distal aspect of the proximal phalanx is the most common technique. It is a rapid and simple procedure and usually provides a wide resection and effective drainage of the affected digit (Figure 11.4-8).

The distal limb is prepared aseptically and intravenous regional anesthesia is administered. The interdigital skin is incised to the level of the distal aspect of the proximal phalanx axially, with a 45-degree angle to the proximal digit abaxially. An assistant can hold the digit to provide more stability when the osteotomy is performed in the same plane. A bandage is applied and left in place for 5 days. The bandage then should be replaced, and the new bandage left in place for another 5 days. A broad-spectrum, systemic antibiotic is administered for 3 to 5 days after the surgery.

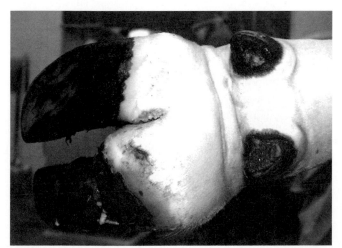

Figure 11.4-7   Chronic septic arthritis of the medial distal interphalangeal joint in cow. Note fibrous enlargement proximal to the coronary band compared to lateral claw.

(Courtesy of Norm G. Ducharme; Cornell University)

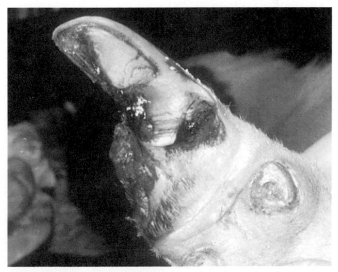

Figure 11.4-8   Digit amputation, a few days after the surgery was performed.

A skin flap could be preserved to cover the stump by continuing the interdigital incision distal and abaxial at the palmar and dorsal aspect of the digit and along the proximal aspect of the coronary band. Although this technique provides a superior cosmetic result and decreases subsequent care of the stump, it may prevent adequate drainage and extension of the infection. The authors therefore recommend this technique for a non-septic process of the digit (pedal fracture, digit luxation) or distal sepsis without extensive soft tissue infection (pedal osteitis).

ARTHRODESIS OF THE DIP JOINT

The techniques for arthrodesis of the DIP joint differ by surgical approach. Choice of a technique should be based on the anatomic structure infected and the location of existing draining tracts. Intact ligaments and tendons should be preserved, when possible, to keep the affected digit stable during the ankylosis procedure.

The advantages of ankylosis of the DIP joint in comparison to digit amputation are that cattle have a longer production life, the outcome is superior for a heavy animal or when the hind lateral or front medial digit is affected, and the healing result is more cosmetic and mechanically more stable. The disadvantages are that it is more expensive and technically demanding, more postoperative care is needed, and cattle have a slower return to previous production because of the pain engendered by the procedure and the long process of ankylosis.

ARTHRODESIS OF THE DIP JOINT BY THE SOLAR APPROACH

The surgery is performed under sedation and intravenous regional anesthesia. Cattle are restrained in a foot-trimming chute or in lateral recumbency with the affected leg uppermost. The plantar or palmar portion of the sole and the heel should be pared away until the sole can be indented easily. In severe and extensive infection of the DIP joint that originates from a solar lesion, the distal sesamoid bone and the joint can be felt through the wound and the sole already can be indented easily. The distal limb is prepared aseptically. A horizontal incision that starts 2 cm proximal to the coronary band is made along the plantar or palmar aspect of the second phalanx (Figure 11.4-9A). The tendinous portion of DDF muscle is cut from its insertion on the distal phalanx and resected proximally at about 2 to 3 inches from its insertion. The distal sesamoid bone is then exposed. If necrotic, it is removed easily with a rongeur (Figure 11.4-9B). If not, the two collateral ligaments and the distal ligaments are resected with a scalpel blade. The DIP joint then is exposed. Debridement of the joint from the solar wound through the dorsal hoof wall, 1 cm distal to the coronary band, is per-formed with a 1.3-cm drill bit. (Figure 11.4-10) The joint is curetted, and copious lavage is performed with isotonic solution. If the tendon sheath or the tendinous portion of the superficial digital flexor muscle is infected and necrotic, the incision is extended 2 to 3 cm proximally to the accessory digit to allow debridement and drainage. Any necrotic tissue at the heel and sole junction is removed. A wooden block is apposed with polymethylmethacrylate on the healthy digit of the affected limb (Figure 11.4-9C), and the claws are wired together with the affected digit in slight flexion. The wound is bandaged, and lavage is performed every other day, if possible. Systemic antibiotics are given for 2 to 3 weeks, and phenylbutazone is given as needed for the first 2 weeks.

Kostlin has reported a success rate of 85% for 281 cattle with this technique. This technique provides good visualization of the DIP joint, excellent drainage, and a good long-term prognosis. However, the approach to the joint is difficult. Even if not affected by the septic process, the tendinous portion of the DDF muscle and the distal sesamoid bone —as well as the tendon sheath —must be resected, which can create instability of the joints.

ARTHRODESIS OF THE DIP JOINT BY A DORSAL APPROACH

Surgery is performed with the cattle sedated and restrained in lateral recumbency. Intravenous regional anesthesia is administered. The surgical site is prepared aseptically. Two arthrostomies are performed either with a trephine that is 5.56 to 14 mm in diameter or by making a circular incision with a scalpel blade. The first arthrostomy is made into the DIP joint on the dorsal aspect of the digit, 0.5 cm proximal to the coronary band, abaxial or axial to the tendinous portion of the common (forelimb) or long (hindlimb) digital extensor muscles. The second arthrostomy is made 0.5 cm proximal to the coronary band caudal to the abaxial ligament of the DIP joint (Figure 11.4-11). When a draining tract communicates with the joint, the tract is enlarged with a trephine if needed, and a second arthrostomy is performed dorsal or palmar at the previously mentioned sides. Cartilage and necrotic bone are curetted through the arthrostomy sites. A wooden block with polymethylmethacrylate is placed on the healthy digit of the affected limb. Joint lavage is performed through the arthrostomies daily for 1 week or until the infection is controlled and the swelling is decreased. From the experience of the authors, cattle were slightly lame postoperatively for 4 months.

This technique is indicated if the distal sesamoid bone and the tendinous portion of the DDF tendon are not affected. The approach to the joint is easy to perform and less invasive. This technique also provides more

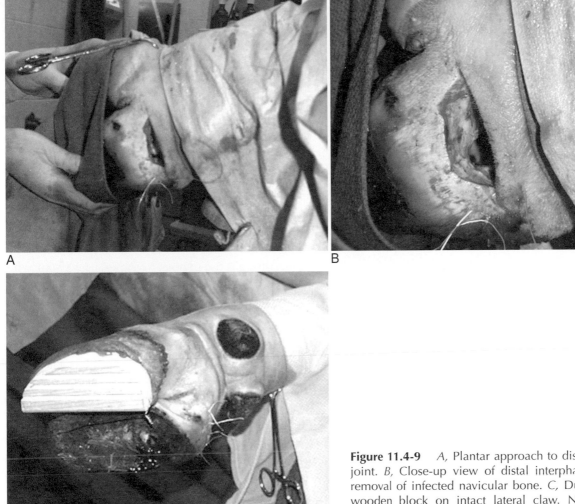

Figure 11.4-9 *A,* Plantar approach to distal interphalangeal joint. *B,* Close-up view of distal interphalangeal joint after removal of infected navicular bone. *C,* During placement of wooden block on intact lateral claw. Note curettage and removal of solar abscess on medial claw.

(Courtesy of Norm G. Ducharme; Cornell University)

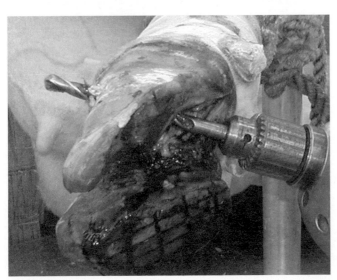

Figure 11.4-10 Facilitated ankylosis of the distal interphalangeal joint—solar approach.

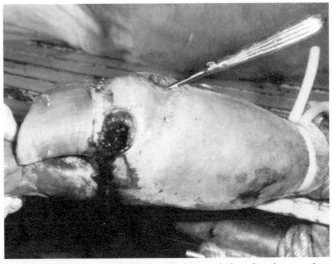

Figure 11.4-11 Facilitated ankylosis of the distal interphalangeal joint—dorsal approach.

stability to the joint, because the tendinous portion of the DDF muscle is not disrupted. Limited visibility of the DIP joint surfaces is attained with this surgical approach; therefore adequate removal of cartilage and necrotic bone is difficult to assess. Drainage is less efficient than with a solar approach.

RECOMMENDED READINGS

Anderson JF et al: Amputation of bovine medial dew claws on hindlegs as an aid in controlling teat trauma, *Vet Med/SAC* 71: 73-76, 1976.

Blikslager AT et al: Excision of the distal sesamoid bone for treatment of infection of the digit in a heifer, *J Am Vet Med Assoc* 201: 1905-1906, 1992.

Choquette-Levy L et al: A study of foot disease of dairy cattle in Quebec, *Can Vet J* 26: 278-281, 1985.

Desrochers A et al: Use of facilitated ankylosis in the treatment of septic arthritis of the distal interphalangeal joint in cattle: 12 cases (1987-1992). *J Am Vet Med Assoc* 206: 1923-1927, 1995.

Greenough PR and Ferguson JG: Alternatives to amputation, *Vet Clin North Am Food Anim Pract* 1: 195-203, 1985.

Kasari TR et al: Use of autogenous cancellous bone graft for treatment of osteolytic defects in the phalanges of three cattle, *J Am Vet Med Assoc* 201: 1053-1057, 1992.

Nuss K, Weaver MP: Resection of the distal interphalangeal joint in cattle: an alternative to digit amputation, *Vet Rec* 128: 540-543, 1991.

Pejsa TG et al: Digit amputation in cattle: 85 cases (1971-1990), *J Am Vet Med Assoc* 202: 981-984, 1993.

Septic Arthritis

André Desrochers

Septic arthritis is the most common condition that affects the joints in cattle (Russel, 1982). It can be caused by direct trauma to the articulation (primary), an adjacent infection to the articulation (secondary), or a systemic infection (tertiary). Direct trauma is a common cause of septic arthritis in adult cattle. Trauma does not have to go through the joint; periarticular infection that results from trauma may progress and extend to the joint at a later time. The distal limb, being less protected by soft tissue, is more susceptible to infection from external trauma, especially if it occurs in a heavily contaminated environment. A good example of a secondary septic arthritis in adults is a foot lesion (abscess/ulcer), which often extends directly into the coffin joint. Calves with umbilical infections or adults with endocarditis are at risk for polyarthritis from a remote site. The most common bacterial organisms isolated from septic arthritis in adult cattle are *Arcanobacterium pyogenes*, *Escherichia coli*, and other environmental bacteria. Cattle affected by *Haemophilus somnus* and *Mycoplasma* spp. usually have

more than one articulation infected. If only one cow is polyarthritic in a herd, endocarditis has to be included in the differential. Cardiac murmur upon auscultation, enlarged jugulars, ventral edema, and a history of recurrent fever should alert the clinician to the diagnosis of endocarditis.

Incidences of lameness related to digital diseases in cattle are well documented. On the other hand, the types and distribution of lameness in general is not well described. In Israel, arthritis accounts for 13.8% of lameness cases (Bargai, 1993). Regardless of the incidence or prevalence of septic arthritis in a herd, it is always potentially serious and detrimental to the productive life of the individual animal. Septic arthritis needs to be addressed quickly with aggressive treatment to control the infection and limit its degenerative action on articular cartilage.

Even though the synovial membrane is somewhat effective in eliminating bacterial contamination (up to 100 colonies of *Staphylococcus aureus*), villi inflammation allows microorganisms to attach and establish themselves. Bacteria directly damage cartilage as well as synovial membrane and fluid, but their immunological effects are the most serious causes of articular degeneration. Microorganisms are destroyed first by neutrophils and their enzymes (elastase, cathepsin, gelatinase, and collagenase). These enzymes destroy cartilage and its components as well as bacteria. Moreover, neutrophils and inflamed tissues release free radicals, which have the same harmful effects on articulation. The inflammation increases capillary permeability and lets other mediators arrive at the site of infection (kinin, factor of coagulation, cascade of the complement, fibrinolytic system). These mediators stimulate the synoviocytes and chondrocytes. The chondrocytes release mediators as MMP (matrix metalloproteinase), which decreases proteoglycan production. The reduced production and increased degradation of proteoglycans deteriorates the physical properties of cartilage, thus decreasing its compressive potential and making it more susceptible to trauma. The presence of fibrin on cartilage and synovial membrane decreases the nutritive effectiveness of synovial fluid and inhibits diffusion of antibiotics used to treat septic arthritis (Bertone, 1996).

Diagnosis

Cattle affected with septic arthritis are severely lame. Direct trauma to the joint is the principal cause of septic arthritis in cattle. Infection may result from external trauma; a wound over a swollen joint should arouse suspicion of septic arthritis (Figure 11.4-12). On closer examination, one may detect synovial fluid flowing freely from the laceration. A wound should be cautiously inves-

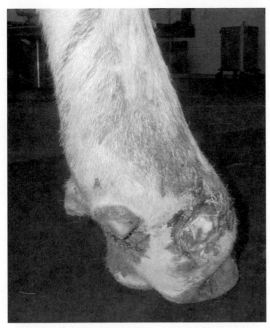

Figure 11.4-12   Contaminated laceration at the pastern area.

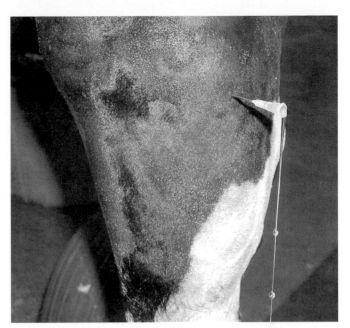

Figure 11.4-14   Arthrocentesis of the tarsocrural joint.

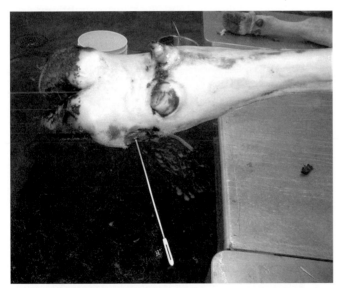

Figure 11.4-13   A malleable probe was inserted through a tract into the proximal interphalangeal joint.

tigated to avoid contaminating the joint if the synovial membrane is still intact. A malleable probe can be used to evaluate a draining tract (Figure 11.4-13). Arthrocentesis is performed in the area away from the wound to avoid contamination. After surgical preparation of the site, synovial fluid is withdrawn and conserved for further analysis. The existence of communication from a wound adjacent to the joint is verified by injecting 10 to 20 ml of a sterile solution into the joint.

Ancillary tests are helpful in differentiating or confirming a diagnosis and finding the causative agent. Arthrocentesis can be easily performed by placing the needle into the area with maximum joint distension (Figure 11.4-14). Macroscopic examination of synovial fluid is often diagnostic (increased turbidity, decreased viscosity, fibrin). If macroscopic changes are subtle, the sample should be submitted for cellular counts and differential. Cell counts greater than 3.0 thousand/μl, a neutrophil proportion higher than 75%, and total protein greater than 40 g/L indicate septic arthritis (Rohde, 2000). Microorganisms are not always seen on cytology. A positive synovial fluid culture provides important information for choosing appropriate antibiotics. Bacterial isolation and identification are obtained in only 50% of the samples submitted. A blood culture medium reportedly increases the likelihood of a positive culture to 70%. Affected animals already on antibiotics have a decreased chance of in vitro bacterial growth. Recently developed sensitive molecular techniques such as polymerase chain reaction (PCR) show promise for increasing the identification rate of microorganisms. Swabbing an open joint through a wound results in multiple bacteria being isolated because of severe environmental contamination and will not be diagnostic.

Radiographic examination helps a clinician specify a diagnosis and establish a prognosis. A portable radiographic machine can be used for the distal limbs, but its power is limited for more proximal articulations like the stifle and coxofemoral joints. It is imperative to take two radiographic views—a craniocaudal and lateromedial. Chronic presentation is common in food animals. For this reason, radiographic lesions are often obvious (Figure 11.4-15). When interpreting radiographic views, the clinician must remember that osseous lesions can only be seen when the actual process is 10 to 14 days old. Therefore the infection can have already begun with no lesions seen until the end of this period. Bone tissues must undergo a demineralization greater than 50% to be visible on radiographs. Cartilage is not visible on radiographs. Soft tissue swelling with gas present can be seen in certain cases, and increased articular space will be observed in acute conditions (Figure 11.4-15). Chronic lesions such as subchondral bone lysis, decreased joint space from articular destruction, osteomyelitis, periosteal reaction, and bony proliferation (Figure 11.4-16) are more visible. These lesions can be focal or multicentric. With chronic septic arthritis, severe bone neoformation is observed more frequently in adults than in calves where bone lysis is more typical (Figure 11.4-17; see Section 15.4 for management of septic arthritis in calves).

Soft tissues are better evaluated with ultrasound examination. Synovial fluid and membrane, joint surface, and surrounding connective tissues are easily seen within

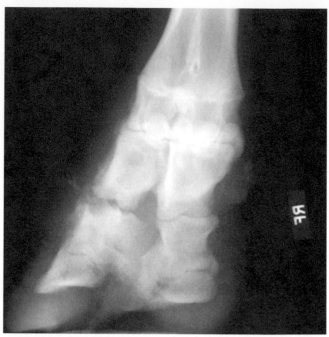

Figure 11.4-16 Dorsopalmar lateral to medial oblique radiographs of infected medial middle interphalangeal joint in an adult cow. Note the lysis at the articular surface and proliferative bone production at the dorsal aspect of P1 and P2.

(Courtesy of Dr. N. Dykes; Cornell University.)

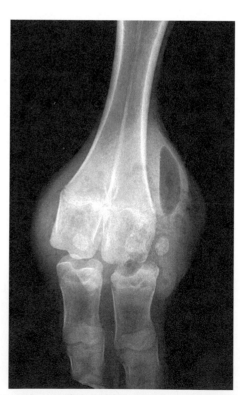

Figure 11.4-15 Radiographic image of a septic fetlock, dorsoplantar view. There is severe soft tissue swelling, presence of gas, and increased joint space.

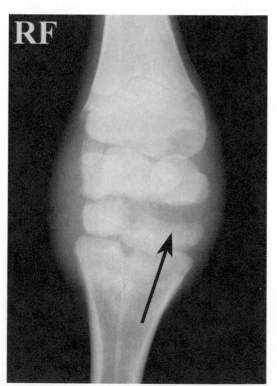

Figure 11.4-17 Dorsopalmar radiographs of a 2-month-old calf with septic arthritis of the middle intercarpal and carpometacarpal joint. Note the severe lysis of the 3rd (arrow).

(Courtesy of Dr. N. Dykes; Cornell University.)

certain limits when ones uses the proper equipment and technique, depending on the joint being ultrasound (see Chapter 2). In acute septic arthritis, the synovial fluid volume increases, and echogenic (grey) material (fibrin) can be seen floating in the joint. Cartilage is anechogenic (black) because of its high water content. Subchondral bone is hyperechogenic (white), and lysis or a defect will change its contour. If a laceration is present, structures surrounding the joint (tendons, ligament, and joint capsule) are evaluated and may help the clinician make a more precise prognosis and apply the appropriate treatment.

Treatment

Before starting any treatment, the owner must be fully aware of the consequences from the condition and the short- and long-term prognoses. A good clinical assessment of the joint is essential in choosing the appropriate treatment. Multiple treatment possibilities exist for septic arthritis, but the following basic principles must be followed: 1) control the infection; 2) remove abnormal joint fluid; 3) control inflammation; and 4) restore joint function. In any case, the primary cause should be treated. Calves with omphalophlebitis have to undergo surgery rapidly before other joint infections occur. A laceration around joints has to be debrided, with the treatment repeated as necessary.

ANTIMICROBIAL USES

In cattle, bacterial infection is the major cause of septic arthritis; therefore antibiotics are used to control the infection. Choosing the appropriate antibiotic is based on the suspected microorganism involved, the antibiotic's ability to work in the presence of fibrin and an acidic environment, route of administration, cost of treatment, and withdrawal time for meat and milk (see appendix). Penicillin procaine is the first choice antibiotic for treating *Arcanobacterium pyogenes,* the most common microorganism isolated in cattle. Antibiotics effective against gram-negative *Bacteroides* should be considered to treat a severely contaminated wound. In general, all antibiotics penetrate and diffuse well into an acute septic joint. The presence of fibrin or necrotic tissue decreases the effectiveness of most antibiotics; therefore adjunct treatments such as joint lavage or drainage (as described in the section on Joint Lavage/Drainage) should be an essential part of the treatment plan. Antimicrobial treatment should be continued 2 to 3 weeks after an animal begins to clinically improve. The standard systemic routes of administration are intravenous, intramuscular, and subcutaneous. Oral medication does not achieve sufficient concentration to

adequately treat joint infections. The clinician should be conscious that any extended treatment duration may change withdrawal time. Other routes should be considered: intraarticular injection, intravenous under tourniquet, and antibiotics incorporated into a slow-release medium.

The main advantage of intraarticular injection is a higher minimal inhibitory concentration (MIC) at the site for a longer time period. Gentamycin injected intraarticularly in horses has shown an antibiotic concentration superior to MIC for 24 hours, but this antimicrobial should never be used in cattle in North America. In cattle, intraarticular injections (IA) have been used empirically based on extrapolation from scientific data in other species. The author recommends intravenous preparation of ceftiofur (150 mg IA). Clinicians must respect the principles of extra-label use of antibiotics when they choose this and other routes of administration. Intravenous injection of cephalosporin has been well investigated in cattle. Regional intravenous perfusion of antimicrobials has many advantages: it reaches infected tissue by diffusion at a far greater concentration (10 fold) than after IV administration. In addition, the local tissue concentrations remain higher than after IV administration; thus a lower dose may be effective. The main disadvantages are the need to apply and maintain a good tourniquet and injection site morbidity. Regional perfusion is performed as follows. A catheter is applied proximal to the joint to medicate and is placed into a local distended vein. Using aseptic technique, the clinician should place a catheter after considering the best protection obtainable. Therefore place the catheter where a bandage can be easily applied and maintained. Alternatively, repeated regional intravenous injection can be given. Appropriate antibiotics are diluted to a 30- to 60-ml volume and administered slowly via a catheter. The following antimicrobial doses have been used: ceftiofur 250 mg, 1 g cephazolin, and 1 million IU of potassium penicillin G.

Implantation of nonabsorbable or absorbable, slow-releasing molecules combined with antibiotics has shown promise. Polymethylmethacrylate (PMMA) in different combinations with antibiotics has been used in horses and humans to treat chronic osteomyelitis. Without a doubt, the slow release of antibiotics for 1 to 2 months at concentrations superior to MIC is an advantage for conditions that necessitate long-term antibiotics. Although PMMA beads are not commercially available in North America, they are easy to make. The antimicrobials are added to the polymer powder and thoroughly mixed before adding the liquid monomer. After the liquid polymer is added, the preparation is mixed until it is uniform. Elongated beads approximately 2 cm long by 5 mm wide are made in a line around a No. 2

nonabsorbable monofilament suture (polypropylene or nylon) to facilitate later removal. Recovery of antibiotics in PMMA beads for years after implantation has been documented, thus necessitating bead removal in farm animals. Typically 1 million units of potassium penicillin or 1 g of ceftiofur are added to the mixture. Unlike PMMA beads, absorbable preparations don't have to be removed. Recent research with gentamycin-impregnated (not allowed in the United States) collagen sponges used to treat chronic septic arthritis in cattle has been promising. Future research will result in new molecules in combination with appropriate antibiotics for cattle.

JOINT LAVAGE/DRAINAGE

Because infected joints are painful, adequate analgesia, anesthesia, and immobilization are necessary for joint lavage and drainage. Most joint lavages are performed under sedation, and the animal should be immobilized in lateral recumbency. If arthroscopy is used to treat septic arthritis, the procedure should be performed under general anesthesia. If available, a trimming chute with the animal standing or in lateral recumbency works very well. Removal of infected tissue, debris, and inflammatory mediators in the joint is essential for normal return to previous function. The goals of joint lavage are to remove debris and dilute the abnormal constituents in the joint with a large volume of sterile fluids. Joint lavage is performed in different ways: tidal, through-and-through, and arthroscopy. Aspiration and irrigation are performed through the same needle in a tidal lavage, which creates a lot of turbulence and dislodges the debris. With this technique, the volume of fluids injected is limited because the tendency is to use the same fluid in the syringe for a long period of time. The author often combines this technique with a through-and-through lavage. The size of the needle used by the author is 16 to 14 g. Using a large volume of fluids is easy with through-and-through lavage. A good knowledge of anatomy and communication between articulation compartments is essential for efficient treatment. Two needles are necessary for this technique. One needle is inserted for ingress and the other for egress. The needles have to be far from each other to avoid direct communication and exit of the fluids without adequate irrigation of the cavity. Intermittently blocking the egress needle distends the joint, thus improving lavage. The volume injected depends on the joint itself and severity of the infection. For example, the distal interphalangeal joint needs 250 ml in comparison to a large articulation like the stifle, with which 3 liters is necessary. If fibrin is present, needles have a tendency to clog; therefore arthroscopy or arthrotomy has to be considered. The fluids used have to be isoosmotic, isotonic, and with a pH close to 7.4. Sterile Ringer's solution, balanced physiological solution, and physiologic saline are types of fluid that are used commonly for joint irrigation. Adding disinfectant or antibiotics to fluids has been debated, but the total volume of the solution injected is more important. Joint lavage is repeated every day or every other day 2 to 3 times, depending on the facility and character of the animal. More articular lavages are often necessary in fibrinous septic arthritis. Macroscopically, the synovial fluids should be clearer with increased viscosity. Leucocyte count and total protein concentration will decrease if infection is controlled. More important, clinical signs should improve 24 to 48 hours after treatment initiation.

Arthroscopy provides a good lavage and drainage of the joint but also helps the clinician visualize the joint for a more precise prognosis. Because athletic performance is not an issue in farm animals, arthroscopy is not routinely performed in cattle for economic reasons.

Arthrotomy is performed if medical treatment has failed (within a few days) or if the joint is full of fibrin or pus so that a through-and-through lavage is impossible. Arthrotomy sites are the same as those for an arthrocentesis. The incision should be long enough to allow adequate drainage and introduction of forceps to remove fibrin. More than one incision per joint is necessary to access the joint compartments completely and improve debridement. To prevent ascending infection, the incisions are covered with a regular bandage or suture stent bandage (Figure 11.4-18), and additional lavages are performed if needed, usually 2 to 4 times. After 24 to 48 hours, the incision often has to be reopened to access the joint cavity because of its tendency to seal with fibrin

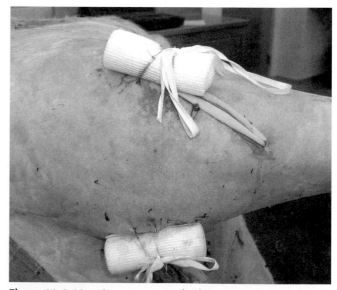

Figure 11.4-18   Stents were applied to protect the arthrotomy incisions of the stifle (cow in lateral recumbency).

or from swollen adjacent tissues. Joint lavage is performed until synovial fluids are clear and the fibrin removed from the cavity is negligible.

ARTHRODESIS

Arthrodesis is the final solution when no treatments have been effective or because chronicity of the disease prevents restoration of joint function. Articulations of the distal limb are easily arthrodesed (fetlock, proximal, and distal interphalangeal joints). Arthrodesis of the distal interphalangeal joint has been described extensively in the literature with a very good prognosis (see Arthrodesis of the of the DIP Joint by the Solar Approach in this Section). Severe carpal and tarsal joint infections have also been treated with arthrodesis. In all cases, the joint is flushed with local antibiotics after debridement, and parenteral antibiotics are continued for 3 weeks.

For high-motion joints such as the carpus and tarsus, the clinician must consider the facilities (stall or small pasture), value, and purpose of the animal before he or she proposes surgery to the owner. In *carpal arthrodesis,* the animal is positioned in lateral or, preferably, dorsal recumbency, and a transverse dorsal skin incision is made at the most distended portion of the joint (Figure 11.4-19). The incision is extended sharply to the joint surface, transecting vessels and extensor tendons. Often the

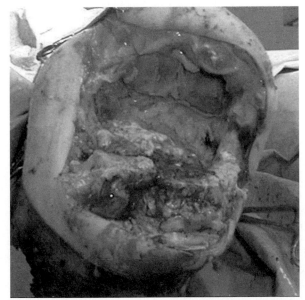

Figure 11.4-19 For arthrodesis of chronic septic arthritis in a calf, a transverse incision is made at the level of the carpal row of the carpal bone to be removed. The entire affected middle row of carpal bone has been removed and the joint thoroughly debrided.

(Courtesy of Dr. N. Ducharme; Cornell University.)

extensor tendon sheaths are infected and need to be debrided. All infected tissue is curetted and removed. If one or more of the carpal bones are severely lytic and infected, they are dissected free, and the entire row of carpal bone is removed. During debridement, one should take care not to disrupt the palmar ligaments and support of the joint or enter the carpal canal. Synovial membrane and surrounding infected tissues are removed through excision or curettage (see Figure 11.4-19). The skin is closed with simple interrupted sutures, and a full leg cast is applied. A cast should be maintained until arthrodesis (usually 3 months) and should be changed at an appropriate frequency (at least every 3 weeks for a calf and every 6 weeks for adults).

In *tarsal arthrodesis,* the animal is positioned in dorsal recumbency. Tarsal joint arthrodesis is performed as follows. For tarsocrural arthrodesis, a vertical skin incision is made on the most distended dorsomedial pouch of the tarsocrural joint. The incision is sharply extended until the joint is reached. A similar arthrotomy is made on the caudolateral-lateral aspect of the joint immediately between the lateral malleolus of the tibia and the tuber calcanei. A final vertical arthrotomy is made on the caudomedial pouch immediately caudal to the medial malleolus; the clinician must be very careful not to enter the tarsal sheath. The skin incision in the final vertical arthrotomy is extended with Mayo scissors to avoid inadvertent entry into the tarsal sheath. Thorough debridement is performed as described earlier. Fascial planes are closed when possible, and the skin is reapposed with simple interrupted sutures.

For *distal tarsal joint* arthrodesis, a vertical incision is made on the craniomedial side, centered on the target joint. The incision is extended to the joint, but it is far more difficult to identify the joint surface. The area is curetted as much as possible, and the infected joint capsule is resected. A 3.2-mm drill bit is placed parallel to the articular surface and used to remove as much surface as possible. The skin is closed with simple interrupted sutures. In both cases, a full leg cast is applied for approximately 12 weeks with regular cast changes (at least every 3 weeks for a calf and every 6 weeks for adults).

Antiinflammatory drug control decreases the harmful effects caused by synthesis of prostaglandins and various cytokines in the joint and the increased stability decreases the pain. Consequently, the animal will be more comfortable, have a better appetite, and carry more weight on the affected limb, which minimizes the harmful effects on the opposite limb (drops of the fetlock, angular limb deformities).

Sodium iodides (30 g/450 kg, IV followed by 60 g of organic iodine P.O. for 2 weeks, discontinue for 2 weeks and reinstitute for 2 weeks until signs of iodism are displayed [i.e., dry skin at the head, neck, and shoulder]) are used for their antiinflammatory and antimicrobial activity. It seems particularly effective when inflammation is chronic and granulomatous (*A. pyogenes*).

Prognosis

In cattle, the prognosis is generally good for return to previous function and productivity. The prognosis depends upon the time of presentation, amount of bone lysis and proliferation (radiographic evaluation), and degree of extracapsular ankylosis. Two studies assess the success rate for treatment of septic arthritis at between 72% and 85%. Cattle with septic tarsi have less chance of recovery. In another study, arthroscopic lavage and implantation of antimicrobial-impregnated collagen sponges was successful in 12 out of 14 animals treated.

After arthrodesis of the carpus, an 87% success rate has been reported if no carpal bone is removed and a 72% success rate if one row of carpal bone needs to be removed, whereas a 35% success rate was seen if both carpal rows were removed. After arthrodesis of the tarsus, an 87% success rate has been reported.

RECOMMENDED READINGS

Bargai U, Levin D: Lameness in the Israeli dairy herd: a national survey of incidence, types, distribution, and estimated cost (first report), *Isr J Vet Med* 48: 88-91, 1993.

Bertone A: Infection arthritis. In McIlwraith CW, Trotter GW: *Joint disease in the horse*, Philadelphia, 1996, WB Saunders.

Farrow CS: The radiologic investigation of bovine lameness associated with infection, *Vet Clin North Am Food Anim Pract* 15: 425-441, 1999.

Gagnon H, Ferguson JG, Papich MG, Bailey JV: Single-dose pharmacokinetics of cefazolin in bovine synovial fluid after intravenous regional injection, *J Vet Pharmacol Ther* 17: 31-37, 1994.

Kopcha M, Kaneene JB, Shea ME et al: Use of nonsteroidal antiinflammatory drugs in food animal practice, *J Am Vet Med Assoc* 201: 1868-1872, 1992.

Meier C: Procedure in purulent arthritis of adult cattle and clinical experience with joint lavage, *Praktische Tierarzt* 78: 893-906, 1997.

Rohde C, Anderson DE, Desrochers A, et al: Synovial fluid analysis in cattle: a review of 130 cases, *Vet Surg* 29: 341-346, 2000.

Russel AM, Rowland GJ, Shaw SR, Weaver AD: Survey of lameness in British dairy cattle, *Vet Rec* 111: 155-160, 1982.

Steiner A et al: Arthroscopic lavage and implantation of gentamicin-impregnated collagen sponges for treatment of chronic septic arthritis in cattle, *Vet Comp Orthop Traumatol* 12: 64-69, 1999.

Van Huffel X, Steenhaut M, Imschoot et al: Carpal joint arthrodesis as a treatment for chronic septic arthritis in calves and cattle, *Vet Surg* 18: 304-311, 1989.

Verschooten F, De Moor A, Steenhaut M, et al: Surgical and conservative treatment of infectious arthritis in cattle, *J Am Vet Med Assoc* 165: 271-275, 1974.

Verschooten F, Vermeiren D, Devriese L: Bone infection in the bovine appendicular skeleton: a clinical, radiographic and experimental study, *Vet Radiol Ultrasound* 41: 250-260, 2000.

Ligamentous Damage and Wounds to the Stifle

William H. Crawford and
Norm G. Ducharme

Lacerations Associated with the Stifle

Puncture wounds to the stifle may result from machinery or cleaning tools, fencing materials, or sticks and horns, all of which carry high levels of environmental bacteria. These wounds need to be assessed to determine whether joints have been penetrated or neurovascular tissues injured. In the bovine, the lateral femorotibial joint compartment reflects distally around the origins of the peroneus tertius and long digital extensor muscles. Therefore deep wounds to the dorsolateral limb in the area of the proximal tibia should be evaluated for involvement of these structures. The joint should be examined to see whether collateral or patellar ligaments have been injured. Radiographs may be useful in determining the involvement of joints or ligaments in a deep wound. The treatment of wounds in the stifle area requires the application of sound principles of wound management. Debridement of traumatized, devitalized, contaminated, and ischemic tissue is indicated. If the wound is contaminated and adequate debridement and lavage is conducted, closure of the wound may be indicated. However, if the wound is chronic (usually greater than 12 hours duration) and untreated, it is likely that bacterial contamination will have progressed to an infection. Under these circumstances, wound culture, debridement and lavage need to be conducted. A provision for wound drainage must be made, and in most cases wound closure is not indicated. Broad-spectrum antibiotics are indicated for deep wounds and should be changed to target-specific antibiotics after wound culture and sensitivity results are obtained. If the joint spaces of the stifle have been invaded by a traumatic incident, large volume joint lavage is necessary to provide the best prognosis. Adequate lavage of a mature cow stifle requires a minimum volume of 5 liters of isotonic electrolyte solution. Appropriate antibiotics may be added to the lavage solution.

In cases where heavy contamination of the joint exists, arthroscopy provides visualization of the joint and is conducive for directing joint lavage, fibrin removal, and debridement to best advantage. If arthroscopic equipment is not available, an arthrotomy has a better chance for successful debridement and lavage than ingress and egress needles (see section on Joint Lavage/Drainage).

To prevent dehiscence, a lateral (or medial) arthrotomy approach should not extend beyond the patellar attachment of the lateral (or medial) patellar ligament. If heavy contamination or septic arthritis is present, the arthrotomy site(s) should be left partially open to allow drainage. The arthrotomy wound left open to drain should be protected from the environment by placing a loop of sutures around the wound, so a stent bandage (see Figure 11.4-18) can be applied and changed as needed until the joint no longer communicates with the environment.

Cranial Cruciate Ligament Injury

Dairy and beef breeds incur injuries to the cranial cruciate ligament (CCL) in males and females. The CCL may completely rupture or be partially torn. The injury often is related to a single traumatic event, but chronic injury may occur in bulls as a result of mounting and thrusting. The instability caused by CCL tears leads to osteoarthritis. However, the reverse is also possible: osteoarthritis leads to synovitis and chronic joint inflammation, which may precede CCL injury.

Cattle with acute CCL rupture are usually nonweight-bearing or partially weight-bearing, but some weight-bearing function is achieved as the injury becomes chronic. Instability between the femur and tibia may be observed in weight-bearing patients; a "snapping" action occurs when the tibia slips forward relative to the femur. If the tibia is displaced cranially relative to the femur, a drawer sign may be elicited as follows: the examiner's knee is placed on the caudal aspect of the hock while the tibia is retracted caudally by placing both hands over the tibial crest (Figure 11.4-20). In addition, internal rotation of the tibia relative to the femur is greater than normal in stifles with CCL rupture. This can be evaluated by having the hock and stifle slightly flexed while the examiner applies outward rotational force to the distal limb (Figure 11.4-21).

Joint effusion is usually present with CCL injury. In acute injuries, there is usually marked distension of the joint because of hemorrhage and increased synovial effusion. In more chronic cases, fibrosis of the periarticular soft tissue may make synovial distension difficult to appreciate.

In a lateral-to-medial radiograph of a normal stifle in a standing animal, the tibial intercondylar eminence is completely overlapped by the femoral condyles. In CCL injuries, the tibia is displaced forward, so the intercondylar eminence will be located cranial to the femoral condyles (see Figure 11.4-22). Additionally, radiographs may provide evidence of fractures of the intercondylar eminence, avulsion fractures at the insertion sites of the

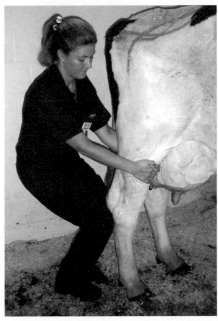

Figure 11.4-20   Drawer test in cattle. The examiner's knee is placed on the caudal aspect of the hock while the tibia is retracted caudally by placing both hands over the tibial crest. Increased laxity and crepitus can be detected with this test.

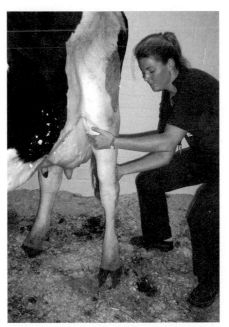

Figure 11.4-21   External rotation of stifle to be followed by internal rotation; this identifies increased range of rotation (because of increase internal rotation) and crepitus in cattle with cranial cruciate tear.

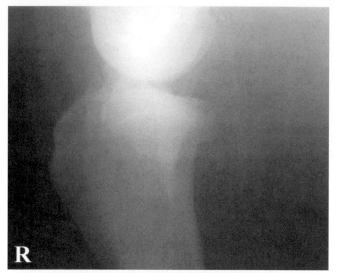

Figure 11.4-22   Mature Holstein-Friesian bull with a cranial cruciate tear of 3 weeks duration. The right tibia is displaced cranially as evidenced by the cranial position of the inter-condylar eminence relative to the middle third of the femoral condyle. Extensive irregular new bone formation associated with the intercondylar eminence and tibial plateau is present.

(Courtesy of Dr. Peter Scrivani; Cornell University.)

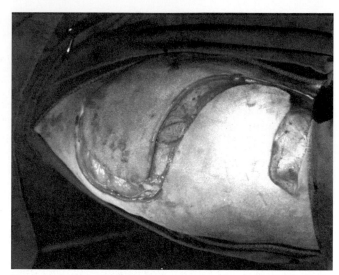

Figure 11.4-23   S-shaped incision used for approach for stifle imbrication.

CCL or medial collateral ligaments, mineralization of the CCL, or other evidence of degenerative joint disease (Figure 11.4-22). Joint instability caused by CCL injury often results in tearing or crushing of the meniscus, which may lead to calcification and/or decreased joint space in the medial femorotibial joint. The caudal-to-cranial radiographic view on a weight-bearing leg provides an evaluation of the meniscal integrity.

Conservative management of CCL disruption is usually unsatisfactory because of the secondary changes that result from joint instability. A degenerative progression occurs, starting with maceration of the medial meniscus, followed by subsequent loss of articular hyaline cartilage, and finally erosion of the subchondral bone of the femoral condyles. Box stall confinement and antiinflammatory medication may be beneficial only in partial rupture of the CCL.

Two surgical procedures are used to provide stability to the femorotibial joint and reduce the progression of osteoarthritis. The simplest procedure is an extraarticular plication of the dorsomedial and dorsolateral retinacular tissues. The second procedure provides intraarticular stabilization of the femorotibial joint.

PREOPERATIVE AND OPERATIVE PREPARATION

Animals are fasted for 36 hours and administered a loading dose of a nonsteroidal antiinflammatory agent (phenylbutazone) and broad-spectrum antibiotics (such

as cephalosporins). The animal is induced and prepared for general anesthesia. Food is withheld for 48 hours and water for 12 hours before anesthetic induction. General anesthesia with halothane, isoflurane, or sevoflurane is recommended with a closed circuit positive pressure ventilation system (see Chapter 6). The animal is placed in lateral recumbency with the affected limb uppermost and elevated at 30 degrees from the horizontal. The limb is aseptically prepared from the hock to 10 cm rostral to the tuber coxae and extending to the dorsal midline.

STIFLE JOINT IMBRICATION
Surgical Procedure

After appropriate draping, an S-shaped incision that starts 5 cm proximal to the patella and extends first medially is made on the cranial aspect of the stifle joint until 5 cm distal to the tibial crest (Figure 11.4-23). The incision is extended with scissors through the loosened areolar subcutaneous tissue and superficial fascia until the strong periarticular fascia is encountered. Synovial fluid must be removed from the stifle joint to achieve maximal imbrication as it interferes with imbrication (Figure 11.4-24). With the limb in nearly full extension, a first row of imbricating suture pattern (Lembert) with a nonabsorbable suture material (no.-5 polyester* or polyblend†) is placed at the level of the lateral femoropatellar ligament and extended from the dorsal aspect of the patella distally to the tibial crest (Figure 11.4-25). The procedure is also performed on the medial aspect of the stifle joint centered over the medial femoropatellar ligament (Figure 11.4-25). A second row is placed over

*Ethibon, Ethicon Inc., Johnson & Johnson; Piscataway, NJ
†Fiberwire, Arthrex, Naples, FL

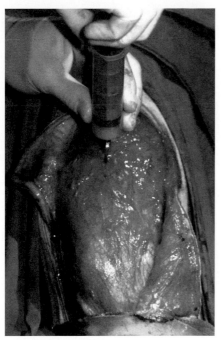

Figure 11.4-24 Exposure of periarticular fascia immediately after skin incision and extending the incision through the superficial fascia. Synovial fluid is being removed before imbrication.

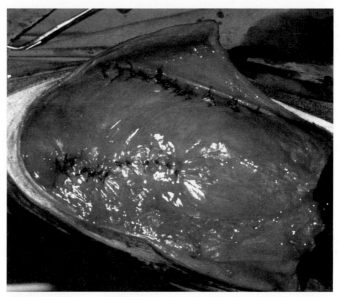

Figure 11.4-25 Intraoperative view after placement of imbrication sutures on the medial and lateral aspect of the stifle joint.

the first row, and a third row is placed if the fascia is strong enough to hold. The number of overlapping rows of imbricating sutures is limited by the strength of the periarticular tissue. If the sutures start tearing the fascia, no further sutures are placed. Placement of an antirotating suture from the lateral attachment of the gastrocnemius muscle on the femoral condyle to the fascia near the tibial crest has been described. Because the common peroneal nerve is located close to the lateral collateral ligament, inadvertent encroachment of the common peroneal nerve can occur; therefore the authors do not recommend placing an antirotating suture.

The superficial fascia is closed with no. 2 absorbable suture material in a simple interrupted or cruciate pattern. The subcutaneous tissue is closed with a simple continuous pattern (1 absorbable suture material), while the skin is closed using a Ford interlocking pattern or a simple cruciate pattern (no. 1 nonabsorbable suture material). A stent is then sutured on to relieve the tension on the incision. The stent bandage is kept in place as long as it is dry, up to a maximum of 7 days.

REPLACEMENT OF CRANIAL CRUCIATE LIGAMENT
Surgical Procedure

The following technique was originally described from independent studies by Moss and Crawford with modifications suggested by Ducharme and Eggleston. In cattle, the superficial gluteal and biceps femoris muscles are continuous and form the gluteobiceps muscle. The medial fascia of the gluteobiceps muscle is 5 to 7 mm thick and approximately 7 cm wide. Distally, the fibers of this fascia are continuous with the fibers of the lateral patellar ligament. A strip of tissue harvested from the medial fascia of the gluteobiceps muscle and the lateral patellar ligament can form a graft. Using a modification of the over-the-top technique, the clinician forms an intraarticular replacement for the disrupted CCL.

After aseptic preparation and draping, a skin incision is made from the major trochanter to the lateral aspect of the patella. The incision is then curved so it is parallel to the lateral distal patellar ligament and extended to the tibial crest. The fascia lata is incised over and parallel to the plane between the vastus lateralis and gluteobiceps muscles. A full thickness strip of fascia 2 cm wide is sharply dissected from the cranial margin of the medial gluteobiceps muscle. The dissection is continued distally through the fibrocartilaginous thickening over the lateral epicondylar bursa. The graft is extended further distally by dividing the lateral patellar ligament (in a cranio/caudal plane) parallel to its fibers down to the tibial crest while maintaining 50 percent of the lateral distal patellar ligament. A continuous graft is thereby formed, attached distally to the tibial crest, which contains the lateral half of the lateral patellar ligament, a portion of the suprabursal fibrocartilage, and approximately

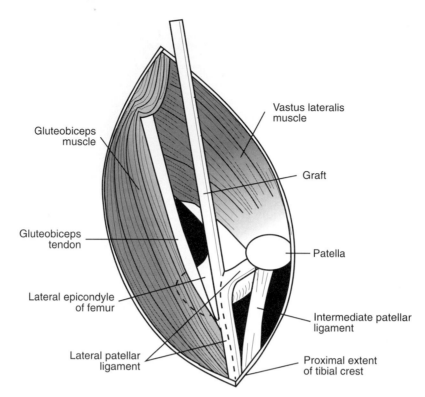

Figure 11.4-26   Lateral view of the right stifle, which shows the autogenous graft formed from the right gluteobiceps fascia and the lateral patellar ligament.

(Redrawn from Crawford WH: Intraarticular replacement of bovine cranial cruciate ligaments with an autogenous fascial graft, *Vet Surg* 19: 380-388, 1990.)

20 cm of the gluteobiceps fascia (see Figure 11.4-26). The femorotibial joint is approached by an arthrotomy between the lateral and middle patellar ligaments. The patellar fat pad is reflected and the insertion of the CCL inspected digitally. Because of the depth of the insertion of the CCL on the tibial eminence, meaningful visual assessment of the joint and ligament damage is difficult. The cranial segments of the menisci may be evaluated. Bone fragments and crushed or torn segments of menisci should be removed if they are accessible. A custom-manufactured, curved graft passer* (Figure 11.4-27A) is passed through the intercondylar space in a cranial-to-caudal direction and is directed through the caudal joint capsule and popliteus muscles to exit through the fibers of origin of the lateral gastrocnemius muscle at the lateral epicondyle (Figure 11.4-27B). A 120-cm length of 8-mm-wide umbilical tape is threaded into the eye of the graft passer and brought out through the arthrotomy incision by retracting the graft passer. Cutting umbilical tape at the graft passer eye leaves two 60-cm lengths of tape in the route taken by the graft passer; one length is designated as a spare in case the first

attempt to pull the graft through the tissue tunnel fails. Pulling the graft through the tissues can be difficult. Because of these difficulties, the following steps are done. First, a length of sterile gauze (soaked in 1% caboxymethyl Cellulose, SCMC) is tied to the umbilical tape leader and pulled through the intercondylar space. With the joint held in 100 degrees of flexion, the gauze is drawn back and forth to enlarge and lubricate the passageway. The graft is then inserted approximately 7.5 cm within the lumen of a 10 mm diameter sterile braided nylon rope (length-2 feet [60 cm]) and is secured to the edge of the graft by using interrupted sutures of no. 1 suture material. The other end of the rope is secured to the gauze. The rope and graft are lubricated with sterile 1% SCMC water-soluble lubricant jelly, and, with the stifle in 100 degrees of flexion, the rope leader and attached graft are pulled through the passageway. The graft enters the intertrochlear space best with the joint in 100-degree flexion while it exits the space best in partial extension. Therefore the stifle is placed in approximately 100 degrees of flexion until it appears to wedge and then is extended 20 degrees while traction is applied simultaneously. Cycling the joint through the range of motion described earlier with continuous traction facilitates graft passing. In this fashion, a 20-mm wide fascial

---

*Messer Innovative Products; Cottage Grove, WI

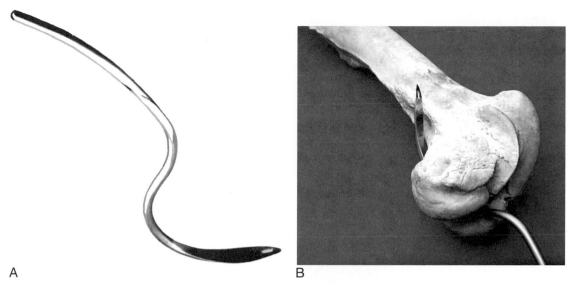

Figure 11.4-27 *A,* Graft passer manufactured by Messer Innovative Products, Cottage Grove, Wis. The overall length is 30 cm and the blade width is 12 mm. The radius of curvature in the instruments varies from 6.5 to 10 cm, depending on the size of the patient. *B,* Anatomical specimen that shows path of the graft passer. The instrument enters between the middle and lateral patellar ligaments and exits through the muscle fibers of the lateral head of the gastrocnemius muscle at the lateral epicondyle.

strip can be pulled through the tissue tunnel. One should evaluate how much of the lateral belly of the gastrocnemius muscle is present between the caudal aspect of the femur and graft. If the graft has exited the caudad aspect of the joint too far from the caudal aspect of the femur, the lateral belly of the gastrocnemius muscle can be partially incised so the graft can be placed against the femur and therefore under greater tension. An attachment site for the proximal segment of the graft is prepared by elevating a 6-cm-wide section of periosteum from the lateral epicondyle. With the stifle placed in approximately 140 degrees of flexion and the tibia slightly externally rotated, the fascial strip is pulled tightly so it lays just proximal to the lateral epicondyle. An assistant holds the graft under tension as it is stapled to the prepared area of the epicondyle with a 1.75 cm bone staple.* The free end of the strip is folded caudad over the stapled attachment, and a second staple is placed to include a double thickness of the strip. Alternatively, a three-hole narrow dynamic compression plate[†] can be placed over the strip to anchor it to the epicondylar bone by using two 44-mm-long, 4.5-mm-diameter cortical bone screws[‡] to compress the fascial strip between the bone and plate (Figure 11.4-28). The free end of the strip is then folded back on itself and sutured in place with #5 nonabsorbable suture material.[†,‡]

The most common postoperative complication is seroma formation and subsequent wound breakdown. A multilayer closure with heavy surgical materials is required to prevent synovial leakage and fascial disruption. The gluteobiceps and vastus lateralis muscles are reapposed by using #2 absorbable sutures (polyglactin 910[§]) in a simple continuous pattern. The joint capsule is closed with similar material placed in a simple cruciate pattern. The transected lateral femoropatellar ligament is reapposed with three interrupted horizontal mattress or interrupted cruciate sutures with #3 polyglactin 910. The distal deep fascia, from the lateral femoropatellar ligament to the tibial crest, is closed with interrupted cruciate sutures of #2 polyglactin 910, and the proximal segment of the deep fascia incision is closed with the same material in a simple continuous pattern. The superficial fascia is apposed with #1 polyglactin 910 in a simple continuous pattern. Skin closure is with #2 polypropylene[||] placed in simple interrupted sutures in the distal one third of the incision and a Ford interlocking pattern in the proximal two thirds. A stent bandage is sutured over the closed incision line and kept in place for 7 days if it remains dry. Perioperative penicillin and cephalosporins are administered for 5 days, with phenylbutazone given every other day. In the first week after surgery the patient should not be fully weight-

---

*Fixation staple, Smith and Nephew; Memphis, TN
[†]Synthes; Paoli, A
[‡]Innovative Animal Products, 6256 34th Avenue NW, Rochester, MN

[§]Vicryl, Inc.; Somerville, NJ
[||]Prolene, Ethicon Inc.; Somerville, NJ

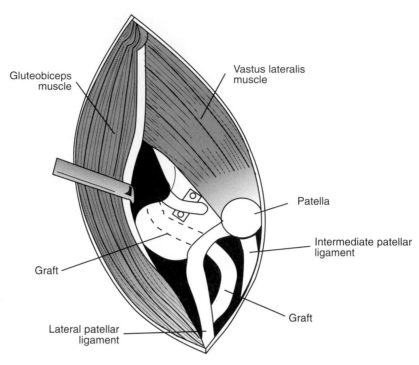

Figure 11.4-28   Schematic drawing demonstrating the placement of the autograft before application of tension and stapling. Graft is continuous behind femur and up over to be fastened by plate.

(Redrawn from Crawford WH: Intraarticular replacement of bovine cranial cruciate ligaments with an autogenous fascial graft, *Vet Surg* 19: 80-388, 1990.)

bearing; therefore the phenylbutazone dosage and duration can be adjusted to achieve the desired amount of pain control.

POSTOPERATIVE CARE AND PROGNOSIS

In both procedures, patients should be kept in a box stall for 6 to 8 months. Skin sutures are removed in 3 weeks because the skin incision is not strong enough to hold in some cattle, given the tension present during joint flexion. Postoperatively, successful animals are toe touching for the first few days with gradually increased weight-bearing. Marked improvement is seen by 2 months, with further improvement up to 6 months after surgery.

Prognosis for return to soundness suitable for breeding function depends on the size of the animal, degree of degenerative joint disease present before joint stabilization, and animal behavior (lying down on good leg, etc.). We have operated on 27 animals (14 bulls and 13 cows) to date. Out of 14 bulls (≥900 kg), 6 bulls developed incisional failure (with 4 developing fatal septic arthritis) and 2 experienced graft failure, which makes a total success rate of 43%. Of the 13 cows operated, 11 (85%) were successful, but two had residual lameness. Cranial crucial rupture has been observed in

the contralateral limb in two cows a few months after repair.

In conclusion, the CCL replacement procedure gives the best results in regard to stability of lameness and return to normal ambulatory function, but catastrophic failure in especially large patients (>900 kg) is a risk. Stifle imbrication is most successful in lighter animals (<400 kg) and has less risk of catastrophic failure.

Damage to the Collateral Ligaments of the Stifle

Injury to the medial collateral ligament (MCL) of the stifle is associated with trauma and may be seen in conjunction with cranial cruciate ligament injury. The ligament may be torn or stretched. Injury to the medial meniscus of the medial femorotibial joint may occur as a result of joint instability created by MCL injury. This is because the medial meniscus is attached to the medial collateral ligament. Injury to the lateral collateral femorotibial ligament is rare and difficult to assess because of the greater musculature and collateral support on the lateral side of the stifle.

Clinical signs of collateral ligament injury include lameness referable to the stifle joint, increased synovial effusion, reduced weight-bearing, and a shortened cranial phase to the stride. Swelling and pain are noted when the site of the MCL is palpated. If the distal limb is passively abducted while palpating the site of the MCL, opening of the medial side of the femorotibial joint can be appreciated if the ligament has ruptured. Caudal-to-cranial radiographs may reveal an avulsion fracture at the origin or insertion of the affected collateral ligament.

Ruptured collateral ligaments of the stifle may heal with 6 to 8 weeks of box stall confinement if the injury is not associated with cranial cruciate ligament rupture or meniscal destruction. In most cases, this treatment is generally unsuccessful; therefore consideration should be made for surgical stabilization.

Surgical Procedure

The animal is positioned in dorsal recumbency with the affected limb placed in a 90° flexion. The diagnosis is first confirmed by arthroscopy, and debridement of a meniscal tear is performed at that time. The incision is extended through the subcutaneous tissue. In cases of detached medial meniscus, a 2-cm skin incision is made dorsal and parallel to the meniscus. Three to four non-absorbable sutures (size 0 suture material) are used to secure the meniscus to the medial joint capsule and collateral ligament. The sutures are placed just proximal to the tibia: starting extraarticularly, entering the joint capsule, proceeding through the wide abaxial edge of the meniscus, and exiting through the joint capsule so the knots can be tied extraarticularly. The procedure's goal is to limit movement of the meniscus. Two options for stabilizing the collateral ligament are available. In the first option, a 5.5-mm cortical screw and appropriate washer are placed at the insertion sites of the collateral ligament on the femur and tibia thru stab incisions. Two or three No. 5 polyester sutures* or polyblend† are placed in a figure-eight pattern. The degree of tension is adjusted to allow a normal flexion range. The second option involves imbrication of the medial periarticular tissues, which is performed by placing four to six Lembert sutures with No. 5 polyester or polyblend sutures.*,†

No leg support is provided postoperatively, but the animal is confined to a stall for 2 to 3 months. Improvement is observed within 2 to 4 weeks postoperatively.

RECOMMENDED READINGS

Arnoczky SP et al: The over-the-top procedure: a technique for anterior ligament substitution in the dog, *J Am Anim Hosp Assoc* 15: 286-290, 1979.

*Ethibon, Ethicon Inc., Johnson & Johnson; Piscataway, NJ
†Fiberwire, Arthrex, Naples, EL

Crawford WH: A surgical technique for the intra-articular repair of cranial cruciate ligament repair in cattle, *Vet Surg* 19: 380-388, 1990.
Ducharme NG: Personal communication, 2001.
Ducharme NG, Stanton ME, Ducharme GR: Stifle lameness in cattle at two veterinary teaching hospitals: a retrospective study of forty-two cases, *Can Vet J* 26: 212-217, 1985.
Eggleston R: Personal communication, 2001.
Hamilton GF, Adams OR: Anterior cruciate repair in cattle, *J Am Vet Med Assoc* 158: 178-183, 1971.
Hofmeyr CFB: Reconstruction of the ruptured anterior cruciate ligament in the stifle of a bull, *The Veterinarian* 5: 89-92, 1968.
Moss EW, McCurnin DM, Ferguson TH: Experimental cranial cruciate replacement in cattle using a patellar ligament graft, *Can Vet J* 29: 157-162, 1988.
Nelson DR, Huhn JC, Kneller SK: Surgical repair of peripheral detachment of the medial meniscus in 34 cattle, *Vet Rec* 127: 571-573, 1990.
Nelson DR and Koch D: Surgical stabilization of the stifle in cranial cruciate ligament injury in cattle, *Vet Rec* 111: 259-262, 1982.

Gastrocnemius Rupture

Norm G. Ducharme

The gastrocnemius muscle consists of a medial and lateral belly with two tendons inserted just dorsal to the point of the hock. This gastrocnemius muscle-tendon unit is responsible for hock extension during weight-bearing and flexion of the stifle while walking. A tear of the gastrocnemius muscle-tendon unit is a rare injury and generally occurs unilaterally in farm animals. Reportedly, prolonged recumbency and bad footing can predispose an animal to slip with a leg extended under the body. In addition, direct trauma with a hard object (wire or shovel) may result in laceration of the Achilles tendon. Damage to the sciatic nerve during misdirected intramuscular injection can result in excessive weight being placed on the gastrocnemius, which will eventually rupture. Finally, this injury can also be seen after partial tibial neurectomy performed to treat spastic paresis if the animal slips during recovery, particularly if the procedure was done under epidural anesthesia.

The gastrocnemius muscle tendinous injury can occur at three sites: the gastrocnemius muscle (tearing of medial and lateral attachment on the femur), the muscle-tendinous junction, or the tendon insertion on the calcaneus bone. Disruption at any of these three locations will lead to a similar gait deficit.

Although clinical signs vary depending on the severity of the injury, partial tearing of the gastrocnemius muscle/tendon structures results in a slightly dropped hock and partially flexed fetlock. Complete disruption results in the plantigrade stance (Figure 11.4-29). The condition may be bilateral (Figure 11.4-30). On physical examination, swelling/hematoma is present at the site

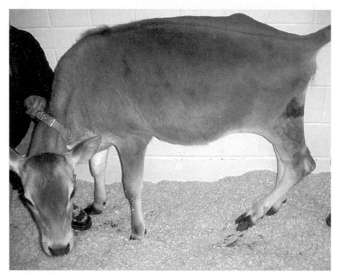

Figure 11.4-29   Jersey calf with acute avulsion of the gastrocnemius muscles after a misdirected intramuscular injection was made near the sciatic nerve. The calf's weight is partially supported by an assistant to prevent complete plantigrade stance, as seen in Figure 11.4-30.

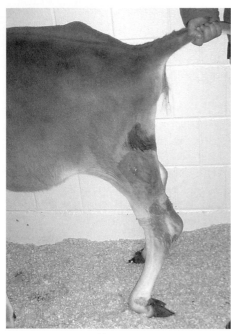

Figure 11.4-31   Same calf as in Figure 11.4-29. Note peroneal nerve deficit resulting in knuckling of the metatarsophalangeal joints.

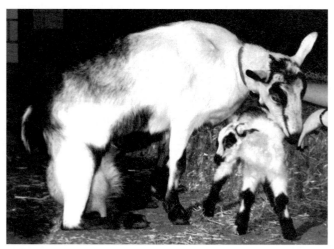

Figure 11.4-30   Female goat with bilateral rupture of the gastrocnemius muscles. Note typical plantigrade stance.

of the tear. In some cases, a complete disruption of the gastrocnemius muscle/tendon unit occurs a few weeks after a partial tear. If sciatic nerve damage is present, peroneal nerve deficit may be observed (Figure 11.4-31).

The diagnosis is made from the appearance of the dropped hock and localized swelling at the disruption site in the gastrocnemius muscle/tendon unit. Ultrasonographic evaluation (5 or 7.5 MHz; see Chapter 2) may allow a precise diagnosis when partial disruption is present, especially if it involves the medial or lateral head of the gastrocnemius muscle. The main differential diagnosis is a tarsal fracture, which should be easy to differentiate radiographically.

In the author's experience, this rare injury often involves the musculotendinous junction or the gastrocnemius muscle attachment on the femur; therefore surgical repair is not an option. Instead, external fixation is the treatment of choice. A full leg transfixation cast is recommended. A cast alone can be used, but the animals have an increased risk of developing plantar cast sores due to the loss of plantar support. Two intramedullary pins (6.35 mm), preferably with a central positive profile, are placed in the distal tibia and proximal third metatarsal bone to fix the hock in a slightly hyperextended position (Figure 11.4-32A and B). The cast should include the hoof and extend up to the stifle joint with good padding at the level of the calcaneus and back of the stifle where mechanical pressure points are present as a result of the injury (Figure 11.4-33). The cast is changed every 3 weeks in young calves (every 6 weeks in older animals whose growth has terminated) unless a laceration that requires more frequent changes to assess the wound is present. External fixation is needed for 6 to 12 weeks; after 6 weeks the transfixation pins are removed and full leg casting alone is used. The animal should be confined to a box stall with excellent footing throughout the healing period.

Alternatively, a 6.5-mm cancellous screw or a 7- or 7.3-mm cannulated screw can be placed to advance and

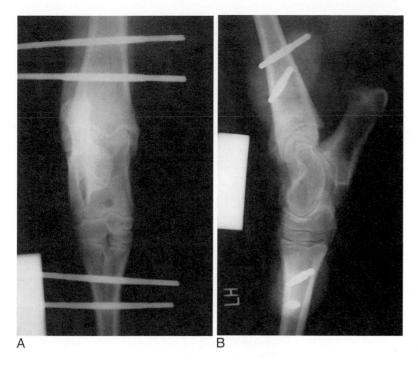

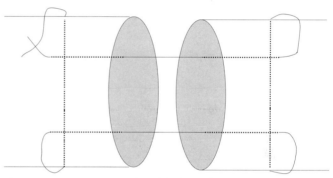

Figure 11.4-32 *A,* Lateral and *B,* dorsoplantar radiographs after application of the intramedullary pins.

(Courtesy of Dr. Tony Pease; Cornell University.)

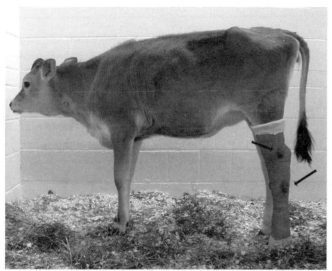

Figure 11.4-33 Calf with transfixation cast applied. Acrylic has been applied over the extremity of the transfixation pin (arrows). Note normal weight-bearing without assistance to the fixation of the hock.

(Courtesy of Dr. Michael Schramme; Cornell University.)

Figure 11.4-34 Principle of locking loop suture in tendon repair.

primary repair of the tendon by using two to three locking loop sutures (Figure 11.4-34) of no. 2 polypropylene or an absorbable monofilament suture is recommended. The degree of contamination influences the choice of suture because absorbable sutures should be used in infected or heavily contaminated wounds.

Although calves may respond to treatment, the prognosis is guarded. Prognosis is grave in adult cattle with a complete tear or laceration. Partial tears carry a better prognosis. Given the prognosis, many animals are euthanized without treatment.

fix the calcaneus to the distal tibia in smaller animals (heifer, sheep, and goats). This locks the hock in extension during healing by fibrosis of the gastrocnemius muscle/ tendon unit. In addition to internal fixation, full limb casting as described earlier is also needed to minimize the cycling of the implant.

Direct surgical repair is possible when two conditions are met: animals that weigh less than 350 kg and cases of tendon laceration. In gastrocnemius tendon laceration,

RECOMMENDED READINGS

Weaver AD: Muscles and neoplasms. In Greenough PR, editor: *Lameness in cattle,* Philadelphia, 1997, WB Saunders.

Wheat JD: Rupture of the gastrocnemius muscle in a cow: a case report, *J Am Vet Med Assoc* 132: 331-332, 1958.

Luxations/Subluxations: Coxofemoral, Patellar, Tarsal, and Scapulohumeral

Norm G. Ducharme and
Steven S. Trostle

Coxofemoral Luxation/Subluxation

Coxofemoral luxations are associated with traumatic episodes and dystocia in adult cattle (falls—sometimes during hypocalcemic episodes) or falling in calves. The luxation is generally craniodorsal, but cranioventral luxation (cranial and ventral to the pelvis) or luxation in the adductor foramen is also seen (Tulleners and Nunamaker, 1987). The clinical presentation varies with the location of the femoral head. Animals with craniodorsal luxation are generally ambulatory with moderate lameness. Part of the lameness component is mechanical in nature because of the associated shortened limb. On further examination, the swelling at the level of the greater trochanter is associated with a shift in the normal gluteal musculature. In addition, the point of the hock on the affected side is displaced dorsally. Animals with a ventral coxofemoral luxation are less able to stand. This is particularly true if the femoral head is in the obturator foramen. The limb is actually longer and held in abduction. In ventral luxation, the area of the greater trochanter is asymmetric because of the associated displaced musculature. Rectal examination can identify the femoral head cranial to the pelvis or in the obturator foramen. Radiographs are useful to get an exact diagnosis plus identify associated damage. Lateral oblique radiographs (Figure 11.4-35A) can usually be obtained with the animal standing and are often sufficient to identify the luxation. A ventrodorsal view under heavy sedation or general anesthesia works best to identify the luxation (Figure 11.4-35B).

In preparation for treatment, hypocalcemia should be treated as adductor muscle damage is likely in the recovery period. Treatment options for coxofemoral luxation involve closed and open reduction techniques. In both cases, significant traction is required. Therefore the animal is anesthetized and placed in lateral recumbency with the affected limb uppermost. Traction and countertraction are applied on the distal limb and inguinal area respectively. Both areas must be appropriately padded. Traction is obtained by placing traction on the distal limb in the opposite direction as the femoral head. External rotation is useful during the traction for craniodorsal luxation. Closed reduction is rarely successful in craniodorsal luxation because the dorsal joint capsule attachment on the acetabulum has a fibrocartilage rim that becomes trapped between the acetabulum and femoral head during reduction. Even if reduction is possible, reluxation occurs at a high rate because of the combined effect from associated muscular damage and the fibrocartilage rim being trapped in the acetabulum preventing proper seating of the femoral head. Therefore open reduction should be considered because of two significant advantages. First, the head of the femur can be seated appropriately in the acetabulum through open reduction because the dorsal joint capsule is prevented from being trapped in—or is removed from—the acetabulum. Second, the dorsal joint capsule can be reinforced to minimize the risk of resubluxation.

Preparation for surgery and approach to the coxofemoral joint is described in section 11.2, Figure 11.2-10. During reduction, traction is applied distally to move the femoral head ventral to the dorsal rim of the acetabulum. At that time, the debris from the acetabulum is removed, and the surgeon ensures that the joint capsule is not within the lumen of the acetabulum. Traction is then released with the limb in slight abduction and internal rotation until the femoral head is seated comfortably in the acetabulum. Sometimes a shoehorn retractor is used to guide the femoral head into place. At this point, the distal limb is manipulated to a full range of flexion and extension and should not be reluxated during these manipulations. If it does reluxate, some debris may be trapped in the acetabulum and prevent correct seating of the femoral head. To minimize the likelihood of reluxation, the dorsal acetabular joint capsule is reinforced as follows: two screws (4.5 mm) and washers are placed in the craniodorsal rim of the acetabulum. A 3.2-mm drill bit is used to drill a guide hole through the rostral aspect of the greater trochanter. Multiple No. 5 nonabsorbable polyester or polyblend sutures are placed between each screw and the pilot hole. The limb is placed in mild flexion, internally rotated, and the sutures tied in place (Figure 11.4-36). These sutures restrict the range the limb can be flexed, so a sufficient degree of flexion (approximately 30 degrees) must be maintained. The various muscle planes are closed by reapposition. Postoperatively, the animal should be stall confined for 3 months.

The success rate for repair of coxofemoral luxation is around 75% for craniodorsal and 30% for ventral. If the animal is down and unable to rise on presentation, a poor prognosis is given. Complicated coxofemoral luxations and fractures are treated by internal fixation with a combination of techniques described earlier (see Figure 11.4-35C) but carry a guarded prognosis.

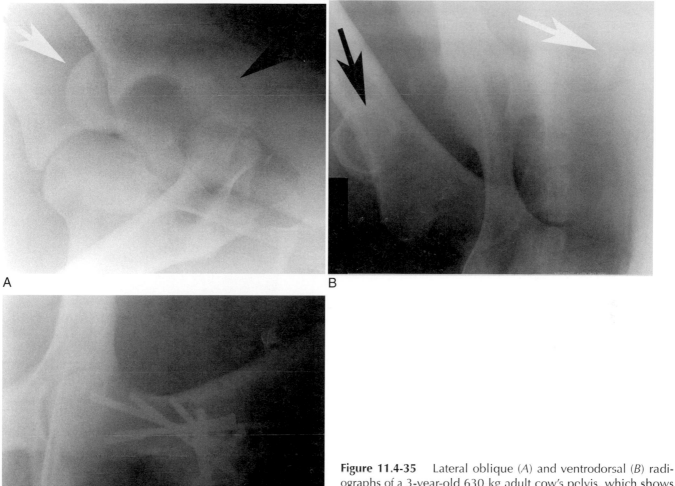

Figure 11.4-35   Lateral oblique (*A*) and ventrodorsal (*B*) radiographs of a 3-year-old 630 kg adult cow's pelvis, which shows a luxated coxofemoral joint (in the adductor foramen). Note how the acetabulum is free of the femoral head in comparison to the contralateral side. In addition to the luxation, there is a greater trochanter fracture (black arrow) and a slipped capital femoral physeal fracture (white arrow). *C*, Postoperative ventrodorsal radiograph after the fractures and luxation are reduced and stabilized with internal fixation.

Dorsal Patellar Luxation

Dorsal luxation (upper fixation) of the patella is a rare anomaly in cattle. It generally presents as an intermittent problem where the patella becomes fixed on the dorsal aspect of the medial trochlea. It has been reported most commonly in beef cattle (Brahma, Angus Simmental, Charbray, Beefmaster, and Chianina), buffalo, and most rarely in Holstein-Friesian dairy cattle. Desmitis of the medial distal patellar ligament associated with work or slippage that results in hyperextension of the limb is believed to be a predisposing factor. Stretching of the medial distal patellar ligament allows it to catch on the medial trochlea, which it normally would not. The con-

dition can be unilateral or bilateral. Historically, it is seen in working dairy cattle but rarely in those less than 2 years old.

Clinical signs include a normal posture at rest with clinical signs, depending on the frequency and permanence of the upward fixation. The limb locks in an extended state, so the animal has to drag the limb to move forward. When the patella returns to its normal position, the release from the extension makes the limb jerk forward. If upward fixation is very frequent, the toe becomes worn down. The condition somewhat resembles spastic paresis (see Spastic Paresis, later in this section). However, spastic paresis is seen in young animals (<2 years of age) with backward movement of

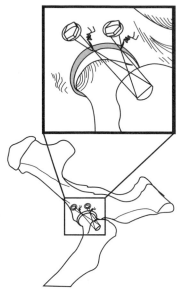

Figure 11.4-36   Schematic showing placement of sutures and screws to reinforce the dorsal joint capsule and prevent craniodorsal reluxation.

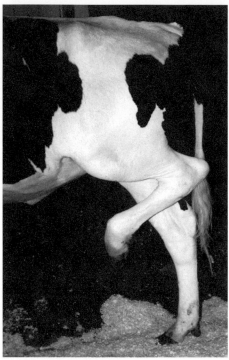

Figure 11.4-37   Heifer with acute luxation of the proximal intertarsal joint. Note the locked position of the hock in a flexed position.

the extended limb, whereas forward movement of the extended limb is associated with upward fixation.

The treatment principle is to transect the medial distal patellar ligament near its attachment on the tibia. The animal is treated standing or preferably in lateral recumbency with casting and sedation. In dairy cattle, lateral recumbency is recommended because the udder interferes with appropriate access to the medial aspect of the stifle joint. With the medial aspect of the affected limb uppermost and the leg tied slightly backward, local anesthetic is applied over the medial patellar ligament attachment on the tibia. Using a 10 Parker-Kerr blade, a 1-cm incision is made over the cranial aspect of the medial patellar ligament just proximal to the tibial crest. A large curved hemostat is passed axial to the ligament to isolate it, and the ligament is clamped. The ligament is transected proximal and distal to the hemostat with a tenotome, and a segment of the ligament is removed. The end of a gloved finger is used to explore the ligament remnant to ensure that no fiber remains. The skin is closed with one or two sutures.

Proximal Intertarsal Luxation/Subluxation

These luxations are rarely seen in farm animals, but their appearance is pathognomonic. They have been reported in young animals (1 year or less) after an acute traumatic episode. Immediately after the traumatic episode, the animal is unable to extend the tarsocrural joint (Figure 11.4-37). Because of the reciprocal apparatus, the stifle

and fetlock are also held in flexion. The animal does not appear to be in pain but simply is unable to extend the limb.

Physical examination reveals a limb locked in a flexed position. Manually, one cannot extend the limb, and little or no swelling to localize the injury site occurs. However, the characteristic appearance of the limb indicates a need to focus on radiographic examination of the hock joint. Radiographically, the luxation involves the proximal intertarsal joint as the calcaneus and centroquartal bone are luxated in a plantar-distal direction. Therefore both the calcaneoquartal and proximal intertarsal joints are involved. The distal displacement of the calcaneus into the groove between the two condyles of the talus appears to be the reason for the locking mechanism. During reduction, the calcaneus tip (coracoid process of calcaneus) is unlocked from the condyles, thus allowing extension of the limb.

Under sedation with xylazine hydrochloride or general anesthesia, the animal is placed in lateral recumbency with the affected limb uppermost. Traction is applied distally and slightly caudally and reduction occurs with little difficulty. A complication of the reduction is a small fracture of the proximal dorsal tip of the calcaneus, but this appears to have no significant consequence. Ideally, the fragment could be removed by arthroscopy, but this has not been performed by the author. Because the limb is stable once the luxation is reduced, no bandage or splinting is required. The animal is confined to a box stall for 6 weeks before resuming normal activity.

Scapulohumeral Luxation/Subluxation

Scapulohumeral luxations are a rare disease in farm animals, and the authors have only observed this in adult cattle. They are generally cranial and lateral and can be recognized by a prominent swelling on the cranial aspect of the shoulder. A severe lameness but no dropped elbow is seen. During examination, one hand is placed on the point of the elbow and the other hand on the proximal end of the humerus to apply internal and external rotation. A humeral fracture should be suspected with crepitus and a lack of movement of the proximal end of the humerus. However, a scapulohumeral luxation is identified by detecting movement of the humeral head. The diagnosis is confirmed by radiography when available.

Reduction is obtained by placing the animal in lateral recumbency under heavy sedation; general anesthesia is preferable. With the affected limb uppermost, traction is applied on the appropriately padded distal limb, with counter traction applied by placing a rope (with appropriate padding) in the pectoral region away from the scapulohumeral joint. The following two manipulation techniques have been reported: 1) traction can be applied caudally with simultaneous manual pressure on the humeral head in a caudal direction; 2) alternatively, traction can be applied distally and slightly cranially and then firm pressure is applied caudally during slow release of the traction. Postreduction, the animal should be confined to a stall for 3 months.

RECOMMENDED READINGS

Arighi M, Ducharme NG, Horney FD, Pennock PW: Proximal intertarsal subluxation in three Holstein-Friesian heifers, *Can Vet J* 28: 710-712, 1987.

Baird AN, Angel KL, Moll HD et al: Upward fixation of cattle: 38 cases (1984-1990), *J Am Vet Med Assoc* 202: 434-436, 1993.

Tulleners EP, Nunamaker DM: Coxofemoral luxations in cattle: 22 cases (1980-1985), *J Am Vet Med Assoc* 191: 569-574, 1987.

Tyagi RPS, Krishnamurthy D, Kharole MU: Studies of the histopathology of ligaments in Bovine animals affected by upward fixation of the patella' *Vet Rec* 93: 362-364, 1973.

Spastic Paresis (Elso Heel)

Norm G. Ducharme

This disease was first reported to be a heritable disease originating from a Dutch bull (Elso II). The pattern of inheritance is generally thought to be multiple recessive genes with incomplete penetrance. Therefore, no affected animals should enter the breeding stock until genomic studies allow identification and possible treatment. The heritability is not known, but one author has reported that 10% of offspring of one bull were affected (Weaver AD).

The clinical presentation expected is spastic contraction of the gastrocnemius muscles. During these spastic contractions, the hock and stifle are hyperextended, and the more affected limb extends caudally (Figure 11.4-38). This stance gives the impression the leg is too short, and this disease has also been referred to as "short leg." If the spasms persist, the hyperextended limb can only be advanced in a swinging motion while walking, because the hock and stifle are extended. The condition can be unilateral or bilateral and is usually first manifested under six months of age. Occasionally, no clinical signs are noted until 1 or 2 years of age. It is unknown whether the disease is first manifested at that time or was previously missed. In unilateral disease, the animal keeps the nonaffected hind limb more axial to support its weight. This increased weight on the nonaffected limb may eventually results in tarsal varus, thus giving a bowed leg appearance.

Physical examination reveals no pain or site of inflammation except in chronic cases in which the persistent hyperextension results in joint inflammation of the hock

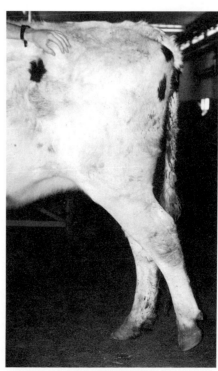

Figure 11.4-38 Young heifer with spastic paresis. During spastic episode, the limb is extended and directed caudally.

and stifle. Chronic hyperextension also results in remodeling of the affected joint, and those signs can be identified radiographically. No resistance to passive manual flexion of the limb occurs, unlike upward patellar luxation. The diagnosis is made based on the stance and gait of the animal. Although upward fixation of the patella looks similar, it is fairly easy to differentiate because of the jerky movement of the patella during unlocking and the absence of caudal movement of the limb in patellar fixation.

Spastic paresis was first thought to be a neurological disease, but the absence of central or peripheral nerve, muscle, or tendinous lesions histologically suggests that it is primarily a functional abnormality. Hypersensitivity of the myotactic reflex is the prevalent hypothesis; thus voluntary movements may stimulate the hyperactivity of the efferent innervation of the gastrocnemius muscles. Because of the stay apparatus (i.e., fibularis tertius or longus), the stifle also is hyperextended. It has been suggested that the caudal thigh muscles may also be affected.

The disease progresses in untreated animals so they become increasingly recumbent, lose body condition, and need to be destroyed between 1 and 2 years of age. Treatment is recommended only to allow the animal to grow normally for slaughter purposes. No medical treatments exist, but two surgical procedures have been described: partial tibial neurectomy and transection of the two insertions of the gastrocnemius tendons on the calcaneus. (For description of the surgical procedure see Section 15.6.)

RECOMMENDED READINGS

Branteghem L: Partial tibial neurectomy in 113 Belgian blue calves with spastic paresis, *Vet Rec* 147: 16-19, 2000.

Ledoux JM: Bovine spastic paresis: etiological hypotheses, *Med Hypotheses* 57: 573-539, 2001.

Vlaminck L, De Moor A, Martens A, Steenhaut M, Gasthuys F, Desmet P, Van Weaver AD: Spastic paresis (Elso Heel). In Greenough PR, editor: *Lameness in cattle*, Philadelphia, 1997, WB Saunders.

CHAPTER 12

SURGERY OF THE BOVINE REPRODUCTIVE SYSTEM AND URINARY TRACT

12.1.1—Surgery of the Male Reproductive Tract

Robert O. Gilbert and Susan L. Fubini

Applied Anatomy and Examination of the Reproductive Tract

The paired testes of ruminants hang vertically in the scrotum with the caput epididymidis dorsally. They are slightly flattened laterally. Testicular blood supply is via the testicular artery, a branch of the abdominal aorta. Testicular lymph drainage is to the medial iliac lymph nodes and reflects the embryonic origin of the testes caudal to the kidneys. Autonomic innervation of the testes is via the renal and caudal mesenteric plexuses.

Cryptorchidism is rare in ruminants. When defects of testicular descent occur, it is usually in the form of incomplete descent, and its subtlety may escape notice in many cases. Instead of its normal attachment to the ventral most aspect of the scrotum, ligament of the tail of the epididymis may attach to a point in the midscrotum. In this case, the testis may appear normal at first observation. When, during examination, it is forced ventrally in the scrotum, its midscrotal attachment becomes apparent as the testis rotates about this point of aberrant attachment, instead of sliding smoothly to the ventral portion of the scrotum. Bulls with this disorder should be culled: testicular thermoregulation is impaired, and

spermatogenesis is rarely normal. It is also likely that the condition is inherited.

The testis is enclosed within two layers of the tunica vaginalis. The inner layer (visceral) is closely applied to the tunica albuginea of the testis. A potential space separates it from the outer (parietal) layer; this space is continuous with the peritoneal space of the abdomen, through the inguinal canal. The sulcus formed by the fold of visceral to parietal layers of tunica vaginalis is occupied by the ductus deferens if approached from the cranial aspect and is attached to the testis along the line of the epididymis if approached from the caudal side. This architecture can be exploited to make midscrotal vasectomy a simple procedure (described later in the chapter).

The testicular artery courses toward the deep inguinal ring of the inguinal canal, where it joins the spermatic cord. The latter structure consists of the testicular artery and vein, the lymphatics, nerves, and the ductus deferens. Together they pass through the inguinal canal. The testicular artery, once external to the abdomen, becomes extremely tortuous. In this area it is in close apposition to the dilated and contorted veins. This complex is known as the *pampiniform plexus*. It serves multiple purposes. The multiple contortions of the artery help blunt the pulsatility of arterial blood flow. (The fibrous outer surface of the testis, the tunica albuginea, is unyielding and extremely sensitive to distension, which means that arterial pulsatility within the testis would be most uncomfortable.) In addition, arterial blood is cooled by exposure to the effluent venous blood, and countercurrent exchange of steroids, especially testosterone, which

351

is produced in the testis and is necessary in high concentrations locally for optimal testicular function. Testicular arterial blood is therefore cooler, is fortified with testicular steroids, and flows with diminished pulsatility.

The testicular artery courses on the surface of the testis in a large S-pattern before entering the parenchyme. The surface of the testis is richly supplied with blood vessels. These are sparsest on the craniolateral surface of the testis, in its upper (dorsal) half. This is of practical significance, because this is the optimal site of testicular biopsy (a procedure with a high possibility of complications caused by hemorrhage and subsequent infarction).

The cremaster muscle is a slip of the internal abdominal oblique muscle. It may contribute to testicular thermoregulation by raising and lowering the testis but the maneuver also functions as a protection mechanism.

The products of spermatogenesis leave the seminiferous tubules (spermatogenic tubules) via tubuli recti into the rete testis. The latter is located in the mediastinum testis, a structure that runs from the proximal to the distal extremity of the testis, and is visible on ultrasonography. Via a number of efferent ductules the newly produced sperm make their way to the epididymal duct at the head of the epididymis. The epididymal duct is a single duct, and multiple connections (efferent ductules) are made to it in the caput epididymis. It is not unusual for one or more of these connecting ducts to end blindly and leave a palpable pealike nodule in the head of the epididymis. If a large number end blindly, they may become large enough to obstruct neighboring, normal ducts. Escape of sperm from these ducts provokes a granulomatous reaction to the foreign material, and further functional blockage may occur. Eventually, the granuloma formation may be sufficient to cause total functional occlusion and render one (or even both) testicular-epididymal unit inoperative. This is occasionally seen in bulls or rams. It is the mechanism of infertility associated with polled goat bucks.

The epididymis is closely applied to the body of the testis. It runs along the caudomedial surface of the testis and ends in the prominent tail (cauda epididymidis). The degree of filling of the epididymal tail is a good indicator of the status of spermatogenesis and an indicator that no blockage of the epididymis exists. The ductus deferens runs medial to the epididymis of its side, enclosed in its own fold of tunica vaginalis, the mesoductus deferens.

The testes and epididymides should be turgid without being hard. Their surfaces should be smooth, and they should be freely moveable within the scrotum.

The ductus deferens enters the inguinal canal, then courses retroperitoneally, medial to the ureters and dorsal to the bladder, where its terminal 10 cm is thickened to form the ampulla of the ductus deferens before it enters the urethra. This thickening is caused by glands in the wall of the deferent duct. The paired ampullae (left and right) are contained within a fold of peritoneum, the plica genitalis, or genital fold. An embryonic remnant, the uterus masculinus, may sometimes be found between the two ampullae.

The scrotal skin is thin, and hair or wool is usually sparse on the scrotum. It is richly endowed with glands. These modifications enhance the thermoregulatory capacity of the scrotum but also make it exquisitely sensitive to insult. Scrotal dermatitis profoundly affects scrotal temperature and spermatogenesis. The tunica dartos is a layer of fibroelastic tissue and smooth muscle that, by contracting, thickens the scrotal skin and raises the testes closer to the body and, by relaxing, lowers the testes and allows the scrotal skin to become thinner. In this way it contributes to thermoregulation. The scrotum (in contrast to the testes) receives its blood supply from the external pudendal artery, and its lymphatic drainage is to the superficial inguinal lymph node. The innervation of the testes is via the genital branch of the genitofemoral nerve, which arises from the second through fourth lumbar roots.

The vesicular glands lie immediately lateral to the ampullae, dorsal to the neck of the bladder. The vesicular glands and ampullae open into the urethra dorsally near the neck of the bladder, on either side of the colliculus seminalis. Four separate openings are present. Very close to the terminations of the ampullae and vesicular glands, and closely applied to the urethra is the body of the prostate gland, which encircles the urethra near the bladder neck. The ampullae actually pass through the parenchyma of the prostate to reach the urethral lumen and open into the urethra via multiple small ducts. In the bull there is also a disseminate part of the prostate gland, which is not palpable, within the wall of the urethra.

The pelvic portion of the urethra and its surrounding thin layer of spongy tissue are covered by the urethralis muscle. At the ischial arch the spongy tissue enlarges to form the bulb of the penis and then continues along the penile urethra as the corpus spongiosum. As the urethra passes over the ischial arch, it runs between the crura of the penis. The penile crura become fused and continue as the corpus cavernosum penis. In ruminants, the corpus spongiosum and corpus cavernosum do not communicate. The ischiocavernosus muscles cover the crura of the penis, and the bulbospongiosus muscle covers the penile bulb. Both muscles are important in the mechanism of penile erection. Partially covered by the bulbospongiosus muscle are the paired bulbourethral glands. The bulb and the crura of the penis and their covering muscles constitute the root of the penis.

The accessory sex glands are palpable per rectum in bulls. The bulbourethral glands can be felt as smooth structures that protrude from under the cranial edge of the bulbospongiosus muscles. The pelvic urethra, surrounded by the urethralis muscle, is prominent in the midline of the pelvic floor. If any doubt exists, the urethralis muscle can be identified by massaging it per rectum; it will respond by contracting rhythmically. As the urethralis muscle is traced forward, a transverse ridge can be felt at its cranial-most end. This is the body of the prostate. Converging on this point, the fairly soft, pliable ampullae can be felt. The ampullae move as a pair within the genital fold and are separated by less than half an inch. They may be displaced to one or the other side by a full bladder. Also converging toward the body of the prostate are the vesicular glands. These lobulated structures project craniolaterally. In young animals they are smaller and softer than in mature bulls.

In rams, the bulbourethral glands are larger and may be palpated by inserting a finger into the rectum. Wethers that graze estrogenic pastures may develop cystic metaplasia of the bulbourethral glands, in which case they may protrude conspicuously as swellings of the perineal area.

The urethral lumen is small, despite the deceptively large diameter of the urethralis muscle. As the urethra turns over the ischial arch there is a dorsal diverticulum formed by a shelf of mucosa. This diverticulum makes urethral catheterization of the bladder virtually impossible, as the leading tip of the catheter invariably finds the diverticulum.

The ischiocavernosus and bulbospongiosus muscles do not extend beyond the fusion of the crura of the penis. The penis is readily palpated through the skin of the perineum. It extends cranially; then turns ventrally and caudally in the first loop of the sigmoid flexure and turns cranially again ventral to the penile root. This distal loop of the sigmoid flexure is also palpable through the perineal skin. Also palpable at this point are the paired retractor penis muscles. They arise from the first two or three coccygeal vertebrae, decussate around the anus, and then pass superficially through the perineal region to attach ventrally to the penis just beyond the distal loop of the sigmoid flexure.

In the resting bull, the tip of the penis lies at a level just cranial to the scrotal neck. The skin of the prepuce (lamina externa) is reflected at the preputial orifice to form the lining (lamina interna) of the preputial cavity. The lamina interna of the prepuce is attached to the penis about 12 cm from the tip of the penis. This integument (it has no glands and is not mucosa) is supported by several layers of loose connective and elastic tissue that allow extension of the penis, during which process the lamina interna comes to lie along the body of the extended penis.

In cross-section, the penis consists of the ventral urethra (dorsal in the middle of the sigmoid flexure) surrounded by the corpus spongiosum and the larger corpus cavernosum (the fusion of the crura of the penis). The corpus cavernosum is encased in a thick, dense, and inelastic tunica albuginea. The corpus cavernosum is supplied by the deep artery of the penis and is drained by the analogous vein. The artery of the bulb of the penis supplies the corpus spongiosum. The dorsal artery of the penis supplies the superficial structures of the penis. The deep artery of the penis, the artery of the bulb and the dorsal artery of the penis are terminal branches of the internal pudendal artery.

The penis of mature bulls is about 120 cm in length, with some breed variation, and extends 30 to 50 cm from the prepuce when erect. Near the free end of the penis is a dorsally located thickened fibrous band, termed the apical ligament. This ligament helps hold the penis straight for intromission. At ejaculation it slips to the side and causes a spiral deviation of the tip of the penis. In some bulls, the ligament slips prematurely, and the spiral deviation arises before intromission, making intromission impossible. The penis of the ram and buck is characterized by a urethral process that extends 4 to 5 cm beyond the glans penis.

The pudendal nerve arises from ventral branches of the second through fourth sacral spinal nerves. Its branches provide motor supply to the retractor penis muscle and, via the dorsal nerve of the penis, sensory innervation of the penis. Penile sensation is important for normal function. Afferent impulses from the glans penis, conducted by the dorsal penile nerve, are essential for ejaculation. Bulls that have lost penile sensation are unable to serve and ejaculate, even if an artificial vagina is used. Care must be taken during surgical procedures to avoid damage to the dorsal nerve of the penis. Fortunately, the nerve divides into plentiful terminal branches near the free end of the penis, and the risk of damage to the entire nerve in this area is small.

Blocking the pudendal nerve achieves relaxation and desensitization of the penis and allows surgical procedures on the penis of the standing, restrained bull, provided the animal's temperament permits. The pudendal nerve can be palpated per rectum. The internal pudendal artery serves as a landmark. It is readily palpable (per rectum) as it courses along the medial surface of the sacrosciatic ligament just dorsal to the ischiatic arch. If the artery is followed caudally, the lesser ischiatic foramen can be identified at the point where the artery divides. The pudendal nerve can be felt about 1 cm dorsal to the artery at the cranial edge of the lesser ischiatic foramen. It is convenient to block the nerve at the foramen and remember that it receives a branch from the caudal cutaneous femoral nerve at that point. The caudal cutaneous femoral nerve runs laterally to the sacrosciatic ligament. To administer a pudendal nerve block, the rectum is evacuated and the skin of the ischiorectal fossa disinfected. A bleb of local anesthetic agent (e.g., 2% lidocaine) is injected under the skin at the notch between the tail fold and the caudal extent of the sacrosciatic ligament, and a 15-cm, 18-gauge needle is inserted. The needle is guided toward the lesser ischiatic foramen with a hand in the rectum and the left hand is used to guide the needle for injection of the right nerve, and vice versa. The author prefers to inject about 10 to 12 ml at the site of the foramen, near the palpable pudendal nerve, and then divert the needle through the foramen to inject about 5 ml on the lateral side of the ligament, thus ensuring that the caudal cutaneous femoral branch is blocked. As the needle is withdrawn, the remaining 3 to 5 ml is injected slowly, in the hope of blocking the caudal rectal nerve. This nerve, although large, is not readily palpable per rectum because it moves with the rectal wall. It provides some innervation to the proximal fibers of the retractor penis muscle. Both pudendal nerves need to be blocked to produce relaxation of the retractor penis muscles and analgesia of the penis. The penis may prolapse out of the prepuce spontaneously after this procedure, but more commonly it is retained within the prepuce by passive mechanisms (loose connective and elastic tissue surrounding the prepuce), and it needs to be extended manually.

The flaccid and insensitive penis should be extended fully, by grasping the free end of the penis with a gauze swab (see Figure 12.1.5-5). Forceps may be used to secure the penis, with care taken not to penetrate the *tunica albuginea* (see Figure 12.1.5-3B). Penetrating towel clamps may be secured to the apical ligament without injury to the penis.

The length of the fully extended penis should be measured from the natural position of the preputial ostium to the tip of the extended penis. For adult bulls of most breeds, this length should exceed 30 cm. An unusually short penis may prevent normal mating, especially in bulls older than 3 or 4 years. Penis extension may be impeded by lesions of the retractor penis muscles (congenital shortness, fibrosis, and calcification). These can be detected by palpating the retractor penis muscles, between the scrotum and the anus, while tension is applied to the tip of the extended penis. Some bulls may be restored to service by myotomy of the retractor penis muscles, performed in the mid to upper escutcheon.

While the penis is extended—and in particular if any impediment to full extension is encountered—the entire penis should be carefully palpated, with particular attention paid to the presence of swellings or adhesions surrounding the penis. The preputial cavity may be examined in more detail by inflating it with gas or fluid. A metal or plastic catheter with rounded tip is inserted into the preputial orifice, and through it compressed air or water (from a regular hose pipe) is carefully introduced, while the preputial orifice is held closed. The normal prepuce is clearly outlined by this procedure and should appear symmetrical and oval in contour. This technique will reveal any irregularity of the preputial lining (scars or adhesions) that may not otherwise be readily detectable.

Another strategy for minor procedures or examination of the free end of the penis is to block the dorsal nerve of the penis. This is especially useful in younger bulls, which are more easily handled. To block the dorsal nerve of the penis, the penis is withdrawn from the prepuce by manual, hand-over-hand action. Working from the left-hand side of the bull, the penis is grasped through the skin of the prepuce and moved forward with the right hand. Then the preputial skin is moved caudally and the penis is anchored with the left hand. With the right hand, the preputial skin is moved caudally, the penis is grasped again and moved forward. (It might be possible to push the penis forward by applying pressure at the distal loop of the sigmoid flexure.) This procedure is repeated until the tip of the penis protrudes from the preputial orifice, where it is grasped by an assistant with sterile gauze sponges. This is only feasible in young (yearling) bulls; the force of the retractor penis muscles is not easily overcome in more mature bulls. Once the penis is extended, lidocaine may be injected beneath the lamina interna of the prepuce dorsally near the preputial orifice. The injection should encompass the dorsal half of the penis. This will provide analgesia of the free part of the penis adequate for minor surgery such as removal of fibropapillomata, correction of persistent frenula, or for more detailed examination.

The preputial orifice should be closely applied to the ventral midline of the bull. Some breeds or individuals have pendulous prepuces that are predisposed to prolapse of the lamina interna. The orifice should permit introduction of three or four fingers but should not be wider than that. The prolapsed lamina interna is predisposed to injury, which may result in local scar tissue formation and stenosis of the prepuce. These lesions can usually be palpated through the skin. If doubt exists, the prepuce of the sedated bull can be inflated by introducing water or compressed air slowly into the prepuce while holding the orifice shut by hand. As the preputial cavity becomes filled its contour is readily discernable, and any stenotic area is easily identified.

Although the surgeon is principally concerned with the structural integrity of the reproductive tract and its surgical restoration, any surgery of the reproductive tract should, wherever possible, be preceded by thorough breeding soundness examination, including assessment of semen quality, to preclude other, nonsurgical problems that would persist after surgical intervention.

Castration

BILATERAL ORCHIDECTOMY

Castration of young ruminants is a common procedure often done by lay people to improve meat quality and render males more manageable. It is appropriate for veterinarians to educate their livestock owners to minimize complications from this procedure. A clean, dry environment as well as fly control is encouraged to prevent postoperative infection.

The desired age at which the animal is castrated varies and depends on an owner's expectation, ease of procedure, and the intended use of the animal. Younger animals are easier to restrain, have a lesser risk of incisional complications, and have decreased aggressive behavior after castration. However, some livestock owners feel that castration at a later age is preferable for improved carcass characteristics and weight gain. In a review of the literature, castration had a mixed effect on weight gain of cattle.

Castration can be done pharmacologically by using immunization against GnRH or by insertion of an estrogen implant. Other techniques include using surgical and bloodless castration techniques. This chapter will focus on the latter two methods of castration.

All small ruminants that are castrated should receive a tetanus prophylaxis (ideally several weeks before the procedure) because tetanus acquisition is one of the main complications of this procedure. This can be in the form of colostral protection, tetanus antitoxin (250 to 500 IU) or two doses of tetanus toxoid (first one 3 to 4 weeks in advance of procedure).

Regardless of the technique used or species involved, it is essential to check that both testes have descended into the scrotum before surgery is contemplated. This prevents unilateral castration of cryptorchid animals, which would give the misleading external appearance of a castrated male. Fortunately, cryptorchidism is rare in calves, rams, and bucks.

CASTRATION OF CALVES AND SMALL RUMINANTS

Lambs and small goats are held, head down, between the operator's knees or head up with the front and hind limbs on each side held together. Calves younger than one month of age are usually restrained in lateral recumbency. Typically, older calves are put into a squeeze chute or stocks. Many operators elect to use a local anesthetic

in the skin and/or spermatic cord, although some young calves and lambs receive operations with only physical restraint. For a standing animal in stocks or head catch, the operator's hand is placed at the base of the tail so that it can be lifted over the animal's back. Lamb or kid sensitivity to local anesthetics necessitates reduction of the concentration of a local anesthetic being administered; lidocaine should be diluted from 2% to 0.5% or 1%. General anesthesia—or heavy sedation (xylazine hydrochloride 0.02 to 0.1 mg/kg IV or 0.04 to 0.2 mg/kg IM) and local anesthesia—are commonly used with larger animals and pets. The lower range should be used on goats and debilitated, aged, young, or depressed animals. Another drug combination that works well on goats is midazolam (0.1 to 0.2 mg/kg IV) in combination with butorphanol (0.02 mg/kg IV).

For animals less than 150 kg, the distal portion of the scrotum is grasped and pulled distally, thus displacing the testes proximally (Figure 12.1.1-1). The distal third of the scrotum is excised to expose the testes (Figure 12.1.1-2). Traction is applied to each testis, and the spermatic cord is freed by stripping the fascia proximally (Figure 12.1.1-3). At this point, the cord can be ligated and transected, emasculated, or stretched until the vasculature ruptures. The latter technique results in vasospasm, which is usually adequate hemostasis for smaller animals but could damage the inguinal ring in lambs and lead to a hernia. For this reason, use of a technique that closes (use of emasculator [Figure 12.1.1-4] or ligation) the spermatic cord is preferable. The wound is usually left open to heal by second intention.

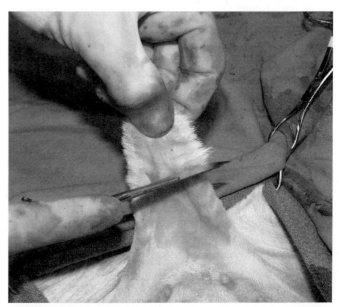

Figure 12.1.1-1 The distal portion of the scrotum of a bull calf in dorsal recumbency is grasped and pulled distally, thus displacing the testes proximally.

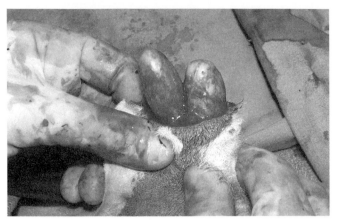

Figure 12.1.1-2   The distal third of the scrotum is excised, exposing the testes.

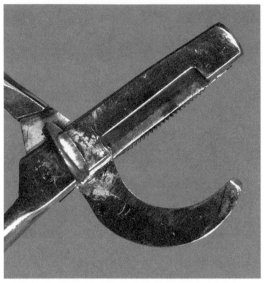

Figure 12.1.1-4   Emasculator. Note the serrated blade used for crushing the spermatic cord to cause hemostasis. When the emasculator is used, the cutting blade must be placed distal to the crushing blade.

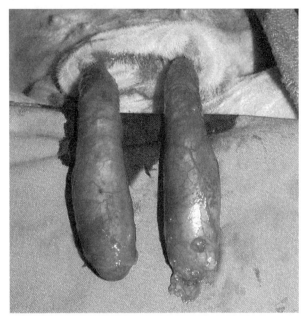

Figure 12.1.1-3   The spermatic cord is exposed by stripping the fascia proximally and applying traction to each testis.

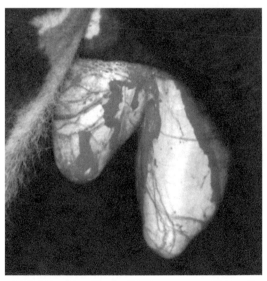

Figure 12.1.1-5   Yearling bull being castrated. The distal end of the scrotum has been removed, exposing the testes.

Another surgical option for calves is to approach the testes by making a vertical incision in the lateral wall of the scrotum with a Newberry knife (Figure 4.4-6A). The Newberry knife blade is placed through the middle of the scrotum (Figure 4.4-6A) and rapidly pulled distally, thus making a cranial and caudal flap of the scrotal skin (Figure 4.4-6A). The same flaps can also be created with a scalpel. The testes are excised as mentioned previously, either with traction, an emasculator, or ligation and excision. The wound is typically left open.

Older animals are occasionally castrated, with the best results obtained when they are restrained in chutes or on a tilt table. Local anesthetic in the scrotal skin and sper-

matic cord is appropriate. The operator's preferences dictate the surgical approach. The distal scrotum can be removed (Figure 12.1.1-5), or vertical incisions can be made on either side of the median raphe. Regardless, the testis is identified and freed from its surrounding fascia with blunt dissection. Once isolated, the spermatic cord is ligated and transected or emasculated. Generally, the vaginal tunic is not incised and is removed *en bloc* with the testis. If the vaginal tunic is incised, the testis and spermatic cord are ligated (or emasculated). Some prefer to split the spermatic vessels away from the pampiniform plexus and ligate (or emasculate) these structures separately. Regardless, the cremaster muscle is ligated with the vaginal tunic, and both are transected approximately 2 cm distal to the ligations. Transfixation sutures help prevent ligature slippage. If primary closure is to be performed, at least a partial resection of the redundant scrotal skin is necessary to minimize dead space. The subcutaneous tissues are closed with a pursestring-type suture (superficial and deep bites) using an absorbable suture material. A subcuticular or skin closure should be done with an absorbable suture if primary closure is elected.

UNILATERAL ORCHIDECTOMY

Injury or illness that involves one testis may detrimentally affect the contralateral tests to the extent that removal of the affected testis provides the best option for returning the bull or ram to fertility. This may be the case in unilateral hydrocele, hematocele, testicular tumor, epididymitis, abscess, varicocele (Figure 12.1.1-6A) or other conditions. In such cases the contralateral testis may be compromised by pressure or increased local temperature. Careful removal of one testis results in preservation of the remaining testis, and some compensatory hypertrophy and increased sperm production by the remaining testis may be expected.

Abnormalities are usually detected during physical and routine breeding soundness examination or may be noticed by an astute owner or herdsman. The abnormality can involve the scrotum, testis, epididymis, ductus deferens, vaginal tunic, or vasculature of the testis. Unilateral disease can result in abnormal semen quality as the heat generated by the abnormal testis affects the contralateral testis. Fortunately, studies have shown the effect on semen quality is reversed after the abnormal testis is removed. Care must be taken to limit postsurgical hemorrhage and inflammation and to prevent the detrimental effects of postoperative pressure or elevated temperature on the remaining testis.

The surgical procedure for unilateral orchidectomy is as follows. The animal is restrained or anesthetized in lateral recumbency. The upper hind limb is abducted and secured in a fixed position; the scrotum may be held by a towel clamp to facilitate preparation (Figure 12.1.1-6B). After preparation of the surgical site, a vertical incision is made on the lateral aspect of the affected side approximately the entire length of the testis. The initial dissection extends the skin incision through the scrotal fascia, and the testis is bluntly dissected within the vaginal tunic. The vaginal tunic is incised the length of the testis, and the spermatic cord isolated, double-ligated, and transected or emasculated. The tunic can be transected and oversewn with an absorbable suture material. It is usually necessary to remove excess scrotal skin. This will help minimize dead space and prevent postoperative seroma formation. The scrotal fascia is closed by using a continuous pattern with an absorbable suture. The subcutaneous tissues and skin are closed routinely.

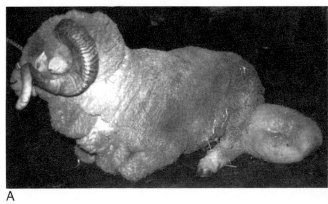

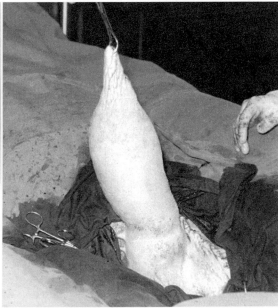

Figure 12.1.1-6 *A,* Mature ram with unilateral varicocele. Note the enlarged asymmetric scrotum. *B,* Intraoperative view before resection.

(Courtesy of Dr. Mary Smith; Cornell University.)

A

B

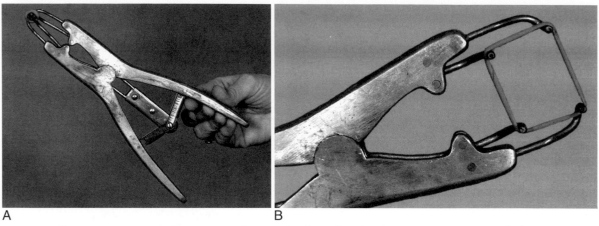

Figure 12.1.1-7   *A,* Elastrator used to apply elastic bands when castrating a young kid. *B,* Close-up view.

Studies have shown that semen quality returned to normal 22 days after unilateral castration in normal bulls. There are other case reports of successful return to production following surgery in several animals with unilateral disease. Currently, surgery is recommended for valuable animals with nonheritable unilateral disorders other than herniation.

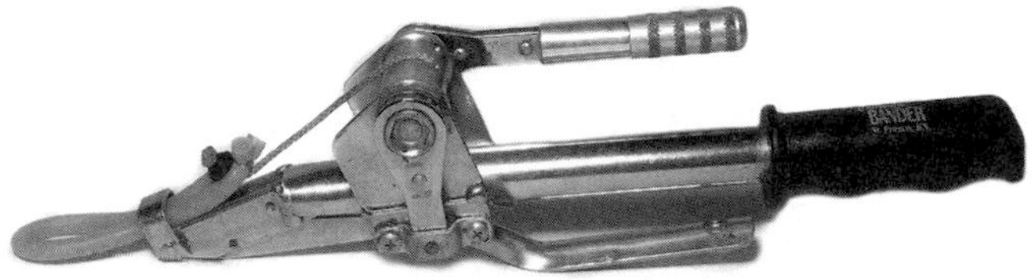

BLOODLESS CASTRATION

Several techniques for castrating farm animals without performing a surgical incision are available. These so-called "bloodless techniques" create ischemia of the testis with subsequent atrophy or necrosis. In very young animals, the most common technique is to use an elastic band. The band and applicator pliers should be soaked in disinfectant before use. Once the animal is restrained, the band is applied around the neck of the scrotum by using the pliers (Figure 12.1.1-7A and B). Other commercially available tools are designed to place heavy-walled latex tubing around the neck of the scrotum in older animals. The scrotum and testes usually slough within 3 weeks of band application. This technique is used quite commonly in small ruminants less than one month of age. Ambulatory clinicians at our institution have been successful with using a callicrate bander* in bulls up to 400 kg (Figure 12.1.1-8). Rare failure has been associated with band breakage. Older, small ruminants should be handled the same as older calves with sedation and surgery; however, one should always be mindful of small ruminant sensitivity to lidocaine. The callicrate bander has been used successfully on older goats after the long hair was clipped from the neck of the scrotum.

Another bloodless technique is to use a Burdizzo emasculatome (Figure 12.1.1-9) to crush the spermatic

*www.nobull.net/bander/

Figure 12.1.1-8   Callicrate bander.

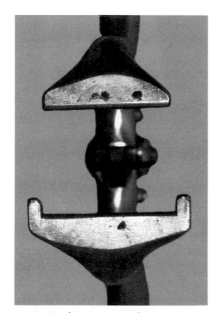

Figure 12.1.1-9   Burdizzo emasculatome.

cord within the scrotum. After this, the testes atrophy but usually do not slough. This instrument is best used by crushing a portion of the scrotum while holding the spermatic cord over the side that is crushed. One can crush the spermatic cord twice while manipulating the cord within the scrotum. These crushes should be staggered without crossing the midline; so no pressure is applied across the entire scrotum, thus minimizing the risk of impairing vascular supply. All animals treated with nonsurgical castration techniques should receive tetanus prophylaxis (ideally several weeks before the procedure) because tetanus acquisition is one of the complications of this procedure.

Postoperative Care

After castration, animals should be observed for abnormalities such as excessive swelling, hemorrhage, and signs of infections such as depression, decreased appetite, and abnormal drainage. When older animals are castrated or with an unclean environment, perioperative antibiotics are administered for 5 to 7 days.

Complications

As mentioned previously, tetanus is a worry in small ruminants and may be of concern in bulls that are castrated with the callicrate bander. Minimal complications—including seroma formation, swelling, and inflammation at the surgery site—are typical. These are usually self-limiting and resolve without further treatment. Other castration complications include infection and hemorrhage. With an open wound, any incisional infection or swelling can usually be handled by simply providing adequate ventral drainage and enlarging the incision bluntly. If appropriate technique is used, hemorrhage is rarely a major problem. If persistent hemorrhage does occur, it may be necessary to pack the scrotum with a sterile towel, laparotomy pad, or gauze roll, with removal in 48 hours. When the sterile packing is removed, any retained blood clot should be gently expressed. If this is elected, antibiotics are appropriate since the packing material can serve as a foreign body in a closed space, thus making a localized infection more likely.

12.1.2—Testicular Biopsy

Robert O. Gilbert and
Susan L. Fubini

Recently, testicular biopsy was performed on six normal bulls to determine whether this would be a useful diagnostic tool for bulls with infertility. The investigators used a 15.2-cm 14-gauge biopsy needle placed through a stab incision in the skin. They determined that there were no long-term changes in semen quality over the course of the 90-day study. Therefore testicular biopsy with histopathological examination may be considered for cases of infertility if time and economic constraints preclude a wait-and-see approach for determining the future breeding ability of a particular bull. It is impor-

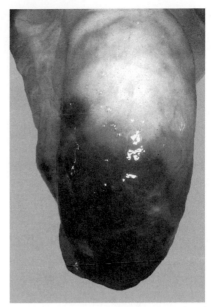

Figure 12.1.2-1 Testicular hemorrhage and infarction after testicular biopsy. To minimize the risk of this complication, needle biopsy should be performed at the dorsolateral, cranial aspect of the testis, where superficial vessels are sparsest (arrow).

tant to obtain the tissue sample from the lateral cranial aspect of the proximal (dorsal) area of the testis where blood vessels are relatively sparse to prevent excessive hemorrhage and infarction. Severe hemorrhage may necessitate removal of the testis (Figure 12.1.2-1). Cultures and sensitivity should be used to assess a testicular condition associated with an inflammatory or infectious process.

12.1.3—Surgical Management of Specific Conditions

Robert O. Gilbert and Susan L. Fubini

Cryptorchidism/Testicular Anomaly

Abnormality of testicular descent results in abdominal, inguinal, or ectopic testes. The left testis is more often retained in cattle, while a predilection for right cryptorchids has been reported in goats. Cryptorchid testes are very rare in ruminants, but ectopic testes are more common. Ectopic testis has been recognized cranial to the base of the scrotum with the long axis parallel to the penis. The physiological implication of an undescended testis is a slight reduction in testosterone production and a decrease in spermatogenesis. Unilateral castration elicits a compensatory hypertrophy in the remaining testis through the pituitary-testis endocrine axis that results in enhanced spermatogenesis. This compensatory hypertrophy is more marked if the animal is castrated unilaterally at an earlier age. Therefore removal of the undescended testis should not interfere with appropriate semen production. However, earlier reports suggest that the condition is heritable. No recent scientific studies have evaluated the cause of this condition. Certainly affected animals with other congenital abnormalities should be removed from the gene pool. It is less clear what recommendation should be made on a bull with an undescended testis that is otherwise normal, but the authors suggest discouraging the owner from breeding the animal.

The clinical diagnosis of undescended testis is made by physical examination where the absence of a testis in the scrotum is detected. To identify the location of the undescended testis one should palpate for (perhaps also search with ultrasound examination) the testis not only on the abdomen and inguinal canal but also in the subcutaneous tissues in the inguinal region, the fold of the flank, and alongside the penis. In addition, rectal examination may identify an abdominal testis. Furthermore, detection of normal size bulbourethral glands would indicate the presence of functioning testicular tissue.

With undescended testes the approach is made directly over the testis, if possible. The bull should be restrained appropriately, usually in dorsal recumbency for testes on the ventral abdomen and inguinal canal. Abdominal testes are best removed via a flank celiotomy. In the latter case, closure of the vaginal ring is needed to prevent formation of an inguinal hernia.

Scrotal Trauma

A common consequence of severe scrotal trauma is rupture of the tunica vaginalis of the testis. This typically results in profuse hemorrhage and formation of a hematocele. The injury may occur when a herdmate trods on the testis of the recumbent bull or when the scrotum is kicked. The scrotum is immediately swollen and painful. No prospect of recovery of the ruptured testis exists, and the only therapeutic concern is preserving the function of the surviving testis. If the condition is presented and diagnosed promptly, drainage of the hematocele after allowing three days for hemostasis helps reduce pressure on the contralateral testis. Hemiorchiectomy may be considered but offers little advantage beyond a better appearance. If the diagnosis is delayed, intervention may offer little advantage. Once the hematoma resolves, if left alone, the ruptured testis is usually replaced with fibrous tissue.

Inguinal/Scrotal Hernia

Inguinal hernia occurs mainly in mature bulls. The internal inguinal ring is palpable per rectum. It should be examined as part of every routine breeding soundness examination. The normal inguinal ring permits insertion of one or two fingers. Bulls with internal inguinal rings sufficiently wide to permit insertion of four fingers are predisposed to herniation, and the owner should be warned.

The overwhelming majority of inguinal hernias occur on the left side of the scrotum, probably a result of the rumen's weight and mature bulls lying in a sternal position with the left rear leg abducted. Most hernias are indirect (the intestinal component is contained within the tunica vaginalis), but occasionally direct herniation occurs when herniated intestine goes through a rent in the vaginal tunic and is contained within its own peritoneal pouch. The hernia is inguinal as long as the contents are within the inguinal canal (most frequent, Figure 12.1.3-1) and scrotal if the hernia extends into the scrotum. A scrotal hernia is rare because anatomic narrowing of the vaginal tunic within the neck of the scrotum (see Figure 12.1.3-1) normally prevents bowel from descending to the scrotum.

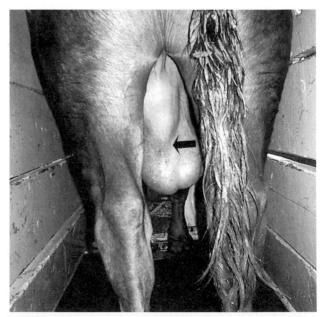

Figure 12.1.3-1   Inguinal hernia in a bull. Note the bulge in the vaginal tunic (arrow) created by the herniated small intestine, thus resulting in an "hourglass" configuration.

(Courtesy of Dr. David Anderson; The Ohio State University.)

Diagnosis may pose a challenge. Inguinal or scrotal hernia has to be differentiated from excess subcutaneous fat at the neck of the scrotum and from pendulous subperitoneal fat passed through the inguinal canal ("pseudohernia"). In pseudohernia, fat accumulates beneath the peritoneum in overconditioned heavy bulls. It may extend through the inguinal canal on a stalk, but it does so outside the tunica vaginalis, which is important information for performing surgery in this area. Passage of this fat mass through the inguinal canal widens the canal, and a true hernia can occur in conjunction with pseudohernia. Hernia can also result when the bull loses some conditioning, thus causing the fat pad to reduce and leaving a large vaginal ring. An accumulation of subcutaneous scrotal fat that occurs in the inguinal region but is bilaterally symmetrical should not be confused with the presence of an inguinal hernia. This subcutaneous fat usually disappears as the bull loses condition. Other abnormalities that can be confused with inguinal or scrotal hernia include hydrocele, aneurysm, neoplasia, and abscesses.

Beef breeds appear to be predisposed, particularly polled Hereford bulls, thus suggesting the condition has a genetic component. Hernia surgery may be combined with hemiorchidectomy of the testis on the involved side (a much easier technique), or an attempt may be made to salvage the testis.

As mentioned, hernias in mature bulls can be direct or indirect and acquired or congenital. An indirect hernia has the bowel within the tunica vaginalis that creates an "hourglass" configuration in an adult bull's scrotum (see Figure 12.1.3-1). This shape can change, depending upon whether the viscera are displaced. The narrowing of the vaginal tunic dorsal to the testis gives the characteristic shape. Inguinal/scrotal hernias are typically chronic and can affect semen quality by altering the bovine scrotum thermoregulatory function.

A true hernia is always palpable per rectum as a mass of abdominal contents that passes through the internal inguinal ring. It may not be possible to clearly identify which tissues are herniating by palpation. The diagnosis is supported if per rectal traction mass results in externally visible movement of the herniated mass. Ultrasonography of the scrotum and inguinal region may confirm the presence of loops of intestine. It is said that auscultation of the region with a stethoscope may reveal intestinal sounds in some cases.

Strangulation of an inguinal hernia is not common but may occur rapidly. Affected bulls show signs of intestinal obstruction, including abdominal pain and decreased fecal output, and the condition must be distinguished from intussusception and volvulus of the root of the mesentery. The hernia may be contained entirely within the inguinal canal without visible scrotal swelling.

Palpation per rectum of the internal inguinal ring is usually diagnostic.

Given a probable genetic component of the etiology of inguinal hernia, owners may elect not to have surgical repair performed.

SURGICAL REPAIR OF INDIRECT INGUINAL HERNIA—FLANK APPROACH

Preparation is the same as for any flank celiotomy. The approach is on the same side as the hernia. The inguinal ring is identified. Traction is applied gently to the herniated contents. Once the hernia is reduced, the internal inguinal ring is closed with blindly placed simple-interrupted or simple-continuous absorbable sutures. This can be difficult to accomplish. Furthermore, bowel adhesions to the vaginal tunic or the presence of inguinal fat pad remnants can make correction difficult or impossible from this approach.

SURGICAL REPAIR OF INDIRECT INGUINAL HERNIA—INGUINAL APPROACH

The bull is placed in lateral recumbency on the side opposite the hernia. General anesthesia is highly desirable. The uppermost leg is elevated and secured to expose the inguinal area. The inguinal area is prepared for aseptic surgery. A sharp 15- to 20-cm skin incision is made over the external inguinal ring. The subcutaneous tissues are divided by using a combination of blunt and sharp dissection to expose the testis, vaginal tunic, and identified anatomic landmarks of the inguinal canal. At this point, determining whether any adhesions exist between the intestine and vaginal tunic is important. If the bowel slides easily and can be replaced into the abdomen without difficulty, it is unnecessary to open the vaginal tunic. Instead, twisting the testis replaces the bowel into the abdomen (Figure 12.1.3-2B). The twisted spermatic cord can be transfixed with no.-2 absorbable sutures and tacked to the sides of the external inguinal ring, effectively occluding the inguinal canal. After this, the testis is emasculated (Figure 12.1.3-2C). Adhesions between the bowel and vaginal tunic make it necessary to incise the vaginal tunic to assess the intestine. If adhesiolysis is required, careful attention to hemostasis and asepsis is essential. The hernia is reduced, the testis emasculated, and the external inguinal ring closed. Removing any inguinal fat pad provides better identification of tissue layers for a more secure closure.

Closing the external inguinal ring enough to prevent intestinal herniation without impairing the testis blood supply has been described as a way to save the testis. The authors prefer to sacrifice the testis on the affected side and close the external inguinal ring with substantial bites

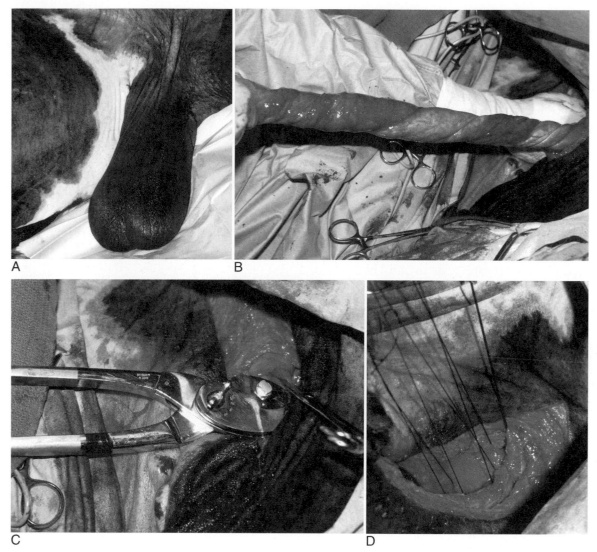

Figure 12.1.3-2   *A*, Bull in lateral recumbency with affected limb abducted. The inguinal area is prepared for aseptic surgery. *B*, Twisting the vaginal tunic to reduce an indirect hernia. *C*, Use of an emasculator. *D*, Placement of sutures in the external inguinal ring (Courtesy of Dr. David Anderson; The Ohio State University.)

of no.-2 absorbable suture (Figure 12.1.3-2D). Subcutaneous tissues and skin are closed routinely in an effort to decrease dead space.

Direct Inguinal Hernia

Direct hernia means the bowel has protruded through a defect in the peritoneum or a tear in the vaginal tunic. The etiology is presumed to be traumatic; less side predisposition occurs and no characteristic "hourglass" shape of the scrotum. If the intestine is incarcerated, the bulls can show signs of intestinal obstructive disease and present as a surgical emergency.

SURGICAL REPAIR OF DIRECT INGUINAL HERNIA—INGUINAL APPROACH

The surgery for direct inguinal hernia is very similar to that described for indirect hernia. However, the status of the bull may indicate the necessity of more intense preoperative care. This would include fluid therapy, nonsteroidal antiinflammatory drugs, and antimicrobials. At surgery, adhesions or devitalized bowel would require resection. A flank laparotomy may be necessary for hernias difficult to reduce or when a large portion of bowel is involved.

Congenital Inguinal Hernia

Repair of congenital inguinal hernia is not recommended unless a bilateral castration is performed. Simple indirect hernias are almost always repaired by twisting the testis as described in the technique above (see section on surgical repair of indirect inguinal herniainguinal approach).

COMPLICATIONS

Considerable postsurgical edema and swelling may occur. This can be controlled with hydrotherapy and diuretics if necessary. If the bull's disposition permits, controlled walking is desirable. If an intestinal resection was performed, antibiotics should be continued for 5 to 7 days.

Epididymectomy

This procedure is performed as the main or supplementary method for producing teaser animals. It may be performed in ruminants of all species; in laterally restrained or standing animals. Local anesthesia of the ventral scrotum and testis is achieved, and the surgical site is prepared. A 2-cm skin incision in the ventral scrotum is extended into the relatively conspicuous tail of the epididymis. The tail of the epididymis is separated carefully from the distal aspect of the testis with blunt dissection, ligated with fine absorbable material, and removed. Care must be taken to avoid injury to the testis, which will bleed profusely if inadvertently incised. The tunica vaginalis is not closed, but the skin incision is sutured. The technique should be performed at least 30 days before intended use of the teaser to allow sufficient time to achieve infertility.

Vasectomy

Vasectomy (removal of a segment of the *ductus* (formerly *vas*) *deferens* to render a male animal infertile) is generally a management technique used to produce teaser males or as an adjunct to such methods. Teasers are used to detect or aid in identification of females in estrus to allow them to be bred by natural or artificial means to males of greater genetic merit than the teasers. Ideal methods for creating teaser animals (see later) involve rendering the teaser both infertile and incapable of mating (to prevent spread of venereal diseases). Vasectomy achieves infertility but does not alter the ability or desire of males to mate; it is best to combine vasectomy with a procedure that precludes mating.

Vasectomy is usually performed with the aid of a local block at the surgical site. It can be done with the animal standing or restrained in lateral recumbency. Rams can be operated on in a sitting position, restrained by an assistant. The conventional technique involves incision of the neck of the scrotum cranially, caudally, or even laterally. Some surgeons prefer a single incision in the median raphe to allow access to both spermatic cords. In bulls and rams, the incisions need to be about 2 cm in length to allow exteriorization of the cord. The skin and parietal layer of the vaginal tunic are incised in a vertical fashion. The ductus deferens is located by palpation because it is firmer than the surrounding vasculature and membranes. It is usually located at the caudomedial aspect of the cord. The ductus deferens also lies within its own fold of vaginal tunic. The cord consists of a mass of arteries, veins, and nerves enclosed by the visceral layers of the vaginal tunic. Incision of the vessels of the cord leads to considerable hemorrhage that is difficult to control and can obscure the other structures of the cord. Care should be taken to identify the ductus deferens, isolate it via delicate blunt dissection, and remove a 3-cm piece of it after 3-0 absorbable ligatures have been placed on each end (Figure 12.1.3-3). The procedure is repeated on the opposite side. For additional security, it is wise to fix and label the removed components to document the removal of the appropriate structure with histopathology. More simply, the excised ductus deferens may be examined under a dissecting microscope to confirm the presence of the characteristic star-shaped lumen. The vasectomized animal should also be permanently identified (e.g., by notching the ear or tattooing) to guard against later confusion of intact and vasectomized animals (particularly important in rams).

Because vasectomy is a common procedure in animals as well as human males, it tends to be regarded as simple. Surgeons who perform a few vasectomies may find pos-

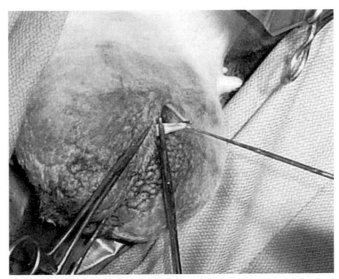

Figure 12.1.3-3   Ductus deferens isolated with Allis forceps.

(Courtesy of Dr. Carlos Gradil; Cornell University.)

itive identification of the ductus deferens amongst the structures of the spermatic cord unexpectedly difficult, especially in fat, meat-breed rams. Fat surrounding the cord may impede identification of the ductus deferens with a conventional (high) approach from the cranial or caudal direction. A novel approach to the procedure, proposed by Lofstedt (1982) is considerably easier to perform, especially for those who do not regularly vasectomize ruminants. The animal is restrained as above. The scrotum is clipped, scrubbed, and draped appropriately, and local analgesia administered. A vertical skin incision is made in the cranial aspect of the scrotum in the middle of the sac. The incision is extended to reach the left or right parietal vaginal tunic, and the cranial aspect of this incision is grasped with Allis forceps. While the testis is stabilized with one hand, a second pair of Allis forceps is inserted in a caudad direction toward the medial reflection of the vaginal tunic (at the body of the corpus epididymidis). The ductus deferens is the only structure in the cul-de-sac created by the reflection of the vaginal tunic (mesorchium), and it is easily identified and grasped with instruments. A section of at least 3 cm is removed to prevent the possibility of reanastomosis. The procedure is repeated on the opposite side. Postsurgical swelling is remarkably limited in scope, and few complications arise from this approach. Administration of tetanus toxoid is wise after vasectomy, especially in rams. Antibiotic therapy is optional.

12.1.4—Surgery of the Accessory Glands

Robert O. Gilbert and
Susan L. Fubini

Seminal Vesiculectomy

Vesiculitis (also called *seminal vesiculitis or vesicular adenitis*) is characterized by palpable changes in the vesicular glands, ultrasonically visible hypoechoic areas in the glandular parenchyma and leukospermia (semen contaminated with leukocytes, particularly neutrophils). During the acute stages, pain may be evident, spontaneously or upon palpation of the gland, but most cases are presented later in the progression of the disease. It occurs most commonly in pubertal bulls or in older bulls. Both types defy treatment with antibiotics. In the pubertal form, spontaneous recovery is quite common. The presence of large numbers of leukocytes impairs fertility, probably by increased oxidative damage to sperm, although most affected bulls are not completely infertile.

Commercial use of the semen for cryopreservation is not possible. Younger (1- to 2-year-old) bulls in which the condition does not resolve spontaneously or valuable mature bulls with vesiculitis are candidates for vesiculectomy, particularly if the condition is unilateral. The presurgical examination should also seek to confirm that the inflammation is limited to the vesicular gland. Involvement of the ampullae may prevent resolution of the leukospermia after surgery and therefore prevent return to normal semen production.

Surgery is performed in the standing bull, confined in an appropriate chute, under epidural analgesia. Prophylactic antibiotic therapy should be administered for two days before surgery. Sedation is not usually needed but should be dictated by the temperament of the bull. The rectum is evacuated, preferably before administration of the epidural analgesic, to prevent rectal "ballooning." A pursestring suture is inserted in the anus to prevent contamination of the surgical field (Figure 12.1.4-1A). The ends of the suture material are left long to facilitate later removal and to remind the surgeon to remove the suture. A crescent-shaped incision is made in the ischiorectal fossa, curved around the anus (Figure 12.1.4-1A). The incision is continued through the skin and subcutis by sharp dissection. With blunt dissection, the loose connective tissue is separated between the rectum medially and sacrosciatic ligament laterally until the vesicular gland is reached. The temptation to use sharp dissection should be resisted once the skin and subcutis is penetrated or profuse hemorrhage may ensue. The inflamed gland is invariably encased in tough connective tissue. The peritoneal reflection covers the cranial most portion of—and always firmly adheres to—the gland. Inflammation in and around the vesicular gland increases the amount of dense fibrous tissue that needs to be broken down blindly with the fingers of one hand. This process takes many minutes—and is tiring—but should be completed patiently and gently. Damage to the rectum or to major blood vessels could potentially be catastrophic. The nerves, vessels, and muscles associated with erection and ejaculation lie close to the operative field. It is important to completely free the vesicular gland as close to its base as possible. Care is taken not to damage the ipsilateral ampulla. In fact, the base of the vesicular gland extends virtually to the urethra, but only the portion of the gland external to the urethralis muscle is freed up and ultimately removed. Experience suggests that the remaining tissue seldom presents a problem; either it is not usually involved in the inflammatory process or postsurgical induration renders it inactive. Once the vesicular gland is completely freed from surrounding adhesions, a sterile écraseur is inserted, and the chain is carefully placed around the freed gland (Figure 12.1.4-1B). The gland is held to ensure the chain is

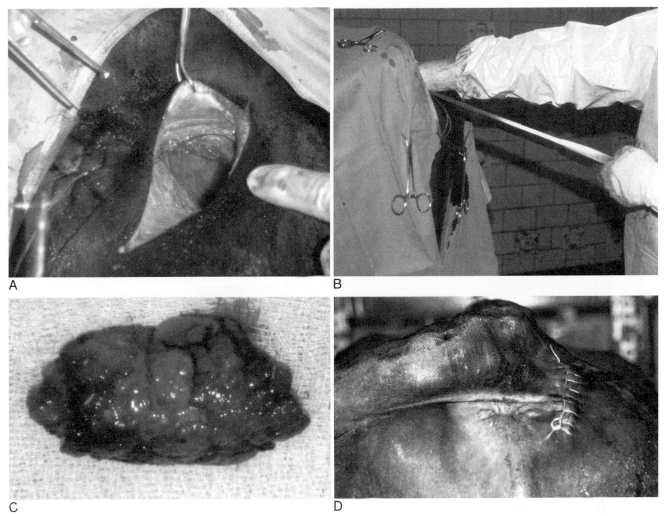

Figure 12.1.4-1 *A*, View of incision site for vesiculectomy. Note pursestring suture in anus (*arrow*). *B*, The incision in the ischiorectal fossa is crescent-shaped, curved around the anus. *C*, Use of écraseur to remove the dissected vesicular gland. *D*, Vesicular gland after removal. *E*, Surgical site after skin closure.

snugly applied to the base of the vesicular gland without encroaching on neighboring structures, and the gland is removed (Figure 12.1.4-1C). Multiple simple interrupted absorbable sutures are used to close as much dead space as possible. The skin is closed routinely (Figure 12.1.4-1D). The pursestring suture is removed from the anus. Postsurgical antibiotics and antiinflammatories should be administered for 3 to 5 days. The skin sutures are removed in 10 days. The bull should be sexually rested for 4 to 6 weeks. Initial semen quality may be disappointing, commonly with numerous detached sperm heads, but gradual improvement in semen quality is the rule.

After unilateral removal of a vesicular gland, the prognosis for return to normal service and fertility by natural service or artificial insemination is excellent. Postsurgical complications may include perirectal hematoma in the

area of blunt dissection. This usually resolves spontaneously, but occasionally becomes infected and forms an abscess which requires drainage. Although success after bilateral vesiculectomy has been reported, the author has had disappointing results with simultaneous and sequential removal of both glands and does not recommend it.

Although the surgical method described above has been very successful, it does require blind operation, and profuse bleeding is a risk. These factors have prompted a search for a method of surgery that allows clear visualization of the operative field. Hull (2001) has described an approach through the floor of the rectum. This procedure is also performed on the standing bull under epidural anesthesia, with sedation if indicated. Again, surgery should be preceded by antibiotic therapy for a day or two. In preparation for surgery the rectum is evacuated, and a tampon made of gauze is inserted about 10 inches into the rectum. The rectum caudal to the tampon is lavaged with an antiseptic solution such as dilute Lugol's iodine. The perineal area is clipped and prepared for surgery. A vertical incision is made in the ventral aspect of the anus and through the connective tissue ventral to the rectum, until the level of the penis is reached. The ventral rectal wall is divided cranially with blunt dissection as much as possible to minimize hemorrhage until the vesicular glands are visible. The incised or separated edges of the rectum are retracted to allow visualization of the surgical site. The affected gland is freed from its peritoneal attachments and any periglandular adhesions, ligated, and removed. The rectal floor is restored by suturing the rectal submucosa and serosa with absorbable inverting sutures in a continuous Lembert pattern, with care taken to not penetrate the rectal mucosa or to leave exposed suture material within the rectum. After removal of the rectal tampon, the anal sphincter is repaired with absorbable suture in a horizontal mattress pattern, and the skin is closed with nonabsorbable sutures. Alternatively, the tampon may be left in situ until closure is complete, when it is withdrawn to occupy the area of surgery, thereby maintaining pressure on the surgical site and preventing hemorrhage, and finally is removed an hour or two later. Antibiotic coverage is maintained for 3 days after surgery.

It is not unusual to encounter a high proportion of morphologically abnormal sperm in the period immediately after vesiculectomy; detached heads usually predominate. A slow return to normal sperm motility and morphology over about 4 to 6 weeks can be expected. Most bulls recover well and return to natural or artificial service. Sperm retain their ability to survive cryopreservation after unilateral vesiculectomy.

12.1.5—Penile Surgery (for Urolithiasis see Section 19.2)

Robert O. Gilbert

Examination of the Penis

Any factor that causes inability to mate is called *impotentia coeundae*. The cause of such impotence may lie outside the genitalia. It is therefore necessary to exclude poor libido or lesions of the neuromusculoskeletal system before exploring the possibility of lesions of the penis or

its adnexa. Note that any lesion that causes *impotentia coeundae* may eventually result in loss of libido, so absence of libido does not guarantee that the original lesion is not one of the penis or other genitalia.

The examination is designed to detect lesions of the penis, retractor penis muscles, prepuce, or connective tissue surrounding the penis, all of which may interfere with the ability to mate successfully. Visual inspection, palpation, special examinations and observation of mating attempts may be required to acquire a comprehensive understanding of the state of the ruminant's penis.

A general physical examination should be done to rule out lesions of the neuromusculoskeletal system that may prevent normal mating or mating behavior. The bull or ram is examined in motion; and particular attention should be paid to the feet, joints, sensation of the skin, muscular development and symmetry, or any other lameness or neurological deficit in the restrained animal.

Visual inspection of the external genitalia and initial palpation do not require any special physical or chemical restraint beyond those readily available in most circumstances. If no cause of impotence can be established, the bull or ram should ideally be observed in one or more mating attempts. For this purpose females in estrus are ideal, but restrained animals may suffice. Some males, especially those of certain breeds (zebu breed bulls) are shy and may not mount or mate readily while under observation. This need not imply a lack of libido or mating ability.

Further examination requires exteriorization of the penis, preferably under pudendal nerve block (as described earlier). Anesthesia of the pudendal nerves achieves sensory block of the free end of the penis as well as relaxation of the retractor penis muscles. It is ideal for penile examination as well as surgical procedures of the penis that can be undertaken in the standing animal.

Penile Hematoma

Perhaps the commonest penile lesion is hematoma or its sequelae (abscessation or adhesion). A hematoma results from sudden or forceful bending of the erect penis. During the peak of erection, blood pressure within the corpus cavernosum penis rises to astronomical levels. Deviation of the penis at this point (by sudden movement of the cow or by thrusting of the bull against the thigh of the cow before intromission is achieved, results in rupture of the tunica albuginea and hemorrhage. The hematoma may be exacerbated by repeated mating attempts by the bull. The site of the hematoma is usually distal to the distal curve of the sigmoid flexure (Figure 12.1.5-1A). At full erection this part of the penis comes to lie at the preputial orifice, which acts as a fulcrum against which the bending force is exerted. Furthermore,

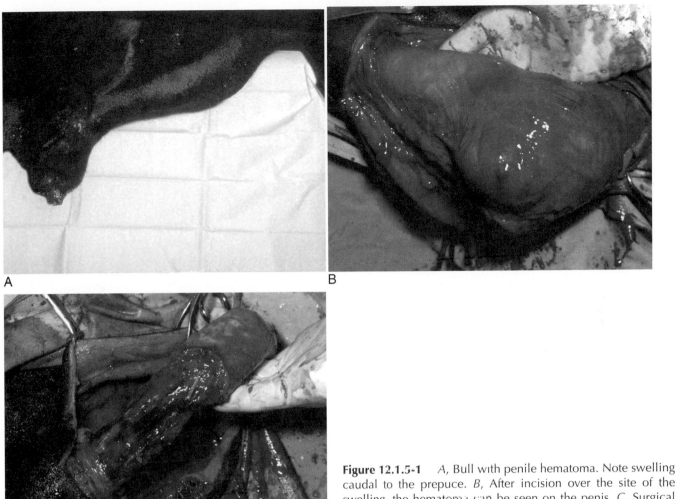

Figure 12.1.5-1 *A*, Bull with penile hematoma. Note swelling caudal to the prepuce. *B*, After incision over the site of the swelling, the hematoma can be seen on the penis. *C*, Surgical site after resection of the hematoma.

(Courtesy of Dr. David Anderson; The Ohio State University.)

this is the site of attachment of the retractor penis muscles. The ventral attachment of the retractor penis muscles results in most ruptures of the tunica albuginea, which occur dorsally or sometimes laterally.

Diagnosis of penile hematoma is usually uncomplicated. The bull may exhibit signs of pain such as an arched back or altered gait, but this is uncommon. The lamina interna of the prepuce may protrude, indicating that the penis is not withdrawn fully to its normal resting position. In some cases paraphimosis (inability to withdraw the penis itself back into the prepuce) may be seen. The swelling is almost always just cranial to the scrotum, reflecting the position of the site of rupture on the partially withdrawn penis. It may not be obvious on inspection, thus requiring palpation to appreciate its full extent.

The prognosis and clinical approach are both influenced by the size of the hematoma. In cases where the swelling is less than 15 cm in diameter, surgery is not usually required. Most of these bulls have a good prognosis for return to normal service behavior with conservative therapy. The bull should be removed from cows for 6 weeks. Daily hydrotherapy with cold water in the acute stage after the injury (about 4 days) and warm water thereafter, coupled with vigorous massage in a deliberate attempt to move the skin, intervening layers of fascia, and the penis to minimize formation of adhesions between these structures, are recommended. The hydrotherapy and massage should be continued for 3 weeks. Nonsteroidal antiinflammatory drugs may be beneficial during the first week. The bull should be reexamined before being returned to service, and his initial mating attempts should be observed to ensure return to copulatory function.

Complications include abscessation or extensive adhesions. These can be corrected surgically but the prognosis is usually poor. If the dorsal nerve of the penis is damaged, the free end of the penis may lack sensation, in which case intromission may be impaired and normal ejaculation is impossible. Semen may be collected from these bulls by electroejaculation for artificial insemination.

When the initial hematoma is over 15 cm in diameter, more extensive damage to the penile adnexa (telescoping fascia) results, making restrictive adhesion formation more likely. Risk of abscess formation is also increased. These factors account for the poorer prognosis and the preference for surgical therapy. Surgery may be performed in the standing animal, but general anesthesia is preferable. The skin covering the area of swelling is clipped and prepared for surgery. The skin incision should be as small as practical, as a larger incision allows more opportunity for firm adhesions to form between the skin and the underlying tissues. Blood, blood clots, and serum are gently removed, with attention paid to hemostasis. The penis is examined (Figure 12.1.5-1B), the area debrided (Figure 12.1.5-1C), and any detectable rent in the tunica albuginea sutured with absorbable material, with care taken to avoid penetrating suture bites through the tunica albuginea that might later become a source of leakage and failure to maintain erection. The skin incision should be left open. Postsurgical treatment should parallel the conservative approach to smaller hematomas.

Most penile hematomas occur in young (3-year-old) bulls, which reflects their inexperience and copulatory exuberance. Recurrence of the injury is common, which suggests that these bulls may have underlying copulatory habits (clumsiness) that predispose them to damage.

Deviations of the Penis

Spiral deviation of the penis ("corkscrew penis," Figure 12.1.5-2) is the most commonly encountered form of

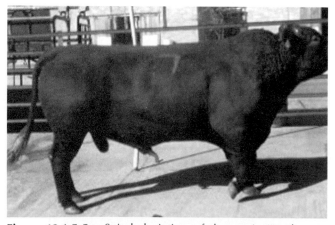

Figure 12.1.5-2   Spiral deviation of the penis ("corkscrew penis").

penile deviation. It results from slippage of the apical ligament of the penis when the penis is erect, but before intromission occurs, and thereby prevents intromission. Formation of a spiral in this way is normal at the point of ejaculation, once the penis is within the vagina. Bulls that suffer from corkscrew penis do not demonstrate this deviation at every service attempt, but it may prevent intromission in 50% to 100% of attempts. This condition is therefore more appropriately regarded as premature spiral formation. Whether the predisposition to this condition is inherited is unknown. The only way spiral deviation of the penis can be diagnosed with confidence is by observation of serving attempts. Reproduction of the corkscrew form during electroejaculation is not diagnostic.

TREATMENT

Surgical repair of spiral deviation of the penis involves anchoring the apical ligament of the penis so it cannot slip laterally and pull the free part of the penis into a spiral or augmenting the apical ligament with an implant. For implantation, one large (Figure 12.1.5-3A) or multiple thin strips of fascia lata may be used; alternatively, synthetic fibers may be implanted.

Surgery to anchor the apical ligament can be performed in standing animals, under pudendal nerve block, although general anesthesia is preferable. The preputial hairs are clipped. The penis is extended and held in place with penetrating towel clamps carefully placed into the distal part of the apical ligament to avoid penetration of the tunica albuginea (Figure 12.1.5-3B). A longitudinal incision is made along the dorsal aspect of the penis for about 10 cm, starting 3 cm from the tip of the penis. (This incision will traverse the preputial reflection.) The incision is deepened until the apical ligament is exposed (Figure 12.1.5-3C). The free edges of the apical ligament are identified, and these edges are carefully tacked to the underlying tunica albuginea, using multiple simple interrupted sutures of synthetic absorbable material. The skin incision is closed with absorbable material. The surgical site is covered with antimicrobial ointment to provide lubrication. Postsurgical care requires inspection to ensure adhesions are not forming; most bulls move the penis a great deal during normal daily activities and adhesion is a rare problem. The bull should be housed alone for 4 to 6 weeks after surgery and not be allowed to be sexually excited.

For implantation of the apical ligament, the bull must be under general anesthesia, and in lateral recumbency. The area of the uppermost thigh (usually left) is prepared for surgery. A 15-cm skin incision is made midway between the tuber coxae and a point about 15 cm caudal to the patella, and the fascia lata identified (Figure 12.1.5-3E). Three or four strips of fascia lata, each about 10 cm long and 0.5 cm wide, are harvested and placed

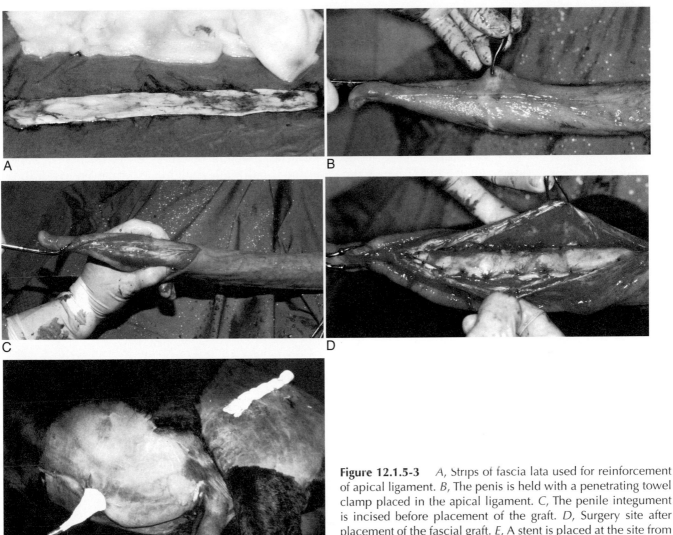

Figure 12.1.5-3 *A,* Strips of fascia lata used for reinforcement of apical ligament. *B,* The penis is held with a penetrating towel clamp placed in the apical ligament. *C,* The penile integument is incised before placement of the graft. *D,* Surgery site after placement of the fascial graft. *E,* A stent is placed at the site from which the fascial graft was harvested.

(Courtesy of Dr. David Anderson; The Ohio State University.)

on moistened cotton sponges. Alternatively, a single strip of fascia lata about 10 cm long and 1.5 cm wide is obtained (see Figure 12.1.5-3A). The defect in the fascia lata is closed with absorbable sutures, and the skin incision is closed in a continuous pattern with nonabsorbable material and a stent sutured in place (see Figure 12.1.5-3E).

The penis is extended and prepared for surgery. Open or closed methods can be used for inserting the fascia strips. The authors prefer the closed method for its simplicity. A 2-cm longitudinal incision is made 3 cm from the tip of the penis, on the dorsal aspect. A fascia strip is threaded through the eye of a blunt needle probe, which is then inserted into the incision and directed proximally along the dorsum of the penis. A small incision is made over the tip of the probe proximal to the preputial reflection, and it is withdrawn, leaving the fascia strip in place.

This is repeated for each strip, and the surgeon should try to spread them evenly across the dorsal aspect of the penis. The incisions in the penile integument are closed with fine absorbable material after cutting off excess length of the fascia implants. The fascia strips need not be sutured in place. Care must be taken to ensure that the fascia strips are not exposed to air since exposed ends may result in local granuloma formation.

For the open method, a longitudinal incision is made along the dorsal aspect of the penis, exposing the apical ligament (see Figure 12.1.5-3C). The ligament is carefully incised, and the tunica albuginea is exposed. The fascial strips are laid carefully on the tunica albuginea, the defect in the apical ligament closed, and the skin incision closed. Alternatively, one large strip is sutured in place (see Figure 12.1.5-3D).

Use of synthetic materials, such as carbon fibers, has been described for each of these procedures. Implantation of fascia lata strips may also be effective for treatment of ventral deviation of the penis.

Erection Failure

Erection failure caused by leakage from the corpus cavernosum penis is a well-described cause of impotence in bulls. In this species, the normal circulation of the corpus cavernosum penis is a closed system. Blood enters the corpus cavernosum penis via the paired deep pudendal arteries at the level of the crura penis and leaves via the homologous veins. The corpus cavernosum penis communicates neither with the corpus spongiosum penis nor with the superficial vasculature of the penis. In the first stage of erection of the bovine penis, musculature that retains the normal resting position of the penis is relaxed. Arterial dilation allows passive filling of the cavernous spaces of the corpus cavernosum penis, and the penis is extended in response to sexual stimulation. During and immediately before mounting, contraction of the ischiocavernosus and bulbospongiosus muscles produces a short-lived but dramatic increase in blood pressure within the corpus cavernosum penis. Full erection is therefore achieved by addition of very little additional blood volume but a great increase in blood pressure. Any leakage of blood from the corpus cavernosum penis can therefore impede erection. Vascular shunts usually communicate with the superficial penile vessels, but in some cases communication between the corpus cavernosum penis and corpus spongiosum penis occur.

Cavernosal vascular shunts must be differentiated from ventral deviation of the penis ("rainbow penis"), which is attributable to a defect of the apical ligament of the penis. In ventral deviation, the penis does not achieve its full length while straight, and it remains rigid. In the case of cavernosal shunts, the penis is usually extended normally, but erection is maintained only momentarily before the penis becomes flaccid and droops. Careful observation is required to make the distinction. Definitive diagnosis depends on contrast cavernosography (Figure 12.1.5-4A).

For contrast cavernosography, the bull is anesthetized and positioned in lateral recumbency. An 18-gauge needle, attached to an extension set, is inserted into the corpus cavernosum penis 10 cm from the tip of the penis. Sterile saline should flow freely when injected. A survey (plain) radiograph is taken to confirm suitability of exposure factors. Following this 10 ml of water soluble contrast medium is injected into the corpus cavernosum penis and a series of radiographs—ventrodorsal, lateral,

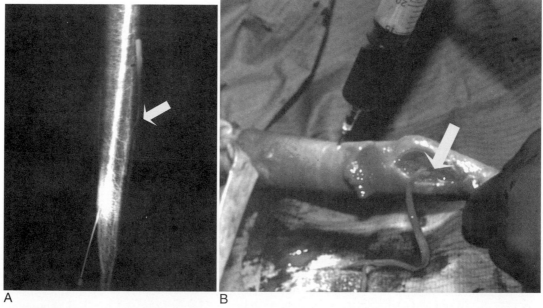

A   B

Figure 12.1.5-4   *A,* Contrast cavernosogram that shows contrast medium escaping from the corpus cavernosum penis (arrow). In normal bulls, the contrast medium remains entirely within the corpus cavernosum penis. *B,* Intraoperative view of correction of cavernosal shunt. Arrow indicates site of leakage from the corpus cavernosum penis. Syringe containing methylene blue is inserted into the corpus cavernosum; injection of a small volume confirms correct identification of the leaking vessel by its blue discoloration.

and oblique—taken. It may be advantageous to place a tourniquet around the base of the penis to achieve elevated pressure of the contrast medium and thereby more closely simulate the normal physiology. In normal bulls the contrast medium remains confined to the corpus cavernosum penis. In the case of shunts, contrast medium can be seen outside of the corpus cavernosum (see Figure 12.1.5-4A). With care, the position of the leakage can be identified. If there is communication between the corpus cavernosum and the corpus spongiosum, surgery is impossible. If the communication is with a superficial vessel, this vessel can be identified at surgery and firmly ligated at its point of emergence from the corpus cavernosum penis (Figure 12.1.5-4B), including superficial bites into the tunica albuginea of the penis with fine absorbable suture material. If doubt exists during surgery as to the correct identification of a communicating superficial vessel, a small (2 to 3 ml) volume of dye (e.g., methylene blue) can be injected slowly into the corpus cavernosum penis; it will be seen escaping from the corpus cavernosum penis via the communicating vessel (Figure 12.1.5-4B). The bull should be allowed 6 weeks of sexual rest.

Cavernosal shunts are believed to arise from congenital presence of communicating vessels. Some cases may follow traumatic or iatrogenic penetration of the corpus cavernosum. At surgery, the communicating vessels appear "normal" and similar vessels can be found upon dissection of slaughterhouse material from presumably normal bulls, leading this author to favor an explanation that leakage constitutes a functional aberration, rather than an anatomical one.

Penile Tumors

The commonest tumor of the bovine penis is fibropapilloma (Figure 12.1.5-5). These are usually encountered

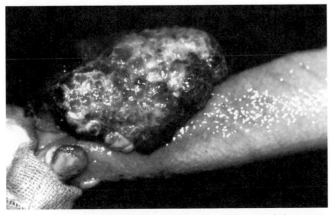

Figure 12.1.5-5   Penile fibropapilloma. The tip of the penis is held by sponge.

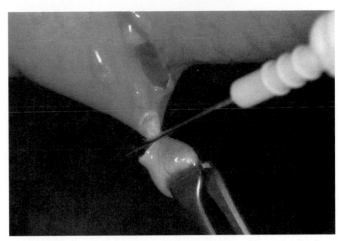

Figure 12.1.5-6   Removal of penile fibropapilloma with electrocautery.

(Courtesy of Dr. David Anderson; The Ohio State University.)

in young bulls. In bulls that are group-housed, as, for example, in a beef bull performance test, penile fibropapillomata may occur in large numbers of animals. Although there is some controversy about this, this author's experience strongly suggests that commercial wart vaccine diminishes the incidence of the condition.

Penile papillomata interfere with breeding by making intromission impossible in some cases or uncomfortable in others. Bleeding interferes with semen quality. The papillomata generally regress spontaneously with time but are usually removed to provide a rapid and certain return to use.

Removal is usually done in the standing bull with appropriate restraint, sedation if necessary, and local (dorsal penile nerve) or regional (pudendal) nerve block. Most penile papillomata are pedunculated. They may be removed by sharp dissection, electrocautery (Figure 12.1.5-6), or cryosurgery. The integumentary defect is sutured if necessary. The bull should be sexually rested for 3 weeks.

When papilloma-like lesions are encountered in mature bulls, histological confirmation of the lesion type by biopsy is indicated; a small number of aggressive, malignant fibrosarcomata may be encountered in the bovine penis. Culling is indicated in these cases.

Penile Procedures for Teaser Bulls

Several methods are used for producing teaser bulls for identification of cows in estrus. These include vasectomy, epididymectomy, and preputial relocation or obliteration, discussed elsewhere. Ideally, teaser bulls should be young, virile, healthy, and the procedure should cause sterility and prevent intromission to limit any potential spread of disease.

Young bulls are generally most active and make the most desirable teasers. With any procedure, particularly those that make intromission impossible, most teaser bulls usually lose interest after a variable time—1 or 2 years. Alternatively, they may become frustrated and very aggressive. It is good practice to use teaser bulls for only one year—or at most two—and plan on regular replacement before bulls become very large or unmanageable.

Penile tie-down is a procedure that creates a permanent adhesion between the penis and the ventral body wall. With the patient in dorsal recumbency, the ventral abdomen is prepared for sterile surgery. A 5-cm longitudinal incision is made midway between the scrotal neck and the preputial orifice, at the level where the prepuce meets the abdomen. The incision is deepened until the linea alba is exposed. Loose connective tissue is dissected from the penis, and the urethra is identified by palpation. The dorsal aspect of the tunica albuginea of the penis (opposite the urethra) is attached to the line alba by multiple interrupted sutures of heavy nonabsorbable suture material placed approximately 1 cm apart and penetrating 1 cm into the body wall and a similar distance into the penis. The skin is closed routinely.

The penis may be attached to the skin of the escutcheon more simply. In the standing bull under epidural analgesia, the skin of the escutcheon, from the scrotal neck to the anus, is prepared for surgery. A skin incision is made over the area where the distal loop of the sigmoid flexure is palpable and is deepened until the penis is identified. Sutures of heavy, nonabsorbable material are placed in the tunica albuginea of the penis and through the skin adjacent to the skin incision. This is done on each side of the incision. Care must be taken to identify and avoid the urethra (closest to the incision) by placing the sutures in the penile tunica albuginea on the (lateral) sides of the penis. It is convenient to include the distal portion of the retractor penis muscles in the sutures, and this helps stabilize the penis.

Penectomy, or phallectomy, may be performed at the same surgical site dorsal to the scrotal neck. A skin incision is made as described above and is deepened until the penis is identified at the level of the distal loop of the sigmoid flexure. The distal portion of the penis can be removed from its abdominal attachments by blunt dissection and firm traction and exteriorized through the incision. The penis is transected about 3 cm ventral to the ventral level of the skin incision. The transection is done at an angle, to provide a ventral flap that can be used to cover the corpus cavernosum to control bleeding. The dorsal artery of the penis is ligated. The urethra is spatulated to provide a suitable aperture for urination and to prevent stricture. The penile stump is attached to

the skin with nonabsorbable suture material. A good mucosa to skin seal is essential. The bull must be observed after surgery to ensure that it is able to urinate.

An alternative method of phallectomy is performed with the bull in dorsal recumbency. The preputial cavity is irrigated with a weak disinfectant solution before surgery, and the ventral abdomen prepared for surgery. A longitudinal skin incision is made, beginning 5 cm cranial to the scrotal neck and extending cranially for about 15 cm. The penis is identified and freed by blunt dissection, until it can be exteriorized through the incision. The sigmoid flexure is straightened, and a tourniquet is applied near the caudal aspect of the skin incision. The penis is transected obliquely (longer ventrally than dorsally) at a point 10 cm from the preputial attachment. The dorsal penile artery is ligated, and the ventral flap of the penile stump is folded dorsally to cover the corpus cavernosum and sutured in place. The urethra is spatulated, and its edges sutured to the penile stump to ensure an adequate orifice for urination. The tourniquet is removed, and adequate hemostasis is ensured by ligation or electrocautery. Then the cranial (free) end of the penis is removed from its preputial attachments and discarded. The prepuce is sutured to the stump previously created with multiple interrupted sutures of fine absorbable material. The skin is closed with nonabsorbable sutures. This method has the advantage that the bull urinates into the prepuce. The bull must be observed after surgery to ensure that urination is possible.

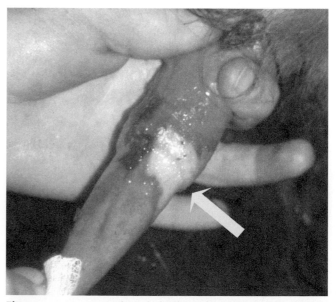

Figure 12.1.5-7   Pubertal bull with ongoing separation between penis and lamina interna of prepuce (*arrow*). This is normal. If separation is incomplete, a persistent frenulum results. Compare with Figure 12.1.5-8A.

Persistent Frenulum

At birth, the integument of the penis is continuous with the lamina interna of the prepuce. Separation occurs at the time of puberty, starting from the tip of the penis and progressing caudally (Figure 12.1.5-7). The last area of separation is the penile raphe, along the ventral edge of the penis. In some bulls this separation is incomplete. Although separation of the penis from the lamina interna of the prepuce is usually complete by about 9 months of age, some incomplete separation will be encountered amongst yearling bulls; this is usually seen as a circumferential zone of pale integument that can be separated with gentle traction. With time, this form of delayed separation usually develops normally. However, some bulls (or rams) retain one or more discrete bands of tissue that connect the free end of the shaft of the penis to the lamina interna of the prepuce (Figure 12.1.5-8A). These connections prevent straight extension of the penis. As erection is achieved, the elongated penis is pulled into a bow shape by the persistent frenulum. Should an entire "curtain" of tissue persist along the raphe, the condition is called *persistent frenum*; *frenulum* is a diminutive form of *frenum*.

Persistent frenulum is an inherited disorder that can be passed on to progeny. Although it is easily repaired, this should be borne in mind. If all progeny are destined for slaughter, the surgery is justified. Otherwise, the owner should carefully evaluate the risks and benefits before electing to use the bull.

In young bulls the penis can often be extended manually with no or little sedation. Application of a dorsal

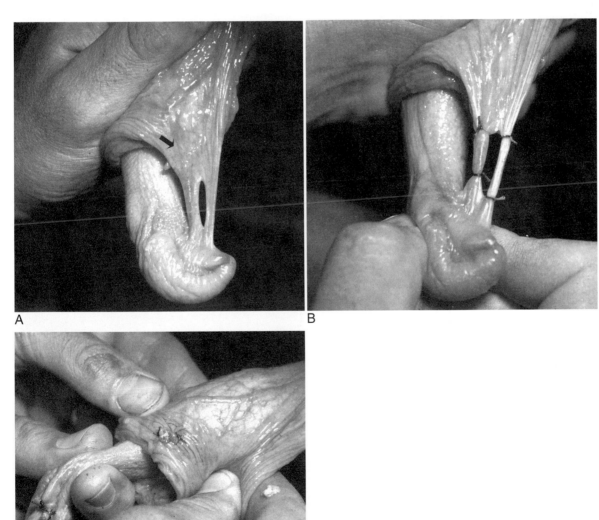

Figure 12.1.5-8 *A,* Persistent frenulum. Note large vessel (*arrow*). *B,* Ligature in place before transection. *C,* Surgical site after transection of the frenulum.

(Courtesy of Dr. Ken Pettey; University of Pretoria).

nerve block is often sufficient to perform this procedure. With the penis extended as far as possible by traction on its free end, a fine needle is inserted through the lamina interna at the dorsal aspect of the preputial orifice. Lidocaine (2%) is injected under the lamina interna and is deposited in a semicircle to cover the dorsal aspect of the penis. This will render the free end of the shaft of the penis insensitive by blocking the dorsal penile nerve before it splits into its terminal branches. Alternatively, pudendal nerve block or administration of xylazine and butorphanol can be used to achieve adequate exposure and anesthesia of the site.

The site of the persistent frenulum is prepared for surgery and then the structure is split between two absorbable sutures (Figure 12.1.5-8B). Although the persistent frenulum is usually a small structure and can be cut quickly without much preparation, this should be avoided, both for the bull's comfort and because it is often endowed with a generous vein and artery that can be the source of disconcerting hemorrhage (see Figure 12.1.5-8B). Repair of a persistent frenulum provides instant cure of this condition (Figure 12.1.5-8C), and bulls may be used a week after surgery.

12.1.6—Preputial Surgery

Robert O. Gilbert

Relocation of the Prepuce and Penis

Relocation of the preputial orifice—and therefore the prepuce and penis to the flank of the animal—allows extension of the penis without intromission and is a common method for production of teaser bulls. The procedure can be performed on bull calves as young as one month old or on more mature animals.

The animal is restrained in dorsolateral recumbency to allow access to the midline and to one flank. Heavy sedation and local block or general anesthesia can be used. A generous area from the umbilicus to the scrotum and extending laterally to beyond the flank fold is clipped and prepared for surgery. The initial incision is circumferential around the preputial orifice, with a radius of about 2 to 3 cm. While this incision is made, the skin remaining around the preputial orifice is notched or marked with a colored suture to preserve the correct orientation and prevent later torsion of the prepuce. The skin incision is extended caudally along the midline to within 5 cm of the scrotal neck. By careful dissection, the preputial lamina interna is freed from the surrounding connective tissue, and larger vessels are ligated as necessary. The operator must be careful not to incise the prepuce. The

lamina should be completely freed from underlying tissue for the entire length of the incision. Some surgeons prefer to insert a sterile glass or plastic speculum into the prepuce to facilitate its dissection. It is important to preserve some connective tissue with the prepuce to ensure sufficient blood supply. Without stretching the prepuce, one moves it to the side and marks a spot lateral to the flank fold to which it can be relocated. A circular piece of skin with a diameter one inch smaller than the freed preputial orifice is resected; note that the removal of the skin leaves a bigger defect than the size of the skin removed. A tunnel toward the base of the scrotum is created by means of blunt dissection with a Knowles cervical forceps or similar large forceps. Once a tunnel of suitable size has been made, the free preputial orifice—covered with a sterile surgical glove and lubricated with antimicrobial ointment—is grasped and withdrawn toward the newly prepared site, with care taken not to twist the prepuce in the process or to allow sharp bends or kinks. The new preputial orifice, former site of the preputial orific, and the longitudinal skin incision are all closed with an appropriate suture pattern.

The prepuce must be relocated to a site lateral to the flank fold. Placement of the preputial orifice more medially allows bulls to achieve intromission in a large number of cases (Figure 12.1.6-1). Some bulls are sufficiently motivated to learn to achieve intromission in spite of correct preputial relocation. This makes it prudent to perform vasectomy or epididymectomy at the same time.

After surgery, the area surrounding the newly relocated preputial orifice should be covered with petroleum jelly to prevent urine scald. This should be reapplied

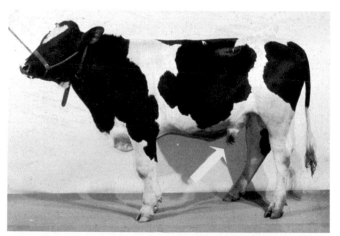

Figure 12.1.6-1   Bull with laterally translocated prepuce. Ideally, the newly created preputial orifice should be adjacent to the fold of the flank (arrow).

twice daily for the first week. Systemic antibiotics should be given for three days after surgery. The bull is observed carefully to ensure that he is able to urinate freely. There is often some swelling of the relocated prepuce, and it may take a day or two before it assumes a normal skin color, which indicates reestablished circulation. Complications are rare.

Preputial obliteration is an alternative method for producing teaser bulls. In this procedure, the preputial orifice is permanently closed, and a fistula created for drainage of urine. The patient is restrained in lateral recumbency and the penis extended. A 1-inch Penrose drain is sutured over the tip of the penis with fine absorbable suture material. A 1- to 2-cm diameter circle of skin is removed ventrally, about 5 cm caudal to the preputial orifice. A corresponding amount of subcutaneous tissue is removed, and the lamina interna of the prepuce is identified and similarly incised. (Insertion of a blunt probe into the prepuce helps identify it.) The preputial lamina interna is sutured to the skin with simple interrupted sutures, thus creating a fistula, and the free end of the Penrose drain is passed through the fistula. The end of the prepuce is removed by cutting through skin, subcutaneous tissue, and preputial lamina interna. These structures are then sutured in three layers. The Penrose drain carries urine past the fresh incision and helps prevent stenosis. The skin sutures and Penrose drain are removed after about 3 weeks.

Individual preference guides the choice of methods for producing teaser bulls. This author prefers preputial relocation combined with vasectomy.

Preputial Avulsion

Avulsion of the lamina interna of the prepuce from its attachment to the penile integument at the fornix, or point of reflection (Figure 12.1.6-2A), is the commonest injury to the penis and prepuce of bulls managed for the collection of semen for cryopreservation. It is observed only in bulls whose semen is collected by artificial vagina, and is not an injury of natural service bulls. This form of injury is costly when it causes temporary suspension of semen collection from extremely valuable artificial insemination bulls that are under considerable pressure to produce semen. These injuries may be left to heal by second intention, but convalescence is prolonged. Surgery, preferably on the same day as injury, is preferred for the bull's more rapid return to use with fewer complications. The etiology of preputial avulsion is not fully understood. This form of injury occurs most often in young bulls newly introduced to semen collection, or reintroduced after a period of layoff (to accu-

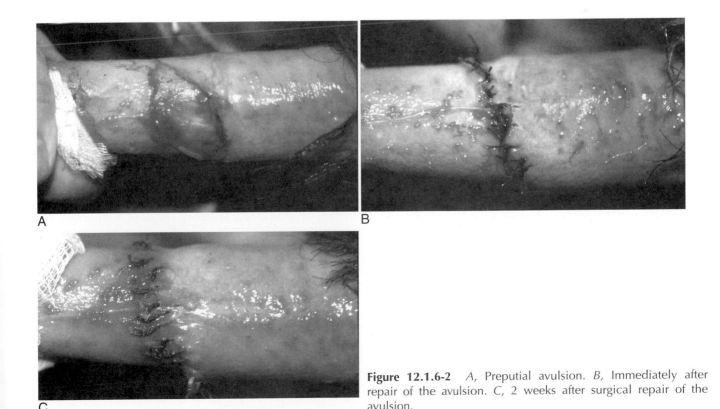

Figure 12.1.6-2 *A,* Preputial avulsion. *B,* Immediately after repair of the avulsion. *C,* 2 weeks after surgical repair of the avulsion.

mulate progeny data) but has been recorded in all breeds and age groups of bulls.

The semen collector or attendant will usually notice bleeding after semen collection. The diagnosis is confirmed by extending and examining the penis. Particularly in young bulls, the penis can be manually exteriorized after administering 5 mg of xylazine. The penis can then be grasped with dry gauze or held by towel clamps placed into the apical ligament (after anesthesia of the penis is established with a dorsal nerve block or pudendal nerve block, see Figure 12.1.6-2A). Surgery may be performed on the standing restrained bull or with the bull in lateral recumbency on a tilt table. The penis, prepuce, and ventral abdomen are thoroughly cleansed for surgery. Dorsal nerve block or pudendal nerve block is performed. The extended penis is held in place by an assistant, who uses sponges or a towel clamp placed in the apical ligament. Ligation of any hemorrhaging vessels is performed before closure of the integument. The integument is sutured with absorbable material on an atraumatic needle, with a simple interrupted pattern (Figure 12.1.6-2B and C). The bull should be withheld from service and housed individually until healing is complete. Ideally, the bull should be isolated from cows or other bulls to prevent sexual stimulation. Spontaneous erection may provoke dehiscence of the surgical site, which is usually indicated by blood-stained bedding. If promptly detected, it may be resutured; otherwise it should be left to heal as an open wound.

The bull is examined approximately 30 days after surgery by extending the penis manually or after sedation. The bull should not be allowed to mount a teaser as this provokes full erection. Return to service is allowed after a further 20 to 30 days, provided the surgical site is fully healed and pliable. Although the etiology is not clear, suspicion that atrophy of the preputial lamina interna with subsequent rupture upon stretching may play a role, suggesting that it would be wise to avoid false mounts upon reintroduction to semen collection. In addition, use of a short artificial vagina appears preferable, and its use at a temperature a few degrees cooler than usual may temper the vigor with which a young bull thrusts into the artificial vagina. Most bulls can be returned to service in about 60 days—a considerably shorter interval than may be expected if surgery is not performed (which may range up to or beyond a year).

Preputial Hair Ring

A ring of preputial hair may occasionally entrap the penis (Figure 12.1.6-3). Although this condition is usually spontaneously resolved, the hair may strangulate and damage the penis. Treatment of the resulting lesion must

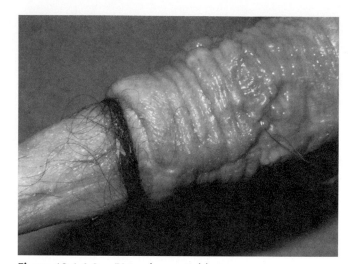

Figure 12.1.6-3   Ring of preputial hair.
(Courtesy of Dr. David Anderson; The Ohio State University.)

depend on the judgment of the surgeon, but many cases can be sutured as for preputial avulsion.

Preputial Prolapse

Preputial eversion is common in some breeds of bulls—particularly polled breeds and Brahman-influenced breeds. This is thought to result from absence or lack of development of the retractor preputii muscles. These muscles are believed to stabilize the lamina interna during movement of the penis and therefore to be instrumental in the prevention of prolapse or eversion. Prolapse of the lamina interna may be constant or may be seen only intermittently, especially during urination and immediately before mating attempts. Prolapse is more common when bulls are stressed. The everted membrane is subject to injury or desiccation. It may become scarred, abscesses may form, and these lesions may be severe enough to prevent penile extension (paraphimosis).

Diagnosis of preputial prolapse is self-evident (Figure 12.1.6-4). Early management includes supporting the prepuce until surgical treatment can be performed (Figure 12.1.6-5). In some cases, preputial damage and scar tissue may be internal and only diagnosable when the entire prepuce is carefully palpated, or inflated with air or water. Sometimes strictures may be located only at the preputial orifice.

If a simple stricture occurs at the preputial orifice, it should be incised longitudinally, beginning at the ventral aspect of the preputial orifices and extending caudally for a few cm. The incision is deepened to the lamina interna, which is then sutured to the skin with simple interrupted sutures of nonabsorbable material.

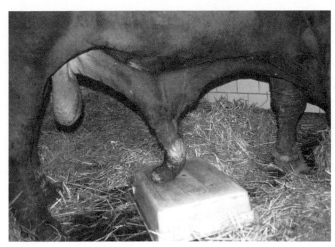

Figure 12.1.6-4 Santa Gertrudis Bull with preputial prolapse.

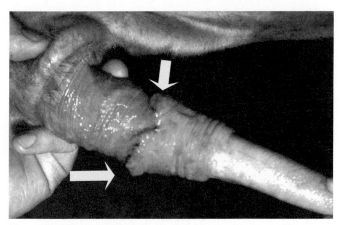

Figure 12.1.6-6 Narrow collar of fibrous tissue causing paraphimosis. Final appearance after a longitudinal incision is made through collar followed by a transverse closure. The dog-eared appearance (arrows) will resolve spontaneously.

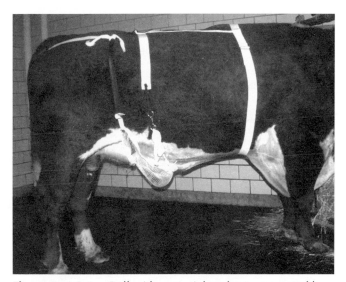

Figure 12.1.6-5 Bull with preputial prolapse supported by a truss.

Stricture caused by a narrow (less than 2 cm) band of connective tissue can be treated by making a longitudinal incision in the affected part of the lamina interna, extending 2 cm into normal tissue on each side of the stricture. The incision is then sutured transversely, by first suturing the cranial and caudal ends of the incision to each other. The resulting "dog ears" can be trimmed slightly while suturing, but this is not necessary, and tissue remodeling soon takes care of them (Figure 12.1.6-6). This procedure results in a wider lumen and free movement of the penis. The procedure can usually be performed in the standing bull, preferably with a pudendal nerve block.

More substantial collars of scar tissue (Figure 12.1.6-7A), whether in the prolapsed part or internal to the prepuce, must be removed by excision ("reefing"). This surgery is best performed under general anesthesia, with the bull in lateral or dorsal recumbency. Circumferential incisions are made at each end (cranial and caudal) of the connective tissue collar, and it is removed (Figure 12.1.6-7B). The edges of the lamina interna are then sutured together (Figure 12.1.6-7C), with care being taken to preserve their original orientation and prevent twisting of the lamina interna. Attaching a Penrose drain over the tip of the penis with a single absorbable suture and passing it through the preputial orifice allows the bull to urinate without irritating the suture site (Figure 12.1.6-8). Occasionally, this procedure will result in restricture along the suture line. Strategies to prevent this include making the original incisions obliquely if there is sufficient preputial tissue to work with, or making a zigzag incision to allow expansion after suturing. When these strictures do recur after surgery, they usually consist only of a narrow band of scar tissue along the incision site. This lesion can usually be treated by longitudinal incision and transverse suturing as described previously. Bulls should be given 6 weeks of sexual rest after surgery.

In rare cases strictures such as those described above prevent retraction of the penis after erection (phimosis), rather than extension of the penis. They are treated in essentially the same way, except that relief of the phimosis is urgent, to allow urination, and to prevent aggravation of tissue damage and swelling of the penis, which complicate subsequent surgery.

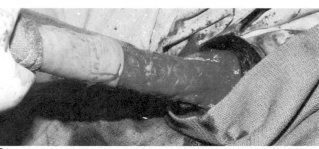

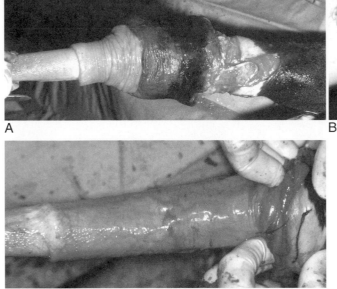

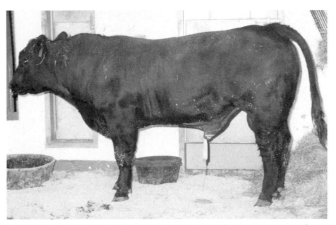

Figure 12.1.6-7   *A,* Preputial mass in a bull. *B,* Circumferential incisions are made at each end (cranial and caudal) of the connective tissue collar, and it is removed. *C,* The edges of the lamina interna are then sutured together.

(Courtesy of Dr. David Anderson; The Ohio State University.)

Figure 12.1.6-8   Bull urinating through a Penrose drain sutured over the tip of the penis.

(Courtesy of Dr. David Anderson; The Ohio State University.)

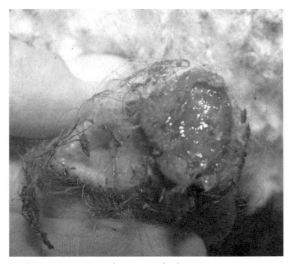

Figure 12.1.6-9   Dorsal preputial ulcer in a ram.

Preputial Erosions

In rams a unique form of decubital lesion occurs dorsal to the preputial orifice (between the prepuce and the abdominal wall) (Figure 12.1.6-9). This occurs only in heavy show rams that are confined in small pens. Because the rams are recumbent much of the time, pressure of the preputial orifice on the body wall results in a chronic ulcer. This lesion is resistant to conservative treatment, and the only successful approach is surgical resection.

Preputial Abscess

Retropreputial abscess may follow injury to the lamina interna of the prepuce (i.e., preputial avulsion or penile hematoma). It is preferable to drain these abscesses into the preputial cavity. Swelling often prevents exteriorization of the penis and access for drainage into the preputial cavity. In these cases, the abscess must be drained by skin incision (Figure 12.1.6-10) in spite of the risk of adhesions, which might prevent normal extension of the penis.

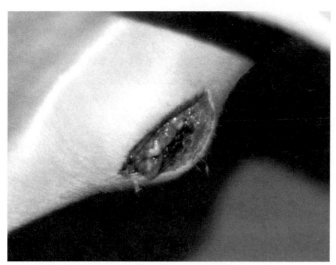

Figure 12.1.6-10   Retropreputial abscess drained through the skin of the prepuce.

RECOMMENDED READINGS

Baird AN, Wolfe DF: Castration of the normal male. In Wolfe DF and Moll HD, editors: *Large Animal Urogenital Surgery*, ed 2, Philadelphia, Williams and Wilkins, 1998, pp 295-320.

Baker JF, Strickland JE: Effect of castration on weight gain of beef calves, *Bov Pract* 34: 124-126, 2000.

Boockfor FR, Barnes MA, Kazmer GW, Halman RD, Bierley ST, Dickey JF: Effects of unilateral castration and unilateral cryptorchidism of the Holstein bull on plasma gonadotropins, testosterone and testis anatomy, *J Anim Sci* 56: 1376-1385, 1983.

Gilbert RO, Lindsay WA, Levine SA: Successful surgical repair of a vascular shunt of the corpus cavernosum penis and penile fibropapillomata in a bull, *J S Afr Vet Assoc* 58: 193-195, 1987.

Gilbert RO, VanderBerg SS: Communication between the corpus cavernosum penis and the corpus spongiosus penis in a bull diagnosed by modified contrast cavernosography, *Theriogenology* 33: 577-582, 1990.

Grings EE, Short RE, MacNeil MD, Roeder RA, Roeder MJ: Interactions in postweaning production of F1 cattle from Hereford, Limousin, or Piedmontese sires, *J Anim Sci* 79: 317-324, 2001.

Heath AM, Baird AN, Wolfe DF: Unilateral orchidectomy in bulls: a review of eight cases, *Vet Med* 8: 786-792, 1996.

Heath AM, Carson RL, Purohit RC, Sartin EM, Wenzel JGW, Wolfe DF: Effects of testicular biopsy in clinically normal bulls, *J Am Vet Med Assoc* 220: 507-512, 2001.

Hull BL: Male reproductive surgery, *Proc Soc Therio* 117-122, 2001.

Huxsoll CC, Price EO, Adams TE: Testis function, carcass traits, and aggressive behavior of beef bulls actively immunized against gonadotropin-releasing hormone, *J Anim Sci* 76: 1760-1766, 1998.

Kohli IS: Cryptorchidism in a herd of Rathi cattle, *Ind Vet J* 49: 241-245, 1972.

Lopez A, Ikede B, Ogilvie T: Unilateral interstitial (Leydig) cell tumor in a neonatal cryptorchid calf, *J Vet Diag Invest* 6: 133-135, 1994.

Lofstedt RM. Vasectomy in ruminants: a cranial midscrotal approach, *J Am Vet Med Assoc* 181: 373-375, 1996.

Methew J, Raja CKSV: Investigation on the incidence of cryptorchidism in goats, *Kerala, J Vet Sci* 29: 47-51, 1973.

Parker WG, Braun RK, Bean B, Hillman RB, Larson LL, Wilcox CJ: Avulsion of the bovine prepuce from its attachment to the penile integument during semen collection with an artificial vagina, *Theriogenology* 28: 237-256, 1987.

Rebhun WC: Bilateral cryptorchidism in a bull, *Cornell Vet* 66: 10-13, 1976.

Saunders PJ, Ladds PW: Congenital and developmental anomalies of the genitalia of slaughtered bulls, *Aust Vet J* 54: 10-13, 1978.

Schanbacher BD: Cryptorchidism and the pituitary: testicular axis in bulls, *J Reprod Fertil Suppl* 30: 67-73, 1981.

Wolfe DF, Hudson RS, Carson RL, Purohit RC: Effect of unilateral orchidectomy on semen quality in bulls, *J Am Vet Med Assoc* 186: 1291-1293, 1985.

12.2.1—Surgery of the Ovary

Susan L. Fubini

Unilateral ovariectomy is performed in cattle for ovarian pathologies such as cystic ovaries, neoplasia, abscess formation, and adhesions. The remainder of the urogenital tract must be normal for a successful return to reproductive performance. Bilateral ovariectomy prevents pregnancy in feedlot heifers, eliminates estrus, simplifies interstate movement of animals from areas of endemic brucellosis and may enable superior fattening of feedlot heifers in conjunction with growth promoters. Because blood supply to the corpus luteum is substantial, the morbidity of ovarian surgeries, such as ovarian pedicle hemorrhage, can be minimized by performing surgery only when the ovaries are in the follicular or early luteal phase. The ovary is approached by abdominal celiotomy through the body wall or colpotomy through the vagina before performing an ovariectomy. Abdominal laparoscopy can also be used.

Surgical Approaches

CELIOTOMY

Most unilateral ovariectomies are accomplished via a flank celiotomy. The cow is restrained in standing stocks or a chute, and the appropriate flank is prepared for surgery. General anesthesia may be especially useful for removing very large (>20 cm) ovaries or those with adhesions to the uterus, omentum, or other gastrointestinal viscus. An incision in the caudal paralumbar fossa gives the best access to the ovary. For small ovaries, it may be possible to "grid" the incision in the internal abdominal oblique muscle by incising the muscle in the direction of its fibers and bluntly extending the incision. This minimizes the incisional defect in the musculature but also limits the manipulations that can be performed. For larger ovaries, a sharp incision through all muscle layers is essential. The ovary is identified and exteriorized (Figure 12.2.1-1). If difficulty is encountered when bringing the ovary out of the abdomen, it may be useful

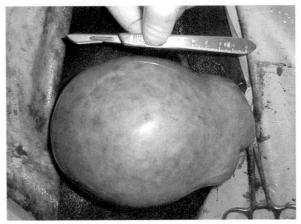

Figure 12.2.1-1   Granulosa cell tumor being removed from the right paralumbar fossa.

to have an assistant hold the ovary in place while the surgeon pushes the body wall around the ovary. If the animal becomes uncomfortable or agitated during manipulation of the ovary, infusing the ovarian pedicle with lidocaine may decrease the painful response while increasing the risk of hematoma formation because swelling in the vascular pedicle makes individual vessels harder to identify. Alternatively, lidocaine-soaked gauze temporarily placed around the pedicle may provide sufficient analgesia. Accessibility to the ovarian vasculature is highly variable. An ovary enlarged for a long period of time may have the broad ligament stretched, thus permitting easier access. Once the ovary has been identified, the vascular pedicle must be ligated. Rarely, can each vessel within the ovarian pedicle be individually ligated. Instead, overlapping bites of no. 2 absorbable sutures are placed across the ovarian pedicle. The author prefers no. 2 polyglactin 910,* which permits use of sliding half hitches when the surgeon is placing wide suture bites for hemostasis. Both sides of the pedicle should be examined to ensure ligation is adequate across the whole pedicle. Alternatively, or in addition to sutures, a surgical stapler† can be used to place staples across the pedicle. Finally, laparoscopic loop sutures can provide a secure ligation of the vascular pedicle. Adequate hemostasis in a smaller ovary may be obtained with an écraseur or emasculator.

If the cow's temperament or medical condition does not permit standing surgery, a caudal flank, ventral midline, or ventrolateral celiotomy can be done in the recumbent cow. The ventral midline approach should be considered in cows with medical conditions that result in chronic ovarian enlargement because it is easy to extend the incision if necessary. The ventral abdominal approach allows good laparoscopic access to the ovary. These approaches are detailed in the chapters on surgical approaches (Section 4.4) and surgery of the uterus (Section 12.2.2).

In cases where bilateral ovariectomy is desired, consideration should be given to colpotomy and laparoscopic ventral midline approaches that allow access to both ovaries. Another option would be to perform a bilateral celiotomy in order to access each ovary and ligate the vasculature on each side. Use of an umbilical clamp across the ovarian pedicle has been suggested in animals intended for slaughter.

COLPOTOMY APPROACH

Because of the risk of hemorrhage and evisceration, a vaginal approach is only recommended for spaying heifers with small, normal ovaries. In all instances, the animal should be healthy and not pregnant. The animal's size must be adequate for rectal and vaginal manipulation. Withholding feed for 24 to 30 hours may improve access to intraabdominal structures. The heifer should be adequately restrained. The ovaries are identified (one at a time) per rectum to ensure their position and size are as expected, and all feces are evacuated. If the urinary bladder is full, the cow should be stimulated to urinate or be catheterized. The perineal area is cleansed with appropriate aseptic technique, and the vagina is lavaged with a dilute antiseptic solution and rinsed with sterile saline. This helps create a pneumovagina, which may aid manipulations. The hand and arm are ensheathed in a sterile, impervious sleeve. The vaginal wall is incised adjacent to the cervix at the 10- or 12-o'clock level with a scalpel blade or instrument designed for an ovariectomy. If a scalpel blade is used, it should be secured to the surgeon's hand with umbilical tape or rolled gauze in case it is inadvertently dropped. The blade is held between the thumb and forefinger with 2 to 3 cm of blade protruding. Entry into the abdominal cavity and avoidance of the retroperitoneal space should be confirmed. The incision is digitally enlarged to first permit entry of several fingers, then the hand and arm.

The surgeon locates the ovaries and uterus before palpating once again for any abnormalities. It may be useful, especially in a fractious animal, to place lidocaine-soaked gauze around the ovarian pedicle before the ovariectomy.

Ovaries can be removed via colpotomy with different commercially available or hand-made instruments. These include a chain écraseur (Figure 12.2.1-2A and B), a Kimberly Rupp‡ spay instrument (Figure 12.2.1-3A and B) or a Willis Rod.§

---

*Vicryl, Polyglactin 910, Ethicon; Somerville, NJ
†TA90 surgical stapler, United States Surgical Corp.; Norwalk, CT

‡K-P® spay instrument, Lane Manufacturing Co.; Denver, CO
§Willis ovariectomy instrument, Willis Veterinary Supply; Chamberlain, SD

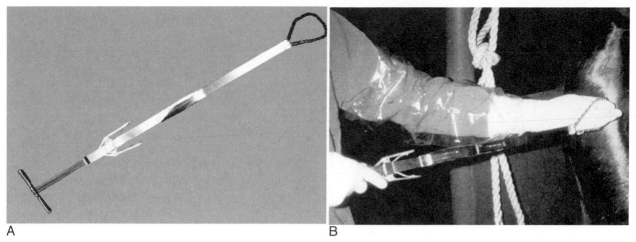

A   B

Figure 12.2.1-2   *A,* Chain écraseur instruments designed for an ovariectomy. *B,* Positioning of the écraseur on the surgeon's hand.

To use a chain écraseur, a gloved hand is passed through the chain loop to grasp the ovary. The chain is then slipped over the ovary and the hand withdrawn. The chain is gradually ratcheted down tightly around the ovarian pedicle. It is essential the surgeon check that only the ovary is ensheathed by the chain and all other intraabdominal structures are free. Once the loop has closed, the ovary and écraseur can be removed. The other ovary is removed in a similar manner through the same vaginal incision. The vaginal incision is left to heal as an open wound.

The Kimberly-Rupp instrument is a long narrow instrument with a trocar point on a tube within a tube (Figure 12.2.1-3A and B). Windows in the tubes are used to introduce the ovary into the inner tube. To use the instrument, the surgeon has one arm in the rectum and the other, gloved hand directs the instrument at the 10- to 12-o'clock range through the vaginal wall into the peritoneal cavity with a short, moderate, anterior thrust. As soon as the peritoneum is penetrated, the near handle is released to retract the trocar point. The instrument is positioned dorsal to the hand manipulating the reproductive tract. The ovary is palpated to be sure it is free from other structures before it is pressed firmly into the indented cutting area on the instrument while the inner cutting tube is rotated. When the ovary passes into the chamber, the inner tube is reversed, thus entrapping the ovary in the chamber. Once it is certain the rectum is not caught in the instrument, the cutting chamber is closed, thereby excising the ovary. The ovary can be pushed forward on the instrument for temporary storage by depressing the plunger with a thumb. The procedure is repeated for the second ovary.

Another instrument used for ovariectomy is the Willis Rod. This is a single flat rod with a keyhole opening for ovary removal. The procedure is initially the same as

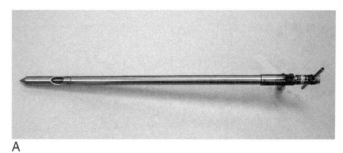

A

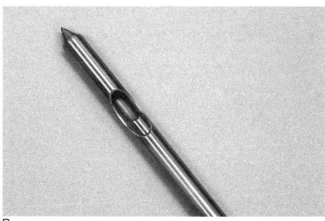

B

Figure 12.2.1-3   *A,* Kimberly Rupp instrument designed for an ovariectomy. *B,* Close-up view.

(Courtesy of Dr. Carlos M Gradil; Cornell University.)

above. Once in the abdomen, the ovary is placed, via rectal manipulation, into the keyhole opening on the spay instrument. The instrument is then forcefully retracted to sever the ovarian pedicle. The procedure is repeated for the opposite side. This technique leaves the ovaries in the peritoneal cavity. It has been reported anecdotally that an ovary with a functional corpus luteum removed in this fashion may have the capacity to revascularize from peritoneal surfaces and maintain a pregnancy.

OUTCOME

A 1992 paper by Drost et al details for research purposes unilateral ovariectomy in 17 cattle, bilateral ovariectomy in nine cattle, and removal of corpora lutea in 11 beef cows via colpotomy. They used either a Kimberly-Rupp instrument, a 70-cm Plexiglas rod with a 2-cm diameter and a 45° pointed end, a 65-cm long piece of polyvinyl chloride pipe with a 50° beveled end, a bloat trocar, or scissors to make the vaginal incision. The ovaries or corpora lutea were removed with an écraseur. They described adhesions in 24.3% of cows examined, although none would have caused any life-threatening problems. The sharp trocar and scissors were not recommended for the colpotomy incision because the resulting incision was too difficult to find. The two rods worked well and were a less expensive alternative to the Kimberly-Rupp instrument.

With all ovariectomy procedures, the biggest risks are hemorrhage, adhesions, and peritonitis. Perioperative antibiotics and analgesics are indicated.

RECOMMENDED READINGS

Drost M, Savio JD, Barros CM, Badinga L, Thatcher WW: Ovariectomy by colpotomy in cows, *J Am Vet Med Assoc* 200: 337-339, 1992.

Habermehl NL: Heifer ovariectomy using the Willis spay instrument: technique, morbidity, mortality, *Can Vet J* 34: 664-667, 1993.

Leder RR, Lane VM, Barrett DP: Ovariectomy as treatment for granulosa cell tumor on a heifer, *J Am Vet Med Assoc* 192: 1294-1300, 1988.

Noordsy JL: Oophorectomy in cattle, *Compend Contin Educ Pract Vet*, 19: 1392-1394, 1997.

Pugh DG, Elmore RG: Granulosa cell tumor in a cow, *Compend for Contin Educ Pract Vet*; 9: F327-F330, 1987.

Ridell MG: Ovariectomy. In Wolfe DF, Moll HD, editors: *Large animal urogenital surgery*, ed 2, Philadelphia, 1999, Williams & Wilkins.

Rupp GP, Kimberling CV: A new approach for spaying heifers. *Vet Med Sm An Clin* 77: 561-565, 1982.

Youngquist RS, Garverick HA, Keisler H: Use of umbilical cord clamps for ovariectomy in cows. *J Am Vet Med Assoc* 207: 474-475, 1995.

12.2.2—Surgery of the Uterus

Susan L. Fubini

Relevant Surgical Anatomy

The cow has a tortuous 20- to 28-cm long uterine tube with a fimbriated infundibulum, which is large and may completely envelop the ovary. A nonpregnant adult cow has 35- to 45-cm long uterine horns that are united closely at the body of the uterus but diverge and spiral ventrally, caudally, and finally dorsally. The horns are joined just before their divergence by an intercornual ligament. The body of the uterus is only about 3 cm long. With repeated pregnancies, the uterus becomes thicker-walled, and the spiral of the horns becomes flatter. The broad ligaments that suspend the uterus from the lateral wall of the pelvic cavity are extensive and become thickened with multiple pregnancies. The round ligaments of the uterus arise from the lateral surface of the broad ligaments. They serve to elevate and lower the uterus.

The cervix is a substantial barrier to the uterine lumen. In addition to the normal layers of viscus, the ruminant cervix is infiltrated with collagenous fibers that make it exceedingly tough. The number and regularity of the annular rings varies with the species: the cow has three to five, the ewe five to six, and the doe five to eight. The cervix rarely dilates except under hormonal influences. The bovine cervix is rarely injured because of its tough and tortuous course.

Cesarean Section

The goal of cesarean section in cattle is to relieve dystocia when vaginal delivery is not possible or is unlikely to produce live offspring. The indications for surgery include maternal reasons such as a relatively oversized fetus, (particularly in heifers that are immature or recipients of embryo transfer calves), inadequate cervical dilation, abnormal pelvic conformation, prepubic tendon rupture, uterine rupture, uterine torsion, uterine inertia, hydrops of the amnion or allantois, and congential or traumatically induced vaginal constriction. Fetal indications include fetal malposition that is not correctable per vagina, absolute fetal oversize, fetal monsters, and emphysematous fetuses. Other, ancillary indications include elective cesarean section for the delivery of embryo transfer calves, the production of gnotobiotic calves, or terminal cesarean sections.

A general physical examination should be performed on the cow, including assessing the animal's attitude, appetite, and hydration status. The mammary gland should be checked for mastitis, and it is appropriate to check ear temperature and rumen motility as indicators of hypocalcemia. More sophisticated laboratory tests, such as determining plasma electrolyte concentrations, are rarely indicated. After a physical examination, a reproductive examination consisting of a rectal exam to assess the uterus and position of the calf and a vaginal exam to determine whether the cervix is dilated and calf presentation is normal should be performed. Ballottement of the abdomen from the right and left side may indicate the side of the abdomen where the calf is located.

SURGICAL APPROACH

Many factors are weighed to determine the best approach for cesarean section, including the experience and preferences of the surgeon, temperament of the cow, available facilities, and whether assistance is available. It is also useful to ascertain if the calf is dead or alive. If the calf is dead, it is helpful to determine the state of the uterus, whether it feels normal or contracted down around the calf, or—even more important—whether the calf is emphysematous. Finally, the vascularity of the cow's ventral abdomen also enters into the decision making.

A rule of thumb is the rumen is easier to manipulate than the rest of the intestinal tract. In most instances, it is easier to deal with the rumen on the left side of the abdomen than manipulating around the intestinal tract on the right side.

When preparing for cesarean section, one should consider the available facilities. A standing chute or stocks are ideal restraint for a standing celiotomy. For recumbent procedures, sedation and a local anesthetic should be used, and there should be a place to secure the head and limbs of the cow. These authors prefer to sedate only animals that are being positioned in lateral or dorsal recumbency because of the risk of the animal becoming recumbent when tension is applied to the uterus and its ligamentous attachments. If the cow is straining, an epidural is appropriate for either standing or recumbent approaches. No more than 5 cc of local anesthetic should be used in the standing cow to avoid the risk of the cow becoming recumbent. Perioperative antibiotics should be administered depending on the cow's value and condition of the fetus. Intravenous fluids are seldom necessary. In most instances, the surgical site can be desensitized with a local anesthetic, and it may be appropriate to administer analgesics (such as flunixin meglumine) to increase likelihood the animal will stay standing. If nonsteroidal antiinflammatory drugs are used, withdrawal times for milk and meat must be considered. Appropriate preparations include an assistant to aid in delivery of the calf, saline lavage of the uterus, chains for delivery of the calf, and oxytocin to administer postoperatively for uterine contraction.

STANDING PARALUMBAR FOSSA CELIOTOMY

The abdominal cavity can be approached via a standing paralumbar fossa celiotomy on the right or left side of the abdomen. The incision should be made in the caudal third of the fossa (Figure 12.2.2-1) to facilitate exteriorization of the uterus (Figure 12.2.2-2). The celiotomy should be large so delivery of the uterus is more easily accomplished. If the right side is elected, the incision

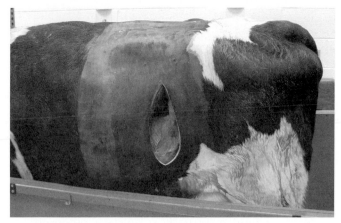

Figure 12.2.2-1   Cow with a caudal left paralumbar fossa celiotomy. The calf has been delivered, the uterus closed and drapes are being changed before closing the abdomen.

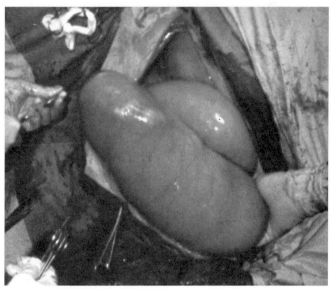

Figure 12.2.2-2   Appropriate left paralumbar fossa celiotomy, allowing exteriorization of the portion of the pregnant horn containing the hind limbs of the calf.

should not extend too far ventrally so there is no problem with intestines prolapsing out of the surgical incision. A sharp skin incision approximately 40 cm long is made in the skin and continued through the subcutaneous tissue as well as the internal and external abdominal oblique muscles. The peritoneum and transversus abdominus should be tented with a forceps and incised with scissors. A finger should be inserted into the abdomen, and the peritoneum should be "swept" for any adhesions before the incision is extended. The peritoneum can be left open or closed with the transversus abdominus. The external and internal abdominal muscles are closed next, followed by the skin. A simple continuous pattern using an absorbable suture material can be used on all muscle layers. The skin is usually apposed with an interlocking pattern by using a nonabsorbable suture. It is recommended the most ventral portion of the skin incision be closed with interrupted skin sutures, so the incision can be drained ventrally if necessary.

VENTRAL MIDLINE CELIOTOMY

Restraint and positioning of adult cattle in dorsal recumbency for a ventral midline approach can be labor intensive. Cattle restrained in this position suffer from cardiovascular and respiratory compromise. Therefore it is ideal to complete surgery as quickly as possible. A 40-cm skin incision is made starting at the udder and extended toward the xiphoid. The subcutaneous tissues and linea alba are sharply incised. The peritoneum is tented and incised with scissors. Some individuals perform the midline celiotomy and then have the cow rotated, so the uterus delivers more easily to one side or the other. There are also large surgery tables that facilitate this procedure by rotating. Some surgeons feel this approach allows better exteriorization of the uterus and subsequent prevention of abdominal contamination. The midline approach is very useful for beef cattle or fractious range cattle that may not tolerate a standing flank laparotomy. A disadvantage in dairy cattle is the large amount of ventral vasculature and udder that may be in the way. To avoid incising a major vessel, it is advisable to trace the vasculature with a marker while the cow is standing and the vessels are distended with blood. A major transverse vein often runs across the abdomen just cranial to the udder and may be inadvertently incised if the incision is made too caudally.

PARAMEDIAN CELIOTOMY

A ventral paramedian celiotomy for cesarean section also requires restraint in dorsal recumbency. It is a multiple layer incision in the caudal abdomen, which may result in more hemorrhage and a poor holding layer for closure. This procedure offers very few advantages and is rarely recommended.

VENTROLATERAL CELIOTOMY

For this procedure, the cow is restrained in lateral recumbency and the "up" hind leg is elevated and secured (Figure 12.2.2-3). The skin incision parallels the superficial mammary vein before cutting up at an angle by the udder (Figure 12.2.2-4). Tracing the vein or marking it with an indelible pen or suture before the animal is cast will prevent inadvertent incision of the vessel because it is no longer prominently distended with blood after casting. Sharp incision is continued through the subcutaneous tissues and abdominal oblique muscles, which

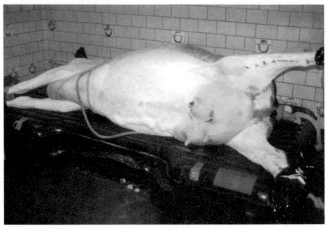

Figure 12.2.2-3   Cow positioned for ventrolateral cesarean section.

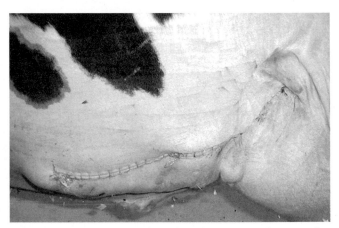

Figure 12.2.2-4   Ventrolateral incision 48 hours after cesarean section. Note typical postoperative edema.

are mostly aponeurotic at this level. The transversus muscle and peritoneum are tented and incised in the same direction as the incision, perpendicular to the direction of the muscle fibers. Because this incision is long and in a vascular area, it is difficult to open and close. However, it allows excellent exteriorization of almost the entire horn of the uterus. If it is hard to move the uterus, the incised edges of the body wall can be grasped on either side and pushed down around the uterine horn. Our hospital reserves this approach for a cow with an emphysematous fetus because the incision length and difficulty in restraining the animal make it more time-consuming and difficult. Closure requires multiple layers, which is also time-consuming. Furthermore, the surgery must be performed by the surgeon kneeling beside the cow so the incision is close to the ground, increasing chances of postoperative wound infection (Figure 12.2.2-5).

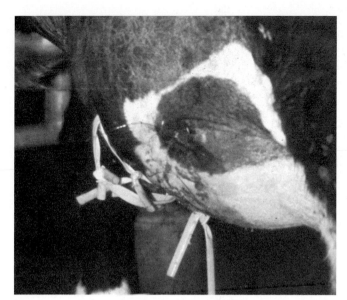

Figure 12.2.2-5 Infected ventrolateral incision.

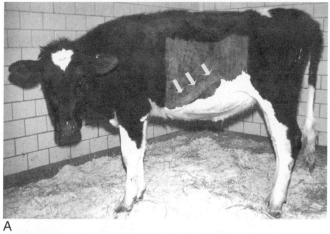

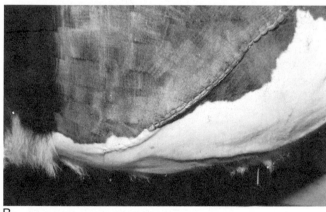

Figure 12.2.2-6 *A,* Left oblique celiotomy for cesarean section outlined by white arrows. *B,* Close-up view of incision.

LEFT OBLIQUE CELIOTOMY

A left oblique celiotomy was described by Parish et al. for a standing cesarean section. The skin incision begins 8 to 10 cm cranial and 8 to 10 cm ventral to the cranial-most aspect of the tuber coxae. It extends cranioventrally at a 45° angle to end 3 cm caudal to the last rib (Figure 12.2.2-6A and B). Subcutaneous tissues and the external abdominal oblique muscle are sharply incised. The internal abdominal oblique and transversus muscles are opened along the direction of their fibers, and the peritoneum is tented and incised. These investigators felt this approach permitted better exteriorization of the uterus than a paralumbar fossa celiotomy. Three of 18 cows did develop incisional complications, and persistent anesthesia of the ventral body wall was apparent.

DELIVERING THE CALF

Regardless of the surgical approach chosen, a large celiotomy should be made. Once entry into the abdomen is accomplished, the position and condition of the calf should be determined. With the exception of the ventrolateral approach, it is very difficult to manipulate the entire uterus. Instead, the surgeon should attempt to manipulate a limb of the calf to the incision. Ideally, the surgeon is able to "lock" a limb in the celiotomy incision (Figure 12.2.2-7), which essentially holds the uterus in place so the hysterotomy is made outside the abdomen and the calf delivered with minimal contamination of the abdomen. If the vertebral column is presented to the incision and it is difficult to reach a limb of the calf, the surgeon should attempt to rotate the uterus. If a clockwise rotation does not bring the limbs within reach of the surgical incision, then a counter-clockwise rotation should be attempted. This is rarely unsuccessful, so another surgical approach normally would not have to be made. Usually it is possible to grasp the limbs, apply traction, and "rock" them up into the incision. If the calf is in anterior presentation, a hind limb is elevated, and the foot and hock are wedged in the incision (see Figure 12.2.2-7). For a posterior presentation, the carpus and flexed fetlock are exteriorized. Once this is done and people are in place to aid with the delivery of the calf, a large uterine incision is made, with care taken not to injure the calf. The limbs of the calf are identified, the placenta incised, the feet delivered, and chains applied around them. While the surgeon stabilizes the uterus, the assistants deliver the calf. If there is no or little assistance available, noncrushing uterine clamps ("Vulsellum Forceps") can be used to hold the uterus in position. It is important the uterus incision be large enough to deliver the calf without tearing the uterus. Once the calf is delivered, whatever placenta comes easily is removed, and the remainder is replaced into the uterus. The surgeon should always check for uterine

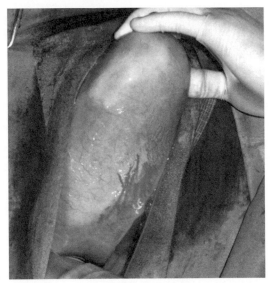

Figure 12.2.2-7   The hind limbs of the calf are delivered through a left paralumbar fossa celiotomy and "locked" in the incision, which helps keep the uterus exteriorized.

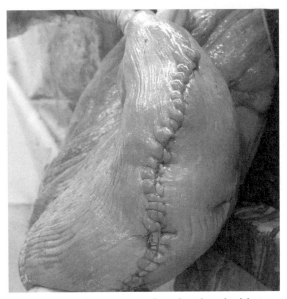

Figure 12.2.2-8   The uterus is closed with a double inverting pattern.

tears, another calf, and proper positioning of the uterus before closing the abdomen.

The surgeon's preference dictates the manner in which the uterus is closed. A popular choice is a simple, continuous pattern incorporating all layers into the closure with a #2 absorbable suture material. Care is taken to avoid incorporating placental membranes. This is oversewn with an inverting suture pattern, usually a Cushing or Lembert, with a #2 absorbable suture material (Figure 12.2.2-8). Others advocate a Utrecht inverting pattern. As long as appropriate technique is used, any inverting pattern is acceptable, although we advocate

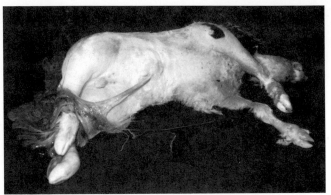

Figure 12.2.2-9   Emphysematous calf necessitated a ventro-lateral approach to the abdomen.

two layers. The sutures should be placed tight enough so the closure remains intact when the uterus contracts. This prevents peritonitis that can result from leakage of uterine fluid. Minimizing exposed suture material may decrease postoperative adhesions. The uterus and surrounding area are rinsed copiously with fluids and replaced in the abdomen in its normal position. Oxytocin (20 IU) should be given intravenously (tail vein) by an assistant upon completion of the uterine closure. The integrity of the uterine incision is then reevaluated. Gloves should be changed.

The abdominal wound should be lavaged and the incision closed routinely. Before the last suture is placed in the first layer, an attempt should be made to eliminate as much air as possible from the abdomen. This decreases pain from pneumoperitoneum and reduces the development of subcutaneous emphysema if the cow continues to strain. For flank incisions, the ventral aspect of the skin incision should be closed with interrupted sutures to permit drainage should a localized wound infection develop (see Section 4.5). After surgery, oxytocin is administered to encourage uterine involution, 20 IU qid until the membranes are passed or for 24 hours. The cow should be monitored to be sure the placenta is passed intact and should receive general medical support, including analgesics if necessary, exercise, and udder care, with fresh water and electrolytes available at all times. Antibiotics are usually continued for 3 to 7 days or until the placenta is passed.

Complications of cesarean section include peritonitis, metritis, and abdominal adhesions. In cattle that have signs of endotoxemia, postoperative sepsis can be life-threatening. Wound infections are a problem, especially when an emphysematous calf is delivered at surgery (Figure 12.2.2-9). These localized infections can often be treated by establishing ventral drainage of the wound and appropriate wound care. Intraabdominal adhesions around the uterus and ovaries may affect future fertility and can be minimized by thoroughly washing the blood off the uterus and burying suture knots. There are very few studies that have followed a large number of cows after surgery to determine postoperative fertility. A 15% decline in fertility was found in one study in which a population of cattle that had cesarean section was compared with a similar group that had "normal" vaginal deliveries. Studies that evaluated cows that have been rebred after cesarean section report a 60% to 80% pregnancy rate with a 5% to 9% loss because of abortion. Cesarean section has been shown to increase the number of services to conception and the days open. If a live calf is delivered at surgery, the cow is in good physical condition, and the procedure goes well, a favorable long term outcome can be expected. If the cow is in poor physical condition at the time of surgery the results are often less gratifying.

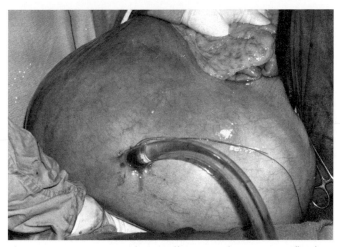

Figure 12.2.2-10   Hydrops allantois. The uterine fluid is being emptied slowly with a stomach tube placed through a purse string suture into the uterus.

Uterine Torsion

Uterine torsion is not an uncommon cause of dystocia in cattle. It usually develops at the end of gestation or during the onset of labor and is suspected after prolonged labor. Rarely it can occur in early gestation and presents as colic.

The diagnosis of uterine torsion is made by rectal palpation. Dorsally, the broad ligament is stretched tightly across the uterus in the direction of the torsion, and ventrally away from the torsion (i.e., with right-sided torsion—clockwise when viewed from behind—the left side of the broad ligament is stretched dorsally across the uterus and the right side of the broad ligament dives down ventrally). Vaginal examination can also indicate a uterine torsion with folds into the vaginal wall pointing in the direction of the torsion.

Correction of a uterine torsion can be attempted vaginally if the cervix is dilated and the calf's feet can be grasped. The calf is rocked until enough momentum is attained to flip the calf into normal position. If vaginal correction is not possible, the cow should be cast into lateral recumbency on the side of the torsion. A large plank is placed in the cow's flank, and a heavy person balances on the plank to minimize uterine motion. The cow is then rolled over on her back and onto her other side. A rectal examination is performed to evaluate uterine position, and the procedure is repeated as necessary. To summarize, for torsion to the RIGHT, the cow is cast on her RIGHT side and is rolled to the RIGHT as viewed from behind.

For uterine torsion that is unable to be corrected with vaginal manipulation or rolling techniques, a celiotomy should be done. It is recommended to correct the torsion before performing a hysterotomy. However, we

have done both (performed the cesarean section before and after the torsion is corrected) and believe either method is equally effective. This is a decision that should be made at the time of surgery and will depend on the condition of the uterus and the difficulty in exteriorizing it. Once the calf is removed, the twist in the uterus is easily corrected.

Hydrops

When hydrops amnion or allantois is present, it is best to drain the large amount of fluid slowly at surgery to decrease the risk of sending the cow into hypovolemic shock. Some surgeons advocate pursestringing a large-bore stomach tube into the uterus to drain the fluid (Figure 12.2.2-10). In this case, it is appropriate to administer intravenous fluids.

Cows that survive hydrops allantois are at increased risk of septic metritis and poor future fertility because of pathologic stretching of the myometrium.

Hydrops amnion is usually the result of abnormal fetal development, and the dam may be a recessive carrier, which should preclude rebreeding.

Uterine Rupture

Uterine rupture/tear can occur after dystocia. Typically, there is a history of extensive manipulations, forced traction, fetotomy, delivery of an emphysematous fetus, or other extensive manipulations.

The tear may be diagnosed on vaginal examination or at the time a cesarean section is performed. If the tear is out of reach during a vaginal examination and the calf is delivered without surgery, it may be up to 5 days before signs become apparent.

Clinical signs are those typical of peritonitis, including depression, inappetence, fever, tachycardia, ileus, and abdominal pain. Cattle with large tears and tenesmus run the risk of prolapsing intestine through the uterine rent. Spontaneous uterine rupture secondary to unattended dystocia has resulted in the calf or fetus being extrauterine in the abdomen.

If the diagnosis is suspected, a vaginal examination should be done following appropriate preparation of the vulva. If the cow is less than 48 hours from freshening, it is usually possible to pass one hand through the cervix. Past 48 hours, it may be necessary to perform an exploratory celiotomy. Most tears are dorsal and just cranial to the cervix. Small dorsal tears may heal with conservative therapy that includes antimicrobials, intrauterine medication, and repeated administration of oxytocin. For a valuable animal, direct, aggressive, surgical therapy may be indicated. This includes repair of the laceration, broad-spectrum antibiotics, and ancillary medical therapy such as calcium solutions, nonsteroidal antiinflammatory drugs, and peritoneal lavage.

If the tear is fresh, it may be possible to close it blindly working through the vagina and cervix. This is difficult, and the cervix closes quickly after parturition. Surgical repair with a caudal laparotomy is the author's first choice. Traction can be placed on the cervix to facilitate exteriorization of the uterus. The tear is identified, and a suture is started. The end of the first knot can be left long or a separate suture placed so traction can be applied. A continuous suture line is placed if possible.

It may also be possible to prolapse the uterus after a slow intravenous infusion of 10 ml of 1:1000 epinephrine. Theoretically, the tear could be repaired and the uterus replaced. This is difficult to accomplish, and there are cardiovascular consequences of intravenous epinephrine.

The prognosis is guarded and will depend mostly on the degree of peritonitis present and adequacy of the repair.

Uterine Abscesses and Adhesions

Isolated inflamed areas of the uterus can result from compromise of the uterine wall during calving, or extension of an endometrial infection. There may be a history of dystocia or an iatrogenic pipetting injury.

Overt clinical signs of a uterine abscess (Figure 12.2.2-11A) or adhesions are not usually present. Instead, they are found on routine rectal examination. Abscesses can vary greatly in size. They may be accompanied by extensive adhesions. A differential diagnosis includes hematoma, cyst, and tumor. The most common

organism isolated is *Arcanobacterium pyogenes (Actinomyces pyogenes)*. The diagnosis is made by rectal palpation and ultrasound examination. There may be elevations in plasma protein levels in some chronic cases. Conservative therapy of parenteral antibiotics (penicillin 20,000 IU/kg sid) for 4 to 6 weeks—possibly in conjunction with 20% sodium iodide (30 gm/450 kg intravenously) followed by daily oral organic iodide (1 oz until signs of iodism are evident)—may be attempted. This is rarely successful, and surgical drainage or resection is recommended. Drainage can be accomplished by performing a celiotomy and placing a 20 French chest trocar into the abscess through a pursestring suture. If the abscess is freely moveable, it may be possible—and preferable—to resect it with a partial hysterectomy.

Adhesions are best treated conservatively. Many will remodel and resolve over time. This may take as long as 4 to 6 months. The same examiner should monitor and follow the cow. If endometritis and a functional corpus luteum are present, the animal may benefit from intermittent injections of prostaglandin (PGF$_{2\alpha}$ or analogues) to encourage uterine involution and evacuation of purulent material. If the adhesions are localized to one side, the cow can sometimes conceive successfully on the contralateral side.

Partial Hysterectomy

Indications for a partial hysterectomy include a localized uterine abscess or tumor, and severe chronic endometritis localized to one horn. Reported tumors include lymphosarcoma, adenocarcinoma, and leiomyoma. The uninvolved horn and ovary should be evaluated by rectal palpation, ultrasound, and uterine biopsy. If normal, the prognosis for return to reproductive performance can be favorable.

SURGICAL TECHNIQUE

Depending on the extent of the pathology and nature of the cow, surgery may be performed in the standing animal or in lateral "recumbency." If lateral recumbency is elected, general anesthesia provides the opportunity for a more controlled environment. The uterus can be approached through a flank or ventrolateral incision in the recumbent cow. In tractable dairy cattle, the authors have had the best results with a caudal flank approach in the standing cow. In small ruminants, dorsal recumbency and a ventral midline incision is another surgical option.

Withholding food for 24 to 48 hours is necessary for recumbency but also improves visibility and provides more room to maneuver in the standing cow. As mentioned, a caudal flank incision is recommended in the standing cow.

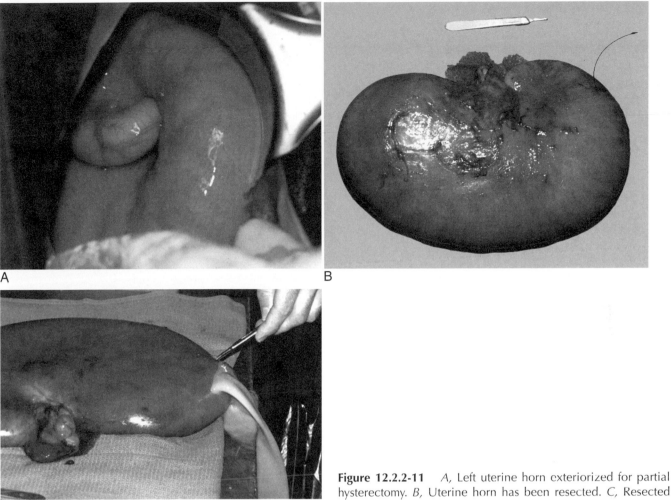

Figure 12.2.2-11 *A,* Left uterine horn exteriorized for partial hysterectomy. *B,* Uterine horn has been resected. *C,* Resected horn is incised revealing purulent contents.

The site is prepared for aseptic surgery and desensitized if the cow is not under general anesthesia. A 20-cm skin incision is made. The muscle layers and peritoneum are sharply incised.

The abnormal horn and ovary are located and gently exteriorized (see Figure 12.2.2-11A). The ovarian pedicle is double-ligated with an absorbable suture material. The ovarian pedicle is transected, and the broad ligament is dissected. The vasculature is ligated as necessary. The transection site on the uterus is chosen, and stay sutures are placed. An intestinal clamp works well as a guide along which to incise. The diseased portion of the uterus is removed and the remaining horn oversewn with a two-layer closure (Figure 12.2.2-11B and C). Another option is to use the TA-90* autosuture equipment, which deposits a double row of staggered stainless steel staples across the uterine horn, and perform the tran-

section distal to the staples. Some surgeons advocate oversewing the staple line with an inverted pattern to avoid exposed mucosa. Closure of the abdomen is routine. The administration of perioperative antibiotics is at the surgeon's discretion. The animal should be given 3 weeks before attempting artificial insemination and 6 weeks before natural service.

COMPLETE OVARIOHYSTERECTOMY
Adult Cattle

Complete ovariohysterectomy is done very infrequently but reportedly has been performed in some cows after uterine rupture, uterine torsion, severe uterine lacerations, or for a heifer with a dead autolyzed fetus. This surgical procedure should be considered for salvage only, and the animal should be culled as soon as it is reasonable.

If possible, the cow is operated on standing. Withholding feed for 24 to 48 hours allows more room for

*Auto Suture®, United States Surgical Corporation; Norwalk, CT

manipulation. At surgery, as much uterus as possible is exteriorized. A loop of umbilical tape or rolled gauze can be placed around the cervix to provide traction. The next step is crude but effective. The entire uterus and its associated vessels are ligated by tightening a 1 m length of 3/16 inch latex tubing or a similar-sized umbilical tape around the uterine body just in front of the cervix. The tubing or tape is pulled snug, and the first knot thrown is held with a hemostat to prevent slippage while the second throw is placed. The uterus is transected 6 to 9 cm cranial to the ligature. If hemorrhage ensues, additional ligatures can be placed. Sutures are passed through the broad ligament creating fenestrations that prevent slippage.

RECOMMENDED READINGS

Barkema HW, Schukken YH, Guard CL, et al: Fertility, production and culling following cesarean section in dairy cattle, *Theriogenol* 38: 589-599, 1992.

Barkema HW, Schukken YH, Guard CL, et al: Cesarean section in dairy cattle: a study of risk factors, *Theriogenol* 37: 489-506, 1992.

BonDurant RH: Examination of the reproductive tract of the cow and heifer. In Morrow DA: *Current therapy in theriogenology,* ed 2, Philadelphia, 1986, WB Saunders.

Campbell ME, Fubini SL: Indications and surgical approaches for cesarean section in cattle, *Compend Contin Educ Pract Vet* 12: 285-291, 1990.

Cattell JH, Dobson H: A survey of cesarean operations on cattle in general veterinary practice, *Vet Rec* 127: 395-399, 1990.

Clark WA: Bovine cesarean section, *Vet Rec* 120: 443, 1987.

Cochran ML, Cochran J: Ovariohysterectomy in complicated bovine cesarean sections, *J Am Vet Med Assoc* 183: 20-121, 1983.

Dawson JC, Murray R: Caesarean sections in cattle attended by a practice in Cheshire, *Vet Rec* 131: 525-527, 1992.

Dehghani SN, Ferguson JG: Cesarean section in cattle: complications, *Compend Contin Educ* 4: S387-S392, 1982.

Frazer GS, Perkins NR: Cesarean section, *Vet Clin North Am Food Anim Pract* 11: 19-35, 1995.

Hoeben D, Mijten P, de Kruif A: Factors influencing complications during cesarean section on the standing cow, *Vet Quart* 19: 88-92, 1997.

Hudson RS: Genital surgery of the cow. In Morrow DA: *Current therapy in theriogenology,* Philadelphia, 1986, WB Saunders.

Noorsdy JL: Selection of an incision site for cesarean section in the cow, *Vet Med Small Anim Clin* 74: 530-537, 1979.

Oehme FW: The ventrolateral cesarean section in the cow, *Vet Med Small Anim Clin* 62: 889-894, 1967.

Pierson H: Uterine torsion in cattle: a review of 168 cases, *Vet Rec* 89: 597-599, 1971.

Rebhun WC: *Diseases of dairy cattle,* Philadelphia, 1995, Williams & Wilkins.

Roberts SJ: Cesarean section in the cow. In *Veterinary obstetrics and genital diseases (theriogenology),* ed 3, Woodstock, Vt, 1986, Edwards Brothers.

Sloss V, Dufty J: Cesarean section. In *Handbook of veterinary obstetrics,* Baltimore, 1980, Williams & Wilkins.

Turner A, McIlwraith CW: Cesarean section in the cow. In Oehme FW: *Textbook of large animal surgery,* ed 2, Baltimore, 1988, Williams & Wilkins.

Turner A, McIlwraith CW: Cesarean section in the cow. In *Techniques in large animal surgery,* ed 2, Philadelphia, 1989, Lea & Febiger.

Vandeplassche M: Embryotomy and cesarotomy. In Oehme FW: *Textbook of large animal surgery,* ed 2, Baltimore, 1988, Williams & Wilkins.

Wenzel JGW, Baird AN, Wolfe DF, Carson RL, Powe TA, Pugh PG: Surgery of the uterus. In Wolfe DF, Moll HD, editors: *Large animal urogenital surgery,* Philadelphia, 1999, William & Wilkins.

Wolfe DF, Baird AN: Female urogenital surgery in cattle, *Vet Clin North Am Food Anim Pract* 9: 69-388, 1993.

12.2.3—Surgery of the Vagina

Susan L. Fubini

Injury of the vagina can result in lacerations. These are best treated by debridement and cleansing, as described in Section 8.1. Most vaginal lacerations heal well by second intention. At times, perivaginal fat must be transected, but surgical intervention is rarely needed to manage vaginal lacerations. Urovagina and prolapsed vagina are two conditions that require surgical correction.

Urovagina

MANAGEMENT

Urovagina is the accumulation of urine in the cranial vagina. This condition is more common in older, multiparous cows with poor conformation. Abnormal function of the constrictor vestibuli muscle resulting from dystocia can result in urovagina. Poor conformation from repeated pregnancies can be manifested by cranioventral tipping of the pelvis, which causes the external urethral orifice to be higher than the adjacent vaginal floor, so urine collects in the vaginal fornix. The urine weight can exacerbate vaginal cranioventral displacement, thus aggravating the problem further. Hormonal influences may be involved in maintaining vaginal conformation. Indeed, the condition has been recognized in heifer cows used solely as embryo donors that have been superovulated and collected several times. Superovulation—or the hormones used in the process—appears to contribute to pelvic ligament laxity, which can lead to cranioventral displacement of the cranial vagina.

The urine accumulation results in vaginitis and cervicitis. Eventually, urine may enter the uterus when the cervix dilates, causing endometritis. These abnormalities combined with the spermicidal nature of urine result in infertility.

DIAGNOSIS

The diagnosis of urovagina can be made by observing urine pooled in the cranial vagina on speculum examination. One study of 14 affected cattle defined a 100 ml accumulation of urine pooled in the vagina as a diagnostic criterion for urovagina. A uterine biopsy may be useful for determining the degree of damage to the uterine wall.

SURGICAL CORRECTION

Surgical descriptions for urovagina in mares and cows can be broadly separated into two categories: vaginoplasty or extension of the urethral tube.

For all procedures, the cow should be restrained in standing stocks and an epidural anesthetic (no more than 5 cc of local anesthetic) administered. The rectum should be evacuated, the vagina rinsed with dilute antiseptic solution, and the tail tied to one side in preparation for surgery. The perineum is prepared for surgery. The vulvar lips are retracted with stay sutures, towel clamps, or a Balfour self-retaining retractor (Figure 12.2.3-1). Incising the vaginal dorsal commissure (while taking care not to invade the rectum) may improve the surgeon's view. A Foley catheter (approximately no. 28) is secured in the urethra. Good lighting of the site provided by a head lamp or a patient, nonsterile assistant who makes constant adjustments to the light is desirable. Taping a flexible light source (such as the endoscope) to the

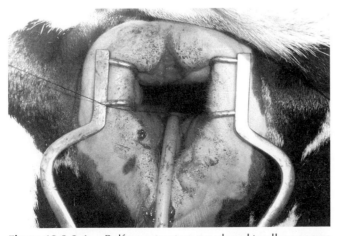

Figure 12.2.3-1 Balfour retractors are placed to allow access to the caudal aspect of the vagina. A 28 French Foley catheter has been placed in the urethra. Note the incision of the vaginal dorsal commissure improves the surgeon's view.

scalpel also provides better visualization. Long-handled instruments facilitate the procedure. Perioperative antibiotics and antiinflammatory agents are indicated until the Foley catheter is removed.

TRANSVERSE FOLD TECHNIQUES

The transverse fold technique used in horses does not allow sufficient urethral extension in cattle. Instead, the urethral extension procedure described below is used. Some authors report additional benefits from creating a thickened transverse urethral fold that acts as a barrier to cranial flow of urine.

To create a more prominent transverse fold that acts like a dam, folds of vaginal mucosa are elevated and held in place by a series of mattress sutures. No long-term report of this technique is available.

URETHRAL TUBE EXTENSION TECHNIQUES

Extending the urethral tube has proven more reliable in managing urovagina. The cow is prepared as described previously. Balfour retractors or stay sutures are used to retract the vulvar lips. A Foley catheter is placed into the urethra before surgery. To start, the transverse fold is grasped and retracted caudally toward the surgeon (Figure 12.2.3-2 A). A U-shaped incision is made in the vaginal mucosa approximately 1 cm cranial to the urethral orifice, continued caudally from the transverse fold junction with the wall of the vestibule to just cranial to the mucocutaneous junction of the vulva (Figure 12.2.3-2B). Using sharp dissection, the incisions are carried parallel with the floor along the walls of the vaginal vault at the 3- and 9-o'clock levels until within 2 cm of the vulvar lips. The dissection of each side is continued by using a combination of blunt and sharp dissection so two mucosal flaps (dorsal and ventral) are created on each side (Figure 12.2.3-2C and D). The ventral flap is first apposed without excessive tension. The incision is closed in the shape of a "y" beginning at the junction of the ventral flap of the transverse fold with the ventral flap of the vestibular wall (Figure 12.2.3-2E). The ventral flaps are sutured with a continuous inverting suture pattern that apposes the raw edges of the mucosal flaps and inverts the free edge into the lumen of the newly created urethral tunnel. The dorsal flaps are then apposed over the ventral flaps. An everting pattern (horizontal or vertical mattress) with 2-0 monofilament absorbable suture is recommended to finish the remainder of the incision. Finally, a Caslick's procedure is done.

The author has had success with the McKinnon technique, which describes closing only the ventral shelf (Figure 12.2.3-3). Furthermore, rather than risk leakage at the sites where the arms of the "Y" join the straight

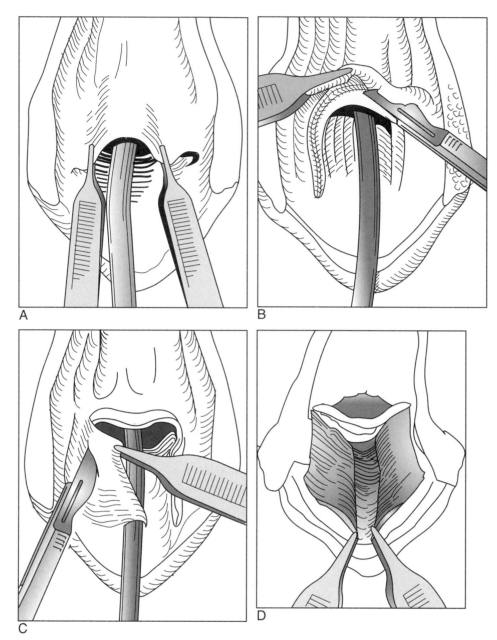

Figure 12.2.3-2   *A,* The transverse fold is grasped and retracted caudally. *B,* A U-shaped incision is made in the vaginal mucosa approximately 1 cm cranial to the urethral orifice and continued caudally, thus creating two parallel incisions along the walls of the vaginal vault at the 3 o'clock and 9 o'clock level. *C,* Using forceps to grasp the incision edge, the surgeon sharply dissects the mucosal flaps from the vagina wall. *D,* Ventral flaps are grasped with forceps and brought into apposition to determine if dissection is adequate (i.e., no tension on the intended suture line).

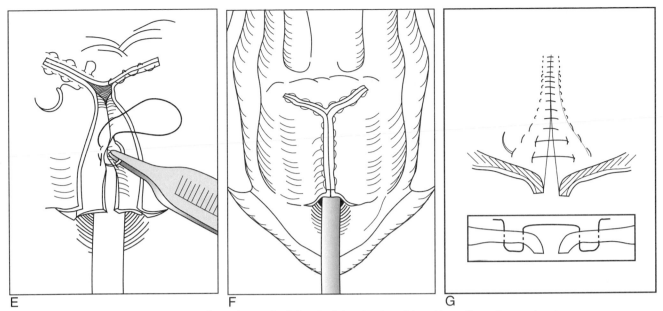

E   F   G

Figure 12.2.3-2, cont'd. *E,* The vaginal flap incision is closed in a Y configuration, using two layers beginning with the ventral flap. The dorsal flap is sutured next. Continuous suture patterns shown apposing the raw edges of the mucosal flaps and inverting the free edges into the lumen. *F,* Completed urethal tube extension. *G,* Alternatively, the U-shaped incision can be closed in a straight line without the arms of the Y, as shown here.

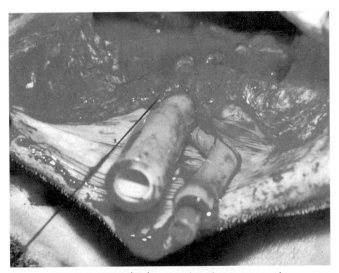

Figure 12.2.3-3   Urethral extension in a cow using a one layer closure. The procedure is almost complete.

long forceps and putting them into apposition before suturing (Figure 12.2.3-4A and B).

Another variation that has been described is to use horizontal mattress sutures to pull folds of vaginal mucosa from each side of the urethral orifice over the Foley catheter. After this, the tissue above the mattress sutures is trimmed creating fresh wound edges. These edges are carefully sutured.

After surgery, some advocate leaving a Foley catheter in place for a minimum of 72 hours. Reports of dysuria have followed surgery, presumably because of swelling or a narrow diameter of the new urethral tube. Another report of 14 cows had no cattle that developed postoperative dysuria. The author advocates leaving a Foley catheter in place for 72 hours after having one cow unable to urinate after surgery despite a patent and seemingly large urethral tube.

Fistula formation is the most common reason reported for surgical failure. Inevitably, these are at the most cranial aspect of the new urethral tube. Some fistulas may be repaired surgically by freshening the edges and suturing the defect, but opening the whole urethral tube and resuturing may be necessary in some instances. Some narrowing of the vaginal vault can be expected after surgery, but the procedure is well tolerated and in most instances the long-term prognosis is favorable.

part, the author usually closes the "U" in a straight suture line that everts the slightly redundant flaps of tissue (Figure 12.2.3-2G). To avoid complications, care should be taken to prevent any excessive tension on the repair. This can be done by lifting the vaginal flaps with

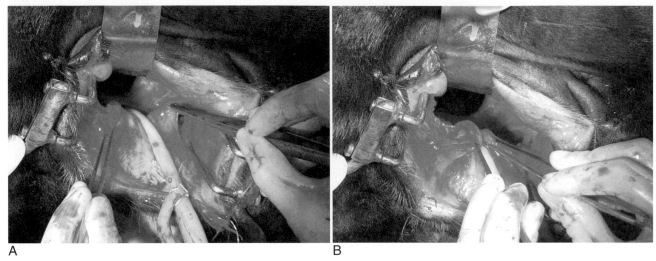

A   B

Figure 12.2.3-4   Urethral extension in a cow. To determine whether the vaginal flaps can be sutured without excessive tension, they are placed into apposition with long forceps. *A,* Flaps are not adequately dissected. *B,* Flaps are brought into apposition without tension.

RECOMMENDED READINGS

Brown MP, Colahan PT, Hawkins DL: Urethral extension for treatment of urine pooling in mares, *J Am Vet Med Assoc* 173: 1005-1007, 1978.

Gilbert RO, Wilson DG, Levine SA, Bosu WT: Surgical management of urovagina and associated infertility in a cow, *J Am Vet Med Assoc* 194(7): 931-932, 1989.

Hudson RS: Surgical procedures of the reproductive system of the cow. In Morrow DA: *Current therapy in theriogenology,* Philadelphia, 1980, WB Saunders.

McIlwraith CW, Turner S: Urethroplasty. In McIlwraith CW Turner AS: *Equine surgery advanced techniques,* ed 2, Philadelphia, 1987, Lea & Febiger.

McKinnon AO, Belden JO: A urethral extension technique to correct urine pooling (vesicovaginal reflux) in mares, *J Am Vet Med Assoc* 192: 647-650, 1988.

St. Jean G, Hull BL, Robertson JT, Hoffsis GF, Haibel GK: Urethral extension for correction of urovagina in cattle: a review of 14 cases, *Vet Surg* 17: 258-262, 1988.

Shires MC: Simple surgical repair for urine pooling in the cow, *Proc World Congress on Diseases of Cattle,* Dublin, 1986.

Wenzel JGW, Baird AN: Female urogenital surgery. In: Wolfe DF, Moll HD, *Large animal urogenital surgery,* Philadelphia, 1999, Williams & Wilkins.

12.2.3.1—Surgery of the Vagina

Robert O. Gilbert

Imperforate Hymen

In contrast to the condition in mares in which fluid accumulates behind the hymen (a thin sheet of tissue that may persist) and is easily remedied by incising the hymen, an imperforate hymen in cows is much more complex. In the bovine, imperforate hymen almost always occurs in conjunction with segmental aplasia of other parts of the reproductive tract—the vagina, cervix or uterine body or horns—as a component of white heifer disease in Shorthorns or other breeds. The vagina ends blindly, and fluid accumulates in portions of the reproductive tract cranial to it. Because of the multiple defects and genetic basis of the condition (believed to be a single, recessive gene linked to the gene for white coat color and sex-limited in its expression), the condition is not amenable to surgery, but offspring may be obtained by heroic intervention in some cases.

Vertical strands in the vagina (remnants of the fusion of the two paramesonephric ducts—and not hymenal remnants) may occasionally cause dystocia by entrapping a portion of the fetus. They may be cut with a blade or scissors to relieve the dystocia. Such cases may be encountered in multiparous cows in which calving has previously occurred without complication. Entrapment of a fetal extremity is a matter of chance and occurs relatively uncommonly even when bands of tissue are present.

CYSTIC MAJOR VESTIBULAR GLANDS

The major vestibular (formally known as Bartholin's) glands are paired glands in the ventrolateral wall of the vestibulum. They secrete a nearly colorless mucus and are usually quite inconspicuous. Blockage of the duct may result in dramatic cystic enlargement of the gland, which in extreme cases causes it to protrude from the vulvar lips, where it becomes susceptible to contamination, desiccation, and physical damage. The cystic gland may be liberally incised to promote drainage. Suturing is not necessary.

12.2.3.2—Dystocia Caused by Stenosis or Constriction of the Vulva and Vestibule

Robert O. Gilbert

Rarely, dystocia may be solely ascribable to inadequate dilation of the vulva and vestibule. This is usually encountered when parturition is assisted by traction and insufficient time is allowed for normal dilation to occur. In some cases it may accompany an inherited condition such as anovestibular stenosis or rectovaginal constriction (in Jersey cattle). Extensive scarring from previous parturient injury may also account for failure of the vulva to dilate.

In all such cases, it is preferable to attempt to achieve dilation of the caudal genital tract by gentle, moderate traction, with plenty of lubrication over a prolonged (30 to 90 minutes) period of time. The vulva can be dilated by traction of the fetal head or rear limbs or by using the hands and wrists of the operator. Should attempts to achieve dilation fail or if time is of the essence, episiotomy may be useful.

After application of epidural analgesia, an incision is made through the skin, subcutaneous tissues, and vestibular mucosa, beginning about 2 to 3 cm from the dorsal commissure of the vulva and proceeding dorsolaterally for up to 10 cm. The dorsolateral direction of the incision is important to prevent tissue tearing in a dorsal direction, which risks creation of a rectovaginal laceration. Immediately after delivery of the calf the episiotomy incision is sutured with deep sutures. This procedure is rarely required, but in the appropriate circumstances, it may be valuable in resolving a stubborn dystocia with minimal injury to fetus or dam.

12.2.3.3—Surgical Conditions of the Postpartum Period

Robert O. Gilbert

Hemorrhage into the Uterus or Vagina

Postpartum hemorrhage may result from trauma, laceration, or rupture of the genital organs—most commonly after forced extraction and cases of uterine torsion. Hemorrhage may be profuse if a major vessel is damaged. Minor bleeding usually resolves spontaneously without treatment. More severe bleeding may be controlled by injecting 20 to 50 IU of oxytocin to promote myometrial contraction. If a bleeding vaginal vessel can be identified, it can be clamped and possibly ligated. If this is impossible, the vagina may be packed to provide pressure on the bleeding vessel. Rarely, catastrophic, fatal bleeding into the abdomen from the uterine arteries may occur at the time of parturition; many afflicted cows have been found to suffer from copper deficiency.

Perivaginal Bleeding and Hematoma

Fetus passage may damage the internal pudendal artery, resulting in formation of a large hematoma lateral to the vaginal wall. In rare cases, this condition may be bilateral. In most instances, these hematomata resolve spontaneously; sometimes they become infected and persist as abscesses. The hematoma or abscess may be drained into the vagina by means of a lateral incision, with care taken not to damage the internal pudendal artery in making the incision. This should not be done until 3 days postpartum to allow complete hemostasis.

Hematomata of the vagina may protrude from the vulva. Hematoma of the vulva is usually obvious. Both may be readily drained after allowing 3 days for hemostasis. Contusions of the vagina and vulva are favored sites for clostridial growth, and affected cows should be treated with antibiotics and vaccinated (against tetanus) to prevent clostridial myositis or tetanus.

Birth Canal Lacerations

Minor lacerations may occur in spontaneous parturition and are usually confined to the area near the vulva. Unless they are severe, these wounds do not require suturing. Lacerations of the vaginal wall may result in prolapse of the bladder or perivaginal fat. Bladder prolapse usually takes place through a tear in the floor of the vagina. The prolapsed bladder fills with urine because the urethra is kinked. It may be necessary to drain the bladder with a fine needle before replacing it. The rent the bladder passed through should be sutured and the animal placed on parenteral antibiotics. Perivaginal fat may prolapse through a very small vaginal laceration and may resemble prolapse of the bladder. The prolapsed mass of fat should be traced to the point where it passes through the vaginal wall, where it may be cut off with minimal bleeding. The vaginal defect should be sutured. A more severe laceration results in second or third degree perineal laceration.

Vaginal and Cervical Prolapse

Eversion and prolapse of the vagina (Figure 12.2.3.3-1)—with or without prolapse of the cervix—occurs most commonly in cattle and sheep. The condition is usually seen in mature females in the last trimester of pregnancy. Predisposing factors include elevations in intraabdominal pressure associated with increased size of the pregnant uterus, intraabdominal fat, or rumen distention superimposed upon relaxation and softening of the pelvic girdle and associated soft tissue structures in the pelvic canal and perineum. These changes are mediated by elevated circulating concentrations of estrogens and relaxin during late pregnancy. Intraabdominal pressure is increased in the recumbent animal. Added to this, sheep tend to face uphill when lying down, so that gravity assists vaginal eversion and prolapse.

The prolapse begins as an intussusception-like folding of the vaginal floor just cranial to the vestibulovaginal junction. In addition to elevated abdominal pressure, dis-

comfort caused by this eversion, coupled with irritation and swelling of the exposed mucosa, results in straining and more extensive prolapse. Eventually the entire vagina may be prolapsed, with the cervix conspicuous at the caudal most extent of the prolapsus. The bladder or loops of intestine may be contained within the prolapsed vagina, resulting in occlusion of the urethra. The bladder then becomes filled and enlarged, which hinders replacement of the prolapsed vagina unless the bladder is first drained. The bladder may even rupture—with potentially fatal consequences.

Although most common in mature animals in late pregnancy, vaginal prolapse can occur in young, non-pregnant ewes and heifers, especially in fat animals. Predisposing factors include grazing estrogenic plants (especially *Trifolium subterraneum*) or exogenous administration of estrogenic compounds (usually in the form of growth-promoter implants). Estrogenic compounds cause relaxation of the structures of the pelvic girdle, which predisposes to the initial folding of the vaginal floor—the common precursor to complete prolapse. Cervicovaginal prolapse is more common in stabled than pastured animals, thus suggesting that lack of exercise may be a contributing factor. Vaginal prolapse may also be a problem in cows that are subjected to repeated superovulation for embryo recovery. A genetic component in the pathogenesis of cervicovaginal prolapse is likely because a breed predisposition exists in cattle (Brahman, Brahman crossbreds, Hereford) and in sheep (Kerry Hill, Romney Marsh). In pigs vaginal prolapse is often associated with estrogenic activity of mycotoxins.

TREATMENT

For replacement of the prolapsed vagina, an epidural anesthetic is first administered. The organ is washed and rinsed, and the bladder is emptied if necessary. This may be achieved by elevating the prolapsus to allow straightening of the urethra; occasionally needle puncture through the vaginal wall may be necessary. The vagina is well lubricated (glycerin provides lubrication and reduces congestion and edema by osmotic action), replaced, and held in position until it feels warm again. Retention is achieved by insertion of a Buhner suture. This is a specific form of deeply buried, circumferential suture placed around the vestibulum to provide support at the vestibulovaginal junction. Its merit is that it provides support at the point at which the initial eversion of the vaginal wall occurs, thus preventing the initiation of the condition. The Buhner suture has largely superseded earlier attempts to prevent prolapse by various patterns of sutures in the vulvar lips (which do not prevent the initial eversion of the vagina into the vestibulum) or methods which relied on placement of a retention device within

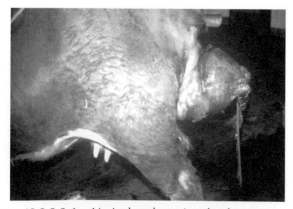

Figure 12.2.3.3-1   Vaginal prolapse in a beef cow.

the vagina (which tend to cause discomfort and further straining). Buhner sutures should generally be removed before parturition to prevent extensive lacerations.

Although the cervical os may be edematous and inflamed, cervicovaginal prolapse seldom interrupts pregnancy and does not specifically predispose to dystocia or *post partum* uterine prolapse, which has a different etiology. Vaginal prolapse in sheep may occur simultaneously in many ewes as a herd problem, making surgery impractical. In these cases, use of a commercially available vaginal retention device (a "bearing retainer") may be useful. Sheep may lamb without mishap while wearing these devices. Permanent fixation techniques (cervicopexy or vaginopexy) have been described in which the cervix or vaginal wall is anchored to other pelvic structures. They may be useful in individual cases.

BÜHNER SUTURE PLACEMENT
Epidural analgesia is administered, the tail tied to the side, and the perineum prepared for surgery. Vertical incisions, each about 2 cm in length, passing through skin and subcutaneous fascia are made dorsal and ventral to the vulva. Dorsally, the incision should be midway between the dorsal commissure of the vulva and the anus. The ventral incision is made a similar distance from the ventral commissure. Both incisions need to be deep enough to allow the suture, once place and tightened, to migrate forward freely. A Görlach needle (a long [approximately 15 cm] sturdy, cutting edged needle on a handle and with an eye at its forward end) is inserted into the ventral incision and passed up and out of the dorsal incision (Figure 4.4-17A and B). The needle should be passed as far cranial and lateral as possible, without damaging blood vessels coursing along the sacrosciatic ligament. If the needle is passed too superficially (relative to the vaginal mucosa), there is a risk that the suture will pull through the mucosa eventually. If the needle is not cranial ("deep") enough, the suture will not support the vestibule-vaginal region (the region of the pelvic diaphragm) and will not serve its purpose adequately.

The needle is passed though the dorsal incision, sterile umbilical tape is threaded through it, and the needle is withdrawn while one end of the umbilical tape is held. The procedure is repeated on the opposite side. The free end of the umbilical tape that was held dorsally is threaded into the needle before it is withdrawn again. This leaves both free ends in the ventral incision. They are tied together, and the suture is tightened until the vestibulum permits passage of two fingers. During tightening, the correctly placed suture should migrate forward so it comes to lie just caudal to the vestibulovaginal junction. Suturing the skin incisions is optional.

If the animal is within 2 months of parturition, the suture ends should be left long, so the suture can be cut and removed to prevent severe laceration at parturition. In any case, the animal should be monitored frequently, and care taken to ensure it is possible for the vestibula to dilate sufficiently to permit passage of the fetus.

CERVICOPEXY AND VAGINOPEXY
In some circumstances pexy of the cranial vagina is used to prevent cervicovaginal prolapse in cows in which the condition recurs frequently. This may be in embryo transfer donors, in which the repeated superovulation, and associated supraphysiological hormone levels, produce softening of the pelvic diaphragm in a way similar to pregnancy. Even in these cases, the condition is usually satisfactorily controlled by correct placement of a Bühner stitch. Rare cases, however, might require fixation of the entire vagina. Before doing this, inherited causes of prolapse (breed predisposition) should be ruled out.

Several methods for vaginopexy have been described. This author's preference is for suturing the cranial vagina to the iliopsoas muscle. This can be done blindly, via the vagina, or by open surgery, with a caudal celiotomy. In the latter case, it is helpful to have an assistant insert a gloved, lubricated hand into the cranial vagina to guide it toward the surgeon. The cranial vagina is secured to the muscle by placement of several sutures through both structures. Another common method involves a through-and-through suture that traverses the gluteal muscles, the sacrosciatic ligament, and the vagina. Usually, the suture is anchored at the skin and in the vagina with a button or similar object to prevent it from pulling through the mucosa or skin. Any pexy should be performed only on one side to prevent chronic pneumovagina.

Uterine Prolapse and Eversion

Prolapse of the uterus may occur in any species; however, it is most common in dairy cows (Figure 12.2.3.3-2) and ewes (Figure 12.2.3.3-3), less frequent in sows. Prolapse invariably occurs immediately after or within several hours of parturition; prolapse more than 24 hours after parturition is extremely rare and is complicated by partial closure of the cervix, thus making replacement difficult or even impossible. Most cases occur in winter and fall, and over half have clinical milk fever. The etiology is unclear, and occurrence is sporadic. Most affected cows are hypocalcemic, and uterine atony seems a likely contributing factor. Prolapse of the uterus usually occurs within a few hours after parturition, when the cervix is open and the uterus lacks tone. The best explanation is that the tip of the post gravid horn becomes invaginated and that the invagination proceeds, either spontaneously,

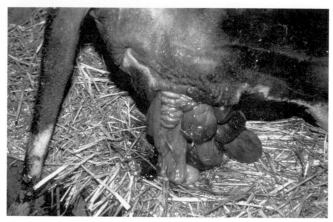

Figure 12.2.3.3-2   Uterine prolapse in a cow.

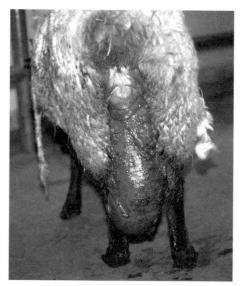

Figure 12.2.3.3-3   Uterine prolapse in a ewe.

or because of abdominal press, until the post gravid horn is completely exteriorized. Prolapse may be precipitated by traction on a fetus or retained placenta. Prolapse of the post gravid uterine horn usually is complete in cows, and the mass of the uterus usually hangs below the hocks. The invagination of the contralateral (formerly nongravid and usually nonprolapsed) horn can be located by careful examination of the surface of the prolapsed organ. In sows one horn may become everted, whereas unborn piglets in the other prevent further prolapse.

Both in its appearance and in its pathogenesis uterine prolapse is quite distinct from cervicovaginal prolapse. Cervicovaginal prolapse usually afflicts pregnant animals, results from relaxation of pelvic structures under hor-monal influence, and begins as a "rollover" of mucosa at the vestibule-vaginal junction. The prolapsed mass is smooth (vaginal mucosa), and the cervix may be visible. In contrast, uterine prolapse occurs immediately post-partum, is predisposed by uterine flaccidity, and starts with invagination of the tip of the formerly gravid uterine horn. Uterine prolapse is recognizable by the presence of visible caruncles (and sometimes placental remnants) on the surface of the prolapsus.

TREATMENT

In cows, treatment involves removing the placenta (if still attached), thorough cleaning of the endometrial surface, and repair of any lacerations. Rubbing the surface of the uterus with glycerol helps reduce edema and provides lubrication so that the uterus can be returned to its normal position. First, an epidural anesthetic should be administered. Replacement of the uterus is much easier if the cow is placed in sternal recumbency, with its rear limbs extended caudally (behind it) so that it is in a "frog-sitting" position. Elevation of the hindquarters is also useful. The cleansed uterus should be elevated to the level of the vulva on a tray or hammock supported by assistants, then replaced by applying steady pressure beginning at the cervical portion and gradually working toward the apex. Another strategy is to locate the opening of the unprolapsed, previously nongravid uterine horn. This appears as an invagination near the base of the prolapsed mass. If it can be identified, pressure can be applied directly to this spot with a clenched fist; this generally permits much easier replacement of the prolapsus than is otherwise possible. Once the uterus is replaced, the operator's hand should be inserted to the tip of both uterine horns to be sure that no remaining invagination could incite abdominal straining and repro-lapse. Instillation (and subsequent removal by siphon) of warm, sterile saline solution is useful for ensuring complete replacement of the tip of the uterine horn without trauma. Once the uterus is in its normal position oxy-tocin (20 IU IV or 40 IU im) is administered to increase uterine tone. Administration of calcium-containing solutions is indicated in most cases, also as a means of increasing uterine tone, and because most cases are hypocalcemic. Caslick sutures or other forms of vulvar closure are not indicated, since they merely obscure recurrence of the prolapse and do nothing to prevent it. Recurrence is prevented mainly by ensuring complete replacement of the uterus, without invagination of the tip of a horn, and restoration of uterine tone.

In sows reposition may be achieved by simultaneously manipulating the uterus from outside with one hand and through an abdominal incision with the other. Resection of the uterus is indicated in long-standing cases in which tissue necrosis has occurred.

The prognosis depends on the amount of injury and contamination of the uterus. Prompt replacement of a clean, minimally traumatized uterus allows a favorable prognosis. The crude recovery rate is about 75%. Of recovered cows, about 85% conceive again—taking 10 days longer to do so than herdmates. No tendency for the condition to recur at subsequent parturitions exists. Prognosis is more favorable if prolapse follows birth of a live calf and if the cow is primiparous. Complications tend to develop when laceration, necrosis, and/or infection occur or when treatment is delayed. Shock, hemorrhage, and thromboembolism are potential sequelae of a prolonged prolapse. In some instances the bladder and intestines may prolapse in to the everted uterus. These require careful replacement of the viscera before replacement of the uterus. The bladder may be drained with a catheter or needle placed through the uterine wall. Elevating the hindquarters and putting pressure on the uterus aids replacement of the bladder and intestines. It may be necessary to incise the uterus carefully (in a longitudinal direction) to replace these organs. In the cow, amputation of a severely traumatized or necrotic uterus may be the only means of saving the animal. Supportive treatment and antibiotic therapy are indicated.

RECOMMENDED READINGS

Gardner IA, Reynolds JP, Risco CA, Hird DW: Patterns of uterine prolapse in dairy cows and prognosis after treatment, *J Am Vet Med Assoc* 197: 1021-1024, 1990.

Houe H, Ostergaard S, Thilaing-Hansen T, Jorgensen RJ, Larsen T, Sorensen JT, Agger JF, Blom JY: Milk fever and subclinical hypocalcemia: an evaluation of parameters on incidence risk, diagnosis, risk factors and biological effects as input for a decision support system for disease control, *Acta Veterinaria Scandinavica* 42: 1-29, 2001.

Jubb TF, Malmo J, Brightling P, Davis GM: Survival and fertility after uterine prolapse in dairy cows, *Austral Vet J* 67: 22-24, 1990.

Risco CA, Reynolds JP, Hird D: Uterine prolapse and hypocalcemia in dairy cows, *J Am Vet Med Assoc* 185: 1517-1519, 1984.

12.2.4—Surgery of the Perineum

Susan L. Fubini

Obstetrical trauma is the most common cause of perineal injuries. These injuries can result from an abnormal position and/or size of the calf in relation to the dam or from overzealous attempts by farmers and veterinarians to aid delivery. Although they can be impressive when the injury first occurs, surgery is usually delayed until bruised tissue swelling has subsided, local tissue necrosis has resolved, and the wound edges have healed.

First- and Second-Degree Perineal Lacerations

Lacerations of the perineal body are classified according to location, extent of injury, and tissues involved. A first-degree perineal laceration involves only the skin and mucosa of the vagina or vestibule. Most of these wounds heal without any invasive therapy, but it is best to follow the repair with a Caslick procedure if there is significant disruption of tissue or deep lacerations.

Protrusion of perivaginal fat through the laceration may require its amputation with an emasculator or scalpel. A Caslick procedure is performed in the standing, restrained cow with epidural anesthesia. The injured area is prepared with appropriate aseptic techniques. A strip of tissue at the mucocutaneous junction is excised in an elongated "U"-shape, starting ventrally at the junction of the dorsal 2/3 and ventral 1/3 of the vulvar lips and proceeding dorsally to the top of the vulva and down the other side. The freshened edges are sutured in a continuous pattern. Enough room (3 cm) is left for urination at the ventral commissure of the vulva (Figure 12.2.4-1A-D).

Second-degree perineal laceration involves disruption of the fibromuscular tissues that separate the rectum and vagina. There is usually considerable swelling and edema of affected tissues. There is no need for emergency surgery. The concern is that loss of functional vulvar and vestibular conformation over time will allow air and fecal contamination of the vaginal vault and eventually lead to infertility through endometritis.

The rectum is evacuated, perineum prepared, and epidural anesthetic administered in preparation to repair these lacerations. A triangular-shaped piece of mucosa and submucosa is removed from each side (Figure 12.2.4-2). The base of the triangle should be located at the dorsal aspect of the mucocutaneous junction of the perineal body. One arm of the triangle is along the dorsal commissure of the vagina while the other arm parallels the rectum. The mucosa is sharply incised and undermined, by carefully using Metzenbaum scissors to lift the mucosa-submucosa flap and leaving a fresh surface on each side. If the tear is asymmetric, this makes it more difficult, and creative modification is needed to design flaps and determine how to appose the tissues. Sutures are first placed deeply, and mucosa and submucosa are apposed in an attempt to create a wide surface like the original perineal body with 2-0 or 3-0 absorbable sutures. Typically a Caslick procedure is done upon completion of the deeper tissues repair.

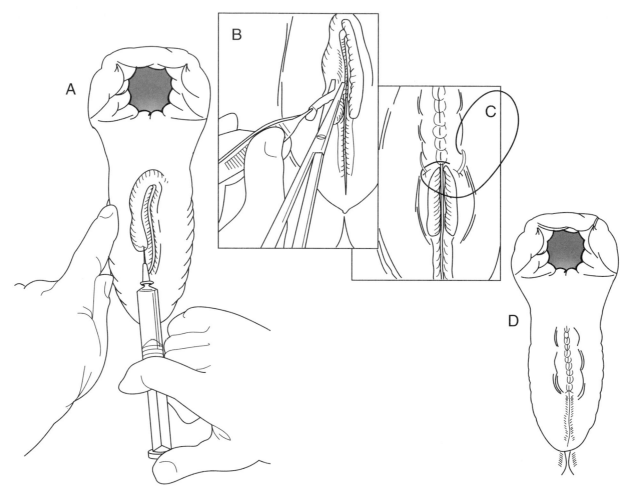

Figure 12.2.4-1   Line diagram of a Caslick procedure. *A*, A local anesthetic is injected at the mucocutaneous junction. *B*, A strip of tissue is removed at the mucocutaneous junction. *C*, The raw edges are apposed, with a continuous suture. *D*, Completed Caslick procedure.

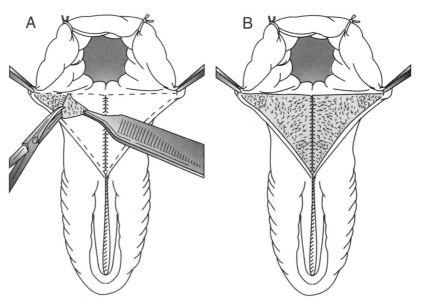

Figure 12.2.4-2   Line diagram of repair of second-degree perineal laceration. Triangular flaps of mucosa and submucosa are resected to rebuild the perineal body.

Third-Degree Perineal Lacerations

Third-degree perineal lacerations result when there is complete disruption of the rectovestibular shelf due to fetal oversize, forced extraction, or some other trauma that leaves a wide opening between the rectum and vagina (Figure 12.2.4-3), often with disruption of the anus. This lesion can result in fecal contamination of the vagina and eventually endometritis and infertility. Unlike some other species, the constrictor vestibuli muscle and cervix of the cow help prevent infection, which allows some cattle with complete perineal lacerations to become pregnant.

Initial treatment after injury consists of local wound care. The wound should be cleaned and debrided the same as any other soft tissue injury. Immediate repair of a fresh tear has been reported but is rare because the swelling results in poor suture holding power. It is also difficult to tell which tissues are viable. Instead, the wound is left alone for 6 to 8 weeks to allow for tissue necrosis and secondary healing (see Figure 12.2.4-3).

For surgical repair the cow is restrained in standing stocks; the rectum is evacuated of feces; and the tail is retracted to one side. Some surgeons like to construct a rectal tampon from an orthopedic stockinette filled with cotton and secured at the ends with umbilical tape (see Figure 12.2.4-3). The authors have not found this to be

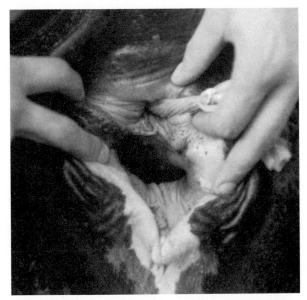

Figure 12.2.4-3 Six-week-old third-degree perineal laceration in a cow. A gauze roll is placed in the rectum to minimize fecal contamination during the repair. Note the complete loss of the rectovaginal shelf.

(Courtesy of Dr. Nigel Cook; University of Wisconsin.)

necessary. After an epidural is administered, the rectum is evacuated and the perineum prepared for aseptic surgery. Perioperative antimicrobials are indicated.

The three steps of the procedure consist of rebuilding the shelf between the rectum and vagina, repairing the perineal body, and performing a Caslick's procedure. The soft consistency of cattle manure eliminates the need for dietary modification.

Retraction is provided by stay sutures, a Balfour self-retaining retractor, or towel clamps. Good lighting is important. The rectovestibular shelf is tented with forceps and divided in a frontal plane, with care taken to avoid penetration of the rectal mucosa. Ideally, the tissues should be divided so the rectal shelf is $\frac{2}{3}$ of the thickness and the vaginal shelf is $\frac{1}{3}$. The dissection should be carried forward and along each side at a 2.5- to 3.0-cm depth. It is critical that the flaps created be brought into apposition to determine whether there is sufficient tissue for suturing without any excessive tension. Reconstruction of the shelf is usually performed with a one-stage technique.

One-Stage Repair (Modified Goetz)

Using this technique, a six-bite vertical pattern is used to rebuild the shelf between the rectum and vagina (Figure 12.2.4-4). Most reports describe using a nonabsorbable synthetic suture and leaving the ends long to facilitate suture removal in 14 days. However, there are several easy-to-handle, nonreactive monofilament absorbable sutures (size #1 or #2) that maintain adequate strength and do not require suture removal. Locating the suture bites through the tissue is described as follows for a right-handed surgeon:

1. Beginning in the vaginal vault, the first bite incorporates 2 to 3 cm of the left vaginal flap directed ventral to dorsal and exiting between the rectal and vestibular flaps.
2. The second bite incorporates the left rectal shelf and exits 2 cm from the edge. Care is taken to ensure penetration of the submucosa—but *not* the rectal mucosa.
3. The next bite is similar to the second bite, which penetrates the right rectal shelf and exits between the rectal and vestibular flaps.
4. The fourth bite is through the right vaginal flap in a dorsal-to-ventral direction that emerges in the vaginal vault.
5. The needle is reversed in the needle holder and "backhanded" for a shallower (1 cm) bite through the right vestibular fold in a ventral-dorsal direction and exits between the two flaps.

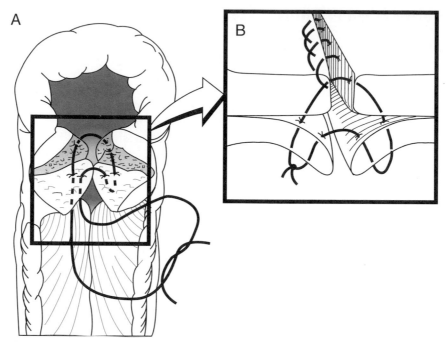

Figure 12.2.4-4   Line diagram showing the six-bite technique to repair a third-degree perineal body.

6. The final bite is similar to the one before, pene-trating the left vaginal flap in a dorsal-to-ventral direction and exiting in the vaginal vault.

The sutures should be placed 1.0 to 1.5 cm apart. They should be tied under tension, and the closure should be palpated after every bite, feeling for any defect that may have been inadvertently created (Figure 12.2.4-5). The author likes to place a simple continuous pattern of 2-0 absorbable sutures (with knots in the rectum) in the rectal mucosa for a better "seal" and to prevent fecal material from contaminating the shelf sutures.

The sutures are continued until the perineal body is reached. If a nonabsorbable suture is used, the ends must be left long to facilitate removal 2 weeks later. The rest of the surgery is performed as described for a perineal body reconstruction (see Figure 12.2.4-2). Finally, a Caslick's procedure is performed (see Figure 12.2.4-1). Four weeks after surgery, healing can be evaluated. Ideally, 6 to 8 weeks should be allowed before breeding or artificial insemination.

Rectovaginal Fistula Repair

Rectovaginal fistulas are not common in cattle but do occur in adults, secondarily to dystocia. During parturi-tion, the front foot of a calf in an anterior, dorsosacral presentation typically perforates the dorsal aspect of the

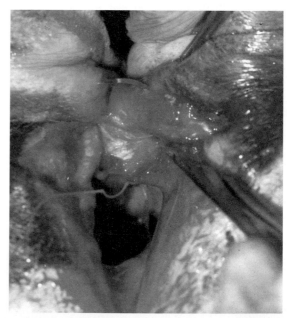

Figure 12.2.4-5   Repair of the rectovaginal shelf is being completed. Note slight eversion of rectal mucosa toward the rectum.

vestibule and enters the rectum. The foot is withdrawn and leaves a defect between rectum and vagina. Recto-vaginal fistulas are also seen in calves with atresia of the anus and cattle with failed, third-degree perineal lacera-tion repair.

If the fistula was traumatic, adequate time (4 to 6 weeks) should be allowed before surgery because the defect size can be reduced markedly as a result of wound contraction. Some smaller defects have been reported to heal completely.

One surgical option (especially with large, deep fistulas) is to convert them to a third-degree perineal laceration before performing the repair. Preparation is the same as for other perineal surgery.

Another option is to repair the fistula primarily. With adequate restraint and preparation, a transverse incision is made between the rectum and vagina. By using a combination of sharp and blunt dissection in a horizontal plane, the fistula is exposed. Ideally $2/3$ of the thickness of the shelf should be with the rectum and $1/3$ with the vaginal shelf. Most fistulas measure 3 to 5 cm. Dissection is continued 3 to 4 cm rostral to the fistula. The rectal defect is closed transversely by using number 0 or 1 absorbable sutures in a simple interrupted pattern placed in the submucosa, with care taken not to penetrate the rectal mucosa. The first suture should divide the defect in half; the next two sutures should be placed to bisect the halves, and so on. Alternatively, one can preplace the sutures. In addition, successful repairs have been reported with longitudinal closure of the rectum. Either technique is adequate if there is good tissue apposition with little tension. The vaginal defect is closed next. Many advocate a continuous horizontal mattress pattern in a longitudinal direction so that the two suture rows are at right angles to each other and the vaginal mucosa is everted. The incised perineal body is closed with multiple interrupted sutures of 2-0 suture; the skin is closed routinely. Complications include dehiscence or fistula formation.

In one review article (Dreyfuss et al, 1990) on perineal surgery in cattle, the prognosis was favorable after surgery. Of the cattle that had surgical repair of third-degree perineal lacerations, 71% ($^{10}/_{14}$) remained fertile; whereas 75% ($^{3}/_{4}$) of cattle were productive after rectovaginal fistula repair.

RECOMMENDED READINGS

Aanes WA: Surgical repair of third-degree perineal laceration and recto-vaginal fistula in the mare, *J Am Vet Med Assoc* 144: 485-491, 1964.

Anderson JF: A modified Caslick's procedure for closure of the dorsal vulva in the cow, *Bovine Pract* 21: 184-186, 1986.

Baird AN: Surgery of the kidney. In Wolfe DF, Moll HD: *Large animal urogenital surgery*, Philadelphia, 1999, Williams & Wilkins.

Beard W: Standing urogenital surgery. In Bertone A, editor: *Standing Surgery, Vet Clin North Am Equine Pract*, Philadelphia, 1991, WB Saunders.

Belknap JK, Nickels FA: A one-stage repair of third-degree perineal lacerations and rectovestibular fistulae in 17 mares, *Vet Surg* 21: 378-381, 1992.

Colbern GT, Aanes WA, Stashack TS: Surgical management of perineal lacerations and rectovestibular fistulae in the mare: a retrospective study of 47 cases, *J Am Vet Med Assoc* 186: 265-269, 1985.

Desjardins MR, Trout DR, Little CB: Surgical repair of rectovaginal fistula in mares: twelve cases (1983-1991), *Can Vet J* 34: 226-231, 1993.

Dreyfuss DJ, Tulleners EP, Donawick WJ, Ducharme NG: Third-degree perineal lacerations and rectovestibular fistulae in cattle: 20 cases (1981-1988), *J Am Vet Med Assoc* 196: 768-770, 1990.

Hilbert BJ: Surgical repair of rectovaginal fistulae in mares, *Aust Vet J* 57: 85-87, 1981.

Hudson RS: Repair of perineal lacerations in the cow, *Bovine Pract* 7: 34-36, 1972.

Moll HD, Stone DE: Perineal lacerations and rectovestibular fistulas (equine). In Wolfe DF, Moll HD: *Large animal urogenital surgery*, Philadelphia, 1999, Williams & Wilkins.

Trotter GW: Surgery of the perineum in the mare. In McKinnon AO, Voss JL: *Equine reproduction*, Philadelphia 1993, Lea & Febiger.

Trotter GW: Surgical diseases of the caudal reproductive tract. In Auer JA: *Equine surgery*, Philadelphia, 1992, WB Saunders.

Wenzel JGW, Baird AN: Female urogenital surgery. In Wolfe DF, Moll HD: *Large animal urogenital surgery*, Philadelphia, 1999, Williams & Wilkins.

Wolfe DF: Surgery of the rectum, perineum, and vulva (farm animal). In Wolfe DF, Moll HD: *Large animal urogenital surgery*, Philadelphia, 1999, Williams & Wilkins.

Wolfe DF, Baird AN: Female urogenital surgery in cattle, *Vet Clin North Am* 9: 369-388, 1993.

12.2.5—Surgery of the Mammary Gland

Susan L. Fubini

Relevant Surgical Anatomy

The udder of the dairy cow can vary in size tremendously, but it can get extremely large and weigh as much as 60 kg. The udder comprises four glands, each of which has one principal teat. A prominent median intermammary groove generally marks the division of the udder into right and left halves. The division between fore and hind quarters of each side is less distinct. The skin covering the udder is thin and freely movable, except in the teats.

The udder is suspended from the body wall by strong fascial medial and lateral laminae that together are termed the suspensory apparatus. The medial lamina is the stronger of the two and is largely made up of elastic tissue. The right and left medial laminae are separated by a small amount of loose connective tissue, which makes it possible to remove one half of the udder fairly easily.

The lateral lamina is composed of dense connective tissue. It arises from the area of the lateral crus of the external inguinal ring and pubic symphysis. It provides protection to the mammary vasculature and superficial inguinal (mammary) lymph nodes. The laminae are thickest dorsally and become progressively thinner at the ventral aspect.

The bulk of the udder is made up of connective tissue mixed with parenchyma. The main arterial supply is the external pudendal artery with a small contribution by the mammary branch of the ventral perineal artery. The external pudendal artery and vein enters the udder after passing through the inguinal canal. The artery first forms a sigmoid flexure before dividing into cranial and caudal mammary branches. The former is large and directed ventrocranially, while the caudal branch supplies the back of the udder. Both vessels branch extensively to supply the parenchyma.

A ring of venous drainage is located above the base of the udder. Contributions come from the external pudendal veins, subcutaneous abdominal ("milk") vein, ventral perineal veins, and udder tributaries. Innervation to the udder is from the lumbar spinal nerves (L1, L2, and the genitofemoral nerve) and sacral spinal nerves (mammary branch of the pudendal nerve).

The udder of small ruminants consists of two glands, which vary from conical and deep in the milking goat to small and spherical in sheep. The structure, suspension, vascular and nervous supply is similar to that of the bovine.

MANAGEMENT OF CHRONIC MASTITIS

Hemimastectomy, or radical mastectomy, is occasionally performed in small ruminants and rarely in cattle. Indications include neoplasia (Figure 12.2.5-1), chronic or gangrenous mastitis (Figure 12.2.5-2), a fibrotic or granulomatous udder, and precocious udder development. In some animals—especially older ones—the suspensory apparatus has weakened, thus allowing the udder to sag and even ulcerate due to contact with the ground (Figure 12.2.5-3). This condition can become inhumane, and surgery is necessary. Ideally, surgery should be performed in a nonlactating animal in good physical condition. This is not always possible, especially

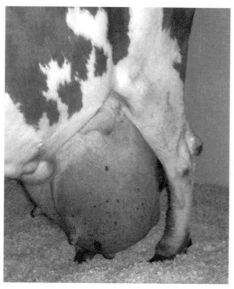

Figure 12.2.5-2   Cow with chronic mastitis resulting in failed mammary suspensory apparatus.

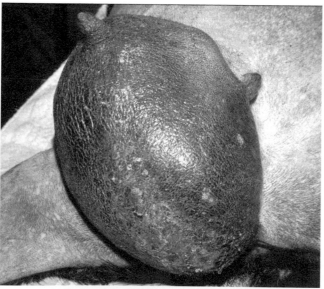

Figure 12.2.5-1   Goat with mammary lymphosarcoma in dorsal recumbency.

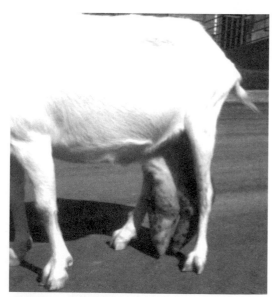

Figure 12.2.5-3   Goat with chronic mastitis resulting in failed mammary suspensory apparatus.

(Courtesy of Dr. Norm G. Ducharme; Cornell University.)

with gangrenous mastitis cases. If septic shock is present because of gangrenous mastitis, the blood loss associated with surgery and removal of a vascular organ such as the mammary gland can overwhelm the animal's defenses. Instead, teat amputation to allow better drainage should be considered (see Section 12.2.3). Chemical destruction of the affected quarter is the medical alternative to chronic mastitis that can be used where the suspensory support of the mammary gland is still intact. Finally, external pudendal artery vein and artery ligation has been used to cause rapid atrophy of the mammary gland, where it would be unwise to perform major surgery on very sick animals.

CHEMICAL DESTRUCTION OF THE MAMMARY GLAND

To perform chemical destruction of the mammary gland, one of several irritating preparations is injected into the affected quarter(s) and not milked out. Significant inflammation (pain swelling and erythema) results, with subsequent atrophy of that part of the gland. If excessive inflammation occurs, it is managed by milking out the preparation 24 to 48 hours after infusion. Chemicals used for this procedure include one of the following: 100 ml of a solution containing 10% formaldehyde diluted in 500 ml of sterile saline, 50 to 100 cc of 3% silver nitrate solution, 20 ml of 5% copper sulfate, 250 ml of a solution containing 1 gm of acriflavine in 500 ml of sterile water, or 60 ml of 2% chlorhexidine.

Mastectomy

Perioperative antimicrobials and nonsteroidal antiinflammatory drugs as well as replacement fluid therapy are indicated, if necessary. Surgery is best performed during fall and winter to avoid fly infestation.

The animal is anesthetized and placed in dorsal recumbency. General anesthesia is recommended because of the risk of aspiration pneumonia and to provide a more controlled environment for vasculature ligation. Should the need arise to administer blood or provide other life support measures, general anesthesia provides better accessibility to the patient. The mammary gland should be cleansed as much as possible and isolated from the rest of the animal with impervious drapes.

An elliptical incision is made around the udder. It is imperative to save as much normal skin as possible so primary closure of the surgical wound can be performed with minimal tension (Figure 12.2.5-4). When an udder is very large, the initial incision should come up the side of the udder, and the skin should be reflected down by the base of the udder as the dissection is continued. Once the skin incision is made, subcutaneous tissues are dis-

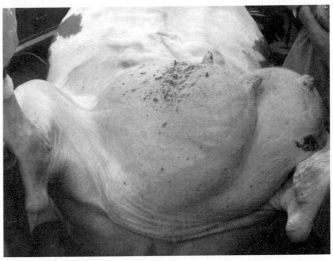

Figure 12.2.5-4   Cow in Figure 12.2.2-1 placed in dorsal recumbency for surgery. Intended line of skin incision preserves sufficient skin for closure.

sected by using a combination of sharp and blunt dissection. Some surgeons suggest that starting the dissection caudally and working in a cranial direction is preferable. Instead, the authors have found starting on the lateral aspect of the udder and establishing a dissection plane before advancing the incision is most useful. After this, the dissection is carried cranially and caudally with a combination of blunt and sharp dissection. The authors prefer to dissect the cranial aspect of the udder first because it is easier to separate the udder from the abdominal wall. This means the vasculature must be isolated to keep from incising it inadvertently as the dissection is carried caudally. Having at least one assistant retract the udder and aid in visualizing the site through suction and sponging of blood is very helpful. The assistant should retract the incised skin edge opposite where the surgeon is working. This allows better exposure of fascial planes and vasculature. Many small blood vessels are encountered, and hemorrhage is controlled with an electrosurgical unit and ligatures. Some surgeons advocate using a carbon dioxide laser for dissection to prevent excessive bleeding. In the author's experience, laser use is only helpful in the subcutaneous tissues; vessel size precludes effective laser use in deeper tissues. The external pudendal artery and veins, smaller mammary branch of the ventral perineal artery, and caudal superficial epigastric vein are the main vessels that require ligation. A number of additional smaller veins emerge from the cranial aspect of the gland and also require ligation, including branches of the external pudendal vessels adjacent to the suspensory ligament of the udder. The dissection is extended first toward the external pudendal artery and veins with the help of an assistant retracting the udder (Figure 12.2.5-7). The artery is double or triple ligated first to minimize vascular loss. Dissection is continued gradually, freeing the entire mammary gland from the body wall (Figure 12.2.5-6). If a hemimastectomy is performed, dissection is continued from the lateral side of the incision to the median lamina of the suspensory ligament of the udder. Then, using a combination of blunt and sharp dissection, the surgeon removes the mammary tissue.

After removal of the udder, the incision is closed. If necessary, tension-relieving sutures in the form of vertical mattress or near-far-far-near sutures can be placed at intervals to appose the deeper tissues. Interrupted

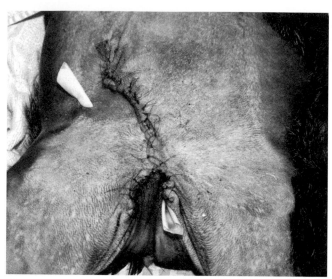

Figure 12.2.5-7 After excising the udder, the incision is closed. A Penrose drain has been placed for drainage.

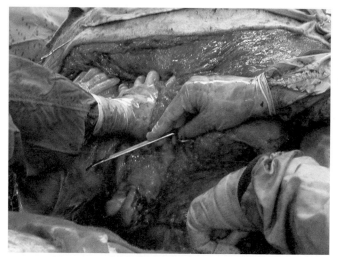

Figure 12.2.5-5 The udder is being pushed laterally to allow the surgeon access to the external pudendal vessels.

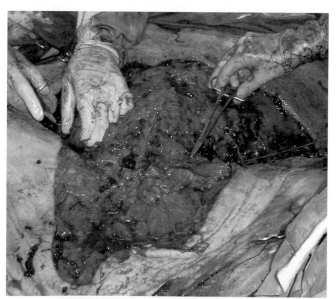

Figure 12.2.5-6 The udder has been removed and the defect will be closed in 2 or 3 layers, thus limiting dead space as much as possible.

sutures can be placed between the tension sutures to bring the remainder of the fascia and subcutaneous tissues into apposition. A Penrose drain may be placed into the defect and exited adjacent to the surgical wound (Figure 12.2.5-7). This allows fluids to drain away from the healing incision. Subcutaneous sutures are carefully placed in an effort to occlude dead space. Individual sutures may be necessary as the skin flaps are pulled into apposition. Finally, the skin is apposed by using a continuous Ford interlocking pattern or other acceptable pattern.

If primary closure is not possible, the wound can be packed with an antiseptic-soaked dressing held in place with a stent, sutures, or bandage. This dressing can be removed 24 to 48 hours later and the area treated like an open wound with daily hydrotherapy and lavage with an antiseptic solution. Fly control is necessary. Antibiotics should be continued for at least 7 to 10 days after surgery. Nonsteroidal antiinflammatory drugs are usually continued for 2 to 3 days. If the wound is left open, diligent wound care is necessary because of possible pockets of fluid and deep recesses that must be flushed. Ideally, exercise is restricted until the wound is at least partially healed.

Ligation of External Pudendal Artery

This procedure is mainly used to treat severe, life-threatening gangrenous mastitis in ruminants, including septic shock cases where the animal's cardiovascular status precludes surgery. Instead, the external pudendal artery and vein are ligated. This decreases toxin absorption into the animal's circulation and leads eventually to atrophy of the affected mammary gland. This procedure is more effective in small ruminants whose major blood supply is from the external pudendal artery. An adult cow's gland also receives blood through the mammary branch of the ventral perineal artery, which may prevent ischemic necrosis and subsequent atrophy of the gland. The procedure is clearly much less invasive than surgery, is not associated with blood loss, and is therefore preferable to udder amputation in a very sick animal. Both the cranial and caudal quarters on the ipsilateral blood supply will become avascular. If both the left and right mammary glands need to be devascularized, the left and right external pudendal vessels must be ligated.

The animal is placed in lateral recumbency with the affected side uppermost. The upper limb is tied upward to allow access to the inguinal region. Sedation is used if needed at a reduced dose, as the patient is generally in a compromised state. After infiltration of local anesthetic over the inguinal area, a 10- to 15-cm incision is made parallel to the external inguinal ring. Using a curved scissor, the surgeon incises superficial fascia. Blunt dissection is used to locate the external pudendal vessels, which are identified as the only two vascular structures exiting the inguinal canal (Figure 12.2.5-8). The external pudendal artery is triple ligated and transected with a double ligation on the cardiac side and a single ligation on the mammary side. The procedure is repeated on the external pudendal vein. The subcutaneous tissues are closed by using three or four pursestring-like sutures. Multiple bites of loose tissue, inguinal fat, and subcutaneous tissue are taken, which reapposes all tissues superficial to the external inguinal ring on either side of the

incision. The skin is closed in a routine manner. After ligation and division of the external pudendal vessels, teats from the affected quarters should be amputated at their bases with curved Mayo scissors to allow drainage.

Postoperative care includes continued systemic antibiotics appropriate for the septic process and continued drainage of the udder until it sloughs off. Appropriate wound care as needed.

Udder Biopsy

For research purposes, it is occasionally necessary to obtain a sample of mammary tissue. The portion of the udder to be biopsied should be clipped and prepared for surgery. An area without visible large vessels is identified. A local anesthetic is used to desensitize the site. A 4-cm skin incision is made through the skin and continued through subcutaneous tissues and fascia. It is critical to go deep enough to sample mammary tissue, not fascia. When mammary tissue is reached, the surgeon should quickly and sharply incise the amount of tissue desired. Substantial hemorrhage will result. Rather than trying to grasp individual vessels, large bites of mammary tissue should be pulled together by using #2 chromic catgut or similar absorbable suture in a simple continuous pattern. As soon as a tight seal is obtained, the pressure will stop the hemorrhage. Subcutaneous tissues and skin are closed with 2-0 absorbable suture material, again in a simple continuous pattern. There may be seepage from the site for 24 to 48 hours and mild swelling. There also may be blood in milk from the operated quarter for several days. The author has used this technique in 20 milking dairy cows with no long-term postoperative problems. Electrosurgical units were ineffective for the degree of hemorrhage encountered.

RECOMMENDED READINGS

The udder of ruminants. In Dyce KM, Sack WO, Wensing CJG, editors: *Textbook of veterinary anatomy,* Philadelphia, 1987, WB Saunders.

Andreasen CB, Huber MJ, Mattoon JS: Unilateral fibroepithelial hyperplasia of the mammary gland in a goat, *J Am Vet Med Assoc* 202: 1279-1280, 1993.

Brewer RL: Mammary vessel ligation for gangrenous mastitis, *J Am Vet Med Assoc* 143: 44-45, 1963.

Bristol, DG: Teat and udder surgery in dairy cattle: part II. *Compend Cont Educ Pract Vet* 11: 983-991, 1989.

Hull, BL: Teat and udder surgery. In *Soft Tissue Surgery, Vet Clin North Am (Food Animal Practice),* Philadelphia, 1995, WB Saunders.

Rebhun WC: Mammary tumors. In Rebhun WC: *Diseases of dairy cattle,* Philadelphia, 1995, Williams and Wilkins.

Rebhun, WC: Diseases of the teats and udder. In Rebhun WC: *Diseases of dairy cattle,* Philadelphia, 1995, Williams and Wilkins.

Mammary gland and milk production. In Smith MC, Sherman DM, editors *Goat medicine,* Philadelphia, 1994, Lea & Febiger.

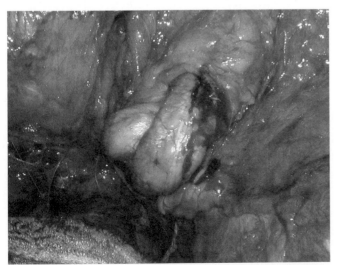

Figure 12.2.5-8 External pudendal vessels are easily identified as they exit the inguinal canal. In an adult cow, the vessels are generally 1.5 cm in diameter.

12.2.6—Teat Surgery

Adrian Steiner

Anatomy

The bovine mammary gland usually comprises four quarters with one teat each. The teat consists of the teat wall, apex with the streak canal, and teat sinus (Figure 12.2.6-1). Proximally, the teat sinus is continuous with the corresponding gland sinus. The annulus (venous ring of Furstenberg) demarcates the teat sinus from the gland sinus. It contains one or more large veins that encircle the base of the teat. The wall of the teat consists of the following layers: innermost is the teat sinus which is lined by a two-layered cuboidal epithelium, followed by the submucosa, connective tissue layer, and smooth muscle layer. Externally, the teat is covered by a stratified squamous epithelium. The connective tissue layer contains numerous large blood vessels that become engorged with blood during milking and suckling processes. In this text, the connective tissue and smooth muscle layers will be called *the intermediate layer*. The streak canal (teat canal, papillary duct) is lined with a stratified squamous epithelium and keratin. It varies in length between 5 to 10 mm and is located at the apex of the teat. It connects the teat sinus to the outside ending at the teat orifice. The rosette of Furstenberg—where the stratified squa-

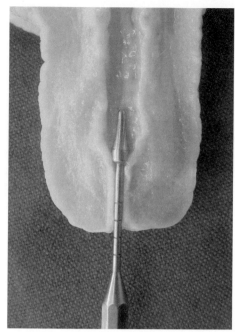

Figure 12.2.6-2   Teat probe shown introduced into the streak canal can be used to measure canal length.

mous epithelium of the streak canal meets the two-layered cuboidal epithelium of the teat sinus—represents the proximal delineation of the streak canal. The teat sphincter is located beneath the rosette of Furstenberg and consists of circularly oriented bundles of smooth muscle fibers. The teat sphincter and keratin lining of the streak canal are responsible for milk continence and preventing ascending infections.

Examination

The teat is examined with the following techniques: 1) visual inspection to describe color, shape, and size of the teat and the type and location of any lacerations present; 2) careful palpation and rolling of the affected teat between thumb and finger to determine any pain elicited as well as location and size of obstructive tissue present; 3) hand and machine milking by using either commercial milking equipment or a custom-made quarter milking machine to determine milk flow; 4) California Mastitis Test or strip test analysis to screen for evidence of mastitis; 5) microbial culture and sensitivity testing of a milk sample from a quarter suspected to be affected by mastitis; 6) probing the streak canal with a teat probe* developed by Fritz to compare its length with the healthy contralateral streak canal (Figure 12.2.6-2); 7) probing the teat and gland sinus with a side opening teat cannula for obstructing tissue in the area; 8) injecting methylene

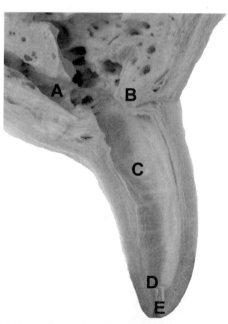

Figure 12.2.6-1   Sagittal section through teat and gland sinus of an adult lactating cow. *A,* gland sinus; *B,* annular ring; *C,* teat sinus; *D,* rosette of Furstenberg; *E,* streak canal.

*Eisenhut-Vet AG; Switzerland.

blue dye into the orifice of a suspected conjoined teat to stain the milk and confirm communication with the primary teat, and 9) ultrasonography, radiography (contrast or double contrast), and endoscopy to visualize size and location of obstructive tissues in the teat and gland sinuses. Ultrasonography and theloscopy have completely replaced radiography for this purpose in recent years. Ultrasonography is noninvasive and allows indirect visualization of the teat and gland. It is a valuable technique for diagnosing pathologies, mainly obstructive tissue, in the teat and gland sinuses. Theloscopy—initially proposed as a diagnostic tool to directly visualize intraluminal pathologies in the teat sinus—soon developed into a surgical tool that allows obstructing tissue to be resected with minimal surgical trauma to the teat.

Restraint, Anesthesia, Preparation of the Surgical Field

Adequate restraint and anesthesia are important prerequisites for surgical interventions in the area of the bovine teat. Success depends on aseptic conditions and meticulous surgical technique. For simple procedures such as cutting the teat sphincter, the cow may be restrained in a chute with the tail held in an upward position and 5 ml of lidocaine hydrochloride injected into the streak canal for local analgesia. This type of restraint and anesthesia is not satisfactory for surgical interventions that require suturing. The physical position with the animal standing is very uncomfortable and may be dangerous for the surgeon, and fecal contamination of the wound is likely to occur. Therefore more invasive surgical procedures require the cow to be restrained on a surgery table or in a trough in lateral or dorsal recumbency with the affected teat positioned uppermost. Depending on the cow's temperament, sedation with xylazine hydrochloride (0.2 mg/kg, IM or 0.1 mg/kg IV) is indicated. If the procedure is to be performed in lateral recumbency, the cow is attached to the table in a standing position, the tranquilizer administered, and the table tilted 10 minutes later. The procedure is similar in dorsal recumbency; the cow is sedated; casting ropes are applied; and the cow is secured into a trough. The limbs are secured to rings on the adjacent wall with hobbles. Once in position, local anesthesia is performed by circumferential injection of 20 ml of a 2% lidocaine hydrochloride solution at the base of the teat in the area of the annular ring (Figure 12.2.6-3). The anesthetic is carefully injected to avoid the circumferential vein and/or the sinus of the teat or gland. The regional block does not interfere with wound healing, and analgesia is adequate for all teat procedures described in this chapter except for proximal lacerations that involve the gland

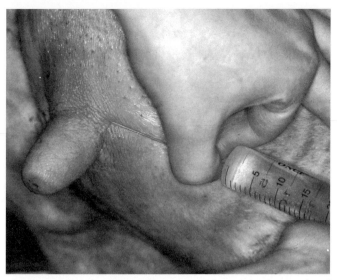

Figure 12.2.6-3 Circumferential injection of 20 ml of lidocaine hydrochloride at the base of the teat for local analgesia.

tissue, where additional local infiltration may be necessary. General anesthesia is not typically necessary for teat surgery. The surgical field is prepared and draped according to aseptic surgery procedures. If the pathology location allows it to be done, a metal tourniquet (teat clamp) is positioned at the base of the teat to reduce intraoperative hemorrhage and prevent milk outflow during the surgical intervention.

Pathologies

Teat pathologies that require surgical intervention include: supernumerary and conjoined teats, pathologies characterized by reduced milk flow, lacerations, and fistulae. Within the *pathologies characterized by reduced milk flow*, congenital obstructions, obstructions uncommonly observed before first milking, and pathologies acquired during lactation or dry period will be discussed.

SUPERNUMERARY TEATS

Supernumerary teats may be surgically removed for the following reasons: interference with milking, increased risk of mastitis, and cosmetics. Because supernumerary teats carry a heritability factor (h^2) of 0.2 to 0.3, some breeding associations do not allow "hidden" removal of these teats. The appropriate technique of teat removal depends on the age of the animal. At 3 to 6 months of age, teats are usually large enough for the veterinarian to distinguish primary teats from supernumerary teats. At this age, supernumerary teats are simply removed with a pair of scissors. The cut is oriented in a craniocaudal direction so the resultant scar blends with the normal folds of the udder. Because of the tendency for increased bleeding at an older age, supernumerary teats in animals older than 6 months are removed with an emasculator. Supernumerary teats removed during the last months of gestation or during lactation require more extensive surgical intervention. The teat is dissected with an elliptical incision performed in the craniocaudal direction at the base, allowing visualization of the mucosa of the accessory gland. Technique of wound closure and type of suture material are similar to those described in the corresponding section of teat amputation. Any evidence of mastitis should be treated aggressively before surgery. Whether removal of supernumerary teats requires local analgesia is determined independent of the animal's age.

CONJOINED TEATS

A conjoined teat (or webbed teat) is defined as a supernumerary teat attached to the side of a primary teat (Figure 12.2.6-4). Conjoined teats do have accessory glands of various volumes. Depending on the degree of fusion, the conjoined teat may be identified as a bulge at the proximal aspect of the primary teat or merely as an extra teat orifice at its side. The latter condition has to be differentiated from the teat fistula described in a separate section that represents a connection to the primary teat. Injecting 20 ml of methylene blue dye into the orifice to stain the milk, or ultrasonography may assist in differentiating a suspected conjoined teat (Figure 12.2.6-5). Surgery is indicated because the conjoined teat's interference with milking and increased incidence of mastitis in the accessory gland represents a permanent risk of infection for the primary gland. The accessory gland's incomplete emptying, chronic trauma to the teat orifice during milking, and insufficient development and

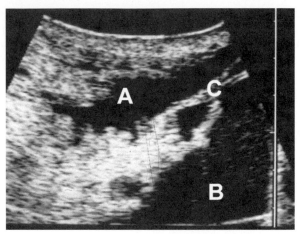

Figure 12.2.6-5   Longitudinal ultrasonographic view of a conjoined teat in a cow. Left, proximal; *A*, sinus of the conjoined gland; *B*, sinus of the primary gland; *C*, septum between primary and conjoined teat sinus.

function of the streak canal and teat sphincter cause the increased incidences of mastitis.

The glandular tissue of the accessory teat usually produces little milk. Therefore surgical intervention mostly consists of resecting the bulging tissue and closing the accessory gland. Elliptical dissection, directed parallel to the long axis of the primary teat, is performed around the contours of the supernumerary teat. The shape of the normal contralateral teat is used as a model. The conjoined teat is carefully dissected to the level of the annular ring to isolate the sinus of the accessory teat. Inadvertent opening of the primary teat sinus should be avoided. A side-opening cannula may be introduced into the accessory teat orifice to aid in the dissection. The accessory tissue is transected at the junction between teat and gland sinus. The wound is closed as described for perforating teat lacerations. Prognosis for undisturbed milking of the primary gland is favorable.

The cisterns of the primary and accessory teats may be connected in those rare cases where the accessory gland has significant milk production. The surgical approach is similar to the one described for resecting the conjoined teat. After the cistern of the accessory teat is opened, a 2 to 3 cm long longitudinal incision is made, with care taken not to sever the circular veins between the accessory and primary cisterns at the level of the annular ring. Wound closure follows the guidelines described for perforating teat lacerations. The respective mucosa wound margins are apposed by using a simple continuous suture pattern. Prognosis for permanent success of this procedure is favorable. The main complications include mastitis development, slow milking, blood clots occluding milk flow, and excessive granulation tissue formation occluding the surgically created

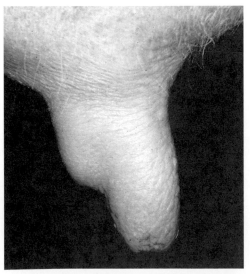

Figure 12.2.6-4   Conjoined teat in a lactating dairy cow.

communication. The heritability of webbed teats is a concern that should be communicated to the owner before surgery.

PATHOLOGIES CHARACTERIZED BY REDUCED MILK FLOW

Reduced or lack of milk flow represent economically important complaints associated with teat problems. Economic losses can be attributed to increased milking time, concurrently increased somatic cell count, treatment costs, discarded milk, clinical and subclinical mastitis, and culling of cows. Reduced milk flow may be caused by various congenital and acquired obstructions, including agenesia, tissue proliferation, and milk stones. A thorough clinical and ultrasonographic examination of the affected teat and mammary gland is indicated because any of the pathologies may require considerably different therapeutic procedures and prognoses. Obstructions not recognized before the first milking commonly are considered congenital. However, many of these obstructions are not congenital, but result from trauma or infection that occurs before first milking.

(Partial) Agenesis of the Streak Canal

Partial agenesis represents incomplete canalization of the streak canal. Considerable variation of incomplete canalization does exist, with the extremes being an imperforate skin membrane at the end of the streak canal and complete agenesis of the streak canal. A bulge may be observed over the area of the teat orifice when milk is squeezed towards the streak canal in a case with an imperforate skin membrane. The skin membrane is opened by using a #11 scalpel blade or a 14-gauge needle. For several days before each milking, the apex of the teat is rolled between thumb and finger. This breaks down fibrinous adhesions and helps open the streak canal. After each milking, a melting teat stent that consists of povidone-iodine in wax is introduced into the streak canal for 5 consecutive days to keep it patent until healing occurs. The prognosis is usually favorable. Lateral theloscopic examination (see Theloscopy) helps determine the degree of agenesis if incomplete canalization involves more than just the distal end. If the rosette of Furstenberg is not developed, prognosis is poor. If the rosette of Furstenberg and the proximal third of the streak canal are developed, a cutting obturator under visual control is used to perforate the skin and connect the teats outside with the canalized aspect of the teat canal. The obturator is replaced by a permanent teat cannula that is sutured to the teat and left in place for 10 days. During this period, milk is passively drained through the cannula once daily. Complications include mastitis, milk incontinence, and hard milking. Long-

term prognosis for undisturbed milk flow after this procedure is fair to good.

Tight Streak Canal

Tight streak canal is usually acquired as a consequence of a self-inflicted injury to the apex of the teat. The cow may crush her teat between its claw and the floor when trying to rise. Chronic trauma as a result of poor function of the milking machine, such as excessive vacuum formation, is considered the second major cause of a tight streak canal. Clinical signs include inflammation at the teat apex, pain elicited by the vacuum, and severely decreased milk flow, which leads to increased milking time. This type of lesion is often self-perpetuating. The traditional owner treatment is to use teat dilators to stretch the streak canal and teat sphincter. Unfortunately, this treatment regimen is often unsuccessful and predisposes the animal to complications such as mastitis and trauma to the teat sinus mucosa. Ideally, the crushed teat is allowed to heal without adding further trauma. The affected teat should not be milked for 7 to 10 days after injury, but milk should be passively drained every second day with a blunt side-opening teat catheter. Hand milking and routine machine milking determines whether milk flow is still reduced. The sphincter is cut with a Hug knife if milk flow is still reduced and ultrasonographic evaluation rules out involvement of a tissue flap in the area of the rosette of Furstenberg. Surgery is best performed before the morning milking to allow proper aftercare during the day. Oxytocin (20 IU) is administered intravenously, the teat is surgically prepared, the streak canal anesthetized with lidocaine hydrochloride, and the Hug knife introduced through the streak canal. The knife is gently pulled out at a 30- to 45-degree angle so only the area of the rosette of Furstenberg (i.e., the teat sphincter and proximal aspect of the streak canal) is cut, but the distal aspect of the streak canal is not severed (Figure 12.2.6-6). Milk flow is assessed by forced hand milking and compared to the contralateral teat. The teat sphincter is cut a second time 180 degrees from the first cut and then repeated each 90 degrees. Milk flow is evaluated after each cut. A fine stream of milk that passively flows out of the teat for at least 30 seconds after cutting indicates sufficient surgical intervention. Aftercare consists of routine morning milking and forceful hand milking of several streams of milk every 1 to 2 hours until afternoon milking. After each routine machine milking, a melting teat stent of povidone-iodine in wax is introduced into the streak canal for 5 consecutive days to keep it patent until healing has occurred. Complications include episodes of acute mastitis, milk incontinence, and recurrence of hard milking. Long-term prognosis for undisturbed milk flow after this procedure is good as long as any inflammation

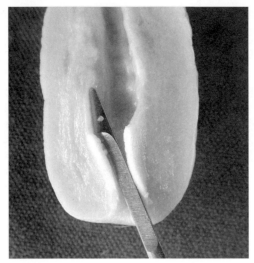

Figure 12.2.6-6   Hug knife introduced into the streak canal at a 30-degree angle.

is allowed to resolve before cutting and stiff traumatic teat dilators are not used during aftercare.

Obstruction in the Area of the Rosette of Furstenberg

This is among the most common causes of reduced milk flow in dairy cows. Similar to the tight streak canal, obstruction in the area of the rosette of Furstenberg is usually acquired as a consequence of a self-inflicted injury to the teat apex. Although the integrity of the skin is preserved, one or more tissue flaps may originate from the proximal aspect of the streak canal and prolapse into the

teat sinus similar to a valve that intermittently interferes with milking. The affected teat should not be milked for 7 to 10 days immediately after the injury, but milk should be passively drained every second day with a blunt side-opening teat catheter. Thereafter, hand milking and routine machine milking determines milk flow. If milk flow is still intermittently reduced, involvement of a tissue flap in the area of the rosette of Furstenberg must be considered. It is diagnosed with the aid of the teat probe and/or ultrasonography (Figure 12.2.6-7). The tissue flap may be removed by blind excision through the streak canal or under visual control during a thelotomy or theloscopy. The latter techniques are described in separate sections. During the postoperative period, milk is drained passively, and the streak canal is kept patent by the daily introduction of a melting teat stent made from povidone-iodine in wax. Stiff teat dilators should not be used for this purpose because doing so may cause severe trauma to the mucous membrane of the teat sinus, as has been described. If milk flow has not returned to normal by the fourth machine milking after surgical removal of the tissue flap(s), the concurrent presence of a tight streak canal must be considered and treated as described for this condition. Prognosis is superior if the flap(s) is removed under direct visual control as compared to blind excision, which is not recommended. Long-term prognosis for return to undisturbed milking is similar with a thelotomy or theloscopy. However, fewer cows treated by theloscopy require the teat sphincter to be cut postoperatively or suffer from episodes of mastitis, and aftercare is less intensive. Therefore minimally invasive theloscopy to remove tissue flaps in the area of the rosette of Furstenberg is preferred.

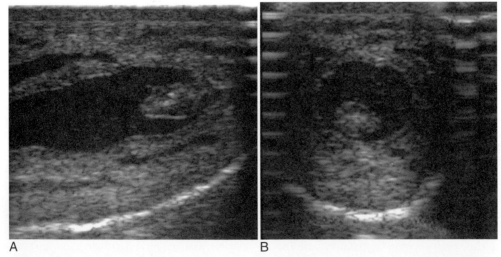

A   B

Figure 12.2.6-7   Longitudinal (A, left, proximal) and horizontal (B) ultrasonographic views of an obstruction in the area of the rosette of Furstenberg in a cow.

Milk Stones

These represent floating calculi that are either completely free or attached to the teat mucosa by a pedunculated stalk. Multiple stones may occur and mechanically interfere with milk flow when forced towards the streak canal during milking. Manual palpation or ultrasonography is used to diagnose milk stones, and forced hand milking usually ejects small stones. A stone that is attached or too large to be milked out is removed or crushed intracisternally with a small alligator forceps introduced through the streak canal. For this procedure, prophylactic intramammary application of an antimicrobial, adequate restraint, local analgesia, and strict aseptic manipulation are recommended. The author has observed recurrence of milk stones.

Obstructions in the Area of the Teat Cistern and/or the Annular Ring

Obstructions in the area of the teat cistern and/or the annular ring are acquired and rarely congenital, although they are not commonly recognized before first milking. Causes of acquired obstructions include acute trauma, chronic trauma from being sucked by herd mates, and unnoticed mastitis during the dry period, which may be spread by flies. Congenital obstructions may result in persistent intraluminal membranes or agenesis of the teat sinus. If mammary secretions cannot be obtained from a primiparous heifer, the quarter must be evaluated for dysgenesis. Obstructions of the teat sinus with less than 30% of the mucosal surface affected are classified as type I lesions (Figure 12.2.6-8), and type II lesions have more than 30% of the mucosal surface affected (Figure 12.2.6-9). Obstructions in the area between the teat and mammary gland sinus are considered type III lesions,

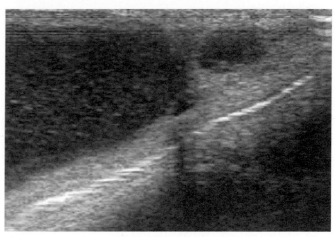

Figure 12.2.6-8   Longitudinal ultrasonographic views of a type I teat lesion in a cow (left, proximal).

and type IV lesions extend from the teat sinus to the gland sinus. Ultrasonographic examination is used to differentiate the four lesion types (see Figures 12.2.6-8 and 12.2.6-9). Surgical techniques currently used to restore patency of the sinus include removal of obstructive tissue by introducing a cutting instrument or cryosurgical probe through the streak canal into the teat sinus and thelotomy with the obstructing tissue excised under direct visual control. After removal during thelotomy, the adjacent mucosa is undermined, and the margins of the mucosa are carefully apposed using a # 4-0 monofilament absorbable suture material. An implant or transplant is considered if insufficient tissue is available to adapt the wound margins. The very loosely attached mucosa and rich tissue blood supply make the

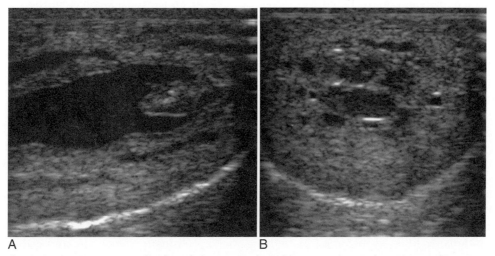

A   B

Figure 12.2.6-9   Longitudinal (A, left, proximal) and horizontal (B) ultrasonographic views of a type II teat lesion in a cow.

teat sinus very prone to granulation tissue formation. Therefore resecting the obstructing tissue through the streak canal is not recommended. New formation of granulation tissue causes the initially good milk flow to decrease and eventually cease within a period of days to a few weeks. A mucosa defect too large to be primarily closed after the obstructing tissue is removed may be covered by transplanting a mucosal graft, implanting a reinforced polytetrafluoroethylene vascular graft, or introducing a silastic tube. However, the long-term success rate for these techniques is guarded to poor. Complications include recurrence of obstruction, implant migration into the gland sinus, implant collapse, increased milking time, implant infection and mastitis. Prognosis of type I and III lesions is good if the defect can be completely covered with mucosal tissue.

Fibrosis of the Gland Sinus

This is characterized by connective tissue replacing normal gland tissue. This can be the results of a congenital disease, or it can occur after infection of the gland sinus before first lactation or during the dry period. Fibrosis is suspected if milk flow at first milking is minimal and palpating the affected mammary gland reveals diffuse induration. Ultrasonographic examination confirms the diagnosis and reveals that fibrous tissue has replaced the secretory tissue, lactiferous ducts, and gland sinus. Currently, no surgical procedure exists to correct this problem. The prognosis for return to milk production is hopeless.

OPEN TEAT LACERATIONS

Teat lacerations can be open lacerations or have skin integrity preserved. Open lacerations are classified as partial or full thickness lacerations that perforate into the streak canal, teat sinus, or gland sinus. Open teat lacerations should be evaluated carefully to determine the prognosis for return of milk flow and normal somatic cell count and the type of surgical reconstruction to initiate. Prognosis depends on various criteria, such as location, size and direction of the laceration, degree of tissue loss, involvement of the streak canal, presence of mastitis and udder edema, age of laceration, and degree of contamination. Longitudinal lacerations heal better than horizontal lacerations because blood flows from the base towards the apex of the teat. Because perfusion is superior at the base of the teat, proximal lacerations heal better than distal lacerations. Partial thickness lacerations at the apex of the teat with the base of the tissue flap located distally may have a poorer prognosis than some full-thickness lacerations perforating into the teat sinus. Streak canal or gland sinus anatomic repair is difficult, which makes the prognosis worse when they are involved. Because the teat generally has good perfusion, age of the laceration is not of primary concern. In our experience, primary repair may be successful for up to 12 hours after the laceration occurred. In older cases, delayed primary closure is recommended.

Surgical Correction of Teat Lacerations

If primary repair is initiated, the cow should be restrained in lateral or dorsal recumbency, the teat anesthetized, and reconstruction performed under aseptic conditions. The wound margins are carefully debrided and rinsed with physiologic saline solution. Any necrotic, contaminated, or infected tissue must be removed. Very little "extra" tissue is available in the teats; therefore preserving as much normal tissue as possible is important. In full-thickness lacerations, a three-layer closure that involves the submucosa, intermediate layer, and skin is appropriate. The submucosa and intermediate layer are apposed separately with a continuous horizontal mattress suture that does not perforate the mucosa using #4-0 monofilament synthetic resorbable suture material with a taper point swaged-on needle. The skin is closed with simple interrupted sutures by using #3-0 or 4-0 monofilament suture material with a reverse cutting swaged-on needle. Partial thickness lacerations are sutured in a similar fashion, but the innermost suture of the submucosa is omitted. Postoperative management includes passive milk drainage every second day and administration of intramammary antimicrobials every 4 days for 10 days. Systemic administration of antimicrobials is rarely indicated. The overall prognosis of teat lacerations that involve the teat sinus is favorable. Complications include partial or total wound dehiscence, necrosis of tissue flaps, fistula formation (Figure 12.2.6-10), impaired milk flow, increased somatic cell count, and episodes of acute mastitis.

If the streak canal is affected, the wound is debrided as described; several simple interrupted sutures are placed in the intermediate layer close to the streak canal; a permanent teat catheter is introduced into the streak canal; and the sutures are tightened and knotted. The skin is closed with simple interrupted sutures. The teat catheter is left in place for 10 days to keep the streak canal patent until healing has occurred. In general, the prognosis for lacerations that involve the streak canal to return to normal milk flow is markedly less favorable in comparison to lacerations that involve the teat sinus.

If reconstruction of a teat laceration is not possible, the teat may be amputated as a salvage procedure. Delayed primary wound healing should be attempted when primary closure and amputation do not represent viable options for repair. Be aware that teat fistula formation is expected in up to 75% of the cases that use secondary healing of full thickness lacerations.

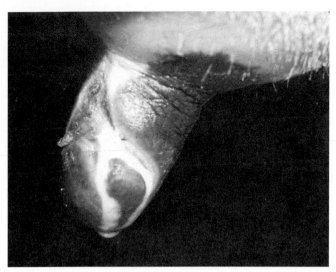

Figure 12.2.6-10 Healed laceration that resulted in the formation of a teat fistula.

(Courtesy of Dr. Norm G. Ducharme; Cornell University.)

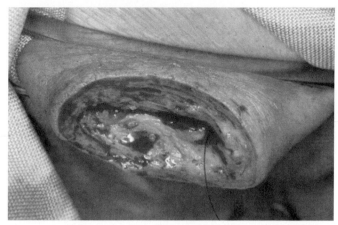

Figure 12.2.6-11 Intraoperative view of the teat stump after amputation of the teat and before suturing is initiated.

TEAT FISTULA

The teat fistula is an accessory opening on the teat that communicates with the primary teat sinus or streak canal. It does not possess a separate streak canal or teat sphincter. It can be congenital but usually results from a full thickness teat laceration and occurs as a complication of secondary wound healing or dehiscence after primary healing. Methylene blue dye injected through a fistula appears in the milk of the main teat. A teat fistula wound should be allowed to granulate until swelling and infection subside and the fistula is well delineated before surgical repair is initiated. The cow is restrained in lateral recumbency with the teat anesthetized, prepared, and draped for aseptic surgery. A longitudinally oriented elliptical full thickness specimen of teat wall centered over the fistulous tract is excised to expose unscarred teat wall. The teat wall is closed as described for full thickness teat lacerations. The prognosis for return to normal milk flow is favorable.

Surgical Interventions

Restraint, anesthesia, and preparation of the surgical field have been described in a separate section and apply to this chapter, unless specified otherwise. Specific surgical teat interventions routinely used in cattle include teat amputation, thelotomy, and theloscopy.

TEAT AMPUTATION

This procedure is performed when teat damage caused by severe trauma is irreversible. Any mastitis present in the corresponding quarter must be treated before surgery. Prophylactic intramammary injections of antimicrobials and milk drainage are performed immediately before amputation. If the laceration does not involve the teat base, a teat clamp is positioned in the area of the annular ring, and the teat is routinely amputated. An elliptical skin incision in the sagittal plane is made around the teat at the junction of the proximal and middle thirds. The teat wall is sharply dissected in a slightly proximal direction and transected, thus creating a fish mouth–like teat stump (Figure 12.2.6-11). Bleeding vessels are ligated separately. With the clamp still in position, the submucosa and intermediate layers are tightly apposed with one nonperforating continuous horizontal mattress suture each and #4-0 monofilament synthetic resorbable suture material with a taper point swaged-on needle. The skin is closed with interrupted sutures accordingly by using #3-0 or 4-0 monofilament suture material with a reverse cutting swaged-on needle. If the laceration does involve the teat base, the amputation is performed just distal to the annular ring. A skin flap attached to the base must be preserved. The wound is curetted and rinsed, margins debrided, and submucosa and intermediate layers routinely sutured. The skin flap is used to cover the defect, which is closed with simple interrupted sutures.

If the corresponding mammary gland did not have mastitis before surgery, prognosis of teat amputation is favorable. The quarter will secrete milk until pressure atrophy of the alveolar tissue occurs and dries up the quarter. The remaining three quarters will produce considerably more than 75% of the previous milk yield because blood flow will bypass the dried up quarter for the secreting quarters.

THELOTOMY

After routine local analgesia, aseptic preparation, and draping of the surgical field, a 3- to 4-cm longitudinal

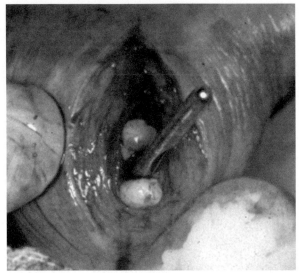

Figure 12.2.6-12   Intraoperative view of obstructive tissue in the area of the rosette of Furstenberg visualized during lateral thelotomy in a cow.

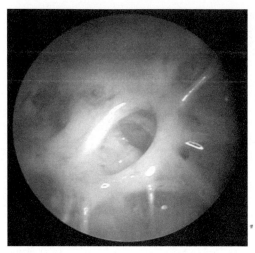

Figure 12.2.6-13   Theloscopic view of a type I lesion situated in the distal third of the teat sinus. The theloscope is introduced through the streak canal into the teat sinus.

incision (depending on the length of the teat) through the skin and intermediate layers is made on the lateral aspect of the teat. A blunt metal probe is introduced through the streak canal into the teat sinus to protect the mucosa of the medial teat wall from inadvertent laceration while the mucosa is being carefully transected with a scalpel blade. The rosette of Furstenberg is exposed and closely inspected (Figure 12.2.6-12), and the obstructing tissue is carefully excised with a pair of fine scissors. The submucosa and the intermediate layer are apposed with one continuous horizontal suture pattern with a size #4-0 monofilament synthetic resorbable suture material with a taper point swaged-on needle. The skin is closed with simple interrupted sutures with #3-0 or 4-0 monofilament suture material with a reverse cutting swaged-on needle. Postoperative management is routine. Formation of scar tissue that reduces milk flow—thus necessitating cutting of the teat sphincter—is the most common complication. A retrospective analysis found that 73% of cows had the streak canal cut during the first week after obstructive tissue in the area of the rosette of Furstenberg was removed during thelotomy. Milk flow returned to normal during the lactation surgery was performed and remained normal during a second lactation in 68% of the cows.

THELOSCOPY

Theloscopy is a diagnostic and surgical procedure (Figure 12.2.6-13) that has replaced thelotomy for removing obstructive tissues in the area of the rosette of Furstenberg under visual control when equipment is available. Theloscopic triangulation or theloresectoscopy with a working endoscope determines the obstruction location. Endoscopy is first performed through the streak canal with an endoscope with an outer diameter less than or equal to 3 mm. The endoscope is introduced into the teat sinus, which is insufflated to a maximum pressure of 200 millibar. The endoscope is then slowly pulled back the mucosa of the teat sinus, the area of the rosette of Furstenberg, and streak canal are inspected closely for superficial lesions and obstructive tissue. If a working endoscope with an outer diameter exceeding 3 mm (theloresectoscope) is used, this inspection is omitted to avoid excessive trauma to the streak canal. For lateral endoscopy, a blunt side-opening teat catheter is introduced through the streak canal, and air is passed through this catheter to insufflate the teat sinus. A perforating stab incision is made in the lateral wall of the teat 10 mm distal to the teat clamp with a #10 scalpel blade. A sleeve and endoscope are introduced through this instrument portal, and the teat sinus is insufflated through the sleeve. The side-opening teat catheter is replaced by a blunt probe. The obstructive tissue in the area of the rosette of Furstenberg is visually examined with the endoscope and manipulated with the probe to determine its size and shape of attachment to healthy tissue. The obstructive tissue is excised and removed using the cautery sling of the working endoscope. If the triangulation technique is used, a pair of endoscopic scissors is introduced into the teat sinus through a separate instrument portal created in the cranial or caudal aspect of the teat approximately 5 mm proximal to the rosette of

Furstenberg. Obstructing tissue is excised with the scissors and removed through the instrumental portal with a pair of endoscopic tissue forceps. After removal of the instruments, the intermediate layer in the area of the portal(s) is closed with size #4-0 monofilament synthetic resorbable suture material and a taper-point swaged-on needle by using one simple vertical adapting suture. Skin incisions are closed by using #3-0 or 4-0 monofilament suture material with a reverse cutting swaged-on needle in a horizontal mattress pattern. Main complications include episodes of acute mastitis and formation of scar tissue that reduces milk flow, thus necessitating cutting the teat sphincter. A retrospective study revealed that milk flow returned to normal during the lactation surgery was performed in 65% and was judged normal during a second lactation in 76% of the cows treated by theloscopic removal of obstructive tissue in the area of the rosette of Furstenberg. Cutting the streak canal after surgery was performed in only 15% of the cows. This was significantly less common than after thelotomy. The rate of complications after theloscopic excision was significantly lower and aftercare less expensive in comparisons to thelotomy removal.

Implantation of Teat Prosthesis (Editors' Addendum)

Teat prostheses have been described for many types of teat obstruction, but they have a high complication rate. They are most successful if used in type I or II teat sinus obstructions in which normal mucosa proximal and distal to the lesion allows the implant to bridge the mucosal defect. When used in other types of teat obstruction, the procedure offers a guarded to poor long-term prognosis for return to normal milk flow.

A thelotomy, as described previously, is performed opposite the lesion to be resected. After careful excision of the obstructive lesion, one needs to determine whether the adjacent mucosa can be slid over the defect. If the lesion's bed can be covered by mucosa, an implant should not be used. If the mucosal defect cannot be covered and the lesion is limited to the teat sinus with normal mucosa proximal and distal to the lesion, an implant is indicated. The morbidity of the procedure— coupled with the milk production potential of three quarters—dictates careful selection of the patient. The implant consists of sterile silastic tubing (7 mm ID, 10 mm OD) without any fenestration. A blunt teat cannula is placed through the streak canal, and the implant placed over the cannula so it rests near the rosette of Furstenberg. The implant is then placed in the teat sinus and the length of the prosthesis selected; the prosthesis must span the teat sinus without entering the gland cistern. The prosthesis is then cut with scissors and replaced in the teat sinus. The implant is secured in place with three

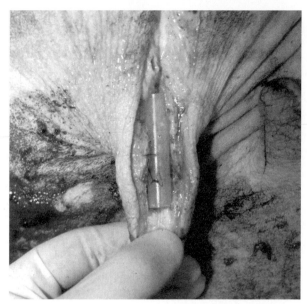

Figure 12.2.6-14 *Post mortem* specimen that indicates position of teat implant. Note the position of retaining sutures and the proximity of the streak canal to the implant.

(Courtesy of Dr. Norm Ducharme; Cornell University.)

vertical equidistant sutures by using nonabsorbable polypropylene 2-0 suture on a cutting needle (Figure 12.2.6-14). These three sutures are placed so that the tubing is pulled distally to rest against the rosette of Furstenberg when they are tightened. The specific bites are placed as follows: the first bite of the suture in the center of the thelotomy incision is placed from proximal to distal into the full thickness of the silastic tubing at the midpoint of the implant. The second bite is placed in the wall of the teat, starting 3 to 4 mm distal to the exit point of the suture in the implant. This suture must be anchored deep in the wall of the teat so the surgeon can feel the needle passing immediately subcutaneously. The suture then exits again a few mm distal to the distal exit point of the suture in the implant. When the suture is tied, the implant is rotated into place. Offsetting the sutures ensures that the implant stays against the proximal aspect of the streak canal (Figure 12.2.6-15). A second suture on the cranial wall of the teat sinus and a third at the caudal wall of the teat sinus are placed similarly. The thelotomy is closed as described earlier.

Postoperative Management

Excluding prosthesis implantation, routine postoperative management includes passive milk drainage for 10 days, except theloscopy requires only 3 days. Frequency of passive milk drainage depends on daily milk yield of the cow and may vary from once a day to every third day.

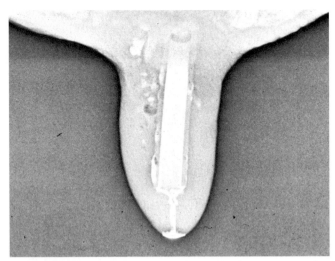

Figure 12.2.6-15 Lateral xeroradiograph of a cow's teat after placement of a teat implant. Note that the implant does not extend into the gland sinus and is directly over the streak canal.

(Courtesy of Dr. Norm Ducharme; Cornell University.)

For this purpose, intermittent introduction of a side-opening metal teat catheter is preferred to temporary implantation of a silastic catheter except for teat lacerations involving the streak canal. Temporary implantation of stiff teat dilators and catheters for several days caused lacerations to the teat sinus mucosa and submucosa. Daily introduction of a melting teat stent into the streak canal for 10 days is indicated to keep the streak canal patent and reduce the formation of scar tissue after dissecting obstructing tissue in the area of the rosette of Furstenberg. Intramammary administration of a broad-spectrum antimicrobial drug as a prophylactic measure against mastitis is performed every four days until 10 days after surgery. Too-frequent intramammary administration of antimicrobials favors growth of fungi. Systemic administration of antimicrobials is indicated in cases of acute mastitis only. Sutures are removed and machine milking resumed on day 11 after surgery. After theloscopy, routine machine milking is resumed by day 4 after surgery. If milk flow has not returned to normal at the fourth milking session, clinical reevaluation of the teat is performed. Cutting the teat sphincter may be indicated if excessive scar tissue has formed in the area of the streak canal.

After placement of a teat implant, the cow is machine-milked in the postoperative period, starting the first day after surgery. Animals that have implants can only be milked by machine or after a teat cannula is inserted. The latter is not recommended because of the risk of ascending infection and the possibility of implant displacement if forceful placement of the teat cannula is necessary.

Complications

The main complications after teat surgery include occurrence of acute mastitis, increased somatic cell count, reduced milk flow, and wound dehiscence. Frequency of episodes of acute mastitis in the postoperative period is markedly reduced if passive milk drainage is performed under aseptic conditions. Somatic cell count depends on the severity of the trauma to the teat and the occurrence of ascending infection in the quarter. Atraumatic surgical technique may help keep somatic cell count low. If reduced milk flow at the fourth session of routine machine milking is evident, thorough examination of the teat is indicated. Slow milking should be avoided because prolonged milking time leads to additional trauma to the teat and decreases milk flow. This development is self-perpetuating. The likelihood of wound dehiscence depends on the degree of wound contamination, age of the teat laceration, and degree of interference of blood supply to the wound. Presence of excessive udder edema markedly interferes with primary healing of teat wounds and is an additional important reason for wound dehiscence. If an implant has been placed, the implant has a tendency to become displaced at 6 to 8 weeks after surgery. This may be of no clinical significance. In some cows, the displaced prosthesis may float into the gland sinus and obstruct milk flow from the gland to the teat sinus. Another complication related to implants is fragmentation of the implant.

RECOMMENDED READINGS

Adams SB, Amstutz HE, Boehm PN: Bovine mammoscopy: a new method for evaluating and treating teat obstructions, *Annual Convention of the AABP*, 1986.

Bristol DG: Treatment of teat obstruction in a cow by transfer of oral mucosa and temporary implantation of an intraluminal tube, *J Am Vet Med Assoc* 195: 492-494, 1989.

Ducharme NG, Arighi M, Horney D, et al: Invasive teat surgery in dairy cattle, I: surgical procedures and classification of lesions, *Can Vet J* 28: 757-762, 1987.

Grymer J, Watson W, Coy C et al: Healing of experimentally induced wounds of mammary papilla (teat) of the cow: comparison of closure with tissue adhesive versus nonsutured wounds, *Am J Vet Res* 45: 1979-1983, 1984.

Hirsbrunner G, Eicher R, Meylan M, et al: Comparison of thelotomy and theloscopic triangulation for the treatment of distal teat obstructions in dairy cows: a retrospective study (1994-1998), *Vet Rec* 148: 803-805, 2001.

Hirsbrunner G, Metzger L, Steiner A: Implantation of a reinforced polytetrafluoroethylene vascular graft for treatment of obstructions of the teat and mammary gland cisternae in cattle, *J Am Vet Med Assoc* 212: 1432-1435, 1998.

Hirsbrunner G, Steiner A: Use of a theloscopic triangulation technique for endoscopic treatment of teat obstructions in cows, *J Am Vet Med Assoc* 214: 1668-1671, 1999.

Johansson I: Untersuchungen über die Variation in der Euter: und Strichform der Kühe, *Züchtungsbiol* 70: 233-270, 1957.

Makady F, Whitmore H, Nelson D et al: Effect of tissue adhesives and suture patterns on experimentally induced teat lacerations in lactating dairy cattle, *J Am Vet Med Assoc* 198: 1932-1934, 1991.

Medl M, Querengässer K, Wagner C et al: Zur Abklärung und Behandlung von Zitzenstenosen mittels Endoskopie, *Tierärztl Prax* 22: 532-537, 1994.

Metzger L, Hirsbrunner G, Waldvogel A et al: Permanent implantation of a reinforced polytetrafluoroethylene vascular graft for traetment of artificial defects of the teat cistern mucosa, *Am J Vet Res* 60: 56-62, 1999.

Rüsch P, Witzig P, Waxenberger M et al: Zur operativen Behandlung von Zitzenkuppenverletzungen mit Durchtrennung des Strichkanals, *Dtsch Tierärztl Wschr* 96: 381-387, 1983.

Schmit KA, Arighi M, Dobson H: Postoperative evaluation of the surgical treatment of accessory teat and gland cistern complexes in dairy cows, *Can Vet J* 34: 25-30, 1994.

Seeh C, Hospes R: Erfahrungen mit einem Theloresektoskop im Vergleich zur konventionellen Zitzenendoskopie bei der Diagnose und Therapie gedeckter Zitzenverletzungen, *Tierärztl Prax* 26: 110-118, 1998.

Seeh C, Stengel KH, Schlenstedt R et al: Endoskopische Prüfung der Schleimhautverträglichkeit eines neuartigen Strichkanalstabes im Vergleich zu konventionellen Zitzenstiften und einer Verweilkanüle, *Tierärztl Prax* 25: 329-335, 1997.

Stocker H, Bättig U, Duss M, et al: Die Abklärung von Zitzenstenosen beim Rind mittels Ultraschall, *Tierärztl Prax* 17: 251-256, 1989.

Trent AM, Smith DF, Cooley AJ et al: Use of mucosal grafts and temporary tube implants for treatment of teat sinus mucosal injuries, *Am J Vet Res* 51: 666-676, 1990.

Trostle SS, O'Brien RT: Ultrasonography of the bovine mammary gland, *Compend Cont Educ Pract Vet* 20: S64-S71, 1998.

Wigger J, Martig J: Verlaufsuntersuchungen nach operativer Behandlung von Zitzenverletzungen beim Rind, *Dtsch Tierärztl Wschr* 92: 247-251, 1985.

Witzig P, Rüsch P, Berchtold M: Diagnosis and treatment of teat stenoses in dairy cattle with special reference to radiography and thelotomy, *Vet Med Rev* 2: 122-132, 1989.

12.3.1—Surgery of the Kidney

Susan L. Fubini

Anatomy

The bovine kidney is large, with distinct renal lobes (Figure 12.3.1-1). The lateral border is convex. The vasculature, nerves, and ureters pass through a hilus on its concave medial border. The kidneys are enveloped in a fibrous capsule surrounded by peritoneal fat. They are contained within the abdominal cavity but are retroperitoneal. The right kidney is enough further forward that it contacts the liver with its cranial pole. It lies just right of midline ventral to the hypaxial musculature, last rib, and first few lumbar vertebrae. The left kidney is further caudad, behind the root of the mesentery. Its position is just right of midline, depending on how much the rumen

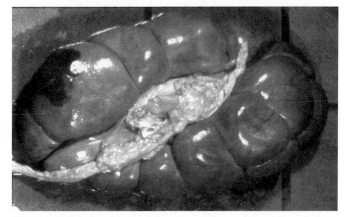

Figure 12.3.1-1 Normal bovine kidney. Note the distinct renal lobes.

(Courtesy of Dr. John King; Cornell University.)

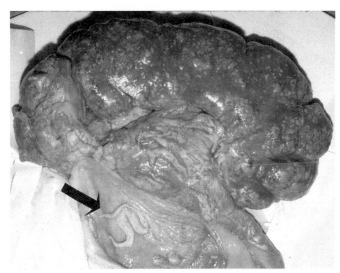

Figure 12.3.1-2 Kidney removed from a cow with pyelonephritis. Note multiple small abscesses in the cortices and pus present in the ureter (arrow).

(Courtesy of Dr. Tom Divers; Cornell University.)

displaces it. Unlike the right kidney, the left kidney is very mobile and easily palpated per rectum. Both kidneys are accessible from the right paralumbar fossa. The left kidney only is accessible from the left paralumbar fossa. Small ruminant renal lobes are fused, thus making the kidneys' external surface appear smooth.

UNILATERAL NEPHRECTOMY

Unilateral nephrectomy is indicated for cattle with unresponsive unilateral pyelonephritis (Figure 12.3.1-2), polycystic kidney (Figure 12.3.1-3) and hydronephrosis, and occasionally indicated for congenital urinary defects

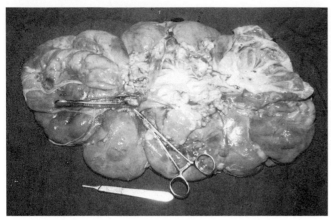

Figure 12.3.1-3   Polycystic kidney. Forceps are outlining the dilated ureter.

(Courtesy of Dr. Tom Divers; Cornell University.)

(i.e., ectopic ureter), neoplasia, abscess formation, and renal lithiasis.

If a unilateral nephrectomy is contemplated, a complete evaluation of the integrity of the remaining kidney is essential. Both kidneys' activity is reflected in laboratory values (creatinine and blood urea nitrogen), although serum elevations are usually not abnormal until 75% of the nephrons are diseased. Ultrasonography and renal biopsy may be indicated to thoroughly evaluate the remaining kidney. Ultrasound examination is performed transabdominally for the right kidney, while the left is best evaluated by rectal probe. Ultrasonographic changes from pyelonephritis include dilation of the renal collecting system; an enlarged kidney with acute disease; or a small, irregular kidney with chronic disease (Figure 12.3.1-4A and B). With urolithiasis, echogenic material

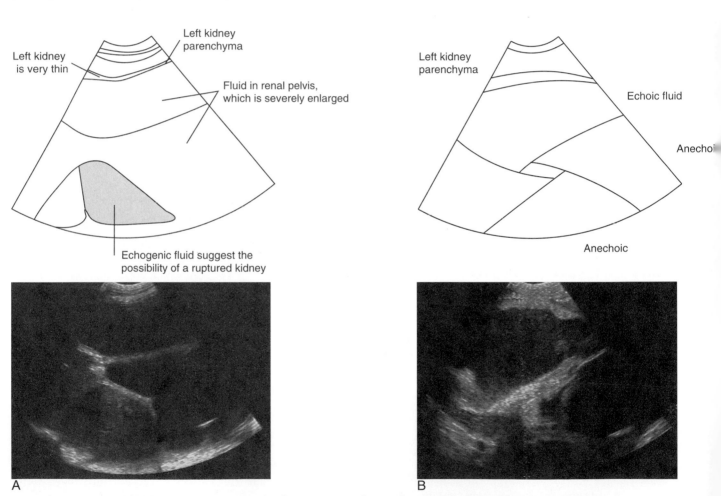

Figure 12.3.1-4   Longitudinal sonograms (schema above) of the left kidney obtained from a 3-year-old Holstein cow with pyohydronephrosis, which was removed surgically. A 4-2 MHz convex probe was used. Both sonograms *(A, B)* show severe renomegaly (greater than 32 × 21 cm) secondary to hydronephrosis. The severely dilated renal pelvis is surrounded by a 1- to 2-cm rim of thin parenchyma or thick capsule. Some of the fluid compartments comprising the dilated renal pelvis are echoic *(B)*. This indicates cellular or high protein fluid, which represents pus in this case.

(Courtesy of Dr. Amy Yeager; Cornell University.)

may be seen within the renal collecting system, and there may be renal enlargement.

Surgery is usually performed in the standing cow, although general anesthesia may facilitate the procedure. Perioperative antibiotics are indicated. Procaine penicillin is an economical choice, and it reaches good concentrations in the urine. Ideally, the cow is restrained in stocks, a chute, or a head gate. The flank is desensitized with regional or local anesthesia. The author prefers not to sedate cattle for standing surgery because of the likelihood they will lay down. Regardless of whether the left or right kidney is affected, a right paralumbar fossa approach is used. A 25- to 30-cm incision is made just caudal and parallel to the last rib to remove the right kidney and a mid-paralumbar fossa to remove the left kidney.

The abdominal oblique and transversus muscle layers are incised sharply. Whenever possible, it is preferable to remove the kidney from the retroperitoneal space, which is easier for the right kidney (Figure 12.3.1-5). It is not uncommon to have a renal abscess (Figure 12.3.1-6) with perirenal adhesions complicate the dissection, thus resulting in inadvertent entry into the peritoneal cavity. Much of the retroperitoneal fat can be removed with blunt dissection. The renal artery, vein, and ureter are individually identified and ligated if possible (Figure 12.3.1-7). Depending on the size of the affected kidney, ligating the renal pedicle may be difficult. Alternatively, the renal vessels and ureter can be identified (Figure 12.3.1-8), securely clamped, transected (Figure 12.3.1-9A and B) and ligated after the kidney has been removed. The vessels and ureter should be double ligated with a nonreactive suture material with good knot security because intraabdominal hemorrhage is the most common complication after surgery. If not performed

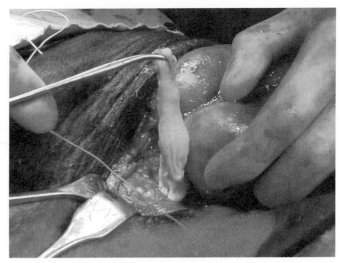

Figure 12.3.1-6 The pyelonephritis has resulted in a perirenal abscess. Purulent material is being removed.

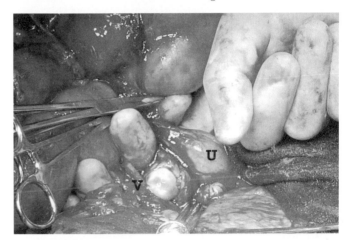

Figure 12.3.1-7 Right flank laparotomy in a cow under general anesthesia. Renal vessels (V) and ureter (U) have been identified.

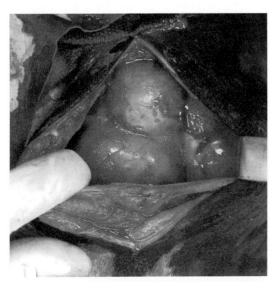

Figure 12.3.1-5 Right kidney (with pyelonephritis) being removed through a right paralumbar fossa incision into the retroperitoneal space in a heifer.

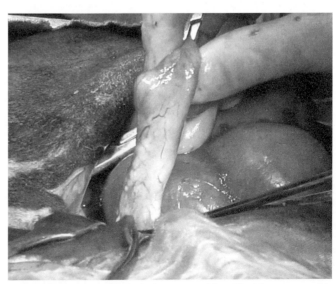

Figure 12.3.1-8 Distended ureter is identified in a cow with pyelonephritis.

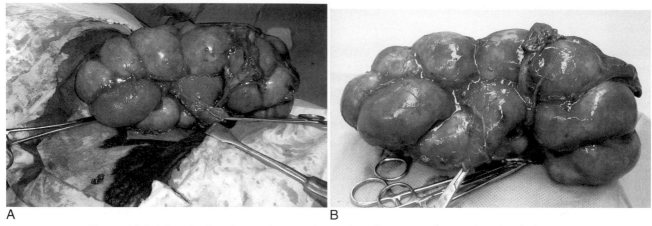

Figure 12.3.1-9 *A,* Renal vessels are clamped and transected. *B,* After the kidney is removed, these structures are ligated.

before surgery, a biopsy of the remaining kidney should be performed before closing the abdomen. If there is a perirenal infection, all (or a portion) of the incision may be left open to allow ventral drainage and granulation of the wound. Some clinicians pack the wound with antiseptic-soaked gauze rolls or towels for a few days after surgery. As the wound granulates, a warm water hose may be used to lavage the wound provided there is no communication with the peritoneal cavity. Owners should be warned these wounds close very slowly, and daily care is required.

The prognosis is favorable if the remaining kidney is viable.

In small ruminants, the surgery is performed in lateral recumbency, typically with the animal under general anesthesia. The kidneys are more mobile, thus making the ligations much easier to accomplish.

RENAL BIOPSY

The left kidney is mobile and easily palpated per rectum, which permits a percutaneous biopsy from either paralumbar fossa. The animal is restrained in a standing stock or chute, and the paralumbar fossa is prepared with appropriate aseptic technique. An epidural anesthetic is useful for a cow that is straining. An assistant palpates the left kidney rectally and positions it against the body wall. The examiner should easily visualize the renal parenchyma with ultrasonography. The biopsy site is chosen, and a bleb of local anesthetic is placed to desensitize the skin. A small, 1-cm incision is made to allow insertion of a Vinn-Silverman* or Tru-Cut biopsy needle.[†] The biopsy needle is thrust into the parenchyma,

---

*J-116V, Vinn-Silverman needle, Jorgensen Laboratories Inc.; Loveland, CO, www.jorvet.com
[†]Tru-Cut, Travenol Inc. (a division of Baxter International); Deerfield, IL, www.baxter.com

avoiding the renal pelvis and vasculature. Once an adequate sample is obtained, it is saved in formalin for histopathology.

The right kidney can usually be visualized well enough ultrasonographically to permit percutaneous biopsy from the cranial right paralumbar fossa. If not, the biopsy can be performed via laparotomy or laparoscopically.

RECOMMENDED READINGS

Fetcher A: Renal diseases in cattle, V: clinical signs, diagnosis, and treatment, *Compend Contin Educ Pract Vet* 817: 5338-5345, 1986.

Hayashi H, Biller D, Rings MD, Miyabayashi T: Ultrasonographic diagnosis of pyelonephritis in a cow, *J Am Vet Med Assoc* 205: 736-738, 1994.

Hooper RN, Taylor TS: Urinary surgery, *Vet Clin North Am Food Anim Pract* 11: 95-121, 1995.

Naoi M, Kokue E, Takahashi Y, Kido Y: Laparoscopic-assisted serial biopsy of the bovine kidney, *Am J Vet Res* 46: 699-702, 1985.

Tulleners EP, Deem DA, Donawick WJ, Whitlock RW: Indications for unilateral bovine nephrectomy: a report of four cases, *J Am Vet Med Assoc* 179: 696-700, 1981.

Wolfe DF, Moll HD: Surgery of the kidney. In Baird AN: *Large animal urogenital surgery*, Philadelphia, 1999, Williams and Wilkins.

12.3.2—Surgery of the Urinary Bladder and Ureters

Susan L. Fubini

Anatomy

The urinary bladder is a muscular organ with a blind apex cranially, the body in the middle, and a neck continuous with the urethra caudally. Remnants of the fetal umbilical arteries give rise to the bladder's round ligaments, which are the thickened portion of the lateral ligaments of the bladder. In the fetus, the apex of the bladder is patent and continuous with the urachus, which empties into the allantoic space. The fetal vessels normally contract during the neonatal period.

The cranial aspect of the urinary bladder has a peritoneal covering; the caudal portion is retroperitoneal. The detrusor muscle is made up of three irregular layers that are continuous with the musculature around the neck of the bladder, which forms the urinary sphincter. As in other species, transitional epithelium lines the bladder. The ureters enter the bladder dorsally at the trigone.

Amputating the urinary bladder apex and manipulating the umbilical vessels' remnants are common procedures performed in umbilical surgery and are discussed in Section 14.3. Isolated reports of urinary bladder and ureter surgery are described in the following discussion.

RUPTURED URINARY BLADDER (ADULT CATTLE)

The most common source of uroperitoneum in cattle is rupture of the bladder secondary to urethral urolithiasis. Steers in feedlot settings are the most commonly affected group, with bulls of all ages less commonly affected. Clinical signs and treatment related to urethral urolithiasis are discussed in Section 18.1. Isolated reports of bladder rupture in heifers and adult cattle that have recently freshened have been made. In young female animals, the presumed cause of bladder rupture is abdominal trauma. In adult females, it is possible the fetus obstructs the pelvic urethra during prolonged dystocia, which leads to eventual compromise of the urinary bladder. Subsequent manipulation of the fetus could result in bladder rupture. Alternatively, the bladder can be trapped under the uterus in the pelvic cavity and be subjected to trauma during parturition.

Leakage from other parts of the urinary system—including kidney, ureter, or (in the neonate) urachus—is much less common. Leakage after incomplete closure of a cystotomy, placement of a transcutaneous bladder catheter, or cystocentesis can also serve as an occasional source of uroperitoneum.

Uroperitoneum does produce mild chemical peritonitis, but infection is relatively uncommon, and cellular changes in the peritoneal fluid are generally limited to a mild to moderate mature neutrophilia. Infection can occur if the original source of contamination contains bacteria or if organisms are introduced during diagnostic or therapeutic procedures by systemic spread or bacterial translocation. Urokinase, a plasminogen activator in urine, tends to limit the development of peritoneal adhesions but may also promote continued leakage by interfering with the development of a fibrin seal.

Diagnosis in a feedlot setting can typically be made with reasonable accuracy based on the presence of progressive abdominal distention with free fluid, dehydration, anorexia, and depression. Anuria, dysuria, and a palpably flaccid bladder support the diagnosis of uroperitoneum, but a temporary fibrin seal may allow intermittent bladder distention and passage of urine. Evaluation of peritoneal fluid is necessary for diagnosis in less commonly affected groups of cattle and can be beneficial in feedlot cattle with less classic presentations. Peritoneal fluid in cases of uroperitoneum is typically clear to slightly turbid and clear to yellow in color. Heating the peritoneal fluid may enhance the odor of ammonia and support the diagnosis. A peritoneal : serum creatinine ratio of 2 : 1 or greater is considered diagnostic for uroperitoneum in both adult and preruminant cattle.

Changes in blood and peritoneal fluid constituents become apparent as urine is deposited in the peritoneal cavity and allowed to equilibrate with blood. Urea nitrogen is a small molecule and equilibrates too quickly across the peritoneal membrane to reliably indicate peritoneal leakage in functioning ruminants. Furthermore, urea excreted in the saliva can be metabolized by bacteria in the rumen, decreasing the blood urea level. Potassium is also concentrated in urine and equilibrates quickly with serum; however, a peritoneal : serum potassium ratio greater than 2.7 : 1 was a consistent finding in experimental bladder rupture in preruminant calves. Serum potassium levels are subject to a variety of systemic factors that may have a greater impact in the functioning ruminant. These include anorexia, aldosterone-induced salivary secretion, gastrointestinal loss in exchange for sodium, and intracellular shifts in exchange for hydrogen ions. As a result, serum potassium levels in adult cattle with uroperitoneum may be high, normal, or low. A hyponatremic, hypochloremic metabolic alkalosis is common in both adult cattle and preruminant calves with uroperitoneum. If left untreated so the animal becomes dehydrated, a metabolic acidosis might develop.

Phosphorous, which is mainly excreted by the salivary glands, may be elevated because of decreased salivary excretion or secondary to hypocalcemia-associated anorexia.

Replacement fluid therapy that consists of 0.9% NaCl is indicated. If hyperkalemia is present, dextrose solutions may be included (2.5% dextrose and 0.45% NaCl is an option). If the rupture occurs in a recently freshened cow, attention should be paid to recognizing and treating hypocalcemia. Theoretically, peritoneal drainage may be useful; however, the authors have had difficulty maintaining patency of abdominal drains in ruminants because of the greater omentum.

It has been reported that some dorsal tears of the bladder will heal spontaneously if a urethral catheter is placed. This is done with a Foley (approximately 12-20 French) catheter in the adult female cow. After adequate restraint and preparation of the perineum, a gloved hand with sterile lubricant applied is inserted into the vestibule. Just under the transverse fold, the urethral opening is identified. The Foley catheter can be slid into the opening with a finger before filling the balloon with sterile saline. If the decision is made to place an abdominal drain, it is very helpful to localize a pool of fluid by ultrasonography. The intended site of drain placement is prepared for surgery, and the skin is desensitized using a local anesthetic. A 2-cm skin incision is made with a scalpel blade, and a chest trocar is directed into the abdomen with a sharp thrust. In the author's experience, these drains function well for a short period of time but then become sealed by omentum or become infected.

Ventral bladder tears usually require surgery and are approached by using local or general anesthesia via a caudal flank or ventrolateral celiotomy in animals with udder development. In heifers or beef cattle, a ventral midline celiotomy may be used.

During surgery, it may be necessary to infuse the urinary bladder to identify the defect. The tear is debrided if necessary and closed in 2 layer—a simple continuous pattern oversewn by an inverting pattern (Cushing or Lembert). Whether to include the mucosa when closing the bladder is somewhat controversial. The authors incorporate mucosa with synthetic absorbable suture and have not recognized any problem to date.

Complications include failure of the repair and adhesions that involve portions of the reproductive or gastrointestinal tract. In a large cow, exposure can be very limited, thus making the repair difficult.

EVERSION AND RETROFLEXION OF THE URINARY BLADDER

Eversion of the urinary bladder is a rare condition in cows because they have a long, narrow urethra. However, this condition has been reported either during or shortly after parturition. One case has been reported in a cow 5 months after calving.

Under excessive abdominal force, the urinary bladder (presumably empty) is forced into the pelvic cavity, where it can enter the vagina either by passing through the urethra (eversion) or by tearing the vaginal wall (retroflexion). External examination reveals a congested and discolored soft mass (sometimes up to 20 cm in diameter) that protrudes downward from the vulva (Figure 12.3.2-1). The displaced bladder can become edematous and necrotic if left unattended.

The diagnosis can be made by examining the protruding mass. The mucosa of the bladder is exposed in bladder eversion, and the serosa of the bladder is evident in retroflexion. The retroflexed bladder can contain urine

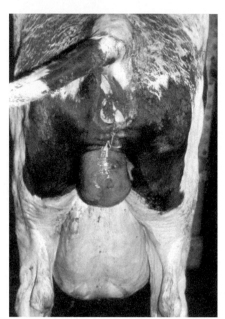

Figure 12.3.2-1   Bladder eversion in a cow. Note the congested and discolored soft mass protruding downward from the vulva.

(Courtesy of Dr. Norm G. Ducharme; Cornell University.)

while the everted bladder has no urine but can contain a serous exudate, thus making differentiation of the two conditions difficult without a cytological exam. Vaginal examination further differentiates the two conditions: the neck of the bladder exits the external os of the urethra in bladder eversion, while the neck of the bladder exits through a defect in the cranial vaginal wall in bladder retroflexion.

Treatment entails manual reposition or amputation of the apex of the bladder. First, an epidural block is performed to arrest straining. The use of a topical hyperosmotic agent such as 40% dextrose may decrease swelling of the bladder and help facilitate repositioning. If multiple attempts to reposition a bladder eversion are unsuccessful, the dorsal aspect of the urethra can be incised (approximately 8 cm) with curved Metzenbaum scissors. After the bladder eversion has been corrected, the urethral incision is sutured with size 0 nonabsorbable suture material in a simple continuous pattern. Another option is to perform a complete epidural block with 100 ml of 2% lidocaine hydrochloride and cast the animal. The cow's hind limbs can be extended caudally, which facilitates repositioning the bladder. Amputating the bladder apex should be considered if necrosis is present or all other attempts at repositioning have failed. If a complete epidural block is performed, one should hobble the hind legs in the recovery period to prevent tearing of the adductor muscles. In the days after repositioning, a standard epidural may need to be repeated to prevent reoccurrence of the condition.

Retroflexion of the bladder is easier to reposition after performing an epidural. However, recurrence or evisceration of the intestine is possible unless the cranial vaginal tear is sutured. This is done blindly as the surgeon places one (or more) cruciate sutures with no 1 or 2 absorbable suture material to close or minimize the vaginal wall defect. Unless treated early, the prognosis for these bladder displacements is guarded because of the difficulty in treating them and the risk of peritonitis.

SURGERY OF THE URETERS

Indications for surgery of the ureters include ureteral calculi and ectopic ureters, both of which are exceedingly rare.

Ureteral Calculi

Ureteral calculi may result from migration of renal calculi. This is a difficult diagnosis to make, but the calculi occasionally can be palpated per rectum or detected by transrectal ultrasonography. Clinical signs of ureteral urolithiasis are dominated by acute abdominal pain (Figure 12.3.2-2). Other signs similar to those of urethral urolithiasis are also present, such as frequent attempts at micturition, occasionally blood-tinged urine, and urine dribbling. A few reports in the literature describe ruminants treated for ureteral calculi. In several cases, the calculi apparently broke up on their own or with palpation and manipulation. Surgical removal has been mentioned (Fabish, 1968) but not described in detail.

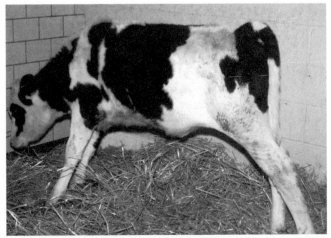

Figure 12.3.2-2 Steer with unilateral ureteral urolithiasis showing abdominal pain. Note stretching.

(Courtesy of Dr. Thomas Divers; Cornell University.)

Ectopic Ureters

Isolated reports describe surgery for ectopic ureters. This condition is more commonly recognized in small animals and horses. It has been reported to be both unilateral and bilateral. Females are overrepresented, but this may be because the incontinence is more easily recognized than in males. If the termination of the ectopic ureter is proximal to the external urethral sphincter in males, retrograde filling of the bladder rather than incontinence may result.

Embryologically, an ectopic ureter results from failure of the metanephric and mesonephric ducts to separate properly. In females, an ectopic ureter may terminate in the urethra, vagina, cervix, or caudal to the trigone of the bladder. In males, ectopic ureters have been reported to empty into the urethra, vas deferens, or seminal vesicles.

The most common clinical signs associated with ectopic ureters are urinary incontinence and urine scalding. Urinary tract infection is common, most likely from urine stasis and ascending infection. Hydronephrosis, hydroureter, and polycystic kidney disease have all been reported secondary to ectopic ureters. Ureteral reflux of urine due to the abnormal course of the ureter may cause a functional obstruction.

Clinical examination through speculum-assisted or endoscopic examination of the vagina and vestibule might allow identification of an abnormal ureteral opening. Parenteral injection of dyes that are concentrated in the urine may facilitate visualization of aberrant ureteral openings. Dyes that have been used include: sodium fluorescein (11 mg/kg IV), neoprontosil (10 ml IV), and azosulfamide (1.9 mg/kg IM). Ultrasonography is helpful in identifying any dilation or abnormality in the kidney or ureter. An intravenous pyelogram may be useful for identifying an ectopic ureter and associated urinary abnormality in young animals or small ruminants (Figure 12.3.2-3).

Either an ipsilateral nephrectomy or vesicoureteral anastomosis can be performed to correct unilateral ectopic ureters. Unilateral nephrectomy is less technically demanding than vesicoureteral anastomosis and has a low morbidity. However, if unilateral nephrectomy is contemplated, the existence and functional status of the contralateral kidney should be determined. Unilateral nephrectomy is discussed in Section 12.3.1.

Ureterovesicular anastomosis or ureteroneocystostomy are the only surgical options for bilateral ectopic ureters. These techniques can be technically difficult. Common postsurgical complications include delayed healing caused by tension on the closure and stenosis of the stoma caused by failure to accurately appose urethral mucosa to bladder mucosa.

Ectopic ureters may be intramural or extramural. An ectopic ureter that bypasses the bladder to enter the

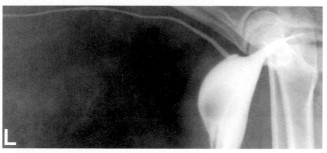

Figure 12.3.2-3 Left lateral radiograph of the caudal abdomen of a 5-year-old goat with urethritis. A positive contrast cystogram and partial normograde urethrogram was performed, and retrograde flow into the ureter is seen. Note normal site of entry ureter.

(Courtesy of Dr. Anthony Pease; Cornell University.)

urinary tract caudal to the trigone is termed extramural. At surgery, the ureter is double ligated and transected caudal to the bladder. The urethral artery must be ligated via a ventral cystostomy. A small circle of bladder wall is excised from the dorsal surface. A mosquito hemostat is tunneled through the circular defect created in the wall, and the ureter is grasped and drawn into the bladder lumen. The end is transected, and the ureter is spatulated by making a 1-cm longitudinal incision on one side. The mucosa of the ureter is sutured to the bladder mucosa with 4-0 synthetic absorbable suture material in an interrupted pattern. Efforts must be made to preserve the blood supply and avoid twisting the ureter. The bladder is closed routinely.

An intramural ectopic ureter appears to enter the bladder serosa in the normal position but runs caudally within the bladder wall and enters the genitourinary tract distal to the bladder. Intramural ectopic ureters are corrected from within the bladder. A cystotomy is performed, and an incision is made through the bladder wall and into the lumen of the ureter. The ureter wall and mucosa are sutured to the bladder mucosa. After this, a catheter is passed caudally through the new ureteral opening. The catheter facilitates identifying the portion of the ureter still connected to the ectopic opening distal to the bladder. This portion of the ureter is identified and double ligated as close as possible to the newly created intravesicular opening.

EXCRETORY UROGRAPHY

The ability to see the kidneys, ureters, and urinary bladder on abdominal survey radiographs is limited by overlying viscera and low subject contrast. Therefore only small animals that weigh less (calves, sheep and goats) can be imaged at this time. Standard urographic

techniques can be used when necessary to examine the urinary system. As for other species, the use of iodinated contrast materials injected intravenously will result in opacification of the urine by virtue of glomerular filtration of an organic iodide compound. After intravenous injection, rapid filtration occurs, and the kidney and ureter should be seen within 3 to 5 minutes. Radiographs should be taken immediately following bolus intravenous dosing. Ideally, ventrodorsal and lateral radiographs are obtained sequentially until anatomical structures are visualized and any abnormalities detected are described. The study may be limited to lateral radiographs because of available equipment and patient cooperation, but some information will be unavailable.

Urographic agents used in veterinary medicine include the ionic compound sodium-methylglucamine diatrizoate (Hypaque®, Renografin®) and the nonionic compounds iohexol (Omnipaque®) and iopamidol (Isovue®). The intravenous dose for all products is 800 mg iodine per kilogram body weight. All are available in various iodine concentrations ranging from 180 to 370 mg iodine/ml solution. A safe guideline for dosing is to start with 2 ml/kg body weight, but twice this dose could be administered under some circumstances. The contrast media should be administered rapidly via an indwelling intravenous catheter, with care taken to avoid extravasation, as the solutions are hypertonic and irritating. Nonionic contrast media are less hypertonic, and fewer local and systemic side effects are reported with these solutions in humans and dogs. The literature has little discussion of dosage or side effects in small ruminants, but the same principles as other species are probably true.

A urographic contrast study for ectopic ureter should ideally combine the positive contrast study of the kidneys and ureters (excretory urography) with pneumocystography. This increases the probability of seeing the location of the ureter at the trigone region. In female sheep or goats, catheterization of the urinary bladder is best performed by direct visualization of the urethral orifice. After removing residual urine, the bladder is insufflated with room air to about 80% volume. This procedure is almost impossible to perform in rams or bucks because of the difficulty in catheterizing the penile urethra (Figure 12.3.2-4A and B). After the urinary bladder is filled with air, the intravenous contrast medium is injected and sequential radiographs are obtained at 3- to 5-minute intervals. Both ventrodorsal and lateral radiographs are useful to follow the ureter(s) to their placement at the trigone. In general, the ureter should course caudally from the kidney then curve ventrally, cranially, and medially to enter the urinary bladder (see Figure 12.3.2-3). The most common congenital malformation is a ureter that bypasses the trigone to enter directly into

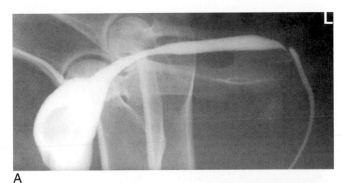

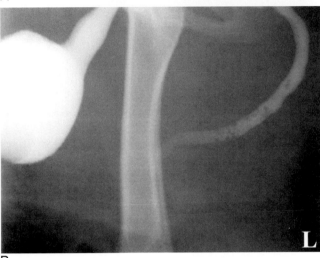

Figure 12.3.2-4 *A,* Left lateral, positive contrast cystogram and urethrogram. The pelvic portion of the urethra is normally distensible and smooth. The area of the urethral diverticulum is clearly seen at the junction of the pelvic and membranous portion of the urethra. Contrast material flows distally and opacifies the entire portion of the membranous penile urethra. No filling defects or irregularities are recognized. *B,* Left lateral, positive contrast, cystogram and normograde urethrogram showing multiple, various-sized filling defects in the urethra consistent with urinary calculi.

(Courtesy of Dr. Anthony Pease; Cornell University.)

the urethra. Anesthesia is recommended to allow catheterization, positioning, and radiography without a struggle.

In larger-sized animals, intravenous injection of indigo carmine* (0.8% ampule use 0.25 mg/kg IV) immediately followed by urethroscopy and cystoscopy

*Taylor Pharmaceuticals, Decatur, IL

can allow identification of an ectopic ureter. Indigo carmine is rapidly excreted through the kidney and gives a blue color to the urine. The ureteral openings are identified by observing the colored urine.

RECOMMENDED READINGS

Barclay WP: Unilateral ureteral ectopia in a Holstein-Friesian heifer, *J Am Vet Med Assoc* 173: 485-486, 1978.

Brobst DF et al: Azotemia in cattle, *J Am Vet Med Assoc* 173: 481-485, 1978.

Brundson JR: A case of urinary bladder prolapse in the cow, *Vet Rec* 73: 437-438, 1961.

Carr EA et al: Ruptured urinary bladder after dystocia in a cow, *J Am Vet Med Assoc* 202: 631-632, 1993.

Divers TJ, Reef VB, Roby KA: Nephrolithiasis resulting in intermittent ureteral obstruction in a cow, *Cornell Vet* 79: 143-149, 1989.

Donecker JM, Bellamy JEC: Blood chemical abnormalities in cattle with ruptured urethras, *Can Vet J* 23: 355-357, 1982.

Ducharme NG, Stein FG: Eversion of the urinary bladder in a cow, *J Am Vet Med Assoc* 179: 996-998, 1981.

Fabisch H: Report on surgical removal of ureteral stones in cows, *Wien Tierarztl Monatsschr* 55: 409-411, 1968.

Fossum TW: Surgery of the kidney and ureter. In Fossum TW editor: *Small animal surgery,* ed 2, Philadelphia, 2002, WB Saunders.

Gaines JD: Postparturient pelvic entrapment of the bladder in two cows, *J Am Vet Med Assoc* 193: 222-223, 1988.

Hojbjerg A: Eversion of the bovine bladder, *Bovine Pract* 25: 120-121, 1991.

McLoughlin MA, Chew DJ: Diagnosis and surgical management of ectopic ureters, *Clin Tech Small Anim Pract* 15: 17-24, 2000.

Roussel AJ, Ward DS: Ruptured urinary bladder in a heifer, *J Am Vet Med Assoc* 186: 1310-1311, 1985.

Silverman S, Long CD: The diagnosis of urinary incontinence and abnormal urination in dogs and cats, *Vet Clin North Am Small Anim Pract* 30: 427-428, 2000.

Smith JA et al: Ruptured urinary bladder in a post-parturient cow, *Cornell Vet* 73: 3-12, 1983.

Sockett D, Knight AP: Metabolic changes associated with obstructive urolithiasis in cattle, *Compend Contin Educ Pract Vet* 6: 5311-5315, 1984.

Sockett DC et al: Metabolic changes due to experimentally induced rupture of the bovine urinary bladder, *Cornell Vet* 76: 198-212, 1986.

Streeter RN, Washburn KE, Higbee RG, Bartels KE: Laser lithotripsy of a urethral calculus via ischial urethrotomy in a steer, *J Am Vet Med Assoc* 219: 640-643, 2001.

Waldron DR: Ectopic ureter surgery and its problems, *Probl Vet Med* 1: 85-92, 1981 Review.

Wallace LL, Bouchard G, Nicholson W, Turk J, Sweeney CL: Polypoid cystitis, pyelonephritis, and obstructive uropathy in a cow, *J Am Vet Med Assoc* 197: 1181-1183, 1990.

CHAPTER 13

SURGICAL DISEASES OF THE EYE IN FARM ANIMALS

Nita L. Irby

Vision is essential for food- or fiber-producing animals to safely exist in their environments and compete for food. Ocular diseases can result in considerable (up to extreme) discomfort to the patient with resultant poor weight gain, decreased milk production, behavioral problems, and poor performance.

A complete history and physical examination should be performed on all patients, even if the complaint concerns "just" the eye. Many ocular problems in food animal species are manifestations of systemic diseases; and these disorders should be ruled out before the ocular examination commences because dehydration, anemia, icterus, and others of these types of physical parameters may affect the ocular findings. Historical information should include the owner's or herdsman's assessment of the patient's visual status. Careful observation of the patient may be necessary if normal vision is questioned and should be performed on a herd animal patient in separate and unfamiliar surroundings. Head carriage should be noted (visually deficient animals often carry their heads close to the ground). Previous ocular diseases should be queried. Current and previous ocular and systemic medications—including conventional and alternative therapeutic modalities—should be noted.

Treatment of any eye problem begins with a proper diagnosis made during a careful, complete eye examination, which every veterinary student learns and available reference textbooks illustrate. However, the difficulties encountered during examination of the eyes of a ruminant patient in a stanchion, chute, barn, or field can make an ocular examination a challenge, even for experienced veterinary ophthalmologists.

Whenever possible, examination of the eyes should be performed in a quiet, dark room. Adequate restraint of the head is essential, and sedation of the patient may be necessary. In addition to an ophthalmoscope,* minimal specialized equipment† is necessary. Box 13-1 lists diagnostic and therapeutic equipment that fits easily inside a small, three-tiered fishing tackle box to make a compact and readily portable unit. In addition, lint-free cellulose sponges‡ are often helpful for fluid absorption but are expensive and only necessary when an eye is ruptured. Finally, a black cloth or cape for shrouding the head of the patient and examiner may be helpful if a darkened area for exam is not available but should be used with care to avoid startling patients.

Examination and Medical Procedures

EYELID AKINESIA

In contrast to the powerful orbicularis muscle of the equine, ruminant species' eyelids are much easier to open. However, any eyelid that is being held firmly shut by a patient should not be forced open for examination purposes unless the underlying disease process is known. Forceful attempts to open eyelids closed over a lacerated cornea may result in all the ocular contents being

---

*Direct ophthalmoscope, Finoff transilluminator, Cobalt filters, see www.welchallyn.com/medical
†Ophthalmic Surgical Instruments, see
www.bausch.com/us/resource/surgical/instruments/index.jsp
‡Weck-Cel®, Solan Ophthalmic Products®, Xomed Surgical Products, Inc., Jacksonville, FL or www.medtronicsolan.com

BOX 13-1

SUGGESTED DIAGNOSTIC AND THERAPEUTIC OPHTHALMIC EQUIPMENT AND SUPPLIES

Portable Ophthalmology Essentials

Welch-Allyn 3.5 V rechargeable halogen direct ophthalmoscope with Finhoff transilluminator

Cobalt blue filter for transilluminator to enhance fluorescein stain fluorescence

20 Diopter or 2.2 D indirect ophthalmoscopy lens

4x magnifying loupe

Sterile cotton-tipped applicators and sterile gauze pads

Fluorescein stain strips—sterile

Mosquito hemostats

Allis, Bishop-Harmon, and Colibri tissue forceps

Small Metzenbaum or Stevens Tenotomy scissors

Small Derf needle holder or large Castroviejo

Lid speculum

2-0 nylon on a straight needle

4-0 to 6-0 Vicryl on small cutting needle

Schirmer Tear Test strips

Xylazine, detomidine, and butorphanol

Mepivacaine or lidocaine

Tropicamide 1%—short-acting mydriatic to dilate pupils

Proparacaine 0.5%—topical anesthetic

10% phenylephrine

Sterile eye collyrium/eye irrigating solution in a spray bottle or sterile saline

5% povidone-iodine solution

Alcohol swabs

Cyanoacrylate tissue adhesive

#11, 12 and 15 BP scalpel blades (#12 is great for suture removal)

Glass slides (cleaned and in carriers)

Matches or lighter

20-g IV catheters for normograde nasolacrimal cannulation and for lavage of the palpebral fissure

Teat cannulae and tomcat catheters for retrograde nasolacrimal duct cannulation

30, 25, 20, and 18 g disposable needles

Tuberculin, 3-cc, 5-cc and two 12-cc syringes

Blood tubes—particularly red top (include 1 to 2 filled with formalin)

Culturettes®—preferably minitip

Broth for bacterial culture

Mila subpalpebral lavage apparatus kits

expelled into the examiner's hand. In every instance, eyelids are most safely opened with the examiner's hand(s) resting securely on the underlying orbit bones while the examiner's fingers "walk" the lids open. Lids should not be forced open by direct application of pressure to the lid margins and thus to the underlying eyeball.

Eyelid akinesia is recommended as the safest way to open eyelids and is essential for standing ocular surgical procedures (nictitans, conjunctival or corneal surgery, etc.). Several methods are available to paralyze the upper eyelids, and akinesia should result within 5 minutes. In thinner-skinned animals (calves, sheep and goats), branches of the palpebral branch of the auriculopalpebral nerve may be palpated at any of a number of sites as branches cross the bony orbit rim dorsocaudal or dorsolateral to the eye along the zygomatic arch. One or more sites are cleansed, and topical anesthetic is injected subcutaneously (SQ, 1-5 ml/site) via a 20- to 25-gauge needle; the needle size and amount injected depend on the patient's size. Nerve branches may not be palpable in adult cattle, but the palpebral nerves can be anesthetized as part of the Peterson Nerve Block (Figure 13-1). A 12-cm needle is inserted subcutaneously at the angle between the frontal and temporal processes of the zygomatic bone. This site is bounded by the zygomatic arch ventrally, the supraorbital process rostrally, and the coronoid process of the mandible caudally. The needle is directed caudally along the zygomatic arch and 10-20 cc of local anesthetic is infiltrated as the needle is advanced.

Complete lower lid akinesia can be difficult to achieve in ruminants, and although specific nerve blocks have been described, the author prefers to use a 20- to 22-gauge spinal needle (7-12 cm) inserted 1 cm ventral to

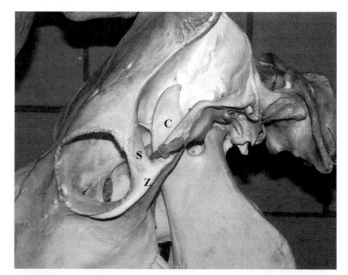

Figure 13-1   Peterson Nerve Block: a 12-cm needle is inserted subcutaneously at the angle between the frontal and temporal processes of the zygomatic bone. This site is bounded by the zygomatic arch (Z) ventrally, the supraorbital process (S) rostrally, and the coronoid process (C) of the mandible caudally.

the lateral canthus and directed medially through the lower eyelid to diffusely infiltrate local anesthetic throughout the lower eyelid. Before injection, topical anesthesia is applied to the ocular surface, and the lower eyelid is supported with finger pressure applied from inside as the needle is advanced, thus also protecting the globe.

Complete akinesia and analgesia of the eye and orbit may be necessary in some cases. A Peterson nerve block can be used or a retrobulbar block can be performed. Pearce et al. showed greater distribution of anesthetic around target nerves and muscles with the retrobulbar block.

TOPICAL ANESTHESIA AND MEDICATION

Although some ruminants are surprisingly tolerant of eye examinations, the use of 0.5% proparacaine solution and other topical anesthetics are essential for certain ophthalmic procedures that require extensive touching or manipulation of the globe or conjunctiva. Topical anesthetic agents cause mild stinging upon installation and hyperemia of the conjunctiva and are mildly toxic to the corneal epithelium, thus resulting in a mild, diffuse corneal epithelial thickening and faint, diffuse fluorescein uptake after topical anesthetic administration. Complete external examination of the eye, including fluorescein staining, should always be performed before anesthetic installation. A repeated administration of topical anesthetic every 15 to 30 seconds for 3 to 5 minutes greatly enhances the depth of topical anesthetic.

Application to the eye of topical anesthetics or any other ocular solutions is most easily performed by *gently* spraying the medication or solution onto the surface of the eye. This technique conserves costly ophthalmic medications, can often be performed without touching the patient's eyelids, and is very hygienic. If the spray device is kept clean, it can be used repeatedly over many days while maintaining sterility of the stock bottle. A very effective "squirt gun" can be made by drawing 1 to 3 ml of the ophthalmic stock solution into a tuberculin or 3-cc syringe. A 25-g needle attached to the syringe *is removed* from the needle hub after the syringe is filled by grasping it between index finger and thumb and bending it until the needle breaks off the hub. The end of the hub is still sharp, so the hub should not be held too close to the patient's eye. The administrator's hand should rest somewhere on the patient's head during administration so that the hand will move away simultaneously to inadvertent movements of the patient's head during spray administration and the patient's eye will not bump the hub. A test spray before administration will ensure the medication is coming straight out of the syringe and is not being diverted to the side as a result of bending during needle removal.

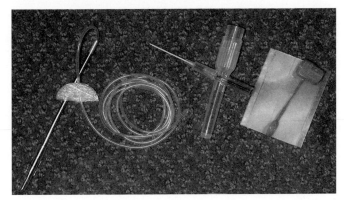

Figure 13-2   Materials necessary to make a transpalpebral ocular lavage apparatus.*

TRANSPALPEBRAL OCULAR LAVAGE APPARATUS

The transpalpebral catheter can be an extremely valuable adjunct to topical ocular therapy in ruminants, notably bulls that are otherwise unsafe to treat. The devices are readily available through commercial suppliers* or can be easily fabricated from polyethylene tubing (Figure 13-2). Medication infusion pumps can be attached to the catheters to help alleviate some handling of intractable patients, especially those with severe ocular disease that might need medication as often as every hour.

The patient is sedated, and the skin at the exit point of the catheter in the area of the dorsolateral orbit rim is cleansed. The upper eyelid is paralyzed as described above and 3 to 5 cc of local anesthetic are infiltrated subcutaneously at the planned exit site. The tubing is secured within a hubless needle or onto a wound drain insertion needle. The needle tip is securely cushioned in the tip of the surgeon's index finger, and the needle with tubing inside is held in the same palm. The surgeon's hand is turned so the index fingernail is toward the cornea and is inserted in the palpebral fissure. The finger with the needle then pushes dorsally until it is touching the inside of the orbit rim (through the palpebral conjunctiva). The opposite hand should simultaneously pull the upper lid out from the globe and over the inserting finger before the needle is advanced from the fingertip to ensure the needle tip does not "buttonhole" a conjunctival fold close to the lid margin, which could prevent proper blinking after the tube is secured. The lid is released, and the same hand is used to push the needle-tubing unit through the upper lid staying just rostral to the bony rim. The tubing is carefully pulled through with the needle until the footplate resistance is felt, taking care that the footplate remains inside the conjunctival sac and is not pulled into the subcutaneous tissues of the dorsal

---

*Eye Lavage Kit—Part #6612, MILA International, Inc., 7604 Dixie Hwy, Florence, KY; (888) MILA-INT (645-2468); milaint@att.net

eyelid. At this point, the eyelid should be manipulated to ensure that it moves freely and is not caught on the tubing. Small pieces of waterproof adhesive tape ("butterflies") are placed around the tube and sutured to the skin just adjacent to the exit point from the lid to prevent retrograde movement of the tubing and footplate into the conjunctival sac. Cyanoacrylate glue is applied over the tape and tube, further securing it to the skin (Figure 13-3). Additional adhesive tape butterflies are placed along the length of the tubing as needed.

Diagnosis of Globe and Orbit Diseases

CONGENITAL
Common congenital abnormalities of the orbit and globe in ruminants include microphthalmos (a smaller-than-normal eye usually with multiple associated ocular defects) and strabismus (Figure 13-4). Patients with microphthalmos (Figure 13-5 A and B) have correspondingly small orbit bones that will not develop normally. Patients with microphthalmos may have associated cardiac, abdominal wall, or caudal spinal closure defects, and a careful physical examination is warranted. Culling may be indicated; a heritable component has been reported in some dairy breeds. Microphthalmos and a wide spectrum of blinding and nonblinding ocular

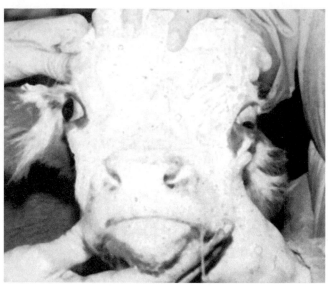

Figure 13-4 A 3-day-old Hereford calf with hydrocephalus, variable strabismus and nystagmus, cardiac and vertebral defects.

anomalies such as cataracts (Figure 13-6) can occur with chronic vitamin A deficiency in pigs.

Unilateral or bilateral congenital strabismus of variable degree and direction may be seen in any species and may be seen associated with other physical and neurologic defects. Bilateral convergent strabismus (esotropia, Figure 13-7 A and B) with or without exophthalmos and nystagmus occurs in dairy cattle and may progress with age. Visual acuity is variable; the condition has been proven to be inherited in some dairy breeds and culling of affected animals may be indicated. If vision is impaired, affected animals may fail to thrive and have difficulty negotiating their environments.

EXOPHTHALMOS
Exophthalmos in adult cattle is usually attributable to either inflammatory disease or neoplasia. A simple history and clinical presentation can often differentiate between these two broad categories. Inflammatory causes of exophthalmos (foreign body, cellulitis, sinusitis, infected tooth, myositis, etc.) are usually peracute to acute in onset, with the patient exhibiting marked pain when the affected eye is retropulsed into the orbit and when the jaw is opened (Figure 13-8). Affected animals are often febrile, depressed, and reluctant to eat. Abnormal ipsilateral nasal odor and discharge may be present with concurrent sinus involvement. In contrast, exophthalmos due to orbital neoplastic diseases is of slower onset, and the patient is rarely in discomfort except in cases of exposure damage to the cornea. Exophthalmos should be distinguished from glaucoma (rare in

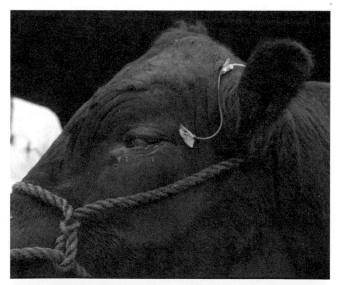

Figure 13-3 Four-year-old Angus bull with homemade transpalpebral ocular lavage apparatus consisting of size #190 polyethylene tubing with footplate flange. This was made by warming tubing over a match flame until it was softened; the tubing was then pressed gently against a metal surface. Footplate size and angulation of the tubing are easily customized.

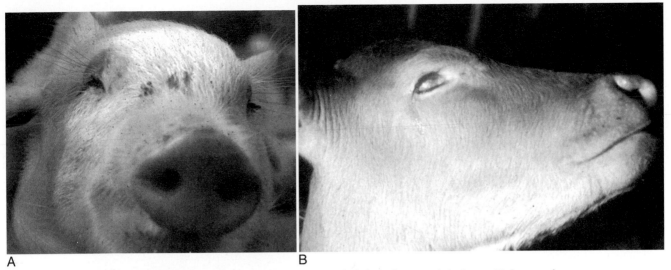

Figure 13-5 *A,* Two-week crossbred piglet with bilateral microphthalmos. Piglet was born to a sow that was fed doughnuts and was severely vitamin A-deficient. *B,* Calf with microphthalmos. Other congenital abnormalities were found in this Jersey calf: wry tail and ventricular septal defect.

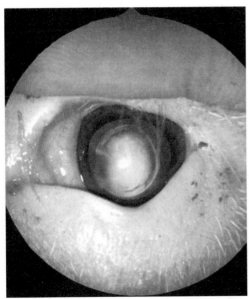

Figure 13-6 Three-week-old crossbred piglet with microphakia, cataract, and other congenital ocular anomalies. Piglet was born to a sow that was fed doughnuts and was severely vitamin A-deficient.

ruminants) and proptosis (protrusion of the eye from the orbit usually due to trauma). In a ruminant, an eye protruding from its orbit associated with trauma often carries a grave prognosis and is usually associated with other craniofacial injuries and possibly neurologic signs. A proptotic eye may require enucleation if it is ruptured or extensive extraocular muscle avulsion exists. Regard-less of cause, an exposed eye requires immediate and frequent cleansing and moistening. The eye and periocular tissues can be moistened in an emergency with sterile saline, sterile eye wash or with any number of contact lens solutions until medical attention is available.

ORBITAL INFLAMMATION AND CELLULITIS

As stated previously, orbit inflammatory disease in cattle usually has peracute to acute onset and may be caused by foreign body penetration, puncture wounds, sinusitis, or extension of a severe infection in the eye (panophthalmitis). Puncture wounds and foreign bodies can enter the orbital space through the facial skin, palpebral fissure, or mouth; all of these areas should be examined carefully, if possible, during the physical examination. However, examination of the oral cavity may be difficult or impossible because of the pain from opening the mouth. Pain with jaw movement may be extremely severe and result in complete anorexia in some patients. The pain is only rarely attributed to temporomandibular joint disease and is more likely a result of movement by the coronoid process of the mandible compressing the retrobulbar tissues. Adjacent muscles of mastication may also be inflamed. Additional physical examination findings may include fever, anorexia, depression, mild-to-severe exophthalmos with possible exposure keratitis, periorbital swelling, and pain (Figure 13-9). Inspection and manipulation of wounds or draining tracts may reveal the presence of a foreign body. Abnormal ipsilateral nasal odor and discharge may be present with concurrent sinus involvement; sinus swelling may be evident

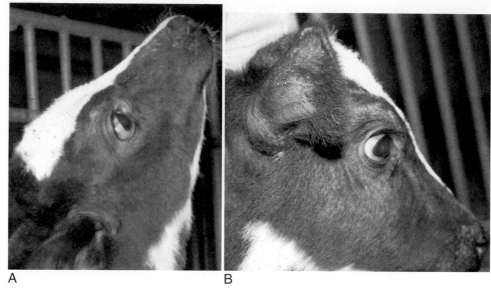

A   B

Figure 13-7   *A,* A 4-week-old female Holstein calf with severe esotropia and a constant "star-gazing" head carriage was unable to walk without stumbling and could not eat from the ground. *B,* Dorsal oblique and lateral rectus muscle shortening procedures were performed with resultant marked improvement in the head position, vision, and behavior. The calf was maintained as a pet and was not bred. Such procedures are best referred to specialists.

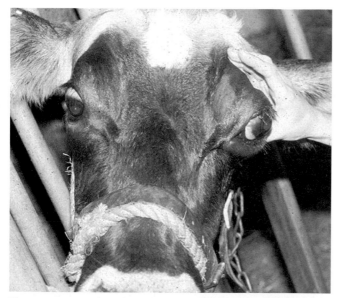

Figure 13-8   Left unilateral exophthalmos in a cow.

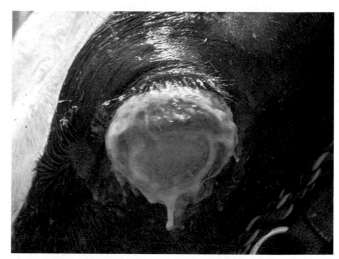

Figure 13-9   Orbit cellulitis with severe secondary exposure keratitis caused by a wooden foreign body found in the retrobulbar tissues in a cow.

and sinus resonance after percussion may be reduced or absent. Ultrasound and radiographic examinations are helpful in locating foreign objects and ruling out fractures, sinusitis, lumpy jaw, or a large mass such as a tumor. Fistulograms can be performed if draining tracts are present. A tissue aspirate for culture and cytology can be useful to confirm the presence of bacteria. Additional

information regarding diagnosis and treatment of sinus disorders can be found in Chapter 9.

Treatment is directed at protecting the cornea, treating inflammation, and correcting the reason for cellulitis. The cornea is treated with sterile artificial tear ointments as often as needed to maintain corneal lubrication; if corneal ulcers are present, standard medical or surgical ulcer treatment is indicated according to the severity of the ulcer. Ophthalmology texts should be consulted for specifics.

Orbit inflammation can be managed with hot packs 4 to 6 times a day, broad-spectrum antibiotics (based on bacterial sensitivity results) and antiinflammatory drugs. If the inflammation persists, surgical drainage may be necessary. Usually, over time, the swelling will localize and ventral drainage can be established. It may be possible to localize a fluid pocket by palpation or ultrasound. The site should be prepped and aspirated with aseptic technique. Ventral drainage is established while vital

structures are avoided. Most orbital abscesses in cattle harbor *Arcanobacter pyogenes* and parenteral penicillin therapy is appropriate.

ORBITAL NEOPLASIA

An adult dairy cow with unilateral or bilateral exophthalmos of subacute to chronic onset is most likely lymphosarcoma (Figure 13-10A and B). Other orbital neoplasias are rare but do occur, primary to the orbit or as extensions from adjacent tissues. Excessive orbital fat or orbital fat prolapse (Figure 13-11A and B) should be ruled out by palpation, cytologic sampling, or biopsy. If

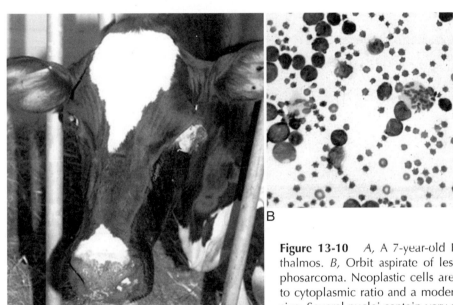

Figure 13-10 *A,* A 7-year-old Holstein with subacute, unilateral exophthalmos. *B,* Orbit aspirate of lesion, showing typical appearance of lymphosarcoma. Neoplastic cells are predominantly large with a high nuclear to cytoplasmic ratio and a moderate variability to nuclear and cytoplasmic size. Several nuclei contain very prominent nucleoli. Centrally, a neoplastic cell is undergoing mitosis.

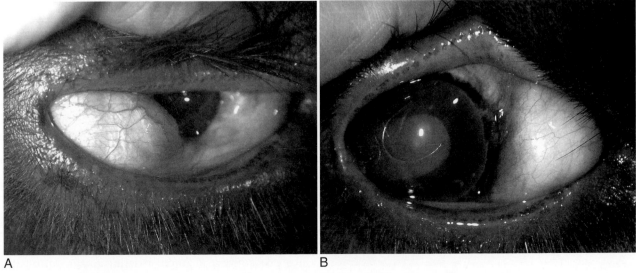

Figure 13-11 *A,* Orbital fat prolapse in an adult Shorthorn cross. *B,* Close-up view.

a biopsy is performed, the conjunctiva must be closed over fat or extensive orbit fat prolapse can occur. Digital palpation of the retrobulbar area through the palpebral fissure after application of topical anesthesia is a useful adjunct examination (Figure 13-12). Orbital fat is soft, fluctuant and nonpainful to palpation; inflammatory lesions usually are painful and firm while lymphosarcoma or other neoplasias are nonpainful but firm.

A complete physical examination should be performed—including careful cardiac auscultation and palpation of peripheral lymph nodes. Rectal examination is done with particular attention paid to uterine palpation and evaluation of regional lymph nodes. In some cases, the orbital mass or swelling may be felt adjacent or caudal to the globe by palpation posteriorly using a finger placed within the palpebral fissure after application of topical anesthesia. Fine needle aspiration of orbital tissues using a 20- to 22-g 7- to 12-cm needle with or without ultrasound guidance may be diagnostic (see Figure 13-10B). Serologic testing may be performed to assist in diagnosing lymphosarcoma.

Cows affected with lymphosarcoma usually die within 3 to 6 months, but a cow in late gestation may survive sufficiently long to deliver a healthy calf. In such cases palliative treatment to protect the eye and reduce ocular pain from exposure may be indicated. If the exophthalmos is mild and only slowly progressive and if parturition is imminent, topical artificial tear ointments 6 to 8 times a day may suffice.

Moderate, progressive exophthalmos or a longer time to parturition may require protection of the globe(s) by permanent complete tarsorrhaphy (Figure 13-13). After sedation and application of local and topical anesthesia, the 2- to 3-mm–wide eyelid margin is trimmed off and

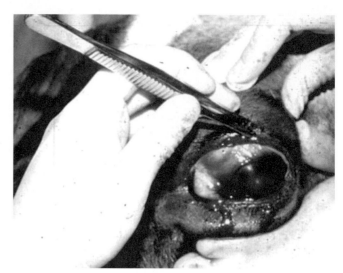

Figure 13-13   Permanent tarsorrhaphy on an 8-year-old Jersey 3 weeks prepartum.

discarded. Lids are closed with 3-0 to 4-0 absorbable sutures in the fibrous tissue layer of the eyelid (tarsal plate) and subcutaneous tissues with or without skin. If exophthalmos is severe, enucleation (Figure 13-14A) or orbit exenteration (Figure 13-14B) may be recommended. In rare instances in very valuable cattle, an evisceration may be performed before placing a prosthesis (Figure 13-14C).

General Surgical Techniques

Indications for enucleation include extensive inflammation or trauma to the adnexa of the eye, orbit, or globe, painful glaucomatous eyes, extensive ocular tumors, or congenital defects that result in exposure damage. The two types of enucleation commonly used are subconjunctival or transpalpebral ablation techniques. In large animal surgery, the transpalpebral technique is recommended.

PREPARATION OF PERIOCULAR TISSUES

Individual surgeons may have strong personal preferences for the type of tissue cleansing and preparation done before surgery, but some basics about periocular surgical preparations should be emphasized. Of utmost importance are protection of the eye and use of prep solutions that do not cause irritation or damage to the eye(s).

Sterile artificial tear ointments are used to protect the cornea before preparation procedures. However, ointments should never be used perioperatively if an intraocular procedure is planned. If artificial tear ointments are not used during preparation, an anesthetized patient's

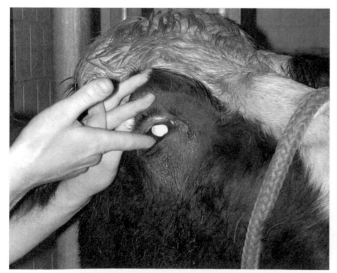

Figure 13-12   Digital palpation of palpebral fissure.

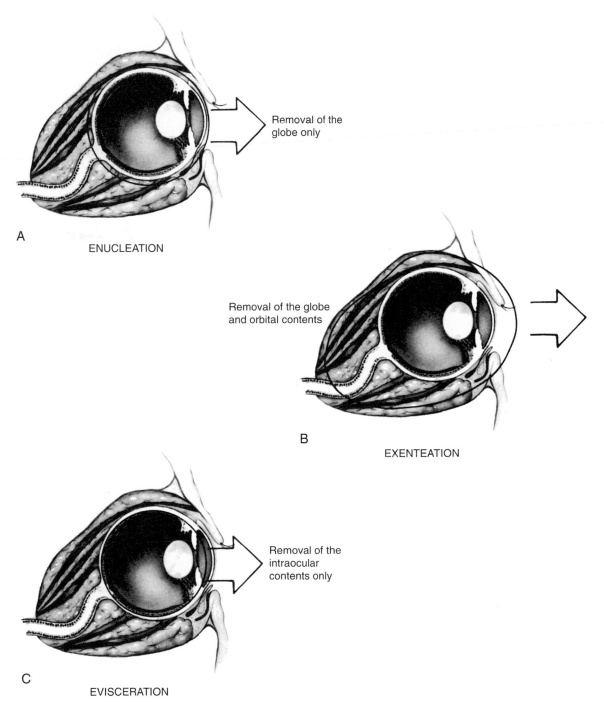

A

ENUCLEATION

Removal of the globe only

B

EXENTEATION

Removal of the globe and orbital contents

C

EVISCERATION

Removal of the intraocular contents only

Figure 13-14   *A,* Diagrammatic representation of enucleation. *B,* exenteration, and *C,* evisceration.

(Reprinted with permission from Slatter D: *Fundamentals in veterinary ophthalmology,* ed 3, Philadelphia, 2001, WB Saunders.)

eyelids should be manually closed whenever they open, and sterile saline or collyrium should be applied frequently to the cornea to prevent corneal desiccation.

Removal of hair from any surgical field is standard presurgical protocol but requires particular care near the eye. Some surgeons do not remove any hair at all before intraocular surgery because of their concern that small pieces of hair may not be completely rinsed from the conjunctival fornices and may enter the open eye during surgery. Other surgeons clip only long or dirty periocular hairs with scissors but do not use electric clippers or razors out of concern for damage and irritation of the sensitive skin of the eyelids. Using care and sharp clipper blades, an experienced surgeon can clip periocular hair without trauma to the patient. Chemical depilatories must not be used near the eye; waxes may cause eyelid swelling and irritation and damage to the eye surface if carelessly applied.

Extreme care must be taken to ensure all hair particles are removed from the conjunctival sac after clipping, particularly if the eye is to be opened during a planned intraocular surgery. A 20- to 22-g, 5- to 7-cm soft, flexible catheter can be attached to a 12- to 20-cc syringe filled with sterile saline and used to repeatedly lavage all of the recesses of the conjunctival sac and the bulbar surface of the membrane nictitans. The author uses the same syringe to thoroughly flush the upper and lower nasolacrimal puncta and ducts. A significant amount of exudate and debris residing within the nasolacrimal duct system can reenter the conjunctival sac during surgery and should be removed before any eye surgery.

Surgical prep detergents, such as povidone-iodine detergent scrubs, alcohol, hydrogen peroxide and chlorhexidine diacetate, should never be used near the eyes or anywhere there is a chance they could drip or run into the eyes. Chlorhexidine diacetate in particular can cause severe ocular disease and should be avoided. Povidone-iodine solutions (10% solution in sterile saline or sterile water) are acceptable sanitizers for the periocular skin. Five or more centrifugal scrubs beginning at the eyelid margins and circling outwards are performed alternating with sterile saline scrubs or rinses. Finally, povidone-iodine should be applied and left in place for several minutes.

Choices of surgical drapes are as varied as the surgeons that use them. The eye can be draped with a standard four-drape technique, a fenestrated drape, or specialized, nonfenestrated, self-adhesive eye drapes. The latter are most highly recommended for any type of intraocular surgery because their fenestration can be customized and the adjacent drape adheres beautifully to the lids and periocular facial skin and hair.

BASIC OPHTHALMIC SURGICAL INSTRUMENTATION

Minimal investment is required to purchase the few additional instruments necessary to perform the surgical procedures discussed in this chapter that would not be found in a standard soft tissue surgical pack.

A basic ophthalmic instrument set (Figure 13-15) suitable for eyelid, conjunctival, and simple corneal surgery includes: small towel clamps such as Schaedel's; Bard-Parker #9 blade handle; small Mayo scissors; general suture scissors; small stitch scissors (Westcott); forceps such as Adson or Brown-Adson suitable for eyelid surgery in large ruminants; Allis tissue forceps useful during entropion surgery; forceps such as fine Bishop-Harmon suitable for eyelid surgery in small ruminants; 4 Hartman curved mosquito hemostats; four 6″ Kelly hemostats; Derf or other small needle holder; large, curved utility scissors with serrated blade (enucleation in adult cattle); small curved and straight Metzenbaum scissors; small ophthalmic scissors such as a Stevens or Westcott tenotomy scissors, a small needle holder appropriate for 5-0 to 6-0 or smaller suture such as an 11 mm, nonlocking, curved Castroviejo needle holder; small tissue forceps suitable for cornea and conjunctiva, such as 0.4 mm Colibri-type 1 × 2 or delicate 1 × 2 Bishop-

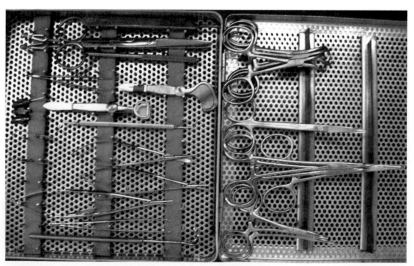

Figure 13-15   A basic ophthalmic instrument set.

Harmon; double-ended Martinez corneal dissector; Snellen or Desmarres lid forceps with solid lower plate; simple eyelid speculum, such as a 20-mm Barraquer; Desmarres lid retractors (2); and nonlinting sponges.* A binocular magnifying loupe (see Figure 13-28A) is extremely useful for eye surgery in the field or hospital if better magnification systems are not available. Suture material appropriate for eye surgery should be available, including 4-0 silk for stay sutures and procedures such as tarsorrhaphies. Synthetic absorbable sutures, 4-0 to 7-0, with the smallest size needle available are suitable for corneal repair in smaller ruminants.

ANESTHESIA

In many instances, these procedures can be done in a standing, sedated (10-20 mg xylazine IV) food animal. However, general anesthesia is certainly advantageous when a cow is fractious or has a severe lesion or for humane concerns.

If the surgery is to be done standing, adequate restraint with local and topical anesthesia is essential. The face is clipped and prepared for aseptic surgery. The cow is put in a chute or stanchion, and the head is tied snugly to the side. Local anesthesia has been described in a variety of ways. If a transpalpebral technique is used, local anesthetic should be deposited circumferentially 4 to 5 cm from the eyelid margins. To anesthetize the eye there are a few options. One possibility is to deposit 35 ml of 2% lidocaine in the retrobulbar cone using an 8.75 cm (3½ in) 18 gauge needle. Another way to provide analgesia to the retrobulbar area is with a Peterson nerve block (described under Eyelid Akinesia; see Figure 13-1). It is also possible to deposit anesthesia at 4 sites around the eye (Figure 13-16).

TRANSPALPEBRAL ENUCLEATION

After appropriate preparation and thorough nasolacrimal duct lavage, the eyelids are sutured together or clamped. A circumferential incision 1.5 cm away from the eyelid margin is made through the skin into the subcutaneous tissues of the eyelid but not through the conjunctiva. The lateral and medial canthal ligaments securing the eyelids to the orbit bones are transected. As traction is applied to the freed eyelids, dissection is continued caudally toward the orbit rim taking care to stay external to the conjunctival sac, which should remain closed. Close to the orbit rim the deep fascia forming the orbital septum is penetrated, and the extraocular muscles and tissues within the orbital cone can be visualized. In cases of panophthalmitis or when enucleation is necessary because of severe orbital cellulitis, the extraocular

---

*Weck-Cel®, Solan Ophthalmic Products®, Xomed Surgical Products, Inc., Jacksonville, FL or www.medtronicsolan.com

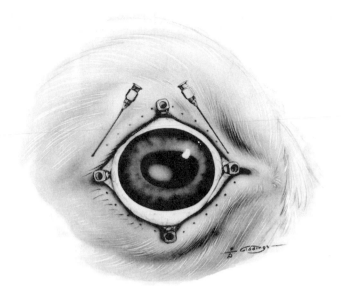

Figure 13-16   Injection sites for local anesthesia before transpalpebral enucleation in cattle. Five to 10 ml of lidocaine is injected at each site to produce anesthesia and proptosis.

(Reprinted with permission from Slatter D: *Fundamentals in veterinary ophthalmology,* ed 3, Philadelphia, 2001, WB Saunders.)

muscles and the other soft tissues within the periorbita should be excised as widely as possible or transpalpebral exenteration should be performed. Significant bleeding will occur in these cases. In other cases in which infection of the eye is not a concern, intraoperative bleeding is considerably lessened if each rectus muscle is transected at its tendon of insertion on the sclera. As each muscle is encountered, one blade of a Metzenbaum scissor is inserted between the muscle and sclera, and the scissor is pulled anterior toward the limbus before cutting, thus ensuring that the transaction occurs through muscle tendons, which bleed much less than the muscle belly. The dorsal and ventral oblique muscle insert deep to each respective rectus muscle and may have very short tendons of insertion. They are transected close to the sclera. After rectus and oblique muscle transection, the globe is grasped, and gentle traction is applied, thus making the retractor muscles that form a cone around the optic nerve easier to visualize. *Traction on the globe should be minimal to decrease vagal nerve stimulation and avoid potential damage to the optic chiasm.* With gentle medial traction on the globe, the surgeon should attempt to "strum" the optic nerve-retractor muscle cone using an approach from the dorsolateral side of the orbit. Once the location of the nerve has been confirmed, the same hand is used to position the blades of a large curved serrated utility scissor around the cone. The cone is rarely visualized directly because of variable amounts of orbital fat and hemorrhage; there-

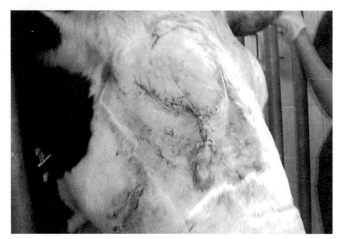

Figure 13-17 Closure of the surgical site following enucleation in a cow.

fore digital palpation is important. One or two cuts of properly placed scissors will almost completely free the globe. It is held in one hand, and the remaining medial attachments severed. The entire third eyelid should be removed at this time. To prevent postoperative lacrimocele formation, it is recommended the lacrimal gland located in the periorbita of the dorsolateral orbit ventral to the orbit rim be surgically removed as well.

Meticulous hemostasis during enucleation is time-consuming, and in most cases not necessary. In the enucleation technique described above, no attempt is made to ligate the optic nerve and muscle cone because ligatures placed around the optic nerve and muscle cone are difficult to place, usually slip, result in tissue trauma in the process, may increase vagal stimulation, and can act as a foreign body inciting an inflammatory response. The orbit is packed with sponges and pressure is applied as closure commences, but all sponges are removed before the subcutaneous tissues are completely closed. An absorbable suture (no. 2-0) is used to close subcutaneous tissues; a nonabsorbable suture is used in the skin (Figure 13-17). A pressure bandage is applied for 24 hours and the pressure of the sutured incision combined with the bandage will almost always be adequate to stop hemorrhage. Drains are not necessary unless there is preexisting infection. Antibiotics should be given for 5 to 7 days after surgery.

TRANSPALPEBRAL EXENTERATION

Exenteration means the globe and as much of the ocular contents as possible are removed. For exenteration surgery, the dissection is done outside the extra ocular eye muscles and conjunctiva, all of which are removed with the globe (Figure 13-18A). For extensive SCC in cattle, this may be the preferred procedure.

The same transpalpebral approach is recommended. The plane of dissection is against the bony orbit. All extraocular eye muscles are removed along with a substantial portion of the optic nerve (Figure 13-18B). If possible, a subcutaneous tissue layer is closed. A drain may be necessary for 48 to 72 hours. Skin is closed routinely.

EVISCERATION

Evisceration is the removal of the contents of the globe, leaving the cornea, sclera, extraocular muscles and adnexal structures in place. This is done before placing a silicon cosmetic prosthesis into the corneoscleral shell.

Surgical Treatment of Specific Conditions

ACUTE HEAD TRAUMA WITH EYE INJURIES

Traumatic injuries to the head, orbit or globe are common in the ruminant. Serious head, ocular and orbital trauma are always emergencies. After injury, the patient's head is restrained, if possible, to avoid additional, self-induced injury that occurs from rubbing the eye and periocular area against the chute, stanchion, stall, wall or forelimb. Examination or manipulation of the ocular or periocular tissues is avoided until adequate restraint and tranquilization are completed.

BLUNT TRAUMA TO THE EYE WITHOUT LACERATION OR RUPTURE

Trauma patients should receive a careful physical, neurological, and ophthalmic examination, including fundus examination and evaluation of direct and consensual pupillary light reflexes. The eye may appear normal or have any combination of injuries. Indirect ophthalmoscopy may be needed for fundus examination through cloudy media. In addition to a routine ophthalmic examination, careful examination of the sclera for occult ruptures should be performed as far posterior on the globe as possible, concentrating especially in the equatorial region. Occult ruptures can lead to phthisis bulbi. Extensive corneal lacerations, corneoscleral avulsions or scleral ruptures require immediate surgical repair, best performed by a specialist. Hyphema is often present acutely. If more than half of the anterior chamber is filled with blood or if spontaneous intraocular rebleeding occurs the eye has a very poor prognosis and phthisis bulbi often results. An initially normal-appearing cornea should be monitored carefully for several days after any blunt traumatic injury because it can slough its epithelium a few days later as a consequence of the contusion.

ORBITAL AND PERIORBITAL FRACTURES

Orbit fractures, common in the equine, are seen less commonly in ruminants. The dorsal (frontal bone) and

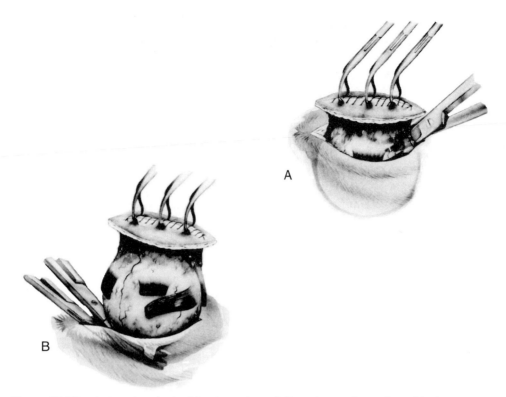

Figure 13-18   *A,* A periocular incision is made and dissection performed outside the extraocular muscles to the orbital apex. *B,* The optic nerve and associated vessels are clamped, ligated, and transected.

(Reprinted with permission from Slatter D: *Fundamentals in veterinary ophthalmology,* ed 3, Philadelphia, 2001, WB Saunders.)

temporal (temporal and zygomatic bones) regions of the bony orbit are most commonly injured. Clinical signs include edema, swelling, pain, blepharospasm, chemosis, subconjunctival hemorrhage that may be accompanied by lacerations, contusions, or other injuries of the face or lids. Subcutaneous emphysema with or without orbital emphysema may be present if the frontal or maxillary sinuses have been fractured and abnormal ocular or nasal discharge may be present. Palpable disruption of the bony orbit rim may be evident if fracture fragments are displaced. The globe may be normally positioned or may be exophthalmic, enophthalmic or have strabismus. Upper eyelid function may be impaired because of tissue swelling or trauma to the palpebral nerve. Rule-outs include orbital cellulitis, orbital extension of sinus disease, orbital neoplasia, and orbital foreign body.

Diagnosis of orbital fractures is generally straightforward if a known traumatic event has occurred. Palpation of the affected area and digital examination of the inside of the orbit rim through the palpebral fissure should be performed once the patient is safely tranquilized and topically anesthetized. Swelling, pain, and the temperament of the animal may prevent complete palpation. Skull radiographs are helpful because orbital fractures are generally much more extensive radiographically than what is evident by palpation. Any combination of skull radiographs, computed tomography, ultrasonography, and MRI may be necessary for full diagnosis.

Eye motility should be thoroughly evaluated by moving the patient's head dorsally, ventrally, laterally and in small circles while simultaneously observing for normal vestibular eye movements, but this may be difficult to accomplish when significant periocular swelling exists. Assessing normal eye movements is important because extraocular muscle entrapment is an indication for surgical repair. Forced ductions of the globe may be necessary for complete evaluation. Forced ductions are performed after moderate sedation and topical anesthesia or under general anesthesia. The limbal conjunctiva is grasped at one or more sites sequentially with small tissue forceps, and the globe is "forced" through all planes of motion.

Symptomatic treatment—including cold compresses, analgesics, and antiinflammatories—is acceptable in cases with normal ocular motility and without fracture fragment displacement. Systemic corticosteroids are used with caution and because of the risks inherent with their use are not recommended unless optic nerve damage is suspected. These include a depressed immune system and the risk of inducing premature labor. Hot compresses may be used after the first 24 hours for 5 to 10 minutes every 2 to 4 hours. Systemic antibiotic therapy is indicated in open fractures, sinus fractures, or skin wounds. Frequent (6 to 8 times or more per day) topical eye lubricants to prevent corneal desiccation are mandatory with any impairment of eyelid function or eyelid integrity. A membrana nictitans flap or tarsorrhaphy may be placed to keep the globe protected. Symptomatic treatment alone is not sufficient if there is significant sinus compromise, displacement of fracture fragments, marked facial deformity, or whenever there is any displacement of the globe or impairment of normal globe movements. Fracture repair is needed urgently in cases of optic nerve compromise.

Fracture repair is most easily accomplished within the first 24 to 48 hours if the condition of the patient permits general anesthesia. Repair may sometimes be accomplished by digital manipulation and bony traction. Many times replacement of the bones close to the original anatomical configuration without fixation is sufficient. If the fractures are unstable more orthopedic manipulation and instrumentation is required such as figure-eight wiring of the bony fragments (see the oral section in Chapter 10 for details on wiring technique).

EYELID AND MEMBRANA NICTITANS DISEASES

Eyelid anatomy varies somewhat across species but there are many common features. Both eyelids should conform and contour perfectly to the globe from the lateral canthus up to the medial 1/6 of the lids where a small separation of lid-to-globe occurs because of the presence of the membrana nictitans or third eyelid. The nictitans should likewise conform perfectly to the globe providing a "squeegee" to the corneal surface with its every excursion. Cilia or eyelashes are present on the upper lids with fewer and smaller lashes present on the lower lids. As the eye is approached from the lashes a flat, hairless lid margin is present that should be perpendicular to the corneal surface over its entire length with no hairs on the lid margin surface (distichia). No eyelid hairs should touch the cornea at any point. If either lid margin is rolled outwards from the cornea ectropion is present, unsightly but not usually irritating or painful to the patient. If either eyelid (usually the lower) is turned inwards, entropion is present and surgical intervention is indicated.

ECTROPION

Ectropion should be corrected in the event of concurrent ocular disease attributable to the eyelid deformation, such as chronic conjunctivitis, keratoconjunctivitis, blepharitis, or facial tear scalding. Ectropion in ruminants is usually secondary to scar tissue formation (*cicatricial ectropion*) but may occur from other causes. True conformational ectropion such as that seen in dogs (Bloodhound) is extremely rare in all large animals. Ectropion may occur in combination with entropion and other eyelid or conjunctival irregularities. A number of corrective procedures have been described, depending on the etiology and degree of disease. Ophthalmic surgical texts should be consulted for details of the surgical procedures. Correction of ectropion can be much more complicated than an entropion correction and may necessitate referral to a specialist.

ENTROPION

Entropion can be congenital, associated with dehydration, particularly in newborns, may occur secondary to microphthalmos or can develop at any age as a result of squinting from eye pain (*spastic entropion*) or secondary to eyelid scarring (*cicatricial entropion*). Entropion is self-perpetuating and must be corrected for patient comfort and corneal and ocular health. Uncorrected entropion can lead to severe keratoconjunctivitis, corneal ulceration, and scarring or possible corneal ulcer perforation. Entropion in some breeds or herds of sheep and goats may have an inherited predisposition and affected animals should be noted, not bred, or culled.

Mild cases of entropion in any species and at any age can be corrected by using a variety of techniques. Newborn animals with entropion secondary to mild dehydration may respond to frequent (every 2 to 3 hours) manual eversion of the eyelid margins in combination with heavy topical lubrication to prevent eyelid spasm while correcting dehydration. If the entropion does not correct within 48 hours or corneal disease develops, additional corrective measures must be taken. Short-term options to effect mechanical eversion of the eyelid margins in cases without corneal disease include injections of saline (very short-term correction) or injections of long-acting antibiotics (3 to 5 days of eversion). These are administered through 22- to 25-g needles placed SQ in the eyelids very close to the lid margins, with care taken to protect the globe during needle placement and injection. A sufficient volume is injected to swell, tense, and evert the eyelid out and away from the cornea (usually 2 to 4 ml).

Entropion of longer duration, spastic entropion associated with corneal disease or entropion in animals that may not be able to be monitored daily (some newborn sheep, goats or calves) necessitate corrections that will maintain longer-term eversion. If only one or two animals are to be treated, horizontal mattress "tacking" sutures of number 3-0 to 4-0 may be placed beginning in the skin of the face, a second bite split-thickness adjacent and parallel to the eyelid margin with the final bite adjacent to the first in the facial skin. As the suture is knotted the lid margin should evert outwards, well away from the cornea (Figure 13-19). The suture ends are trimmed short, and care is taken to ensure that they cannot touch the cornea. If absorbable suture material is

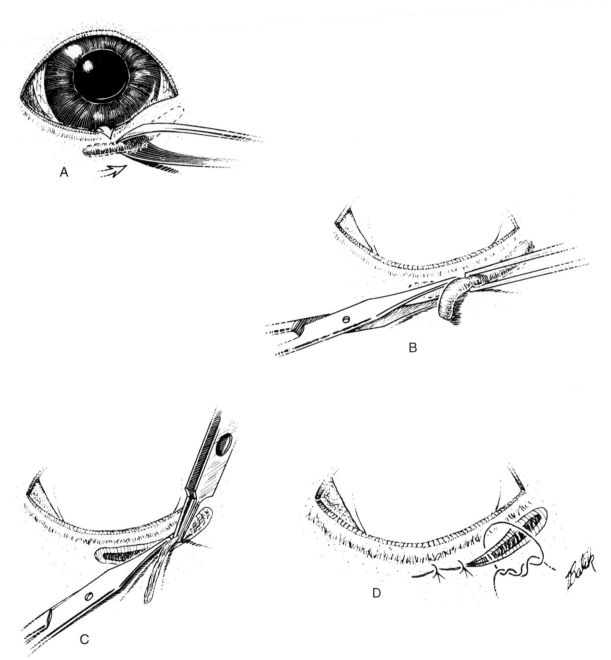

Figure 13-19   Hotz-Celsus procedure for treatment of entropion. *A,* Tenting of skin with Allis tissue forceps 2 mm away from eyelid margin. *B,* Removal of the ridge of skin. *C,* Removal of strip of orbicularis oculi muscle. *D,* Closure of skin: as the suture is knotted, the lid margin should be everted outward.

(Reprinted with permission from Bistner SI, Aguirre G, Batik G: *Atlas of veterinary ophthalmic surgery,* Philadelphia, 1977, WB Saunders.)

used, the sutures will fall out in a few weeks. Suturing is not practical where a large number of animals must be treated and is performed with some risk the needle will injure the eye of a struggling newborn or youngster. Skin staples or wound clips have been used in such cases with good success and are highly recommended. The patient is restrained, and one or more staples are clipped over a fold of skin adjacent to and paralleling the eyelid margin, which that is pinched up using Allis or other tissue forceps. If a clip is improperly placed it can be immediately removed and corrected. Sufficient staples (usually 2-4) are placed to correct the length of turned-in lid margin. The staples will fall out in a few weeks and do not require removal. Concurrent corneal or ocular disease can be treated with topical or subconjunctival medications.

Ruminants rarely require skin removal techniques to correct entropion such as the Hotz-Celsus (see Figure 13-19) and other procedures described in small animal ophthalmology textbooks. These techniques mandate general anesthesia and are reserved for valuable or show stock animals or for cases of cicatricial entropion.

Periocular Fat Pad Hypertrophy in Pot-Bellied Pigs

Entropion in the Vietnamese pot-bellied pig can be extremely difficult to correct and commonly recurs days to months later, particularly in cases with excess periocular fat and conformational enophthalmos. In some cases, true entropion is not actually present, since the lid margin is in normal position. In these cases, the periocular fat pads become thickened, hypertrophied, hardened, heavy, and vision is impaired. Affected pigs are unable to open their eyelids and because of this develop a wide range of related behavior and physical changes including lethargy, apprehension, aggression, loss of interactive capabilities, fear biting, dermatitis, and weight gain. Modified Hotz-Celsus and other skin-removal procedures can be used in the lower eyelid but are almost uniformly unrewarding in the upper eyelid because of the weight or mass of the dorsal fat pad.

The periocular fat pads are most severely enlarged dorsally and most prominent on the dorsolateral aspect of the orbit. Andrea et al. reported that most of the dorsal fat pads measured 2 to 4 cm in width and 4 to 6 cm in length. A few pigs also had fat accumulation along the ventral aspect of the orbit. Attempts at controlling the condition with dietary management were unsuccessful, in part because affected animals are reluctant to move. The authors had good results performing a resection on the hypertrophied fat pad and redundant skin.

The pig is positioned in sternal recumbency under general anesthesia. The periocular skin is prepared for aseptic surgery. To prepare the area the fat pads may need to be lifted so that the underlying skin can be thoroughly cleansed; the tenacious greasy exudates hidden in the heavy thickened folds are very difficult to remove.

A sharp skin incision is made in the cleavage line at the ventral aspect of the fat pad, beginning just rostral to the tragus, extending rostrally, crossing the upper eyelid and redirected dorsomedially to the midline dorsal to the nose. The incision continues toward the midline, crossing the upper eyelid, until it meets the corresponding incision from the other side. The resulting large flap of forehead skin is elevated from the frontal bone, incorporating the fat pad but sparing the muscles of the face—including the parotidoauricularis, the frontoscutularis, and the levator anguli oculi muscles. To allow improved skin pliability the dorsal flap can be tensed and everted by using penetrating bowel or towel clamps while slices of subdermal fat (2 to 4 mm at a time) are removed until the bases of the hair follicles in the overlying skin are visible. Once the skin is freed and all dermal fat debulked to the level of the front of the ears, the skin flap is put back into place and the now pliable excessive skin of the brow is trimmed to create a snug fit between the undermined skin flap and the ventral wound edge. The skin is sutured in an interrupted pattern with No. 0 polypropylene suture material. In some pigs it will be necessary to remove an ellipse of additional redundant skin and fat ventral to the eye and over the bridge of the nose. Perioperative antibiotics and nonsteroidal antiinflammatory drugs are indicated. In the report it was mentioned all nine pigs had a favorable outcome, with minor postoperative discomfort. Vision was restored in all animals, and all owners responded that the outcome was favorable in regards to postoperative appearance and improvements in behavior (Andrea et al., 1999).

EYELID LACERATIONS

Eyelid lacerations usually occur because the individual has caught the upper or lower eyelid on a hook, nail, or other pointed object; the apparent laceration may actually be an avulsion or rupture of the tissue that occurs as the patient pulls the head away. Some apparent lid lacerations are actually a result of blunt compression or crushing and in such cases tissue trauma may be very extensive.

The diagnosis is usually obvious. The wound may be a simple laceration perpendicular to the lid margin, a flap of eyelid hanging from a pedicle, or a laceration that has removed the lid margin. The wound is usually edematous and bloody, with tears and mucoid to mucopurulent ocular discharge apparent in the periocular area. The individual is usually in mild to moderate pain. A fluorescein dye test must be performed to assess the integrity of the cornea. A complete ocular examination, including intraocular exam, should be performed as soon as possible. Any corneal or other ocular injury should be treated appropriately. The eye is lubricated and protected from self-trauma before, during, and after the examination. If the etiology is unknown, skull radiographs may be indicated to rule out metallic foreign bodies.

Any eyelid laceration that breaches the eyelid margin should be repaired as soon as possible, depending on the condition of the patient, to ensure normal eyelid function and corneal health. Many eyelid lacerations in ruminants can be repaired under sedation and local anesthesia, but general anesthesia may be needed for the best cosmetic and functional result and for extensive injury cases. Owners or veterinarians tend to treat eyelid lacerations by simply trimming away the thin flaps of tissue hanging from the remaining eyelid. This should not be done. Seemingly redundant eyelid tissue or flaps of eyelid margins should be incorporated into the closure. No other tissue in the body can substitute for missing eyelid margin and removal of these thin strips of tissue can result in a lifetime of chronic discomfort for the animal because of irritation from hairs present at the edge of the wound that will become the new eyelid margin. Removal or improper repair of an eyelid margin leads to chronic corneal disease from irritation by eyelid hairs (trichiasis), exposure keratitis due to improper spreading of the tear film over the cornea, and chronic keratoconjunctivitis due to an inability of the eye to properly cleanse itself.

Perioperative antibiotics are indicated. Lid lacerations can be repaired under local anesthesia and sedation if the patient is cooperative and the repair is a simple one. General anesthesia should be used in all cases of complicated repairs or if the patient is difficult to manage. In either case, repeated topical anesthetic applications may be helpful during surgery. Clipping the lid hair around the wound may be necessary in many cases but not all and can be troublesome because the small cut hairs are difficult to eliminate from the wound. Coating the wound before clipping with sterile gel may prevent hair contamination, but the lubricant must be washed carefully away during wound preparation. The periocular tissues should be thoroughly cleansed with 10% povidone-iodine solution with sterile saline rinses. The wound should be checked carefully for any foreign bodies. Wound debridement should be extremely minimal to preserve as much eyelid tissue as possible, and eyelid margin must be conserved whenever possible. Tissue that appears hopelessly desiccated, inflamed, and/or infected may heal well if properly repaired. Wound debridement is best performed by simply rubbing with dry gauze until bleeding is noted, but wounds that are more than 24 hours old may require scarification with a #15 scalpel blade, taking care not to remove tissue, only to restore a liberally bleeding surface.

Full-thickness wounds should be closed in 2 to 3 layers with 3-0 to 5-0 absorbable sutures according to the size of the patient and thickness of the eyelid. The fibrous tarsal plate and orbicularis oculi muscle should be incorporated in the deep layer and the subcuticular tissues in a second layer. Careful examination of the deeper layers of the eyelid may be needed to identify the thin connective tissue layer of the eyelid, the tarsal plate, but this is the most important layer to incorporate in the deep sutures. The first suture placed is the most important; it should appose the eyelid margins perfectly. Figure-8 sutures in this fibrous muscle layer are very useful and highly recommended because they allow excellent wound apposition and position the knot well away from the eyelid margin. This suture is tightened but not tied. If placement is not exact and a "step" develops in the eyelid margin, the suture is replaced. This suture should be preplaced to facilitate placement of other sutures. Additional deep sutures are placed as necessary, depending on the length of the laceration. Skin closure is routine, but the ends of skin sutures placed near the eyelid margin must be secured well away from the lid margin to prevent corneal irritation. Synthetic absorbable sutures (4-0) can be used successfully in the skin and do not require removal. Regardless of the suture pattern chosen, the surgeon should always ensure that sutures do not penetrate the full thickness of the eyelid at any point, and suture knots and ends must not touch the cornea.

Severe lacerations may need stent support during healing. Eyelids can be successfully stented to the opposing eyelid via tarsorrhaphy, using split-thickness horizontal mattress sutures in the eyelid margins. If the eyelids must be closed, a transpalpebral lavage apparatus should be preplaced for administration of topical medications (if needed) before the lids are closed (see Transpalpebral Ocular Lavage Apparatus, Figure 13-3), or a sufficient opening should be left at the medial or lateral canthus to allow instillation of medications. Lacerations in the area of the medial canthus require careful assessment of the nasolacrimal system. If the canaliculi have been lacerated and full restoration to function is desired such as in show animals, microsurgical repair is indicated as soon as possible after the injury.

Postoperative medical management should include warm compresses, if possible, for 10 minutes every 2 to 3 hours for 2 to 3 days. Topical corticosteroids should be avoided. Topical broad-spectrum antibiotic six times a day for 24 hours, then four times a day for 7 to 10 days is indicated if excessive tissue injury is present or if corneal integrity is in doubt but otherwise is not necessary. If the cornea is injured, topical medications are chosen more judiciously and administered more intensively. Caretakers should be advised to avoid placing unnecessary tension or stress on the eyelid during the application of topical medications. If this is not possible, topical ophthalmic antibiotic solutions may be sprayed onto the cornea via medication in a tuberculin syringe with the needle hub attached but with the needle broken off the hub. This makes a very effective, simple, medication "squirt gun." Systemic antibiotics are indicated for 5 to 7 days; systemic antiinflammatories are indicated if excessive inflammation or discomfort is present. Self-trauma should be prevented, and the periocular area should be cleansed as often as exudates and discharges accumulate. After cleansing and drying, the area of the face beneath the eye should be coated with a film of petrolatum jelly to prevent hair loss from irritation by ocular secretions. The eye should be examined daily to ensure normal eyelid function and no suture irritation.

PALPEBRAL NERVE PARALYSIS

The palpebral nerve is a branch of the auriculopalpebral branch of the facial nerve. Palpebral nerve paralysis and the resultant inability to blink the eyelids in one or both eyes is usually of traumatic origin as a result of stanchion or chute trauma to the palpebral branch of the auriculopalpebral nerve(s). Chronic otitis media or brainstem diseases should be ruled out, especially if the entire facial nerve is involved. The absence of a palpebral reflex is diagnostic.

The initial clinical sign is ptosis of the affected eye(s) followed subacutely by tearing and chronically by exposure keratitis, corneal ulceration, and corneal hyperkeratosis. Corneal ulcers are usually central to ventrotemporal paracentral and may be superficial to deep.

Acute treatment includes antiinflammatories, hot compresses, topical DMSO at the site of trauma and systemic steroids unless contraindicated. Topical ophthalmic lubricants should be applied at least 4 to 8 times daily until lid function returns. Topical antibiotics are given four or more times daily in cases that have corneal ulcers. Membrana nictitans flaps or temporary tarsorrhaphy may be indicated if topical medications cannot be applied at sufficient frequency to maintain corneal health.

A temporary tarsorrhaphy can be performed under sedation, local and topical anesthesia. Nonabsorbable suture, 3-0 or 4-0, is placed first through a stent (rubber band piece, portion of 3.5 French red rubber feeding tube, button, etc.), and then a bite is made partial thickness through the eyelid, with the needle entering the skin 4 to 5 mm posterior to the lid margin and exiting beneath the lashes through the central hairless portion of the eyelid margin. The suture should be inspected to ensure that at no point does it penetrate the conjunctiva, where it could contact the globe. While the cornea is protected, the suture is continued across the palpebral fissure to the opposite lid margin and enters on the margin and exits the skin in a similar manner. Another stent is placed, the needle direction is reversed, and the mattress suture completed, ending with a final bite through the stent. Several sutures may be preplaced, and while the cornea is protected, the sutures are tightened and knotted. A bow-type knot may be placed, if desired, to allow the lids to be opened intermittently for corneal examination, but in such cases care must be taken so the long suture ends do not rub the cornea. This is accomplished most easily if the sutures are begun in the lower lid with the resultant knots and suture ends ventral to the eye.

The temporary tarsorrhaphy is a useful procedure but is reserved for cases that require temporary corneal protection (few days to a few weeks, at most). The procedure requires careful attention by the caregiver so that loose sutures do not rub the cornea, a common complication as initial swelling of eyelids decreases. A large amount of ocular and suture-induced exudate tends to accumulate on the sutures over time, is esthetically displeasing and may cause ocular or skin irritation.

If eyelid function is not expected to return in a short time, a reversible split-lid tarsorrhaphy (Figure 13-20A-C) can be performed. This is an extremely useful procedure for cases of unilateral or bilateral facial nerve palsy or paralysis which can be left in place permanently or which can be opened gradually from medial to lateral as nerve function returns—in 6 weeks or in 6 years. Reversible split-lid tarsorrhaphy is a very simple, useful procedure that closes the temporal $\frac{1}{2}$-$\frac{3}{4}$ of the palpebral fissure to provide permanent protection to the cornea but can be opened at a later date if there is return of normal lid function. If needed, this tarsorrhaphy has also been left in place for months to years. As the focal wounds heal some tissue stretching occurs, and the lid margins will separate sufficiently medially and possibly between the focal tarsorrhaphies to allow the patient to see. With sufficient time, full return of normal facial nerve function occurs in many cases of VII nerve paralysis, the reversible split-lid tarsorrhaphy can be opened gradually from medial to lateral simply with sedation and a snip of small scissors. Because the lid margins are not removed, there is minimal lid scarring and excellent lid function.

General anesthesia is preferred for this procedure, but it has been performed many times under heavy sedation with local anesthesia. With a #64 Beaver or #15 Bard-Parker scalpel blade, two 6- to 7-mm incisions are made perpendicularly through the upper eyelid margin, following the Meibomian (or tarsal) gland orifices, incising to a depth of 4 to 6 mm, that splits the lid into inner and outer layers (see Figure 13-20 A and B). One incision

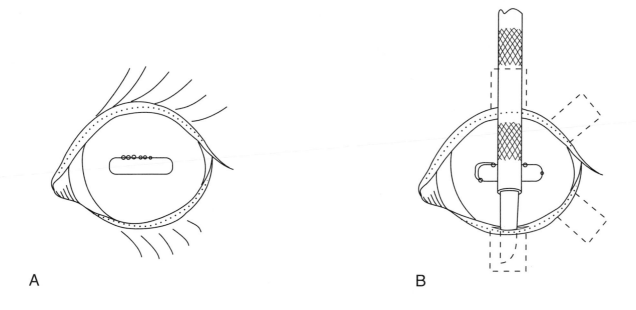

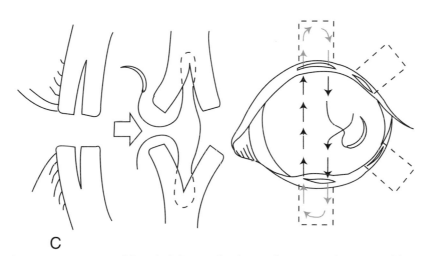

Figure 13-20   Reversible split lid tarsorrhaphy. *A,* Illustration of upper and lower lid margins slightly everted to show the "dotted line" of tarsal gland openings. *B,* A no. 64 Beaver blade is used to incise just inside the tarsal gland splitting the tissues into 2 layers: skin-orbicularis muscle layer externally and tarsal plate-conjunctiva layer internally to a depth of 5 to 7 mm. Four incisions are made at two apposing sites on each lid as shown. *C,* With a 5-0 Vicryl, a single simple interrupted suture is preplaced into the apex of each "pocket." After both bites are placed, they are tied securely to ensure that the knots are buried. For extra security or in lids with normal tone, the sutures are placed through the outer skin-orbicularis layer.

should be placed centrally in the upper lid and the second in the temporal $\frac{1}{3}$ of the upper lid. The eyelid margins are not removed; the lids are merely split into two layers: inner and outer. Corresponding incisions (same position, length and depth) are made in the lower lid margin. The lower lid margin is less well-defined than the upper and careful attention must be paid to ensure that the lid is

split properly into outer skin/muscle layer and inner tarsal plate/conjunctiva. The inner layer (upper or lower lid) must not contain any hairs or hair follicles because it will be everted towards and touching the cornea after closure. Using 5-0 absorbable suture, the surgeon places a single suture deep in the apex of each pocket paralleling the lid margin (see Figure 13-20C). When these sutures are tied they bring the corresponding upper and lower eyelid wounds together in a "kiss" that everts the inner (tarsal plate/conjunctiva) layers towards the cornea and the skin/muscle layers externally. The knots should bury easily within the "kiss" and suture ends are trimmed short. Several horizontal mattress absorbable sutures are placed in the skin-muscle layer, further everting all hairs and ensuring wound security. Sutures do not require removal if absorbable and 4-0 or smaller.

The lids will look over-corrected or almost completely closed initially due to lid swelling, but the medial portion of the palpebral fissure will open in a few days. As healing completes and tissue stretching occurs, small openings may be present centrally and laterally and these allow seemingly excellent vision. Medications can be applied through the open medial portion of the palpebral fissure.

Depending on the cause of the paralysis, normal eyelid function may not return for weeks or many months, if ever. Eyelid function should be assessed regularly by the owner. If a palpebral reflex returns, the medial spot tarsorrhaphy can be opened initially with small scissors; the more temporal spot can be opened once normal function is present or can be left in place for life. Vision is usually normal through the enlarged medial canthal opening.

EYELID TUMORS

Eyelid masses often are seen in cattle but are less common in other ruminants or pigs. Papillomas (warts), benign skin masses of probable viral origin, are commonly seen periocularly in cattle but are also seen in sheep and goats. They are usually self-limiting, and spontaneous regression is likely. Papillomas that involve the eyelid margins, or are of sufficient size in the periocular area to cause irritation to the eye, should be removed. Small ruminants with self-limiting wartlike masses should be evaluated for contagious ecthyma, a zoonotic disease.

Depending on the type of tumor, its location, and the equipment available, the tumors may be removed surgically, or by cryotherapy, hyperthermia (see Figure 4.4-24A), or radiofrequency. A combination of these modalities can also be used.

The most common eyelid tumor seen in cattle is squamous cell carcinoma (SCC). It can involve the eyelid(s) (Figure 13-21), the membrane nictitans (Figure 13-22A and B), conjunctiva (Figure 13-23), or cornea (Figure 13-24). The tumor is locally aggressive in almost all cases and metastasizes late in the course of the disease. Pre-

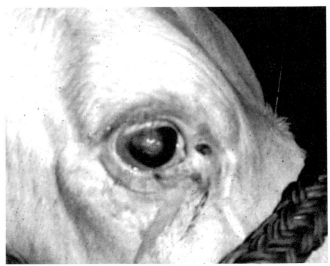

Figure 13-21   Squamous cell carcinoma of lower eyelid in a cow.

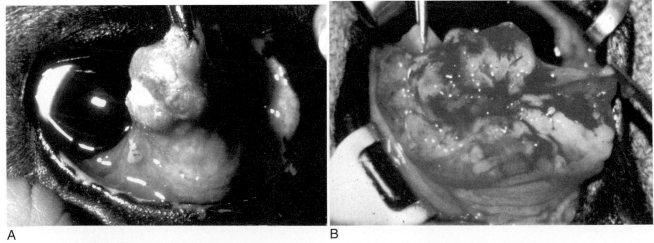

A   B

Figure 13-22   *A,* Squamous cell carcinoma of the membrane nictitans suitable for a standing nictitans excision. Note the wide border of normal nictitans below (and above) the lesion. *B,* More extensive SCC nictitans and conjunctiva lesion, which require more dissection, thus making the lesion unsuitable for a standing surgical procedure.

cursor lesions (Figure 13-25) (e.g., carcinoma in situ) can resemble papillomas, granulomas, or epithelial inclusion cysts. The diagnosis is based on the appearance of the tumor and is confirmed by histopathological evaluation of the scraping or biopsy of the lesion.

Many therapeutic modalities are used to treat squamous cell carcinomas. Different therapeutic approaches are used in feedlot cattle in comparison to those used in valuable breeding animals. Early recognition of small tumors less than 2.0 cm in diameter allows consideration of some less invasive therapeutic techniques for SCC.

Small tumors of the eyelids may be removed by sharp excision if sufficient functional lid margin remains (Figure 13-26 A and B). In an adult bovine, this usually means the tumor should be less than 1 centimeter in

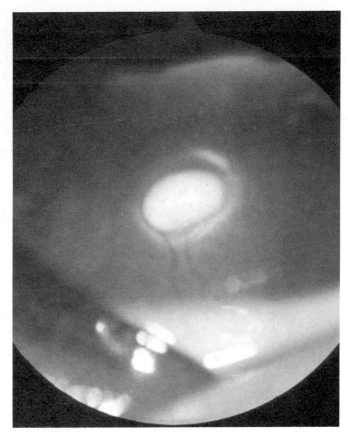

Figure 13-25   Corneal dyskeratosis—a precancerous lesion in a 2-year-old bull.

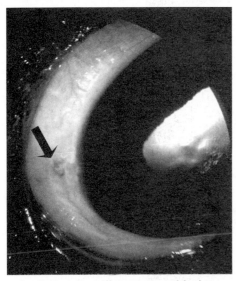

Figure 13-23   Squamous cell carcinoma (black mass at arrow) of the conjunctiva in a cow.

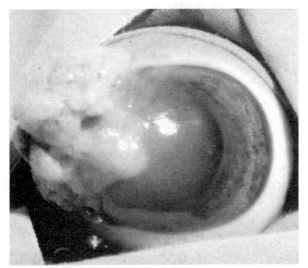

Figure 13-24   Squamous cell carcinoma of the cornea in a cow.

diameter. Although a "wedge" excision of the eyelid is described in many older references as appropriate to remove lid margin tumors, a wedge removal should not be used because maximum eyelid marginal tissue is removed. A "tent"-shaped excision is preferred because it maximizes the amount of eyelid preserved (Figure 13-27). After routine preparation of the eye and periocular tissues, the eyelid is first inspected carefully to confirm the extent of the tumor. A lid forceps or clamp with a solid lower plate such as a Snellen Entropion forceps or Demarres Chalazion forceps, if available, is placed around the lesion and tightened to gently compress the lid tissue. The use of such clamps is a significant aid to hemostasis, and the solid lower plate provides a firm surface for incision. Two sharp incisions are made with a #15 Bard-Parker scalpel blade, one on either side of the tumor, and as much eyelid margin as possible is conserved. These incisions are perpendicular to the eyelid margin and extend into the affected lid just as far as the tumor (see Figure 13-27). These two incisions are then connected in a "v" so the excised piece of lid is shaped somewhat like a tent, with the lid margin being the base. The wound is closed as described for lid lacerations; a figure-8 suture is preferred in the connective tissue layer. Postoperative management includes cold compresses if

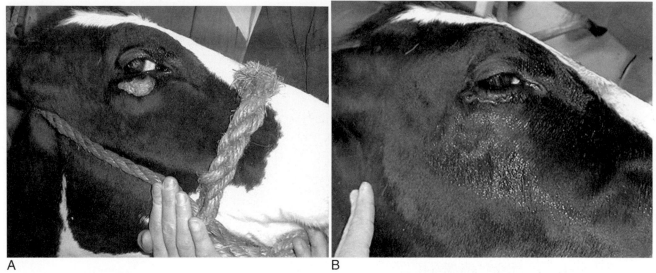

Figure 13-26   *A,* Papilloma on the lower eyelid of a calf. *B,* Calf after surgery to remove lower eyelid lesion. An elliptical incision was made and the skin closed primarily.

(Courtesy Dr. Norm G. Ducharme; Cornell University.)

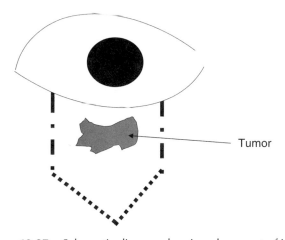

Tumor

Figure 13-27   Schematic diagram showing placement of incisions for removal of larger eyelid tumor.

needed for 24 hours and topical antibiotics 3 times a day. The eye should be examined daily for increased squinting, tearing, clouding, redness or pain. If these occur, veterinary attention will be needed. Suture irritation should be ruled out.

Cryosurgery can be appropriate for small- to moderate-sized lesions. The cow is sedated, restrained, and the surgical site desensitized with a local (and/or topical) anesthetic. The area to be frozen is identified. Adjacent areas are protected by petroleum jelly. The eye itself is carefully covered with a shield. Two freeze-thaw cycles are performed with a probe, cup, or spray. The periph-

ery of the lesion should reach −40.0°C. Effective time of cryodestruction is 10 to 20 minutes once temperature equilibrium has been reached. To maximize results with cryosurgery, the operator strives for two quick-freeze/slow-thaw cycles. Frozen tissue sloughs in 7 to 14 days; new hair growth can come in white. The eye should be monitored carefully for 2 to 3 weeks afterwards to ensure that sloughing tissue does not cause corneal irritation. Topical antibiotics may be needed for 7 to 14 days.

Radiofrequency hyperthermia* is ideal for small tumors that can be debulked before application of this device. Penetration is only 0.5 to 1.0 cm; therefore it is not an appropriate procedure for larger masses. Reports in beef cattle are encouraging, although multiple treatments may be necessary.

As is the case with many carcinomas, SCC is a radiosensitive tumor. Very small lesions less than 2 mm in depth can be treated with 7,500 to 10,000 rads of β radiation with a strontium applicator[†] (Figure 13-28 A and B). However, β particles do not penetrate deeply and a strontium probe is not useful for penetrating larger mass lesions. Other radiation treatments such as implanted radon seeds (Brachytherapy) may be effective, but radiation laws limit their practicality.

---

*Hach RF 22A Thermoprobe Device, Hach Chemical Co., Loveland, CO
[†]AmerSham International, AmerSham Laboratories, White Lion Road, Bucks, UK; or the American subsidiary, American Corporation, 2636 Clearbrook Drive, Arlington Heights, IL

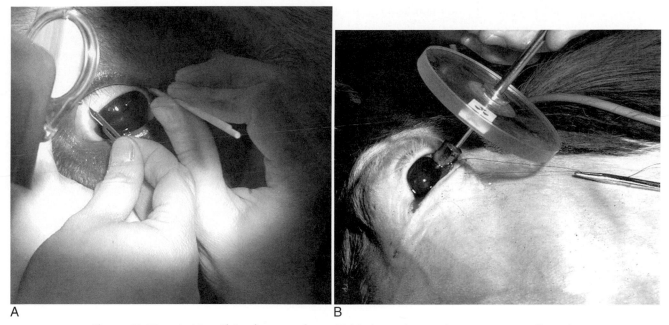

Figure 13-28 *A,* Magnifying loupe and no. 15 blade used to excise squamous cell carcinoma from the lateral limbus in a cow before beta radiation. Q-tips are used in the opposite fornix to position the globe. *B,* Use of the strontium applicator.

MEMBRANA NICTITANS EXCISION

SCC also commonly develops on the membrana nictitans. If the tumors are less than 2 to 2.5 cm in diameter and involve only the free margin of the nictitans like the mass in Figure 13-22A, they can be successfully removed by excising the entire nictitating membrane with the animal standing. Although this procedure can result in keratoconjunctivitis sicca in a dog or cat, large animal species depend less on the secretions of the membrana nictitans gland, and it can usually be removed without consequence.

The patient should be premedicated for 24 hours with topical antibiotics. After sedation, the eyelids are paralyzed and topical anesthesia applied. The conjunctival sac is lavaged with sterile saline. The eye is retropulsed, and the nictitans is grasped with a hemostat on the free margin. The nictitans is everted, and the extent of the tumor on the bulbar surface of the nictitans is confirmed. The surgeon ensures sufficient normal nictitans tissue dorsally and ventrally to allow complete removal. As the nictitans is stretched across the cornea towards the lateral canthus, curved Kelly hemostats are clamped across the folds of normal nictitans conjunctiva dorsal and ventral to the tumor so their tips almost touch each other medially at the base of the "T" cartilage. Scissors or a scalpel blade held in the fingers are used to cut along the clamps, leaving the clamps on the patient. A third clamp is then placed across the base of the "T" cartilage and the remainder of the nictitans excised. The clamps should remain on the patient for at least 5 minutes, longer if possible. The eye and lids must not be manipulated after the procedure is completed except to remove the clamps.

Complications are uncommon but include incomplete excision, excessive hemorrhage, and, rarely, orbit fat prolapse. Incomplete excision should not occur if the clamps are carefully applied. If clear margins sufficient for clamp placement beyond the tumor are not available, the procedure should be aborted and removal under general anesthesia planned. Hemorrhage and orbit fat prolapse occur rarely if the clamps remain in place for at least 5 minutes. Hemorrhage can be controlled by manual direct pressure or a pressure bandage applied to the head and left in place for 24 hours. Orbit fat prolapse is of more concern and will worsen as the patient wakes up and retracts the eyeball. If possible, the clamps should be replaced and the conjunctiva oversewn with 5-0 synthetic absorbable suture. Prolapsing fat should not be removed because chronic enophthalmos will result. General anesthesia may be required to replace severe fat prolapses.

OTHER CONDITIONS INVOLVING THE MEMBRANA NICTITANS

Other than SCC, major diseases of the nictitating membrane are rare. Lacerations of the nictitans can occur and, if extensive, should be repaired or the nictitans can be excised as described above, although there may be some loss of normal tear production. Traumatized nictitans require careful examination to ensure the cartilage is not exposed on the bulbar surface, which could cause chronic corneal irritation.

Orbital fat may prolapse into the nictitans and resemble a neoplastic swelling; lymphosarcoma should be ruled out in these cases. The lacrimal gland surrounding the cartilage at the base of the nictitans can become hypertrophied. This may resolve with topical or intralesional steroids or may require clamping and excision. Normal tear function should be ascertained before this procedure. The nictitans is a common site for seclusion of foreign bodies (usually plant material) and the bulbar surface of the nictitans must be examined in all cases of refractory corneal ulcers. In sheep and goats, intense follicular hyperplasia of the nictitans may occur with conjunctivitis caused by *Chlamydia* spp., *Mycoplasma* spp., or *Rickettsia* spp.

CONJUNCTIVAL AND CORNEAL DISEASES

Dermoids are a common congenital problem that affects the cornea and conjunctiva of large animals (Figure 13-29). In cattle and other large animal species, they are readily diagnosed because they appear as a piece of skin attached to the cornea, conjunctiva, sclera, and/or eyelids (Figures 13-30 and 13-31).

Affected animals may be asymptomatic for a short time after birth if the dermoids are small or nonhaired. Most cases quickly develop chronic conjunctivitis, epiphora, blepharospasm, and ocular discomfort. Corneal ulceration may occur as a result of poor distribution of the tear film. Large dermoids of the cornea may cause visual impairment or blindness. Given the chronic irritation and discomfort associated with the dermoid, excision is warranted if the affected animal is to be kept. Dermoids may be associated with other intraocular anomalies and a careful ophthalmic examina-

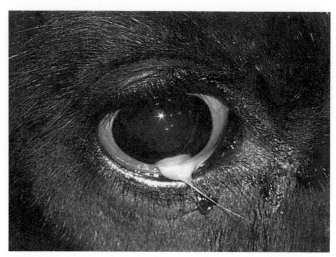

Figure 13-30   Epiphora and chronic conjunctivitis in the right eye of same patient.

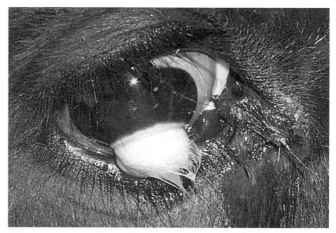

Figure 13-31   Dermoids originating from cornea in a cow.

tion concentrating on the anterior chamber, iris, and lens is warranted, particularly if surgical removal is planned. A slit lamp biomicroscopic examination by a trained individual may be helpful in these cases (Figure 13-32).

Dermoids that do not involve deeper layers of the eye may be removed by lamellar superficial keratectomy using conventional sharp excision or removed via CO_2 or excimer laser ablation. CO_2 lasers can cause extensive damage to normal corneal tissue and should be used with caution. Cryosurgery is not recommended because of the potential for extensive damage to adjacent corneal endothelial cells with resultant chronic corneal edema.

A superficial lamellar keratectomy is most easily performed with an operating microscope but can be done using a simple magnifying loupe. Specialized instrumentation—including an operating microscope—allows a quicker, more precise surgery with less postoperative

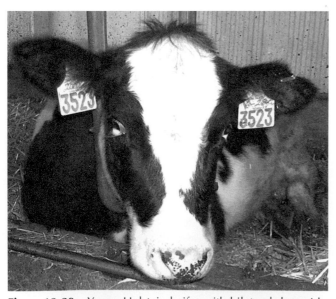

Figure 13-29   Young Holstein heifer with bilateral dermoids.

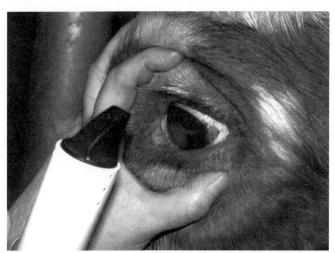

Figure 13-32   Slit lamp biomicroscopic examination of temporal limbal squamous cell carcinoma.

scarring. Minimal instrumentation should include an eyelid speculum or retractors, 1 × 2 mm toothed Bishop-Harmon or Colibri forceps, a #64 Beaver blade or #15 Bard-Parker blade, a Castroviejo needle holder and Stevens' tenotomy scissors. A Martinez corneal dissector is highly recommended to facilitate undermining the lesion by lamellar corneal separation.

General anesthesia is strongly recommended because precise, controlled corneal incision and dissection is extremely difficult to perform on an eyeball that is moving. The eye is clipped and prepped, previously mentioned. The cornea is incised circumlesionally; extreme care is used to avoid incising too deeply and breaching the anterior chamber. Hand stability is much improved if the surgeon is sitting with forearms supported. The base or sides of the surgeon's palms should be resting on the patient's head anytime the cornea is incised or held. Most dermoids are quite superficial and involve the epithelium and very superficial stroma; the initial circumlesional incision should extend to the superficial stroma. Incisional depth can be difficult to judge without an operating microscope, but a good guideline is to carry the incision just deep enough to see a clear separation of the wound edges. The beginning surgeon usually makes too shallow an incision so only the epithelium is incised and the wound margins do not separate even though the incision is visible. When the epithelial basement membrane and the most superficial stroma are incised, the wound edges relax because of the looser intracellular connections present in the stroma.

If the dermoid extends beyond the limbus, the surrounding conjunctiva should be incised with tenotomy scissors. After the initial incision surrounding the whole lesion, the corneal wound edge to be removed is grasped

with a small-toothed tissue forceps and elevated slightly while the corneal dissector is introduced. If a Martinez dissector is not available, a #64 Beaver blade can be used to undermine the lesion, but extra care should be taken because the blades are much sharper than the dissector. The corneal dissector is gently rotated while it is advanced beneath the lesion and separates the corneal lamellae; it should advance easily if it is in stroma. Once the dissector has been introduced and the lamellar dissection begun, the surgeon should take care to keep the dissection in the same plane. If the corneal dissector does not advance easily the dermoid may extend into the deeper corneal tissues or the initial plane of dissection may be too shallow. As dissection progresses, bleeding may be encountered if the lesion and dissection cross the limbus and the corneal dissector will fail to advance easily. Tenotomy scissors or scalpel incision may be necessary to remove the remaining lesion. The wound bed is inspected to ensure complete removal; any excess bleeding from the conjunctiva and sclera can be controlled with gentle pressure applied for a minute or so or with a spray of 1:10,000 epinephrine. The cut conjunctival edge can be secured to the limbus by using a simple continuous pattern of 5-0 synthetic absorbable suture with the knots trimmed short. If, during surgical excision, the lesion is found to be deeper than expected, the cornea may require reinforcement with a conjunctival flap.

The eye is treated postoperatively as for a corneal ulcer by using 1% atropine BID-TID to control the uncomfortable ciliary muscle spasm that occurs with corneal disease and topical broad spectrum antibiotics four times a day. The eye should be inspected daily for a few days to ensure the cornea is stable and infection or corneal malacia do not develop. Recheck at 1 week should reveal that a lesion initially 1 cm in diameter is no longer retaining fluorescein stain; larger lesions will heal in 10-14 days in almost all cases.

LACERATIONS AND RUPTURES OF THE CORNEA AND/OR SCLERA

If any suspicion of laceration of the cornea or sclera exists, the owner should be instructed not to touch or attempt to examine it and to prevent the patient from causing self-trauma to the eye. Examination of the eye or periocular area by the owner or veterinarian should not be performed until the patient has been heavily sedated and the eyelids paralyzed. Failure to follow these guidelines can result in a simple laceration becoming a hopeless evisceration. Instruct the owner that not even eye medications should be applied to the eye until the examination has been completed. No ophthalmic ointment should be placed in a lacerated eye during the examination, preoperative preparation, or surgery, because it can cause chronic intractable inflammatory disease if it gets inside the eye.

The diagnosis of a corneal laceration is usually obvious with a corneal and/or scleral defect of variable size that is usually "plugged" with fibrin, iris, or other uveal tissue. The globe may appear smaller than normal because of leakage of aqueous humor from the eye, and the anterior chamber, if visible, may be shallow or collapsed. Small to large amounts of fibrin, hypopyon, and/or hyphema may be present in the anterior chamber. Fluorescein stain should be applied to determine wound leakage (a clear stream of aqueous in fluorescein-stained tears) and to assess for other corneal damage; fluorescein will stain the wound margins and may cause fluorescence of the aqueous humor if the wound is not yet sealed. During the examination, it is important to assess the nature and extent of the eye injury and to evaluate for neurologic or other injuries elsewhere on the body. A complete extraocular and intraocular examination of both eyes should be attempted, but examination of the inside of the affected globe can be difficult if fibrin, hyphema, miosis, severe corneal edema, or anterior chamber collapse are present. A focal, very bright light should be used to assess the consensual papillary light response. The dazzle reflex (a subcortical response of partial, bilateral blinking of the eyelids in response to a quick, very bright light stimulus) should be assessed because it can indicate an intact visual pathway to the level of the midbrain. Transpalpebral ultrasonography can be performed to assess lens integrity and position and to assess and characterize posterior segment damage and can be a valuable supporting tool for prognosis in many cases. It should only be performed under very heavy sedation or general anesthesia. If the animal is awake and resistant to the procedure, ocular movements or retractor bulbi contractions can cause further prolapse or distortion of intraocular contents. A heavy coating of sterile ultrasound coupling gel should be applied to the closed lids, and a transpalpebral scan should be performed with no pressure applied to the globe. Gel must not enter the palpebral fissure. A stand-off pad is not recommended because its use applies further weight/pressure to the eye.

All lacerations of the globe have a guarded prognosis because of the possibility for infection, but certain lacerations carry a guarded to grave prognosis; enucleation or intrascleral prosthesis placement should be discussed with the owner instead of repair. Restoration of a visual eye is extremely unlikely in these cases, and many will develop phthisis bulbi, a shrunken and often painful eye. Any laceration associated with proptosis, 50% or greater hyphema, lens rupture/dislocation or as a result of severe blunt trauma carries a very guarded prognosis. Cases with ruptured lenses require phacoemulsification to remove all lens cortical material or chronic uveitis results in most cases. Lacerations of greater than 24-hour duration with a flat anterior chamber have a guarded prognosis. An eye ruptured from blunt trauma carries a grave prognosis because the intense blunt force required to rupture the eye usually results in multiple, severe intraocular damage. Extensive laceration with prolapse of intraocular contents other than aqueous or iris tissue carries a poor prognosis, but the examiner should be sure that suspected vitreous prolapse is not just clotted aqueous. Lacerations that extend across the limbus into the sclera have a poor prognosis if a large amount of uveal tissue has prolapsed through the scleral wound. Prolapsed uveal tissue in these cases usually includes the ciliary body, and damage to the ciliary body results in decreased aqueous humor production, hypotony, and phthisis bulbi. The uveal tissue prolapse through the sclera can occur beneath an intact overlying conjunctiva, and if the conjunctiva is swollen or hemorrhagic, the prolapse can be difficult to confirm by visualization. Because many of these types of injuries develop phthisis bulbi, if the client wants to preserve the appearance of a somewhat normal eye, an intraocular prosthesis can be placed through the wound at the time of the initial surgery after complete removal of intraocular contents or as a second procedure performed immediately upon recognition of shrinkage of the globe. Lacerations that are heavily contaminated or are caused by a perforating injury have a high likelihood of infection and are not candidates for prosthesis placement.

Lacerations with a fair prognosis include those that are not full-thickness, those with a formed anterior chamber, and those with only a small amount of hemorrhage or fibrin in the anterior chamber or on the surface of the cornea. Iris may protrude through and close the wound, but there is minimal distortion of intraocular structures. Full-thickness lacerations require immediate surgical repair under general anesthesia. Wounds that are not full thickness but with margins separated by more than 2 to 3 mm also need surgical repair under general anesthesia. Referral to a veterinary ophthalmologist is recommended for all but the simplest cases. Surgery should not be attempted unless standard ophthalmic surgery instruments and appropriately sized suture are available. The repair is usually more difficult than anticipated. Magnification is essential, but only a few specialized instruments are needed, most of which are described above for lamellar keratectomy.

Repairs should always be performed under general anesthesia. Ketamine is to be avoided for general anesthesia or induction, and muscle relaxants are sometimes needed as part of anesthetic protocol to eliminate nystagmus. The eye must be protected during induction so that further injury and tissue prolapse does not occur.

After preparation of the surgical field, the wound should be cultured.

The eye should be gently lavaged and cleansed, and any healthy-appearing prolapsed uveal tissue (usually iris) should be replaced into the anterior chamber in acute injuries. The surgeon must understand that postoperative uveitis is proportional to the degree of uveal damage/handling. Necrotic, desiccated, macerated uveal tissue is carefully excised if necessary. A rule of thumb is to always excise uveal tissue that is clearly contaminated or that has been prolapsed longer than 24 hours. Uveal excision can result in severe hemorrhage. Battery-operated microcautery* devices are extremely helpful in these cases. The anterior chamber is irrigated and then reformed with balanced salt solution or lactated Ringer's. The lens is inspected if possible. Viscoelastic substances are used to assist chamber formation and dissection of uveal tissue but may require removal before complete wound closure or postoperative ocular hypertension can result.

Wound apposition should be precise and is greatly improved if binocular magnification is used. Appropriate suture size varies somewhat with the size of the patient; 7-0 or 8-0 polyglactin 910 ophthalmic suture may be the most practical since it does not require removal. Sutures should be placed 1 to 1.5 mm apart—as deep as possible in the stroma—but must not be full-thickness; entry and exit points of the suture should be perpendicular to the corneal surface and wound edge, respectively. Sutures should be tightened just to the point of tissue apposition; overly tight sutures can cause deep wound gapping. The chamber is reformed after wound closure with lactated Ringer's or BSS through a 27- to 30-gauge needle inserted at the limbus. Wound integrity should be confirmed by applying fluorescein to the corneal surface while applying gentle external pressure to the globe. Unstable, irregular wounds or repairs may be reinforced with a conjunctival flap, but this is not usually necessary unless the security of the wound closure is in doubt. Conjunctival flap placement almost always results in a denser, more opaque corneal scar postoperatively. Ophthalmic texts should be consulted for details on conjunctival flap placement. A transpalpebral lavage device should be placed at this time if desired. The eye should not be covered by a tarsorrhaphy or membrana nictitans flap except during the immediate postoperative and recovery period unless there is a strong indication for the procedure. Nictitans flaps and temporary tarsorrhaphies can cause corneal irritation. Furthermore, nictitans flap placement can increase intraocular pressure, thus resulting in wound leakage, and both preclude direct examination of the globe, which is important postoperatively.

The eyes should be monitored daily or more often for 7 to 10 days postoperatively. Profound secondary uveitis is common and will require management; endophthalmitis may develop. Postoperative treatments are greatly facilitated by placement of a transpalpebral lavage apparatus as discussed in the introduction while the patient is under general anesthesia. Topical 1% atropine solution should be used to effect or 3 to 4 times a day, to facilitate pupil dilation and cycloplegia and to stabilize the blood aqueous barrier. Topical broad-spectrum antibiotic solutions should be used every 1 to 2 hours for 24 hours, then every 2 to 4 hours for 3 to 7 days, and then every 4 to 6 hours, depending on the condition of the eye, for 3 or more weeks. Systemic broad-spectrum antibiotics with a good gram-positive spectrum are indicated; systemic nonsteroidal antiinflammatory agents may be indicated in some cases to help control postoperative uveitis. Topical nonsteroidal medications may be used with caution if needed, but the eye should be observed daily for progressive keratomalacia.

Superficial nonpenetrating, nongaping lacerations can be treated like corneal ulcers and monitored carefully every 1 to 2 days for secondary infection, particularly if the laceration was caused by plant matter. Medications should include topical 1% atropine bid-tid or to effect to maintain pupil dilation, topical broad-spectrum antibiotics every 2 to 4 hours for 3 days then 4 to 6 times a day, depending on the condition of the eye. Systemic nonsteroidal antiinflammatories may be needed occasionally until the wound is healed and any associated uveitis controlled. The wound should be monitored for enzymatic digestion by tissue collagenases or proteases, which would cause the cornea to develop a jelly-like or mucoid consistency. Topical 10% acetylcysteine should be added every 2 hours to the treatment regimen if in doubt.

Some corneal injuries result in deep flap wounds of varying thickness that are still attached to the cornea, and these should be repaired the same as lacerations. Flaps that are very thin with minimal edema can be carefully replaced over the wound bed by rolling a cotton swab over the flap to press it firmly in place. After this, the flap is secured at the wound edges with points of tissue adhesive or sutures. If the flap subsequently detaches, it may need to be excised, but corneal tissue should be preserved whenever possible.

CORNEAL FOREIGN BODIES

Corneal foreign bodies are found frequently in food animals with painful, irritated eyes and are usually foodstuffs, although other plant material, hairs (eyelash or tail), metallic, glass, shot or other substances have been

---

*Acuderm, Inc 5370 NW Terrace, Ft. Lauderdale, FL; (800) 327-0015; or Aaron Medical, 7100 30th Avenue North, St. Petersburg, FL; (800) 537-2790, www.acuderm.com

found. Rebhun (1995) reported corneal foreign bodies commonly occurred after windstorms and were associated with tail switching. In such cases, hairs can be imbedded in the cornea or intraocularly. If a corneal foreign body is suspected, the owner should keep the patient quiet and prevent self-trauma to the eye.

Clinical signs initially include squinting, tearing and photophobia; a mucopurulent ocular discharge may develop after 1 to 3 days in some cases that develop secondary infection. Signs can vary with the size, location, nature, and extent of the injury and the type of foreign body. The patient may rub the affected eye, blink it frequently and forcefully, and have frequent extrusions of the membrana nictitans. Ocular examination with a focal light source and magnification is usually diagnostic if the foreign bodies are imbedded in the cornea. Sedation, eyelid block, and topical anesthesia may be necessary for diagnosis because most affected animals are in a lot of pain with intense blepharospasm. Corneal or ocular foreign bodies may be readily visible or very small and difficult to see, even with good magnification and lighting. The depth of the foreign body should be assessed carefully. The iris and anterior chamber are examined very carefully for evidence of foreign body penetration—including aqueous flare, fibrin, hyphema, and so on. These may be obvious to very subtle. Fluorescein stain should be applied to determine the extent of associated corneal ulceration and to assess aqueous humor leakage in the case of deep stromal foreign bodies (leaking aqueous humor appears as a clear stream in the fluorescein-stained tears). Foreign body penetration into the anterior chamber has a guarded prognosis. The examiner should also use care examining anything that appears as a black foreign body in the cornea, because what appears to be a foreign body may be a piece of iris or corpora nigra that is sealing a corneal perforation. These are approached with caution because disturbing the lesion may cause the aqueous humor to leak. Careful anterior chamber and iris examination should be diagnostic. Cases with large, deep or penetrating foreign bodies or corneal perforations require general anesthesia before removal and may need referral to a specialist trained in microsurgical technique who is capable of managing a potential perforation.

All foreign bodies should be removed as soon and carefully as possible to prevent further patient discomfort and penetration of the object through the corneal layers. Regardless of the type of correction used, it is critical to make certain all foreign material is removed. This requires a very bright focal light source, magnification, time and patience. Superficial foreign bodies can often be removed by using a strong spray of sterile saline from a syringe directed tangentially at the foreign body through a 20- or 22-g needle hub while the eyelids are held open. If the lids cannot be maintained open, a palpebral nerve block should be performed. If spraying does not dislodge the offending material, topical anesthesia can be applied and a 25-gauge needle or small, toothed forceps (e.g., Bishop-Harmon $1 \times 2\,mm$, Colibri or other) can be used to gently remove the material. All foreign particles should be sent for bacterial and fungal culture and sensitivity. Postoperatively, the eye is managed topically as a complicated corneal ulcer, including 4 to 6 times daily broad-spectrum antibiotics and topical atropine twice a day to effect pupil dilation.

Prognosis is fair if all foreign material can be removed and no severe secondary infection is found. Prognosis for penetrating foreign bodies is guarded because of the high incidence of secondary endophthalmitis, particularly if the perforation was caused by plant material or hair.

CORNEAL ULCERS REQUIRING SURGICAL INTERVENTION

Corneal ulcers seen in cattle and small ruminants most commonly occur from trauma, foreign bodies under the lids or nictitans, or primary or secondary infectious agents. The corneal disease in cattle caused by *Moraxella bovis* is certainly the most economically significant disease in the world in veterinary ophthalmology; *Chlamydia* spp. (Figure 13-33), *Mycoplasma* spp., and *Rickettsia* spp. can also cause serious individual or herd problems with resultant economic losses to sheep and goat producers or owners. Corneal ulcers require immediate veterinary attention, frequent topical and often systemic medications, and careful follow-up. Veterinary ophthalmology textbooks or species-specific medical texts should be consulted for the details of proper medical management of corneal ulcers.

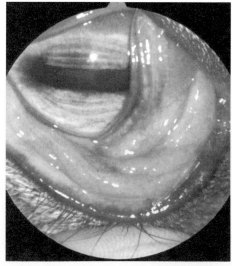

Figure 13-33.   Acute *Chlamydia* sp. conjunctivitis in a heifer.

Corneal ulcers that are extremely large or deep on initial examination (e.g., descemetoceles), do not respond, or worsen with medical therapy may require surgical intervention. A simple procedure that provides some protection and support to the healing cornea is the membrana nictitans, or third eyelid flap, which secures the nictitans to either the dorsotemporal bulbar conjunctiva or to the upper lid. Both procedures can be performed under heavy sedation, topical anesthesia, and eyelid akinesia, but for best results and to reduce the risk of rupturing a deep ulcer, general anesthesia may be necessary. The preferred techniques are described by Severin. Although securing the nictitans to the bulbar conjunctiva may provide more support and less movement of the nictitans against the healing corneal epithelium, the preferred procedure in large animal patients is to secure the third eyelid into the fornix of the upper eyelid. Although there is more movement of the eye independent of the nictitans and potentially less direct corneal epithelial support with this procedure, there is much less risk of a suture penetrating the globe during placement and of corneal irritation from the sutures. This type of flap can be left in place for a longer time than those secured to the bulbar conjunctiva.

To perform the procedure the nictitans is gently, carefully grasped at the free margin and stretched across the cornea to determine the normal direction of movement for that patient. In general, most flaps will be secured to the dorsotemporal fornix, but occasional cases are best secured laterally, according to the anatomy of the individual patient. The preferred suture is 3-0 to 4-0 silk because of ease of handling and knot security, but silk must be removed at a later date. Bovine surgeons may prefer 2-0 chromic catgut, which will dissolve over time and loosen the flap without suture removal but may leave irritating suture ends during the process. Three horizontal mattress sutures are planned and bites spaced accordingly. The surgeon should remember to place each suture first through a stent of tubing or other material if the flap is to be left in place for several weeks. The upper lid is grasped and pulled away from the globe as the needle is passed first through the skin and conjunctiva approximately 1 cm from the lid margin. During needle passage in the standing animal, the cornea should be protected with a lid plate or fingers. The next bite is a horizontal mattress-type bite through the palpebral or front surface of the nictitans, 2 to 3 mm from the free edge. The bite may partially penetrate the cartilage—but not the caudal or bulbar surface of the nictitans—and should not be placed around the base of the "T"-shaped cartilage. The suture is completed by passing it back through conjunctiva and skin so that the final bite is 3 to 5 mm from the first. Three sutures are preplaced. Before tying, the bulbar surface of the nictitans is inspected and

mucous and exudates are washed from the eye. The sutures are pulled in unison as the nictitans is guided under the upper lid. The free margin of the nictitans should be tucked well under the upper lid before knots are tied on the outside of the eyelid. Sutures should be slightly over-tightened before knotting if there is excessive tissue swelling to ensure the sutures remain tight and well-away from the cornea as swelling decreases.

Although unsightly for owners to look at, third eyelid flaps cause minimal discomfort to the patient, can be a useful adjunct to healing, can reduce pain, and can prevent further injury (e.g., from exposure), but they are not without problems. One of the most serious concerns is a flap precludes daily examination of the eye, which is critical in rapidly deteriorating corneal ulcers. If the flaps are placed improperly or the sutures loosen or pull out, corneal ulceration may result. The flaps should be removed immediately for careful eye examination if increased rubbing, squinting, exudates (pus, mucous or tears), pain, fever, or depression is noted.

Conjunctival flaps are the treatment of choice for many rapidly deteriorating or deep corneal ulcers. They support the ulcer, provide immediate blood supply, release beneficial blood components over its surface, provide a source of fibrovascular tissue to reinforce the healing wound, and increase the concentration of systemically administered drugs that reach the site. They should be used judiciously and only when necessary for ulcers located in the central cornea; the resulting scar can be quite dense and permanent in some cases and will impair vision. Conjunctival flaps are also useful to reinforce the cornea after laceration or foreign body removal.

Many types of conjunctival flaps have been described including 360 degrees (total), hood, bridge, pedicle, rotational, peripheral, advancement, tongue, and others. The type of flap used varies with the location, depth and etiology of the ulcer; the available instrumentation, proper lighting and magnification, and experience of the surgeon are other variables that should be considered before surgery.

A total (360 degree) flap is the simplest of the described procedures and requires the least instrumentation. Conjunctiva is dissected as described below, 360 degrees around the limbus and extended a sufficient distance toward the equator of the globe to allow conjunctiva from opposing hemispheres to be sutured together centrally by using mattress sutures of 4-0 to 6-0 synthetic absorbable suture. Corneal sutures are not usually placed, and the procedure does not necessarily require use of a microscope or magnifying loupes. All of the other described flap procedures require 6-0 to 8-0 accurately placed corneal sutures, mandating good magnification.

A properly performed conjunctival flap dissects only the conjunctiva and does not incorporate the thick, underlying, somewhat gelatinous, and quite elastic Tenon's capsule. Conjunctiva is extremely thin and almost transparent. During proper dissection of the conjunctiva one should be able to clearly visualize the tips of your scissors at all times—not just imagine their presence or see their impression through the tissue. Tenon's capsule is hard to exclude from the dissection, but care should be taken to do so. A too-thick flap is ultimately harder to place, harder to secure, more likely to retract after placement, and will eventually result in a more dense scar that can be blinding in the central visual axis. Severin recommends a subconjunctival injection of sterile saline before dissection to make the tissues easier to separate. Care must be taken at all times during dissection to avoid severing any of the extraocular muscles deep to the Tenon's capsule and superficial to the sclera.

Some disadvantages of the 360 degree flap are the same as for a nictitans flap, with prevention of a complete examination of the cornea and other structures inside the eye due to obstruction by the total flap being the most significant. In addition, the 360 degree flap is often much thicker and opaque than other types of flaps, and corneal scarring may be more severe. In most cases, the author prefers pedicle or rotational flaps, the details of which can be found in any ophthalmology text. Whenever possible, the flap should be positioned so the nictitans can move smoothly over the flap rather than "bumping" against its margins. The appearance of the final scar can be improved if pigmented conjunctiva can be transposed.

Corneoscleral transposition, lamellar keratoplasty, and penetrating keratoplasty are additional surgical procedures that can be used in some cases of corneal ulcers, abscesses, or some degenerative diseases. All of these procedures require highly specialized instrumentation and operating microscopes and may require referral to veterinary ophthalmologists trained in the procedure(s).

CATARACT SURGERY

Cataracts are not reported as commonly in food animals as they are in horses and small animals, but they do occur. Cataract removal may be indicated in select cases and is performed with phacoemulsification (Figure 13-34). Replacement intraocular lenses suitable for food animals are not available. Moderately severe hyperopia may result but successful cases show mild to marked improvement negotiating what should be a controlled environment. The surgery is best performed at specialty referral centers.

INTRASCLERAL PROSTHESIS

In select cases in which enucleation might ordinarily be recommended, an intrascleral prosthesis can be placed

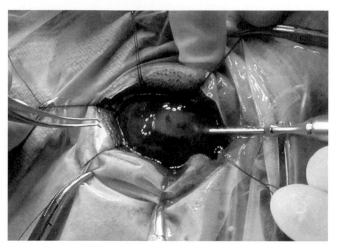

Figure 13-34   Phacoemulsification of a cataract in a water buffalo.

and results in a painless, moderately cosmetic appearance of the eye after 6 to 8 weeks of healing. In general, prostheses are placed to benefit the owner or public, who may prefer the presence and appearance of even a gray-white eye to an empty orbit.

Indications for the procedure are chronic glaucoma or any other blinding painful ocular disease where neoplasia and infections have definitely been ruled out. Perioperative antibiotics should be administered. The procedure must be performed under general anesthesia. After a routine clip, prep, and nasolacrimal lavage, an eyelid speculum is placed or stay sutures or hand-held retractors are used to retract the eyelids. Stay sutures of 4-0 silk are placed at 3 and 9 o'clock in the limbus, with care taken so that they do not penetrate the globe. The dorsal conjunctiva is sharply incised dorsally at the 12 o'clock position anterior to the equator and approximately 0.4-1.5 cm from the limbus (increasing the distance from the limbus according to the size of the globe). The conjunctival incision parallels the limbus and is continued from the 12 o'clock to the 2 o'clock and 10 o'clock positions on the globe so the final incision encompasses 120 degrees. Using a #11 blade, the surgeon makes a sharp incision through the sclera at 12 o'clock in the same manner; vitreous and aqueous will exit the wound, thus collapsing the globe, and can be suctioned as needed. The incision is extended 120 degrees to the same 2 and 10 o'clock positions as the conjunctival incision with thermocautery or scissors. If care is taken at this point to incise only sclera and not the underlying choroid, bleeding will be reduced. Suction and pinpoint cautery can be used as needed for hemostasis.

Bleeding will be significant as the choroid is removed from the eye; and suction, always directed caudally in the globe to avoid the cornea, is highly recommended. A small blunt spatula, such as a lens or cyclodialysis spatula, is inserted between the sclera and choroid and directed forward to separate the choroid from its scleral attachments in the area of the iridocorneal angle. The surgeon must use extreme care now and throughout the entire procedure to insure the corneal endothelium is not injured. The choroid is then bluntly separated from the sclera. Finally, the surgeon uses two-tissue forceps to grasp and remove the choroid from the eye in a hand-over-hand manner. The choroid may tear during removal, with remnants inside remaining attached to the sclera. They will continue to bleed and should be removed as completely as possible using suction and blunt dissection.

The implant is then placed inside the corneoscleral shell. The implant size should be determined and several sizes made available before surgery according to Severin: the same, 1 to 2 mm greater, and 1 to 2 mm less than the horizontal diameter of the cornea of the normal eye. If neither eye is normal, an approximation can be made by measuring the normal eyes of an animal of the same species. The preferred implants are black silicon balls,* which should be cleansed, sterilized, and rinsed again before placement. Implants less than 30 mm in diameter can be introduced via a Carter Sphere Introducer.† Larger implants require placement of 4 to 6 stay sutures around the wound margins that are used to elevate the cut sclera up, out, and over the ball as it is pushed gently through the wound. The wound may be lengthened slightly if needed to avoid tearing during insertion, but the 3 and 9 o'clock positions should be avoided. The sclera is closed with 4-0 to 6-0 synthetic absorbable sutures in a simple interrupted pattern; suture size varies according to the size of the eye. The sclera is oversewn with the same suture in a simple continuous pattern. The conjunctiva is closed with 5-0 to 6-0 suture in a simple continuous pattern. A temporary tarsorrhaphy is placed in the lids as described previously.

Postoperative discomfort should be controlled, and nonsteroidal antiinflammatories are indicated; systemic and topical antibiotics should be continued for 10 to 14 days. A considerable amount of tissue swelling is present, and cold packs are recommended qid for 24 hours. They are followed by hot packs as needed.

Client education is important during the postoperative period. The eye will be filled with blood for several weeks, and the red blood will gradually degrade to a greenish color—similar to the color changes seen in a bruise. Beginning at 5 to 7 days, a 360 degree interstitial keratitis develops as the cornea accommodates itself to the silicon inside and the lack of nutrition provided by the aqueous humor. At 4 to 6 weeks (time varies with corneal diameter), the cornea is markedly red and heavily vascularized. At approximately 8 weeks the cornea will begin to clear to its final dark gray marble appearance. Rarely, central corneal ulceration (which may actually be central corneal necrosis) develops and may require reinforcement with a conjunctival flap or extrusion of the implant may occur.

RECOMMENDED READINGS

Andrea CR, George LW: Surgical correction of periocular fat pad hypertrophy in pot-bellied pigs, *Vet Surg* 28: 311-314, 1999.

Bistner SI, Aguirre G, Batik G: *Atlas of veterinary ophthalmic surgery*, Philadelphia, 1977, WB Saunders.

Gelatt KN: Food animal ophthalmology, *Veterinary ophthalmology*, ed 3, Philadelphia, 1999, Lippincott Williams & Wilkins.

Pearce SG, Kerr CL, Boure LP, et al: Comparison of the retrobulbar and Peterson nerve block techniques via magnetic resonance imaging in bovine cadavers, *J Am Vet Med Assoc* 223: 852-855, 2003.

Rebhun WC: Inflammatory and traumatic disorders. In *Diseases of dairy cattle*, Baltimore, 1995, Williams & Wilkins.

Severin GA: *Severin's Veterinary Ophthalmology Notes*, ed 3, Fort Collins, Colo., 1996, self-published.

Slatter D: Infectious bovine keratoconjunctivitis. *Fundamentals in veterinary ophthalmology*, ed 3, Philadelphia, 2001, WB Saunders.

Smith MC, Sherman DM: Ocular system. In *Goat medicine*, Philadelphia, 1994, Lea and Febiger.

*Jardon Eye Prosthetics, Inc., 17100 W. 12 Mile Road, Southfield, MI, (248) 424-8560
†Storz Instruments available from Bausch & Lomb, see www.bausch.com/us/resource/surgical/instruments/index.jsp

PART III

Calf Surgery

CHAPTER 14

SURGERY OF THE CALF GASTROINTESTINAL SYSTEM

14.1—Abomasal Disease

Ava M. Trent

A few noteworthy physiological differences exist between calves and adult cattle (see Section 10.4). The parietal cells in the fundic region responsible for secretion of HCl are essentially inactive in the neonate, and abomasal fluid has a pH near 6.0. The neutral pH, lack of proteolytic enzymes, and diversion of milk through the reticular groove are all essential to allow colostrum to pass rapidly through the abomasum into the duodenum, where immunoglobulins can be absorbed intact. However, parietal cells are active, and the pH of fundic secretions reaches adult pH levels by 36 hours after birth. Suckling also stimulates rennin and pepsin secretion from chief cells in the fundus of the abomasum, which is essential for clot formation in the diverted milk. The volume of milk consumed and the nature of duodenal chyme regulate abomasal emptying in the milk-fed calf. Somatostatin, secretin and cholecystokinin are hormones that inhibit abomasal emptying in calves. Introduction of hyper- or hypotonic solutions can also depress abomasal motility in milk-fed calves in which normal abomasal contents are essentially isotonic.

In comparison to adults, preruminant calves with abomasal diseases have fluid and electrolyte disturbances that are more difficult to predict and more rapidly detrimental. The body fluids of all neonate species represent a higher percentage of their body weight, and fluid loss or sequestration can result in rapid dehydration. Abomasal outflow disturbances can produce the hyponatremic, hypochloremic metabolic alkalosis seen in adult cattle, but mixed metabolic and respiratory disturbances may obscure this change. Outflow disturbances with vascular compromise may also lead more rapidly to ischemic lactic acidosis. Finally, severe abomasal distension can interfere with ventilation, thus adding a component of respiratory acidosis to the clinicopathological picture.

Abomasal Displacement

The clinical presentation of abomasal disease seen in calves varies. The abomasum can displace without volvulus to the left or right (LDA or RDA) of its normal position by swinging, folding, or stretching the lesser omentum and attached structures. Figure 14.1-1 shows that the abomasum and its attachments can stretch to the point at which the abomasum can be exteriorized almost completely through the left paralumbar fossa. In addition, dilation without apparent displacement is also described in calves. Abomasal volvulus (RVA) is seen in calves and seems to progress quickly if untreated. Finally, abomasal perforations secondary to abomasal ulcers are prevalent in calves.

461

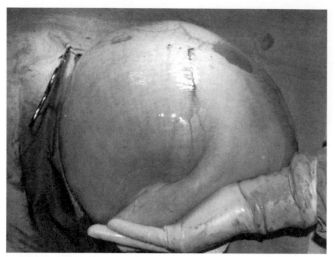

Figure 14.1-1 Standing left paralumbar fossa celiotomy in a 6 month old calf with LDA. The abomasum is exteriorized before decompression.

(Courtesy of Dr. Norm G. Ducharme; Cornell University.)

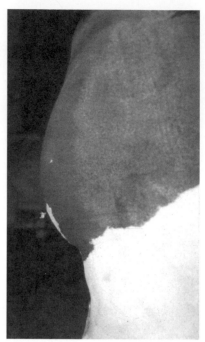

Figure 14.1-2 3-month-old calf with large LDA viewed from above. Note the prominent left-sided abdominal distention.

(Courtesy of Dr. Thomas Divers; Cornell University.)

Left displacements are recognized occasionally in beef and dairy calves, most commonly between 3 weeks and 4 months of age, but the dietary predisposing factors are different; high amounts of starch in milk replacer and abomasal ulcers have been reported as factors in the pathogenesis of LDAs. The prevalence of abomasal ulcers in veal calves has been estimated at 39% of LDA cases.

DIAGNOSIS

Clinical signs of left displacement are less well-described in calves but are more variable than in adults. They include nonspecific signs such as reduced appetite, poor weight gain, recurrent tympany, and variable fecal consistency. Unlike adult cattle, the distended abomasum typically fills the left flank in affected calves and can cause distinct asymmetry when viewed from behind or above (Figure 14.1-2). The ping detectable by simultaneous auscultation and percussion may be less high-pitched than in adult cattle, thus making it easily confused with ruminal distention. This may be why the diagnosis is sometimes delayed in calves. Sometimes the area of percussion is lower than one would expect adding to the diagnostic difficulty (Figure 14.1-3). Calves may also have concurrent diseases typical of their age group including pneumonia and diarrhea. As noted above, calves do not consistently demonstrate the hypochloremic metabolic alkalosis shown by adult ruminants with LDA, and laboratory evaluation is highly recommended if possible. Ultrasound evaluation can be very useful as well.

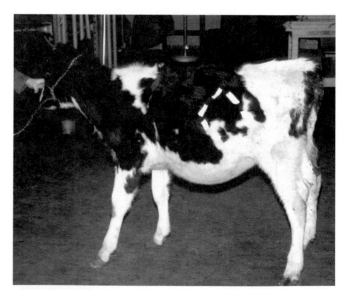

Figure 14.1-3 LDA in a 3-month-old calf. The "ping" is outlined with white markers.

(Courtesy of Dr. Thomas Divers; Cornell University.)

TREATMENT

Some aspects of medical therapy are valuable adjuncts to surgical correction of gastrointestinal disturbances in calves. The potential for rapid dehydration dictates that systemic therapy begin before laboratory results can be obtained, even in calves with mild dehydration. Isotonic saline or lactated Ringer's solution with supplemental dextrose is generally a safe choice until laboratory analysis is available. Oral supplementation should not be used as the primary method of rehydration. Oral and systemic intestinal stimulants have not been well evaluated in calves with abomasal displacement and are not recommended. Initiation of oral or systemic therapy for abomasal ulcers may be appropriate because of the association of displacement with ulcers in calves (see Chapter 5 for more details on fluid therapy). Appropriate medical therapy for other concurrent calf diseases such as pneumonia should be initiated.

MEDICAL MANAGEMENT

Contrary to the relatively poor outcome in adult cattle, rolling may be more effective in managing abomasal dilation as well as right and left displacement in calves. Successful management in 19 out of 21 calves without distinction between left and right displacements was reported in one study after rolling (see Section 10.4 for a description of the procedure). However, the editors feel that this should be a temporary measure to be used only in sick calves that cannot tolerate immediate surgery.

SURGICAL TREATMENT

Standing procedures are not generally recommended in small calves because of their tendency to lie down mid-procedure and the difficulty for the surgeon. However, larger calves may tolerate standing surgery. An omentopexy can be performed from a right flank approach in a calf in left lateral recumbency or standing; however, the omentum is fragile in calves and other approaches that directly stabilize the abomasum are preferable. A left paralumbar fossa abomasopexy is another surgical option (see Figure 14.1-1). This can also be done in the standing or recumbent animal. If the clinician is unsure whether the left-sided viscus is rumen or abomasum this is an attractive surgical option.

A right paramedian abomasopexy can be performed in calves positioned in dorsal recumbency with appropriate reduction in incision length and suture material size. Indications and contraindications are similar to those in adult cattle. Particular attention to the animal's respiratory status is important because pneumonia is a common finding in calves. The lack of access to intestinal structures distal to the abomasum is potentially a greater concern in calves with signs of generalized intestinal distention. The ability to directly stabilize the abomasum is a distinct advantage of this approach.

A modified abomasopexy via a right paracostal approach with the calf positioned in left lateral recumbency offers several advantages over the right paramedian approach. The lateral position places less stress on the respiratory system, and the paracostal incision provides better access to evaluate other intestinal structures. Furthermore, if the abomasum needs to be emptied, it can be accomplished better from this lateral approach.

Abomasal Volvulus

Calves with either an RDA or RVA typically present to the herdsman with signs very similar to those described for LDAs (i.e., partial or complete anorexia, abdominal distension, and decreased fecal output with altered consistency [fluid or pasty]). However, in the case of an RVA, the progression of signs may be very rapid, and a subset of affected calves will first present with signs of severe depression, anorexia, and dehydration.

The presence of a tympanic area (ping) centered over the 10th to 13th ribs and on a line from elbow to tuber coxae is the primary diagnostic sign of an RDA or RVA. This ping must be differentiated from other sources of right-sided pings, which include cecal dilation/torsion, gas accumulation in the duodenum, spiral colon, ascending colon or small intestine, or right flank abscess. An abomasal ping generally can be differentiated from pings associated with other structures by combining information about ping location, size, and pitch. The cecum, colon, and small intestines are limited in their mobility by their mesenteric attachments to the dorsal body wall, whereas the abomasum and ascending duodenum are limited by more cranial attachments at the duodenal sigmoid flexure and the reticular connection to the diaphragm. Cecal, colonic, and small intestinal pings will generally be centered on a point in the paralumbar fossa, more caudal than that for the abomasum or duodenum. The cecum is the only structure that has the potential to dilate to the maximum size possible for the abomasum and is the primary differential for single-pitched pings greater than 10 cm in diameter. In addition, to differentiate the ping's center by location, the outline of the cecum can usually be seen through a right paralumbar fossa with the calf in lateral recumbency (see Figure 14.2.3-1). Small intestinal pings are typically a collection of small diameter pings of varying pitch. Spiral colon pings also tend to involve multiple areas that vary in pitch. Ultrasound evaluation may be very useful to differentiate the right sided viscus. The presence of tachycardia (>130/min) and colic have been reported to be more consistent with RVA in calves; however, controlled studies are lacking.

A right paracostal approach can be used to perform an abomasopexy (preferred procedure) in calves positioned in left lateral recumbency. A rolling procedure with percutaneous decompression (as described for LDAs previously) has been reported to be effective in calves with right-sided pings; however, this is risky should the calf have an RVA or involvement of

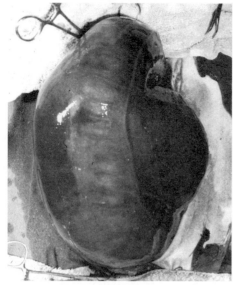

Figure 14.1-4   Abomasal volvulus in a calf viewed from a right paralumbar fossa. Note the distended omasum *(O)* and abomasum *(A)* with the abaxial surface covered by greater omentum which is seen only if a volvulus is present.

(Courtesy of Dr. Mary Smith; Cornell University.)

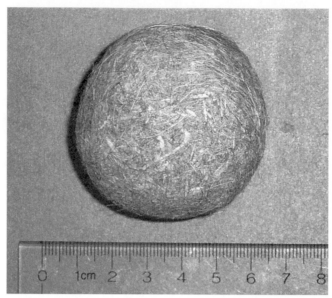

Figure   14.1-5   Trichobezoar   removed   from   a   calf's abomasum.

(Courtesy of Dr. Brad L Njaa; Cornell University.)

another right-sided viscus. The veterinarian should be prepared to move to an open approach within 2 to 3 hours if clinical signs do not improve. A modified right flank or right paracostal omentopexy (Figure 14.1-4) can be used to correct abomasal displacement or volvulus in calves in left lateral recumbency. However, the limited holding power of the omentum in calves makes this a less desirable approach than the right paramedian or right paracostal abomasopexy described earlier.

Luminal Obstruction

Intraluminal obstructions are more common in calves than in adult cattle. Grooming behavior in group-housed calves can result in multiple cases of trichobezoars (hairballs) (Figure 14.1-5). As for LDAs in calves, the specific acid-base and electrolyte changes that result from outflow obstruction are more variable.

Ileus can lead to abomasal dilatation. Excessive milk consumption and changes in nutrition from milk to solid feed have also been suggested as a cause of abomasal distention without displacement in calves. Abomasitis is recognized as an inflammatory condition in young calves presumably as a result of infection with *Clostridium perfringins, Sarcina* sp., or *Salmonella typhimurium*. Affected calves present with signs of toxemia, including dehydration, abdominal distention, tachycardia, and a fluid filled abomasum in normal position on ultrasound examination (Figure 14.1-6).

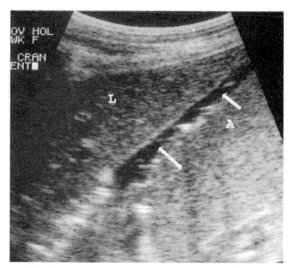

Figure 14.1-6   An ultrasound image of a calf with abomasitis presumed to be caused by *Clostridium perfringens*. The liver is imaged *(L)*; the abomasum *(A)* is distended with fluid, and the abomasal wall is thickened and edematous (arrows).

(Courtesy of Dr. Thomas Divers; Cornell University.)

Surgical access to the pyloric area in calves can be achieved from a right flank, right paracostal, or right paramedian approach with the calf positioned in left lateral recumbency (flank or paracostal) or dorsal recumbency (paracostal or paramedian). This allows an incision over or near the site of obstruction and extraction of the obstructing material with minimal contamination.

Abomasal Ulceration

In one study of calves with clinically apparent abomasal ulceration, 17 of 118 animals had bleeding ulcers. Perforating ulcers (Types 3 and 4) appeared to be most common in veal calves, beef calves, and yearling feedlot cattle (Figure 14.1-7). The incidence in beef and veal calves was highest at 4 to 8 weeks of age, with most cases occurring by 12 weeks of age. Of clinically apparent ulcers in a 3-year study of calves, 81 of 118 were perforating. The occurrence of perforating ulcers in beef calves is highest in the spring, reflecting the age of greatest risk. The incidence of fatal ulcers (Types 2, 3, and 4 combined) was highest in the winter in yearling feedlot cattle but occurred throughout the year. Ninety-three percent of 209 fatal ulcers in beef calves were perforating.

A variety of factors have been proposed as causative, including nutritional deficiencies, bacterial and fungal agents, abrasive agents, and stress. Copper deficiency has been the primary mineral incriminated, although a large study of western Canadian beef herds found a higher fatal ulcer incidence in calves in herds with adequate mineral supplementation. The incidence of ulcers in general increases 20% to 30% when calves are allowed access to roughage. Transition to solid feed and/or transition in abomasal function have been attributed with predisposing and protective effects in beef calves. *Clostridium perfringens* type A has been the pathogen most commonly incriminated in calves, although fatal ulceration may remain as a problem in herds that use consistent vaccination programs. Hairballs in extremely cold weather conditions and poor-quality roughage are the most commonly suggested abrasive agents. However, hairballs were as common in calves of the same age dying of other causes as they were in calves dying of perforating ulcers. Although nonspecific stress is commonly associated with development of diffuse nonpenetrating ulcers

(Type 1), the association with focal perforating ulcers is less clear.

DIAGNOSIS
Type I Ulcers
Type I ulcers often lack any detectable clinical signs. However, the presence of Type I erosions/ulcers may be suspected in those groups of calves known to be at risk and showing signs of poor appetite and decreased weight gain.

Type II Ulcers
Calves are identified by loss of appetite; weakness; depression; occasional mild colic; and black, tarry, foul-smelling feces. Pale mucous membranes are common. Aspirated ruminal fluid may be visibly contaminated with blood or may be occult blood positive.

Type III and IV Ulcers
Clinical signs of perforating ulcers appear to be more severe and rapidly progressive in calves than in adult cattle. In a controlled study of veal calves, many calves showed normal development until the day before perforation. Herdsmen report progression from a normal nursing calf to recumbency within 12 hours. Seventy-five percent of surveyed herdsman indicated that most calves affected by fatal abomasal perforation were found dead without preceding clinical signs. The rapid progression of clinical signs in calves compared to adult cattle may reflect the tendency for perforating ulcers in calves to occur in the pyloric antrum and fundus of the abomasum that is not covered by omentum, thus resulting in generalized peritonitis. In addition, calves are more susceptible to dehydration and infection. Clinical signs when present include depression, colic, anorexia, hypothermia, tachycardia, pale mucous membranes, dehydration, a tense abdominal wall with pain on deep palpation, and an expiratory grunt consistent with abdominal pain. Mild-to-moderate abdominal distention may be present in some cases, with detectable free fluid on ballottement and auscultation in approximately half of affected animals.

Feces were positive for occult blood in 20% of calves with perforating ulcers. Abdominocentesis may be useful in confirming diffuse or localized peritonitis in some cases, but false negatives are common. In one study of 50 veal calves, abdominocentesis was diagnostic for peritonitis in 30% of calves with perforating ulcers, and non-diagnostic in 70%. A strong acid or putrid odor, low pH or high chloride content in the peritoneal fluid suggests abomasal perforation. Ruminal fluid pH may be decreased below 6.0 and rumen chloride levels may be increased above 60 mmol/L. If left untreated, death occurs from diffuse fibrinopurulent peritonitis, toxemia and systemic shock within 48 hours.

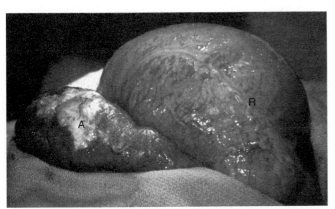

Figure 14.1-7 Type III abomasal ulceration in a calf. Note distended rumen covered by greater omentum (*R*). Note fibrin surrounding abomasum (*A*).

(Courtesy of Dr. Susan Fubini; Cornell University.)

MANAGEMENT

Treatment of individual animals with Type I or multiple Type II ulcers with systemic agents such as clenbuterol and H_2 receptor antagonists such as cimetidine have been tested as prophylactic and therapeutic agents in calves with little beneficial effect.

The small size of the abdomen, limited development of the omentum, ease of visceral manipulation, and relatively rapid rate of systemic deterioration make surgical intervention a viable proposition for calves with perforating ulcers. The preferred approaches in calves are low right paracostal incisions with the animal positioned in left lateral recumbency as described earlier. The goal of surgery is surgical exploration with identification of the ulcer. The ulcer may require resection and closure, or it may be possible to simply oversew the affected portion of the abomasal wall. Aggressive abdominal lavage and systemic fluid and antibiotic therapy are appropriate ancillary therapy.

Calves should be positioned in left lateral recumbency for a 20-cm right paramedian or right paracostal approach. The right paracostal approach provides adequate access to the entire abomasum in most calves of this age and is generally preferred. The abomasum should be exteriorized and stay sutures placed cranial and caudal to the ulcer site. Using laparotomy sponges to pack off the abdominal cavity, the surgeon should resect the ulcer site, if necessary, and the contents of the abomasum, including any hairballs, should be drained away from the incision. The abomasal surface should be vigorously lavaged and the resection site closed with a double inverting pattern using an absorbable suture material as described previously for adult cattle. If contamination from the ulcer appears to be restricted to the right body wall, then lavage should be restricted to this area by exposing contaminated tissue for lavage. If this is not possible or if signs of inflammation extend beyond this area, it is possible to effectively lavage the entire abdominal cavity in calves. Care should be taken to use a sterile pH-balanced isotonic solution for lavage and to remove as much fluid as possible from the abdominal cavity after lavage. If the ulcer is small and focal it may be possible to simply invert it into the lumen of the abomasum and oversew it with a double inverting pattern.

If a localized abscess is adjacent to the abomasum or within the omental bursa, it may be marsupialized for drainage as described for adult cattle (see Section 10.8).

Prognosis

Information on the prognosis for surgical management of calves with perforating ulcers is limited. In one study of ten 4- to 6-week-old calves with perforating fundic and greater curvature ulcers, four were successfully treated with surgical intervention and aggressive supportive care.

RECOMMENDED READINGS

Carlson SA, Stoffregen WC, Bolin SR: Abomasitis associated with multiple antibiotic resistant *Samonella enterica* serotype Typhimurium phagetype DT 104, *Vet Microbiol* 85: 233-240, 2002.

Dirksen G: Ulceration, dilatation and incarceration of the abomasum in calves: clinical investigations and experiences, *Bov Pract* 28: 127-135, 1994.

Frazee LS: Torsion of the abomasum in a 1-month old calf, *Can Vet J* 25: 293-295, 1984.

Grymer J, Johnson R: Two cases of bovine omental bursitis, *J Am Vet Med Assoc* 181: 714-715, 1982.

Jelinski MD, Janzen ED, Hoar B et al.: A field investigation of fatal abomasal ulcers in western Canadian bred calves, *Agri-Practice* 16: 16-18, 1995.

Jelinski MD, Ribble CS, Campbell, Janzen ED. Investigating the relationship between abomasal hairballs and perforating abomasal ulcers in unweaned beef calves, *Can Vet J* 37: 23-26, 1996.

Kümper H: A new treatment for abomasal bloat in calves, *Bov Pract* 29: 80-82, 1995.

Roeder BL, Chengappa MM, Nagaraja TG, Avery TB, Kenncdey GA: Experimental induction of abdominal tympany, abomasitis, and abomasal ulceration by intraruminal inoculation of *Clostridium perfringens* type A in neonatal calves, *Am J Vet Res* 49: 201-207, 1988.

Roeder BL, Chengappa MM, Nagaraja TG, Avery TB, Kennedey GA: Isolation of *Clostridium perfringens* from neonatal calves with ruminal and abomasal tympany, abomasitis, and abomasal ulceration, *Am J Vet Res* 190: 1550-1555, 1987.

Tulleners EP, Hamilton GF: Surgical resection of perforated abomasal ulcers in calves, *Can Vet J* 21: 262-264, 1980.

Welchman D de B, Baust GN: A survey of abomasal ulceration in veal calves, *Vet Rec* 121: 586-590, 1987.

14.2—Ruminal Distension in Calves

Norm G. Ducharme and
Susan L. Fubini

Diet inadequate in roughage can prevent normal growth of ruminal flora and is the most common cause of indigestion in calves. Undigested roughage accumulates and ruminal distention develops. It has been suggested that exclusively milk (or milk replacer) diets can cause hyperkeratosis of the rumen and recurrent ruminal distention. A similar syndrome is called *ruminal drinkers* where a calf's esophageal groove partially or completely fails to close, so ingested milk is diverted to the rumen instead of the abomasum. This leads to fermentation and ruminal distension (Figure 14.2-1). Why this syndrome develops is unclear, but the following factors must be

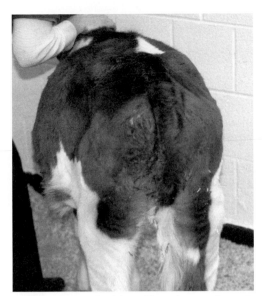

Figure 14.2-1 4-week-old calf with esophageal groove closure failure, resulting in abdominal distention when fed (so-called *ruminal drinker*).

(Courtesy of Dr. Thomas Divers; Cornell University.)

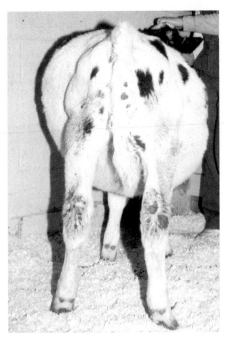

Figure 14.2-2 "Papple-shaped" abdomen in a calf with chronic bronchopneumonia and presumed vagal nerve damage.

(Courtesy of Dr. Thomas Divers; Cornell University.)

present for the esophageal groove to close normally. The fluid drunk by a calf must contact the pharyngeal receptors, be consumed voluntarily, and have no unpleasant taste or odor; and the general status of the calf should not be disturbed. Altering the method of intake or weaning the calf can be curative.

Another source of ruminal distention in calves is vagus nerve impairment due to pharyngeal disorders or chronic severe bronchopneumonia. The vagus nerve can apparently become inflamed or compressed by enlarged lymph nodes or severe pulmonary parenchymal damage. Because this nerve provides innervation to the forestomach compartments, an abomasum outflow obstruction develops with distention of the dorsal and ventral sacs of the rumen (Figure 14.2-2).

Clinical Findings

Pharyngeal trauma can be diagnosed by physical examination findings that include swelling, dysphagia, and excessive salivation (see Section 10.1). Thoracic lesions can be identified based on physical examination and imaging studies. For example, signs of bronchopneumonia, such as coughing, tachypnea, abnormal auscultation (wheezes, squeaks, crackles or decreased lung sounds), and dullness on thoracic percussion, help identify a primary respiratory problem requiring treatment. Imaging of the head or thoracic cavity by ultrasonography or radiography could confirm a diagnosis of trauma or bronchopneumonia.

Rumen Fistula

Rumen fistulas are indicated to relieve free-gas bloat in calves. The procedure is most effective in calves free from other disease that respond to a stomach tube passed to relieve gaseous accumulation. Fistulas are also placed to allow alimentation for calves unable to eat because of another disease process (i.e., tetanus, pharyngeal trauma).

Calves that have had severe bronchopneumonia and subsequently develop free-gas bloat, presumably from vagal nerve damage, may benefit from a rumen fistula that gives gas an escape route until the thoracic inflammation subsides.

Commercial trocars can be used in free-gas bloat or in an emergency situation. For longer-term use, surgically placing a fistula is recommended.

Surgical Technique

The purpose of surgery is to allow decompression of the rumen, thus giving the primary condition an opportunity to resolve. The fistula should not be too ventral, or ingesta will tend to occlude the fistula, thus allowing ruminal distension to recur. The fistula is placed in the dorsal aspect of the left paralumbar fossa. However, the fistula should not be too dorsal if the rumen is empty (i.e., an animal with tetanus), or it will cause excessive tension on the suture line. The appropriate area on the left flank is identified, desensitized with a local block, and prepared for surgery. A 6-cm vertical skin incision is made. The external abdominal oblique and transversus muscles are incised sharply. The peritoneum is tented and incised.

Several surgical options are available, including the three-layer technique the authors use. We recommend the transversus abdominis (which is mostly fascia) and peritoneum be sutured to the dermis on each side of the incision for the first layer. This protects the muscle layers and is usually done with a size 0 absorbable suture on a cutting needle. For the second layer, the rumen wall is sutured circumferentially to the dermis to provide a "seal" between the rumen and the skin. For this layer, a cutting needle is required; and the suture line is "broken" several times to avoid a pursestring effect. For the third layer, the rumen is incised, and the wall is sutured to the skin in a simple interrupted pattern with size 0 nonabsorbable sutures. The ends are left long to facilitate removal. To keep the fistula patent, an appropriate-sized syringe case (with four holes in its collar) is fitted into the incision site. The syringe case is secured to the skin with umbilical tape placed through the pre-placed holes in the collar to four separate "loops of sutures," placed in the skin at four corners approximately 5 cm from the fistula (Figure 14.2-3).

The syringe case is capped when the primary cause of the ruminal distension appears to have resolved. If the ruminal distension does not recur after a few weeks, the syringe case is removed. In some calves, the fistula will close over the ensuing weeks. In other calves, the fistula

will need to be resected en bloc and the rumen and body wall closed separately as described in Section 10.3 for a rumenotomy closure.

RECOMMENDED READINGS

Dirr L, Dirksen G: Dysfunction of the esophageal groove ("ruminal drinking") as a complication of neonatal diarrhea in the calf, *Tierarztl Prax* 17: 353-358, 1989.

Ducharme NG: Surgical considerations in the treatment of traumatic reticuloperitonitis, *Compend Contin Educ Pract Vet* 5: S213-S224, 1983.

Ducharme NG: Surgery of the bovine forestomach compartments, *Vet Clin North Am (Food Anim Pract)* 6: 371-397, 1990.

Habel RE: A study of the innervation of the ruminant stomach; Cornell *Vet* 46: 555-633, 1956.

Neal PA and Edwards GB: "Vagus indigestion" in cattle, *Vet Rec* 82: 396-402, 1968.

14.2.1—Small Intestinal Surgery in Calves

Susan L Fubini

Small intestine surgery in calves is much the same as adult cattle, although intestinal accidents due to congenital abnormalities are more common in calves. In addition, intestinal accidents caused by urachal remnants or related to adhesions (Figure 14.2.1-1) and umbilical infections are prevalent in the calf age group. Intussusceptions occur in the calf small intestine (Figure 14.2.1-2) as they do in adults, but calves also suffer from intussusceptions

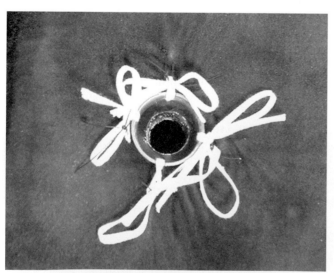

Figure 14.2-3   Completed rumen fistula in a calf.

(Courtesy of Dr. Brett Woodie; Cornell University.)

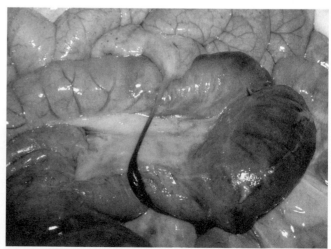

Figure 14.2.1-1   1-month-old calf opened at surgery from a right paralumbar fossa celiotomy in lateral recumbency. Note the fibrous band incarcerating a section of small intestine.

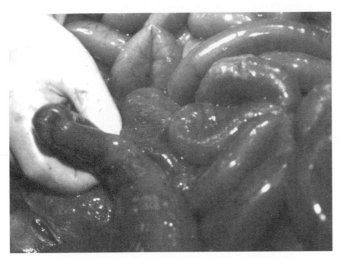

Figure 14.2.1-2 Small intestinal intussusception in a one month old calf. Note distended small intestine proximal to the lesion and the intussusception in the surgeon's hand.

(Courtesy of Dr. Ryland B. Edwards III; University of Wisconsin.)

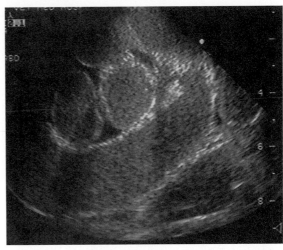

Figure 14.2.1-3 Distended small intestine in a calf with intussusception.

(Courtesy of Dr. Amy Yeager; Cornell University.)

throughout the intestinal tract. This may be because calves have less substantial mesenteric fat.

Signs of small intestinal obstruction are similar to those in an adult and include abdominal pain, abdominal distention, scant manure, succussible fluid on the right side of the abdomen, and small variable areas of tympanic resonance on the right. It can be very difficult to distinguish between an ileus secondary to enteritis and a small intestinal obstruction. A digital rectal examination is rarely beneficial. Ultrasound examination can confirm the bowel distention, and, sometimes, image the actual obstruction (Figure 14.2.1-3). Subjectively, we think abdominal pain in young calves is more often seen with obstructive bowel disease than with enteritis.

Surgical preparation is as described for adult cattle. Local anesthesia and sedation is an option, but general anesthesia is preferable. A right flank celiotomy is the approach of choice. Upon entry into the abdomen, one should be aware of the more common causes of small intestinal obstruction: intussusception, volvulus and intestinal entrapment in adhesions, or umbilical remnants (Figure 14.2.1-4A and B). The bowel in small ruminants is thin-walled and easily traumatized, thus making gentle tissue handling essential. A 1% carboxymethylcellulose[a] application is recommended before

beginning surgical manipulation to avoid serosal trauma or drying (see Section 10.9). Once the lesion is identified, it should be corrected if possible, and the viability of the bowel should be assessed.

If an area requires resection, it should be kept exteriorized while the remainder of the bowel is replaced into the abdomen. The bowel to be resected should be packed off from the rest of the abdomen with sterile bath towels or laparotomy pads. Penrose drains can be used to occlude the lumen of the bowel proximal and distal to the site of resection. The drains should be carefully placed to minimize the defect created in the mesentery. The vasculature is easier to see in calves because the mesentery is not as fat-filled as in adults. Vessels should be ligated close to the bowel. The authors recommend using small (# 3-0) absorbable suture material for anastomosis or enterotomy closure to avoid leakage through the needle tracts. For an end-to-end anastomosis, the mesenteric and antimesenteric sutures are placed first and tagged. The anastomosis is completed with a simple interrupted or simple continuous pattern. After anastomosis, the mesenteric defect is closed. To minimize peritoneal adhesions, liberal lavage with sterile isotonic fluids or 1% carboxymethylcellulose during surgery is indicated. Gloves and instruments are changed, and closure is routine.

After surgery, strict attention must be paid to keeping the calf warm and adequately hydrated. Antimicrobials are indicated for 5 to 7 days if a resection and anastomosis were performed.

[a]Solution of high molecular weight carboxymethylcellulose (700 to 1000 kd) is prepared as follows. The carboxymethylcellulose (Grade 7HFPH; Aqualon, Delaware) is added to isoosmolar PBS solution of pH adjusted to 7.1 and pressure-filtered first through a 410-μm filter mesh, then through a 10-μm filter mesh to remove gel bodies. The solution is then placed in a 1-L bottle and sterilized by autoclaving at 115° C for 25 minutes by using a liquid slow-release cycle.

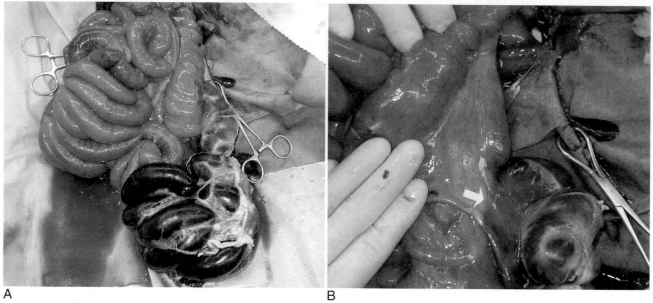

A   B

Figure 14.2.1-4   1-month-old calf opened at surgery from a right paralumbar fossa celiotomy in lateral recumbency. *A,* A portion of the small intestine was entrapped in an adhesion. Distinct demarcation is seen between necrotic and healthy small intestine. *B,* The line of vascular demarcation is shown (arrow).

RECOMMENDED READINGS

Baxter GM, Darien BJ, Wallace CE: Persistent urachal remnant causing intestinal strangulation in a cow, *J Am Vet Med Assoc* 191: 555-558, 1987.

Constable PD, St. Jean G, Hull BL, Rings DM, Morin DE, Nelson DR: Intussusception in cattle: 336 Cases (1964-1993), *J Am Vet Med Assoc* 210: 531-536, 1997.

Murphy DJ, Peck LS, Detrisac CJ, Widenhouse CW, Goldberg EP: Use of high-molecular weight carboxymethylcellulose in a tissue protective solution for prevention of postoperative abdominal adhesions in ponies, *Am J Vet Res* 63: 1448-1454, 2002.

14.2.2—Cecal Intussusceptions

Adrian Steiner

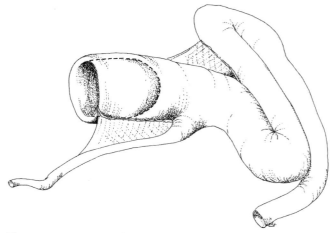

Figure 14.2.2-1   Schematic representation of cecocecal intussusception.

Occurrence

One suggestion as to why adult cattle have a low occurrence of intussusception (IS) in the cecal region is that they have a fat-filled mesentery that maintains the relationship of the various segments of the intestine. Calves' mesenteric fat is usually minimal, which allows increased mobility of the slings of the intestine. This may partially explain why IS in general, and specifically IS of the cecum, is significantly more common in calves less than 2 months of age than in older cattle. Four different types of IS involving the cecum have been described. They include cecocecal (Figure 14.2.2-1), cecocolic (Figure 14.2.2-2), ileocecocolic (Figure 14.2.2-3), and ileocecal (Figure 14.2.2-4) IS. In a retrospective study of 48 cases of IS diagnosed over a 9-year period that involved the cecum, the breakdown of cases was found to be 46% cecocolic and 25% cecocecal IS. Seventy-eight percent of the cases occurred within the first 4 weeks of life, and 80% had a

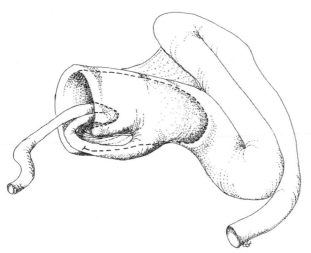

Figure 14.2.2-2 Schematic representation of cecocolic intussusception.

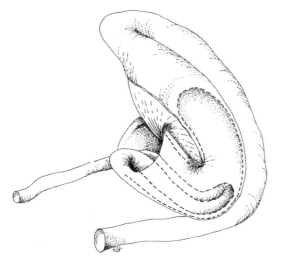

Figure 14.2.2-3 Schematic representation of ileocecocolic intussusception.

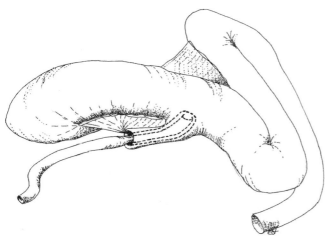

Figure 14.2.2-4 Schematic representation of ileocecal intussusception.

history of severe diarrhea with a mean duration of 1 week. Intussusception that involves the cecum rarely occurred spontaneously without concurrent disease.

Symptoms and Diagnosis

Symptoms include moderate to severe depression, partial to complete anorexia, abdominal distension accentuated in the right flank, and mild signs of abdominal pain. Scant amounts of dark-red feces and mucus strands may be present. Tachycardia and dehydration may be evident. Auscultation performed simultaneous with percussion identifies variable small "pings" and superficial splashing sounds of fluid-filled bowel in the right flank when performed simultaneously with succussion. Radiography and ultrasonography may be used as diagnostic aids to identify distended bowel in young calves where a rectal examination cannot be performed. The definitive diagnosis is usually made during exploratory celiotomy.

Therapy and Prognosis

Dehydration and acid/base imbalances should be corrected before surgery. Perioperative antimicrobials should also be administered. The calf is restrained in left lateral recumbency and an exploratory celiotomy performed in the right flank under local or general anesthesia. The affected bowel is exteriorized, and the IS manually reduced if possible. Depending on the type of IS, cecal amputation (see Section 10.6 for details on cecal amputation) and resection of the ileum and proximal loop of the ascending colon (PLAC) may be indicated (Figure 14.2.2-5). The high recurrence rate of IS necessitates cecum amputation, even if the compromised bowel is viable. The ileocecal junction is left intact if it

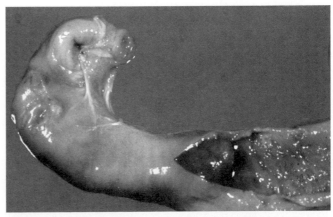

Figure 14.2.2-5 *En bloc* resection of cecocolic intussusception in a calf.

(Courtesy of Dr. Donald Smith; Cornell University.)

is not compromised by the IS. Postoperative measures include correcting electrolytes, acid/base, and energy imbalances/losses and aggressively treating the primary disease (e.g., diarrhea).

The prognosis is guarded after treating cecal IS because affected calves are frequently in poor general condition before surgery. Rate of survival is mainly influenced by the prognosis for the concurrent diarrhea.

RECOMMENDED READINGS

Bristol D, Fubini S: Surgery of the neonatal bovine digestive tract, *Vet Clin North Am (Food Anim Pract)* 6: 473-493, 1990.

Constable P, St. Jean G, Hull B, et al: Intussusception in cattle: 336 cases (1964-1993), *J Am Vet Med Assoc* 210: 531-536, 1997.

Doll K, Klee W, Dirksen G: Blinddarminvagination beim Kalb. *Tierärztl Prax* 26: 247-253, 1998.

Julian R, Hawke T: Cecal colic intussusception in a calf, *Can Vet J* 4: 54-55, 1963.

Pearson H: Intussusception in cattle, *Vet Rec* 89: 426-437, 1971.

Steiner A, Oertle C, Flückiger M, et al: Was diagnostizierten sie? Welche Massnahmen schlagen sie vor? *Schweiz Arch Tierheilk* 131: 577-578, 1989.

14.2.3—Surgery of the Colon

Adrian Steiner

Intussusception of the Spiral Colon

Intussusception of the spiral colon is rare. The history of affected animals may include diarrhea, which presumably leads to irregular motility patterns and the intestinal accident. Affected calves present with distension of the abdomen, which is especially evident on the right side of the abdomen as the cecum and colon proximal to the obstruction distend with fluid and gas (Figure 14.2.3-1). Other presenting signs are vague but include a decreased appetite, mild abdominal pain, and progressive dehydration. There may be an area of tympanic resonance in the right paralumbar fossa and succussible fluid. Ultrasound examination confirms the cecal and colonic distension.

Treatment consists of reduction with or without resection of the intussusceptum (Figure 14.2.3-2); resection *in situ* is required if the intussusception cannot be manually reduced. Manual reduction of intussusception without subsequent resection may only be performed successfully if the bowel is not compromised and the presence of any predisposing causes, such as intraluminal or intramural masses, is excluded. Because intussusceptions are typically relatively short, resection of a short segment may be all that is needed to revitalize the bowel,

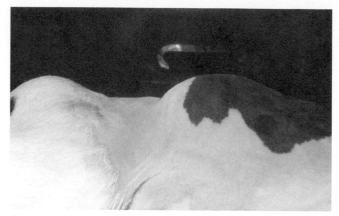

Figure 14.2.3-1   Holstein-Friesian calf in left lateral recumbency. Note the distended paralumbar fossa secondary to cecal distension proximal to a spiral colon obstruction.

(Courtesy of Dr. Susan Fubini; Cornell University.)

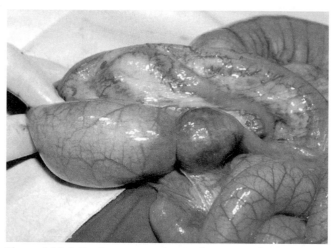

Figure 14.2.3-2   Intussusception in the proximal spiral colon of a 3-week-old calf. Note the distended bowel proximal to the obstruction, and the empty bowel distally.

(Courtesy of Dr. Brett Woodie; Cornell University.)

and only minimal mesenteric dissection may be necessary. When a resection is performed, it behooves the surgeon to stay close to the bowel, thereby avoiding any major disruption of the mesentery. This prevents disturbance of the vascular supply to the colon.

Luminal Obstruction of Spiral Colon

Calves with severe diarrhea may slough their intestinal mucosa. This may result in a fibrinous cast that can obstruct the spiral colon. An affected animal shows signs of abdominal distension, progressive depression, and decreased appetite. Exploratory celiotomy through a

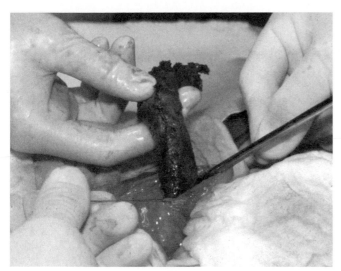

Figure 14.2.3-3 Intraoperative view of a fibrinous cast obstructing the midspiral loop of the ascending colon. The cast is being removed through an enterotomy.

(Courtesy of Dr. Susan Fubini; Cornell University.)

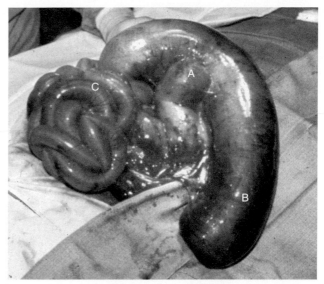

Figure 14.2.3-4 Intraoperative view of a 3-day-old calf with atresia coli in the mid-spiral loop of the ascending colon. *A*, blind end of spiral colon; *B*, cecum; *C*, distended small intestine.

(Courtesy of Dr. Susan Fubini; Cornell University.)

right paralumbar fossa reveals distension oral to the obstruction. The obstruction is felt as a firm object within the lumen of the spiral colon. After isolating the spiral colon with sterile towels, an enterotomy is made along the longitudinal axis of the affected segment of spiral colon (Figure 14.2.3-3). The intraluminal obstruction is removed and the longitudinal enterotomy is closed transversely to prevent stricture, using a one-layer simple interrupted suture pattern with 2-0 polyglactin or similar absorbable suture material.

Atresia Coli

OCCURRENCE AND ETIOLOGY
Intestinal atresia is the complete absence of a portion of the intestinal lumen. The ascending colon is one of the most commonly affected segments in the calf. Atresia of the colon is most frequently located in the mid spiral loop of the ascending colon (Figure 14.2.3-4). The cause of atresia coli in calves is not well understood and represents a matter of scientific controversy. In a retrospective study, Holstein-Friesian calves were identified significantly more often with atresia coli than would have been expected from the hospital population. Supporting this finding, in a Holstein-Friesian herd, atresia coli was found to be inherited autosomally recessive with a single locus displaying two alleles being responsible for the disease. On the other hand, atresia coli was found in one of identical twin calves—but not the other. In addition, purposely mating five affected cows and two affected bulls produced 23 calves but failed to create a single offspring with atresia coli. The heritability of atresia coli was

estimated to be 0.0875, which implies other, non genetic etiologies, such as early manual pregnancy testing. Rectal palpation of the amniotic vesicle at 42 days of age or earlier was associated with increased incidence of colonic and jejunal atresia. At this time, we consider this a non genetic disease because of the above observations and the low heritability factor.

Clinical Signs and Diagnosis

Affected calves are usually born without incident and have a normal appetite until 12 to 48 hours later when they develop inappetence, abdominal distension, signs of abdominal pain, and progressive depression and weakness. The hallmark of the disorder is that no manure is passed. At clinical examination, tachycardia, hyperpnea, and normal to reduced rectal temperature are evident. Calves have a normal appearing anus and rectum. On digital palpation per rectum, a clear to yellow mucus, sometimes blood-tinged is identified. A well-lubricated flexible catheter may be passed through the descending colon without resistance. However, this is not recommended because of the risk of trauma to the bowel. The abdomen becomes severely distended, and percussion (ping) and succussion auscultation in both flanks are positive. The contours of distended large intestinal loops may be detected by visual examination or palpation in the right paralumbar fossa. A presumptive diagnosis can be made with an accurate history and physical examination. Imaging studies can confirm the distended viscera. Lateral radiographic examination of the standing animal reveals gas distension of the small and large intestine. Distended small (Figure 14.2.3-5) and large (Figure 14.2.3-6) intestinal loops are routinely observed at ultrasonographic examination of the ventral and dorsal aspects of the right flank, respectively. Dehydration with normal to low plasma protein concentration and neutrophilia with left shift are typically observed at hematological analysis. The diagnosis is confirmed by a right paralumbar fossa exploratory celiotomy.

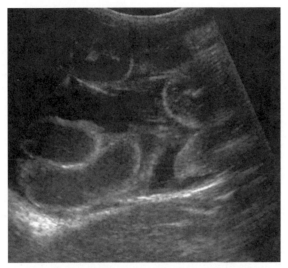

Figure 14.2.3-5   Ultrasonographic view from the ventral aspect of the right flank showing distended small intestinal loops in a calf with atresia coli.

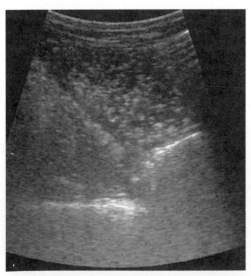

Figure 14.2.3-6   Ultrasonographic view from the dorsal aspect of the right flank showing distended large intestinal loops of the same calf as Figure 14.2.3-2.

SURGICAL MANAGEMENT

Because immediate surgical intervention is rarely considered necessary, supportive medical treatment—including rehydration, correction of acid-base imbalances, and antimicrobial treatment—is initiated before subjecting the calf to additional stress. Plasma may be necessary because failure of passive transfer can be present in these calves either because of intake failure or poor absorption. Surgery is performed under local or general anesthesia through the right paralumbar fossa with the calf in left lateral recumbency. Gas is evacuated from the distended cecum and spiral colon. Digesta are removed from the intestine proximal to the site of atresia through an enterotomy at the apex of the cecum or through the dissected proximal blind end of the colon (Figure 14.2.3-7). If the enterotomy site is in the cecum, it is closed with two layers by using at least one inverting pattern. The compromised segment of the dilated blind end is resected, and continuity is established to the descending colon by either an end-to-side or side-to-side anastomosis. It is usually recommended to perform an end-to-side anastomosis because two calves that had a side-to-side anastomosis developed a volvulus of the blind end, which grew in length; this is presumably because of the growth potential of the bowel in the neonate. However, retrospective studies have not found a significant difference in survival rate between end-to-side and side-to-side anastomosis. The descending colon is best identified by passing a flexible catheter into the rectum and then isolated with two umbilical

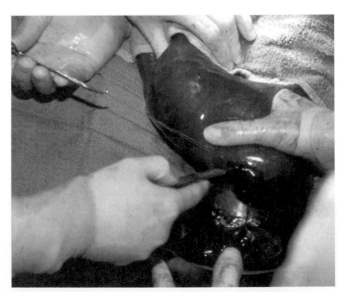

Figure 14.2.3-7   Intraoperative view of a calf with atresia coli. A typhlotomy is being performed to remove ingesta and meconium.

(Courtesy of Dr. Norm Ducharme; Cornell University.)

tape loops placed carefully through the mesocolon (Figure 14.2.3-8). The surgeon must be careful not to puncture the friable descending colon when passing the umbilical tape. Anastomosis is achieved by either a single layer of apposing simple interrupted sutures or a GIA 55* stapling instrument (Figure 14.2.3-9). Postoperative management includes maintenance of appropriate electrolyte and fluid therapy, antimicrobial treatment for 5 to 7 days, and gradual resumption of oral feeding within 12 hours after surgery.

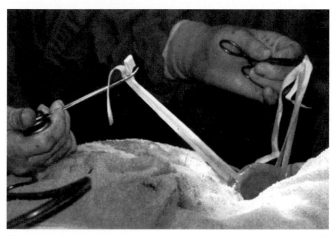

Figure 14.2.3-8 Intraoperative view of a calf with atresia coli. The descending colon is identified by passing a stallion catheter gently per rectum and isolated with two umbilical tape loops placed carefully through the mesocolon.

(Courtesy of Dr. Susan Fubini; Cornell University.)

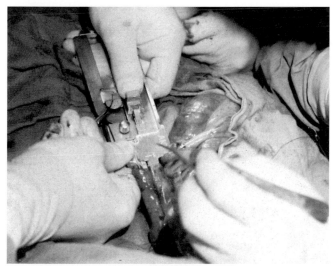

Figure 14.2.3-9 Intraoperative view of a calf with atresia coli. The ascending colon is being anastomosed to the descending colon using a GI-55 stapling instrument.

(Courtesy of Dr. Susan Fubini; Cornell University.)

---

*Gastrointestinal anastomosis stapler, U.S. Surgical Corp., Norwalk, CT 06856

PROGNOSIS

Prognosis depends mainly on acid-base and electrolyte status at admission; an anion gap exceeding 24 mEq/L predicting death. Calves that "do well" are bright, alert, and hungry by 12 to 24 hours after surgery. Feces are passed by this time and are initially loose but firm up over the next few days. If problems are going to develop, they usually are evident in the immediate postoperative period. The most commonly reported complications after surgery include peritonitis, failure of anastomosis, diarrhea, impaction at the anastomosis site, incisional infection, chronic cecal dilation, functional obstruction of the spiral colon, and adhesive bowel obstruction. An astute observer will note abdominal distention and decreased fecal output, followed by inappetence and loss of appetite in calves developing complications related to the gastrointestinal tract. Some of the complications related to the anastomosis can be resolved with additional surgery, although it becomes an expensive undertaking. The overall long-term survival rate, defined as reaching reproductive age, varies from 12% to 37%. Long-term survivors are likely to have loose feces and not to grow as well as otherwise expected. As an alternative procedure to intestinal anastomosis, cecostomy in the right flank may be performed. This technique allows bypass of the colon and fattening of the calf to a final body weight of 130 to 140 kg.

The current knowledge is that atresia coli is not a heritable disease in Holstein Friesian calves, but caution should still be used in breeding affected animals. The author judges surgical treatment of an affected calf as questionable because of economical and ethical reasons.

Atresia Ani (Et Recti)

OCCURRENCE AND ETIOLOGY

Atresia ani is found less often in dairy than beef cattle breeds. Lack of tail, fistula formation between the rectum and the reproductive tract, and abnormalities of the urinary tract may accompany atresia ani. In females, the rectum may communicate with the vagina, in males with the urethra or the bladder. Inheritance is reported in swine and lambs, and is possible in calves—but not documented. Surgical treatment of animals with breeding potential, presence of a fistula, and/or other abnormalities is ethically and economically questionable.

CLINICAL SIGNS AND DIAGNOSIS

Affected calves show signs within the first day of life because they are unable to pass feces. An exception to this is the affected female with a rectovaginal fistula that passes some feces through the fistula. Other congenital defects—including cleft palate, polydactyly, and abnormalities of the urogenital tract—can be seen (Figure

14.2.3-10). They exhibit progressive abdominal distention, straining, signs of abdominal pain, depression, and weakness. If only the anus is involved, the rectum usually bulges subcutaneously in the normal region of the anus during straining and when the abdomen is manually compressed. If no bulge is observed, atresia of the caudal rectum is suspected (Figure 14.2.3-11). The degree of involvement of the rectum may be determined radiographically. In newborn infants, ultrasonography was found to be an adequate noninvasive method to determine the distance between rectal pouch and perineal skin.

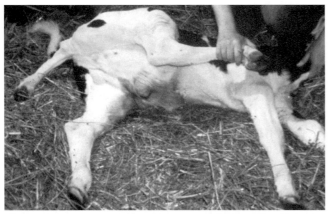

Figure 14.2.3-10   Polydactyly in a newborn calf with multiple congenital defects including atresia ani.

(Courtesy Dr. Susan Fubini; Cornell University.)

SURGICAL MANAGEMENT AND PROGNOSIS

For surgical correction, 1 ml of 1% lidocaine solution is injected epidurally, and the hind part of the calf is directed toward the edge of the surgery table in sternal recumbency with the hind feet pulled slightly craniad. After routine aseptic preparation of the surgical field, a 1-cm diameter circular incision is made through the skin and subcutaneous tissue at the site where the anus would normally be located. Careful blunt dissection in a cranial direction is used to identify the rectal pouch, which is gently pulled caudad with a pair of tissue forceps (rectal pull-through procedure). If this does not allow the rectum to be identified, it may be grasped during left flank exploratory celiotomy and moved in a caudal direction by simultaneous traction through the pelvic canal and manipulation in the abdomen. The rectum is sutured to the subcutaneous tissue with four to six interrupted sutures, the rectal pouch is incised, and the rectal mucosa is sutured to the skin using a broken simple continuous or interrupted suture pattern (Figure 14.2.3-12). Intraoperatively, the presence of anal sphincter muscles is rarely evident. Fecal incontinence is therefore a frequent complication of surgical correction of atresia ani (et recti). A single stab incision through the perineum into the rectum is not successful, as stricture and obstruction are likely to occur. If there is a sizable portion of rectum (and descending colon) missing, surgery is exceedingly difficult because the short mesocolon does not readily stretch. In these cases, surgery should be discouraged.

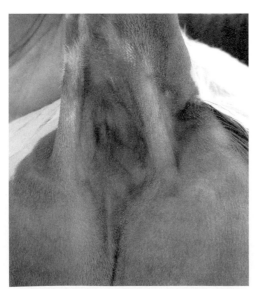

Figure 14.2.3-11   Atresia ani et recti in a 1-day-old calf before attempted surgical reconstruction.

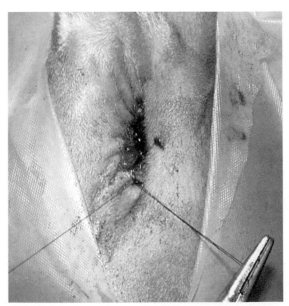

Figure 14.2.3-12   Surgical reconstruction of atresia ani (et recti) in a 1-day-old calf.

Before suturing the rectum to the perineal skin, any rectovaginal or urethral fistula needs to be located and transected in the female. This is usually done most easily by exploring the vaginal opening and fistula with a blunt instrument.

RECOMMENDED READINGS

Berchtold M, Mittelholzer A, Camponovo L: Atresia coli beim Kalb, *Dtsch Tierärztl Wschr* 92: 395-398, 1985.

Bristol D, Fubini S: Surgery of the neonatal bovine digestive tract, *Vet Clin North Am (Food Anim Pract)* 6: 473-493, 1990.

Constable P, Rings D, Hull B, et al: Atresia coli in calves: 26 cases (1977-1987), *J Am Vet Med Assoc* 195: 118-123, 1989.

Ducharme N, Arighi M, Horney F et al: Colonic atresia in cattle: a prospective study of 43 cases, *Can Vet J* 29: 818-824, 1988.

Hamilton G, Tulleners E: Intussusception involving the spiral colon in a calf, *Can Vet J* 21: 32, 1980.

Hoffsis G, Brunner R: Atresia coli in a twin calf, *J Am Vet Med Assoc* 171: 433-434, 1977.

Johnson R, Ames N, Coy C: Congenital intestinal atresia of calves, *J Am Vet Med Assoc* 182: 1387-1389, 1983.

Leipold H, Saperstein G, Johnson D et al: Intestinal atresia in calves, *Vet Med Small Anim Clin* 74: 1037-1039, 1976.

Oppenheimer D, Carroll B, Shochat S: Sonography of imperforate anus, *Radiol* 148: 127-128, 1983.

Saperstein G: Congenital abnormalities of internal organs and body cavities, *Vet Clin North Am (Food Anim Pract)* 9: 115-125, 1993.

Sharratt R: The surgical correction of a case of anorectal agenesis in a calf, *Vet Rec* 79: 108-109, 1966.

Smith D, Ducharme N, Fubini S et al: Clinical management and surgical repair of atresia coli in calves: 66 cases (1977-1988), *J Am Vet Med Assoc* 199: 1185-1190, 1991.

Steenhaut M, De Moor A, Verschooten F et al: Intestinal malformation in calves and their surgical correction, *Vet Rec* 98: 131-133, 1976.

Syed M, Shanks R: Atresia coli inherited in Holstein cattle, *J Dairy Sci* 75: 105-111, 1992.

Syed M, Shanks R: Incidence of atresia coli and relationships among the affected calves born in one herd of Holstein cattle, *J Dairy Sci* 75: 357-364, 1992.

Syed M, Shanks R: What causes atresia coli in Holstein calves? *Cornell Vet* 83: 261-263, 1993.

14.3—Hernias/Umbilicus

Gary M. Baxter

The umbilicus in calves consists of the urachus, umbilical vein, and paired umbilical arteries. These latter structures are often referred to as the umbilical remnants. The urachus, umbilical vein, and umbilical arteries normally regress after birth to become a vestigial part of the bladder apex, round ligament of the liver, and lateral ligaments of the bladder, respectively. Infection (subcutaneous abscess or disease within the umbilical remnants),

herniation (nonstrangulating or strangulating), or a combination of infection and herniation are the primary problems associated with the umbilicus in calves. Each of these problems usually cause enlargement of the umbilicus; therefore an umbilical mass is not always synonymous with an umbilical hernia. Infection of the umbilicus or umbilical cord remnants often occurs in the neonatal period as a result of environmental contamination, but the umbilicus may also be seeded with bacteria from a generalized septicemia/bacteremia. Common bacterial isolates from umbilical infections in calves include *Arcanobacterium pyogenes* and *Escherichia coli*. Umbilical hernias are the most common bovine congenital defect and can occur in any breed, although they appear to be most common in Holstein-Friesian cattle. They are often classified as uncomplicated versus complicated, depending on whether a secondary infection exists.

Umbilical Hernias/Masses

Umbilical masses in calves may be divided into five categories:

1) uncomplicated umbilical hernias
2) umbilical hernias with subcutaneous infection/abscesses
3) umbilical hernias with umbilical remnant infection
4) umbilical abscesses/chronic omphalitis
5) urachal cysts/ruptures

Calves with an umbilical abscess or enlarged umbilical stalk may not have concurrent umbilical hernias but may have clinical signs similar to calves with hernias because of the enlarged umbilicus. However, a combination of the history, signalment and physical examination of the animal is usually sufficient to accurately diagnose the problem and differentiate between calves with and without hernias. Visual inspection of the mass should be performed to evaluate the size, shape, color, and presence of drainage. Palpation of the mass for consistency, temperature, and presence of pain should be performed. The presence of a complete or incomplete hernial ring and reducibility of the contents within the mass should also be determined. Placing the calf in lateral or dorsal recumbency may facilitate deep palpation of the mass. Additionally, ultrasound may be performed to evaluate the umbilicus, which is especially beneficial in documenting abnormalities in the umbilical remnants. There is usually a good correlation between ultrasonographic and surgical findings of infected umbilical remnants in calves.

UNCOMPLICATED UMBILICAL HERNIAS

Uncomplicated umbilical hernias are considered hereditary in cattle and most commonly occur in the Holstein-

Friesian breed. Beef cattle appear to be at lower risk of developing umbilical hernias than dairy cattle. These hernias are usually present during the first few days of life and typically enlarge uniformly as the calf grows. The umbilical mass is completely reducible with a palpable circumferential hernial ring. The hernial sac may contain intestines (enterocele), abomasum (most commonly) omentum, or both (Figure 14.3-1). Calves with these hernias are usually in good condition and rarely show signs of gastrointestinal dysfunction.

Strangulation of the small intestine, omentum, or abomasum within the hernial sac is possible, although rare. Affected calves usually demonstrate signs of abdominal pain and have metabolic derangements (hypochloremic, hypokalemic metabolic alkalosis) caused by sequestration of chloride and hydrogen ions within the abomasal lumen. Chronic hernias may also develop an abomasal-umbilical fistula in which chloride is lost from the abomasal lumen, resulting in dehydration and metabolic abnormalities. Depressed, sick calves with metabolic abnormalities should be stabilized with fluids to correct the metabolic problem before surgery is performed.

Most calves presented for repair of umbilical hernias are less than 6 months old and have hernias less than 10 cm in length. Conservative treatment options for uncomplicated hernias include hernial clamps, elastrator bands, abdominal support bandages, local injection of irritants around the hernial ring and daily digital palpation to irritate the ring. Hernial clamps, elastrator bands, and support bandages are only recommended when the hernia is less than 5 cm long, completely reducible, and

free from evidence or history of infection. Support bandages are more effective in calves than foals because the bovine umbilicus is more cranial and the abdomen more pendulous, preventing caudal slippage of the bandage. Most umbilical hernias longer than 5 cm or demonstrating any evidence of pathology should be repaired surgically with an open herniorrhaphy.

UMBILICAL HERNIAS WITH LOCALIZED ABSCESSES/SUBCUTANEOUS INFECTION

Calves have a higher prevalence of infection associated with umbilical hernias than do foals. This difference may be related to improper care of the umbilicus, increased environmental contamination, and partial or complete failure of passive transfer. Unlike foals, calves with umbilical infections do not usually develop septicemia or a patent urachus. Instead the infection remains localized to the umbilical area. In one study 45% of calves presented for repair of umbilical hernias had evidence of concurrent infection, such as umbilical remnant infections, omphalitis, and subcutaneous abscesses and cellulitis. Calves with an umbilical hernia associated with subcutaneous infection usually have a history of an enlarged umbilical cord since birth, but the umbilical mass is not present until the calf is several weeks old. The calves are generally in good condition, and careful palpation of the mass reveals a reducible dorsal hernia and a firm, nonreducible ventral portion attached to the skin. Although there may be local evidence of inflammation, drainage is usually absent and the hernial ring is palpable. Many of these hernias may be acquired secondary to infection-induced weakening of the body wall.

Surgical removal of the abscess or area of cellulitis or fibrosis, together with repair of the hernia, is the treatment of choice. An open herniorrhaphy is recommended because the subcutaneous abscess may extend into one of the remnants of the umbilical cord, necessitating more extensive excision. In addition, adhesions that involve the greater omentum or abomasum may be present and require resection. An open herniorrhaphy also facilitates closure of the abdomen by eliminating redundant soft tissue (the hernial sac) in the suture line and the need to invert the umbilical remnants.

UMBILICAL HERNIAS WITH INFECTION OF THE UMBILICAL CORD REMNANTS

Umbilical cord remnant infections include omphalophlebitis, omphaloarteritis, and infection/abscessation of the urachus. More than one umbilical cord remnant may be infected, and not all animals have a concurrent umbilical hernia. *Arcanobacterium pyogenes* is the most commonly isolated organism from infected umbilical cord remnants; but *E. coli*, *Proteus*, *Enterococcus*, *Streptococcus* and *Staphylococcus* species may also be identified.

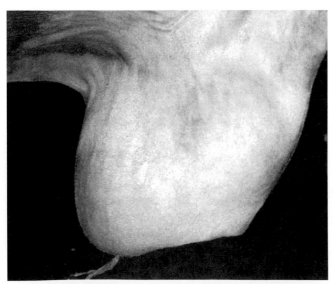

Figure 14.3-1 This large umbilical hernia was present in a 7-day-old beef calf. The mass was completely reducible and nearly the entire abomasum was within the hernial sac.

Consequently, draining tracts should be cultured before surgery or the infected umbilical remnant or abscess cultured after excision.

The usual history in calves with umbilical hernias and remnant infections is intermittent purulent drainage from the umbilicus beginning at 1 to 2 weeks of age. The drainage is often followed by a rapidly enlarging mass several weeks later. These calves are often unthrifty and small for their ages and may have concurrent infectious diseases, such as septic arthritis, pneumonia, peritonitis or bacteremia. A complete blood count may indicate hyperfibrinogenemia, hyperproteinemia, neutrophil-lymphocyte reversal, and mild anemia. The umbilical mass is usually large, broad-based, painful to palpation, and only partly reducible, and the hernial ring is incompletely palpable. In small calves deep palpation of the abdomen with the animal in lateral or dorsal recumbency may reveal an enlarged, infected umbilical remnant. An infected enlarged umbilical vein courses dorsocranially toward the liver; and the infected urachus or umbilical arteries course caudodorsally toward the urinary bladder and internal iliac arteries, respectfully. However, ultrasound of the ventral abdomen is the ideal method to document an abnormality in the umbilical remnants (Figures 14.3-2 and 14.3-3). In one study there was good-to-excellent correlation between ultrasound findings and actual physical (surgical or postmortem) findings of the umbilical structures. However, ultrasound was unreliable in documenting concurrent intraabdominal adhesions associated with these infec-

tions, which were present in 47% of the animals in the study. In foals there are reports of using laparoscopy to evaluate and, in some instances, ligate and/or resect umbilical cord remnants.

Umbilical hernias in calves complicated by infections of umbilical cord remnants have been reported to occur in approximately 24% of cases. This figure was calculated from animals presented for surgical repair on umbilical hernias and does not include calves that were successfully treated with conservative measures in the field. Therefore this percentage may reflect an overestimation of the true prevalence of infections of umbilical cord remnants among all calves with umbilical masses. However, umbilical remnant infection should be suspected in calves with large umbilical masses, especially if the animal is unthrifty.

The urachus is the most frequently infected umbilical remnant associated with umbilical masses in calves (Figure 14.3-4). Dysuria, pollakiuria, pyuria, and cystitis are all sequelae to urachal abscesses/infections in calves. These clinical signs may occur because of direct communication between the abscess and bladder lumen or by mechanical interference with normal bladder filling and emptying. For all surgery that involves umbilical remnant infections, the surgeon should be prepared to extend the incision and drape the site accordingly.

In some of the urachal infections that extend to the bladder, the urachal stalk and lumen of the bladder are distinctly separated. Surgical excision of the infected urachus combined with repair of the hernia is the treatment of choice. Urachal infections that extend to the bladder require excision of the apex of the bladder and ligation of the umbilical arteries. The entire urachus, umbilical arteries, hernial tissue, and overlying skin are removed en bloc to prevent contamination of the abdomen (Figure 14.3-5).

Omphalophlebitis may be localized along the umbilical vein or may extend the entire length of the vein and involve the liver. Infection that progresses to the liver can result in multiple liver abscesses, septicemia, bacteremia, and unthriftiness. Localized umbilical vein abscesses that do not involve the liver can usually be surgically ligated and removed en bloc (Figure 14.3-6). Umbilical vein abscesses that extend to and involve the liver are handled by a marsupialization technique. The abscess is exited from the abdomen through a separate incision in the right paramedian area, or through the cranial aspect of the ventral median incision. With either technique, the wall of the infected umbilical vein must be secured to the ventral body wall in a two- or three-layer closure to prevent leakage and peritonitis. The advantages of incorporating the vein within the existing ventral incision are that only one abdominal incision is required and the infected umbilical vein does not need to be passed

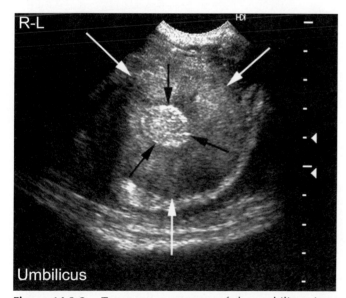

Figure 14.3-2 Transverse sonogram of the umbilicus in a 5-month-old Holstein heifer calf with an umbilical abscess. Images were obtained using a 5-3 MHz phased array sector probe. Note the thick umbilicus (white arrows) and the echoic (purulent) material present within the lumen (black arrows).

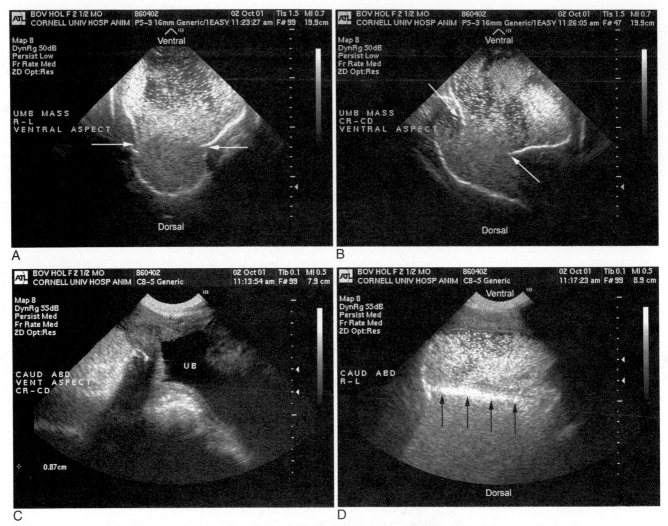

Figure 14.3-3   Sonograms of the umbilical hernia sac and caudal abdomen obtained from a 2.5-month-old Holstein heifer calf with an umbilical hernia and urachal abscess. A 5-3 MHz phased array sector probe and an 8-5 MHz convex probe were used. The transverse (A) and longitudinal (B) sonograms illustrate the hernia sac containing a 7-cm, well-circumscribed, thick walled, fluid cavity mass (abscess). The arrows denote the hernia ring in the body wall. The longitudinal sonogram of the caudal abdomen (C) illustrates the urachal abscess extending ventrally to the apex of the urinary bladder. Note the caliper markers indicate the urachus and **UB** represents urinary bladder. In the transverse sonogram of the caudal abdomen (D), the mass contains a fluid/gas interface or gas-cap (black arrows). This finding is pathognomonic for an abscess.

intraabdominally to a paramedian position, whereas the disadvantage is the entire incision could become contaminated. After surgery, the marsupialized tract is irrigated with dilute povidone-iodine until closure by second intention. However, the tracts should not be lavaged under pressure, especially in calves younger than 2 months of age; because the lavage solution may enter the systemic circulation through the liver and cause serious adverse reactions. Both marsupialization techniques have been reported to be very successful at resolving umbilical vein infections in calves. In addition,

the umbilical vein stalk may be subsequently removed en bloc at a second surgery once the infection has completely resolved.

Omphaloarteritis is the least common infection of an umbilical cord remnant. Normally, the umbilical arteries retract into the abdomen at birth, thus minimizing the risk of infection. One or both arteries may be infected anywhere along their course. Intestinal strangulation is reported to be an uncommon sequela of omphaloarteritis. Surgical ligation and resection of the involved arteries, umbilical mass (and, at times, resection of the apex of

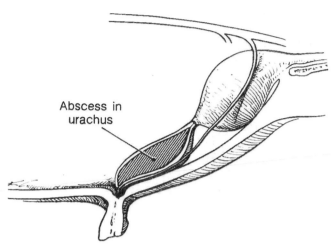

Figure 14.3-4 Schematic illustration of an infection within the urachal remnant. The urachus is the most commonly infected umbilical remnant and usually does not communicate with the lumen of the bladder.

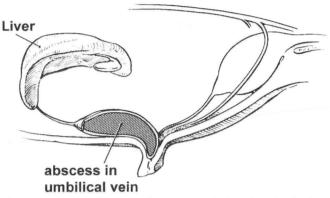

Figure 14.3-6 Schematic illustration of a localized infection within the umbilical vein. This abscess could be completely resected at surgery. Abscesses extending to and involving the liver cannot be resected en bloc and should be marsupialized to the ventral body wall.

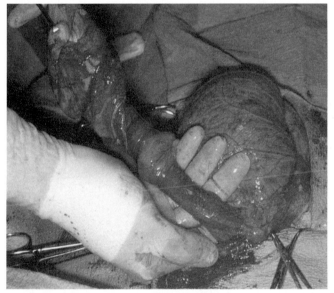

Figure 14.3-5 Surgical isolation of the external umbilicus (top left of slide) and a large, infected urachal stalk. This tissue was removed en bloc by excising and closing the apex of the bladder in this calf.

the urinary bladder), and overlying skin during repair of the umbilical hernia is the treatment of choice. The omentum may be adhered to the arteries, requiring careful dissection and ligation.

UMBILICAL ABSCESSES/CHRONIC OMPHALITIS

Umbilical abscesses are common sequelae to circumscribed omphalitis. The umbilical mass often occurs shortly after birth but may develop anytime between birth and 2 years of age. Similar to calves with infections of umbilical remnants, these calves are often unthrifty and may have evidence of infectious diseases in organs remote from the umbilicus. The umbilical mass is usually warm, painful to palpation, nonreducible, and firm or fluctuant. No hernial ring is palpable, and drainage is uncommon. Diagnosis of an umbilical abscess is based on physical examination, characteristics of the umbilical mass, and aspiration of purulent material from the mass. Ultrasound may also be used to document the presence of purulent material within the umbilicus. Most umbilical abscesses will respond to drainage and lavage of the abscess cavity. Systemic antimicrobials may or may not be indicated. Chronic infection of the umbilicus may lead to a thickened, fibrotic umbilical stalk that may appear similar to an abscess. The need for surgery depends on how well the infection responds to medical treatment and the cosmetic appearance required. If the abscess recurs, the possibility of the infection extending into the umbilical cord remnants must be considered, and surgical removal is indicated. However, initial drainage of purulent material is essential.

An open herniorrhaphy with complete removal of the abscess is recommended. A fusiform incision is made around the border of the abscess, and the subcutaneous tissue is sharply dissected to expose the linea alba. The abscess cavity should not be entered. A small incision is made into the abdomen either cranial or caudal to the base of the abscess to permit digital palpation of the umbilical cord remnants. If the infection extends intra-abdominally, the abdomen is opened further, and the involved umbilical remnants are removed along with the abscess. If the abscess is localized, the capsule and all adherent tissue are extirpated. The incision is closed as described for a routine herniorrhaphy.

URACHAL CYSTS/RUPTURES

Several anatomical abnormalities of the urachus may occur in all species and have been reported in cattle. Urachal cysts have been found in calves with umbilical masses/hernias and should be included as a differential diagnosis in calves with nonreducible umbilical masses. Urachal cysts can be imaged with ultrasound and the diagnosis confirmed at surgery. In one calf, the urachal cysts ruptured into the subcutaneous tissues around the umbilicus subsequent to attempts to reduce the umbilical swelling. The subcutaneous urine caused severe tissue inflammation around the umbilicus with necrosis of a small area of skin. Rupture of the urachus into the subcutaneous space occurs in foals, but is usually not associated with an urachal cyst. It is thought to be a result of traumatic foaling, with evidence of umbilical swelling and subcutaneous urine accumulation very soon after birth. The other main urachal anatomical defect is failure to involute or disappear after birth. The typical noninfected patent or persistent urachus with dribbling of urine seen in neonatal foals is very uncommon in neonatal calves. A persistent urachus consisting of a thin band of tissue has been reported to cause small intestinal strangulation in an adult cow. Additionally, rupture of a persistent urachus that communicated with the lumen of the bladder resulted in uroperitoneum in a yearling bull. Similar anatomical or congenital abnormalities of the umbilical vein and arteries in calves have not been reported.

Diagnosis

A tentative diagnosis of the cause of an umbilical mass in most calves can be determined from physical examination of the animal and close inspection of the umbilical region. Calves placed in lateral recumbency relax their abdomen, which permits deep palpation of intraabdominal structures. However, ultrasonography of the umbilicus is recommended in most cases to document the diagnosis and determine the site(s) and severity of the infection preoperatively in cases of concurrent infection. Enlargement of the internal umbilical structures and the presence of echogenic material (fluid and/or gas) usually confirms the diagnosis of infection within the umbilical remnants. However, normal ultrasonographic findings do not always indicate the absence of infection, and ultrasound cannot be relied on to always accurately assess the presence of intraabdominal adhesions.

Surgical Management

The appropriate management of patients with umbilical masses/hernias depends on accurate preoperative diagnosis. As previously stated, small, uncomplicated umbilical hernias and many umbilical abscesses may not require surgery. Uncomplicated umbilical hernias requiring surgery can often be repaired with the calf in dorsal recumbency using sedation (xylazine hydrochloride) and a local anesthetic. If infection or some other problem associated with the umbilical mass is identified or likely, surgery should be performed with the animal under general anesthesia because of the increased surgery time and potential for complications. Inhalation general anesthesia is preferred; but IV combinations such as xylazine hydrochloride-ketamine hydrochloride, valium-ketamine hydrochloride, or xylazine hydrochloride-ketamine hydrochloride-guaifenesin may be used to help reduce expense.

Proper preoperative management of abscesses, omphalitis, and infections of umbilical cord remnants may decrease the potential for contamination and the duration of surgery. Large abscesses should be drained or aspirated and treated medically with antimicrobials for several days before surgery to decrease their size and minimize the number of bacteria. Draining tracts should be lavaged and given time to heal before surgery, if possible. Otherwise, they should be oversewn at the beginning of surgery to minimize contamination. Infected umbilical remnants and abscesses should be resected en bloc if possible to prevent contamination of the abdomen and incision. If infection is confirmed or possible, antimicrobials should be given before surgery and continued after surgery if needed. Antimicrobials should be based on the results of a culture and sensitivity, but procaine penicillin and/or ceftiofur should be effective against most bacteria associated with umbilical infections in calves.

Small, uncomplicated hernias in calves can be repaired with a closed herniorrhaphy (peritoneum is not opened) similar to that performed in foals. However, compared to a closed herniorrhaphy, an open herniorrhaphy often takes less time, is less traumatic, allows inspection of the abdominal viscera, and permits removal of the umbilical remnants if considered necessary. Before surgery, the external opening of the umbilicus and prepuce are oversewn to prevent contamination of the surgery site. A fusiform incision is made around the umbilicus, and the abdomen is entered cranial to the umbilical stalk to permit digital palpation of intraabdominal structures. The scarred edge of the hernial ring is sharply incised together with the peritoneum. In cases with umbilical remnant infections, the umbilical vein and arteries are ligated above the site(s) of infection, and the urachus is excised along with the apex of the bladder. The bladder is closed routinely. Complete removal of the infected umbilical remnants in situ can usually be performed except with severe infections of the umbilical vein. Simple apposition of the unscarred hernial ring with minimal tension is thought to lead to ideal healing. Several suture patterns may be used but simple interrupted, interrupted cruciate, or simple continuous patterns are used most commonly. In most cases absorbable suture material such as polyglactin 910, polydioxanone,

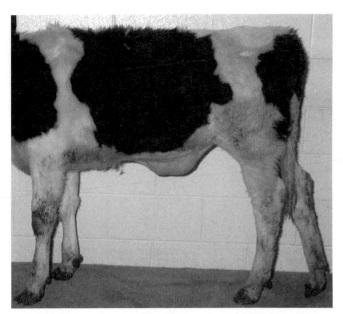

Figure 14.3-7 The umbilical hernia in this Holstein calf had been repaired two previous times without success. The hernia was large and a mesh implant was used to close the defect.

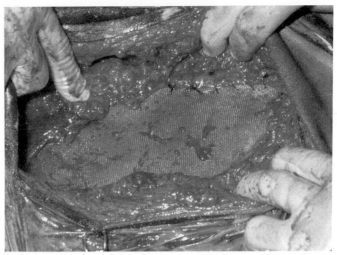

Figure 14.3-8 Placement of the mesh within the hernial defect in the calf in Figure 14.3-5. The plastic mesh was doubled, placed retroperitoneal, and secured to the hernial ring with nonabsorbable suture material. A fascial overlay technique was used for the mesh herniorrhaphy in this calf.

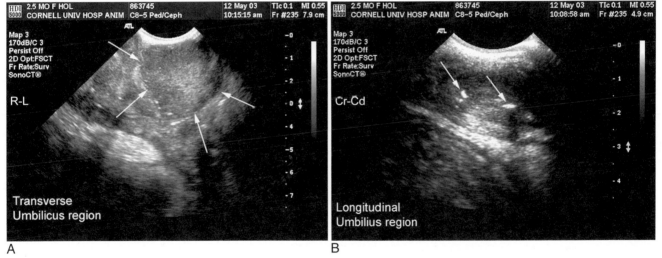

Figure 14.3-9 Transverse (A) and longitudinal (B) sonograms of the umbilical region in a 2.5-month-old Holstein heifer calf one month after an umbilical abscess resection. Images were obtained using an 8-5 MHz convex probe. (A) Arrows outline abscess cavity that has formed at the previous resection site. (B) In the abscess cavity, there are hyperechoic foci that cast acoustic shadows representing suture material (arrows).

or polyglycolic acid is recommended to close the body wall. In larger defects, tension-relieving sutures such as near-far-far-near placed at regular intervals may help appose the two sides. In an older animal, withholding solid food for 36 to 48 hours reduces the rumen volume and greatly facilitates body wall closure.

Large hernias (greater than 15 cm) and hernias unsuccessfully repaired previously are often candidates for mesh herniorrhaphy (Figure 14.3-7). Polypropylene (Marlex) or plastic (Proxplast) mesh products are the most commonly used, although plastic mesh is less expensive than polypropylene. In addition, plastic mesh is less elastic and decreases the amount of sagging seen after surgery. A fascial overlay technique is recommended for placing the mesh (McIlwraith and Robertson, 1998). Briefly, a semielliptical incision is made along one side of the hernial ring. The skin, subcutaneous tissue, and fibrous hernial sac are reflected across the hernial defect to expose the opposite hernial ring. Usually the peritoneum is adhered to the hernial sac and is incised. A double layer of mesh is placed either retroperitoneal or between the incised edges of the hernial ring (Figure 14.3-8). The mesh is secured circumferentially around the hernial ring with interrupted horizontal mattress sutures, making certain the mesh is taut. The reflected hernial fascia, subcutaneous tissue, and skin are placed over the mesh and closed routinely. Antimicrobial therapy should be used for mesh herniorrhaphies because of the increased risk of infection associated with mesh implantation.

Complications

Postoperative complications of umbilical herniorrhaphy are more numerous in calves than in foals, probably because concurrent infection is more common in calves with umbilical hernias (Figure 14.3-9). Most complications are related to incisional problems such as suture abscesses, seromas, hematomas, and dehiscence. The majority of these problems usually do not affect the success of the surgery unless the local infection is severe enough to cause failure of the body wall closure and recurrence of the hernia. The more ventral location of the suture line and the greater weight distributed across it in calves compared to foals may lead to a higher risk of incisional dehiscence in calves. Abdominal support bandages may help prevent re-herniation if the abdominal wall appears weak at surgery; however, good surgical technique and limited postoperative activity are the most important factors in preventing body wall dehiscence. Peritonitis is a more serious potential complication and

is usually associated with severe contamination of the abdomen during surgery or with foci of intraabdominal infection that were incompletely removed at surgery. This complication is most likely in calves with umbilical vein infections involving the liver. Although these complications are possible, most calves do very well after umbilical herniorrhaphy with a favorable prognosis for a productive life.

RECOMMENDED READINGS

Baxter GM: Umbilical masses in calves: Diagnosis, treatment, and complications. *Compend Contin Educ Pract Vet* 11: 505-513, 1989.

Boure L, Marcoux M, Laverty S: Laparoscopic abdominal anatomy of foals positioned in dorsal recumbency. *Vet Surg* 25: 1-6, 1997.

Edwards RB, Fubini SL: A one-stage marsupialization procedure for management of infected umbilical vein remnants in calves and foals. *Vet Surg* 24: 32-35, 1995.

Fischer AT Jr: Laparoscopically assisted resection of umbilical structures in foals. *J Am Vet Med Assoc* 214: 1813-1816, 1999.

Lischer CJ, Iselin U, Steiner A: Ultrasonographic diagnosis of urachal cyst in three calves. *J Am Vet Med Assoc* 204: 1801-1804, 1994.

McIlwraith CW, Robertson JT: Herniorrhaphy using synthetic mesh and a fascial overlay. In *Equine surgery advanced techniques*, ed 2, Philadelphia, 1998, Williams & Wilkins, pp 365-370.

Staller GS, Tulleners EP, Reef VB, Spencer PA: Concordance of ultrasonographic and physical findings in cattle with an umbilical mass or suspected to have infection of the umbilical cord remnants: 32 cases (1987-1989). *J Am Vet Med Assoc* 206: 77-81, 1995.

Steiner A, Lischer CJ, Oertle C: Marsupialization of umbilical vein abscesses with involvement of the liver in 13 calves. *Vet Surg* 22: 184-189, 1993.

Trent AM, Smith DF: Surgical management of umbilical masses with associated umbilical remnant infections in calves. *J Am Vet Med Assoc* 185: 1531-1534, 1984.

Watson E, Mahaffey MB, Crowell W, et al: Ultrasonography of the umbilical structures in clinically normal calves. *Am J Vet Res* 55: 773-780, 1994.

CHAPTER 15

SURGERY OF THE CALF MUSCULOSKELETAL SYSTEM

Norm G. Ducharme

Numerous musculoskeletal system diseases in farm animals exist—ranging from the more rare congenital abnormality (malformation, angular or flexural deformity) to acquired diseases such as septic arthritis and fractures. This section will describe diseases seen mainly in calves, such as angular and flexural deformity as well as other congenital abnormalities. The readers are directed to Chapter 11 for the principles of diagnosing and managing fractures).

15.1—Polydactyly

The etiology of this disease has been reported in Simmental cattle to a mixed dominant (one locus) and recessive gene (another locus). This congenital malformation is rare in farm animals, and treating it should be seen only as a salvage procedure for food production. Indeed, the possibility of inheritable diseases in all breeds argues against adding these animals to the genetic pool.

The clinical diagnosis is straightforward. The front limbs are generally affected. Radiographic examination helps determine the extent of the abnormalities (Figure 15.1-1). Surgical removal is done with the animal under general anesthesia with the abnormal digit uppermost. Consideration of placement of surgical incisions should allow sufficient skin for closure. In addition to skeleton being removed (Figure 15.1-2A and B), the flexor tendons associated with a deformity must also be removed. One should carefully dissect the flexor tendons to ensure that the remaining flexor tendons are left as a functional unit.

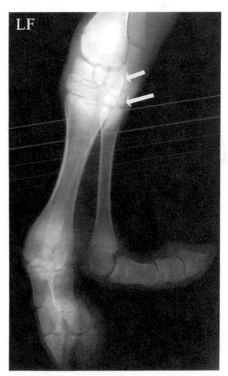

Figure 15.1-1 Lateral radiographs of a 10-day-old Holstein-Friesian heifer calf with polydactylia and flexural deformity. Supranumary carpal, metacarpal, sesamoids, and phalangeal bones are present. Note the two additional carpal bones (arrows).

(Courtesy of Dr. Markus Wilke; Cornell University.)

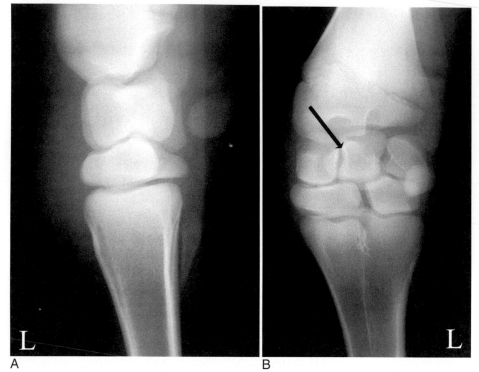

Figure 15.1-2   Postoperative radiographs of calf in Figure 15.1-1 after removal of the supranumary phalangeal, sesamoid, metacarpal, and distal carpal bones. *A*, lateral view. *B*, Dorsopalmar view; note remaining proximal carpal bone (arrow).

(Courtesy of Dr. Markus Wilke; Cornell University.)

RECOMMENDED READINGS

Johnson JL, Leipold HW, Schalles RR: Hereditary polydactylia in Simmental Cattle, *J Hered* 72:205-208, 1981.

15.2—Flexural Deformities

Norm G. Ducharme

Calves present with flexural deformity (i.e., contracted tendons) either as a congenital or acquired problem. Congenital flexural deformities are seen within 1 or 2 weeks of birth. Flexural deformity ranges in severity from mild knuckling at the fetlock to being unable to walk, stand, and nurse. The etiology of congenital flexural deformity in cattle is generally unknown, but cattle seen with additional congenital abnormalities may have a heritable condition and should be removed from the breeding pool. Other congenital abnormalities sometimes seen simultaneously with flexural deformity are cleft palate, dwarfism, and arthrogryposis. Lupine ingestion by the dam between 30 and 70 days of gestation may result in arthrogryposis. In addition to congenital flexural deformity, acquired flexural deformity is seen secondary to reduced weight bearing associated with a primary painful orthopedic disease.

Clinical Presentation

Usually, calves present with mild metacarpophalangeal (MP) or carpal flexural deformity. The condition is mild and usually bilateral. In a more severe presentation, the calves have constant knuckling of the fetlocks; the carpus sometimes is also involved (Figure 15.2-1). Rarely, the metatarsophalangeal joints are affected. Owners report that calves are born with this condition or develop it within a few days to a week of birth. The deformity may be so severe that calves are unable to stand, so failure of passive immunity transfer may be a complicating factor. Abnormal hoof wear is present as a result of irregular weight bearing. Depending on the housing situation and disease chronicity, affected calves that must compete for feed may have poor body condition.

Acquired flexural deformity seen in older calves is generally unilateral and secondary to a severe orthopedic injury where the animal cannot bear any or only minimal weight on the affected limb (Figure 15.2-2). A

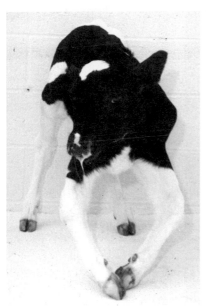

Figure 15.2-1 Newborn calf with bilateral carpal and metacarpophalangeal deformities.

(Courtesy of Dr. Mary Smith; Cornell University.)

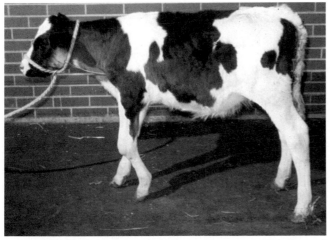

Figure 15.2-2 Heifer calf with unilateral carpal flexural deformity secondary to a primary carpal orthopedic disease. Note enlarged carpus.

dropped fetlock and varus deformity at the carpus of the contralateral limb is evidence of excessive weight bearing.

A chronic deformity may have associated skin ulcerations on the dorsum of the fetlock with the wound extending into the joint, resulting in septic arthritis.

Anatomical Considerations

The relevant anatomy of the flexor tendons and suspensory ligaments is important in relation to surgical

transection. The level of the incision is influenced by the number of structures that need to be transected to release the flexural deformity.

The superficial digital flexor muscle arises from the medial epicondyle of the humerus and divides in two parts, forming two distinct tendons: a deep tendon that passes through the carpal canal and a superficial tendon that passes outside the carpal canal. Both tendons fuse in the midcannon bone but divide at the fetlock into the medial and lateral digit, forming a sleeve that encircles the deep flexor tendon. Each divided superficial flexor tendon inserts on the proximal palmar aspect of their respective middle phalanx.

The deep digital flexor tendon passes into the carpal canal and lays dorsal (deep) to the superficial flexor tendon until near the fetlock, where it divides to insert on the palmar aspect of the distal phalanges of the medial or lateral digit, respectively.

The suspensory ligament (interosseus muscle in young animals and ligamentous in adults) on the palmar aspect of the metacarpal bone lies deep to both flexor tendons. It originates from the proximal aspect of the metacarpal bone and divides at the midmetacarpal region, sending a band that joins the superficial flexor tendon. A few centimeters distally, the suspensory ligament divides into three branches: two abaxial and one in the middle. The two abaxial branches further divide distally into two branches that each attach to the corresponding medial and lateral sesamoid bone before continuing to their insertion on the palmar aspect of each proximal phalanx. In addition, each suspensory ligament abaxial branch continues into an extensor branch that joins the abaxial aspect of the extensor tendons on the dorsal aspect of each digit. The middle branch passes through the intertrochlear notch and divides into two branches that each join the axial aspect of the extensor tendons of each digit.

The ulnaris lateralis and flexor carpi ulnaris both insert on the accessory carpal bone. The ulnaris lateralis originates from the lateral epicondyle of the humerus, and the flexor carpi ulnaris originates from the medial epicondyle of the humerus and ulna.

Diagnosis

The diagnosis can be easily made when the abnormally flexed position of the limb with the deformity centered on the affected joint is observed (see Figure 15.2-1). One should use palpation in an attempt to identify a cause for the deformity, such as a swollen joint, ruptured extensor tendon, or other orthopedic lesions (see Figure 15.2-2). This is especially true in acquired flexural deformities of calves. One should flex and extend the affected limb to identify a painful process that may be contributing to the deformity. The veterinarian should also evaluate how much of the deformity can be corrected by manually extending the limb. Although radiographs illustrate the deformity of the axial skeleton well, they rarely add to the diagnosis. Radiographs only help identify the extremely rare orthopedic malformations (i.e., deformed joints that cause a deformity).

Management

Mild cases of flexural deformity respond well when patients are placed in housing with good footing. In addition, rather than spending extended periods standing, daily walking exercise is preferable. Treatment for more affected calves depends on whether the leg can be straightened manually so that the calf can walk. Medical treatment is indicated when no predisposing orthopedic anomaly is present and the limb can be manually extended so the toe's ventral aspect can touch the ground. A splint should be placed on the palmar aspect of the limb, starting at the heel (leaving the claws out) and extending to the proximal metacarpal (or metatarsal) III bone (for MP flexural deformity) or proximal radius (for carpal flexural deformity). The splint is changed every 2 to 3 days. Alternatively, a cast may be placed and removed/changed 2 to 3 weeks later (Figure 15.2-3). Although oxytetracycline IV (3 g in 250 ml of physiological saline) can be given to relax the muscles for more rapid correction of the limb, it should be avoided whenever possible in calves. Tetracycline is very nephrotoxic in calves, so a single treatment may result in significant renal damage.

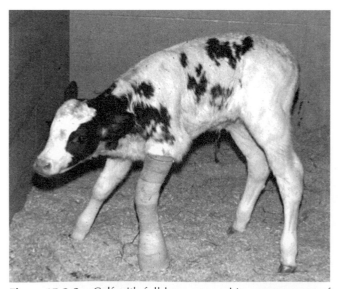

Figure 15.2-3   Calf with full leg cast used in management of carpal flexural deformity.

The splint is placed as follows: 3 to 4 cotton sheets (or roll) are placed around the limb for sufficient padding to minimize skin ulceration at the pressure points of the splint. Alternatively, reusable quilt material can be used. The splint should be light so as to cause as little interference as possible with movement. Satisfactory splint materials include a piece of wood or polyvinyl chloride (PVC) piping (10 cm in diameter cut into quarters or halves). The splint is placed at the palmar aspect of the limb, starting at the heel and extending to either the proximal cannon bone or radius, depending on the location of the deformity. A splint terminating at the proximal end of the cannon bone should be placed to allow maximum flexion of the carpus. If palmar skin sores develop, the splint should be placed on the dorsal aspect of the limb. Young calves with bilateral splinting may require assistance to stand at first. Surgical treatment should be considered if an animal does not respond within a few weeks of treatment.

Surgical correction is indicated for calves not responding to splinting or with insufficient correction of the deformity to allow weight bearing. MP flexural deformity is treated by sequentially transecting the superficial flexor tendon, deep digital flexor, and suspensory ligament until the deformity is released. The number of tendons transected is decided during surgery. The tendons of the flexor carpi ulnaris and ulnaris lateralis muscles are transected to treat carpal flexural deformity.

The surgical procedure is performed under sedation (xylazine hydrochloride 0.1 mg/kg IM) and infiltration of local anesthesia at the intended surgery site or under general anesthesia. The calf is placed in lateral recumbency with the affected limb uppermost. This is critical for tenotomies of the flexor carpi radialis and ulnaris lateralis, but the digital flexor tendons can be transected from either a medial or lateral approach. Anatomically, two superficial digital flexor tendons each receive a branch from the suspensory ligament, two deep digital flexor tendons, and two abaxial suspensory ligaments, each with two branches. When a structure is transected, the specified flexor tendons and/or suspensory ligaments for both medial and lateral digits must be transected. Antibiotic prophylaxis is optional, but the animal should receive NSAID (i.e., flunixin meglumine 1 mg/kg sid IV or aspirin 100 mg/kg bid po) preoperatively and for 2 to 3 days after surgery.

To correct a MP flexural deformity, a 7.5-cm incision is made over the lateral (or medial) aspect of the deep digital flexor tendon at the level of the midcannon bone. The fascia surrounding the flexor tendon is incised in the same plane, with care taken not to injure the lateral (or medial) palmar (or plantar) digital artery, vein, or nerve. The superficial digital flexor tendons and the connecting branches from the suspensory ligament are identified and elevated with curved hemostats. The superficial digital flexor tendons should be carefully elevated and isolated to prevent injury to the contralateral vessels. The superficial digital flexor tendons and the connecting branches from the suspensory ligament are transected after they are isolated. The surgeon then extends the fetlock to evaluate the degree of correction achieved. The goal is to obtain sufficient correction so that the hoof contacts the ground without the fetlock knuckling. Exercise and the calf's body weight will place the joint in a normal position when the calf is walking if the knuckling is corrected. If the deformity is not sufficiently corrected after the superficial digital flexor muscle is transected, the tendons of the deep digital flexor muscle are isolated and transected as described previously. If the deformity is still not sufficiently corrected, the suspensory ligament is identified immediately caudal to MC (or MT) III, isolated with a curved hemostat, and transected. The peritendinous fascia and subcutaneous tissues are closed separately with nonabsorbable sutures in a simple continuous pattern. The skin is closed with an acceptable pattern.

The limb is bandaged, and a decision is made as to whether a splint is needed. When the superficial digital flexor tendons and their connecting branches from the suspensory ligament are transected, a splint is not needed postoperatively unless tension from the splint is needed to force additional extension for optimum correction. In rare cases, a splint is needed after surgery if the animal appears painful. If the deep digital flexor tendons are also transected, the limb(s) may need splint support up to 30 days. In addition, if the deep and superficial flexor tendons (tenotomies) plus the suspensory ligament are transected, destabilization of the palmar aspect of the carpus occurs. Therefore a splint that extends to the radius to give palmar support to the carpus needs to be placed on the back of the limb.

For carpal flexural deformity, a 10-cm incision starting at the accessory carpal bone and extending proximally is made on the lateral aspect of the carpus over the tendon of the ulnaris lateralis. The incision is extended bluntly until the tendons of the ulnaris lateralis and flexor carpi ulnaris tendon are identified, isolated with a curved hemostat, and transected. The subcutaneous tissues are closed separately with nonabsorbable sutures in a simple continuous pattern. The skin is closed with an acceptable pattern. A splint is placed postoperatively on the palmar aspect of the knee unless full correction is obtained. The care of splints is described under Medical Management.

In calves with flexural deformity secondary to an orthopedic injury, one must first address the primary problem. Splints, as described previously, are used to combat secondary flexural deformities.

Prognosis

The prognosis for calves with flexural deformity is usually good. Secondary healing after transection of flexor tendons and even the suspensory ligament usually results in a functional gait. The low athletic demand on farm animals explains the fairly good success in treating primary flexural deformity.

RECOMMENDED READINGS

Anderson DE, St Jean G: Diagnosis and management of tendon disorders in cattle, *Vet Clin North Am Food Anim Pract* 12:85-116, 1996.

Dyce KM, Sack WO, Wensing CJG: The forelimb of ruminants. In Dyce KM, Sack WO, Wensing CJG, editors: *Textbook of veterinary anatomy*, Philadelphia, 1996, WB Saunders.

Van Huffel X, De Moor A: Congenital multiple arthrogryposis of the forelimb in calves, *Comp Cont Ed Pract Vet* 9:F333-F339, 1987.

Verschooten F, De Moor A, Desmet P et al: Surgical treatment of congenital arthrogryposis of the carpal joint associated with contraction of the flexor tendons in calves, *Vet Rec* 85:140-171, 1969.

15.3—Angular Deformities

Norm G. Ducharme

An angular deformity originates from many sources: growth plate abnormality, fracture, and ligament rupture. The angular deformity is called *valgus* if the distal limb extremity (distal to the site of angulation) deviates laterally and *varus* if it deviates medially. In addition, rotational deformities are often seen as part of an angular deformity. For instance, the claws usually rotate outward with a valgus and inward with a varus deformity except in cases of multiple angulations in a limb.

Etiology

Congenital angular deformity is very rare in cattle and reportedly is in the middiaphysis of the affected long bone when it occurs. The exact etiology is unknown but has been attributed to in-utero bending stresses early in gestation.

Growth plate differential growth commonly seen in horses is rarely seen in farm animals. More accurately stated, angular deformity is a common event in cattle in that most calves have a mild carpal valgus deformity of approximately 7 degrees (Figure 15.3-1), which is within the normal range for most farm animals and does not require treatment. Orthopedic injuries such as fracture and its healing process, collateral ligament tear, physeal

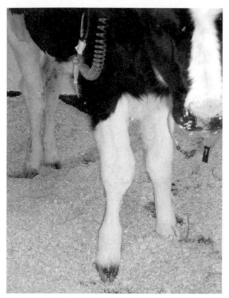

Figure 15.3-1   The forelimb of a 1 week old calf is examined. The observer needs to be aligned with the center of the front claws to determine if the pastern area, third metacarpal bone, and radius are in line. Note the slight normal divergence of the line between the metacarpal bone and the radius.

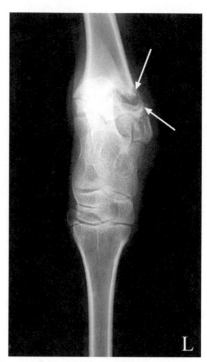

Figure 15.3-2   Septic physitis in a ewe with angular deformity. Note the lytic area at the physis (arrows) (Courtesy of Dr. Anthony Pease; Cornell University.)

infection (Figure 15.3-2), or physeal fracture commonly cause secondary angular deformity.

Wolff's law (1872) states that gradual or repetitive load changes due to trauma or change in activity cause functional remodeling so that trabeculae are reoriented to align with new stress axes. This plays a role in misaligned fracture healing and an animal's ability to remodel the area to correct or improve the deformity. The effect of pressure and shear force on longitudinal growth varies and depends on the degree of pressure and whether it is intermittent or constant. Intermittent pressure allows the growth plate to respond to the line of stress. Partially through reduced blood flow, constant pressure reduces longitudinal growth from the affected physis plate. The uncompressed side of the physis maintains normal growth, which results in an angular deformity (usually varus). This is often seen at the hock or carpus on the contralateral limb of a limb affected with a painful orthopedic problem.

Clinical Presentation

Animals presented for evaluation of angular deformities are easy to recognize. For an accurate diagnosis, one should align himself or herself with the claws and evaluate whether all the long bones are in line (see Figure 15.3-1). This perspective is important because differentiating an angular deformity from a rotational deformity is difficult when one is observing the animal from the front or back. Standing directly in the center front of the claws eliminates the rotational deformity as a confounding factor.

Further examination should focus on the area where the limb loses linearity. Physical examination can assess whether pain or other signs of an orthopedic injury—including the following—are present: increased laxity, swelling and its characteristics, degree of lameness, and presence of muscle atrophy. Although valgus deformity is relatively common (it may be normal for cattle), varus deformity is abnormal (Figure 15.3-3). If varus deformity is found unilaterally, the contralateral limb should be examined for a significant orthopedic injury as a cause for excessive weight bearing in the deformed limb/joint. Obtaining radiographic evaluation is important in investigation of orthopedic injuries, which are often important causal factors in angular deformity in farm animals.

Diagnosis

The diagnosis is made based on the clinical signs, but an exact etiology may not be determined unless radiographic examination is done. A dorsopalmar view is needed for examination of the anatomical location of the deformity and its measurement (Figure 15.3-4). Like the visual examination, the dorsopalmar view must be taken

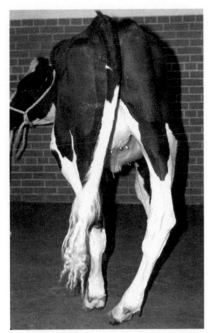

Figure 15.3-3 Calf with varus deformity of the right hock secondary to excessive weight-bearing.

with the radiographic beam in line with the claws. To estimate the degree of angular deformity, a long cassette is needed so that more accurate lines overlying the center of the longitudinal axis can be drawn. The area of divergence (pivot point) of these lines confirms the angular deformity site, and the radiographic abnormality helps identify the causes (see Figure 15.3-4). Further radiographic views may be needed, depending on the nature of the injury or problem.

Management

MEDICAL MANAGEMENT

Trimming the claws of a young calf creates growth plate response to stress applied opposite the deformity, so self correction occurs. The trimming and other hoof manipulation is based on the principle that the hoof will turn in the direction of the longer claw or toward the side of the wider wall (Figure 15.3-5). To correct a valgus deformity, the lateral claw is trimmed so that it is shorter than the medial claw. To correct a varus deformity, the medial claw is trimmed so that it is shorter than the lateral claw. Acrylic can also be applied. Acrylic is applied over the lateral aspect of the lateral claw of a varus deformity to make the claw wider with more lateral contact with the ground. The lateral claw must not extend more than 1 cm; otherwise the stress on the lamina may cause inflammation and pain. The procedure is reversed for a valgus deformity (extend the medial wall of the medial

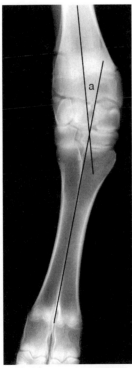

Figure 15.3-4 Dorsopalmar view of a radiograph of a calf forelimb. Lines overlying the center of the longitudinal axis have been drawn. The pivot angle (a) marks the degree of angular deformity (Courtesy of Dr. Anthony Pease; Cornell University.)

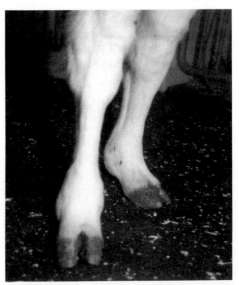

Figure 15.3-5 Animal with valgus deformity of the right hind. Note that the inside claw is shorter than the outside claw, contributing to the lateral deviation and external rotation. (Courtesy of Mr. Michael Wildenstein, Farrier; Cornell University.)

claw). Finally, a shoe may be glued onto the claw to extend the lateral or medial claw.

Primary treatment is directed at the orthopedic injury if a varus deformity is present secondary to a contralateral limb orthopedic injury. Preventing a secondary varus abnormality is far more effective than treating it. Resolving excessive weight bearing, trimming the medial claw, and sometimes applying acrylic over the lateral aspect of the lateral claw may help correct a varus deformity.

SURGICAL MANAGEMENT

When significant marked angular deformity is associated with growth plate disturbance, periosteal stripping and growth retardation can help correct the deformity. It is important to note that no significant studies have documented the results of periosteal stripping in calves. This technique was extrapolated from its use in horses, which is itself controversial. Furthermore, no known data exists regarding when the various growth plates of cattle functionally close. The general belief is that cattle growth plates close a few months later than their equine counterpart. The author and others have used this procedure with apparent success in a few calves under 6 months of age with carpal valgus.

Periosteal stripping is performed on the concave side of the limb: medial aspect for a varus deformity and lateral aspect for a valgus deformity. Periosteal stripping is performed as follows. The procedure is performed under general anesthesia or sedation with infiltration of local anesthesia over the intended surgical site. In a unilateral case, the calf is placed in lateral recumbency with the affected limb uppermost. In a bilateral case, the calf is placed in dorsal recumbency with the affected limb tied in an extended position. The lateral aspect of the affected growth plate is aseptically prepared, and a 23-gauge needle is inserted into the prominence of the physis to identify the growth plate. A 5-cm skin incision is made from the growth plate, extending proximally along the longitudinal axis of the affected long bone. The incision is extended through the periosteum in the same plane. Using a curved hemostat to retract the skin and extensor tendons, the surgeon makes a second periosteal transection 1 cm parallel to the growth plate and perpendicular to the first periosteal incision, while he or she carefully avoids injury to the extensor tendons at the dorsal aspect of the limb. Using a periosteal elevator, the surgeon elevates the periosteum so it forms two triangular flaps of periosteum. The periosteum on the smaller ulna is next elevated in the same fashion. Note that the distal growth plate of the ulna is not at the same level as the distal radius (Figure 15.3-6). The subcutaneous and skin incisions are closed separately in a simple continuous pattern.

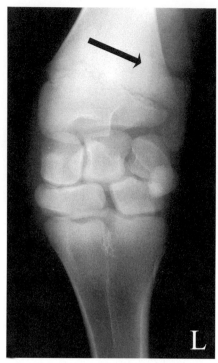

Figure 15.3-6   Dorsopalmar radiograph of a calf left carpus. Note the ulna size and location of the distal ulnar growth plate *(arrow)* versus the distal growth plate of the radius.

Growth plate retardation procedure is performed under general anesthesia with the position described for periosteal stripping. This procedure can be performed on either the medial or lateral aspect of a given growth plate. Although no studies have documented its use in calves, this procedure is effective if sufficient growth is left in the affected growth plate. The procedure (best done under radiographic control) is performed on the convex side of the limb: lateral aspect for a varus deformity and medial aspect for a valgus deformity. After the growth plate is identified, a 1-cm stab incision is made midway between the growth plate and radiocarpal joint distal to the physis. A pilot hole is drilled with a 3.2-mm drill bit, and a 4.5-mm tap allows a threaded 4.5-mm screw (usually 32 to 36 mm in length) to be placed distal and parallel to the growth plate (see Section 11.2 for details on general orthopedic techniques). The screw is inserted for 95% of its length. A second stab incision is made 5 cm proximal to the first screw, and a second screw is placed with its tip directed 20 degrees toward the physis. Using a curved hemostat, the surgeon creates a subcutaneous path between the two screws, and the proximal stab incision is extended proximally to facilitate wire placement and knot tying. A 15-cm length of 1- to 1.2-mm orthopedic wire is bent in its middle, and the leading edge of the bent wire is inserted through the most proximal stab incision and tunneled subcutaneously until hooked on the distal screw. The wire is then secured around the proximal screw in a figure eight pattern, and a knot is made after twisting the wires on the front of the proximal screw. In calves greater than 100 kg, a second wire is placed similarly, and the knot is placed on the back of the proximal screw. The screws are then fully tightened. It is important to note that the screws should be almost completely inserted before tightening the wires, otherwise bone thread damage leading to screw stripping will occur. The stab incisions are then closed in an acceptable manner.

The area is bandaged postoperatively. The bandage is removed 3 days later, and the skin sutures are removed 10 to 14 days postoperatively. The calf is allowed normal exercise after the sutures are removed. If growth retardation was used, the implant must be removed as soon as the leg is acceptably straightened, or overcorrection that causes the radius to curve (because of retarded growth in the ulna growth plate) will occur. If the procedure was done bilaterally, the implants must be removed from each leg as soon as it straightens. Under general anesthesia, a needle is used to palpate and locate a screw head; the proximal screw is usually the most readily detected. A stab incision is made when the screw head is located, and the screw is removed. A ruler is used to measure 5 cm from the screw that was found, and the surgeon palpates to locate the remaining screw. After a stab incision is made and the screw is removed, a large curved hemostat is placed in the proximal stab incision to hook both orthopedic wires. After elevating the knots out of the skin incision, proximal traction allows the wires to be removed. This last step requires significant force because of the fibrous tissue associated with the surgical procedure.

Finally, a closing wedge osteotomy or a step osteotomy can be performed (if financially justifiable) when an angular deformity is related to a malunion or physis closure or damage prevents further growth. To prepare the location and site of the osteotomies, the preoperative radiographs should be measured. These measurements are used to determine the pivot point and angle of angulation by measuring the angle between the intersecting lines.

Preoperative Measurements

These measurements and radiographic markings serve only as guides because adjustments for magnification error must be made intraoperatively.

Closing Wedge Osteotomy

Sufficient bone should be left when the closing wedge osteotomy (Figure 15.3-7) is designed for appropriate

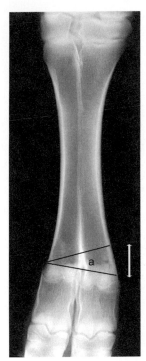

Figure 15.3-7   Radiographic manipulation creating a metaphyseal deformity to illustrate the intended preoperative measurement for a closed wedge osteotomy. The pivot angle (a) was previously calculated as indicated in Figure 15.3-4, which determines the height of the wedge (white arrows). The black lines illustrate the intended line of the two osteotomies.

purchase of the screws through the plate being used to immobilize the osteotomy site. A line is drawn parallel to the joint at the level of the pivot point. The height of the second osteotomy site is calculated by using the angle of deviation at the pivot point.

Step-Wise Osteotomy

A horizontal osteotomy line is drawn parallel to the joint, starting again at the pivot line but extending only through half the diameter of the affected bone in the dorsopalmar (plantar) plane (Figure 15.3-8). A line is drawn from the axial end of the horizontal osteotomy line and extends 5 cm proximally along the long axis of the bone. A second vertical line the same length is drawn from the same starting point but angled to represent the previously measured pivot angle; the width of that wedge is measured. The last osteotomy line is drawn horizontally from the proximal aspect of these two vertical lines and extending perpendicular to the long axis of the proximal bone.

SURGICAL TECHNIQUES

A skin incision is made over the dorso or dorsolateral aspect of the affected long bone. The incision is extended

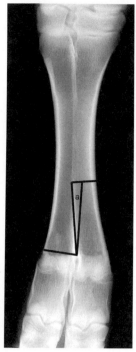

Figure 15.3-8 Same radiographs as Figure 15.3-7 to illustrate the intended preoperative measurement for a step osteotomy. The pivot angle (a) was previously determined as indicated in Figure 15.3-2, and it determines the width of the vertical wedge to be removed. The black line illustrates the intended line of the osteotomies.

to the affected bone, and subperiosteal dissection exposes the bone before the osteotomies.

Closing wedge osteotomy is performed as follows. Using a reciprocating saw, the surgeon transects the affected bone parallel to the joint surface immediately distal to the level of the pivot point while carefully protecting all surrounding soft tissue. The height of the second osteotomy is measured from the radiographs. Starting on the convex side, the second osteotomy is extended to the opposite side of the bone until it meets the first osteotomy site (see Figure 15.3-7). The bone fragments are fixed after the wedge removal is performed (see Section 11.2).

To perform a step wedge osteotomy a 3.2-mm hole is drilled from dorsal to palmar (plantar) in the center of the bone at the intended start of the longitudinal osteotomy lines. A second hole is drilled 5 cm proximal. These two holes prevent inadvertent longitudinal fissures associated with the creation of the longitudinal (i.e., vertical) osteotomies. Using an oscillating saw or Gigli wire, the surgeon joins two holes by a longitudinal osteotomy. Using the width measurement of the wedge needed, another hole is placed proximally; and the surgeon performs the second longitudinal osteotomy. The horizontal osteotomies are made by cutting the bone

parallel to the joint without extending any further than the distal aspect of the longitudinal osteotomies. The proximal osteotomy site is done perpendicular to the long axis of the proximal fragment. The distal osteotomy is made parallel to the distal joint. Reduction to correct a rotational deformity can be enhanced by removing an additional bone wedge at the dorsal or palmar (plantar) aspect of the vertical bone segment created. During the repair, lag screws are applied across the vertical component created as part of the internal fixation repair. Appropriate surgical closure is done. Depending on the weight of the animal, a cast may be needed for further support.

PROGNOSIS

The prognosis is reasonable for angular deformities associated with growth plate imbalance, such as most valgus deformities. Both of the surgical procedures described (periosteal stripping or growth plate retardation) result in production of significant fibrous tissue, and gross enlargement of the surgery site is evident for 2 months after surgery. The fibrous tissue remodels after two months, which makes the surgical site cosmetically acceptable in most cases. Wedge osteotomies carry a fair prognosis for functionality, although a cosmetic defect due to enlargement at the surgery site is expected.

The prognosis for angular deformity secondary to contralateral orthopedic injury (such as most varus deformities) is generally poor because it is usually centered over a joint (carpus or tarso crural joint) and is also dependent on the prognosis of the primary orthopedic injury.

RECOMMENDED READINGS

Baird AN, Wolfe DF, Bartels JE, Carson RL: Congenital maldevelopment of the tibia in two calves, *J Am Vet Med Assoc* 204:422-423, 1994.

Edinger H, Kofler J, Ebner J: Angular limb deformity in a calf treated by periosteotomy and wedge osteotomy, *Vet Rec* 137:245-246, 1995.

Steiner A, Hirsbrunner G, Geissbuhler U: Management of malunion of metacarpus III/IV in two calves. *Zentralbl Veterinarmed A* 43:561-571, 1996.

Ferguson JG. Surgery of the distal limb. In Greenough PR and Weaver AD, editors: *Lameness in cattle*, Philadelphia, 1997, WB Saunders.

15.4—Septic Arthritis

André Desrochers

Systemic or remote infection has to be considered when a calf is diagnosed with septic arthritis, especially if more than one joint is affected and no wound can be seen. The umbilicus is a very common route of infection. Inadequate hygiene, not disinfecting the umbilicus after birth, and passive immunity transfer failure are the most important factors that contribute to umbilical infection. Calves with omphalophlebitis are at high risk of septicemia and consequently, septic arthritis. Pneumonia, diarrhea, septicemia, and passive immunity transfer failure must also be considered when physical or ultrasound examination reveals a normal umbilicus. Systemic origin rather than local trauma increases the probability of more than one joint being infected. Calves with septic arthritis must have a thorough physical examination to find a remote infection site until proven otherwise. Other causes include direct trauma to the carpi seen when calves are kept on inadequate flooring, have flexural deformities, or are unable to stand adequately.

Frequency of septic arthritis in a herd is generally low. *Mycoplasma* and *Haemophilus somnus* should be considered as possible causes when the incidence of septic joints increases in a herd without umbilical involvement. Incidences of septic arthritis increase in the presence of *Mycoplasma* pneumonia and mastitis in a herd (Adegboye 1996).

Diagnosis

Onset of clinical signs in calves is acute and severe. The differential diagnosis of swollen joints in calves should include septic arthritis, ligament injury, osteochondrosis, articular fracture, and idiopathic arthritis. Septic arthritis should remain high on the list of possible diagnoses for swollen joints in calves. Lameness will vary, depending on the duration and severity of the infection and number of joints affected. During the physical examination, investigating the origin of septic arthritis should be emphasized—with a very special focus on the umbilicus. All of the joints should be palpated, and particular attention should be paid to the most commonly involved joints in septic arthritis (carpus, tarsus, stifle, and fetlock). A low serum total protein (less than 55 g/L) or immunoglobulin level indicates that passive immunity transfer has failed, which helps determine the calf's immune status. If passive immunity transfer failure is diagnosed, plasma or whole blood can be administered to the animal.

A blood culture improves the chance of finding bacteria in a febrile calf. *Mycoplasma* should be considered if the calf's umbilicus is within normal limits at the physical examination, especially if multiple animals are affected. Intrauterine transmission of *Mycoplasma bovis* is suspected in neonates. Therefore suspected *Mycoplasma* arthritis should be a test specified on the laboratory request.

Arthrocentesis can be performed to confirm diagnosis. Macroscopic examination of the synovial fluids is

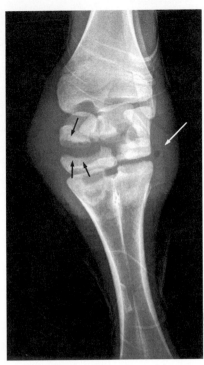

Figure 15.4-1 Craniocaudal radiographic view of a carpus from a young calf. There is severe soft tissue swelling with air (white arrow). The intercarpal joint space is increased with lysis of the subchondral bone (black arrows).

usually diagnostic. If doubt exists, the specimen is submitted for cytologic examination. Culture of the synovial fluids helps the clinician confirm or modify the choice of antibiotic. Cytologic examination and bacterial culture of the synovial fluid can be repeated if the animal does not respond well to initial treatment.

Radiographs of the infected joint confirm the diagnosis and prognosis. Radiographic lesions in calves have a tendency to be more lytic, with less new bone formation occurring in comparison to older animals (Figure 15.4-1).

Treatment

Antibiotics, antiinflammatory drugs, joint lavage or drainage, and physical therapy are the principal components of septic arthritis treatment (Figures 15.4-2 and 15.4-3). The treatment will vary based on the severity and duration of the disease, location and number of joints infected, microorganism isolated in the septic joint, primary disease (umbilical infection), and economic value of the animal. These factors should be considered to give the owner an accurate prognosis and establish a treatment. An infected umbilical vein with liver involvement should be surgically removed

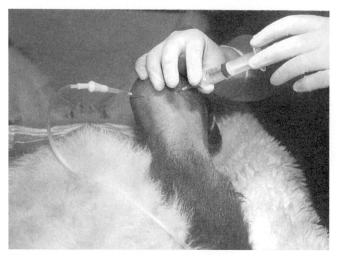

Figure 15.4-2   Articular lavage of the antebrachiocarpal joint on a Hereford calf.

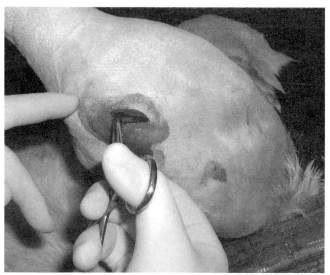

Figure 15.4-3   Arthrotomy with debridement of the antebrachiocarpal joint.

promptly after diagnosis to stop the potential spread of microorganisms.

In the author's opinion, the antibiotic chosen for calves with septic arthritis should be aimed at effecting *Mycoplasma* if no organism is isolated and the umbilicus is unlikely to be the cause. Otherwise, antibiotics should be effective on gram-negative organisms. The duration of antibiotic treatment is empirical. Therapy should be continued for 2 to 3 weeks after clinical improvement (decreased lameness, improved quality of the synovial fluid). Conservative treatment with systemic antibiotics and antiinflammatory drugs alone is indicated if the course of the disease is short (less than 5 days). Other treatment alternatives have to be considered when the

disease lasts more than 5 days. Local administration of antibiotics (intra-articular) has to be considered because of its capacity for providing concentrations above MIC for a long period of time. Administering local antibiotics also requires a smaller volume, which is an advantage for toxic or expensive drugs. A local antibiotic is chosen based on the organism isolated and its innocuousness for the joint. Besides intraarticular administration, local intravenous administration under tourniquet (Figure 15.4-4) and antibiotic-impregnated collagen implants are being used sporadically. Slow-release impregnated absorbable implants have shown promise in providing high local concentrations for an extended period of time, which would certainly improve therapeutic efficacy by minimizing use of systemic antibiotics.

Clinical signs from acute septic arthritis should improve between 2 to 4 days after treatments are started. An arthrotomy should be performed to provide better drainage if the animal does not improve after two joint irrigations or the synovial fluids still have fibrin. General anesthesia is considered when treating more than one joint. Knowledge of each different articulation's anatomic boundaries and communication is essential before starting local intervention. If calves do not respond to arthrotomy, arthrodesis—as described in Chapter 11 (see the section on arthrodesis) is recommended.

Calves can be administered nonsteroidal antiinflammatory drugs (NSAIDs) (i.e., flunixin meglumine 1 mg/kg sid IV or aspirin 100 mg/kg bid po) for a few days to decrease the harmful effects caused by synthesis

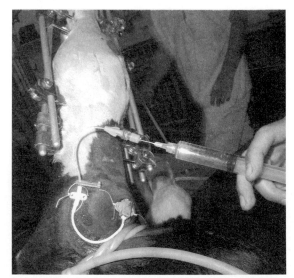

Figure 15.4-4   Regional perfusion of the carpus of a calf with chronic septic arthritis: local antibiotics were administered IV distal to a tourniquet. An arthrodesis was performed, and an external fixator was used to stabilize the joint.

of inflammatory mediators in the joint and to minimize the pain. If NSAID treatment is prolonged, calves should be monitored for abomasal ulcers, especially if they are not eating or drinking properly.

Prognosis

Rapid intervention after the onset of clinical signs increases the chance of recovery. The prognosis is poor with more than two infected joints. Joint lavage is very effective in acute cases. Eighty percent of 20 calves responded to joint lavage that required two or more flushes (Jackson, 1998). Chronic septic joints contain a lot of fibrin that is not easily removed, even through multiple arthrotomy sites. Ankylosis of the joint, muscle atrophy, and tendon deformities (contraction) complicate an animal's rehabilitation, even after the infection is controlled. This should be considered before establishing a treatment plan. An animal with chronic septic arthritis with bony lesions does not have a good prognosis for complete recovery and becoming a productive animal. Arthrodesis is an option for full recovery in low-range motion distal joints like the interphalangeal and fetlock joints. Pain-free arthrodesis of the carpus that permitted full weight bearing was obtained in 69% of 72 cattle treated (Huffel, 1989).

RECOMMENDED READINGS

Adegboye DS et al: *Mycoplasma bovis*-associated pneumonia and arthritis complicated with pyogranulomatous tenosynovitis in calves, *J Am Vet Med Assoc* 209:617-649, 1996.

Huffel X van et al: Carpal joint arthrodesis as a treatment for chronic septic carpitis in calves and cattle, *Vet Surg* 18:304-311, 1989.

Jackson P: Treatment of septic arthritis in calves, *In Pract* 21:596-601, 1999.

Jackson PGG et al: Treatment of septic arthritis in calves by joint lavage: a study of 20 cases, *Cattle Pract* 6:335-339, 1998.

Smith JA, et al: Drug therapy for arthritis in food-producing animals, *Compend Contin Educ Pract Vet* 11:87-93, 1989.

Ryan MJ, et al: Morphologic changes following intraarticular inoculation of *Mycoplasma bovis* in calves, *Vet Pathol* 20:472-487, 1983.

15.5—Patellar Luxation

Norm G. Ducharme

Patellar luxation causes a significant gait deficit, which brings it to the attention of the veterinarian early in the course of disease. It may be a congenital condition associated with malformation of the femoropatellar joint—most commonly hypoplasia or osteochondrosis of the lateral trochlea. A femoral nerve deficit is associated with difficult parturition, especially breech presentation, and will present with a similar gait deficit because of the loss of quadriceps function. Additionally, loss of normal quadriceps muscle activity coupled with the normal lateral pull of the gluteobiceps muscle may also result in lateral patellar luxation. Finally, direct trauma to the stifle joint that tears the femoropatellar ligaments or causes a distal femoral fracture may also result in patellar luxation.

CLINICAL PRESENTATION AND DIAGNOSIS

Affected calves are unable to extend the stifle joint, and the pelvis is lowered on the affected side (Figure 15.5-1). While walking, the animal is able to bear weight but cannot normally extend the stifle, thus creating an obvious gait deficit with the calf in a unilateral or bilateral crouch position. The animal prefers to lie down, and weaker calves will be unable to rise without assistance. The ability to stand and walk depends on the calf's age and strength, the quadriceps muscle function, and whether the condition is unilateral or bilateral. Even calves with bilateral disease are often able to stand and be somewhat ambulatory.

Femoral nerve damage and trauma (femoropatellar ligament rupture, patellar fracture, or distal femoral fracture) may result in a dysfunctional quadriceps unit. On physical examination, one should attempt to differentiate patellar luxation from femoral nerve damage or trauma. Femoral nerve damage generally has a history of difficult assisted birth; excessive pulling stretches the nerve and causes various degrees of nerve damage, ranging from neurapraxia to axonotmesis. Given this etiology, the condition is often bilateral. On clinical examination, there may be a small area of skin denervation on the medial aspect of the distal femur, which is the dermatome of the femoral nerve through the saphenous branch. This can be detected by pinching the skin in the

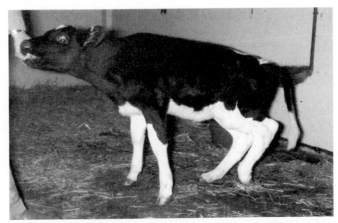

Figure 15.5-1 Holstein-Friesian calf with grade III patellar luxation. Note the crouch position in the affected limb.

(Courtesy of Dr. Michael Schramme; Cornell University.)

area with a hemostat. However, because of the femoral nerve "blurred" dermatome and the general hyposensitivity of young calves, this clinical sign is difficult to detect. As time progresses, either return to function occurs or the quadriceps muscle progressively atrophies. A dysfunctional quadriceps unit usually has femoral nerve damage diagnosed as the cause by exclusion. Absence of function of the quadriceps can lead to patellar luxation. Recognizing this diagnosis is important because either surgical treatment is not needed or would have a very poor prognosis if femoral nerve function does not return.

Direct trauma to the stifle joint is a rare cause of patellar luxation and is usually easily identified by marked periarticular edema and by fibrous tissue production as part of the normal healing process in response to injury in chronic cases. Sonographic examination helps establish the loss of femoropatellar ligament integrity. In addition, radiographic anomaly can also be detected if a fracture is present. The amount of pain the calf exhibits and the periarticular swelling are key hallmarks of trauma-induced patellar luxation or dysfunction of the quadriceps unit. Also, congenital luxation of the patella is almost exclusively lateral, while luxation associated with direct trauma can result in lateral or medial luxation. Pain is not a feature of congenital patellar luxation or femoral nerve deficit.

Patellar luxation is identified by first localizing the patella between the index and thumb and noting its position more lateral (or medial) to the lateral (or medial) trochlea. Normally, a patellar luxation should not be inducible. In grade I and II patellar luxation, luxation can be induced with the stifle in full extension (see the section on classification of patellar luxation in this chapter). Likewise patellar luxation can usually be reduced with the stifle in full extension. In more severe case, the patella can be observed or felt to luxate laterally during flexion of the stifle.

Radiographic examination (lateral, craniocaudal, Figures 15.5-2A and B) of the stifle joint allows confirmation of the diagnosis and an estimation of the degree of osteoarthritis. If present, distal femoral fractures can be identified. In addition, the anatomical conformation of the lateral and medial trochlea and the trochlear grove can be assessed through a skyline view (Figure 15.5-3).

CLASSIFICATION OF PATELLAR LUXATION

In small animals, the patellar luxations are classified from I to IV. The following classification modification is proposed for farm animals:

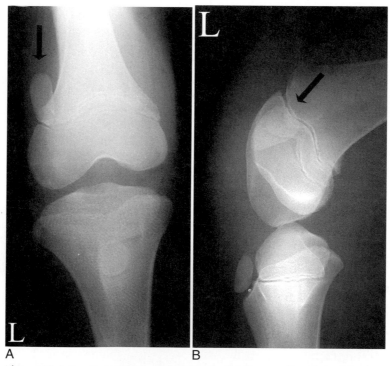

Figure 15.5-2 Radiograph of a 2-month-old Bison calf with patellar luxation in the left hind. *A*, Craniocaudal view; note lateral position of the patella (arrow). *B*, Lateral view; patella (arrow) is not seen dorsal to the trochlea groove but overlaps the trochlea because of its lateral position.

(Courtesy of Dr. Lisa Fortier; Cornell University.)

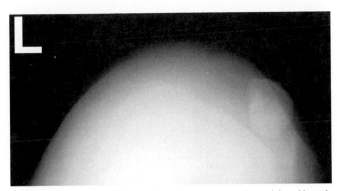

Figure 15.5-3 Skyline radiographs of a 2-day-old calf with luxated patella. Note the normal shaped medial trochlea and absence of trochlear groove and lateral trochlea.

(Courtesy of Dr. Anthony Pease; Cornell University.)

I. Intermittent patellar luxation causes the calf to crouch occasionally on the affected limb while the animal walks. The patella easily luxates manually at full extension of the stifle joint, but returns to the trochlea when released.

II. There is occasional patellar luxation with the associated gait deficit described in I. The animal is capable of full stifle extension most times. On physical examination, the patella can be easily luxated manually at full extension and does not readily return to normal position.

III. The patella is permanently luxated. The animal is unable to extend the stifle, so it walks in a crouch position. During physical examination, one can reposition the patella, but it does not stay in place when the joint is flexed. The depth of the trochlear groove varies.

IV. The patella is permanently luxated. The animal is unable to extend the stifle, so it walks in a crouch position. During physical examination, one cannot reposition the patella. Radiographically, the trochlear groove is flat or absent, and the lateral trochlea has been deformed by the overlying patella (see Figure 15.5-2B).

MANAGEMENT

Patellar luxations due to femoral nerve damage are managed differently. The femoral nerve deficit may resolve within 30 days. The calf should be placed in a box stall with excellent footing or in a small outside pen so that it gets limited physical activity. An antiinflammatory agent such as flunixin (1 mg/kg sid IV) can be administered for a few days. Because the prognosis is poor if the quadriceps function does not return, surgical treatment is not recommended if the muscular function does not improve.

In other cases of patellar luxation, the grading system can serve as a guideline for a treatment plan. Grades I and II are left untreated because most animals can have a normal productive life without treatment other than good footing and avoiding competition for food. Grades III and IV require surgical treatment.

The timing of surgery to treat patellar luxation is influenced by several factors. The patella, femoral trochlea, and trochlear groove ossify over the first 3 months of a calf's life. The presence of the patella within the patellar groove appears important to developing a normal depth to the patellar groove. Therefore grade III luxation should be treated early, so normal femoropatellar joint development occurs. Furthermore, untreated patellar luxation does lead to degenerative osteoarthritis and progression to grade IV luxation, so early treatment is preferable. However, delaying surgical treatment in a newborn calf for a few weeks may be wise because of the risk of neonatal infection. If femoral fracture or other direct trauma to the stifle joint is the cause of luxation, surgical treatment should be done as early as allowed by soft tissue condition.

Surgical management through lateral release and medial imbrication is preferable in early grade III. However, a trochleoplasty should be performed in chronic grade III where the patellar groove did not form normally and is too shallow. Lateral release, medial imbrication, and recessive trochleoplasty are always required in grade IV luxation. In addition, tibial crest repositioning to reestablish the line of tension of the quadriceps axial to the femoropatellar joint can also be done in a grade IV luxation, especially in smaller weight animals. The morbidity of tibial crest transposition (i.e., implant failure and/or nonunion) dictates avoidance of this procedure in heavier animals.

The surgical procedure is done with the calf in lateral recumbency under general anesthesia with the affected limb uppermost. Preoperative use of antibiotics (cephalosporin and penicillin) is recommended. The affected limb is placed in an 80 degree abducted position because access to the medial and lateral aspect of the femoropatellar joint is required. After appropriate draping, an S-shaped incision that starts 5 cm proximal to the patella and extends first medially is made on the cranial aspect of the stifle joint until 5 cm distal to the tibial crest (see Figure 11.4-23). The incision is extended with scissors through the loosened areolar subcutaneous tissue and superficial fascia until the strong periarticular fascia is encountered. The goal of the procedure is to release lateral traction and reinforce medial soft tissue pull on the patella. The attachment of the gluteobiceps tendon on the lateral aspect of the patella is identified and transected (Figure 15.5-4A and B). Immediately underneath the gluteobiceps tendon (which joins with

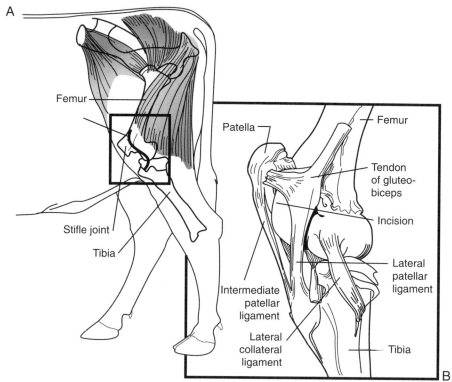

Figure 15.5-4   Schematic representation of *A,* lateral release and *B,* medial imbrication techniques.

the lateral distal patellar ligament) is the lateral femoropatellar ligament (note: this is *not* the lateral patellar ligament). At this point, the patella should be easy to replace in its normal anatomical position, but it will probably not stay if the joint is flexed.

The medial aspect of the joint is then imbricated as follows. With the limb in full extension, a first row of nonabsorbable suture material (no. 2 or 5 polyester) is placed in an imbricating suture pattern (Lembert pattern) at the mid level of the medial femoropatellar ligament and extended from the dorsal aspect of the patella distally to the tibial crest (Figure 11.4-25). The limb is then placed in the normal unabducted position and flexed through a complete range of motion multiple times to confirm the absence of luxation. The joint should be able to flex almost completely without luxation. If luxation still occurs, a second row of imbricating sutures is placed over the first row. Additional medial imbrication sutures can be placed in a stepwise fashion to maintain the stifle joint's range of motion. Often the lateral joint capsule is opened during transection of the lateral femoropatellar ligament because of its close proximity to the joint capsule. The joint is closed with simple interrupted or cruciate sutures after the medial imbrication is complete.

Additionally the patellar groove should be deepened if a very shallow patellar groove is present. The pitfall of these procedures is that the lateral or medial trochlea may fracture if too much bone is resected abaxially. Trochleoplasty may be performed using a recession trochleoplasty (wedge or rectangular) or by curettage of the trochlear groove. The femoropatellar joint capsule is incised between the middle and lateral distal patellar ligaments. The joint is opened from the insertion of the lateral patellar ligament on the patella to the tibial crest between the middle and lateral patellar ligaments. The limb is placed in extension, and the patella is luxated medially. For the wedge resection technique, a reciprocating saw is used. Two angle osteotomies are created in the femoropatellar groove to create a triangular fragment of bone that is excised and placed in a moist sponge. A second set of osteotomies are created 4 to 5 mm parallel and abaxial to the first ones. This creates two bone sections (one lateral and one medial) for removal and disposal. The previously excised triangular bone fragment is replaced into the patellar groove without fixation. The rectangular trochleoplasty is performed by creating two parallel incisions on the abaxial surface of the trochlear groove. One should make sure the wall of the osteotomies is 90 degrees to the floor of the trochlear groove while carefully maintaining 75% of the medial and lateral trochlea width to prevent postoperative trochlear fractures. Using an osteotome, the surgeon joins two vertical osteotomies by a 90-degree osteotomy at the floor of the trochlear groove, and the rectangular segment of bone is removed. Using a burr or curette, the surgeon deepens the floor of the trochlear groove, and the previously removed rectangular segment of bone is replaced. The advantage of the rectangular recession trochleoplasty is that the medial and lateral trochlea width is more accurately preserved.

If chondromalacia of the patellar groove is present, preserving its overlying cartilage is no longer needed. In those cases, the trochlear groove is deepened with an air-powered surgical instrument.

Closure

Upon completion of the procedure, the joint capsule and overlying retinaculum are closed with a simple interrupted or cruciate pattern. The subcutaneous fascia is closed with a simple continuous pattern, and the skin is closed in an appropriate pattern. A stent is sutured on the skin to decrease tension on the incision, and an adherent impervious drape is placed over the incision.

Postoperative Care

The stent is kept on for 7 to 10 days if dry. If not, the area is protected from the environment with sponges covered with an adhesive drape or other acceptable bandage. Antibiotics are continued for 5 to 7 days because of the tendency to develop seromas and the possibility of ascending infection associated with incisional leakage. Postoperatively, skin sutures are not removed until 14 days, and the animal is restricted to a box stall for 2 to 3 months.

The prognosis is fair to good in unilateral cases. Bilateral cases are operated 8 weeks apart and have a less favorable prognosis because of the increased morbidity associated with bilateral procedures. Femoral nerve degeneration associated with patellar luxation carries a grave prognosis unless neural regeneration restores normal quadriceps function.

RECOMMENDED READINGS

Baron RJ: Laterally luxating patella in a goat, *J Am Vet Med Assoc* 191:1471-1472, 1987.

Ferguson JG: Luxating patella and femoral nerve degeneration. In Greenough PR and Weaver AD, editors: *Lameness in cattle*, Philadelphia, 1997, WB Saunders.

Hobbs MT, Kenward JK: Surgery for luxating patella in a calf, *Vet Rec* 133:508, 1993.

Kobluk CN: Correction of patellar luxation by recession sulcoplasty in three foals, *Vet Surg* 22:298-300, 1993.

Leitch M, Kotlikoff M: Surgical repair of congenital luxation of the patella in the foal and calf, *Vet Surg* 9:1-4, 1980.

Shettko DL, Trostle SS: Diagnosis and surgical repair of patellar luxations in a flock of sheep, *J Am Vet Med Assoc* 216:564-566, 2000.

Vasseur P: The stifle joint. In Slatter, D ed: *Textbook of small animal surgery*, Philadelphia, 1993, WB Saunders.

Weaver AD, Campbell JR: Surgical correction of lateral and medial patellar luxation in calves, *Vet Rec* 90:567-569, 1972.

15.6—Spastic Paresis (Elso Heel)

Norm G. Ducharme

The clinical presentation, pathophysiology and diagnosis of spastic paresis are described in Chapter 11.(see section on spastic paresis) This section will focus on surgical treatment of the condition. Treatment allows the animal to be fattened as salvage for beef production because affected animals should not be allowed to enter the breeding stock. General anesthesia is preferred for performing the surgical procedures, but sedation with xylazine hydrochloride and local anesthesia administered at the intended surgical site or epidural anesthesia are both also acceptable in young calves (see Chapter 6 for details on anesthesia). The owner should be made aware that in unilateral cases the disease may be manifested in the contralateral limb at a later date and require further treatment.

For *partial tibial neurectomy*, the calf is placed with the affected limb uppermost, and the caudal aspect of the stifle is prepared for aseptic surgery. A 15- to 20-cm incision is made on the caudal aspect of the stifle between the junction of the semimembranous and gluteobiceps muscles (Figure 15.6-1A). The incision is extended through the fascia. The branches of the tibial nerves that innervate the gastrocnemius muscles are identified after retracting the semimembranous and biceps femoris muscles (Figure 15.6-1B). An alternative approach to the branches of the tibial nerves splits the biceps femoris muscle overlying the nerves longitudinally. Identifying the correct branches to transect is crucial. First, the peroneal nerve is identified as it courses over the lateral head of the gastrocnemius muscle (Figure 15.6-1B); this nerve must be preserved. The branches of the tibial nerves to the lateral and medial belly of the gastrocnemius muscles are identified for careful dissection and their function verified using electrostimulation (sterile electrodes connected to an electrical current source). The belly of each gastrocnemius muscle is stimulated separately and observed to detect whether it contracts and hock extension occurs during stimulation. All nerve

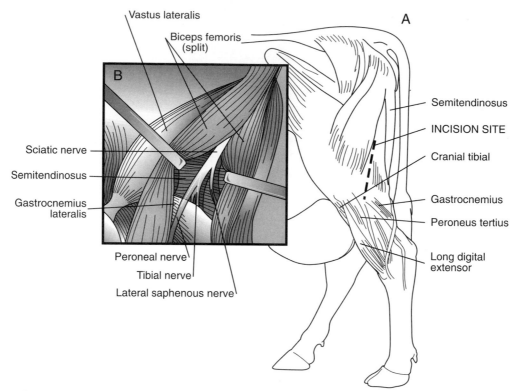

Figure 15.6-1   Schematic representation of partial tibial neurectomy. *A,* The incision is made over the junction of the semimembranous and biceps femoris muscles at the caudal aspect of the stifle. *B,* After splitting the biceps femoris muscles, the tibial and peroneal nerves are identi..ed.

branches to these muscles are transected, and a 2-cm section is removed. The nerves are ligated proximally with a nonabsorbable suture material to prevent axonal regeneration. The muscles and subcutaneous tissue are reapposed by using an appropriate-sized absorbable suture in a continuous pattern. Skin closure is routine. If general anesthesia or epidural anesthesia was used, the limb should be hobbled during recovery to prevent slipping and gastrocnemius rupture. Postoperative activity is restricted until suture removal at 14 days.

Reportedly, the problem is improved or completely resolves in nearly 80% of the animals. A slight chance of recurrence remains, presumably because some branches were missed or reinnervation occurred. Complications after the procedure are rare but include dropped hock and ruptured gastrocnemius tendon.

A *tenotomy/tenectomy* procedure's advantage is a simpler, less invasive technique with less chance of recurrence. The procedure can be performed with the animal standing under local anesthetic but is preferably done with the animal lying down under sedation or general anesthesia. If the animal is recumbent, the affected limb should be uppermost. The lateral aspect of the distal tibia over the Achilles tendon is prepared for aseptic surgery. A 7-cm skin incision is made over the craniolateral aspect of the Achilles tendon, a hand's width proximal to the point of the calcaneus (Figure 15.6-2A). The incision is extended through subcutaneous tissue until the Achilles tendon is reached. The superficial digital flexor tendon and superficial tendon of the medial head of the gastrocnemius muscle cross at the proximal level of the incision (Figure 15.6-2B). The superficial flexor tendon is identified (the gastrocnemius tendon attaches on the tuber calcaneus while the superficial flexor tendon continues past the tuber calcaneus toward the digit) and preserved. The fascia surrounding the Achilles tendon is incised longitudinally, and the superficial and deep tendon of the gastrocnemius muscle are elevated separately and transected to remove a 2- to 3-cm section of tendon (identifying and separating the tendon is easier with the leg in extension.) The tendinous sheet around the tenectomy site must also be transected and resected while the surgeon takes care to preserve the superficial digital flexor tendon and relevant vessels (tibial nerve and lateral saphenous vein). The subcutaneous tissues are

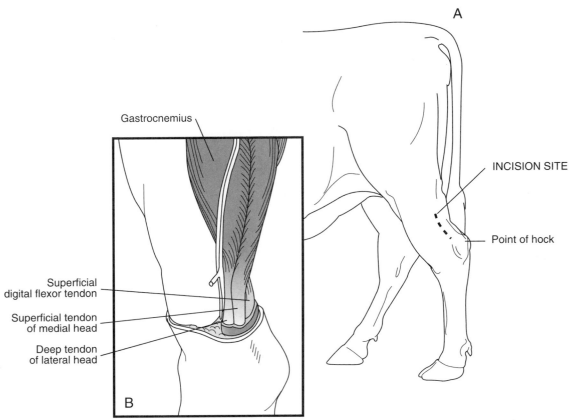

Figure 15.6-2   Schematic representation of a partial tenectomy of the gastrocnemius muscle. *A*, The incision is made above the hock over the cranial and lateral aspect of the Achilles tendon. *B*, The superficial digital flexor tendon is identified and avoided. The deep and superficial tendons of the gastrocnemius are identified and a section removed.

reapposed by using an appropriate-sized absorbable suture in a continuous pattern. Skin closure is routine. Postoperative activity is restricted until suture removal at 14 days.

Complications associated with this procedure are rupture of the gastrocnemius muscle during recovery. Therefore a bilateral procedure should not be performed, but the procedure can be performed on the contralateral limb after 6 weeks. If gastrocnemius muscle rupture occurs, the hock must be immobilized in a cast for at least 6 weeks to allow sufficient fibrosis for repair (see Chapter 11, the section on gastrocnemius rupture).

The tendon transection procedure is also highly successful and can be done more rapidly without the need for electrostimulation.

RECOMMENDED READINGS

Bouckaert JH, De Moor A: Treatment of spastic paralysis in cattle: improved denervation technique of the gastrocnemius muscle and post-operative course, *Vet Rec* 79:226-229, 1966.

Pavaux C, Arnault G, Baussier M, Dumont M: Treatment of spastic paresis in cattle with Goetze's technique, triple tenectomy, *Point Veterinaire* 20:41-50, 1988.

Pavaux C, Saulet J, Ligneux IY: Anatomy of the bovine gastrocnemius muscle as applied to the surgical correction of spastic paresis, *Vlaams Diergeneeskd Tijdschr* 54:296-312, 1985.

Vlaminck L, De Moor A, Martens A, Steenhaut M, Gasthuys F, Desmet P, Van Branteghem L: Partial tibial neurectomy in 113 Belgian blue calves with spastic paresis, *Vet Rec* 147:16-19, 2000.

Weaver AD: Modified gastrocnemius tenectomy: a procedure to relieve spastic paresis in dairy cattle, *Vet Med* 86:1234-1239, 1991.

Weaver AD: Spastic paresis (Elso Heel). In Greenough PR, ed: *Lameness in cattle*, Philadelphia, 1997, WB Saunders.

CHAPTER 16

OTITIS MEDIA

Thomas J. Divers, J. Brett Woodie

Otitis Media/Interna: Calves

Otitis media interna (M/I) is a very common disorder of young dairy calves. The majority of cases seen are in calves 3 to 6 weeks of age. It can be a farm problem and may occur concurrently with respiratory disease. *Mycoplasma* spp. are the organisms most often implicated in the disease process, and the disorder is particularly common in herds with mycoplasma positive bulk milk cultures.

ANATOMICAL AND PHYSIOLOGICAL CONSIDERATIONS

The middle ear comprises the tympanic cavity and auditory tubes lined by mucous membrane. The tympanic cavity, located between the tympanic membrane and internal ear, consists of three parts: the atrium, the epitympanic recess—which contains most of the auditory ossicles—and the large tympanic bulla (Figure 16-1A and B). The function of the middle ear is to transmit sound waves that reach the tympanic membrane through the auditory ossicles to the internal ear. The internal ear consists of two cavities (membranous and osseous labyrinth) in the petrous part of the temporal bone that enclose a complex membranous membrane containing the auditory cells and distal ramification of the auditory nerve. The osseous labyrinth, immediately medial to the tympanic cavity, has three parts: the cochlea, vestibule, and semicircular canals. The membranous labyrinth lies within the osseous labyrinth; it contains supporting cells and hair cells. The distal extremities of the cochlear nerves are located at the base of the hair cells.

Chronic suppurative otitis media results first from a bacterial infection. The latter may be primary or secondary to a viral infection. This causes inflammation, ulceration, and production of granulation tissue within the middle ear (Figure 16-2B). The cycle of inflammation described above leads to destruction of the bony margins of the middle ear (Figure 16-2A and B).

CLINICAL SIGNS

Facial nerve paresis and/or vestibular signs are the clinical signs of otitis M/I. The signs may be unilateral or bilateral. Facial paresis can be easily missed in the affected calf because, unlike in other species, no deviation of the muzzle is associated with facial paresis in the bovine. Instead, ear droop, diminished eyelid tone, and "packing" feed in the cheek area are typical signs of facial paresis in the calf. Fortunately, exposure keratitis is not common. Signs of vestibular disease include balance dysfunction (especially ataxia) and head tilt. Lateral vestibular disease may cause abnormally low head carriage without a head tilt. Dysphagia commonly is observed in affected calves, but the pathogenesis of this is unclear. Discharge from the ear (otitis externa) is rare. A cough, nasal discharge, and other signs of pneumonia may be found in many of the affected calves.

DIAGNOSIS

The diagnosis is based upon clinical signs and signalment. Mycoplasma is commonly cultured from a tracheal wash sample. Confirmation of the diagnosis is seldom necessary but could be gathered by performing a CAT scan (see Figure 16-1) or radiographs. Fluid density and lysis of the surrounding bones (e.g., scrolls) confirms the diagnosis.

TREATMENT

The treatment is antimicrobial therapy and supportive care in most cases. Tetracycline is the most commonly

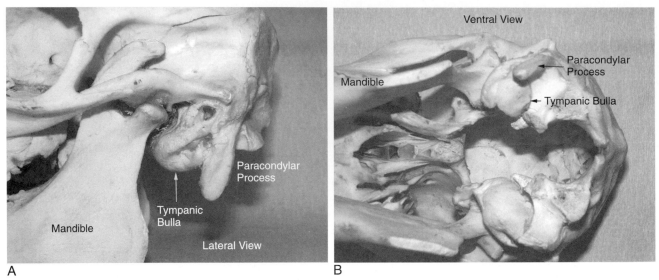

Figure 16-1   Anatomical specimen that shows position and relationship of tympanic bullae in calves: *A,* lateral view; *B,* ventral view.

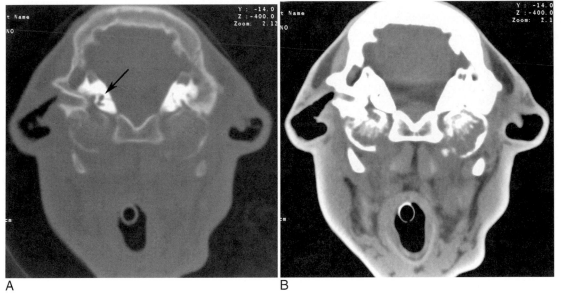

Figure 16-2   CT scan of a calf with otitis media. This is a transverse CT image of the temporal region, acquired using a standard algorithm. *A* is displayed in a bone window (3200 window, 250 level) and *B* in a soft tissue window (375 window, 40 level). This examination illustrates bilateral otitis media with bilateral bulla osteitis and right otitis interna. Evidence of otitis media: note the lysis of the wall of the tympanic bullae (*A*) and presence of purulent exudate and granulation tissue (soft tissue density instead of air density) in the affected tympanic bulla (*B*). Evidence of otitis interna: lysis right petrous temporal bone (arrow, *A*).

(Courtesy of Dr. Anthony Pease; Cornell University.)

used antibiotic, although some *Mycoplasma* spp. may be resistant. Enrofloxacin would be a more effective drug but can only be used in beef cattle. Erythromycin and Florfenicol are additional options. Regardless, 4 or more days of antimicrobial therapy is generally required before

any improvement in clinical signs is noted. Supportive therapy includes feeding from the ground to help prevent aspiration pneumonia, flunixin meglumine for 1 to 3 days for antiinflammatory/antipyretic properties, good nutrition, and good ventilation. Antibiotic ophthalmic ointment should be applied to the eye on the affected side(s) three or more times daily. Surgery should be considered for those cases that do not show improvement within 7 days.

VENTRAL TYMPANIC BULLA OSTEOTOMY

The calf is positioned in dorsal recumbency with the neck extended and the head secured to the operating table with adhesive tape. The caudal aspect of the vertical ramus of the mandible is palpated, and the paracondylar process of the occipital bone is identified. The tympanic bulla is located dorsal and medial to these structures. A 6-cm paramedian skin incision is centered between the vertical ramus of the mandible and the paracondylar process of the occipital bone. The platysma muscle is incised longitudinally the entire length of the skin incision. The mandibular lymph node is identified, and deep dissection is continued on the medial aspect of the node. Blunt dissection is used to separate the digastricus muscle from the hyoglossal and styloglossal muscles. The hypoglossal nerve is located on the lateral aspect of the hyoglossal muscle and must be avoided. Deep digital palpation confirms the ventral aspect of the bulla. It is a raised rounded structure. A periosteal elevator can be used to remove any soft tissue and muscle fibers from the ventral aspect of the bulla, if necessary. The external carotid artery is ventral and lateral to the tympanic bulla, and the glossopharyngeal nerve is medial to the bulla. Both of these structures must be avoided. Blunt self-retaining or handheld retractors are necessary to provide exposure of the tympanic bulla. The entire ventral aspect (floor) of the tympanic bulla should be removed with rongeurs or an air drill. Samples for cytological and microbiological examination are taken. Any exudate present is removed with a curette. The tympanic cavity is lavaged with warm saline and suctioned. Care must be taken to avoid damaging the dorsal aspect of the bulla. A drain should be placed into the tympanic cavity and allowed to exit through the incision so that postoperative lavage can be performed. The drain can be secured with an absorbable suture in the deep layers of the incision and secured to the skin using a nonabsorbable suture. Absorbable sutures placed in a simple interrupted pattern are used to appose the digastricus, hyoglossal, and styloglossal muscles. The skin incision is partially closed to allow drainage.

Postoperatively the drain is removed on day 2 or 3, and the skin sutures are removed on day 14. Antibiotics are continued for 10-14 days. Dysphagia can be associated with the primary disease or result from inadvertent damage to the hypoglossal nerve. Treatment includes antiinflammatory agents such as flunixin meglumine and, if necessary, intravenous nutrition if the calf is already ruminating or forced intubation feeding for younger calves.

RECOMMENDED READING

Ellenport CR: The ear. In Getty R, ed: *Sisson and Grossman's anatomy of domestic animals*, ed 5, Philadelphia, 1975, WB Saunders.

PART IV

Sheep and Goat Surgery

C H A P T E R 1 7

SURGERY OF THE SHEEP AND GOAT INTEGUMENTARY SYSTEM

Scott R. R. Haskell

Primarily, three integumentary surgical considerations occur in sheep and goats: skinfold ablation in certain sheep breeds, tail docking or amputation, and wound care that responds to predator attacks in both sheep and goats.

Skinfold Ablation

Skinfold ablation is of primary concern in Merino and Rambouillet sheep breeds. Genetic selection for wool production over time has resulted in gross enlargement of skin folds, primarily in the neck region. Veterinary practitioners are occasionally requested to perform skin fold ablation surgery of these folds. Environmental factors such as increased temperatures, precipitation, humidity, shearing cuts, and myiasis commonly lead to moist skin fold dermatitis and secondary fly strike. Both bacterial and fungal invaders commonly populate these lesions. Mulesing (removal of skin from caudal thighs) is commonly performed in Australia and New Zealand.

As always, the owner and practitioner need to consider the value of an individual animal before undertaking this surgical procedure. In most instances, the surgical procedure is cost-prohibitive, and flock genetic selection needs to be evaluated. Procedural hemorrhage

is generally minimal with rapid healing time. If possible, the surgery should be performed in young stock during the fly-free months. Skin folds are clipped and surgically prepared. Surgical incisions are made to ablate the skin fold with subsequent reapposition. Subcutaneous tissues are closed, if necessary, to appose the skin and obliterate dead space. Generally, nonabsorbable suture material is used in the skin with a simple interrupted suture pattern. Pain medication is indicated for the first 2 days. If aseptic surgical procedures are followed, antibiotic use is rarely indicated.

Predator Attack

Sheep and goats are commonly preyed upon by a multitude of carnivores. Sheep are generally attacked more often than goats, just by the nature of production practices and species temperament. Sheep and goat livestock operations near urban areas more often see attacks by domestic dogs. Dogs seem only interested in the chase of a flock or herd and are generally not hunting for food. On the other hand, wild carnivores generally kill livestock for food. It is not common to find survivors from carnivore attacks by any species other than dogs. Also, livestock carcasses are generally partially consumed and dragged to a distant site from the kill. Occasionally an owner will interrupt wild carnivores before they kill their prey, and the veterinary practitioner is called to evaluate the survivors.

Three physiologic systems seem to be of primary concern: cardiovascular (exhaustion, shock, and blood loss), penetrating wounds to the musculoskeletal system, and punctures of the gastrointestinal system. When evaluating sheep and goats maintaining heavy fleece, the initial physical examination should be thorough. Fractures and serious lacerations are extremely common in survivors. Myopathy can be a common secondary sequela. It is often difficult to thoroughly examine individuals maintaining a dense fleece.

Wounds seem to focus in two areas: the ventral cervical region and head, rear limbs, and anus (Figure 17-1 A and B). Repairing fractures and lacerated ligaments in most cases exceeds an animal's value. All but "pet" animals are many times destroyed. The veterinary practitioner should take adequate precautions to determine the most likely predatory species involved, as hostile litigation and pet destruction is a common outcome. It is

common for predator (wild carnivores and domestic dogs) visits to the flock to continue. Rabies in the attacker should always be considered as a possibility, and protective gloves should be worn when dealing with saliva.

Tracheal and esophageal punctures are common and easily missed on animals maintaining a full fleece. Generally, "sucking sounds" are evident as well as subcutaneous emphysema and dyspnea. Subcutaneous emphysema may be a common sequela to all traumatic wounds from predator attack. The potential for abscesses, myopathies, tissue necrosis, nerve and ligament damage as well as secondary osteoarthritis should be discussed with owners.

Aseptic wound care is the cornerstone of patient healing. Clipping hair and wool from wounds, debriding devitalized tissues and foreign material, and cleansing the area are the initial steps of treatment. If a wound is less than 8 hours old and is easily cleaned, it may be indicated to attempt primary closure. Good aseptic technique and apposition of tissues without excessive tension gives primary closure the best chance of success. For wounds with a lot of dead space, placement of a drain may be useful.

For lacerations missing a large quantity of skin, second intention healing is indicated. Surrounding hair should be clipped, and any pockets should be drained ventrally. The wound should be cleaned often, and allowed to heal "from the inside-out." On the same animal, some wounds may be able to be sutured while others are left open. Tetanus vaccination status should be assessed and tetanus antitoxin (500 IU) is indicated in all but the most recent vaccinates. Neurologic deficits, rectal lacerations and ligament avulsion maintain a poor prognosis and generally require that the animals be destroyed.

Supportive care of the patient is extremely important for healing success. Keeping the animal warm, dry and relatively stress-free are necessary considerations. If the animal is moderately dehydrated, jugular catheter placement and subsequent fluid therapy or blood transfusion is used. If shock is extreme, corticosteroid therapy is indicated (dexamethasone 2 mg/kg IV). Myopathy and orthopedic trauma require the use of nonsteroidal antiinflammatory drugs. Flunixin meglumine (1-2 mg/kg IV or IM) or oral aspirin (100 mg/kg) (use not indicated in hemorrhaging patients but fairly economical with short drug withdrawal time) therapy is also employed. Broad spectrum antibiotic therapy is indicated where slaughter is not an issue. Antibiotic choices include: penicillin (20,000 IU/kg bid), florfenicol (20 mg/kg IM EOD or 40 mg/kg SQ) and sulfadimethoxine (55 mg/kg IV or po initially then 27.5 mg/kg sid) for 5 days. Clients should always receive a written

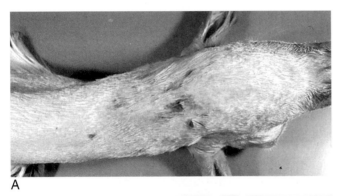

A

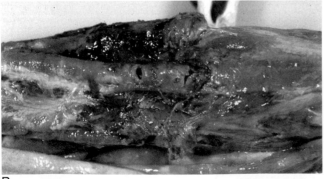

B

Figure 17-1   *A,* This goat was attacked by dogs. Note bite wound on the ventral neck area. *B,* At *post mortem,* the skin has been removed to show the extensiveness of the injury; note tracheal defects and muscle lacerations.

(Courtesy of Dr. John King; Cornell University.)

statement concerning withdrawal times and animal care in the advent of adverse drug reactions.

Consistent wound cleaning and fly control should be emphasized to the owner. Appetite and water consumption are important for the client to monitor. Animals are encouraged to stand and walk several times a day to avoid tendon contraction in the front limbs; otherwise physical therapy should be done to keep tendons stretched is indicated. Environmental stress should be minimized as much as possible.

Tail Docking

Tail docking (amputation) is usually performed in sheep (not goats) in Western nations, excluding Europe. This procedure is done to prevent fly strike, improve ram-breeding efficiency, and provide a more balanced carcass to the meat packer. Docking is typically performed in the first two weeks of the lamb's life. However, it is not uncommon for the veterinary practitioner to dock the tail on a mature ewe overlooked at a younger age. The 1- to 2-week-old lamb is docked with little or no hemorrhage. Techniques include the following: hot chisel, electric hot docker, emasculator, Burdizzo, elastrator, and blade amputation. The tail is amputated at the mid to distal limit of the caudal tail fold found on the ventral aspect of the tail. The remaining "dock" or stump should cover the anus. The recent producer trend of extremely short tail docks has led to an outbreak of a number of secondary health problems, most notably rectal prolapse.

An assistant holding the patient upside down with each hand locking the respective front and rear limbs usually accomplishes restraint of a lamb. Surgical clipping and cleaning is not generally employed if the tail is clean and free of fecal debris. Tetanus antitoxin (250 IU SQ) is indicated if previous dam vaccination has been ignored. The practitioner should not recommend elastrator/rubber bands. They function through ischemic necrosis, and tetanus is a common sequela.

Amputation of a mature tail is a serious surgical procedure. General anesthesia is recommended, but many practitioners use physical restraint accompanied by either a caudal epidural perfusion block or local infusion with 2% lidocaine. Postsurgical analgesia is always indicated. The tail is surgically clipped and cleaned. A tourniquet is applied at the base of the tail for hemostasis. The mature tail is amputated at the mid to distal limit of the caudal tail fold found on the ventral aspect of the tail. The loose skin should be retracted proximally before incision and amputation to allow adequate reapposition. The skin is incised in a "V" pattern to permit easy closure. The vertebra are either incised interdigitally or crushed and cut with an emasculator for added hemo-

stasis. Closure is completed with nonabsorbable 0 to 2-0 suture material in a simple interrupted or horizontal mattress suture pattern. Tetanus prophylaxis (antitoxin 500 IU SQ), seasonal fly control, and appropriate antibiotics are given after surgery.

RECOMMENDED READINGS

Acorn RC, Dorrance MJ: *Methods of investigating predation of livestock*, Edmonton, Alberta, 1990, Alberta Agriculture Agdex 684914.

Dille SE: Care of the flock after a predator attack, *Proc Regional Symp, Am Assoc Sheep Goat Pract*, Feb 27, 1985, University of Minnesota, College Vet Med.

Guthery FS, Beasom SL: Effects of predator control on Angora goat survival in south Texas, *J Range Management* 31: 168-173, 1978.

Geske J: Predators. In Haskell SH et al: *Sheep care and management*, Minneapolis, 2002, University of Minnesota Extension Service.

Long J et al: Fox attacks on Cashmere goats, *J Agric West Aust* 29: 104-106, 1988.

Reilly LK et al: Diseases of the musculoskeletal system. In Pugh DG: *Sheep and goat medicine*, Philadelphia, 2002, WB Saunders Company.

Rollins D: Interpreting physical evidence of predation on hoof stock and management alternatives for coping with predators. In Van Metre DC: *The Veterinary Clinics of North America, Food Animal Practice* 17: 265-281, 2001.

Smith MC, Sherman DM: *Goat medicine*, Philadelphia, 1994, Lea and Febiger.

17.1—Caprine Dehorning

Eugene C. White

When deciding whether to dehorn a goat, one must consider several factors. Goats with horns pose a threat to other animals and the people that work with them. Some goat breeds cannot be registered or shown until they are dehorned. Goats without horns are less destructive to farm facilities and are less likely to become entangled in fences. In addition, dehorning can be combined with descenting in males. However, dehorning is not appropriate for all goats. Goats that range or are kept on tethers should be allowed to keep their horns as a defense mechanism. In addition, dehorned bucks may be less able to compete with horned herdmates for breeding purposes and dehorning in adulthood may have secondary complications that include delayed healing, decreased milk or sperm production, and possibly death.

Given the complications and costs associated with dehorning, select breeding for polled goats would seem to be advantageous. However, goats have a dominant polled gene closely linked to an infertility recessive gene.

Goats homozygous for the polled condition are less fertile because of conditions such as sterile intersex females and a predisposition toward sperm granulomas in males. Breeding programs should account for this possibility, and polled goats should not be interbred to avoid these complications.

Disbudding

Removal of horn buds in young goats is most appropriately termed *disbudding* and should be performed within the first week of life. European breeds of buck kids should be disbudded between 3 and 5 days of age while doe kids should be disbudded between 5 and 7 days of age. The horns of Nubian kids grow more slowly than European breed kids, which allows disbudding in Nubians to be delayed until two weeks of age. Some goat kids are polled and will not need to be disbudded. Polled goats can be recognized by a single whorl of hair on top of their heads, whereas horned goats have a whorl of hair over each horn bud.

RESTRAINT AND ANESTHESIA
Several methods of restraint and anesthesia are available for disbudding kids. Although some prefer to use physical restraint alone, others use a combination of physical restraint, local anesthesia, sedation, and general anesthesia. If physical restraint is used alone, a goat disbudding box can be useful. The boxes are roughly 24 inches long, 18 inches tall, and 7 inches wide, with a lid and small opening at the front of the box for the kid's head. Kids dehorned with physical restraint alone resume normal behavior immediately after the disbudding process has been completed, which some think is justification enough for this method.

The cornual branch of the infratrochlear and lacrimal nerves innervate the horn bud of the goat. A subcutaneous line block along the dorsomedial rim of the orbit blocks the cornual branch of the infratrochlear nerve. The site to block the cornual branch of the lacrimal nerve is located halfway between the lateral canthus of the eye and the posterior edge of the horn along the cornual ridge behind the supraorbital process. Local anesthesia is performed in kids by injecting 1 milliliter of a solution (1 milliliter of 2% lidocaine diluted with 3 milliliters of sterile water) into each of four sites required to block the two horn buds (Figure 17.1-1).

In the field, xylazine (0.06 mg/kg IV) can be used to provide sedation. A 2% to 3% halothane gas can be used to anesthetize kids when dehorning is performed in an office. The high oxygen content of the halothane gas may make the goat's hair prone to combustion in the presence of a hot iron; therefore it must be removed before the iron is applied.

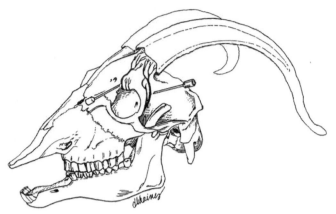

Figure 17.1-1   Injection sites for anesthesia of the horn in goats.

(From Riebold TW, Geiser DR, Goble DO: *Large animal anesthesia, principles and techniques*, ed 2, Ames, Iowa, 1995, Iowa State University Press.)

SURGICAL TECHNIQUE
Heat cautery is the most commonly used technique to disbud kids. A 200-watt dehorning iron with a $^3/_4$ to 1-inch tip is used for heat cautery. Lower wattage dehorning irons do not get as hot and must be applied to the head longer to burn the same degree as the higher wattage models. The hair over the horn bud should be clipped before disbudding to improve visualization and decrease the amount of smoke inhaled by the person performing the disbudding.

Once the dehorner has become cherry red, it should be applied to the horn bud for 3 to 4 seconds while being rocked around the bud. The head should be allowed to cool before reapplying the iron for another 3 to 4 seconds. Two applications of the iron should be adequate to completely destroy the horn corium, and this is assured if a ring of copper-colored skin that encircles the horn bud and cannot be scraped off with a fingernail has formed. The circle of skin inside the ring should be burned as well. Buck kids require a larger ring of burnt skin than doe kids do, and bucks can also be descented at this time by burning an additional crescent of skin caudomedial to each horn bud (Figure 17.1-2).

The most common mistakes associated with using heat cautery include inadequate burning that leads to scur formation (Figure 17.1-3) and excessive burning that leads to heat meningitis. The frontal bone's thinness and the absence of a frontal sinus at the age kids are disbudded make them prone to heat meningitis. Signs of heat meningitis include unresponsiveness and an inability to nurse. Treatment with antibiotics, antiinflammatory agents, supplemental heat, and tube feeding may allow some affected kids to recover from this condition.

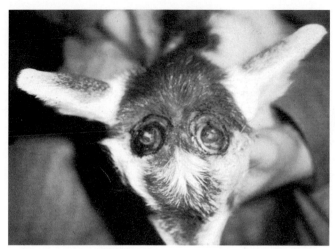

Figure 17.1-2 Dehorning in a young male goat using a dehorning iron. Note that the caudomedial surface adjacent to the horn bud has been burned to descent the goat at the same time.

(Courtesy of Dr. Mary Smith; Cornell University.)

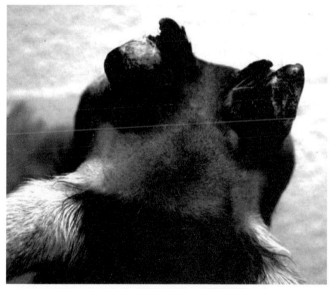

Figure 17.1-3 Scur formation in a young goat that had insufficient extent of burn when dehorned with cautery.

(Courtesy of Dr. Mary Smith; Cornell University.)

An alternative method for disbudding kids has been described using a 1-inch diameter stainless steel tube with a cutting edge. The instrument is centralized over the horn bud and rotated back and forth to cut through the skin. Once the incision has reached the skull, the bud is scooped out, thus leaving a clean surgical wound. The superficial temporal artery located laterally is sealed with electrocautery, and a pressurized aerosol of antibiotic powder is applied to the surgery site.

Dehorning paste should not be used in kids. The paste can injure the eyes, burn holes in the skin of herd mates that contact the paste, and burn through the calvarium underlying the horn bud, permitting bacteria to penetrate the brain.

POSTOPERATIVE CARE

After disbudding, a pressurized aerosol of antibiotic powder should be applied to the wound, and kids should be kept warm, in sternal recumbency, until the anesthesia has worn off completely. Tetanus prophylaxis should be given at this time—including both 250 IU of tetanus antitoxin and two doses of tetanus toxoid using separate syringes in two different locations. Colostrally derived antibodies for tetanus prophylaxis will not be adequate for kids that have failure of passive transfer.

Dehorning Older Kids

The horn of kids will become large enough within a couple of weeks to prevent a dehorning iron from reaching the skin around the base of the horn. To dehorn these older kids, the tip of the protruding horn must be removed before the dehorning iron can be applied to skin around the base of the horn. The tip of the horn can be removed with hoof nippers, shears, or a small Barnes dehorner, with care taken so that the dehorners do not penetrate deep enough to reach the brain cavity.

Once the tip of the horn has been removed, heat cautery is applied to the edges of the wound to burn the skin around the horn base as described for disbudding. Postoperative care is similar to that described earlier except the dose of tetanus antitoxin should be increased to 500 IU. By the time kids have reached 6 to 8 weeks of age, they should be treated as small adults described below.

Dehorning Adults

The risks and benefits of dehorning adult goats must be fully considered before attempting this procedure. In addition to the risks of tetanus, sinusitis, myiasis, abortion, ketosis, and death associated with dehorning the adult dairy goat, the wound left after this procedure will leave a large defect in the frontal sinus. This defect may take months to close, if it closes at all. After the procedure, the goat will need to be isolated from other goats to avoid injury until healing is complete, and the goat may lose its social status within the herd.

ANESTHESIA

Adult goats should be withheld from feed for 12 to 24 hours before surgery. Although adult goats can be anesthetized with xylazine at the dose discussed earlier, general anesthesia with inhaled halothane gives more satisfactory results if available. Two local blocks per horn should be performed by using 1 milliliter of 2% lidocaine in each of the sites as described earlier. A ring block can be performed around the horn as well, being careful not to exceed the toxic dose of 13 mg/kg of lidocaine.

SURGICAL TECHNIQUE

After anesthesia and surgical preparation, the skin is incised 1.5 cm from the base of the horn, with care taken to leave at least a 1-cm strip of skin between the two horns. While an assistant supports the goat's head, a Gigli wire saw is seated into the caudomedial aspect of the skin incision, and the horn is sawed off in a craniolateral direction to avoid cutting too deeply into the skull and entering the cranial cavity (Figure 17.1-4). The horn must be supported during the cutting process to prevent the frontal bone from fracturing. Once the horn has been removed, the superficial temporal artery (located laterally) should be pulled, cauterized, or ligated.

The scent glands of male goats located at the caudomedial base of each horn can also be removed at this time.

When done correctly, dehorning will leave a large opening in the frontal sinus. The procedure must be performed as aseptically as possible with any clots or bone dust removed from the sinus to avoid developing sinusitis.

The cosmetic dehorning of an adult goat previously described reduces the risk of myiasis and sinusitis. However, too large a defect as a result of the size of the horn base will prevent the skin over the dehorning wound from being closed.

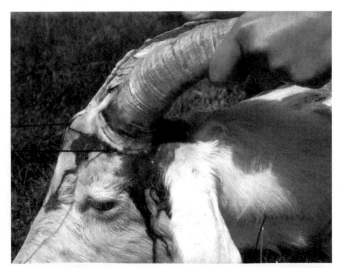

Figure 17.1-4 Adult goat dehorned with a Gigli wire placed to ensure a margin of haired skin around the horn is removed.

(Courtesy of Dr. Mary Smith; Cornell University.)

In some cases, owners may elect to simply remove the distal end of horns, such as when a horn's tip has grown into the side of the goat's head. The tip of the horn can be removed by using Gigli wire under light sedation. The amount of horn to be removed can be determined by taking a radiograph to discern the extent of horn, sinus and bony cornual process, or small sections of the horn can be removed until a satisfactory length is obtained or the horn first begins to bleed if radiographs are unavailable.

POSTOPERATIVE CARE

After dehorning, adult goats must be kept isolated until the wound has healed completely. Antibiotics should not be necessary unless complications such as sinusitis or myiasis develop, but a 50-mg dose of intravenous flunixin postoperatively may make the goat more comfortable. The goat should be fed off the ground rather than an overhead hayrack and housed in a barn with a clean ceiling to avoid foreign matter falling into the wound. Tetanus prophylaxis should be provided by using either tetanus toxoid or 500 IU of tetanus antitoxin as determined by the previous vaccination history of the goat.

While not all clinicians apply a bandage to the wound, many apply an initial bandage that is changed in 2 days, followed by a second bandage left in place for 1 week. To wrap the wound, antiseptic powder and nonadhesive dressing is applied to the dehorning site. An orthopedic stockinet with eyeholes can be pulled over the goat's head and taped in place to hold the dressing in place. Alternatively, an elastic bandage can be taped to the head and wound around the ears in a figure-eight pattern.

Postoperative Complications

Dehorning goats of any age is not a benign procedure, and the chance of postoperative complications becomes more severe the longer the procedure is delayed. In addition to the complications of tetanus, thermal meningitis, sinusitis, myiasis, loss of social status, and scar formation previously mentioned, the stress of dehorning may lead to other complications such as abortion, listeriosis, and ketosis. These possibilities must be discussed with owners before dehorning, and this is especially important for dehorning adults. Owners should be instructed to watch for signs of complications and inform the clinician if any signs are noted.

Descenting Bucks

The scent glands of the buck are situated under the skin on the caudomedial aspect of the horns, and their location can be identified as a shiny, hairless, crescent-shaped patch of skin with pores. Descenting is usually performed in conjunction with dehorning as described earlier but can be performed without dehorning if the client desires. Although removing the scent glands decreases a buck's odor, owners should be warned that only castration entirely removes the buck's smell. Bucks have other scent glands in addition to those located behind the horns, and intact males continue to urinate on their heads, beards, and forelegs during the breeding season.

To remove the glands, the buck should be sedated and the skin to be removed infiltrated with lidocaine. Once the glands have been located, a crescent-shaped piece of skin can be removed and the area closed surgically. Alternatively, if the scent glands extend further from the horn base, a triangular flap of skin with the apex located on midline 3 to 4 centimeters in front of the rostral aspect of the horns can be reflected caudally to fully expose the scent glands. The scent glands can then be removed and the skin flap sutured back into place.

RECOMMENDED READINGS

Boyd J et al: Disbudding of goat kids, *Goat Veterinary Society Journal* 8: 77-78, 1987.

Brent AH et al: Cosmetic dehorning in goats, *Veterinary Surgery* 26: 332-334, 1997.

Buttle H et al: Disbudding and dehorning of goats, *In Practice* 8: 63-65, 1986.

Hull BL: Dehorning the adult goat, *Veterinary Clinics of North America: Food Animal Practice* 11: 183-185, 1995.

Mobini S: Cosmetic dehorning in adult goats, *Small Ruminant Research* 5: 187-191, 1991.

Riebold TW, Geiser DR, Goble DO: *Large Animal Anesthesia, Principles and Techniques*, ed 2, Ames, Iowa, 1995, Iowa State University Press.

Skarda RT: Local and regional anesthesia in ruminants and swine, *Veterinary Clinics of North America: Food Animal Practice* 12: 579-626, 1996.

Smith MC, Sherman DM: *Goat medicine*, Philadelphia, 1994, Lea & Febiger.

Williams CF: Routine sheep and goat procedures, *Veterinary Clinics of North America: Food Animal Practice* 6: 737-758, 1990.

17.2—Lumps and Bumps of Sheep and Goats

Paul J. Plummer

Small ruminant practitioners are commonly faced with diagnosing and treating a subcutaneous mass on the body of a goat or sheep. Many etiologies are associated with these masses, with some carrying significant economic and management consequences while others pose only a cosmetic nuisance. When writing certificates of veterinary inspection (health certificates), one must consider these different etiologies to accurately assess the effect of the mass on an animal's transport and exhibition. The accurate diagnosis begins with determining the distribution of the lesions as well as any lymph node involvement.

Lesions Associated with Lymph Nodes

CASEOUS LYMPHADENITIS

By far the most common cause of abscesses associated with lymph nodes of small ruminants is caseous lymphadenitis (CL). The responsible organism is *Corynebacterium pseudotuberculosis*, a facultative anaerobe. Gram stains reveal a gram-positive to gram-variable coccoid rod from culture, although gram-stained smears of abscess material may yield a longer rod. The organism is endemic in all of the Americas, Australia, New Zealand, Europe, and South Africa. These hardy bacteria can persist for weeks to months in the environment and bedding, feed bins, or on wood. For this reason, affected animals should be immediately removed from the herd and isolated in an area not used for general housing.

Transmission of CL occurs via ingestion or inhalation of infective bacteria from the environment. Management practices can have a significant effect on an animal's abscess distribution because the organism often gains access to the body via a break in the skin. In sheep, the most common sites associated with infection result from trauma during shearing or dipping for external parasites. Inhalation of these organisms plays a definite role when animals are held in close confinement, like that typically seen in shearing sheds of large sheep operations. Thus sheep lymph nodes of the hind legs and neck often have abscesses. In contrast, goat abscesses, more commonly found on the head or neck, become infected by breaks in the neck skin or ingesting contaminated feed utensils.

The clinical signs depend on the extent of abscessation and route of entry. Most commonly, goats present for abscessation of the parotid, submandibular, retropharyngeal (Figure 17.2-1) prescapular or mandibular lymph nodes, with the pre-femoral or popliteal lymph nodes less commonly involved. These swellings start out firm and progress to flocculent swellings with a very soft center when "ripe". The incubation period from exposure to abscess formation seems to be roughly in the 2- to 6-month range. The cutaneous form seen in sheep presents with similar findings except that they occur more often in the lymph nodes of the neck and hind legs. The appearance of the abscess material in goats is a characteristic cheesy consistency and is greenish-white with no odor. In contrast, sheep abscesses form a firm mass that can be expressed intact and often has a laminar appearance when cut in cross section (Figure 17.2-2).

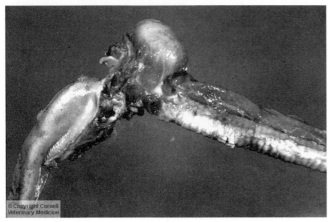

Figure 17.2-1   Retropharyngeal abscess in a sheep.

(Courtesy of Dr. John King; Cornell University.)

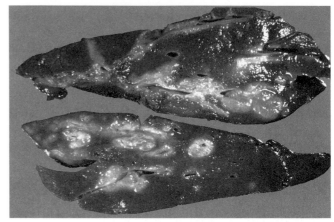

Figure 17.2-3   Liver abscessation due to *Corynebacterium pseudotuberculosis*.

(Courtesy of Dr. John King; Cornell University.)

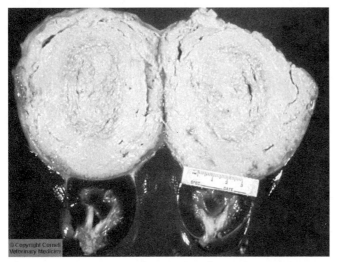

Figure 17.2-2   Caseous abscessation due to *Corynebacterium pseudotuberculosis* in a sheep. Note the laminar pattern.

(Courtesy of Dr. John King; Cornell University.)

The visceral form of CL may range from no clinical signs to severe weight loss and systemic disease. This is the most common form seen in sheep, and it is estimated a large percentage of goats with external abscesses also form some internal abscesses (Figure 17.2-3).

Diagnosis of CL is generally made based on the clinical signs and history of the herd or flock. Significant historical findings might include the following: a new animal purchased from an unknown source, a history of abscesses in the herd or flock, or a herd where the animals are moved often and have significant contact with outside animals (i.e., a show herd). If necessary, the abscess can be aspirated with a needle and syringe for cytology and culture. Very often, the needle tract will allow continuous drainage and should only be performed

after the animal has been isolated from the rest of the herd. If the abscess is "ripe" (i.e., mature with a soft area), the clinician might opt to lance the abscess. This is generally accomplished by clipping any hair over the swelling and performing an aseptic preparation of the area before using a scalpel to incise the abscess. Opening the infected pocket is important so that its most ventral extent is drained. If the abscess is mature, very little innervation is usually left on the soft part of the abscess, and local anesthetic is often not necessary. The material in the abscess should be collected and burned to minimize contamination of the area. The abscess cavity can be flushed with dilute povidone-iodine or hydrogen peroxide. The external opening should be kept clean and open, with the lesion allowed to heal from the inside out. This generally takes several weeks, and a small scar may remain in place of the abscess. During this time, the animal should be isolated.

Surgical removal of the abscessed lymph node provides the advantage of decreased contamination to the environment. Unfortunately, the lymph nodes most commonly involved lie in areas with many other vital anatomical structures, making surgical dissection complicated (i.e., the carotid arteries, esophagus, and parotid lymph node). If surgery is to be performed, meticulous dissection of the soft tissues should be performed after a sharp skin incision. The surgeon should stay as close to the mass as possible, which usually makes it easier to establish a plane of dissection. If possible, the entire abscess is removed. It may be necessary to close with a drain, depending on the amount of dead space created. If the abscess cavity is inadvertently incised, it can be drained and allowed to heal as an open wound. It also may be possible to marsupialize the abscess by suturing the capsule to the skin, thereby protecting the soft tissues.

Diagnosis of internal abscesses often poses a considerable challenge. Ultrasound of the abdominal organs and radiographs of the thorax can reveal abscess formation in the internal lymph nodes or organs. Several serologic tests have been developed for use; however, few are good at differentiating ongoing disease versus previous exposure. Maternal antibodies may yield false-positive results to serologic testing on animals less then 6 months of age, while previous vaccination or well walled-off abscesses may yield erroneous results in older animals. A fourfold rise in titer over a 2- to 3-week period would be consistent with active infection; however, lack of this response may not rule out a chronic shedding situation. The test would be most useful in accessing exposure and screening new animals being brought into a herd.

In most field situations, treatment consists of monitoring lymph nodes, isolating infected animals, and draining abscesses as they mature. If the herd does not have a history of CL and an animal develops clinical signs, one must be vigilant in minimizing exposure to the rest of the herd. Culling based on clinical signs of CL is warranted in herds or flocks with no history of disease.

If the economic value of the animal does not allow culling and treatment as described earlier is not acceptable, several other possible treatments offer variable success. As mentioned before, surgical excision of the abscesses may be feasible but is often a difficult dissection and requires considerable surgical skill to minimize complications. Long-term treatment with systemic antibiotics that provide good abscess penetration has been used but is often unsuccessful. Antibiotic choices would include potassium penicillin with rifampin or erythromycin and rifampin. None of the drugs are approved for use in goats and only some are in sheep; therefore use involves extra-label requirements and all of the paperwork associated with it. In addition, no withdrawal times have been established for these drugs in small ruminants.

Recently, some veterinarians have been promoting the use of intra-lesional formalin. Theoretically, formalin injected into the abscess sterilizes it and forms a type of autogenous vaccine. Many people report the abscesses resolve once injected with formalin; however, the affect on internal abscesses is less certain. Other formalinized vaccines for CL are commercially available and have shown questionable success at resolving established infections, and it seems hard to believe that intraabscess formalin would be any different. The technique involves aspirating 10 to 20 ml of exudate through a 14-g needle in the dorsal part of a soft abscess. The material is mixed with 10-20 ml of formalin, and part of this mixture is reinjected into the abscess. This procedure is repeated five times, and the abscess, reportedly will often resolve in several weeks. Aside from the concern about continued internal abscess formation, liability is also associated with this technique. Formalin may be carcinogenic to people and is not approved by the FDA for use in food-animal species. The veterinarian is responsible to the FDA (regardless of any signed agreement between the owner and veterinarian) if the animal yields residues in meat or milk. Some argue that formalin will be contained in the abscess; however, this has not been demonstrated experimentally.

Control of CL within a herd or flock consists of vigilance when moving animals into the herd and during times of exposure to animals of unknown status. If the herd does not have a history of disease, all precautions should be taken to prevent introduction; early detection paired with aggressive culling may be warranted. Several inactivated whole cell wall vaccines are commercially available in the United States. At this time, all of them primarily activate a humoral response, which is more likely to prevent an acute case dissemination than resolve an established case. Lethargy, pain, sterile abscess formation, and a drop in milk production are vaccination side effects that appear to be more severe in goats than sheep. Animals previously exposed to CL tend to react more severely. It is recommended that veterinarians inform goat owners of the vaccine's limitations and potential side effects before using it.

OTHER CAUSES OF LYMPHADENOPATHY

Although the large majority of lumps and bumps associated with lymph nodes of the small ruminant represent CL lesions, other differentials should be considered if the diagnostics or clinical presentation do not support a CL diagnosis. Any inflammatory process associated with a cellulitis or regional infection can cause swelling of a regional lymph node. Additionally, caprine arthritis-encephalitis, lymphosarcoma, and melioidosis (*Pseudomonas pseudomallei*) can cause a lymphadenopathy. These often do not progress to abscesses, and the inciting cause is usually obvious after a complete physical exam, and, in some cases, aspirating the affected lymph node. These lesions may or may not represent infectious processes that warrant isolation of the affected animal.

Lesions not Associated with Lymph Nodes

THORAX AND ABDOMEN

Lumps and bumps on the body wall of the thoracic cavity or abdomen typically represent noninfectious lesions secondary to trauma, congenital, or acquired defects. Perhaps the most common cause of this type of lesion is formation of a hematoma or seroma secondary to trauma. These lesions can vary in size but are generally associated with a history or evidence of trauma and are located in the subcutaneous or muscle layers of the body wall with an acute onset. They can be aspirated to aid in diagnosis. However, a significant risk of seeding the hematoma or seroma and inducing an abscess exists if aseptic technique is not used.

If the lump is associated with the umbilicus or is in the flank, a hernia should be considered. Intestine entrapped in a hernia that is not reducible may represent a surgical emergency. If no intestine is involved, these lesions can be allowed to mature for several months until the ring fibroses, making them easier to repair surgically.

Although seeing caseous lymphadenitis abscesses on the chest or abdomen is unusual, other causes of abscesses present in these regions. A sterile abscess associated with vaccination in the axillary region is one common cause. These abscesses seldom mature and usually resolve over a period of months.

NECK

Wattle cysts (Figure 17.2-4) are one of the most commonly misdiagnosed causes of neck masses. These masses are typically similar in size to a CL abscess and occur in the throat latch area of the neck where there are no prominent lymph nodes. They appear to be localized accumulations of lymphatic fluid in the area where wattles originate from the neck. These cysts can be found in the same area on animals that do not have wattles.

Diagnosis can generally be made based on location and palpation. The lesions are flocculent and reveal a cyst with hypoechoic noncellular fluid when imaged with ultrasound. Following a sterile scrub, the swellings can be easily aspirated through an 18-20g needle with a syringe. The fluid is a yellowish transparent fluid with low cellularity but often contains some flocculent-type floaters. When aspirated, the cyst generally collapses on itself. Some of these cysts seem to resolve and disappear after several years. If aseptic technique is used and the cyst is not seeded with bacteria, it can be aspirated as needed for cosmetic concerns. The cysts can also be excised when the animal is restrained with sedation and a local anesthetic (Figure 17.2-5). The underlying jugular vein should be carefully avoided during surgery.

Swelling of the neck can involve the thymus and/or thyroid glands located on either side of the trachea at the level of the larynx. In young goats, the thyroid glands are commonly buried in a portion of thymic tissue (that is felt to be accessory thymus or remnants of embryonic thymus). It is not uncommon for healthy, growing kids to get some swelling associated with the thymus that spontaneously regresses over a period of time. Typically these kids are healthy in other respects and have a nice looking hair coat. If the kid is unhealthy, not growing properly, or has a poor-looking hair coat, thyroid hyperplasia associated with goiter may be the cause. Goiter is more commonly seen in areas of the country with soils deficient in iodine. The goiter seen in kids is generally associated with either a nutritional iodine deficiency or feeding of food sources containing materials that block digestive uptake of iodine. Dietary iodine can be

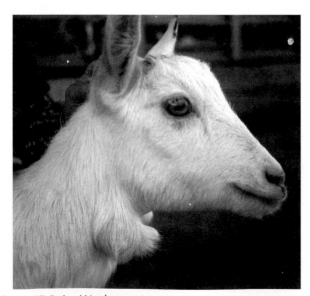

Figure 17.2-4   Wattle cyst in a goat.

(Courtesy of Dr. Mary Smith; Cornell University.)

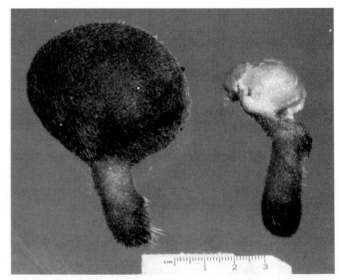

Figure 17.2-5   Excised wattle cyst in a goat. There is a large cyst on the left and a smaller cyst on the right.

(Courtesy of Dr. Mary Smith; Cornell University.)

supplemented in the ration or as free-choice iodinated-salt. Although T_4 levels can be run on these animals, normal ranges of goats are not well defined at this time. As in other species, unhealthy animals may have a low T_4 associated with euthyroid sick syndrome, not thyroid disease. The general health of the kid should be accessed before supplementation, because iodine toxicity has been documented in kids that received an iodine supplement when they had a thymus, not thyroid, enlargement.

HEAD

If swellings or bumps that occur on the head are not associated with lymph nodes; the first diagnostic steps should include a good oral exam. Packing the cud in the buccal cavity lateral to the molars is commonly associated with a missing tooth or severe dental abnormalities but poses no significant problem for the animal. One will also see abscesses associated with trauma to the buccal surface at the level of the molar occlusion. These are often associated with sharp points on the teeth, and floating the teeth may be beneficial. The abscesses generally resolve without therapy. If the swelling is located more on the ventral aspect of the ramus of the mandible, a thorough evaluation for missing, loose, or fractured teeth in that area should be included in the exam. This presentation is common for a tooth-root abscess that will gradually swell the ramus of the mandible and eventually open and drain. Radiographs of the head and dental arcade may be helpful in a definitive diagnosis. Once confirmed, removing the tooth may help achieve a complete resolution. However, unless decay allows the tooth to be easily extracted via the mouth, surgical extraction will be required. This can be difficult, and mandibular fracture is a risk during the procedure. The animal should be placed in lateral or dorsal recumbency to approach the mandible overlying the affected tooth. The bone of the mandible is carefully removed with a small, motorized burr until the tooth root is exposed. The tooth is then repelled into the oral cavity. Because of the risks, extraction via the mouth is preferable.

Other possible causes of swellings on the head include salivary mucoceles (Figure 17.2-6) and edema. Salivary mucoceles form along the salivary ducts, usually secondary to trauma. Aspiration of the swelling yields thick, clear yellow mucoid saliva, which confirms the diagnosis. These cysts rarely cause problems but can be removed if desired (see Section 10.1).

If surgery is to be performed the animal is positioned in lateral recumbency under general anesthesia. A sharp incision is made in the skin between the maxillary and linguofacial veins directly over the swelling. A combination of blunt and sharp dissection is used to free both the mandibular and sublingual glands. The duct, which

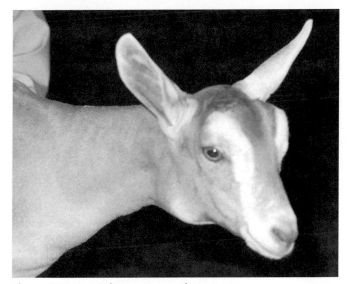

Figure 17.2-6   Salivary mucocele in a goat.

(Courtesy of Dr. Mary Smith; Cornell University.)

is at the most rostral portion of the gland, should be ligated carefully to avoid chronic drainage. It may be necessary to place a drain, depending on the amount of dead space created.

Young kids will sometimes present for edema in the intermandibular space. This is commonly called *bottle jaw* and is generally associated with hypoproteinemia due to severe endoparasitism.

Conclusions

Although potential causes of lumps and bumps in small ruminants are many, the diagnostic key is determining the distribution and extent of the lesions. The first step is to determine if lymph nodes are primarily involved, and if so suspect CL until proven otherwise. If the lymph nodes are not involved, a list of differential diagnoses should be made based on the location of the lesions and appropriate diagnostics chosen to arrive at a final diagnosis.

RECOMMENDED READINGS

Anderson DE, Rings DM, Pugh DG: Diseases of the integumentary system. In Pugh DG: *Sheep and goat medicine*, Philadelphia, 2002, WB Saunders.

Fubini SL, Campbell SG: External lumps on sheep and goats, *Vet Clin North Am: Large Anim Pract* 5: 457-476, 1983.

Smith MC, Sherman DM: Subcutaneous swellings. In *Goat medicine*, Philadelphia, 1994, Lea & Febiger.

Williamson LH: Caseous lymphadenitis in small ruminants, *Vet Clin North Am: Food Anim Pract* 17:359, 2001.

CHAPTER 18

SURGERY OF THE SHEEP AND GOAT DIGESTIVE SYSTEM

Scott R. R. Haskell

Gastrointestinal surgeries in sheep and goats are not commonly performed by the private veterinary practitioner but should always be considered for individual patients of economic worth. Surgeries that are performed most commonly include drainage or resection of pharyngeal abscess (traumatic, foreign body, caseous lymphadenitis), surgeries of the forestomach (reticulorumen) and abomasum, rumen and esophageal fistula placement, correction of intestinal obstruction, or intestinal accident.

Pharyngeal trauma and subsequent abscess formation in small ruminants is a common finding. If undiagnosed, this condition can lead to cellulitis, severe tissue necrosis, dyspnea, and subsequent bloat. Radiographs, ultrasound, and endoscopic examination can help confirm and localize the lesion. If the animal is severely dyspneic and the swelling is compressing the trachea, a temporary tracheostomy is indicated. Organisms typically isolated from abscesses include: *Arcanobacterium pyogenes,* *Yersinia pseudotuberculosis,* *Staphylococcus* species, and *Pseudomonas* species. Medical therapy can be attempted, but surgical intervention may be needed if the abscess is large and the animal is symptomatic. If economically feasible, general anesthesia is warranted because of the large number of vital structures in the area, including the vagosympathetic trunk, carotid vasculature, and esophagus. Antibiotic and antiinflammatory pharmaceutical utilization should be determined by culture and sensitivity results and the severity of the lesion.

When deciding on surgical points of entry, the practitioner should always consider the location of vessels and nerves in the area. An abscess should be entered from the oral cavity whenever possible (and when attached to the oropharynx) (see Figure 10.1-5) and lanced so that it drains into the digestive system. This is best accomplished by aspirating the contents first with an 18-gauge needle and syringe. A larger gauge needle will be needed in those instances when the abscess capsule may be thick.

Either a left lateral or ventral approach is indicated for surgical drainage. The use of a blindfold in sheep and goats may accent the anesthetic effects or, in many cases, lessen the stress to the surgical patient. The surgery site is surgically prepared. It is imperative that the esophagus, carotid artery, and jugular vein be initially visualized and shielded from possible incision. Dissection should be done bluntly to avoid vital structures. Ideally the abscess is isolated and removed in its entirety. Alternatively the capsule can be sutured to the skin and the abscess marsupialized. If neither of these options is possible, the abscess can be drained by aspiration and the animal kept on long-term antibiotics.

Surgery of the Rumen

Disease of the forestomach (reticulorumen) can be fairly common in sheep and goat practice. Ruminal distention, rumen acidosis, rumen impaction, bezoar formation, and foreign body consumption (Figure 18-1) with subsequent impaction and rumenitis/reticulitis are conditions that may require surgical intervention. Advanced rumenitis generally has a poor surgical prognosis. Rumenotomy and/or trocar placement can be required to correct the other conditions.

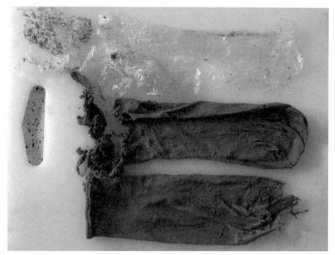

Figure 18-1   Foreign bodies (plastic bags) ingested by a goat resulting in ruminal obstruction.

(Courtesy of Dr. Mary Smith; Cornell University.)

If a rumenotomy is not performed under emergency conditions, the patient should be held off feed for 12 to 24 hours before surgery. General anesthesia helps control animal movement and maintains a clean surgical field. However, if economics preclude general anesthesia use, a rumenotomy can be done with a local anesthetic and manual restraint. The practitioner should be aware that sheep and goats are highly susceptible to the toxic effects of lidocaine; therefore low volumes of diluted (1%) lidocaine should be used.

The patient is placed in lateral recumbency with the right side down and the left flank prepared for aseptic surgery. For a rumenotomy, a 15-cm vertical skin incision is made parallel and 5 cm caudal to the last rib. The underlying muscle layers can either be sharply incised or bluntly dissected along their fascia planes ("grid technique") if a small incision is needed. Sheep and goat muscle layers are much thinner than those in cattle, and there is a more prominent cutaneous trunci muscle. Surgeons not used to small ruminants need to be careful not to make the common mistake of being too aggressive on the abdominal approach or incising over the kidneys. Once the rumen has been visualized, 10 cm should be exteriorized and sutured to the skin of the wound margin with a Lembert-type pattern around the entire incision margin. A bite is taken through the skin; then a bite is taken through the rumen (see Figure 10.3-10). This suture pattern forms a seal that prevents rumen fluid from entering the abdomen and is important to the surgery's success. Once the suture placement is inspected and found intact, the rumen wall is incised within this margin. The surgeon should avoid traumatizing the rumen wall as much as possible.

Examination of the lumen of the rumen is now possible. Any foreign material is removed, and the cardia and reticuloomasal orifice are inspected and checked for patency. The abomasum can be palpated through the rumen wall for distention and normal location. The ventral floor of the rumen can be swept, checking for any adhesions.

It is best to close the rumen wall with two rows of continuous sutures. The second row should be an inverting pattern, such as a Cushing or Lembert, created with an absorbable suture material. Once the rumen has been closed, gloves, surgical instruments, and gowns should be changed. The wound should be flushed with copious warm saline to remove any remaining debris. Once wound cleansing has been accomplished, the rumen to skin suture should be removed and the rumen lavaged again before it is replaced into the abdomen.

Closure of the abdomen is routine, although much smaller suture material (#0 or 1) can be used than in an adult cow. Each layer is closed in a simple continuous pattern with an absorbable suture, and lavage is performed between each layer. The skin is usually closed with a nonabsorbable suture. The most ventral sutures should be placed in an interrupted fashion in case drainage of the wound is necessary. Appropriate antibiotics should be used for at least 5 days after surgery. Anti-inflammatory drugs are commonly used, especially in goats (flunixin meglumine 1 to 2 mg/kg IM or butorphanol 1 mg/kg IM bid for no more than 48 hours). Clients should receive written notification of drug withdrawal times.

Rumenotomies to remove a foreign body have the most favorable prognosis. The most common items found in the rumen are plastic bags, rope, and large foreign bodies. A rumenotomy can also be performed for toxic indigestion; however, the prognosis is guarded for conditions longer than 12 hours' duration. Medical management of these cases through intravenous fluids, electrolyte monitoring and replacement therapy, probiotics, and orogastric introduction of alfalfa meal or feed mill "fines" is usually as—or more—successful. Alkalizers* may also be helpful. Stabilization of the rumen pH and transfaunation can be important tools for successful case management. Transfaunation per os generally requires 250 to 500 ml of collection fluid 2 to 3 times daily for 3 to 5 days. This fluid should be kept anaerobic, at rumen temperature, and out of light until inoculation occurs. Ideally, the time from collection to transfaunation should be less than 30 minutes.

ABOMASAL SURGERY

Disease of the abomasum is much less common than in cattle and decidedly more difficult to manage surgically.

*Carmalax®: www.qcsupply.net/carbolpfiz1.html, Pfizer, NY

Abomasal impaction, abomasitis, perforating abomasal ulcers, abomasal foreign bodies and abomasal emptying defect (AED) in Suffolk sheep can potentially be managed with surgical intervention. However, in most instances medical management should be attempted initially.

Generally, genetics are of extreme importance regarding abomasal impaction in sheep. Depending on an individual animal's value and owner preference, ancillary diagnostic tools may be helpful. Ultrasound of the abomasum in the standing patient is simple and noninvasive. The abomasum is generally packed tightly with sand and ingesta. On physical examination, heart and respiratory rates are elevated. Normal rumen movements with scant feces are evident. Commonly, abomasal outflow obstruction results in hypochloremic hypokalemic metabolic alkalosis and eventually dehydration, uremia, and tachycardia. Renal excretion of $NaHCO_3$ and $KHCO_3$ with secondary hypovolemia occurs. Serum electrolytes should be monitored and managed before surgery. Radiology is generally of limited value and inconclusive as a diagnostic tool, although ultrasound examination may be helpful. Medical management may include the following: large volume fluid replacement, correction of electrolyte imbalance, cholinergic drugs, and IV calcium and vitamin E/selenium—all of which have been used with limited success. Abomasal impaction is much more common in goats than in sheep. Pregnancy, poor quality hay, and feeding a total pelleted diet can predispose goats to impaction. Abomasal impaction can also occur in goats confined to semidesert grazing of grassland/brush forage that contains a high percentage of awns, which form phytobezoars ranging in size from 2 to 10 cm. Patients present with inappetence, malaise, weakness, scant feces, and cranial right abdominal swelling/distension. An abomasotomy is generally corrective.

Abomasal emptying disease in Suffolk sheep commonly presents as impaction, but the etiology is different and has not been elucidated. Pregnant sheep on a diet high in concentrates are commonly affected with AED. Medical management seems to be the most common treatment course, but an abomasotomy is occasionally attempted. The flock's genetic merit needs to be evaluated.

Abomasotomy

Two surgical approaches can be used for abomasotomy: the right paracostal and ventral midline approaches. Both approaches give good visualization. However, the right paracostal approach makes exteriorization of the abomasum easier and is recommended. General anesthesia is ideal, although sedation and a local anesthetic may be adequate for a tractable animal. If the animal is greatly distended, risk of aspiration pneumonia is considerable. The patient is positioned in left lateral recumbency and the right paracostal region prepared for aseptic surgery. A 15-cm incision is made parallel to and 3 cm away from the last rib and is extended along the costochondral junction. Subcutaneous tissues and muscle layers are sharply incised. The peritoneum is tented and entered sharply. A finger is inserted to check for adhesions and then the incision is extended. The greater curvature of the abomasum should be evident upon entry into the abdomen as the greater curvature normally lies in the paracostal position. The abdomen is quickly explored. If a distended abomasum is the only abnormal finding, the abomasotomy is performed. The greater curvature is exteriorized as much as possible and isolated from the rest of the abdomen with sterile towels. A generous curved incision is made in the abomasal wall, and the impacted contents are emptied. Once the abomasum is empty, the site is rinsed with sterile fluids. The abomasum is closed in two layers with an inverting pattern in the second layer. Time is spent rinsing with copious fluids to free the area of debris as much as possible. Gloves are changed and the abdomen closed routinely. Attempts to perform an abomasojejunostomy to encourage abomasal emptying have not met with success.

The prognosis is guarded. With AED, medical therapy is currently recommended.

Rumen, Abomasal and Esophageal Fistulization (Cannulization)

Rumen fistula placement may occasionally be requested for nutritional studies as well as the development of animals for herd/flock transfaunation. Most fistulas (cannulas) are commonly made from inert plastics; however, rubber, PVC and stainless steel are also occasionally used. The thinness of the abdominal wall requires a lightweight cannula. Currently, one company* manufactures fistulas for small ruminants and cattle in the United States. Abomasal cannulization for research purposes in sheep and goats is generally performed with a Pezzar[†] (mushroom head) urinary catheter.

Surgical Procedure

The left paralumbar fossa region is prepared for surgery and a local anesthetic administered. A circular skin incision site approximately 1 to 1.5 cm smaller than the diameter of the cannula to be used is the difference between this procedure and a rumenotomy (Figure 18-2). Muscle dissection is blunt, so the holding capacity

---

*Bar Diamond Parma: *www.bardiamond.com*, Parma, ID
[†]Pezzar®, Davol, Arista Surgical Supply Co., NY

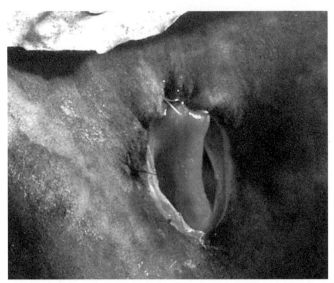

Figure 18-2 For placement of a rumen cannula, a circular skin incision site approximately 1- to 1.5-cm smaller than the diameter of the cannula to be used has been removed. The rumen is being secured to the skin.

of the muscle layers is retained. The rumen is exteriorized and sutured first to the dermis and subcutaneous tissues using an absorbable suture material. A broken continuous pattern is appropriate. Once a good seal of rumen to skin is obtained, the rumen is incised and the mucosa sutured to the skin using a simple interrupted pattern of nonabsorbable sutures. Most often, the cannula is warmed in hot water before insertion to make the plastic more pliable. Postsurgical antibiotics are indicated as with the rumenotomy procedure described earlier.

Esophageal cannula placement is a less common request. These are used primarily for grazing experiments. The surgery tends to be problematic in sheep because of wool growth. Myiasis and wool irritation are both common sequela that need to be addressed.

The surgical technique is similar to rumen cannulization. General anesthesia is indicated, with tracheal intubation mandatory. Stomach tube placement is maintained as a landmark for the incision site. The surgical site is in the midcervical region just ventral to the jugular furrow and left of midline. The practitioner should palpate the stomach tube and incise the skin directly over the tube. Blunt dissection of the sternomastoideus and cleidomastoideus muscles allows visualization of the esophagus. It is important to remember the jugular vein, carotid artery, and vagosympathetic nerves all run close to the surgical site. Careful dissection is imperative. The esophagus should be incised for 2 to 3 cm. At this time, the stomach tube should be retracted and the esophageal cannula positioned for suture. The esophageal wall should be sutured caudal

and cranial up to the cannula using an inverting suture pattern. The suture material should be absorbable and small in diameter (2-0). Pursestring suturing can also be used. A three-layer closure is indicated to obliterate dead space. In this region, it is important the sutures not be too tight as tissue necrosis can be a common sequela. Skin closure is cranial and caudal to the cannula and is created with a nonabsorbable suture material using a simple interrupted pattern. Generally, antibiotics are indicated. The owner should be instructed to shear the wool regularly from around the cannula site.

Abomasal cannulization of sheep and goats with the Pezzar (mushroom head) urinary catheter can be a challenge. The site selection and procedure is as previously described in the abomasotomy, except the abomasum is exteriorized but not sutured to the wound margin. The catheter is a 36 to 40 French Pezzar catheter that is inserted into the ventral aspect of the abomasum.

The midventral aspect of the abomasum can be exteriorized from a ventral or paracostal approach. Once the desired site is located, a circular pursestring suture pattern is placed with a 3-cm diameter using a 2-0 to 3-0 absorbable material. A small incision, just large enough to insert the mushroom head of the Pezzar catheter (approximately 1 cm), is made into the lumen of the abomasum. The pursestring suture can then be tightened around the catheter. The catheter is exteriorized through the abdominal wall (right of midline) separate from the primary incision. Enough slack should be allowed so the abomasum can be replaced in normal position. As previously described, the incision sites are closed in three layers. Before repelling the abomasum back into normal position in the abdomen, the surgeon should flush the wound field with warm sterile saline. Gloves and instruments should be changed before closure. The catheter is sutured to the skin with nonabsorbable suture material. The catheter should be supported with a body bandage for the first 10-14 days. Antibiotics and nonsteroidal antiinflammatory drugs are also indicated.

Surgical Management of Intestinal Obstruction

Management of intestinal obstruction in sheep and goats is determined by the economics of the situation. Symptoms of digestive system disease are often very vague. Inappetence, abdominal distension, diarrhea, melena, and a history of foreign body consumption are typical. Many field practitioners do not have the capabilities for abdominal radiographs or ultrasound, or clinical pathology data. In these animals, exploratory surgery could be indicated for diagnostic purposes. General anesthesia with intubation is appropriate for an exploratory examination in small ruminants, although much can be done with sedation and regional anesthesia if necessary. Suspected foreign body obstruction, intussusception, ileus, cecal volvulus, and torsion of the mesenteric root can all be indications for surgical intervention. Cecal volvulus and concomitant mesenteric torsion is a medical/surgical emergency. The patient is usually in extreme pain and rapid hypovolemic shock occurs. It is imperative emergency surgery be implemented. On the other hand, many times intestinal ileus can be managed medically. Ileus can be a common sequela to anesthesia in small ruminants. Generally, supportive care for pain and fluid therapy is corrective without the need for surgery.

Exploratory Laparotomy

The patient is placed in left lateral recumbency, and the right paralumbar fossa is prepared for aseptic surgery. A 10- to 12-cm vertical skin incision is made in the mid-paralumbar fossa. The muscle layers, which are much thinner than in the cow, are incised sharply in a vertical direction. The peritoneum is tented and incised.

Upon entering the abdominal cavity, the organs should be inspected in a thorough and organized manner. Great care should be taken manipulating the intestinal tract, as it can be quite friable and much less forgiving in small ruminants than in adult cattle. Bowel resection for foreign body removal, intussusception and ileus are performed as described in calves (see Section 14.2.1). The small ruminant needs special attention to prevent contamination of the abdominal cavity. They are highly susceptible to peritonitis. Instillation of sodium carboxymethylcellulose may decrease adhesion formation. Closure of the laparotomy site is in three or four layers. Both sheep and goats usually require postsurgical antibiotic therapy as well as pain control. Transfaunation or the use of probiotics may be indicated when long-term antibiotic use has been implemented.

Rectal Prolapse

Rectal prolapses are very common in sheep (Figure 18-3). Inciting causes include the following: short tail docks, diarrhea with tenesmus, grazing clover fields and other high estrogen feed stuffs, chronic bronchitis/pneumonia with cough, urolithiasis, coccidiosis, overcrowding, and feeding stock uphill. Two types of prolapse—mucosal prolapse and complete anatomic prolapse—can occur. Mucosal prolapse generally is secondary to mucosal edema accumulation and requires medical rather than surgical management. With complete prolapse, a caudal epidural or local infusion anesthesia with more aggressive therapy is indicated.

Most rectal prolapses present in a fairly chronic state, so simple replacement with a pursestring suture is

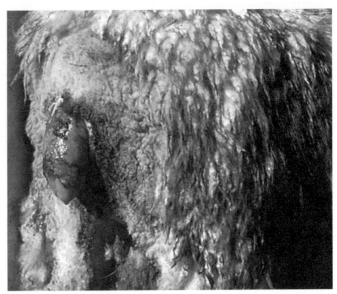

Figure 18-3   Rectal prolapse in a sheep.

(Courtesy of Dr. John King, Cornell University.)

generally ineffective. Amputation of the prolapsed segment and correction of the primary problem usually yields the best results. In the field, many practitioners commonly employ swine rectal prolapse rings with elastrator bands in the anchor groove. This technique is rapid and inexpensive with a high success rate. However, direct amputation is the most definitive procedure. Before surgery, the prolapsed segment is palpated to ensure that none of the intestinal tract is included in the prolapse. Mucosal resection is accomplished after prolapse stabilization by using transfixation needles through the proximal part of the prolapsed tissue. Sutures that are nonirritating to tissues, such as 2-0 or 3-0 synthetic absorbable sutures, are used. Generally, an interrupted horizontal mattress suture pattern with light-to-moderate suture tension is indicated. Hemostasis is primarily required dorsally because of the internal pudic vein and artery. Removal of the stabilizing needles is accomplished after surgery. If the mucosa is so severely traumatized that mucosal resection is not possible, the entire segment can be amputated as described for cattle (see Section 10.7). Pursestring sutures placed in the anus are commonly employed in conjunction with the amputation to maintain reduction of the prolapse for the first several days. It should be noted that the probability of success is limited if the inciting cause is not rectified before surgery. Postsurgically, the surgeon should insert a digit into the rectum to assure patency. Generally an alcohol sacral nerve/paravertebral block at S-3 through S-5 will control tenesmus and edema, common postsurgical sequelae.

RECOMMENDED READINGS

Akerajola OO et al: A simplified abomasal cannulization technique in sheep, *Vet Med/Sm Anim Clin* 69: 1110-1111, 1974.

Cook CW et al: Use of an esophageal fistula cannula for collecting forage samples in grazing sheep, *J Anim Sci* 17(1): 189-193, 1958.

Guard C: Abomasal dilation and emptying defect of Suffolk sheep. In Smith BP, editor: *Large animal internal medicine,* ed 2, St Louis, 1996, Mosby.

Guard C: Obstructive intestinal diseases. In Smith BP, editor: *Large animal internal medicine,* ed 2, St Louis, 1996, Mosby.

Hooper RN: Abdominal surgery in small ruminants. *Proceedings of the 1998 Symposium on the Health and Disease of Small Ruminants,* 1998, Las Vegas, NV.

Hooper RN: General surgical techniques for small ruminants: part II. *Proceedings of the Small Ruminants for the Mixed Animal Practitioner,* Western States Veterinary Conference, 1998, Las Vegas, NV.

Kimberling CV: Diseases of the digestive system. In Kimberling CV: *Jensen and Swift's diseases of sheep,* ed 3, Philadelphia, 1988, Lea and Febiger.

Kline EE et al: Abomasal impactions in sheep, *Vet Rec* 113: 177, 1983.

Linklater KA and Smith MC: *Color atlas of diseases and disorders of the sheep and goat,* London, 1993, Wolfe Publishing.

Mitchell WC: Intussusception in goats, *Agri-Practice* 12: 1918, 1983.

Navarre CB, Pugh DG: Diseases of the gastrointestinal system. In Pugh DG: *Sheep and goat medicine,* Philadelphia, 2002, WB Saunders.

Smith MC, Sherman DM: *Goat medicine,* Philadelphia, 1994, Lea and Febiger.

VanMetre, DC et al: Diagnosis of enteric disease in small ruminants, *Vet Clin North Am: Food Anim Pract* 16:87, 2000.

CHAPTER 19

SURGERY OF THE SHEEP AND GOAT REPRODUCTIVE SYSTEM AND URINARY TRACT

Ahmed Tibary and David Van Metre

19.1—Anesthesia and Restraint

Ahmed Tibary

Most elective surgeries in small ruminants can be done by using a combination of chemical and physical restraint. In nonemergency situations (e.g., teaser preparation in rams and bucks, laparoscopy), food should be withheld for 24 to 48 hours and water for 12 to 24 hours. Broad-spectrum antibiotics should be given 2 hours before surgery. Mild sedation can be obtained with 0.05 mg/kg xylazine. Chemical restraints most commonly used include a combination of xylazine, telazol, and ketamine. A xylazine (0.11 mg/kg) and telazol (13.2 mg/kg) IV combination provides 90 to 120 minutes of anesthesia with good smooth muscle relaxation. Telazol (6.6 mg/kg IV) and ketamine (6.6 mg/kg) IV provide 20 to 40 minutes. Telazol (6.6 mg/kg), ketamine (6.6 mg/kg), and xylazine (0.11 mg/kg) IV provide 60 to 90 minutes of anesthesia time.

A lumbosacral epidural is a good choice for pain relief for more involved surgery (i.e., penile translocation, cesarean section). This is accomplished by injecting 2 ml of 2% lidocaine hydrochloride per 10 kg or 1 ml of 0.75% bupivacaine per 4 kg in the space between the last lumbar vertebra and the sacrum (lumbosacral foramen). An 18- or 20-gauge, 4-cm disposable needle is used for small-sized animals. Larger sheep may require a 9-cm spinal needle. No blood or cerebrospinal fluid should be seen. Onset of anesthesia is within 5 to 15 minutes and lasts 60 to 120 minutes.

Epidural anesthesia in sheep and goats achieved with 2 ml of 2% lidocaine hydrochloride induces perineal anesthesia 1 to 3 minutes after injection and lasts 60 minutes. Ataxia may be seen with a larger volume of lidocaine.

General anesthesia is preferred for abdominal surgery (cesarean section, ovariectomy, hysterectomy), although sedation and regional anesthesia (achieved with a line block of 10 to 20 ml of 1% lidocaine) can be used. Higher doses of lidocaine may cause toxicity (apnea, respiratory depression, hypotension, and hypothermia). An inverted L block can be used for flank cesarean section.

Surgery of the Female Reproductive Tract

CESAREAN SECTION

Cesarean section should be considered to manage dystocia when vaginal delivery is not possible (oversized

527

fetus or failure of cervical dilation "ring womb"). Occasionally the technique can be used to terminate pregnancy in ewes that are suffering from pregnancy toxemia or ketosis.

RESTRAINT AND ANESTHESIA

Cesarean section can be performed via either a ventral abdominal paramedian or midline incision with the animal in dorsal recumbency or via a left flank (paralumbar) incision with the animal in right lateral recumbency. Ventral midline or paramedian techniques are the preferred methods in sheep because the area does not have as much wool. This technique also provides easy access to both horns of the uterus, which is important because most ewes carry more than one fetus. Cesarean section can be performed in the field under lumbosacral epidural and local anesthesia, although use of lumbosacral epidural anesthesia has been associated with a risk of shock as a result of pooling of blood in the viscera. Epinephrine (0.02 mg/kg IM) may be administered intramuscularly as a prophylactic measure.

VENTRAL ABDOMINAL PARAMEDIAN APPROACH

After anesthesia, the ewe is restrained in a dorsal position in a cradle with her legs extended. The surgical area, which extends from the umbilicus to the base of the mammary gland and externally toward mid flank, is prepared by clipping the wool and aseptic preparation of the skin.

The 25-cm skin incision extends from the base of the udder toward the umbilicus. The incision should be made between the linea alba and subcutaneous abdominal vein, which is very prominent in late pregnancy. The approach is continued by using a combination of blunt and sharp dissection through subcutaneous tissues. The external rectus abdominis sheath is sharply incised, the rectus muscle bluntly separated along its fibers, and the internal rectus sheath tented, along with the peritoneum, and incised. The abdominal incision may be extended, if necessary, to allow easy exteriorization of the uterine horn. The operator should be careful not to incise the greater omentum, which lies deep into the peritoneum. The greater omentum and abdominal viscera are retracted cranially to expose the uterus. The uterine horn is grasped and exteriorized gently to avoid perforation (Figure 19.1-1). Hysterotomy is performed on the greater curvature of the uterine horn, starting at the upper third and extending towards the uterine bifurcation. Care should be taken to avoid incising through cotyledons, which prevents excessive bleeding. In most cases, ewes carry more than one fetus. Therefore a uterine incision large enough to allow a fetus in the other horn to be exteriorized through the same incision should be placed along the caudal aspect of the horn. If this is

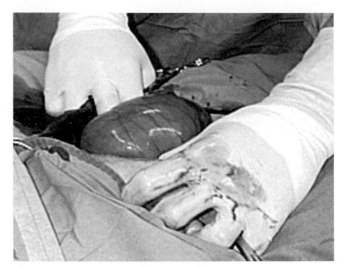

Figure 19.1-1   Paramedian ventral cesarean section: exteriorization of the uterus.

too difficult, a second hysterotomy may be performed on the other uterine horn. Depending upon the presentation, the fetuses are exteriorized by traction on the front legs and head or on the hind legs. During exteriorization of the fetus, the surgeon should be careful not to tear the uterine wall. Excess fetal fluid should be removed from the uterus. The placenta should be removed only if it is already detached. The uterus is sutured with an atraumatic needle with chromic catgut (No. 0 or 1-0) or similar synthetic absorbable suture in a continuous inverting suture pattern (Figure 19.1-2). If the uterus is compromised, a two-layer closure may be

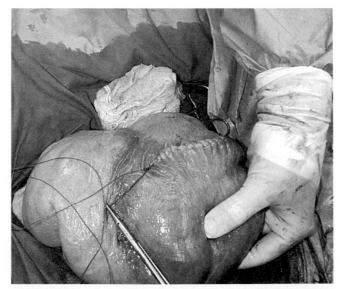

Figure 19.1-2   Cesarean section: closure of the uterus using a continuous inverting suture pattern.

indicated. The sutured uterus should be checked for tears and lavaged copiously with sterile fluids before it is replaced into the abdominal cavity. Some authors suggest intrauterine and intraabdominal antibiotic therapy, but this is not usually necessary if the surgery is performed under aseptic or very clean conditions and systemic antibiotics are provided.

The peritoneum and internal rectus sheath are sutured in a single layer with synthetic absorbable sutures in a continuous pattern. It is not necessary to include the peritoneum, it just depends on the surgeon's preference. The rectus abdominis muscle may be closed to decrease dead space. The external rectus sheath is the "holding layer." This should be closed carefully with an absorbable suture. Subcutaneous tissues and skin are closed routinely. The size of the suture varies with the weight of the animal. Some advocate the use of nonabsorbable sutures to decrease the risk of herniation and provide better security.

Postsurgical care includes oxytocin if the cervix is open and systemic antibiotics when indicated. The udder should be examined for milk let-down. During the surgery, there should be an assistant designated to attend immediately to the newborn and provide neonatal care.

Left Flank Laparotomy
This technique is recommended under field conditions and can be done quite easily with sedation and a line or an inverted "L" block anesthesia. In some cases, epidural anesthesia may help restrain the animal. The skin incision may be vertical or slightly oblique. All muscle layers can be opened by blunt dissection in a grid fashion. The peritoneum is incised in the manner described earlier. The author prefers a flank laparotomy for cesarean section in goats.

Ventral Midline Approach
The ventral midline approach to cesarean section in small ruminants differs from the paramedian approach in that the skin and abdominal incisions are made directly over the linea alba. Incision of the skin starts at the base of the udder and is extended about 20 cm cranially towards the umbilicus. The subcutaneous tissue is incised to expose the linea alba, which should be evident as a small concave line. The abdominal wall is grasped with tissue forceps and tented, and a small incision is made on the linea alba (Figure 19.1-3). The incision is continued through the linea alba and peritoneum, with scissors guided by the operator's index and middle fingers to avoid damaging the omentum or intestinal loops. Exteriorization of the uterus and delivery of fetuses is done in the same manner as described for the paramedian approach. The linea alba and peritoneum are sutured in an interrupted or continuous pattern with synthetic

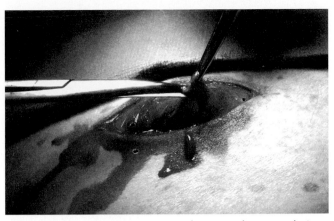

Figure 19.1-3 Cesarean section by ventral approach in a goat; the internal rectus sheath and peritoneum are tented before they are incised.

absorbable or nonabsorbable sutures (again, the choice is surgeon's preference). Subcutaneous tissues and skin are closed routinely. Postsurgical care is similar to the paramedian technique.

OVARIECTOMY AND OVARIOHYSTERECTOMY
Exteriorization of the female reproductive organs is required for many reproductive techniques such as embryo collection and transfer, oocyte collection, uterine tube flushing, etc. An ovariectomy or ovariohysterectomy is usually performed for convenience to prevent sexual activity and eliminate pregnancy or to remove diseased organs (ovarian masses, chronic pyometra, uterine neoplasm, etc.).

An ovariectomy or ovariohysterectomy performed as an elective surgery should be done during the luteal phase of the cycle or during anoestrus so that the uterus is relaxed and bleeding problems that would be associated with a toned, well-vascularized uterus during estrus are prevented. Ovariectomy is easily performed on the anesthetized animal placed in dorsal recumbency. A small 6- to 8-cm incision is made in the ventral midline just cranial to the udder and continued into the abdominal cavity as described for cesarean section. The surgeon introduces two fingers into the abdominal cavity. The urinary bladder is identified, and the uterus is recognized in its dorsal aspect by following one of the horns to the uterine bifurcation. Once the uterine horn is grasped between the fingers, it is pulled towards the surgical incision. Both horns are exteriorized by gentle traction (Figure 19.1-4).

For ovariectomy, the vascular pedicle of the ovary is isolated by passing forceps through the mesovarium and making sure to incorporate the ovarian artery and vein. A size "0" absorbable suture material is used to transfix the ovarian pedicle before transection.

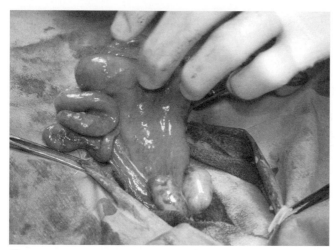

Figure 19.1-4 Ovariectomy/ovariohysterectomy: exteriorized uterine horns and ovaries.

For hysterectomy or ovariohysterectomy, the mesometrium and round ligament of each uterine horn are transected after ligation of small blood vessels. Transfixation ligatures are placed proximal to the cervix; the surgeon should make sure to include the large uterine vessels located on each side. The uterus is transected at the level of the body between two hemostatic forceps (Figure 19.1-5). A circumferential transfixation ligature of absorbable suture material is placed close to the cervix. If the remaining portion of the uterine body is large, it should be closed with an inverting suture pattern before replacing it in the abdomen. Removal of one horn or part of a uterine horn, a partial hysterectomy, is some-

times used in reproductive experimentation or for pathology confined to one side of the abdomen. The technique is similar to a total hysterectomy, although a flank approach would be possible. The vasculature supplying the ovary and horn on one side are ligated and transected. The remaining uterus is closed with an inverting pattern. Some advocate a two-layer uterine closure. For successful reproductive performance, it is essential the remaining ovary and uterine horn are normal.

Laparoscopy

Laparoscopy is widely used in small ruminants as a tool for reproductive studies and application of reproductive technologies such as intrauterine insemination, embryo transfer, oocyte collection, and ovulation rate determination. This technique can also be used for direct visualization of ovarian abnormalities, diagnosis of periuterine abnormalities, and evaluation of abdominal organs. Laparoscopic procedures to visualize and manipulate the female reproductive tract in small ruminants are easy to learn and present the advantage of being less invasive than complete exteriorization of the genital tract. The technique requires use of a rigid laparoscope with a diameter of 6 to 10 mm and various lens angles, depending on the use. For most reproductive techniques, a 6-mm diameter laparoscope with a 30° angle is sufficient. This allows a minimal size for entry portals.

Laparoscopy is usually performed on the sedated animal in dorsal recumbency on a cradle that can be tilted. Animals should be fasted for at least 12 hours to reduce rumen fill and the possibility of regurgitation. Withholding food and water for 24 hours or more reportedly almost guarantees no regurgitation. Many practitioners prefer 3 to 4 hours emptying in spring (green feed) or no fasting if ewes are on dry feed.

An area 25 cm by 25 cm cranial to the mammary gland is prepared by clipping and surgical scrubbing. For most reproductive procedures, two or three portals are necessary: one each for the laparoscope, a manipulation instrument, and special instruments (insemination gun, suture material) (Figure 19.1-6). For insemination and embryo transfer, only two portals are necessary: one each for the laparoscope and insemination gun. The site of the desired portals is infiltrated with local anesthetic before introducing a trocar and cannula. For simple techniques, the portals are created by making a small skin incision to allow trocar introduction. The trocar is advanced 4 cm subcutaneously before the abdominal cavity is penetrated by applying pressure on the abdominal wall muscle and peritoneum. This provides portals into the abdomen not directly aligned with the skin incision, which helps to prevent contamination of the abdominal cavity. This

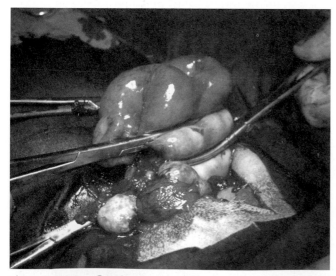

Figure 19.1-5 Ovariectomy/ovariohysterectomy: transection of the uterus at the level of the uterine body between two hemostatic forceps.

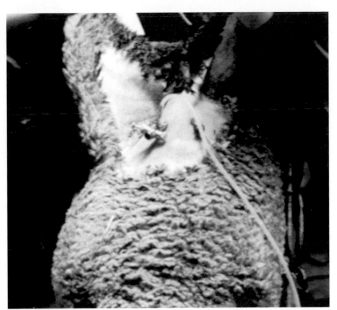

Figure 19.1-6 Laparoscopic artifical insemination: location of the portals for the light source *(left)* and insemination gun *(right)*.

technique does not require suturing the abdominal muscle. Visualizing the abdominal viscera requires insufflation with CO_2 and elevating the hindquarters to a 40° angle.

For embryo transfer, a sedation dose is obtained with xylazine and ketamine. The recipient is placed in a cradle at 45 degrees. A 2-cm incision is made on the ventral midline about 5 to 6 cm cranial to the udder. Babcock forceps 18 cm in length are introduced alongside the scope and used to grasp the uterine horn and bring it to the incision. The scope is removed, and the embryo is placed in utero by using a micropipette mounted on a tuberculin syringe to penetrate the uterine wall. The uterine horn is replaced gently, and the abdominal wall is closed.

SURGICAL EMBRYO COLLECTION

Embryo collection generally is done under general anesthesia. An area similar to that described for cesarean section is prepared for surgery and draped. A ventral midline incision is made just cranial to the base of the udder and extended for 6 to 8 cm towards the umbilicus. The linea alba is exposed by blunt dissection and then incised. The uterus and ovaries are located and exteriorized as described earlier. The ovaries are inspected for numbers of corpora lutea. During the procedure, the uterine horn is lavaged repeatedly with sterile saline, so it does not dry out. Each horn is flushed separately. A small incision is made at the base of the horn, and a Foley or Argyle silicon No. 10 catheter is introduced and

maintained in place by inflating the cuff. The uterine horn is flushed from the uterotubal junction towards the base. Suturing the uterus is unnecessary if the endometrium is not prolapsing through the uterine incision. The linea alba is apposed carefully. Subcutaneous tissues and skin are closed routinely.

Surgery of the Male Reproductive Tract

CASTRATION

Most small ruminants are castrated early at 2 to 3 weeks of age. Techniques used at this age are usually bloodless (see Bloodless Castration Techniques). Surgical castration of rams can be done under sedation/analgesia and local anesthesia. General anesthesia is recommended for adult goats or castrations performed because of testicular disease. Because of the large size of the testicular cord in these species, hemostasis is best accomplished with emasculators or by placing a transfixion ligature proximal to the pampiniform plexus. The distal third of the scrotal sac should be removed.

Young animals are usually sedated and restrained in a sitting position with the legs on the same side held together. The bottom third of the scrotal sac is excised, and the testes are removed by stripping while maintaining pressure on the inguinal ring (Figure 19.1-7).

In the adult ram or buck, general anesthesia is recommended. The animal is placed either in lateral or dorsal recumbency. The scrotum and surrounding area are clipped and prepared for surgery. An incision is made

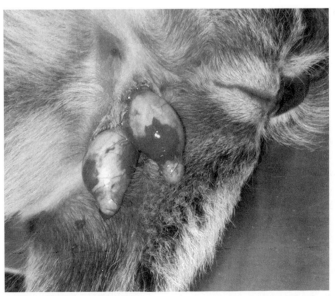

Figure 19.1-7 Castration in a billy goat. The bottom third of the scrotum has been resected and the testes are stripped.

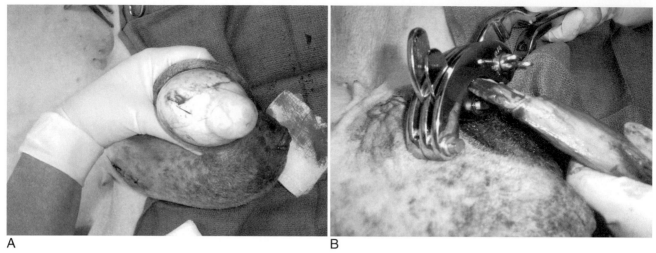

A   B

Figure 19.1-8   Castration in an adult ram. **A**, Exteriorization of the testis; **B**, castration using an emasculator.

on the lateral surface of the testis through the skin and tunica dartos. The testis and its envelopes are separated by blunt dissection. The vaginal tunic is excised to expose the testis. The cremaster muscle is separated from the vascular testicular cord. Each of these structures is ligated by transfixation suture. Some practitioners prefer to ligate the spermatic artery and vein separately. The cord is transected distal to the ligatures. Use of an emasculator can be indicated if the testes are normal size (Figure 19.1-8, *A* and *B*). The vaginal tunic is transected distally enough to allow the tunics to be closed over the remaining cord. An inverting suture pattern is used with an absorbable suture material. The tunica dartos muscle is closed over the wound with a simple continuous pattern. Excess skin may be trimmed. The subcutaneous tissues and longitudinal skin incision are closed. Bandaging the scrotum is recommended if bleeding is observed. Alternatively the incisions can be left to close by second intention if preferable or if the conditions are unsanitary.

VASECTOMY

Vasectomy is a management technique in bucks and rams used to provide teaser animals and estrus synchronization through the "ram effect." The surgery can be performed on rams after sedation and local anesthesia. General anesthesia is recommended for bucks because of their tendency to become agitated and vocal, which may disturb owners if surgery is done on the farm. Vasectomy has also been performed in rams after lumbosacral spinal analgesia. Rams can be restrained in the sitting position. Dorsal recumbency is the preferred position in goats.

The scrotal skin is prepared by clipping and surgical scrubbing. Surgical drapes are placed around and under-

neath the scrotum. A 3- to 4-cm vertical incision is made slightly medial on the cranial surface of the scrotal skin above the testicular cord. The spermatic cord is freed by blunt dissection and exteriorized with the help of hemostatic forceps (Figure 19.1-9). The vas deferens can be easily identified by palpation or visually by its white color and the presence of adjacent vein and artery. The vas deferens is exteriorized by using forceps or a spay hook through a small nick made in the vaginal tunic. A 3-cm portion of the vas deferens is removed after ligating each end (Figure 19.1-10, *A* and *B*). The vaginal tunic does not need to be sutured. The skin is sutured or stapled, and the same procedure is repeated on the other side. Excised tissue should be submitted for histological con-

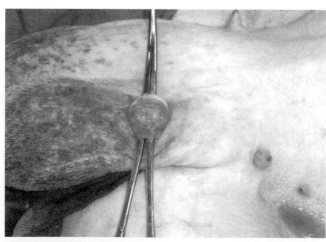

Figure 19.1-9   Vasectomy in a ram: exteriorization of the spermatic cord and identification of the vas deferens.

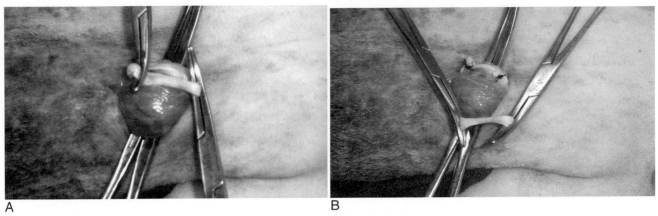

Figure 19.1-10   Vasectomy in a ram. **A**, Ligature and **B**, removal of a portion of the vas deferens.

firmation. Flushing and observing spermatozoa under the microscope is another quick way to confirm the excised tissue was in fact the vas deferens.

EPIDIDYMECTOMY

The animal is prepared as for castration. A local block is provided by infusing 2% lidocaine in the ventral scrotal skin directly over the caudal epididymis. The testis should be held firmly within the scrotum to better visualize the prominent tail of the epididymis (Figure 19.1-11). The skin is incised (2.5 to 3 cm) on the ventral, posterior aspect of the scrotum (just above the caudal

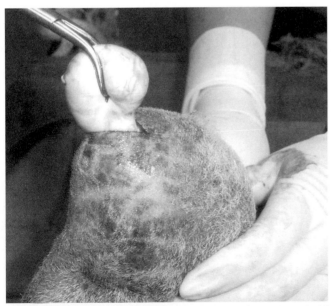

Figure 19.1-11   Epididymectomy in a ram: the testis is held firmly within the scrotum and an incision is made over the prominent tail of the epididymis.

epididymis). Using blunt dissection, the veterinarian isolates the epididymis and holds it with an instrument or stay suture. The tail of the epididymis is transected after ligating each border with a nonabsorbable suture material. The skin is sutured by using a simple interrupted suture pattern. Semen should be collected at least three times before the male is used as a teaser.

TRANSLOCATION OF THE PENIS

The objective of this surgery is to translocate the preputial opening laterally to render vaginal intromission of the penis impossible during normal erection and mounting behavior. It is preferable to perform penile deviation under general anesthesia or deep sedation/analgesia. The animal is placed in dorsal recumbency, and the area from the umbilicus to the base of the scrotum is clipped, scrubbed, and draped for surgery. Special attention should be given to thoroughly flushing the prepuce with diluted iodophor. A skin incision is made about 1.5 to 2 cm around the preputial orifice and continued caudally towards the sigmoid flexure (Figure 19.1-12). The prepuce is entirely freed from the skin and surrounding tissue with blunt scissors dissection. Placing a catheter in the prepuce helps orient the surgeon. Once the desired length of the prepuce is completely freed, a site is selected on the abdominal wall at a 45° angle from the base of the penis to create the new preputial location. A circular skin flap is removed at this site (Figure 19.1-13). A closed long forceps is used to create a subcutaneous tunnel that extends from the circular skin incision to the base of the scrotum. The freed prepuce is placed in a sterile plastic sleeve, grasped with the forceps, inserted into the subcutaneous tunnel, and transferred to the new location. The surgeon must be sure that the organ does not twist. The preputial opening is sutured to the skin with synthetic nonabsorbable suture material

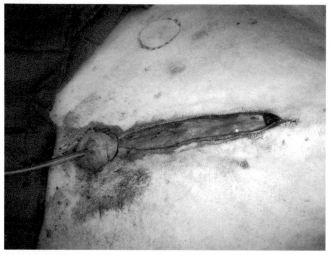

Figure 19.1-12   Translocation of the penis: skin incision around the preputial orifice continuing caudal towards the sigmoid flexure.

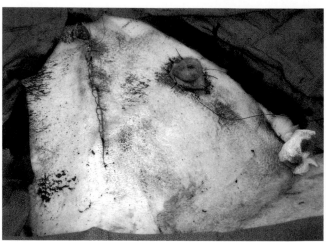

Figure 19.1-14   Translocation of the penis: skin suture and appearance after translocation of the organ.

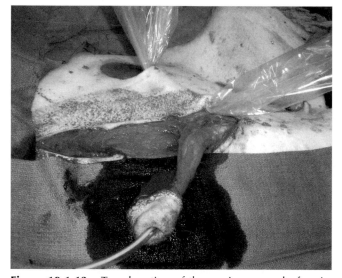

Figure 19.1-13   Translocation of the penis: removal of a circular flap of skin at the site where the preputial opening is to be relocated.

in an interrupted simple or horizontal mattress pattern. The midline abdominal skin incision is closed routinely (Figure 19.1-14). Postoperative care includes systemic antibiotics. Ventral edema may develop in some animals and persist, generally for a few days. Urination should be verified, and the patient should be examined carefully if there is a large amount of persistent preputial edema. Skin sutures may be removed 10-to-14 days after surgery.

RECOMMENDED READINGS

Boundy T, Cox J: Vasectomy in the ram, *Practice* 18: 330-334, 1996.

Harrison FA: Laparotomy and hysterotomy. In *Surgical techniques in experimental farm animals,* ed 1, New York, 1995, Oxford University Press.

Janett F, Hussy D, Lischer C, Hassig M, Thun R: Semen characteristics after vasectomy in the ram, *Theriogenology* 56: 485-491, 2001.

Mobini S, Heath AM, Pugh DG: Theriogenology of sheep and goats. In Pugh D, editor: *Sheep and goat medicine,* Philadelphia, 2002, WB Saunders.

Riddle MG: Castration of the normal male. In Wolfe DF and Moll HD, editors: *Large animal urogenital surgery,* ed 3, Philadelphia, 1999, Williams and Wilkins.

Riddle MG, Wolf DF: Embryo transfer. In Wolfe DF and Moll HD, editors: *Large animal urogenital surgery,* ed 3, Philadelphia, 1999, Williams and Wilkins.

Smith M and Sherman D: Reproductive system. In *Goat medicine and surgery,* ed 1, Baltimore, 1994, Lea and Febiger.

Williams CSF: Routine sheep and goat procedures. *The veterinary clinics of North America: food animal practice* 6: 737-758, 1990.

Wolfe DF: Surgical preparation of estrus detector males. In Wolfe DF and Moll HD, editors: *Large animal urogenital surgery,* ed 3, Philadelphia, 1999, Williams and Wilkins.

19.2—Urolithiasis

David Van Metre

Urinary calculi, or uroliths, cause disease in ruminants through trauma to the urinary tract and obstruction of urine egress. Calculi are mineral/mucoprotein aggregates that may be a single or multiple mass(es) that measures several millimeters in diameter or numerous fine, sandlike particles that pack together to fill the urethral lumen.

Obstruction of the urinary tract typically occurs in the urethra of male and castrated male ruminants and swine. The distal sigmoid flexure is the most common obstruction site in steers and bulls. Uroliths tend to obstruct the urethra at the level of the sigmoid flexure and/or the distal penile urethra of swine. In sheep and goats, the urethral process or vermiform appendage is the most common site of urethral obstruction. The distal sigmoid flexure is also often obstructed in small ruminants, commonly by multiple calculi.

Obstruction of the ureter and/or renal pelvis is very uncommon in ruminants and swine. Urinary tract infection is not a common concurrent finding in ruminant and porcine urolithiasis, although prolonged partial urethral obstruction, prior urethrostomy, or urethral catheterization may increase the risk of concurrent infection.

Preoperative Considerations

Evaluation of the hemogram as well as the acid-base and electrolyte status of urolithiasis patients is warranted if the animal is debilitated or if general anesthesia is planned. Ruminants with acute (<24 hours) urethral obstruction, without bladder or urethral rupture, typically show mild hemoconcentration secondary to dehydration and mild-to-moderate prerenal and postrenal azotemia. If present, derangements of acid-base balance and serum electrolytes are usually mild in these animals.

Animals with rupture of the urinary bladder or urethra are more debilitated and dehydrated and typically have more profound hemoconcentration and azotemia. Hyponatremia and hypochloremia are consistent derangements. However, acid-base status and serum potassium and calcium concentrations tend to vary and are less easily predicted. Animals with a history of long-standing (>24-48 hours) urinary obstruction may also show severe electrolyte and acid-base abnormalities. These abnormalities should be corrected before general anesthesia because they may precipitate potentially fatal cardiac arrhythmias. Intravenous administration of 0.9% saline, supplemented with calcium or potassium if indicated, is recommended to obtain stabilization. Electrolyte changes with uroperitoneum are discussed in more detail in the chapter on urinary bladder surgery (see Section 12.3.2). Serum potassium concentration is unpredictable and should be evaluated, especially if general anesthesia is necessary.

Administration of intravenous fluids to an animal with urethral obstruction may induce diuresis and increase the likelihood of bladder or urethral rupture. However, this risk is acceptable when it is weighed against the need to stabilize an animal before general anesthesia. Cystocentesis may be performed in small ruminants, calves, and swine if the surgeon decides to postpone surgery and administer intravenous fluids. The advantages of cystocentesis include improved patient comfort and temporary reduction of the risk of necrosis or rupture of the bladder. The disadvantages include uroperitoneum, induced by persistent urine leakage from the bladder at the cystocentesis site. With cystocentesis, the clinician controls the location and size of the bladder defect to a focal stick point; otherwise the bladder could rupture in a less manageable location or in a larger area if fluids are given without cystocentesis. Another option is percutaneous, ultrasound-guided placement of a Foley catheter into the bladder with subsequent fluid diuresis. Unfortunately, this runs the risk of peritonitis and adhesions to other viscera.

If possible, ultrasonographic evaluation of the kidneys is warranted for animals with chronic (>24 hour) urethral obstruction. The presence of severe hydronephrosis with a loss of visible cortical tissue in both kidneys warrants a poor prognosis for restoring normal renal function.

Preoperative administration of an antimicrobial agent that concentrates in the urine (e.g., beta-lactams, sulfonamides) is prudent. Examples of appropriate choices are: procaine penicillin G, 22,000 IU/kg IM or SC q12h; ampicillin 11 mg/kg IM q24h; and sulfadimethoxine 55 mg/kg IV or PO loading dose, followed by 27.5 mg/kg IV or PO q24h. Postoperative antimicrobial therapy should be dictated by the procedure chosen, slaughter withholding considerations, the status of the patient, and the tissues involved. Administration of potentially nephrotoxic antimicrobials should be avoided, and nonsteroidal antiinflammatory drugs should be used with caution.

In cases requiring general anesthesia, preoperative administration of epidural anesthesia may reduce the concentration of inhalant anesthetic required for surgery. In cases of urinary bladder rupture, slow drainage of urine from the abdomen prior to surgery may decrease abdominal volume and facilitate ventilation in the recumbent or anesthetized animal.

If an animal is to be culled, slaughter should be delayed for 4 to 6 weeks after surgery for animals that are suffering from bladder or urethral rupture. This delay allows debilitation and uremia to pass and provides ample time for healing of tissues damaged by urine. In cases of urethral rupture, small stab incisions into the skin of swollen areas around the perineum, prepuce, and ventral abdomen may facilitate urine drainage. A sterile instrument can be inserted into the stab incisions to gently spread the skin apart, thereby opening fascial planes for better drainage of extravasated urine.

Potential Complications

The owners of the animal should be informed that urolithiasis may reoccur postoperatively, and the risk of recurrence increases if the dietary and management changes needed for prevention are not consistently practiced. Relevant anesthetic and surgical complications should be described when counseling owners before surgical intervention. Although rare, postoperative renal failure due to hydronephrosis and/or severe volume depletion should be mentioned in a discussion of potential complications. Uremic animals may have impaired coagulation. Two months of postoperative sexual rest must be enforced in breeding males undergoing urethral surgery because earlier return to sexual activity may result in dehiscence of a urethral closure.

Surgical Treatment

URETHRAL SURGERY
General Considerations

Most surgical procedures that involve the urethra can be performed under local or epidural anesthesia in field conditions. All are usually appropriate for animals intended for slaughter. However, stricture of the urethra in breeding animals may occur as a complication of a urethral incision, and fibrosis in the tissues surrounding the penis may limit penile extension during erection. Except for urethral process amputation and urohydropulsion, surgical procedures involving the urethra carry a guarded-to-poor prognosis for breeding.

In cases of bladder rupture, urethral surgical procedures do not allow direct repair of the bladder defect. Bladder wall defects, particularly those located on the bladder dorsum, may seal within 2 to 4 days without primary repair, provided the urethral obstruction is relieved or bypassed to allow urine egress. Aggressive fluid and electrolyte therapy—as well as intermittent abdominal drainage—are necessary supportive measures in such cases. Laparotomy and bladder wall repair are indicated if uroperitoneum persists for several days after urethral surgery.

Urethral Process Amputation

The urethral process, or vermiform appendage, is a 1- to 2-cm extension of the urethra and integument off the distal aspect of the glans penis of sheep and goats. It is essential to examine the urethral process during clinical evaluation of a small ruminant with potential urethral obstruction. The diagnosis can be confirmed visually or by palpating a calculus within the urethral process. If a calculus is found in the process, amputation may result in restoration of urine outflow. Removal of the urethral process does not adversely affect fertility in the long term, although hemorrhage from the amputation site may adversely affect semen viability for several days. Therefore 1 to 2 weeks of sexual rest is warranted in breeding animals that undergo this procedure. Prepubertal animals may possess a persistent frenulum large enough to limit exteriorization of the penis.

Urethral process amputation can be expected to restore urine outflow in approximately one half of small ruminant urolithiasis cases, according to data from two reports (Haven et al., 1993; Van Metre and Smith, 1991). Failure to restore urine outflow after amputation indicates the presence of additional calculi in the lower urinary tract, frequently located in the area of the sigmoid flexure and bladder. If the process is not obstructed, the owner may elect removal to prevent future obstruction at that site. Urethral process amputation also facilitates retrograde passage of a urinary catheter to determine the site of urethral obstruction.

If needed, sedation can be performed with intravenous diazepam (0.1-0.2 mg/kg IV). The sheep or goat is propped on its rump. The penis is grasped through the skin at the level of the sigmoid flexure immediately caudal to the sheath and cranial to the scrotum or castration scar. The penis is forced cranially while the preputial orifice is forced caudally. The glans is thus exteriorized and grasped with a gauze sponge. If manual exteriorization fails, Allis tissue forceps or long hemostats can be introduced into the preputial cavity and used to grasp and exteriorize the penis. In larger rams and bucks, epidural anesthesia may facilitate exteriorization by eliminating penile sensation and the pull of the retractor penis muscles.

Once the glans penis is exteriorized and secured, the surgeon can use scissors or a scalpel blade to amputate the process at its base, while the surgeon carefully avoids damage to the glans. The hemorrhage that results from amputation is self-limiting. After amputation, urination is usually spontaneous and voluminous if the obstructing calculus or calculi have been removed. If urination does not occur, the surgeon may pass a urinary catheter to determine the location of the obstruction. Lidocaine infusion into the urethra before catheterization—as well as lubrication of the catheter—may reduce patient discomfort during catheter passage. Catheter passage within an inflamed urethra may be difficult, and the surgeon should weigh the benefits of catheterization against the potential added trauma and risk of urethral rupture. In ruminants, swine, camelids, and cervids, retrograde passage of a urinary catheter into the bladder is extremely difficult because the catheter usually enters the urethral diverticulum at the level of the ischium.

When urethral process amputation is successful in restoring urination, the animal owners should be cautioned to monitor the animal closely because recurrent urethral obstruction caused by additional calculi appears to be common. Imaging studies (ultrasonography, radiography) of the bladder and urethra may aid in detecting additional uroliths in these cases.

Urohydropulson

Retrograde passage of a urinary catheter into the urethra, followed by sterile saline flushing (urohydropulsion), is commonly used in small animals to dislodge urinary calculi and flush the obstructing calculi or mucoid plug retrograde into the bladder. In farm animals, passage of a catheter in the retrograde direction allows the surgeon to determine the location of the urinary obstruction, which may guide subsequent surgical management, particularly if urethrotomy or urethrostomy is anticipated. However, use of urohydropulsion has inconsistent, limited data about the relief it gives from urethral obstruction in farm animal species. This procedure may be more successful if a solitary calculus is responsible for the obstruction.

The catheter size used varies with the size and species of the animal involved. For mature bucks, wethers, and rams, a 5-8 French polypropylene catheter is usually appropriate, although the length of most standard canine catheters may not be adequate to reach the perineal segment of the urethra in larger breeds. A 10 or 14 French, rubber or polypropylene catheter or 100- to 200-cm long, sterilized polypropylene or rubber tubing may be needed to catheterize the urethra of larger bulls and steers. The catheter tip should be coated with sterile lubricant before introduction. In small ruminants, amputation of the urethral process facilitates catheter introduction and passage. A small volume of lidocaine may be flushed into the urethra to reduce discomfort during passage. If urohydropulsion is to be attempted, the surgeon should compress the urethral orifice with his or her fingers during gentle flushing with saline to prevent the saline from leaking out of the orifice. Potential complications of catheter passage and urohydropulsion include traumatic urethritis and urethral rupture.

Passage of a urinary catheter into the bladder is difficult in ruminants and swine. These animals have a urethral recess (urethral diverticulum) (Figure 19.2-1) that extends from the dorsum of the urethra at the level of the ischium. During retrograde urethral catheterization,

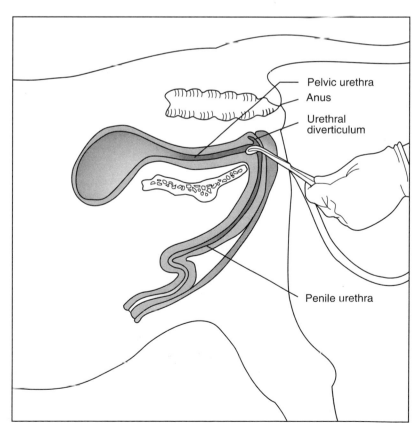

Figure 19.2-1 Diagram of the urethral diverticulum.

it almost invariably enters the recess and cannot be redirected into the bladder. To confirm that the catheter has reached the urethral recess, the surgeon can introduce a hand or finger into the animal's rectum and palpate the catheter tip at the caudal aspect of the pelvic urethra while the catheter is gently moved back and forth.

Penectomy (Penile Amputation)

Penectomy is considered a salvage procedure for intact and castrated ruminants and swine intended for slaughter. Bulls and steers are restrained in a squeeze chute or stocks; the rectum is emptied of feces; and sacrocaudal epidural anesthesia is administered. Calves, sheep, goats, and swine are typically restrained in dorsal or lateral recumbency. Sacrocaudal or lumbosacral epidural anesthesia, local infiltration with 2% lidocaine, or general anesthesia can be administered. The tail is tied to the side. The perineum, which extends from the anus to the scrotum or castration scar, is clipped and disinfected.

The skin incision should be located in the lower half of the prepared area, where the vertical surface of the perineum begins to curve cranioventrally. Placing the surgical site here will facilitate urine egress from the transected penis and minimize urine scald. A vertical skin incision is made on the midline. The incision length should be approximately 10-20 cm or more in bulls and steers and 3-6 cm in calves, small ruminants, and swine. The subcutaneous tissue and fascia are incised to reveal the pink, paired, strap-like retractor penis muscles that extend dorsal to ventral beside the midline of the deep subcutis. The retractor penis muscles can be traced distally to identify their insertion point, which is the distal bend of the sigmoid flexure of the penis. These muscles may be ligated and excised if the surgeon desires to clear the surgical field. Alternatively, the dissection is continued between the retractor penis muscles to reveal the penis. The penis is firm and covered by the smooth, white tunica albuginea.

Blunt digital dissection is used to free the entire circumference of the penis. Blunt dissection is continued ventrally and cranially to free the distal bend of the sigmoid flexure. Traction should be applied to the penis in a caudodorsal direction to exteriorize enough of the penis so the distal sigmoid flexure is held external to the incision under minimal tension. This is relatively easy to accomplish in urethral rupture cases because the peripenile tissues and preputial attachments of the penis are necrotic from extravasated urine. If urethral rupture does not exist, sharp dissection with heavy scissors is often necessary to free the distal penis from its attachments to the prepuce.

If still present, the retractor penis muscles are ligated and excised. In bulls and steers, the transection point for the penis should be located approximately 5 to 10 cm distal to the dorsal aspect of the skin incision. In calves, small ruminants, and swine, the transection point should be located 2 to 4 cm distal to the dorsal aspect of the skin incision. The transection site should be located so that the resultant proximal penile stump can be easily oriented in a caudal and slightly ventral direction.

The surgeon should then decide if the distal penis is to be excised. Excision of the distal penis greatly facilitates drainage of urine-damaged tissues in cases of urethral rupture. If the surgeon prefers to excise the distal penis, the vessels on the dorsum of the penis should be ligated immediately proximal to the selected transection site. The penis is then transected perpendicular to its long axis, and the distal penis is excised. If the distal penis is to be preserved, the vessels on the dorsum of the penis are carefully dissected free from the tunica albuginea of the penis at the level of the proposed transection site. A pair of hemostatic forceps is placed between the vessels and the dorsal surface of the tunica albuginea of the penis. These forceps are intended to protect the vessels from transection. The penis is transected at the appropriate site, leaving the dorsal vessels and distal penis intact.

Heavy monofilament suture (e.g., nylon) is preferred for suturing the proximal penile stump to the skin because monofilament suture is expected to hold less exudate, debris, and bacteria in the wound than braided suture or umbilical tape holds. The proximal stump is composed of the urethra and corpus spongiosum within the dorsal third of the stump and the corpus cavernosum located in the ventral two thirds of the stump. The stump is oriented to face caudoventrally and is fixed to the skin with a horizontal mattress suture. To create the first limb of this suture, the suture is passed through the skin at a point 1-3 cm lateral to the right side of the skin incision. The suture is then passed through the entire body of the penile stump, passing through the corpus cavernosum. The surgeon should take care not to incorporate the urethra into this suture. The suture is exited from the skin on the left side of the incision, equidistant from the incision edge as placed on the right side. The second limb of the horizontal mattress suture is created by returning the suture through the skin on the left side of the incision, passing through the ventral aspect of the penile stump, and exiting on the right side of the incision at a point ventral to the suture entry point (Figure 19.2-2). The suture is then pulled tight and tied to secure the penile stump in place. If needed, additional interrupted sutures may be placed through the ventral aspect of the tunica albuginea of the stump and the ventral apex of the skin to add security to the penile stump fixation.

The urethra is then incised along its long axis from the end of the stump to the dorsal aspect of the incision.

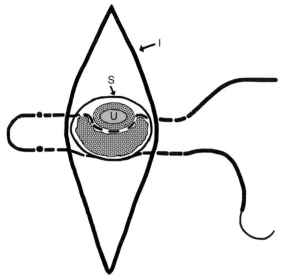

Figure 19.2-2 Securing the penile stump to the skin in a penectomy. *U,* urethra; *I,* skin incision; *S,* tunica albuginea of the penile stump.

The urethra is thus "spatulated" to provide a larger opening for urine egress. To create a secure urethral spatula, the dorsal aspect of the resulting urethral mucosal flaps may be sutured to the adjacent skin edges (i.e., left urethral flap to left skin edge) by using monofilament, nonabsorbable suture in a simple continuous pattern. The distal 1 to 2 centimeters of the urethral flaps, which protrude well away from the skin edge, should not be sutured to the skin. This technique has been termed *urethral fistulization.*

Hemorrhage from the corpus spongiosum penis may be heavy, particularly in larger animals. To limit hemorrhage, a short length of rubber tubing can be introduced into the urethra to exert outward pressure on the corpus spongiosum. This tube can be sutured in place at the edge of the stump. The tube is removed in 3 to 5 days. Alternatively, the corpus spongiosum can be closed by placing closely spaced, simple continuous 2-0 absorbable sutures through the edge of the urethral mucosa and corpus spongiosum penis, thereby sealing the cut edge of the spongiosum. Hemorrhage from the corpus cavernosum is usually less of a problem because of the compressive effect of the mattress fixation suture. If hemorrhage from the cavernosum of the stump is problematic, a horizontal wedge of the cavernosum can be excised from the distal aspect of the stump and the edges sutured together to seal the cavernosum shut.

Postoperative antimicrobial therapy is warranted for 5 to 7 days in cases of urethral rupture. Application of petroleum jelly to the skin ventral to the incision and on the medial surface of the hind limbs may help to limit urine scald. Myiasis may be limited through application of fly repellant around the surgical site or by taping a fly repellant ear tag to the tail. Suture removal is performed 2 weeks after surgery.

Perineal Urethrostomy

In perineal urethrostomy, the penile urethra is opened and sutured to the skin of the perineum to create a permanent stoma for urine egress. This procedure is preferred over penectomy for pet animals or animals with several more months before their slaughter weight is achieved; our experience indicates that the stoma tends to remain patent for a longer period of time than for a penectomy. Perineal urethrostomy is a valid option in cases of urethral rupture. This procedure results in loss of natural breeding ability.

Recurrent obstruction is possible if large calculi obstruct the urethra proximal to the stoma. Stricture of the stoma is a common complication following this procedure; in some studies, stricture severe enough to cause stranguria occurred within a few weeks to months after surgery. This is most likely a result of the urethra's small size, the animal's size, and how deep the urethra is located, all of which cause tension on the repair. Therefore the surgeon should place the initial urethrostomy site in the ventral half of the perineum to allow for repeat urethrostomy at a site more dorsal in the perineum. Placing the urethrostomy site in the ventral half of the perineum also minimizes urine scalding. Placing the incision at the site where the vertical surface of the perineum begins to curve cranioventrally is appropriate; this site lies immediately proximal to the scrotum or castration scar.

Anesthesia, preparation, and the approach to the penis are performed as for penectomy. Adequate blunt and sharp dissection is necessary to allow the penis to be exteriorized without excessive tension. To avoid placing the urethrostomy in tissues likely damaged by sharp calculi, the site chosen for urethrostomy should lie proximal to the distal bend of the sigmoid flexure.

In cases of urethral rupture, it may be advantageous to transect the penis distal to the urethrostomy site; this will facilitate drainage of urine from the tissues of the inguinal region and prevent infection in devitalized tissue. The dorsal penile vessels should be ligated immediately proximal to the transection site. As described for penectomy, the penis is transected and the distal segment excised, a horizontal wedge resection of the cavernosum of the stump is performed, and the cavernosum is closed to limit hemorrhage. The penis is then positioned so the stump is located at the distal apex of the skin incision. If the distal penis is not to be excised, the dorsal penile vessels should be left intact.

To hold the exteriorized segment of penis in place, a horizontal mattress suture of monofilament, nonabsorbable material is placed through the skin and into the tunica albuginea of the penis on each side of the distal apex of the skin incision. Alternatively, the tunica albuginea can be secured with absorbable suture to the subcutis of the apex of the distal incision. The urethra is incised a vertical length of approximately 10 to 15 cm in steers and bulls and 3 to 6 cm in small ruminants and swine. With proper positioning of the penis, the urethral incision should lie immediately adjacent to the skin incision. If the skin incision is judged to be of excessive length, it can be closed to create a skin incision that more closely aligns with the edges of the incised urethra. A 0 to 3-0 monofilament, nonabsorbable suture material is used to appose the edges of the urethral mucosa to the adjacent skin edges, thus creating a spatulated urethral orifice. The dorsal and ventral apices of the urethral incision are sutured to the corresponding apices of the skin incision. A simple interrupted pattern, or several small sections of simple continuous pattern, can be used. Meticulous apposition of the urethral mucosa to the skin is necessary to limit hemorrhage from the corpus spongiosum, prevent urine leakage into the subcutis, and create a permanent stoma.

Stab incisions into edematous tissue will facilitate urine drainage in cases of urethral rupture. Postoperative care is similar to that for penectomy. In obese animals, excision and closure of small strips of skin lateral to each side of the stoma may help keep the stoma open and limit interference with urine egress by skin folds (Figure 19.2-3). Suture removal is performed two weeks after surgery.

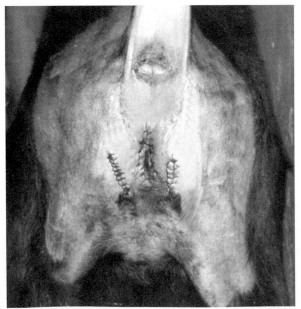

Figure 19.2-3   Perineal urethrostomy in a wether goat. Strips of skin on each side of the urethrostomy have been resected and sutured closed to facilitate urine outflow from the stoma.

Ischial Urethrostomy

In this procedure, a proximal perineal urethrostomy is created, and an indwelling catheter is inserted into the bladder via the urethrostomy site. Ischial urethrostomy can be used in animals intended for slaughter and in cases of bladder or urethral rupture.

The procedure is most easily accomplished with the animal standing. Epidural anesthesia is applied; the rectum is emptied of feces; and the perineum is clipped and aseptically prepared from the anus to the scrotal base. The perineal skin incision is made on the midline of the perineum at a point immediately dorsal to the level of the tubera ischiadicum. The incision is continued distally along the perineal midline for approximately 10 cm in steers and bulls and 4 to 6 cm in small ruminants and swine. A thick layer of fascia is encountered deep to the subcutis; this should be incised on the midline to reveal the retractor penis muscles. These muscles are separated bluntly and retracted laterally to reveal the slightly rounded surface of the underlying bulbospongiosus muscle. On the midline raphe of this muscle, a groove is detected by palpation. The urethra lies within this groove. A 1- to 2-cm vertical incision is made through the raphe of the bulbospongiosus and into the urethral lumen. Hemorrhage from the corpus spongiosum is often profuse and can be limited by applying firm digital pressure dorsal to the incision. A finger or set of hemostatic forceps can be inserted into the incision to confirm that the smooth urethral lumen has been entered.

A sterile Foley catheter* is introduced into the urethra and passed retrograde into the bladder. The appropriate Foley catheter diameter is dictated by the size of the animal, but the largest catheter possible should be used. A well-lubricated polypropylene catheter or disinfected wire guide can serve as a stylette for guiding the catheter into the bladder. Passage may be facilitated by placing a slight curve in the stylette; the curved tip of the catheter is then maintained in a cranioventral direction during passage. Alternatively, the catheter can be grasped with curved forceps and guided into the pelvic urethra, from which point it can be advanced into the bladder. The proximal location of the incision typically allows the catheter to avoid entry into the urethral recess (diverticulum).

Once the catheter tip is in the bladder, the stylette is removed, and the Foley catheter balloon is inflated with the appropriate volume of saline. The catheter should be directed ventrally from the incision and securely sutured to the perineal skin. The siphoning effect of the catheter is improved if the catheter opening is secured so it lies ventral to the catheter tip in the bladder. To improve the siphoning effect of the catheter, a small length of rubber

---

*Sherwood Medical; St. Louis, Mo.

tube can be attached to the catheter opening to extend the effective outside length of the catheter, so the external opening lies well ventral to the level of the bladder. This is particularly useful in bladder rupture cases where effective drainage is desired.

To prevent aspiration of air into the bladder, a Heimlich valve or a slit finger from a latex glove is fastened or glued to the catheter opening. A square rubber flap can be fashioned from an inner tube and sutured or glued to the perineal skin between the anus and dorsal apex of the incision. The flap covers the surgical site and Foley catheter, thereby limiting fecal contamination. The catheter is maintained in place until the time of slaughter.

Ischial Urethrotomy

For breeding bulls, a surgical approach identical to that for ischial urethrostomy is combined with an alternate method of catheter placement to preserve urethral patency along the entire urinary tract and maintain breeding ability. Primary closure of the urethra is performed; therefore the procedure is termed an *ischial urethrotomy*. Adaptation of this technique to breeding males of other species is possible, provided the penis can be exteriorized and catheterized during surgery. This procedure is less likely to restore breeding ability in animals affected by urethral rupture.

The approach to the urethra and urethral incision are performed as described for ischial urethrostomy. The distal penis is exteriorized from the sheath by an assistant, and a retrograde urinary catheter introduced into the urethral orifice and passed to the level of the obstruction. Retrograde urohydropulsion is performed with large volumes of sterile saline to expel the calculus or calculi from the urethral incision. Once the obstruction is dislodged and the urethra can be flushed freely, the retrograde catheter is removed.

One end of a 200 cm sterile polyethylene tube 3 mm in diameter is lubricated and inserted into the bladder from the urethral incision. The opposite end is then passed normograde (down the urethra) to exit the urethral orifice. Passage through the sigmoid flexure is facilitated by extending the penis. The catheter is then flushed with saline to set up a siphon from the urinary bladder. The catheter is held in place by friction. The urethra is closed with 2-0 or 3-0 monofilament, absorbable suture in a simple interrupted pattern. The bulbospongiosus muscle and fascia are closed with 0 or 2-0 absorbable suture in a simple continuous pattern. Skin closure is performed. The catheter is flushed with saline to initiate siphoning of urine from the bladder. Although the catheter typically remains in place for 4 to 5 days postoperatively, it may be allowed to remain in place for as long as 10 days.

In cases of urethral rupture, it is optimal to maintain the catheter in place for 2 to 3 weeks to provide the best chance for healing the urethral defect(s). To accomplish this, the penis is exteriorized, and the distal 3 to 5 cm is inserted into the lumen of a latex rubber Penrose drain. The drain is sutured to the distal penis with 2-0 nonabsorbable, monofilament suture. The distal end of the drain should extend 3 to 4 inches from the tip of the glans. The urethral catheter can be sutured to the Penrose drain to provide a flexible external fixation point for the catheter. The catheter should be cut off so it does not protrude too far out of the preputial orifice.

Completion of this procedure requires that urohydropulsion successfully relieve the obstruction. If retrograde urohydropulsion is not successful, alternate methods of calculus removal, such as basket catheters and laser lithotripsy, may be used. If these options are not available, the incision can be closed and another procedure that preserves breeding ability (e.g., tube cystostomy, urethrotomy) can be performed. Alternatively, the surgery can be completed as an ischial *urethrostomy,* as described above. In such cases, the obstruction may resolve spontaneously or may be dissolved by flushing the urinary tract with sterile, mildly acidic solutions (see tube cystostomy, below). Although a guarded prognosis for breeding should be made if an ischial urethrostomy is performed, relief of the urethral obstruction, maintenance of the urethral wall integrity, and complete, second intention healing of the urethrostomy site might render the animal eventually able to breed.

Urethrotomy

In this procedure, the skin and subcutis are incised directly over the obstruction. The obstructing calculus or calculi are massaged or flushed out of the urethra, shattered or crushed by applying an instrument to the urethra, and/or removed through a urethral incision. If the urethra is incised, it may be sutured for primary closure or left open to heal by second intention. If the urethra is compromised, it may be advisable to avoid primary closure.

Identifying the urethral obstruction location is necessary to ensure proper incision placement. Palpation of the penis through the skin, ultrasonography, urethral catheterization, or positive contrast urethrography can be used to identify the obstruction location. Alternatively, in cattle, the surgeon may simply orient the incision over the distal bend of the sigmoid flexure, thereby relying on the tendency for calculi to obstruct steers and bulls at this level.

Urethrotomy may allow breeding ability to be maintained. However, a guarded-to-poor prognosis is warranted because adhesion development at the surgical site may limit normal extension of the penis. Urethral stricture is another potential complication of this procedure. Urethrotomy is not a productive endeavor in cases of urethral rupture because the ruptured urethral wall is usually too friable for repair by primary closure. At least 60 days of sexual rest must be enforced to prevent dehiscence of the urethral repair during breeding.

The following description applies to cases in which the urethral obstruction is located at the level of the distal sigmoid flexure. In small ruminants and swine, lumbosacral ("high") epidural anesthesia may be used. In steers and bulls, sacrocaudal epidural anesthesia alone is often insufficient for complete anesthesia of this region, so it is combined with lidocaine infiltration of the subcutis at the incision site. The animal is placed in dorsal or lateral recumbency with the upside hind limb abducted. The skin immediately cranial to the scrotum is clipped and prepared, and if needed, local anesthetic is injected subcutaneously on the midline to create a "line block."

The penis is grasped through the skin, and a 5- to 10-cm longitudinal skin incision is made over the penis on the midline. The subcutis and peripenile elastic tissue are incised. Hemostasis should be meticulous, as hematoma/seroma formation will promote infection and fibrosis. Blunt dissection in a caudal and dorsal direction is performed to free the distal sigmoid flexure of the penis, which can be identified by finding the insertion of the retractor penis muscles. Blunt dissection should be limited to the minimum necessary to exteriorize the distal bend of the sigmoid flexure of the penis. A longitudinal groove is located on the ventral penis that overlies the urethra, and the obstruction can usually be located by careful palpation along the length of this groove.

If packed, sand-like calculi comprise the obstruction, retrograde urethral catheterization and urohydropulsion can be combined with digital massage of the urethra to clear the obstruction. Large calculi may need to be crushed into smaller fragments before massage and urohydropulsion can promote their passage. A towel clamp, hemostatic forceps, or Allis tissue forceps is positioned over the calculus. Pressure applied to the calculus through the urethral wall is slowly increased to crush the calculus. Calculus fragments may be massaged to promote passage or flushed out of the urethral orifice by injecting saline through a small-gauge needle placed into the urethra proximal to the obstruction. Calculus crushing carries the potential complication of inciting urethral rupture or necrosis, and repeated attempts at crushing may damage the urethral wall.

If the calculus is not passed after two crushing attempts or the surgeon elects not to attempt crushing, a small incision is made into the urethral lumen with a #15 blade. The incision should be located directly over the calculus if the urethral wall at that site appears normal. If the urethral wall over the calculus is discolored or crushing attempts have traumatized the wall, the urethral incision should be placed in relatively healthy tissue adjacent to the calculus. The calculus is gently removed from the urethral lumen. A urinary catheter is introduced into the urethral lumen, and the urethra is flushed in both directions to ensure patency before closure. If an additional obstruction is located in the urethra distal to the incision, passage of a urinary catheter into the urethral orifice and urohydropulsion can be used to expel the calculus or calculi from the urethral incision. If additional calculi are encountered in the proximal urethra, these can be flushed retrograde into the bladder or—failing that—can be removed through a separate urethrotomy site. The urethra is closed with 3-0 monofilament, absorbable sutures in a closely spaced, simple interrupted pattern. The incision should be flushed copiously with sterile saline. The penis is returned to its normal position, and the subcutaneous tissues and skin are closed routinely.

Moderate swelling of the incision site is expected during the first few days after surgery. However, urine accumulation in the tissues surrounding the incision site manifests as severe, progressive swelling and indicates dehiscence of the urethral incision. Urethrostomy revision or an alternative procedure is to be considered in such cases, particularly if the animal is intended for breeding.

SURGERY OF THE URINARY BLADDER
General considerations
In breeding animals with urolithiasis, surgical procedures of the bladder allow the surgeon to avoid making a urethral incision, thereby reducing the likelihood of postoperative urethral stricture and peripenile fibrosis. The surgeon is able to repair defects in the bladder wall in cases of bladder rupture, and calculi within the bladder lumen may be removed. Bladder surgery is generally more difficult to accomplish under field conditions than urethral surgery. General anesthesia greatly facilitates patient positioning and restraint for these procedures, although local anesthesia with or without concurrent epidural anesthesia can be used.

Cystotomy
Cystotomy is combined with retrograde and normograde urohydropulsion to clear the lower urinary tract of calculi. General anesthesia is usually required for this procedure. Local anesthesia of the abdominal wall combined with lumbosacral (high) epidural anesthesia will provide adequate anesthesia. However, local anesthesia of the abdominal wall alone does not provide sufficient anesthesia because the discomfort resulting from penile

extension, urinary catheter passage, and repeated urohydropulsion is not eliminated. This procedure has been used most often for small ruminants and swine because it is very difficult to achieve adequate access to the bladder in large steers and bulls with this procedure.

Retrograde urohydropulsion requires exteriorization of the penis, which is difficult to do if the penile frenulum is intact. An intact frenulum may be present in prepubertal animals or, less commonly, in animals castrated at an early age. Because bidirectional urethral catheterization and flushing are required to clear the urethra, this procedure carries the risk of iatrogenic urethral rupture or stricture. An assistant is needed to perform retrograde urohydropulsion during the surgery.

The animal is placed in dorsal recumbency, and the ventral abdomen and inguinal area are clipped and prepared. The penis is exteriorized from the prepuce; the urethral process is amputated; and the penis is secured with towel clamps to one side of the abdomen. A 5 to 10 French polypropylene urinary catheter is passed into the distal urethra and left in place. The penis and urinary catheter are covered with sterile towels and a waterproof drape.

A paramedian skin incision, measuring 10 to 30 cm as dictated by the patient's size, is made in the caudal abdomen on the side opposite the exteriorized penis. The incision should be placed 1-3 cm lateral to the prepuce, with its caudal apex located even with the level of the rudimentary teats in small ruminants or the last row of teats in swine. The subcutis is incised to expose the external rectus sheath. At this point, the surgeon can enter the abdominal cavity by continuing the paramedian approach or can undermine the subcutis over the ventral midline and enter the abdomen through the linea alba.

Sterile laparotomy sponges are used to pack off the bladder from the surrounding viscera. Exteriorization of the bladder is facilitated by first aspirating urine from its lumen. The bladder should be inspected carefully for areas of necrosis or leakage. Stay sutures are placed and a 3-4 cm cystotomy incision is made in the ventral wall of the bladder. Calculi within the bladder and pelvic urethra are removed by suction, with a finger, and/or a bladder spoon. A sample of calculi should be submitted for mineral analysis.

A 5-10 French polypropylene urinary catheter is introduced into the bladder and guided through the trigone into the pelvic urethra. Multiple saline flushes through this catheter are used to dislodge calculi from the pelvic urethra and propel them back into the bladder for retrieval.

An assistant reaches underneath the drapes to attach a syringe filled with sterile saline to the retrograde catheter to perform retrograde urohydropulsion. Aseptic technique should be used for handling the saline and urinary catheter. During retrograde flushing, the assistant should squeeze the urethral orifice to prevent loss of saline to the exterior. Meanwhile, the surgeon can place a finger through the bladder trigone to digitally occlude the lumen of the pelvic urethra. As the urethra dilates, the finger is withdrawn, and calculi are flushed from the urethra into the bladder lumen where they can be retrieved. Repeated flushes are usually needed to clear the urethra. Injecting saline into the retrograde catheter is difficult if the catheter has been advanced into the urethral recess, so this catheter should be kept in the distal urethra during retrograde urohydropulsion. However, it can be advanced intermittently to assess urethral clearance.

If retrograde flushing can be performed readily without evidence of saline filling the bladder, a rupture of the urethra should be suspected. In such cases, passage of a normograde urinary catheter should be attempted and left in place for 10 to 14 days, if successful, to limit urine contact with the ruptured urethra. Regardless of the success of normograde catheterization, a tube cystostomy should be performed (see the following discussion) to reduce the volume of urine passing into the ruptured urethra.

The urethra can be considered patent if saline can be flushed in the normograde and retrograde directions and be recovered at—or seen to exit readily from—the opposite end. The bladder incision is then closed with two layers of a monofilament, absorbable suture in an inverting pattern. If bladder tears or necrotic areas of bladder wall are present, they should be debrided and closed, or resected and closed, respectively. The abdomen should be lavaged with sterile saline before closure. The abdominal wall is closed routinely.

Because the animal must void urine through the traumatized urethra, postoperative dysuria may be severe. Judicious administration of antiinflammatory drugs is indicated if azotemia does not exist and hydration status is normal. Postoperative antibiotic therapy should be continued for 3 to 5 days. For valuable animals, urethroscopy and laser lithotripsy can be used to clear distal urethral stones that are refractory to urohydropulsion. Urethroscopy provides an assessment of the urethral mucosa.

Tube Cystostomy

In this procedure, a Foley catheter is placed into the bladder lumen via a laparotomy. Tube cystostomy is a valid option for animals intended for breeding as well as castrated males kept as pets or intended for slaughter. Because this procedure involves a laparotomy, primary repair of bladder rupture is possible. This procedure is also an option for breeding males with urethral rupture, as it allows urine to bypass the urethral defect to facilitate urethral healing (Haven et al, 1993; Rakestraw et al, 1995). Local, epidural, or general anesthesia may be used, and the animal can be placed in dorsal recumbency (ventral midline/paramedian approach), lateral recumbency (low paralumbar fossa approach), or lateral recumbency with the upside hind limb abducted (ventrolateral approach). When the animal is in lateral recumbency, ruminal gas distension may hinder bladder visualization and make closure of the body wall difficult, so repeated decompression is necessary.

Tube cystostomy can be performed on a variety of ruminants and swine of diverse sizes. In bulls and large steers, the low paralumbar or ventral oblique approaches are preferred, and two assistants are often needed to retract the sides of the incision for adequate visualization of the bladder. However, exposure of the bladder is limited in large bulls, even with assistants present to provide retraction.

The size of the Foley catheter needed will vary somewhat with the animal's size. The author prefers to err on the side of a larger catheter because the opening of the catheter tip is larger and less likely to become obstructed with blood or calculi. A 14-22 French catheter is commonly used in adult small ruminants, and a 26-32 French catheter is used for bulls. A 12-18 French catheter is usually adequate for smaller sheep, goats, and swine. A new catheter should be used for this procedure because the balloons of used, resterilized catheters appear to deflate prematurely in some cases.

If local anesthesia is used, the surgeon will need a sterile syringe filled with 5 to 10 ml of 2% lidocaine and a sterile needle added to the surgical tray to anesthetize the body wall for a stab incision for passage of the Foley catheter.

Once the surgeon is scrubbed in, he or she should fill the Foley catheter balloon with the appropriate volume of saline to test it for leaks. Usually, the maximum saline volume for the balloon is indicated on the wrapper. If not, the balloon is filled with enough saline to make it approximately 2 cm in diameter (Figure 19.2-4). Catheters that leak saline from the balloon or its injection port should not be used. The balloon is then deflated until the catheter has been placed into the bladder lumen.

For a paramedian approach, the animal is placed in dorsal recumbency, and the ventral abdomen and inguinal region are clipped and prepared. A paramedian skin incision of 10 to 20 cm is made in the caudal abdomen. The incision should be placed 1 to 3 cm lateral to the prepuce, with its caudal apex located even with the level of the rudimentary teats in small ruminants or the last row of teats in swine. The subcutis is incised to expose the external rectus sheath. Careful hemostasis should be practiced. The surgeon can enter the abdominal cavity by continuing the paramedian approach or can

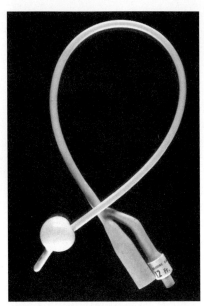

Figure 19.2-4   A Foley catheter shown with the balloon anchor inflated with sterile saline.

undermine the subcutis over the ventral midline and enter the abdomen through the linea alba.

For a low paralumbar approach, the patient is restrained in lateral recumbency with the hind limbs extended and secured behind the animal. A 15- to 40-cm vertical incision is made in the caudal aspect of the paralumbar fossa, 1 to 4 cm cranial to the level of the tuber coxae, with the incision length made proportional to the animal's size. Careful hemostasis should be practiced to limit hematoma/seroma formation. The incision is continued through the muscles of the paralumbar fossa, and the abdomen is entered.

For a ventral oblique approach, the animal is placed in lateral recumbency with the upside hind limb extended behind the animal and secured in an abducted position. The caudal apex of the skin incision should lie even with the rudimentary teats. The incision is oriented on a line that lies just medial to the fold of the flank, extending from the inguinal area caudally on an oblique line toward the umbilicus cranially. A 15- to 40-cm incision is made along this line through the skin; the incision length is adjusted to the animal's size. Careful hemostasis should be practiced because persistent incision hemorrhage may promote hematoma/seroma development. The external rectus sheath is incised, the underlying muscle is opened with scissors, and the internal rectus sheath and peritoneum are incised.

The bladder is identified, and urine is aspirated from its lumen to ease handling and exteriorization. The bladder is inspected for tears and areas of necrosis. Laparotomy sponges or moistened towels are used to pack off the bladder from the rest of the viscera. A pair of stay sutures are placed 3 to 5 cm apart in the ventral bladder wall immediately caudal to the apex of the bladder. A 0.5 to 1.0-cm long incision is made into the bladder between the stay sutures. Repeated suction and lavage are used to remove calculi from the bladder lumen; any calculi retrieved should be saved for mineral analysis.

A stab incision is now made in the body wall, through which the Foley catheter will be passed. For all approaches, the stab incision in the body wall should be placed even with the transverse plane of the bladder incision. The stab incision should be situated at a point so the bladder can be easily apposed to the ventral abdominal wall. For the paramedian/ventral midline approach, the site for the stab incision is typically located 2 to 4 cm lateral to the laparotomy incision. For the low paralumbar fossa approach, the stab incision should be located immediately medial to the flank fold. For the ventral oblique approach, the stab incision is located 2 to 4 cm ventral to the incision. If local anesthesia is being used, the proposed stab incision site should be infiltrated with 2% lidocaine. The stab incision should measure approximately 1 to 2 cm in length and should be oriented in a craniocaudal direction. The stab incision is extended through the skin and muscle to the level of the peritoneum. The peritoneum should be punctured with a blunt instrument, such as hemostatic forceps. The jaws of the forceps are spread apart repeatedly to spread open the peritoneum. The surgeon should manually protect the underlying viscera during this step.

Large forceps are then introduced into the abdomen via the laparotomy incision, with the jaws extended through the stab incision. The tip of the Foley catheter is then gently placed into the forceps and pulled into the abdomen. The tip of the Foley catheter, including the deflated balloon, is placed through the bladder incision and into the bladder lumen. The balloon is filled with the appropriate volume of saline. The balloon should be palpated through the bladder wall to ensure that it is properly filled.

A pursestring, monofilament, absorbable suture—size 0 or 00—is placed in the bladder wall to secure the catheter in place and prevent urine leakage. Care should be taken to avoid puncture of the catheter or its balloon during suture placement. The external end of the catheter is then pulled gently to appose the bladder wall to the body wall at the interior aspect of the stab incision of the body wall. Nonabsorbable suture in a Chinese fingertrap or pursestring pattern is used to secure the Foley catheter to the skin surrounding the stab incision in the body wall.

Tears in the bladder wall are then repaired, and any devitalized areas of bladder wall are resected and closed.

The laparotomy sponges or towels are retrieved, and the abdomen is lavaged with sterile saline. The body wall and skin incision are closed. To reduce dead space, each muscle layer can be intermittently sutured to the layer immediately interior to it. The Foley catheter should be sutured to the skin in several sites so that it lies close to the abdomen when the animal stands up (Figure 19.2-5). This will prevent the animal's hind feet from pulling out the catheter. A Heimlich valve can be fashioned from a finger cut from a latex glove and fastened to the catheter opening to limit aspiration of air.

The Foley catheter should be checked for patency several times per day. Urine should drip slowly but consistently from the catheter opening. If obstruction of the catheter is suspected, ultrasonography should be performed to ensure the catheter is still within the bladder lumen. Rarely, deflation of the catheter balloon results in displacement of the catheter from the bladder lumen. If the catheter is in place, the outer end of the catheter can be disinfected and sterile saline flushed into the catheter to dislodge blood clots or calculi that may occlude the catheter opening in the bladder. Radiopaque dye can be introduced into the tube to evaluate urethral patency and locate the level of obstruction created by radiolucent calculi or urethral stricture (Figure 19.2-6).

In the days to weeks after surgery, while urine is diverted from the bladder through the catheter, the calculi remaining in the urethra are most likely passed spontaneously from the urethral orifice after urethral spasm and swelling subside. Beginning 3 to 4 days after surgery, the Foley catheter can be clamped shut or plugged for 1 to 3 hours each day to determine whether

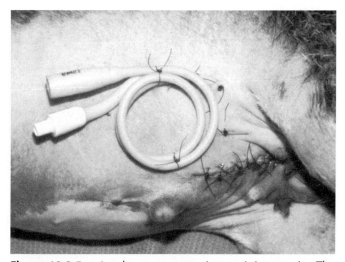

Figure 19.2-5 A tube cystostomy in a miniature pig. The catheter has been sutured to the abdominal skin in several sites to prevent it from being stepped on. Note the latex glove finger glued to the catheter port to serve as a Heimlich valve.

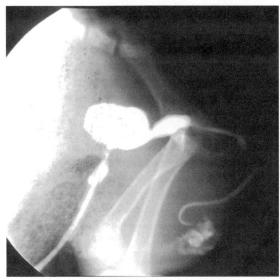

Figure 19.2-6   Normograde, positive contrast cystourethrogram was performed in a goat via a cystotomy tube. Extravasation of the contrast medium is detected at the ventral aspect of the sigmoid flexure in the penile urethra, thus indicating a urethral rupture.

the urethra has become patent. The patient should be observed closely while the catheter is occluded. If the animal shows signs of colic or stranguria, the catheter can be unclamped or unplugged to allow urine egress; the process is repeated on the following day. In 15 small ruminants treated by tube cystostomy, urine began to drip from the urethral orifice after an average of 7.5 days (range, 1 to 20 days) postoperatively (Rakestraw et al, 1995).

Infusion of a mildly acidic, polyionic solution into the urinary tract via a tube cystostomy was used to promote urolith dissolution in a ram (Cockroft, 1993). Acetic acid can be added to sterile saline to create an acidic flush solution. One drop of glacial acetic acid added to 500 ml of nonbuffered sterile saline creates a solution with a pH between 4.5 and 5.5. Measurement of the pH and, if needed, adjustment until it is within this range is recommended before infusion.

Once urine is seen dripping from the preputial orifice, the length of time the catheter is occluded can be gradually extended until normal micturition occurs. If the animal continues to void normally with the catheter completely occluded for 1 to 2 days, the catheter can be removed; however, catheter removal should be delayed until at least 7 days after surgery to ensure that a fibrinous or omental seal develops around the bladder incision. Catheter removal took place an average of 14 days after surgery (range, 4 to 36 days) in the aforementioned study (Rakestraw et al, 1995). Thus the duration of postoperative care can be considerable with this procedure.

To remove the catheter, the skin around the tube entry site is disinfected; the balloon of the catheter is deflated fully; and the catheter is gently pulled out. Urine will usually drip for 1 to 2 days from the body wall fistula created by the tube. Ultrasonography often reveals the bladder is adhered to the interior of the body wall at this site, but this adhesion appears to either break down or stretch in most cases, and no observable effects on the animal's ability to void urine usually result.

Postoperatively, antimicrobial therapy should be continued until at least one week *beyond* the date of catheter removal. Ascending infection of the bladder is likely with this procedure; the interior of the tip of the Foley catheter was found to culture positive upon removal in 10 of 10 animals treated with tube cystostomy (Van Metre and Gnad, 2001). However, treatment of these animals with a beta lactam or sulfonamide antibiotic as described above resulted in no cases of persistent urinary tract infection.

Bladder Marsupialization

In this procedure, a permanent stoma is created between the bladder mucosa and the skin of the ventral abdomen, thus allowing direct urine outflow from the bladder to the exterior. Although originally described for use in goats, this procedure could be used in other animals. It is a valid option as a primary corrective procedure for urolithiasis. Bladder marsupialization is also useful as a salvage option for animals that have developed stricture of the urethra or a perineal urethrostomy. Postoperative urinary incontinence is inevitable, and urine scalding of the ventral abdomen may occur. Although uncommon, stricture of the marsupialization site and ascending urinary tract infection are potential complications (May et al, 1998).

Local, epidural, or general anesthesia can be used. The animal is placed in dorsal recumbency, and the ventral abdomen and inguinal region are clipped and disinfected. A 10-to-15-cm-long skin incision is made 3 cm lateral to and parallel with the sheath. The incision is continued through the external sheath of the rectus abdominus muscle, the rectus abdominus muscle, the internal rectus sheath, and peritoneum. The bladder is identified, and urine is aspirated from the bladder to facilitate exteriorization.

Two stay sutures are placed beside the bladder apex, approximately 4 to 6 cm apart. A 3- to 4-cm longitudinal cystotomy incision is made on the ventral aspect of the bladder apex. Copious lavage and suction are used to clear the bladder lumen of urine and calculi.

The apex of the bladder is then positioned against the peritoneal surface on the contralateral side of the ventral abdominal wall, equidistant from midline as for the laparotomy incision. The bladder apex is positioned as far cranially as possible without producing excessive tension on the bladder. This step allows the surgeon to determine the optimal location for the marsupialization incision. At this site, a second 4-cm paramedian, longitudinal celiotomy incision is made, which will be called the *marsupialization incision*. The stay sutures are used to reposition the bladder apex through the marsupialization incision. The interior of the marsupialization incision is carefully inspected to ensure that bowel is not entrapped with the bladder apex.

Four simple interrupted sutures of absorbable, 0 or 00 monofilament material are placed through the external rectus sheath of the marsupialization incision and into the seromuscular layer of the bladder, immediately dorsal to (deep to) the cystotomy incision. These sutures should be placed to position the edges of the cystotomy incision even with the level of the skin. These sutures are placed at 12, 3, 6, and 9 o'clock in the marsupialization incision.

Next, the entire circumference of the seromuscular layer of the bladder immediately dorsal to (deep to) the cystotomy incision is secured to the external rectus sheath with 2-0 monofilament, absorbable material in an interrupted horizontal mattress pattern. The edges of the cystotomy incision are then sutured circumferentially to the skin with 3-0 monofilament, absorbable material in a simple continuous pattern. The abdomen is lavaged, and the laparotomy incision is closed routinely.

Postoperative antimicrobial therapy is continued for approximately one week. The hair on the abdomen may need to be clipped periodically to limit urine scald. The marsupialization site may require periodic cleaning.

Postoperative Care

Fluid therapy is continued for azotemic animals or those with significant acid-base or electrolyte derangements. Periodic assessment of body weight and hydration status is necessary to maintain normal fluid balance; occasionally, postobstructive diuresis results in large volume fluid losses that require aggressive therapy. With the return of the patient's appetite, salt can be gradually added to the diet to promote water intake and production of dilute urine. Dietary manipulations for prevention of urolithiasis have been reviewed (Van Metre and Divers, 1996).

RECOMMENDED READINGS

Cockcroft PD: Dissolution of obstructive urethral uroliths in a ram, *Vet Rec* 132: 486, 1993.

Haven ML et al: Surgical management of urolithiasis in small ruminants, *Cornell Vet* 83: 47-55, 1993.

May KA et al: Urinary bladder marsupialization for treatment of obstructive urolithiasis in male goats, *Vet Surg* 27: 583-588, 1998.

May KA, Moll HD, Duncan RB, Moon MM, Pleasant RS, Howard RD: Experimental evaluation of urinary bladder marsupialization in male goats, *Vet Surg* 31: 251-258, 2002.

Rakestraw PC et al: Tube cystostomy for treatment of obstructive urolithiasis, *Vet Surg* 24: 498-505, 1995.

Van Metre DC, Divers TJ: Ruminant renal system. In Smith BP: *Large animal internal medicine,* ed 2, St Louis, 1996, Mosby.

Van Metre DC, Gnad DP: Unpublished data. Colorado State University, Kansas State University, 2001.

Van Metre DC, Smith BP: Clinical management of urolithiasis in small ruminants, *Proc 9th Ann Forum, ACVIM*, 1991.

Wolfe DF: Urolithiasis. In Wolfe DF, Moll HD: *Large animal urogenital surgery*, ed 2, Baltimore, 1999, Williams & Wilkins.

CHAPTER 20

CONGENITAL ANOMALIES IN THE SHEEP AND GOAT

Paul J. Plummer

Numerous congenital abnormalities have been reported in both sheep and goats. As in other species, these abnormalities generally result from a genetic defect (spontaneous or inherited) or an in utero environmental exposure of the fetus. Included in the list of recognized environmental causes are a number of viruses, toxic plants, and teratogenic drugs. With the exception of congenital defects involving the genital organs, very little research into the chromosomal genetics of defects has been conducted. In many cases, the genetic basis of a defect is founded on the increased incidence or expression of the defect in a given family of animals. When the defect involves the genitalia of the animal (particularly the external genitalia), then alteration in its ability to mature and reproduce often leads to an increased recognition of the abnormality. A defect that involves a specific enzyme deficiency is much more difficult for a breeder to recognize and thus may not be identified as a congenital problem. For the purposes of this chapter, we will focus on two of the more commonly recognized genital abnormalities of sheep and goats.

Intersex

As in many other species, the genotypic sex of sheep and goats is determined by the X and Y genes. The genotypic code for males is the XY karyotype while the XX karyotype is for females. Unlike many other body systems in which genotypic and hormonal control of embryonic differentiation are independent of outside influences, the differentiation of the genital system is highly influenced by local endocrinologic events. Genital differentiation is basically controlled by the formation of gonadal and ductal tissues. Before differentiation, the gonadal tissues (gonocytes that migrate from the endoderm of the yolk sac) have the ability to form either testicular or ovarian tissue. The differentiation of the gonadal tissue is for the most part regulated by the chromosomal sex of the fetus determined at fertilization. The XY karyotype code expression of the H-Y antigen pushes differentiation of the gonadal cells to early testicular cells. If no H-Y antigen is expressed, as would be the case in a chromosomal XX fetus, the cells differentiate into ovarian tissue by default. Once gonadal tissue differentiation occurs, the ductal formation is driven by expression of hormones in the local and systemic environment. Thus defects in hormonal expression, receptor expression, or presence of exogenous hormones can all have a profound effect on ductal formation and genital development.

The intersex congenital abnormality involves the presence of both male and female characteristics in the same animal (Figure 20-1). A variety of presentations can be seen. When female and male gonads are both present, this intersex condition is called *hermaphrodite*. When the gonads of one sex are present with the phenotype of the opposite sex, this condition is called *pseudohermaphrodite* (Figure 20-2); a male pseudohermaphrodism has the male gonads, whereas the female has the female gonads. Although the condition of intersex is recognized in both sheep and goats, the incidence is highest in the goat species, whose genetics has been extensively studied. The incidence of the intersex condition is higher in polled goats. Animals that are polled (congenital absence of horns) have the dominant mutation of the polled gene

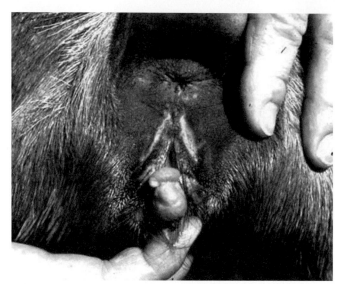

Figure 20-1 Vulva of a goat; note vestigal penis typical of a female pseudohermaphrodite.

(Courtesy of Dr. John King; Cornell University.)

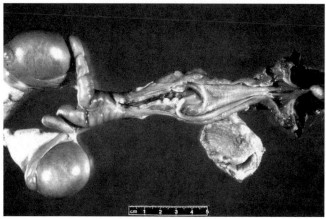

Figure 20-2 Male pseudohermaphrodite in a goat. Note the presence of the uterus and testes but no ovaries. The additional presence of ovarian tissue would have made the animal a true hermaphrodite.

(Courtesy of Dr. John King; Cornell University.)

coded at the horn locus. Thus the mutated gene (P) in either a homozygous (PP) or heterozygous (PP) state codes for a polled animal, and the homozygous recessive state (pp) codes for horns. Because many breeders would prefer to have polled kids that do not require disbudding or dehorning, various attempts have been made to breed polled animals. However, it appears that the polled locus is in close proximity to a gene that effects sexual differentiation. This autosomal gene has functions similar to a Y chromosome, thereby inducing masculinization. As

such, females (XX) that are homozygous for the polled gene have the intersex condition (female pseudohermaphrodite), and the males are predisposed to stenosis of the epididymis. No such association has been reported in polled sheep.

As with other species, some female small ruminants born as a twin to males may have an intersex condition termed *freemartinism*. This condition occurs as a result of the chorioallantoic circulation of the twins fusing and exchanging leukocytes and fetal hormones. These hormones presumably cause a masculinization of the female co-twin. Unlike cattle, in which twins have a very high rate of freemartinism (11 of 12 pairs of twins), small ruminants have a much lower incidence (about 1% of twins in sheep). This difference in incidence is most likely attributable to a low frequency of vascular anastomoses in small ruminants. The condition is characterized by severe ovarian hypoplasia and absence or hypoplasia of the tubular genitalia of the female. External genitalia may demonstrate clitoromegaly or increased anogenital distance. The male twins are generally normal, although fertility may be subnormal and unilateral or bilateral cryptorchidism occurs.

Because of the profound effect the intersex condition has on fertility, these animals should be culled. Surgical procedures to correct these conditions are not recommended because of the potential transmission of some genetic component. However, it should be mentioned that some affected animals have the potential to be used as teaser animals as long as the abnormality is of sufficient severity to assure the animal is not fertile. Hormone assays should detect the presence of androgens, even in genotypic XX animals that have no external male genitalia. These animals are prime candidates for teaser animals. There have been reports of surgical correction of specific urethral and genital abnormalities in intersex goats if the animal is of great emotional value to the owner.

Cryptorchidism

Cryptorchidism is defined as one or both testes not descending into the scrotum. Early in genital embryogenesis, the testis is located in the fetal abdomen adjacent to the caudal pole of each kidney. It migrates caudally through the inguinal canal into the scrotum, preceded by the epididymis. The migration is directed in part by the gubernaculum and vaginal process; however, defects in these tissues are not always associated with cryptorchidism. It appears that hormones, particularly Mullerian inhibiting substance (MIS) and testosterone, may also play an important role in testicular descent. MIS is produced by the Sertoli cells of the fetal testis. During embryogenesis production, the MIS induces a local (restricted to the side of production) regression of the paramesonephric ducts (precursors of the female genitalia) and initiates intraabdominal migration. Goats with a deficiency of MIS production by the Sertoli cells or lacking the receptor for MIS on the paramesonephric ducts develop a reproductive defect known as persistent Mullerian duct syndrome (PMDS). Clinically, these bucks have a well-developed penis but are bilaterally cryptorchid. Surgery or *post mortem* examination demonstrates the presence of both male and female internal genitalia. These bucks have a XY karyotype, and PMDS is generally considered distinct from the intersex conditions. In dogs and humans, PMDS is inherited as an autosomal recessive trait, and this may be true for goats as well.

Once the testis reaches the inguinal canal, the descent appears to be controlled by local testosterone production. The epididymis relies on testosterone for maturation, so incomplete maturation due to testosterone deficiency may impair testicular descent. In some circumstances, the epididymis may be located in the inguinal canal while the testis is still intraabdominal.

The incidence of cryptorchidism in small ruminants is estimated at 1% but may reach levels of 10% in some herds. It is likely cryptorchidism in the sheep and goat is inherited as an autosomal sex-linked gene. It is unclear whether the gene for cryptorchidism is a recessive or dominant gene with incomplete expression. Affected testes are generally smaller and firmer then normal testes

(Figure 20-3). They can be located in either the abdomen or inguinal canal or both. If they are in the abdomen, they are generally located somewhere along the path of migration from the caudal pole of the kidney to the inguinal canal. The left testis appears to be more commonly retained than the right testis in most species. Histopathology of retained testes generally reveals marked fibrosis of the tissue. If the animal is a unilateral cryptorchid, the normal testis may be enlarged and show cellular evidence of compensatory hyperplasia. Bilateral cryptorchids are invariably sterile, whereas unilateral cryptorchids may still be fertile. Given the inherited nature of this congenital defect, affected animals should not be used as breeding animals. Castration of cryptorchid animals should be recommended if the owner wants to retain the animal in the herd. Before starting a cryptorchid castration, the side of the retained testis should be determined. The normal testis should be removed after the retained testis to avoid confusion should attempts to remove the cryptorchid testis fail. A thorough palpation of the inguinal area and canals should be performed to determine whether the testis is intraabdominal or inguinal. Sometimes it is best to administer a sedative or general anesthesia before performing palpation. Ultrasound evaluation of the inguinal region and inguinal canal may also provide useful information about the location of the testis. Transabdominal ultrasound to evaluate an intraabdominal testis is generally performed through a right paralumbar fossa because

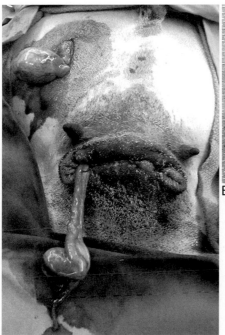
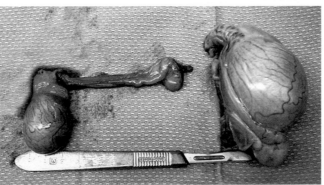

Figure 20-3   *A,* Intraoperative view of a pygmy goat in surgery for a right cryptorchid testis. The normal testis is the larger one seen through a scrotal incision. Only the epididymis could be delivered through the scrotal incision. A right paramedian celiotomy incision was made to deliver the cryptorchid testis seen at the top of the figure. *B,* Both testes are shown after resection. Note the normal larger left testis on the right of the figure and smaller right cryptorchid testis on the left of the figure.

(Courtesy of Dr. Brett Woodie; Cornell University.)

of the difficulty of imaging the kidneys around the rumen in the left paralumbar fossa. The area between the caudal pole of the kidneys and the inguinal canals should be evaluated. It should be mentioned that many intraabdominal testes are small and structurally abnormal, thus making them difficult to identify by ultrasound. If the testis is located in the inguinal canal, a surgical approach similar to that described for horses may be used to exteriorize the testis and facilitate castration. Briefly, an incision is made over the external inguinal canal of the effected side. Digital palpation of the inguinal canal should reveal the presence of the epididymis. Once the epididymis is located, a clamp can grasp it firmly, so gentle outward pressure can be applied to exteriorize the testis. In some cases, the vaginal tunic inverted up into the inguinal canal can be used to blindly locate the testis as described in the equine.

In most cases, a ventral celiotomy and exploratory are required to locate the intraabdominal testis because the inguinal canal is too small to permit any surgical manipulations. Laparoscopy is the preferred method of accessing and removing the abdominal testicles (see Section 4.6 for laparoscopic techniques). Once the testis is located, all vessels should be ligated and the testis completely removed. Once the retained testis is removed, the normal testis can be removed with normal castration techniques.

It should be noted that retained testes have been associated with an increased risk of tumor formation or torsion of the spermatic cord. Therefore surgical removal of the retained testis may be warranted if an animal is not being culled. In any case, the owner should be informed of the genetic association of cryptorchidism in goats and should be encouraged not to breed the animal. As mentioned earlier, some of these animals make suitable teaser animals if their infertility is certain (i.e., after performing an epididymectomy of the normal testis).

RECOMMENDED READINGS

Basrur PK: Congenital abnormalities of the goat, *Vet Clin N Am Food Anim Pract* 9:183-202, 1993.

Dennis SM: Congenital defects of sheep, *Vet Clin N Am Food Anim Pract* 9:203-217, 1993.

Karras S et al.: Surgical correction of urethral dilation in an intersex goat, *J Am Vet Med Assoc* 201:1584-1586, 1992.

Ladds PW: Congenital abnormalities of the genitalia of cattle, sheep, goats, and pigs, *Vet Clin N Am Food Anim Pract* 9:127-144, 1993.

Mueller E: Developmental conditions of the scrotum and testes. In Wolfe DF Moll HD, editors: *Large animal urogenital surgery*, Philadelphia, 1998, Williams and Wilkins.

CHAPTER 21

SURGERY OF THE SWINE DIGESTIVE SYSTEM

Guy St. Jean, David E. Anderson

Swine industry economics often limits veterinarians' options for surgical management of disease. The main task is to relate production unit economics and disease control to increase profits. Veterinarian services should meet enterprise needs because the individual pig versus the population in large-scale operations often has a minimal value. Surgery on an individual pig is not always cost-effective. However, some conditions—like hernia, prolapse, dystocia, and atresia—that can occur in large numbers of animals can be very costly and need to be investigated so a solution and treatment can be applied. In a commercial swine operation, the veterinarian often teaches the manager and experienced personnel how to perform minor surgical procedures, including castration, ear notching, canine teeth clipping, and tail amputation in a cost-effective fashion. The veterinarian's role is to ensure these procedures are properly and humanely performed. Among purebreds, pets (such as Vietnamese potbelly pigs), or biomedical research animal model pigs, the individual animal often has a high perceived value, and surgery is often requested. Also, genetically valuable breeding stock allow for more

This chapter's discussion of tusk removal was written by J. Brett Woodie.

sophisticated treatment of disease. A veterinarian who offers excellent surgical service to swine producers will have greater credibility as a herd consultant.

Digestive tract

Infected mandibular canine teeth (tusks) result in local swelling and purulent drainage. The local swelling along the mandible is difficult to detect on physical examination because of the normally thick jaw of pigs. Purulent drainage can be seen at the lateral aspect of the mandible, generally over the caudal aspect of the tooth root. Some animals have decreased appetite and drooling of saliva from the affected side. Halitosis can be a feature if the infected tooth is draining into the oral cavity. The diagnosis is confirmed by radiography under general anesthesia or heavy sedation. On radiography, one can document the soft tissue swelling and areas of lysis surrounding the affected canine tooth (Figure 21-1A and B.) CT examination is more precise and allows confirmation of osteitis surrounding the infected tusk (Figures 21-2 and 21-3A and B.)

Treatment of an infected tooth requires removal. However, this is a difficult surgery and should only be undertaken if one can definitively confirm the diagnosis.

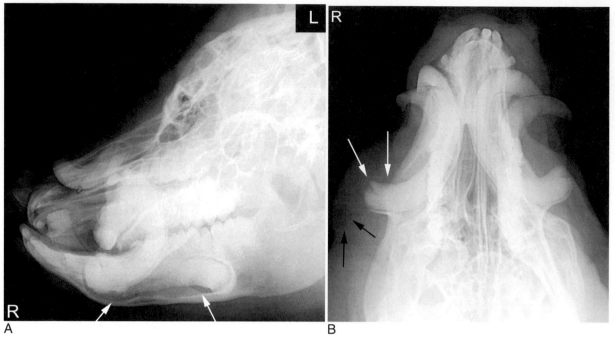

Figure 21-1   Right dorsal-left ventral oblique (A) and ventrodorsal radiograph (B) of an adult castrated-male potbelly pig with a draining tract on the right lateral aspect of the mandible. Note the area of bone lysis with loss of the normal lamina dura *(white arrows)* and the associated soft tissue swelling with gas *(black arrows.)* This pig was diagnosed with a tooth root abscess of the right mandibular canine tooth.

(Courtesy of Dr. Anthony Pease; Cornell University.)

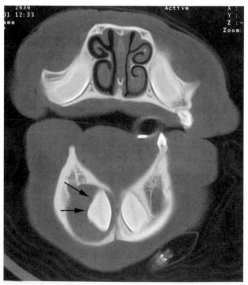

Figure 21-2   Transverse CT of the mandible in an adult pig with a tooth root abscess. An area of fluid density surrounds the right canine tooth (tusk). There are small gas densities (arrows) within the fluid density.

(Courtesy of Dr. Anthony Pease; Cornell University.)

The owners should be warned of the possibility of mandibular fracture, and appropriate equipment should be ready if repair is necessary. After induction of general anesthesia, the animal is placed in sternal recumbency. Lateral recumbency can also be used. To give access to the crown of the affected tooth, a mouth gag (block of wood or a canine mouth gag) (Figure 21-4) is placed between the contralateral cheek teeth. A dental elevator is placed around the crown as far caudal as possible to separate the tooth from the alveolus. A second approach is made over the most caudal aspect of the root as follows. First, a 3- to 4-cm vertical incision is made over the most caudal aspect of the affected tooth. Electrocautery is helpful in providing hemostasis. A Gelpi retractor is placed, and the incision is bluntly extended to the root. A dental elevator is used to free the root circumferentially as far rostrally as possible. Using a mallet and 1-cm tooth punch, the veterinarian gently taps the tooth while the assistant applies traction on the crown. The tooth's comma shape necessitates moving it in a semicircle for extraction (Figure 21-5). The extraction is difficult, and repulsion and traction must be applied in the correct direction to minimize the possibility of mandibu-

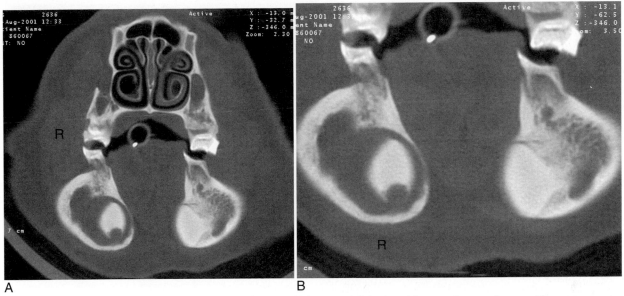

Figure 21-3 *A,* Transverse CT of the mandible in an adult pig with a tooth root abscess. The right canine tooth (tusk) has a concave area of lysis and is surrounded by an area of fluid density. *B,* Close-up image showing an area of lysis on the right tusk that is compared to the normal left tusk.

(Courtesy of Dr. Anthony Pease; Cornell University.)

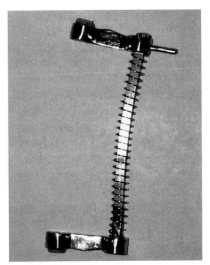

Figure 21-4 Spring-loaded mouth gag to be placed in contralateral side.

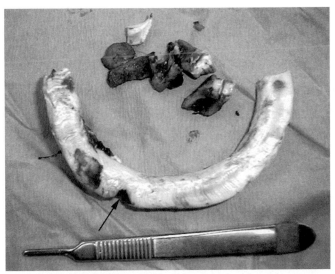

Figure 21-5 Photograph of a right canine tooth (tusk) with tooth root abscess removed from an adult pig. Note the area of lysis (arrows) that was seen on the associated CT.

lar fracture. If the tooth was draining caudally, the incision is left open to heal by second intention. If no drainage is present caudally, the incision can be closed in two layers with absorbable suture material, preferably monofilament.

If the tooth cannot be extracted, the caudal incision is extended rostrally along the lateral aspect of the tooth. The dissection is quite extensive until the mandible is reached. The lateral wall of the mandible over the tooth is removed using an air drill while carefully avoiding the parotid duct and facial artery. Once the lateral wall has been removed, the tooth can be pried out. The incision is closed in an acceptable manner after removal of the tooth.

Postoperatively, antimicrobials are continued for 2 weeks, and the draining tracts are kept clean with warm water and dilute Betadine solution. Vitamin A and D ointment is placed around the draining tract to prevent scalding.

If a mandibular fracture occurs, the latter is fixed with wires placed in a figure-eight pattern around the crown of teeth adjacent to the fracture site (see Chapter 10 for further details.) These wires will need to be removed 2 to 4 months later.

GASTROINTESTINAL TRACT

Surgery of the swine gastrointestinal system is not commonly performed. This may be the result of low individual economic value and difficulties in diagnosing a surgical digestive abnormality rapidly enough to allow successful intervention. A ventral midline celiotomy under general anesthesia is the surgical approach of choice for most digestive surgery in swine. A celiotomy is used to explore the abdomen to confirm a diagnosis and possibly correct the problem.

Ulcers

Gastric ulcers are common conditions of the swine gastrointestinal tract. Clinical signs are pale mucous membranes and dark, tarry feces. Decreased feed intake, vomiting, and weight loss may be observed. In valuable pigs, gastrotomy, partial gastrectomy, or oversew of the ulcer may be performed. With the animal in dorsal recumbency, an incision is made on the ventral midline starting at the xiphoid cartilage. The stomach is isolated from the rest of the abdomen, and the serosal surface is evaluated for changes in color and appearance that would indicate an ulcer. A gastrotomy is performed, and the stomach contents are removed. If an ulcer is found, it can be surgically dissected and the edges electrocoagulated or ligated. The incision in the stomach is then apposed with a simple continuous suture pattern followed by an inverting pattern (e.g., Cushing's type.) If multiple bleeding ulcers are present, the prognosis is poor.

Intestinal Obstruction

Intestinal obstructions may occur because of feed impaction, intussusception (Figure 21-6), foreign bodies, or intestinal volvulus (Figure 21-7.) Clinical signs observed may include depression, vomiting, abdominal distension, and a decrease in the amount of feces, sometimes with blood and/or mucus. These conditions are rarely diagnosed in live animals. If surgery is an option a ventral midline exploratory celiotomy is performed. Feed impactions may be disrupted manually with massage and infusion of saline solutions or may be removed via an enterotomy. An enterotomy may be performed to remove a foreign body obstruction. An intestinal resection and anastomosis may be done to resect ischemic bowel or an intussusception.

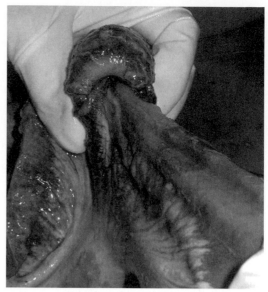

Figure 21-6 Photograph of the ileum of a 3.5-year-old castrated male pig found dead. Note ileal intussusception.

(Courtesy of Dr. Donald H. Schlafer; Cornell University.)

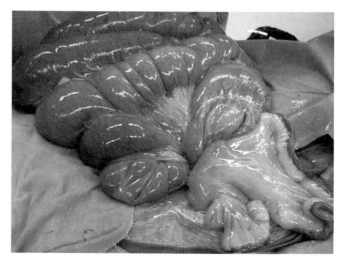

Figure 21-7 Photograph of a 7-year-old female pig with a volvulus of the spiral colon. The pig had been off feed for 9 days.

(Courtesy of Dr. Vanessa Cook; Cornell University.)

In one series of cases, acute abdominal accidents were characterized clinically by sudden death and were observed more commonly in dry sows. It was proposed that feeding dry sows in large breeding units once a day or every other day might be an important provoking factor. This feeding method often makes sows ingest large quantities of feed and water rapidly. Gastric torsion in swine results in death preceded by a short period of anorexia, abdominal distension, shortness of breath, cyanosis, and salivation (Morin et al, 1984.) Clockwise torsions are more common than counterclockwise torsions. These torsions occur along the longitudinal axis of the organ, and the stomach is distended with fluid, gas, and food. In some sows, the spleen rotated with the stomach; affected spleens were severely congested; and some had ruptured, thus causing hemoperitoneum. Liver torsion was also seen occasionally. For the eight sows in that study, an intestinal volvulus diagnosis was more commonly observed in young sows. The entire small intestine was included in the volvulus of four sows, the posterior half of the small intestine in one, the small intestine and colon in one, and the cecum and colon in another.

Atresia Ani

Atresia ani is possibly the most important cause of intestinal obstruction in the pig and occurs more commonly than in any other species. This congenital defect may be transmitted genetically. The diagnosis is made based on the following findings: absence of anal opening, abdominal distension, slower growth rate, lack of defecation, and vomiting. Because pigs vomit, thus decompressing their intestinal tract, the diagnosis of atresia ani is sometimes not made until 3 to 4 weeks of age. A fistula may occur between the rectum and vagina of a female piglet, so the feces may be voided through the vulva. Surgical treatment of atresia ani is necessary for the pig's survival. After anesthesia, a circular piece of skin is excised below the tail over the bulging rectum. Ideally the rectal pouch is mobilized and tacked to the subcutaneous tissues before it is opened. Once the pouch is opened feces are usually discharged immediately. The area is cleaned and the rectal mucosa sutured to the skin in an interrupted pattern making an effort to provide a large stoma. Pelvic dissection may be necessary if there is no rectum present at the skin opening. Atresia of the rectum and anus (atresia ani et recti) may make surgical correction impossible. Surgical treatment with a celiotomy and colostomy or rectal pull-through may be necessary but is rarely justifiable economically for these extreme cases. After correction of atresia ani or recti, the pigs should be fed until they reach slaughter weight.

Rectal Stricture

Pigs with rectal stricture often show clinical signs similar to pigs with atresia ani, except they have an anus and are generally older. One series of pig cases with rectal stricture were 16 to 18 weeks of age (Saunders, 1974.) These pigs suffered from weight loss in comparison to their herdmates, no feces were passed, and the abdomen continued to distend. These pigs were slaughtered or killed by other pigs. Most cases of rectal stricture result from rectal prolapse that has constricted after repair or are an

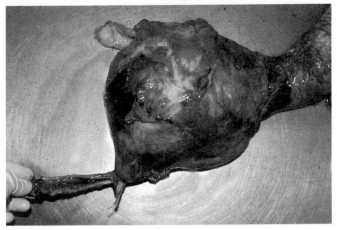

Figure 21-8 *Post mortem* photograph of a pig with chronic rectal stricture. Note distended descending colon proximal to the stricture area.

(Courtesy of Dr. Michael Schramme; Cornell University.)

end result of Salmonella colitis. At necropsy, these pigs show a distended cecum and colon. The rectum is usually severely constricted by fibrous tissue. It is speculated that rectal mucosa inflammation leads to rectal scar formation with subsequent stenosis and eventually possible complete obstruction (Figure 21-8). Surgical treatment is similar to atresia ani. An elliptical incision is made around the anus and the dissection is extended perirectally to the rostral aspect of the stricture (Figure 21-9). If the strictured segment is short, the narrowed portion is resected rostrally, and the rectum is sutured to the circular skin incision using absorbable sutures of 00 or 0. If the stricture extends more cranially, a ventral midline celiotomy can be performed to complete the resection. In some instances, the proximal end of the descending colon can be anastomosed to the perianal skin incision. A loop of spiral colon may need to be dissected (with its vascular supply) for use in the colonic pull-through because stretching the descending colon interferes with the vascular supply. The pull-through is accomplished by temporarily occluding the segment of spiral colon with a continuous suture or intestinal staples. The mesenteric and antimesenteric sides are tagged with stay sutures that are used to deliver the bowel through the pelvic inlet to the perianal region. The segment of bowel used in the pull-through procedure must also be sutured to the dorsal body wall to prevent volvulus of the segment. Alternatively, pigs with rectal stricture may respond to left flank celiotomy with colostomy.

Rectal Prolapse

Rectal prolapse is a common occurrence in swine. Prolapse of the rectal mucosa occurs after straining to

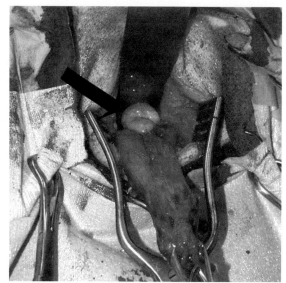

Figure 21-9 Intraoperative photograph of perirectal dissection. With the pig in dorsal recumbency, Gelpi and malleable retractors are used to provide the surgeon greater visibility. Holding the anus with a Lahey thyroid clamp provides traction on the rectum and facilitates dissection. Pelvic fat is seen (arrow).

(Courtesy of Dr. Michael Schramme; Cornell University.)

defecate. The mucosa rapidly becomes edematous and often shows bleeding lesions. Many factors have been associated with rectal prolapse development including: genetics, a birth weight less than 1 kg, being male, diarrhea, coughing, short tails, autumn and winter piling as a consequence of chilling, chronic water shortage, certain antibiotics, zearalenone toxicosis, and a diet that contains 20% more lysine than required. Diagnosis of rectal prolapse is obvious on physical examination, but the prolapse should be carefully assessed to identify other organs it contains.

The simplest procedure to reduce rectal prolapse is gentle massage, and retention obtained by applying a purse-string suture pattern using umbilical tape around the anus. The suture is passed in and out through the skin around the anal opening 1 cm from the anus. A one-finger opening should be left when tying the purse string. The suture usually is left in place for 5 to 10 days. This should be done only if the rectal mucosa is viable and close inspection does not reveal any lacerations. If the mucosa is too necrotic to replace, alternative methods of correction are available. One technique is surgical amputation, which requires hemostats, scalpel blade, scissors, thumb forceps, two 18-gauge needles 3 or 4 inches long, suture material, and a small-diameter rubber tube. After anesthesia, the rubber tube is inserted in the rectum until 2 or 3 inches protrude. To fix the rubber tube in the rectum, two needles are inserted through the rectum at

right angles to each other, so they pass through the rectum and tube and emerge from the opposite side (see Figure 10.7-4.) The entire circumference of the exposed rectal mucosa is dissected down to the serosa of the inner wall about a centimeter from the mucocutaneous border where mucosa is still healthy (see Figures 10.7-5 to 10.7-7.) The usually minor hemorrhaging is controlled with gauze until all the layers have been dissected and the dorsal artery of the rectum is cut. Once the dissection around the prolapse is complete, the rectum is attached to the rubber tube with needles to hold it in place. A size 0 absorbable suture material in a cruciate pattern is suggested to suture the rectum ends together. After the rectum has been sutured, the needles are pulled from the tube before removing it from the rectum. The rectum is allowed to retract into place. An alternative method of rectal amputation is to use a prolapse ring, PVC tubing, syringe case, or corrugated tube. The ring or tubing is placed in the rectum with the tube's halfway point inserted as far as the anal sphincter. A ligature or rubber band is applied over the prolapse as near as possible to the anus. The ligature or rubber band must be tight enough to disrupt blood supply to the prolapse. Feces may go through or may block the tube. Usually, the necrotic prolapse falls off in 5 to 7 days with the implant in place, and fecal production returns to normal (Figure 4.4-21A to E).

Three possible complications seen with rectal prolapse are bladder retroversion, eventration of the small intestine, and rectal stricture. In a 1-month-old castrated pig, eventration of the small bowel was seen concurrently with a rectal prolapse. The rectal prolapse was 5 cm in length, edematous, and purple-black. A small tear was found in the rectum in the pelvic area, and eventration of small intestine was observed. It was speculated that the long duration of the prolapse allowed necrosis to occur. This provided a friable area, and the small intestine perforated this necrotic area during straining to defecate. Surgical correction of small intestine eventration in a pig is usually not economically feasible. If treatment is requested, preoperative medical management is necessary to treat shock and dehydration. Under general anesthesia, the intestine is examined, cleansed, and resected if necessary. A ventral midline incision is made to isolate the intestine segment remaining within the abdominal cavity. The portion of intestine involved in the rectal laceration is resected close to the rectum. The viable end of intestine is then exteriorized through the ventral midline incision and a single-layer, simple interrupted, end-to-end anastomosis performed. Bladder retroversion with rectal prolapse has been observed in a sow 2 days after normal farrowing. The sow had a grapefruit-sized rectal prolapse with protrusion and tension of the perineal area. The bladder was drained by passing a catheter. One week *post partum*, the prolapsed rectum was amputated. The sow reared nine

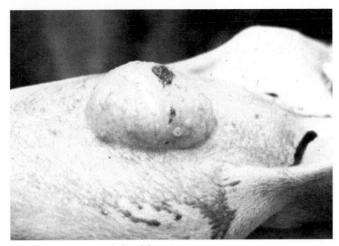

Figure 21-10 Umbilical hernia in a pig.

piglets to 6 weeks of age and was sent for slaughter 1 week after weaning the piglets.

Umbilical Hernia

Umbilical hernia is a developmental defect of pigs. An umbilical hernia is a discontinuity of the abdominal wall at the umbilicus with protrusion of abdominal content into a hernia sac formed by the skin and surrounding connective tissue (Figure 21-10). In swine herds, the frequency of umbilical hernias ranges from 0.4% to 1.2% and varies with breed and sex (Searcy-Bernal et al, 1994). In addition to heredity, the etiology of umbilical hernia may be umbilical infection or abscess. After birth, iodine or similar antiseptic agents are applied to the umbilicus to decrease the likelihood of infection. Pigs with umbilical hernias may suffer from growth retardation and die from intestinal strangulation. In one study, pigs sired by American Spotted and Duroc boars were more likely to develop hernia than those sired by Yorkshire boars. Umbilical hernias often were detected in pigs between 9 and 14 weeks of age. Possibly the condition was recognized at that age because the rapid growth of pigs, combined with increased weight of the abdominal contents, leads to a hernia of significant size. Females had a higher risk of developing umbilical hernia. As with many other swine surgical conditions, the cost of treatment may preclude surgical correction. In that case, pigs should be consigned to an early slaughter, usually within 1 month after hernia detection, before evisceration, intestinal strangulation, or fistula occurs. A case of intestinal umbilical fistula has been described in a 30- kg castrated pig (Lewis, 1973). The risk of intestinal incarceration and strangulation is higher with an umbilical hernia of small dimension.

The reduced growth rate in untreated pigs with umbilical hernias may encourage surgical correction of the defect. However, whether surgical correction of umbilical hernia will restore the growth potential is unknown. In purebred, show animals, and pet pigs, surgical correction is often indicated. Herniorrhaphy should be performed early in life. After anesthesia, the pig is restrained in dorsal recumbency in a "V"-shaped trough. The surgical area is cleaned and prepared for surgery. If surgical correction is performed on a male, the prepuce, preputial diverticulum, and penis should be reflected posteriorly or to one side (e.g., inverted "V" or "J" incision.) The hernia sac is isolated, and dissection is performed to the hernia ring. The hernia sac and any abscesses should be removed and the edges of the ring freshened. If intestinal contents adhere to the hernia sac, the adhesions are separated, and bowel viability is assessed before replacing it in the abdomen if judged acceptable. If intestinal viability is compromised, resection and anastomosis of viable intestine should be performed. If no infection is present, the hernia sac can be inverted into the abdomen, but this procedure has a higher postoperative hernia risk in comparison to open herniorrhaphy techniques. The abdominal defect is closed in an overlapping or simple continuous pattern. The prepuce, preputial diverticulum, and penis are repositioned and sutured to the abdominal muscle with absorbable suture material. The skin is sutured using a simple interrupted pattern of nonabsorbable suture material. For surgical correction of umbilical hernia in the female, an elliptical incision is made around the hernia sac, and the excess skin is discarded. With a combination of sharp and blunt dissection, the hernia sac is cut and removed, and the abdominal muscle is closed as in the male. The subcutaneous tissue and skin are then closed. Systemic antibiotic should be administered for 5 days, and the skin suture removed in 10 days.

RECOMMENDED READINGS

Amass SF, Schinckel AP, Clark LK: Increased prevalence of rectal prolapses in growing/finishing swine fed a diet containing excess lysine, *Vet Rec* 137: 519-520, 1995.

Douglas RGA: A simple method for correcting rectal prolapse in pigs, *Vet Rec* 117: 129, 1985.

Greenwood J: Treatment of bladder retroversion with rectal prolapse in sow, *Vet Rec,* Oct: 405-406, 1989.

Lewis AM: An intestinal umbilical fistula in the pig and its surgical treatment, *Vet Rec* 93: 286, 1973.

Morin M, Sauvageau R, Phaneuf JB, Teuscher E, Beauregard M, and Legace A: Torsion of abdominal organs in sows: a report of 36 cases, *Can Vet J* 25: 440-442, 1984.

Peyton LC, Colahan PT, Jann HW, and Granstedt ME: Prolapsed rectum and eventration of the small intestine in a pig: surgical treatment, *Agri-practice VM-SAC,* Aug: 1297-1330, 1980.

Saunders CN: Rectal stricture syndrome in pigs: a case history, *Vet Rec* 94: 61, 1974.

Searcy-Bernal R, Gardner IA, and Hird DW: Effects of and factors associated with umbilical hernias in a swine herd, *J Am Vet Med Assoc* 204: 1660-1663, 1994.

CHAPTER 22

SURGERY OF THE SWINE MUSCULOSKELETAL SYSTEM

Guy St. Jean, David E. Anderson

Digit Amputation

Digit amputation is indicated when severe foot abscesses or septic arthritis of the interphalangeal joints have caused unmanageable damage to a single digit (Figure 22-1). Radiography, if elected, may show the extent of the lesion (Figure 22-2A and B). These injuries are most commonly caused by wounds from trauma on concrete flooring or metal side panels. The decision for amputation should not be delayed. Digit amputation will not be curative if the infection extends to the fetlock or more proximally on the limb. Also, the soundness of the opposite digit should be assessed to determine whether the pig will be able to ambulate on the remaining digit after amputation.

After induction of general anesthesia, the affected digit is cleaned and prepared for surgery. A tourniquet is placed proximal to the surgery site to prevent extensive hemorrhage during surgery. A circumferential incision is made through the skin and soft tissues at a 45-degree angle to the coronary band, starting at the axial aspect of the digit and continuing proximally to the abaxial surface. The skin is reflected proximal to the site being amputated, and a sterile obstetrical wire is used to amputate the digit. The distal phalanx and a portion of the middle phalanx are removed by this procedure. The remaining tissues are debrided and cleaned thoroughly. The foot is placed in a padded bandage for 10 to 14 days. The foot is cleaned daily with water until the wound is healed. Perioperative antibiotics and antiinflammatory drugs are indicated.

Ankylosis of the Proximal or Distal Interphalangeal Joint

Septic arthritis of the proximal or distal interphalangeal joint is an indication for digit amputation. However, the lateral claw of the hind limb is important for normal ambulation and breeding activity. Salvage of the digit by facilitated ankylosis is an option to preserve normal ambulation. The affected pig is placed under general anesthesia and the digit prepared for surgery. A 1-cm incision is made into the affected joint. A 3.75-cm-long needle is inserted distally immediately proximal to the coronary band for an approach to the distal interphalangeal joint. The proximal interphalangeal joint may be located by palpation or inserting the needle into the midpastern region. After the arthrotomy has been made, a 4- or 6-mm diameter drill bit is used to destroy the articular surfaces of the joint. Curettes are used to debride the joint and remove all infected subchondral bone. A distinct difference in texture and hardness will be noted between the necrotic (gritty and irregular) and healthy (smooth and hard) bone. Thorough curettage of all infected bone is critical to establishing effective joint ankylosis. The tissues are extensively lavaged with normal saline, and antibiotics are administered for 10 to 14 days. Strict confinement for 6 to 8 weeks is needed for ankylosis to occur. A cast extending from the ground to the carpus or hock will hasten convalescence.

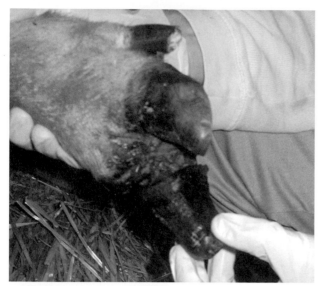

Figure 22-1   Pig with severe septic arthritis of the distal interphalangeal joint. Note that the claw is sloughing.

(Courtesy of Dr. Christopher Beinlich; Cornell University.)

Fracture Repair

Swine with fractured long bones are often salvaged because economic considerations preclude treatment. However, veterinarians may be asked to treat fractures in swine of potential value for genetic improvement.

Treatment of fractures can be rewarding, and Vaughan reported clinical experiences with fracture fixation in commercial swine. Fracture injuries were associated with breeding (two pigs), slipping on concrete flooring (three pigs), fighting (one pig), and unknown causes (five pigs). The most common fractures treated were tibia and fibula (five pigs), femur (three pigs), humerus (two pigs), and tibiotarsal joint luxation with fracture of the fibula (two pigs). Affected pigs weighed between 64 and 168 kg and were 6 months to 2 years old. Fracture of the tibia and fibula were treated by open reduction and internal fixation by using a bone plate and a full limb cast (three pigs) or by using only a full limb cast (two pigs). Fracture of the femur was treated by applying a bone plate (three pigs). Humerus fractures were treated by confinement (one pig) or applying a bone plate (one pig). A tibiotarsal joint luxation—combined with a fractured fibula—was treated by applying a bone plate and using a full limb cast (two pigs). Ten out of twelve pigs returned to normal production use, and two were salvaged (one pig with tibiotarsal joint luxation developed *E. coli osteomyelitis;* one pig with a humeral fracture repaired by internal fixation suffered permanent radial nerve damage).

Surgical repair of an articular fracture of the humeral condyles has been reported for miniature pigs. Fractures were repaired by using lag screw and Kirschner wire fixation. Five pigs were reexamined two months after

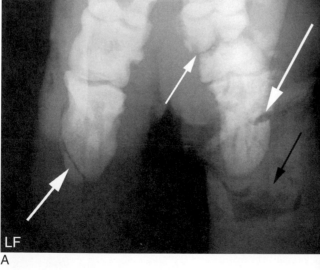

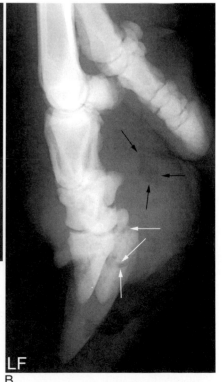

Figure 22-2   *A,* Dorsoproximal and *B,* lateral radiographs of the left thoracic-limb digit in a 2-year old female-intact porcine with left thoracic-limb lameness. Note the fractures in the middle and distal phalanges of the third digit and the distal phalanx of the fourth digit *(white arrows).* Also, in the soft tissues of the claw, there are multiple gas opacities *(black arrows).* The diagnosis in this patient was chronic pathologic fractures secondary to osteomyelitis and cellulitis.

(Courtesy of Dr. Anthony Pease; Cornell University.)

surgery, and all were walking soundly at that time. Femoral fractures were diagnosed in 20 pigs over a 6-month period. Nutritional analysis revealed inadequate calcium and phosphorus (both in absolute concentration and calcium to phosphorus ratio) in the feed. Affected pigs were approximately 20 weeks old and weighed between 80 and 90 kg. Pigs walked with a stilted gait and arched back. Necropsy found separation of the proximal femoral epiphysis from the femoral neck. After correction of dietary calcium and phosphorus, clinical evidence of a femoral fracture was not observed in any additional pigs. Femoral, pelvic, and vertebral fractures have been found in pigs after accidental electrical shock. Pigs with multiple trauma injuries and fractures associated with nutritional deficiency are poor candidates for surgical repair. Fracture of the greater trochanter of the femur has also been identified as a cause of lameness in pigs.

RECOMMENDED READINGS

Bildfell RJ, Carnat BD, Lister DB: Posterior paresis and electrocution of swine caused by accidental electric shock, *J Vet Diag Investig* 3: 364-367, 1991.

Blowey RW: Trochanter fracture and patellar osteochondrosis as causes of lameness in pigs, *Vet Rec* 134: 601-603, 1994.

Payne JT, Braun WF, Anderson DE et al: Articular fractures of the distal portion of the humerus in Vietnamese pot-bellied pigs: six cases (1988-1992), *J Am Vet Med Assoc* 206: 59-62, 1995.

Rousseaux CG, Gill I, Payne-Crosten A: Femoral fractures in pigs associated with calcium deficiency, *Austral Vet J* 57: 508-510, 1981.

Vaughan LC: The repair of fractures in pigs, *Vet Rec* 79: 2-8, 1966.

CHAPTER 23

SURGERY OF THE SWINE REPRODUCTIVE SYSTEM AND URINARY TRACT

Guy St. Jean, David E. Anderson

Male

CASTRATION OF PIGLETS

Castration of pigs is routinely performed in attempts to improve performance, feed conversion, carcass traits, and make management easier than for intact pigs. Boar meat becomes tainted with an unpleasant odor and taste at the onset of puberty. However, age recommendations for pig castration vary. The stress of pig castration was evaluated at 1, 2, 4, 8, 16, and 24 days of age (White, et al, 1995). This study indicated that pigs castrated after administration of lidocaine anesthetic subcutaneously and around the spermatic cords had a lower heart rate and less vocalization than pigs castrated without local anesthesia. This effect was greatest for pigs castrated after 8 days of age. Behavioral changes associated with castration were evaluated in pigs castrated at 1, 5, 10, 15, and 20 days of age. Castration caused reduced suckling, reduced standing, and increased lying time in comparison to intact male pigs at all ages. Pigs castrated at 14 days old were heavier at weaning and had a higher gain rate in comparison to pigs castrated at 1 day old. Administration of aspirin or butorphanol failed to improve castration-associated reduction in feeding time and weight gain. Administration of lidocaine anesthesia before castration prevented castration-induced nursing behavior suppression in 2-week-old pigs. This effect was not observed for pigs castrated at 7 weeks old. Pigs castrated at 2 weeks of age had less pronounced behavioral changes than pigs castrated at 7 weeks of age. Therefore we recommend piglets be castrated at 2 weeks of age to minimize castration stress and maximize performance until weaning.

Two-week-old pigs can be castrated by suspending them by the hind limbs while they are laid across a smooth rail. The surgical site is prepared for aseptic surgery. If used, lidocaine anesthetic is injected subcutaneously (0.5 ml per site) into tissue overlying each testis and spermatic cord (0.5 ml per site) in the inguinal canal. A 1-cm incision is made over each testis, and the testes are pulled from the scrotum. Hemorrhage is minimal at this age. Ligation of the spermatic cord is recommended for older pigs (see Castration of Older Pigs). Topic antiseptic ointment or spray may be applied at this time. Systemic antibiotics are usually not required, except for castration of older pigs. Castrated piglets are placed under a heat lamp in the farrowing crate for convalescence.

CASTRATION OF OLDER PIGS

Veterinarians may be asked to castrate older pigs intended for show or mature boars that will no longer be used for breeding. Castration of older pigs is best performed with the pig sedated or under general anesthesia. The boar is restrained in lateral recumbency, and the surgical site is aseptically prepared (Figure 23-1A). A 4- to 6-cm incision is made overlying the testis at the ventral aspect of the scrotum. The testis should be removed with the vaginal tunic intact (Figure 23-1B). Inguinal fat and

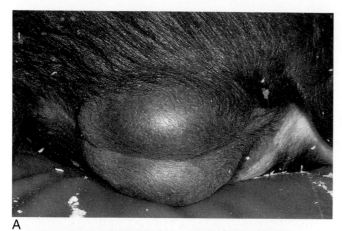

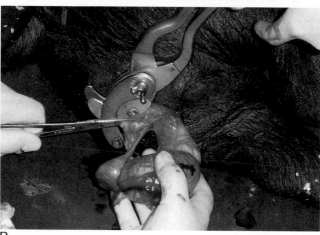

Figure 23-1   A, Boar under general anesthesia in lateral recumbency prior to castration. B, The testes are removed within the vaginal tunic.

(Courtesy of Dr. Christopher Beinlich; Cornell University.)

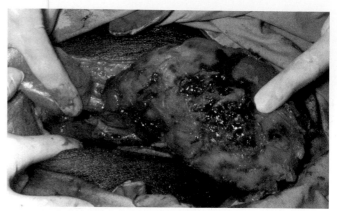

Figure 23-2   Boar with testicular torsion. Note swollen hemorrhagic testis.

(Courtesy of Dr. Andre Desrochers; University of Montreal.)

soft tissue are stripped from the spermatic cord and evaluated for the presence of an inguinal hernia. The vaginal tunic and spermatic cord are twisted until the cord is tightly compressed to the level of the external inguinal ring (see Figure 23-6). Two circumferential ligatures (No. 1 synthetic absorbable suture material) are placed around the vaginal tunic and spermatic cord. An emasculator (see Figure 4.4-8A and B) is used to complete the castration (see Figure 23-1B). Closure of the surgical wound is rarely done and should only be performed if asepsis has been maintained. We prefer to administer antibiotics for 3 days, beginning the day of surgery, to reduce the incidence of postoperative infection. Also, the animal should be kept in a clean, dry stall during this period.

The most common complications after pig castration are hemorrhage, abscess, scirrhus cord, inguinal hernia, and seroma or hematoma formation. Fatal hemorrhagic shock has been reported after castration of 7 week old

pigs by a lay person. The testes had been pulled through a 10-cm incision and cut using a knife. Fatal hemorrhage occurred into the pelvic canal and abdomen; therefore the cause of death was not recognized until necropsy. This report emphasizes the need for routine necropsy to determine the cause of all non-apparent deaths. Meat inspection of 131 pigs with postcastration abscesses revealed that *Actinomyces pyogenes, β-hemolytic Streptococci, Streptococcus viridans, Staphylococcus aureus,* and *Pasteurella multocida* were the most common bacteria isolated. Approximately 65% of the abscesses were monomicrobial, and 35% were polymicrobial infections. Of the 131 pigs inspected, 11% were judged to be unfit for human consumption. Bilateral hydronephrosis also has been reported as a complication of castration in a Hampshire pig castrated at 8 weeks old. A ventral midline incision was used to remove both testes and tincture of iodine applied after castration. Infection of the soft tissues occurred, and the ensuing infection resulted in progressive occlusion of urethra at the level of the sigmoid flexure. Chronic resistance to urine outflow caused hydronephrosis, and the pig died 4 weeks after castration. This case illustrates the importance of adequate ventral drainage after castration.

UNILATERAL CASTRATION

Indications for removing only one testis include testicular trauma, torsion (Figure 23-2), hematoma (Figure 23-3), seroma, and orchitis or periorchitis. The damaged testis may cause enough swelling, heat, and pressure to reduce fertility. The boar is placed under general anesthesia, a 6-cm incision is made over the testis starting at the most ventral aspect of the scrotum, and the testis is removed by circumferential ligation and excision. The wound should be left open for drainage and second

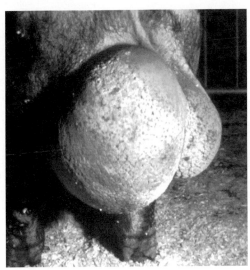

Figure 23-3   Boar with testicular hematoma. Note swollen scrotum.

(Courtesy of Dr. Andre Desrochers; University of Montreal.)

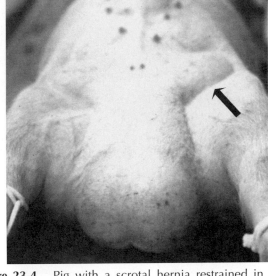

Figure 23-4   Pig with a scrotal hernia restrained in dorsal recumbency. Note swelling in left scrotum and left inguinal area (arrow).

intention healing. Antibiotics are administered for 5 to 7 days, and daily hydrotherapy is used to minimize postoperative swelling. Affected boars may return to productive service 30 to 60 days after surgery.

INGUINAL HERNIA

Inguinal hernia results when a defect permits intestines or other abdominal organs to pass into the inguinal canal. The hernia develops when an abnormally large and patent vaginal ring allows free communication between the vaginal tunic and peritoneal cavities. Organs protrude into the scrotum to form a scrotal hernia, a more exaggerated form of the defect (Figure 23-4). These hernias are common in swine. The frequency of inguinal hernia among the porcine population varied between 0% and 15.7%, with a realistic estimate of approximately 1%. The development of these hernias seems to be genetically influenced. One study indicated that the variation associated with anatomic structures relevant to scrotal hernia is influenced polygenically. In that study, the heritabilities of susceptibility to scrotal hernia development were estimated to be 0.29, 0.34, and 0.34 in Duroc, Landrance, and Yorkshire-sired pig groups, respectively. Inguinal (see Figure 23-4) and scrotal hernias need to be differentiated from hydrocele, scirrhous cord, and hematoma (see Figure 23-3) of the testis. Diagnosis is made by historical data (e.g., a pig that has been castrated before is more likely to have a scirrhous cord) and direct manipulation. If necessary, ultrasonography and needle aspiration can be used. Inguinal hernias often are encountered at the time of castration. Some of these

hernias will reduce spontaneously but recur later. With chronic inguinal hernia, intestinal incarceration and strangulation may be observed.

Surgical repair of an inguinal or scrotal hernia is easier before the pig is castrated. With the pig restrained in dorsal recumbency and its rear quarters elevated, the inguinal and scrotal area is thoroughly cleaned and prepared for surgery. An oblique incision is made over the affected superficial inguinal ring (Figure 23-5). Once the incision pierces the skin, the subcutaneous tissue is dissected bluntly. The tunica vaginalis is also isolated by blunt dissection (see Figure 23-5). The tunica vaginalis should be kept intact, because this will keep the intestine contained. While external pressure is put on the scrotum, the tunics are gently pulled free from their scrotal attachment. The tunic and testis are then twisted to force the intestines into the peritoneal cavity (Figure 23-6). The tunics and spermatic cord are transfixated as close to the superficial inguinal ring as possible. The tunic and cord are cut, and the superficial inguinal ring is closed with interrupted or horizontal mattress sutures. The herniorrhaphy site is checked by applying external pressure on the abdomen. The skin is closed using absorbable sutures. The authors recommend checking the opposite inguinal ring for possible bilateral herniation before performing a castration. If the surgery was done to repair a large hernia in which marked serum accumulation in the scrotum is expected, an incision in the most ventral aspect of the scrotum should be performed to provide ventral drainage. If intestinal adhesion and incarceration are observed during surgical correction, the vaginal tunic

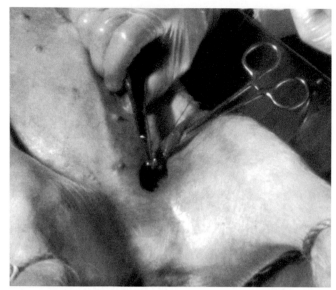

Figure 23-5 Pig restrained in dorsal recumbency; an oblique incision is made over the affected superficial inguinal ring and the vaginal tunic isolated.

(Courtesy of Dr. Andre Desrochers; University of Montreal.)

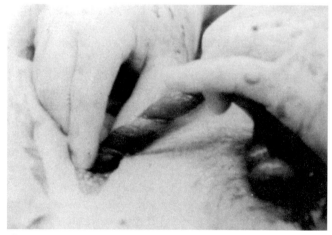

Figure 23-6 Surgical repair of an inguinal hernia showing the tunic and testis being twisted to force the intestines into the peritoneal cavity.

should be opened and the intestine dissected free or an intestinal resection and end-to-end anastomosis performed. If an inguinal hernia occurs after castration, one needs to clean and lavage the herniated bowel, enlarge the vaginal and superficial inguinal ring, and replace the prolapsed intestine (if it is judged still viable) before suturing the superficial inguinal ring closed.

CRYPTORCHIDISM

Veterinarians may be presented with barrows (male hogs castrated before sexual maturity) that demonstrate boar-

like traits for removal of retained testicular tissues. The testes of swine descend in the last 30 days of gestation and should be palpable at birth. True cryptorchidism (testis not descended at birth) is a common congenital defect in swine. A homozygous recessive trait involving two gene loci has been postulated based on a breeding trial of cryptorchid Duroc swine. Cryptorchid testes are usually intraabdominal and are found midway between the ipsilateral kidney and deep inguinal ring. However, the affected testis may be located within the inguinal canal and not readily palpable from either the inguinal region or peritoneal cavity. Previous removal of the descended testis makes surgical removal of the retained testis more difficult because the incision is best made over the affected superficial inguinal ring. Often, determining which testis has been removed is difficult. The authors prefer to perform cryptorchid surgery with the pig under general anesthesia. A 6-cm incision is made over the appropriate superficial inguinal ring. Laparotomy may be performed by making an incision 1- to 2-cm medial to the inguinal canal (parainguinal incision), or the superficial inguinal ring may be enlarged by starting the incision at the cranial commissure of the superficial inguinal ring. The fingers of one hand are used to perform an exploration of the abdominal cavity, starting at the pelvic brim and searching along the dorsal and lateral abdominal wall until the kidneys are encountered. For show pigs, we prefer to perform laparoscopic exploration and removal of abdominal testes because better cosmesis, fewer incisional complications, and more rapid incisional healing are achieved.

True cryptorchidism should be differentiated from ectopic testicular tissue. Ectopic testicular tissue has been observed in numerous pigs at the time of slaughter. These tissues occur as smooth, pink, or tan nodules on the surface of the liver, spleen, mesentery, and other abdominal viscera. Initially, these masses may be interpreted as metastatic neoplasia, but histology reveals the presence of convoluted seminiferous tubules and interstitial cells. No evidence for neoplasia is seen. Ectopic testicular tissues may be found in castrated or intact male pigs.

PREPARATION OF TEASER BOARS

Vasectomy or epididymectomy is done to produce teaser boars—which are used to detect sows in heat for artificial insemination or breeding to valuable boars—or to promote onset of cyclicity in confined gilts (young females). For vasectomy, the boar is placed in dorsal recumbency under general anesthesia, and a 4-cm incision is made over each spermatic cord approximately 6 cm cranial to the ventral aspect of the scrotum. Each spermatic cord is elevated and incised, and the ductus deferens isolated. The ductus deferens is firm and pale, and an arterial pulse is not present (see Figure 19.1-10). A 3- to 4-cm segment of the ductus deferens is excised and each end ligated. The incision through the tunic is sutured with No. 2-0 PDS synthetic absorbable suture material, and the skin is sutured with No. 0 nonabsorbable suture material in a simple interrupted pattern. Epididymectomy is done by making a 2-cm incision in the scrotum overlying the tail of the epididymis. The tail and 1 cm of the body of the epididymis is isolated. Ligatures are placed between the testis and the tail of the epididymis and around the exposed portion of the body of the epididymis. The epididymis is excised between these two ligatures. The skin is closed with No. 0 nonabsorbable sutures in an interrupted pattern.

PROLAPSED PENIS

Penile and preputial prolapse have been seen after administration of neuroleptic drugs but also may occur as a result of trauma to the penis. The authors diagnosed congenital penile prolapse in a litter of Vietnamese pot-bellied pigs. All males in the litter were affected. While prolapsed, the penis is at great risk of further injury. The penis and prepuce must be returned to their normal position as soon as possible after prolapse. Treatment of penile prolapse usually requires the boar be placed under general anesthesia. The penis is thoroughly cleaned with cold water and a topic antiseptic ointment applied to its surface. If a penile wound is present, debridement may be done. Penile wounds typically are not sutured closed unless they have occurred within 2 to 4 hours because of the likelihood an abscess will form. The penis and prepuce are gently massaged until reduction into the sheath is completed. Use of hydroscopic agents (e.g., anhydrous glycerin) may help reduce the swelling by resolving edema. After the penis and prepuce have been repositioned, a pursestring suture may be used to prevent reoccurrence of the prolapse. The purse string should be removed in 5 to 7 days. If wounds or abrasions are present, daily preputial lavage or administration of systemic antibiotics and antiinflammatory drugs is indicated. If wounds are not present, sexual rest should be enforced for at least 14 days. If wounds that require treatment are present, sexual rest should be enforced for 30 to 60 days. Reevaluation of the penile injury is advisable before use for mating. In cases of congenital penile prolapse, penopexy was used to maintain normal penile retention, but all males were castrated and used as pets.

PERSISTENT FRENULUM

The epithelial attachment of the penis and prepuce atrophies and these tissues separate between 4 and 6 months old in boars. Sexual maturity is achieved by 7 to 8 months of age. Persistence of the frenulum attachment between the penis and prepuce beyond sexual maturity causes failure of breeding soundness. Surgical removal of the persistent frenulum is performed with the boar under general anesthesia or during a hand mating exercise. Resection of the tissue may be performed with scissors. Ligation is not required in most cases, but can be done, and minimal bleeding is observed after excision (Figure 12.1.5-8A to C). Sexual rest should be enforced for 7 to 10 days after surgery.

PREPUTIAL PROLAPSE

Prolapse of the internal lamina of the prepuce may occur with penile prolapse or may result from preputial injury and swelling. If wounds to the prepuce are not present, the internal lamina may be repositioned within the sheath, as described for penile prolapse, and a pursestring suture used to maintain the reduction. Careful evaluation of the preputial swelling should be done to ensure that urination is possible. Preputial edema may be reduced by application of hydroscopic agents. A preputial retaining tube, constructed from rubber or polyurethane tubing, may be placed into the preputial cavity to prevent prolapse but allow exit of urine.

Often, the prolapsed internal lamina has been traumatized, and surgical removal of the affected tissues is indicated. Preputial amputation may be performed, but the opening to the preputial diverticulum must be maintained. Alternatively, the preputial diverticulum may be removed at the time of surgery. The boar is placed under general anesthesia, the internal lamina is pulled cranially until normal preputial epithelium is exposed and stay sutures or crossed pins (7.6-cm, 18-gauge needles) are placed through the exposed internal lamina to prevent premature retraction into the sheath. The damaged tissues are amputated, and the two layers of internal lamina are sutured closed in an interrupted suture pattern. After anastomosis, antiseptic ointment is placed on the internal lamina, and it is replaced into the sheath. A pursestring suture is placed at the preputial orifice for 7 to 10 days and sexual rest is enforced for 30 to 60 days. Systemic antibiotics should be administered perioperatively.

RESECTION OF PREPUTIAL DIVERTICULUM

Abnormalities of the preputial diverticulum may cause reproductive unsoundness. Preputial diverticulitis (Figure 23-7A), diverticular ulcers, urine retention, and penile deviation into the diverticulum may be found. Preputial diverticulectomy may restore breeding soundness to affected boars. The boar is placed under general anesthesia and prepared for surgery. Any of the following three procedures for diverticulectomy (Figure 23-7B) may be performed: 1) preputial diverticulectomy via the preputial orifice is done by passing forceps through the preputial orifice, into one lobe of the bilobate diver-

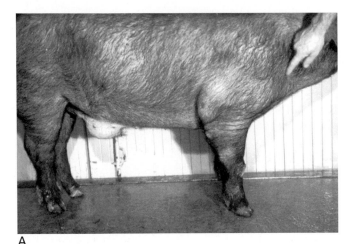

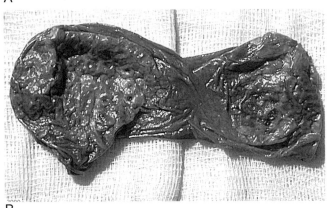

Figure 23-7 *A,* Preputial diverticulitis in a boar. *B,* Excised diverticulum.

(Courtesy of Dr. Andre Desrochers; University of Montreal.)

ticulum, while gently everting the lobe out through the orifice, and repeating this procedure for the remaining lobe. After both lobes of the preputial diverticulum are everted, the diverticulum is excised. Suturing is not required for young boars, but the opening to the diverticulum may be sutured closed in adults. 2) A 6-cm incision is made overlying the lateral aspect of one lobe of the preputial diverticulum. The diverticulum is everted through the preputial orifice, excised, and sutured closed. 3) A 6-cm incision is made as described previously, but the diverticulum is dissected free from the surrounding soft tissues, excised, and sutured closed. For methods 2 and 3 above, extreme care must be taken not to perforate the diverticulum before removal because contamination will result in incisional infection. Flushing the preputial diverticulum with antiseptic solutions before surgery is recommended to reduce this possibility. Also, filling the diverticulum with antiseptic solution or gauze pads before surgery makes identification of the diverticulum easier at the time of surgery.

Female

VAGINAL PROLAPSE

Vaginal prolapse occurs as a prepartum event (Figure 23-8). The cause of vaginal prolapse is unknown, but straining to urinate or defecate may be involved. Sows with lateral deviation of the bladder and difficulty urinating or with inflammation associated with cystitis and urethritis may develop vaginal prolapse because of straining. When the cause can be found, treatment should be aimed at resolving the initial lesion. After appropriate anesthesia of the sow, the prolapsed vagina is cleaned with cold water; hydroscopic agents are applied; a towel is wrapped around the prolapsed portion; and constant gentle pressure is used to reduce the edema and swelling. The prolapse can usually be reduced in 15 to 20 minutes. The vagina should be cleansed and topical antibiotic or antiseptic ointments used to reduce the secondary bacterial vaginitis that invariably occurs. Administration of antiinflammatory drugs may reduce straining and shorten convalescence. The bladder should be evaluated to ensure it is in a normal position. A Buhner suture (see Figure 4.4-17A-C) is placed around the vagina to prevent reoccurrence of the prolapse. The sow should be closely monitored and the Buhner suture removed at the first indication of farrowing. If excessive swelling of the soft tissues in the pelvic cavity has occurred, a cesarean section is indicated and should be performed early in the process of farrowing.

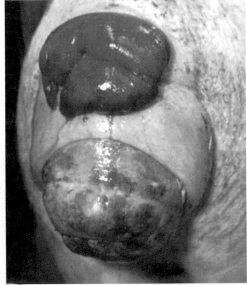

Figure 23-8 Sow with vaginal and rectal prolapse.

(Courtesy of Dr. Mary Smith; Cornell University.)

BLADDER DISPLACEMENT OR RETROVERSION

Displacement of the bladder occurs in multiparous sows in the latter stages of gestation. The bladder is displaced laterally and occasionally may become displaced caudally. The displaced bladder results in a swollen appearance to the vagina (Figure 23-9A and B). Bladder displacement results in difficulty with urination. The displaced bladder may give the appearance of a vaginal prolapse when the sow is lying down. Affected sows may be seen straining because of the difficulty urinating, and this may lead to true vaginal prolapse or rectal prolapse (see Figure 23-9A and B). Decompression of the urinary bladder by cystocentesis or catheterization may allow permanent replacement of the bladder. When displacement recurs, an indwelling urinary catheter may be used to allow urination until after parturition (Figure 23-9C). Ascending bacterial cystitis is a complication of the indwelling urinary catheter.

OOPHORECTOMY

Removal of the ovaries is rarely indicated in swine. However, oophorectomy may be requested to facilitate research or for pet pigs. For pet pigs, removal of the ovaries is easier, faster, and has less risk of fatal hemorrhage than ovariohysterectomy (OVX). The blood vessels of the broad ligaments of the uterus are extensive and require ligation when OVX is chosen. Both ovaries may be removed from a paralumbar (flank), ventrolateral, paramedian, or ventral midline incision. In large, obese pigs, we prefer to perform ovariectomy via a left or right flank incision with general anesthesia. For a paralumbar approach, the incision is started ventral to the transverse processes of the lumbar vertebrae, midway between the tuber coxae and the last rib. In young pigs, the ventral midline laparotomy approach is preferred because of owners' cosmetic concerns. Each ovary is elevated through the incision; two hemostatic forceps are placed on the ovarian pedicle; two ligatures (No 2-0 absorbable suture material) are placed proximal to the first hemostat; the pedicle is cut between the two hemostats; and the ovary removed. Each ovarian artery must be observed for hemorrhage prior to closure. Paralumbar incisions are closed in three layers (transversus abdominis m + peritoneum, internal + external abdominal oblique m, skin). Ovariectomy alone may be performed in pet pigs that have not begun normal estrus cycles. Uterine atrophy is expected to occur after ovariectomy. We recommend OVX in sexually mature pigs because of the potential risk for pyometra in a uterus in which the cervix has been open.

HYSTERECTOMY

Elective hysterectomy is rarely done in commercial swine. However, hysterectomy may be requested for research purposes or for pet pigs. When hysterectomy is performed for pet pigs, the ovaries also are removed.

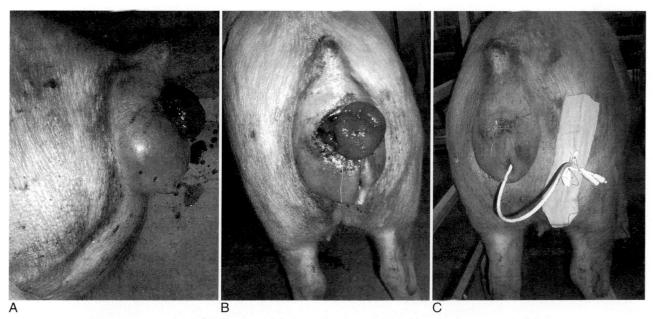

A   B   C

Figure 23-9   *A,* lateral and *B,* caudal view of a sow with bladder displacement and associated rectal prolapse. *C,* Treatment involves catheterization of the bladder until farrowing.

(Courtesy of Dr. Mary Smith; Cornell University.)

General anesthesia should be used during hysterectomy. The uterus may be removed via a flank, ventrolateral, paramedian, or ventral midline incision. We prefer to perform hysterectomy via either flank or ventral midline incision. The uterus is elevated through the incision; the ovaries are removed as described earlier; the mesometrium (broad ligament of the uterus) is ligated with two to four overlapping simple interrupted sutures for mass ligation of the blood vessels; and transfixation ligatures are placed in the uterine body immediately cranial to the internal os of the cervix. The uterus and ovaries are removed and the incision closed as described previously. All sutured pedicles should be checked for adequate hemostasis before closure.

CESAREAN SECTION

Cesarean section is required when transcervical extraction of pigs from the uterus is not possible and to obtain gnotobiotic or specific pathogen-free pigs. Cesarean section for gnotobiotic pigs is usually performed with the sow under general anesthesia. Cesarean section for dystocia is usually chosen as a last resort procedure for fetal extraction because of economic pressures. Therefore the mortality rate among sows and gilts that have cesarean section is expected to be higher than for other species. This is not surprising because affected swine suffer extreme physical exhaustion, stress, and shock by the time the decision for cesarean section is made. Owners and veterinarians may become reluctant to perform cesarean section because of expense, previous experiences with fatalities, and the high rate of dead pigs delivered. Our opinion is that unnecessary delays in the decision for surgery is the principle cause of sow and baby pig mortality associated with cesarean section. When the veterinarian is presented with a sow in dystocia, it should be ascertained as early as possible during the initial examination whether the owner is willing to incur the costs of cesarean section. Other factors that influence the decision for cesarean section include the cause of dystocia, how long the sow has been in labor, how long the owner has tried to manually extract the pigs, and how swollen or traumatized the sow's pelvic canal has become. Many owners are adept at extracting pigs, and their failure to successfully remove pigs may justify immediate cesarean section if the cause of dystocia is not apparent. In our experience, cesarean section performed at the earliest indication has a high success rate for sow survival and rate of live pigs obtained.

Swine that are physically exhausted, stressed, or in shock must be stabilized before cesarean section. Among sows necropsied after sudden death, retained fetuses and toxemia were found in approximately 10%. Stabilization of the sow often is simple and readily achieved. We rou-tinely place a 16- or 18-gauge, 2-inch (5.08-cm) intravenous catheter in an ear vein. This catheter is sutured or glued in place and intravenous fluids (0.9% saline or Lactated Ringer's Solution) administered rapidly (initially 20 to 40 ml/kg of body weight/hour, then 4 ml/kg/hour once stabilized) and continued for the duration of the surgery. The authors prefer to add dextrose (1.25% final solution) and calcium (1 ml/kg) to intravenous fluids *after* the patient has been stabilized. The metabolic shock status of the sow may be improved further by administration of flunixin meglumine (1 mg/kg IV). Because extensive manipulation of the intrauterine environment before cesarean section increases the risk for postoperative septic peritonitis, we prefer to administer preoperative antibiotics (procaine penicillin G, 10,000 IU/kg IM or ceftiofur HCl, 3 to 5 mg/kg IM). In severely compromised sows, sedation and local or regional anesthesia may be adequate for surgery. Epidural anesthesia (lumbosacral level) also may be useful.

Multiple surgical approaches have been described for cesarean section. Selection of the surgical approach depends upon the preference of the surgeon, the condition of the patient, and means of restraint and anesthesia used for surgery. The most common approaches are paralumbar fossa, ventrolateral (horizontal low flank), ventral midline, or paramedian. With a ventral or paramedian approach, movement by the sow must be prevented because of the risk for contamination of the incision. Also, the mammary veins must be carefully avoided or ligated to prevent excessive loss of blood during the procedure. In our experience, ventral and paramedian incisions have the highest risk for development of postoperative incisional infection. The ventrolateral incision is made parallel and axial to the fold of the flank and lateral to the mammary chain. The sow is placed in lateral recumbency with the uppermost hind limb tied in abduction and extension. The incision is started approximately 10 cm cranial to the inguinal region and extended cranially for 15 cm. For paralumbar fossa incision, the sow is placed in lateral recumbency, and the incision is made in the middle of the paralumbar fossa ventral to the transverse process (Figure 23-10A). The incision is extended ventrally to a point approximately 5 cm dorsal to the cranial skin fold of the flank. Ventrolateral and paralumbar incisions are relatively easy to perform, have little blood loss during surgery, and are less likely to become infected after surgery. After exteriorizing the closest uterine horn (Figure 23-10B), a 6- to 8-cm incision is made along the greater curvature of the uterus (Figure 23-10C) and as close to the bifurcation of the uterine horns as possible. All piglets may not be able to be removed from a single incision in the uterus; if necessary a second incision can be performed on the other uterine horn.

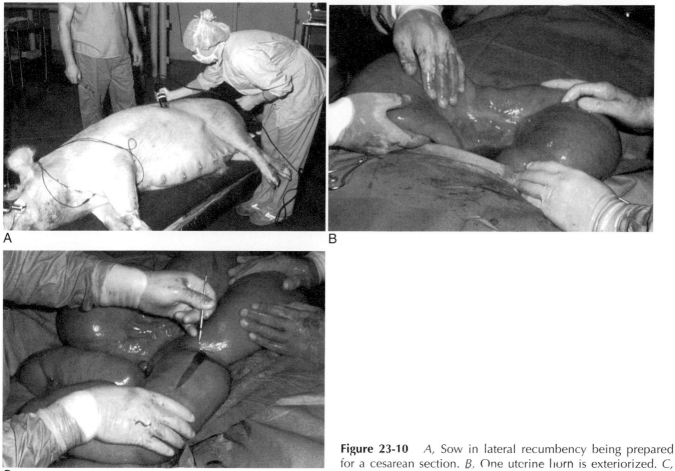

Figure 23-10 *A,* Sow in lateral recumbency being prepared for a cesarean section. *B,* One uterine horn is exteriorized. *C,* Longitudinal uterine incision.

Closure of the uterine incision is done with #1 synthetic absorbable suture material placed in a Cushing or Utrecht pattern. The authors close the transversus abdominis muscle and peritoneum together and the external abdominal oblique and internal abdominal oblique muscles together with synthetic absorbable suture material placed in simple continuous pattern. For closure of ventral midline or paramedian incisions, the authors use synthetic absorbable suture material placed in a simple interrupted or interrupted cruciate pattern in the linea alba or external rectus sheath. The subcutaneous tissues and skin are closed in a routine fashion. The sow should remain confined for a minimum of 14 days after surgery.

The production of gnotobiotic or specific pathogen-free pigs is an accepted model for scientific research. The selected sow should be placed under general anesthesia and the surgery site aseptically prepared. Several methods have been described for obtaining gnotobiotic pigs including hysterectomy, closed hysterotomy (using a sterile chamber attached to the side of the sow through which surgery is performed), and open hysterotomy with

germicidal trap. All methods are expected to have a baby pig mortality rate of less than 15%. When a hysterectomy technique is selected, baby pig survival is better when the surgery is performed with the sow under general anesthesia rather than euthanasia of the sow before hysterectomy.

UTERINE PROLAPSE
Prolapse of the uterus is occasionally seen in sows during or up to several days after parturition. Excessive straining (because of fetal malpositioning, fetal:maternal disproportion, or trauma with swelling and inflammation in the birth canal) is thought to cause uterine prolapse. Prolapse of the entire uterus has the greatest potential for a life-threatening crisis because of profuse hemorrhage, but partial prolapse also may occur. The sow must be stabilized before attempts to replace the uterus into its normal position. If hemorrhage, hypovolemia, or shock is present, the sow should be placed into a warm environment, an IV catheter placed into an auricular vein, and intravenous fluids administered. For replacement of

the prolapse, the sow may be placed on an inclined floor or platform in sternal recumbency with the hindquarters elevated. Epidural anesthesia (administered at the lumbosacral space), sedation, or general anesthesia may be required to eliminate struggling, straining, and agitation of the sow. The prolapsed uterus is thoroughly cleaned with physiologic warm saline and assessed for the presence of lacerations and necrosis. Small lacerations may be cleaned, superficially debrided, and sutured closed. Hemorrhage may be stopped by ligating affected vessels or by performing en bloc tissue imbrication. Sutures may be placed over stents to increase the region of pressure to control hemorrhage. Hydroscopic agents may be applied to the uterus to assist in reducing edema. The uterus is wrapped in a towel and gentle pressure applied, starting from the tip of the uterine horn and working toward the body of the uterus. After approximately 15 minutes, the edema should be sufficiently reduced to allow manipulation of the uterine horns. Each horn should be inverted starting with the tip and gradually reduced until the uterine body has been reached. The extensive edema and soft tissue swelling of the pelvic canal often impedes progress. When this occurs, a left paralumbar fossa laparotomy is indicated. After appropriate preparation of the surgical site a 10-cm, vertically-oriented incision is made in the middle of the left paralumbar fossae. The clinician's left arm is passed through the peritoneal cavity and into the everted uterus. One of the uterine horns is grasped and pulled back into the peritoneal cavity. The clinician's right arm or an assistant helps by applying gentle pressure on the everted horn from the outside. After the uterus has been repositioned, all remaining fetuses should be removed. The laparotomy incision should be closed in three layers (transversus abdominis m + peritoneum, internal + external abdominal oblique, skin). Antimicrobial and antiinflammatory medications are desirable, but strict attention should be paid to drug residues in the meat before slaughter. Finally, a Buhner suture should be placed around the vulva to prevent recurrence of the prolapse. The Buhner suture (6.4-mm wide sterile cotton tape) (Figure 4.4-17A and B) should be deeply placed at the junction of the labia and skin of the perineum to recreate the function of the vestibular sphincter muscle. The Buhner suture may be removed in 7 to 10 days with minimal risk of prolapse. Oxytocin (20 units) is routinely administered to facilitate contraction and involution of the uterus and cervix. If prolapse reduction using laparotomy is not used as a last resort treatment, sows should survive partial prolapse of the uterus (>75 % survival rate), but complete prolapse carries a guarded prognosis (<50 % survival rate).

Amputation of the uterus is indicated when excessive bleeding, extensive laceration, trauma, or necrosis of a uterine prolapse is found. Before amputation, the uterus should be closely inspected to ensure the bladder or small intestine is not entrapped. Hypovolemic or hemorrhagic shock may be present and should be addressed during the course of treatment. If the uterus is swollen, it should be elevated above the pig to encourage drainage of venous congestion. We recommend placing towels around the uterus so that pressure may be applied without further trauma to the wall of the uterus. Hydroscopic agents may be used to help resolve edema of the uterine tissues. After venous congestion has been reduced, amputation is more easily performed. Transfixation ligatures are placed around the circumference of the uterus. Heavy suture material (0.5-cm sterile cotton tape, #3 polymerized Caprolactam) is used because the thickness of the uterus requires extreme tension to completely occlude the uterine arteries. Stay sutures or cross pins (with 15-cm, 18-gauge needles) are placed in the vital uterus and the prolapsed portion amputated. Then any bleeders are ligated before the remaining tissues are released and placed back into the pelvic canal. A Buhner suture or pursestring suture should be placed into the labia at the level of the vestibular sphincter to prevent prolapse of the remaining tissues. Affected sows are salvaged as soon as possible or after weaning of the litter.

MASTECTOMY

Mastitis caused by *Actinomyces suis* may cause formation of abscesses, granulomas, and mammary fistulas. The swellings may become large and problematic for the sow (Figure 23-11). Surgical removal of the mammae is indicated for the sow's return to production soundness. Sows with at least 12 intact mammary glands that are not in the first week or last four weeks of gestation are suitable

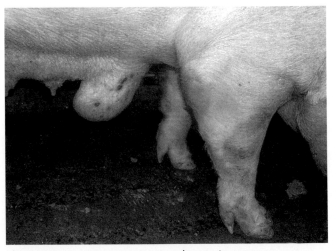

Figure 23-11   Mastitis-associated mass in a sow.

(Courtesy of Dr. Mary Smith; Cornell University.)

candidates for surgery. In pet pigs, mammary adenocarcinoma has been diagnosed. These tumors are found on routine health examination, including palpation of the mammary tissue. Tissue biopsy confirms diagnosis. The authors have performed partial mastectomy and complete mastectomy in several pet pigs. In no case, has metastasis been observed. The sow is placed under general anesthesia and the affected mammary gland prepared for aseptic surgery. An elliptical incision is made approximately 1 cm from the base of the swelling around the mammary gland so enough tissue remains to allow closure of the tissues with minimal tension. A combination of sharp and blunt dissection is used to extirpate the gland, granuloma, and abscesses. The cranial superficial epigastric vein should not be compromised, but hemostasis is essential. The subcutaneous tissue and skin are closed. Administration of perioperative antibiotics is indicated.

RECOMMENDED READINGS

Libke KG: Gross and histopathologic lesions in a field case of fatal hemorrhagic shock following orchectomy in young pigs, *Vet Med Sm An Clin* 62: 551-554, 1967.

McGavin MD, Schoneweis DA: Porcine bilateral hydronephrosis secondary to castration, *Cornell Vet* 62: 359-363, 1972.

McGlone JJ, Hellman JM: Local and general anesthetic effects on behavior and performance of two- and seven-week-old castrated and uncastrated piglets, *J Anim Sci* 66: 3049-3058, 1988.

McGlone JJ, Nicholson RI, Hellman JM, et al: The development of pain in young pigs associated with castration and attempts to prevent castration-induced behavioral changes, *J Anim Sci* 71: 1441-1446, 1993.

Miniats OP, Jol D: Gnotobiotic pigs: derivation and rearing, *Can J Comp Med* 42: 428-437, 1978.

Rothschild MF, Christian LL, Blanchard W: Evidence for multigene control of cryptorchidism in swine, *J Heredity* 79: 313-314, 1988.

Sanford SE, Josephson GKA, Rehmtulla AJ: Sudden death in sows, *Can Vet J* 35: 388, 1994.

Százados I: Judgement of castration-induced abscesses in pigs at meat inspection, *Acta Veterinaria Hungarica* 33: 177-184, 1985.

Todd GC, Nelson LW, Migaki G: Multiple heterotopic testicular tissue in the pig: a report of seven cases, *Cornell Vet* 48: 614-619, 1968.

Van Straaten HWM, Colenbrander B, Wensing CJG: Maldescended testis: consequences and attempted therapy in pigs, *J Fertil* 24: 74-75, 1979.

Vogt DW, Ellersieck MR: Heritability of susceptibility to scrotal herniation in swine, *Am J Vet Res* 51: 1501-1503, 1990.

White RG, DeShazer JA, Tressler CJ et al: Vocalization and physiological response of pigs during castration with or without a local anesthetic, *J Anim Sci* 73: 381-386, 1995.

APPENDIX 1

NORTH AMERICAN ANTIBIOTIC OPTIONS FOR PREVENTION AND TREATMENT OF FARM ANIMAL BACTERIAL INFECTIONS

Ava M. Trent and Norm G. Ducharme

DESCRIPTION	AMOXICILLIN	AMPICILLIN	CEFTIOFUR	FRYTHROMYCIN
TRADE NAME(S):	Amoxi-Bol (Bolus oral) Amoxi-Inject	Polyflex	Naxcel, Excenel	Gallimycin
MANUFACTURER(S):	SK Beecham	Fort Dodge	Pharmacia & Upjohn	Biomeda
DOSAGE(S):				
Cattle	6-10 mg/kg (2-5 mg/lb) SQ or IM q 24 hrs <5 days	6-10 mg/kg (2-5 mg/lb) SQ or IM q 24 hrs <7 days	1.1-2.2 mg/kg IM q 24 hrs 1.1-2.2 mg/kg SQ SID– Excenel	4-8 mg/kg IM SID or BID
Calves	7 mg/kg PO q 8-12 hrs			100 mg/ml females <14 days
Sheep, Goats				2.2 mg/kg IM SID
Swine				2.2-6.6 mg/kg IM SID
PRODUCTION STATUS/AGE				
All	X	X	X	
Nonveal calves <20 mos.	X (nonruminating)			X
Calves <20 mos.				
Dairy calves <20 mos.	X (nonruminating)			X
Beef cattle				X
Dairy bulls				
Dairy cows (lactating)				X[1]
SPECTRUM:				
Broad				
Anaerobes	<penicillin	<penicillin		X
G+ Aerobes	X	X		X
G– Aerobes	Some	Some	X	Some
Staphylococcus	Variable	Variable	X	

DESCRIPTION	AMOXICILLIN	AMPICILLIN	CEFTIOFUR	ERYTHROMYCIN
WITHDRAWAL:	Depends on formula			
Cattle				
Milk	0	48 hrs	None	72 hrs
Meat	20 days calves, 25 days	6 days	0 Naxcel, 48 hrs Excenel	14 days
Sheep, Goats	A	A	A	A
Milk				
Meat				
Swine	A	A	A	A
Milk				
Meat				
ADVANTAGES:				Active in fibrin and abscess. Injectable 100 mg/ml Gallimycin approved for cattle.
RESTRICTIONS:			Efficacy uncertain with pus, fibrin and necrotic debris.	Significant tissue damage and pain at injection site. Oral forms risk severe diarrhea. No advantage over other agents.

DESCRIPTION	FLORFENICOL	OXYTETRACYCLINE	PENICILLIN	ENROFLOXACIN
TRADES NAME(S):	Nuflor	100 mg/ml[B] 200 mg/ml[B]	penicillin K injection[D] procaine penicillin G[B]	Baytril
MANUFACTURER(S):	Schering-Plough	The Butler Co, Columbus, OH Pfizer Animal Health, Exton, PA	Pfizer, New York GC Hanford, Syracuse, NY	Bayer
DOSAGE(S):				
Cattle	20 mg/kg IM (neck)	5-10 mg/kg IM SID or 20 mg/kg q 48-22 hrs 2.5-5 mg/kg IV SID 10-20 mg/kg PO SID	44,000-66,000 Units/kg IM SQ SID	2.5-5 mg/kg SQ single dose 2.5-5 mg/kg q 24 hrs × 3 days IM
Calves				
Sheep, Goats		6-11 mg/kg IV or IM BID 10-20 mg/kg PO QID		
Swine		Same as sheep, goats	40,000 IV/kg SID	
PRODUCTION STATUS/AGE				
All		X	X	
Nonveal calves <20 mos.	X			X
Calves <20 mos.				
Dairy calves <20 mos.				
Beef cattle	<Breeding age			X
Dairy bulls				X
Dairy cows (lactating)	<20 mos			
SPECTRUM:				
Broad	X (treat BRD)			
Anaerobes			X	Poor
G+ Aerobes			X	Variable
G- Aerobes				X
Staphylococcus				X
WITHDRAWAL:				
Cattle				
Milk	NA	96 hrs (LA 200)[2]	48 hrs[2]	NA[3]
Meat	28 (IM) or 38 (SQ) days	28 days[2]	10 days[2]	28 days
Sheep, Goats	A	A		A
Milk			48 hrs[2]	
Meat			9 days[2]	

DESCRIPTION	FLORFENICOL	OXYTETRACYCLINE	PENICILLIN	ENROFLOXACIN
Swine	A	A		A
Milk			48 hrs[2]	
Meat			7 days[2]	
ADVANTAGES:		Infrequent use is helpful. Some penetration and activity in abscess.	Combined gives good broad spectrum. Aqueous IV fast initial high levels.	
RESTRICTIONS:	Little abscess efficacy.	Do not use first half of pregnancy. IV chelation of calcium exacerbates hypocalcemia.	Fibrin and necrotic debris limits efficacy. Aqueous costly and short half life. Benzathine inadequate serum or tissue levels.	Use allowed in beef cattle only. Dairy cattle use illegal. Cartilage abnormality is risk.

DESCRIPTION	POTENTIATED SULFONAMIDES
TRADES NAME(S):	Trimethoprim sulfa Albon
MANUFACTURER(S):	Schering-Plough Roche
DOSAGE(S):	
Cattle	TMS: 48 mg/kg IV or IM q 24 hrs Albon: 5.5 mg/kg IV initial dose; 27.5 mg/kg IV q 24 hrs thereafter
Calves	
Sheep, Goats	
Swine	
PRODUCTION STATUS/AGE	
All	
Nonveal calves <20 mos.	X
Calves <20 mos.	
Dairy calves <20 mos.	
Beef cattle	
Dairy bulls	
Dairy cows (lactating)	
SPECTRUM:	
Broad	X
Anaerobes	
G+ Aerobes	
G− Aerobes	
Staphylococcus	
WITHDRAWAL:	
Cattle	
Milk	60 hrs—Albon
Meat	5 days—Albon
Sheep, Goats	A
Milk	
Meat	
Swine	A
Milk	
Meat	
ADVANTAGES:	
RESTRICTIONS:	

[A]No data available.
[B]Current manufacturer used out of many available.
[1]Some products approved for use in lactating cows.
[2]Check label for this information.
[3]Extra label use of drug (ELUD) prohibited.

INDEX